Mosby's

Comprehensive Review of

PRACTICAL NURSING

for the

NCLEX-PN®

Examination

14th Edition

Mosby's

Comprehensive Review of

PRACTICAL NURSING

for the

NCLEX-PN®
Examination

14th Edition

Editor

Mary O. Eyles, Ph.D., RN
Director of Nursing/Wellness Services
Independence Manor at Hunterdon
Flemington, New Jersey

Adjunct Assistant Professor
Department of Physical Medicine
and Rehabilitation
University of Medicine and Dentistry of New Jersey
New Jersey Medical School
Newark, New Jersey

(formerly) Director of Continuing Education
National Association for Practical Nurse
Education and Service, Inc. (NAPNES)

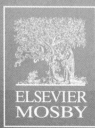
ELSEVIER
MOSBY

ELSEVIER
MOSBY

11830 Westline Industrial Drive
St. Louis, Missouri 63146

NOTICE

Pharmacology is an ever-changing field. Standard safety precautions must be followed, but as new research and
clinical experience broaden our knowledge, changes in treatment and drug therapy may become necessary or
appropriate. Readers are advised to check the most current product information provided by the manufacturer
of each drug to be administered to verify the recommended dose, the method and duration of administration,
and contraindications. It is the responsibility of the licensed health care provider, relying on experience and
knowledge of the patient, to determine dosages and the best treatment for each individual patient. Neither the
publisher nor the editor assumes any liability for any injury and/or damage to persons or property arising from
this publication.

International Standard Book Number 0-323-01952-8

Executive Editor: Loren Wilson
Senior Developmental Editor: Nancy L. O'Brien
Publication Services Manager: John Rogers
Project Manager: Kathleen L. Teal
Designer: Paula Ruckenbrod

Printed in the United States of America

Last digit in the print number: 9   8   7   6   5   4   3   2   1

*This text is dedicated to all individuals
and organizations, who by their
commitment to practical/vocational
nursing, have given of their
knowledge, skills, and abilities
in promoting and providing
excellence in patient care within the
United States and Canada.*

Contributing Authors

Sandra G. Brewer, BA, RN
Coordinator and Professor of Nursing
Georgian College
Owen Sound, Ontario, Canada
Canadian content for Chapter 1 and Chapter 2

Kathy K. Clark, MSN, RN, CPN
Director of Quality Improvement and Education
CareMed Chicago Home Health Agency
Chicago, Illinois
Chapter 8, Pediatric Nursing

Mary O. Eyles, PhD, RN
Director of Nursing/Wellness Services
Independence Manor at Hunterdon
Flemington, New Jersey
Chapter 1, Introduction for Students Preparing for the Licensure Examination

Patricia M. Jacobson, MSN, BSN, RN
Nursing Instructor
Bullard Havens RVTS
Bridgeport, Connecticut
Chapter 3, Pharmacology
Chapter 7, Maternity Nursing

Linda Kerby, BSN, MA, BA, RNC
Mastery Educational Consultations
Leawood, Kansas
Chapter 4, Nutrition
Chapter 10, Emergency Nursing

Linda F. Lucot, BSN, RN
Instructor, Practical Nursing
Jefferson County-Dubois A.V.T.S.
Reynoldsville, Pennsylvania
Chapter 9, Nursing Care of the Aging Adult

Sharon Powell-Laney, MSN, RN
Coordinator of Practical Nursing
Jefferson County-Dubois A.V.T.S.
Reynoldsville, Pennsylvania
Chapter 2, Review of the Basics
Chapter 5, Medical-Surgical Nursing

Kim Inman Smith, MSN, MA, BSN, RN
Instructor, Practical Nursing Program
Shelton State Community College
Tuscaloosa, Alabama
Chapter 6, Mental Health Nursing

Contributing Item Writer

Nuha Hababo, MPA, BSN, RN
Nursing Administrator/Educator
Millville, New Jersey

Reviewers

Julie Barry, PhD, RN
Director, Nursing Education
John Wood Community College
Quincy, Illinois

Sally J. Flesch, PhD, RN
Professor
Black Hawk College
Moline, Illinois

Cecilia Jane Maier, MS, RN, CCRN
Assistant Professor
Mount Carmel College of Nursing
Columbus, Ohio

Nola Ormrod, MSN, RN
Nursing Director, Associate Professor
Centralia College
Centralia, Washington

Vicky Mack Penn, BS.Ed, BSN, RN
Practical Nurse Instructor
Flint River Technical College
Thomaston, Georgia

Pat Recek, MSN, RN
Department Chair, Vocational Nursing
Austin Community College
Austin, Texas

Frances M. Warrick, MS, RN
Program Coordinator, Vocational Nursing
El Centro College
Dallas, Texas

Preface

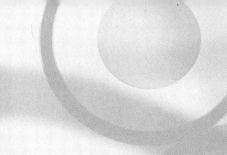

Mosby's Comprehensive Review of Practical Nursing for the NCLEX-PN® Examination has been developed to provide individuals preparing for entry or reentry into nursing at the practical/vocational nurse level with a dependable source of information as they prepare to become valued members of today's health care team. The most current, up-to-date developments in health care and in the field of practical/vocational nursing are incorporated in the text as each contributor has recently been or is currently active in practical/vocational nursing education.

In this, the fourteenth edition of *Mosby's Comprehensive Review of Practical Nursing for the NCLEX-PN® Examination,* the basic practical/vocational nursing curriculum is addressed, from concepts basic to all levels of nursing to the complexities of specialty areas, while incorporating the nursing process throughout. This text also refers to the approved listing of NANDA International Nursing Diagnoses (see Appendix A for a complete listing). Although the LP/VN is not solely responsible for the formulating of a nursing diagnosis, the practical/vocational nurse does assist the registered professional nurse by collecting data essential to formulating a nursing diagnosis.

The text is comprised of ten chapters: Chapter 1 is an introduction to the use of the text and its contents, while offering ways in which one can improve their test-taking abilities; Chapter 2 covers basic skills, fundamental nursing concepts of the practical/vocational nurse curriculum, and today's trends in nursing and health care in the United States and Canada; Chapters 3 and 4 cover Pharmacology and Nutrition completing coverage of basic content found in the NCLEX-PN examination. Chapters 5 through 10 cover the more complex nursing concepts encountered in the various specialty areas of nursing, such as medical-surgical nursing, obstetrics, pediatrics, mental health, and emergency nursing.

The fourteenth edition has been thoroughly revised and updated to reflect current nursing practice. Each chapter's content is organized in a concise outline format to enhance study, and is followed by review questions to help the reader determine what was learned and what areas need additional work in that particular subject area before advancing to the next chapter. Answers and rationales for correct and incorrect answer options follow the review questions.

Two comprehensive examinations are included at the end of the text, each containing 250 questions following the format of those on the National Council Licensure Examination for Practical Nurses (NCLEX-PN®). The correct answer and rationales for both correct and incorrect answer options are also provided following the examinations.

The fourteenth edition of *Mosby's Comprehensive Review of Practical Nursing for the NCLEX-PN® Examination* has significantly increased the total number of practice questions available with this text. Along with the chapter review questions and the two comprehensive examinations, a CD-ROM containing all of the test items printed in the text as well as 1,200 bonus test items is packaged with this book. The bonus questions on the CD-ROM are *not* repeated in the text. The CD-ROM provides both review and test modes of content-specific or comprehensive exams. To reinforce study and build confidence, it is suggested that students practice answering questions on a computer to simulate the NCLEX-PN® computer adaptive test.

For the sake of clarity and consistency, the word *nurse* is used to indicate a practical/vocational nurse. The recipient of care is termed the *patient* to provide consistency as well, although we acknowledge that the term *client* may be preferred and used, in some cases, within this text.

The editor and contributors of this text have the utmost respect for and recognize the LP/VN as a valued member of today's health care team, providing quality nursing care to patients nationwide. It is because of this respect and recognition that this text has been developed, with the hope that individuals preparing for entry or reentry into nursing at the practical/vocational nurse level will find a dependable source with which to prepare to become that valued member of today's health care team.

As coordinating editor, I would like to thank all of those individuals who have worked so diligently in the preparation of this text, that is, all of the contributors and item writers, as well as those at Mosby, especially Nancy O'Brien, without whom this text would not have been possible. I would also like to extend a special thank you to my loving husband, Robert, for being so supportive of our efforts during the revision of this text.

To those who will use this text, we wish you the very best as you enter into a service that will offer you both challenge and satisfaction, the greater of which is the satisfaction of extending care and a helping hand, your hand, to those in need.

Welcome to the caring profession: *welcome to nursing.*

Mary O. Eyles, Ph.D., RN

Contents

Mosby's

Comprehensive Review of

PRACTICAL NURSING

for the

NCLEX-PN®

Examination

14th Edition

CHAPTER 1 — Introduction for Students Preparing for the Licensure Examination

The practice of nursing is regulated by law in each state, the District of Columbia, Guam, Puerto Rico, and the Virgin Islands for the express purpose of protecting the public. The state board of nursing in each of these entities is charged with upholding the regulation of such law. To do so, each state board requires that qualified individuals take a licensing examination prepared by the National Council of State Boards of Nursing (The National Council). Puerto Rico has developed its own licensing examination and does not use the one prepared by The National Council. However, content covered in its examination closely parallels that in the National Council Licensure Examination for Practical Nurses (NCLEX-PN® examination). This book provides a valuable review tool regardless of the licensure examination taken. A special note appears at the end of the chapter for Canadian readers.

The NCLEX-PN examination covers all areas of the practical/vocational nursing curriculum and has been designed to test your nursing knowledge and the application of the principles of that knowledge to given clinical situations in a safe and effective manner. Periodic revision of the NCLEX-PN examination test plan can be expected because of the continually changing face of nursing. Nevertheless, such changes do not compromise your use of this text as you prepare for the licensing examination.

WHY REVIEW?

The purpose of this text is threefold: (1) to assist you in determining the extent of your nursing knowledge relative to your areas of specific strengths and weaknesses, (2) to increase your understanding of nursing knowledge through additional study, and (3) to increase your familiarity with and ability to respond to written test questions and corresponding clinical situations similar to those presented in the NCLEX-PN examination.

The National Council's test plan for the NCLEX-PN examination consists of one essential content dimension (framework): *client need*. This framework serves to provide a structure that is universal in defining the skills and competencies necessary to provide safe and effective nursing care. The dimension of *client need* is therefore critical to ensure the final intent of the examination: to protect the public through safe practitioners. A more detailed description of the test plan, is provided in Box 1-1.

The test plan for the NCLEX-PN examination will be revised in 2005. While major revision is not anticipated, there may be revisions of what is now termed the "subcategories" under each major client need category. Please note that while the test plan may undergo change, all content and related concepts will remain intact.

EFFECTIVE STUDY AND THE USE OF THIS TEXT

The key to effective study and the use of this text can be determined only by you. The review is presented in a manner that is easily adaptable to various forms of study habits, in addition to familiarizing you with timed tests or examinations.

Each chapter outlines a specific content area within the practical/vocational nurse curriculum, followed by a set of questions relative to that particular content area. The correct answers and the rationales for both the correct and the incorrect responses are found at the end of the chapter. Rationales are provided for all four answer choices for each question. The rationale for the correct answer is listed first, followed by the other rationales.

All questions have been classified by *cognitive level, nursing process, client need,* and *level of difficulty.* These classifications follow the question number in the Answers and Rationales portion of the chapter:

First classification or word—the *cognitive level* of the question
   Knowledge, comprehension, application, or *analysis*
Second classification or word—the *phase of the nursing process*
   Assessment, planning, implementation, or *evaluation*
Third classification or word(s)—one of the 4 *client need* categories
   Health Promotion and Maintenance
   Physiological Integrity
   Psychosocial Integrity
   Safe, Effective Care Environment
   (See Box 1-1 for a more detailed outline of *client need* categories and related concepts.)
Letters in parenthesis—the *difficulty of the question*
   The letter (a) signifies that more than 75% of students should answer the question correctly.
   The letter (b) signifies that between 50% and 75% of students should answer correctly.
   The letter (c) signifies that between 25% and 50% of students should answer correctly.

You may want to start with the chapter questions first to determine areas in which you need more study time, then return to review the outline of that particular chapter in its entirety, and then review the chapter questions again. Concentrate study efforts on those areas in which you scored low (i.e., less than 80% to 85% of the questions answered correctly) during your first assessment of the chapter questions. Should you need more in-depth study, you may refer to texts from the Suggested Readings list found at the end of each chapter, your own nursing texts, or current nursing journals.

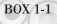

BOX 1-1   Test Plan for the National Council Licensure Examination for Practical/Vocational Nurses: Major Client Need Categories and Related Concepts

Safe, Effective Care Environment
Coordinated Care
Includes all collaborative efforts with other members of the health care team necessary to facilitate delivery of effective patient care

Safety and Infection Control
Includes all means taken to protect patients and health care personnel from environmental hazards

Health Promotion and Maintenance
Growth and Development Through the Life Span
Includes all efforts taken to assist the patient and his or her significant others in the normal expected stages of growth and development from conception through advanced old age

Prevention and Early Detection of Disease
Includes efforts taken to provide patient care relative to prevention and early detection of health problems

Psychosocial Integrity
Coping and Adaptation
Includes efforts taken to promote the patient's or significant other's (or both individual's) ability to cope, adapt, and problem solve situations related to illnesses or stressful events

Psychosocial Adaptation
Includes all participatory efforts in recognizing and providing care for patients with maladaptive behavior and assisting with behavior management of patients with acute and chronic mental illness and cognitive psychosocial disturbances

Physiological Integrity
Basic Care and Comfort
Includes all means to provide comfort and assistance in the performance of activities of daily living

Pharmacological Therapies
Includes all means by which to provide care relative to administering medication and monitoring of patients receiving parental therapies

Reduction of Risk Potential
Includes all measures taken to reduce the patient's potential for development of complications or health problems relative to treatments, procedures, or existing conditions

Physiological Adaptation
Includes all participatory efforts taken to provide care to patients with acute, chronic, or life-threatening physical health conditions

Additional Considerations
Integrated throughout the four *client needs* categories, as identified in the test plan, are additional concepts and processes that are essential to the safe and effective practice of entry-level practitioners. These concepts and processes are the *nursing process, caring, communication, cultural awareness, documentation, self-care,* and *teaching and learning.* Entry-level scope of practice, relative to these integrated concepts and processes, is determined by the laws and statutes of each jurisdiction or state

Modified from the NCLEX-PN® Examination Test Plan for the National Council Licensure Examination for Practical Nurses, April 2003. Adapted with permission of the National Council of State Boards of Nursing, Chicago, Illinois. Detailed information about the NCLEX-PN® Test Plan and the NCLEX® Examination Candidate Bulletin is available from the National Council of State Boards of Nursing on their web site: www.ncsbn.org.

Once you have completed the review and corresponding questions of all chapters, you are ready to take the two comprehensive examinations. Each comprehensive examination contains 125 questions and should take 2 hours to complete. Time yourself with an alarm clock, or have someone else monitor your time.

In April 1994 the National Council began administering the NCLEX-PN examination via computerized adaptive testing (CAT), a change from the traditional paper-and-pencil method of testing. To use this text effectively in preparation for CAT, we suggest that, using a pencil or pen with erasable ink, you darken your answer choice on the chapter review questions and the comprehensive examination questions. Marking your answers in this manner allows you to concentrate on answering the questions much as you would during the actual examination.

CAT allows candidates to take the examination at their own pace. No set minimum amount of time has been established for the examination; however, a maximum time of 5 hours is available. Each candidate's examination is essentially unique to him or her because it is created interactively as the candidate is being tested.

In addition to the questions at the end of each chapter, this review book contains two examinations, each having two parts, simulating the NCLEX-PN examination content. Each part of the examinations contains 125 questions, which should be completed within 2 hours. Even though time may no longer be a major concern, becoming more proficient in time-management skills will be to your advantage during the actual examination. Proper use of this text increases not only your nursing knowledge, but also your self-confidence in your test-taking abilities.

Remember, intelligence plays a vital role in your ability to learn. However, being *smart* involves more than just intelligence. Being practical and applying common sense are also part of the learning experience.

Regardless of how you choose to study, you may find the following simple study guides helpful:

1. Establish your study priorities and the goals by which to achieve these priorities.
2. Enhance your organizational skills by developing a checklist and creating ways to improve your ability to retain information (e.g., index cards, which are easy to carry and review whenever you have a spare moment).
3. Enhance your time-management abilities by designing a study program that best suits your needs and current daily routines by considering the following:
   - Amount of time needed
   - Amount of time available
   - "Best" time to study
   - Allowance for emergencies and free time
4. Prepare for study by reflecting on the following:
   - An environment that will be conducive to learning
   - The appropriate study material
   - Planned study sessions alone, with a friend, or group
   - A formal review course

A note of warning: *do not* expect to achieve the maximum benefits of this text by cramming a few days before the examination. It does not work. Instead, organize planned study sessions, by yourself or with others, over a reasonable period of time in an environment that you find relaxing, stress free, and supportive of the learning process.

TEST-TAKING SKILLS

By now you more than likely have been exposed to a variety of testing in both objective and subjective forms. The licensing examination contains primarily the objective, multiple-choice form of testing. However, after April 2003, the examination will contain innovative item formats that may include fill-in-the-blank items, multiple-choice items that require the choosing of two or more responses, or items that include charts, tables, or graphic images. **DO NOT PANIC!** At some point in your nursing program, you have taken tests that included these formats. Whether this form of testing is familiar to you or not, the following *common sense* pointers will help you to avoid some common test-taking errors:

1. Answer the question that is asked. To do so, you need to read, not scan, the situation and the question carefully, looking for key words or phrases. Do not read anything into the question or apply what you did in a similar situation during one of your clinical experiences. Think of each question as pertaining to an ideal situation. No one is trying to trick you. Let us take a closer look at two of the more familiar formats:

Multiple-choice format: each question contains a stem (the main intent of the question), followed by four plausible answers or alternatives that either complete a statement or answers the question. Only one of the alternatives is the best answer; the remaining three alternatives are known as distracters, so named because they are written in such a way that they might be the correct answer and so distract you to a certain degree. However, your nursing knowledge will lead you to the correct answer.

For example:

Which of the following hormones is secreted only during early pregnancy?
   1. Estrogen
   2. Progesterone
   3. Follicle-stimulating hormone (FSH)
   4. Human chorionic gonadotropin (HCG)

The correct answer is 4. HCG. The alternatives are female hormones and are intended to distract you. However, the key phrase, "only during early pregnancy," is the clue to the correct answer.

Fill-In-the-blank format: each situation contains the main focus of the situation, followed by essential information about the patient or situation (or both) and a question. From the given situation and the information given, you will be able to answer the question and actually fill in the blank.

For example:

The physician orders diazepam (Valium) 7.5 mg IV. Diazepam is supplied in a 10 mg (2-ml) Bristojet container. How many milliliters should the nurse administer?

Answer: 1.5 ml

The correct answer is determined by using the following formula:

$$\frac{(\text{Desired Dose [D]} \times \text{Quantity [Q]}}{\text{Dose on Hand [H]})} = \text{Amount Given}$$

2. Listen to the examiner, and follow directions carefully. All candidates will be given a short training session, which includes a keyboard tutorial complete with a practice session. No prior computer experience is necessary. Should you have any question regarding the directions, ask the examiner for clarification.
3. Have confidence in your initial response to a question because it probably is the correct answer. If you are unable to answer a multiple-choice question immediately, eliminate the alternatives you know are incorrect, and proceed from that point. The same goes for a multiple-choice question that requires you to choose two or more of the given responses. If a fill-in-the-blank question poses a problem, read the situation and essential information carefully, then formulate your response. Although a time factor is not involved, do not spend an excessive amount of time on any one question. One minute is the recommended time allotted to any question. Not all questions will take a full minute; some may take only 20 or 30 seconds to read and answer.

   *It is important to note that with CAT, skipping questions or going back to review a response or change a response (or both) is not possible. In fact, you must answer the question because you **will not** be able to continue with the examination until you do so.*
4. Avoid taking a wild guess at an answer. However, should you feel insecure about a question, eliminate the alternatives you believe are definitely incorrect and reread information given to make sure you understand the intent of

the question. This approach increases your chances of randomly selecting the correct answer or getting a clearer understanding of what is being asked. Although no penalty is applied for guessing on the NCLEX-PN examination, the subsequent question will be based, to an extent, on the response you give to the question at hand; that is, if you answer a question incorrectly, the computer will adapt the next question accordingly based on your knowledge and skill performance on the examination to that point.

5. Above all, begin with a positive attitude about yourself, your nursing knowledge, and your test-taking abilities. A positive attitude is achieved through self-confidence gained by studying effectively. Stated simply, this point means (a) answering questions (assessment), (b) organizing study time (planning), (c) reading and further study (implementation), and (d) again answering questions (evaluation).

Emotional Preparedness

Being emotionally prepared for an examination is also a key factor to your success. However, proper use of this text over an extended period (at least 5 to 6 months before the actual examination) ensures your understanding of the mechanics of the examination, as well as increases your confidence about your nursing knowledge. Your lifelong dream of becoming a nurse is now within your reach! You are excited, yet anxious. This feeling is normal. Although a little anxiety can be good because it increases our awareness of reality, a lot of anxiety has the opposite effect and keeps us from reaching our goals. Your attitude about yourself and your goals will help keep you focused, adding to your strength and inner conviction to achieve success. What happens if you find yourself in a slump over the examination? Take a "time-out" to refocus and reenergize! Talk to friends and family who are supportive of your efforts, and remember one of your major accomplishments in life. This effort will help you regain confidence in yourself and get you back on the right path toward the realization of your long-anticipated goal.

> "There are two ways to face the future. One way is with apprehension; the other is with anticipation." Jim Rohn

Practicing a few relaxation techniques may also prove helpful, especially on the day of the examination. Relaxation techniques such as deep breathing, imagery, head rolling, shoulder shrugging, rotating and stretching of the neck, leg lifts and heel lifts with feet flat on the floor can effectively reduce tension while causing little or no distraction to individuals who are around you. The recommendations are that you do one or two of these techniques intermittently to avoid becoming too tense. The more anxious and tense you become, the longer it will take you to relax.

Test Wise Cues

Before you begin review of the questions, consider the following test cues as well because they may prove quite helpful to you during the licensing examination:

- Many times, the correct answer is the longest alternative given, but do not count on it. Individuals who prepare the examination are also aware of this fact and attempt to avoid offering you any such *helpful hints*.
- Avoid looking for an answer pattern or code. Many times, four or five consecutive questions have the same letter or number for the correct answer.

- Key words or phrases in the stem of the question, such as *first, primary, early, or best,* are also important. Similarly, words such as *only, always, never, and all* in the alternatives are frequently evidence of a wrong response; as in life, no real absolutes exist in nursing. Of course, every rule has its exceptions, so answer with care.
- Be alert for grammatical inconsistencies. If the response is intended to complete the stem (an incomplete sentence) but makes no grammatical sense to you, it might be a distracter rather than the correct answer. However, test developers try to eliminate such inconsistencies.
- Look for options that are similar in nature; if all are correct, you should know that it is either a poor question or that all are incorrect, the latter of which is more likely. For example, if the answer you are seeking is directed to a specific treatment and all but one option deals with signs and symptoms, then you would be correct in choosing the treatment-specific option because it totally excludes the other three options.
- Identify option components as correct or incorrect; being alert for correct or incorrect option components (parts) can help you eliminate a wrong answer. For example, if you were being asked to identify a specific diet, your knowledge about that condition would help you choose the correct response, even though you are unable to recall the exact diet (cholecystectomy = low fat, high protein, low calorie).
- **Identifying content and what is being asked about that content is critical to your choosing the correct response.** Be alert for words in the stem of the item that are the same or similar in nature to those in one or two of the options. For example, if the item relates to and identifies stroke rehabilitation as its focus and only one of the options contains the word stroke in relation to rehabilitation, you are safe in identifying this choice as the correct response.
- Be aware that information from previously asked questions may help you respond to other examination questions.
- Be alert for details. Specific details given in the stem of the item, such as *behavioral changes or clinical changes (or both) within a certain time period,* can give you a clue regarding the most appropriate response or responses.
- You have at least a 25% chance of selecting the correct answer. Should you feel uncertain about a question, eliminate the choices you think are wrong, and then call on your knowledge, skills, and abilities to choose from the remaining responses.
- Above all, do not panic! Panic will only increase your anxiety. Stop for a moment, close your eyes, take a few deep breaths, and resume review of the question.
- Read every word of each option before answering the question. Glossing over the questions just to get through the examination quickly can cause you to misread or misinterpret what the question is really asking. Equally important is the amount of time you take to read an item. The maximum amount of time a person should spend on an item is 60 or 70 seconds. Spending more time on an item can lead to overanalyzing, thereby losing the intent of the question.

READY! SET! GO!

The night before the examination, you may wish to review some key concepts that you believe need a bit of extra time, but then relax and get a good night's sleep. Remember to set your alarm, or have someone wake you. In the morning, allow yourself plenty of time to dress comfortably (preferably in layers, depending on the weather), have a good breakfast (your colleagues will not appreciate an organ recital during the examination), and arrive at the testing site at least 15 to 30 minutes early. Be sure you know where to park and where the test will be given. If the testing site is in an area with which you are not familiar, you should consider a test run a week before the date of the examination. Additionally, remember to take eyeglasses (if needed), your admission card, and second proof of identity. Being prepared will reduce your stress or tension level and help you *remember that **positive attitude.***

"What the mind can conceive and believe, the mind can achieve." Napoleon Hill

THE NCLEX-PN EXAMINATION

The number of questions will vary in CAT and will be based on the candidate's performance, which measures knowledge, skills, and abilities. All successful candidates will answer no fewer than 85 questions or a maximum of approximately 205 questions within the 5-hour time frame. Rest periods (one mandatory after the first 2 hours of testing and one optional following the next 90 minutes of testing) and the computer tutorial are included as part of the 5-hour testing session.

The goal of CAT is to find the point at which a candidate answers 50% of the items correctly. Initially, the computer asks a relatively easy question, and if it is answered correctly, the candidate will receive a more difficult question to answer. Items will continue to become more difficult until such time as the candidate answers incorrectly, and then the items will become less difficult. This process continues until the computer can identify the point at which the candidate answers 50% of the items correctly, thus indicating the candidate's ability level. Once the candidate has answered the minimum number of questions, the computer compares the candidate's ability level to the standard required for passing. Candidates definitely above the passing standard pass, while those definitely below the passing standard do not pass. If a candidate's ability level is close to the passing standard but is questionable as to which side of the passing standard his or her ability level falls, the computer continues the process until it has enough information to make a proper pass-fail determination. At this point, the examination will end.

In some instances, candidates' ability level is so close to the passing standard that all items in the item pool may not provide adequate information to ascertain their ability level. In such instances, these candidates will complete the maximum number of items, and the computer will make a pass or fail decision based on equating of the final ability level.

A candidate who fails will receive a diagnostic profile, which will assist him or her to focus further study efforts for retaking the examination.

The examination has been developed with the basic knowledge necessary for the practice of practical/vocational nursing. Test items reflect the cognitive levels of knowledge, comprehension, application, and analysis.

Although the test plan focuses on one major dimension, that of client need, keep in mind that the elements of accountability, nutrition, anatomy and physiology, growth and development, documentation, communication, fundamentals, and patient education are included throughout the examination (see Box 1-1).

Please note that the NCLEX-PN examination may contain test items (questions) that are being validated for future NCLEX-PN examinations, which are not identifiable to the test taker. Whether you answer these questions correctly or incorrectly, you do not gain or lose points. As already stated, these test items are being validated (tested) for use in future NCLEX-PN examinations.

In all likelihood, no two candidates will be given the same questions to answer because the examination is individualized according to the candidate's knowledge and skills while meeting test plan requirements.

A SPECIAL NOTE FOR CANADIAN CANDIDATES

Nursing is regulated in each province and territory in Canada. Regulations require that a designated body of nurses in each jurisdiction has the responsibility for setting minimum standards of safe practice for practical nurses (PNs), thus ensuring the client and the public a consistent standard of nursing care in any setting. To be allowed to practice as a PN, qualified individuals are required to take a registration or licensure examination before receiving a certificate of registration. All provinces, except Quebec, use the Canadian Practical Nurse Registration Examination (CPNRE). The CPNRE is prepared by Assessment Strategies Incorporated (ASI), previously known as the Canadian Nurses Association Testing (CNAT) division. Examinations are available in both English and French. The Quebec government regulates the licensure of practical nurses in the province of Quebec.

The CPNRE is offered three times a year, over the course of one day. The examination is comprehensive in nature, integrating all clinical areas and age groups. The examination has also been adapted over the years to meet the changing requirements for registration as a practical nurse in Canada. The first administration of the newest version of the CPNRE took place in September 2001.

The CPNRE is composed of two parts: Part A and Part B. Part A is a competency-based examination written by all candidates taking the examination. The test is divided into two Books, Book I and Book II. Book I is written in the morning and Book II in the afternoon. Part A consists of approximately 260 multiple-choice questions (Book I containing approximately 145 questions and Book II containing approximately 115 questions). All candidates will write Part A, while Part B is written only in the jurisdictions in which competencies measured by Part B apply. Part B, also a competency-based examination, consists of Book III, containing approximately 40 multiple-choice questions. The content of Part B measures competencies such as performing auscultation and percussion, preparing and administering intramuscular injections, and assessing and administering infusion therapy, inclusive of blood administration.

Approximately 20% to 40% of the questions on the CPNRE are presented in a case-based format (i.e., a group of approximately five questions that are associated with a brief introductory text or scenario). The remainder of the examination (60% to 80%) consists of independent questions not directly associated with the scenarios or other questions on the examination. The test books for the CPNRE also contain some experimental questions, which are being validated to determine suitability for use on future examinations. Although candidate responses to these questions do not count toward their score, candidates should do their best on all questions because they do not know which questions are being validated for future examinations.

Each question on the examination, whether in the scenario or independent format, contains a stem and four options, as do the majority of questions in this text. Of the four options, one is the correct (or best) answer, and the remaining three are incorrect (or less correct) options. Each correct answer is worth one mark.

The CPNRE is the end result of many test development activities that took place over a 2-year period. PN educators, clinicians, and administrators from across Canada created and evaluated examination questions with assistance from ASI test consultants who ensure the CPNRE meets testing specifications. A thorough review was done of the competencies expected of practical nurses beginning to practice throughout Canada during 2000 and 2001. This review led to a new set of competencies, which form the basis of the present CPNRE.

The CPNRE tests fundamental core competencies an entry-level PN is required to have to practice safely and effectively. These competencies represent outcomes of combined knowledge, abilities, skills, attitudes, and judgments that PNs possess. The examination reflects common health problems encountered across the life span that are representative of PN educational curricula across the country.

The content and specifications for the CPNRE are described in the *Blueprint for Canadian Practical Nurse Registration Examination* (2001). A total of 112 competencies are examined, with each question on the examination linked to one of the competencies. Success on the CPNRE depends on two main factors: (1) your knowledge of practical nursing principles and content and (2) your ability to apply this knowledge in the context of specific health care scenarios presented in the CPNRE.

The *Blueprint for the Canadian Practical Nurse Registration Examination* (2001) identifies major concepts, as well as content areas covered in the examination, outlining the competencies on which the examination is based. The following has been adapted with permission from Assessment Strategies, Inc., Ottawa, Canada, and is also available on the Internet at www.asitest.ca/PN:

Framework for the Development of the Examination
Assumptions Established for Development of the Examination

The competencies represent the combined nursing knowledge, skills, attitudes, and judgment that entry-level practical nurses require for safe and effective practice.

1. Practical nurses are educated to practice in a variety of settings or contexts that influence their role and scope of practice.
2. Practical nurses practice collaboratively, within interdisciplinary health care teams, to meet the physical, psychosocial, and spiritual needs of clients.
3. Practical nurses are accountable for their own actions within their scope of practice.
4. Practical nurses care for clients throughout the life cycle.

5. Practical nurses follow a systematic approach to nursing care by applying their knowledge base in assessment, planning, implementation, and evaluation.
6. *Standards of practice* and the *code of ethics* form the foundation of practice.
7. Practical nurses are committed to the principles that their primary purpose is to serve the public in a safe and effective manner.

Competency Categories

Please note that the number of competencies in each category is not necessarily reflective of the importance that each category has in the practice of practical nursing.

PART A	
Professional, Ethical, and Legal Responsibilities (32 competencies)	25% to 30%
Holistic Caring Practice (45 competencies, inclusive of assessing, planning, intervening, and evaluating)	40% to 60%
Partnerships (28 competencies)	15% to 30%

PART B	
Holistic Caring Practice (7 competencies)	

Cognitive Domain (Level) of Examination Questions

Knowledge and comprehension	10% to 20%
Application	50% to 70%
Critical thinking	20% to 30%

Contextual Variables

1. Client type: individual, families or groups
2. Client age and gender:
   Neonate (0-1 years)
   Child (1-12 years)
   Adolescent (13-18 years)
   Adult (19-64 years)
   Older adult (65 years or more), divided into independent older adult and dependent older adult
3. Client culture: questions represent a variety of cultural backgrounds encountered while providing nursing care in Canada
4. Client health situation: the client's biophysical, psychosocial, and spiritual dimensions form the basis of every health situation; therefore the examination questions reflect a cross section of these situations
5. Health care environment: because the PN works in a variety of settings and contexts in which competencies are equally applicable, the examination specifies health care environment only when it is required to provide guidance to the candidate.

In your review, study all areas to be tested, and budget your time appropriately. This text has three main purposes: (1) to assist you in determining the extent of your nursing knowledge relative to your specific areas of strength and weakness, (2) to increase the understanding of your nursing knowledge through additional study, and (3) to increase your familiarity with and ability to respond to written test questions and corresponding clinical situations. Although the questions in this text assess similar competencies to the American NCLEX-PN examination, the majority of questions are directly applicable to all Canadian practical nurses. Using this text with your notes and other textbooks will focus your attention on the material applicable to your program, which is the bulk of this text. This book should not be used for last-minute cramming, but rather should be used as an adjunct to planned study and for practicing examination questions with instant feedback. Refer to sections on effective study and test-taking skills presented earlier in this chapter.

CONCLUSION

You started preparation for the licensing examination the day you began your nursing program. Every lecture, quiz, examination, term paper, and clinical experience had definite purpose and meaning. This fourteenth edition of *Mosby's Comprehensive Review of Practical Nursing for the NCLEX-PN Examination* has been developed as a culmination of this preparation process. It is now in your hands, because only your persistence and commitment will motivate you to achieve your long-awaited goal.

"Part of success is preparation on purpose."

Jim Rohn

Before you move on to the review chapters, answer the test questions on the following page to find out just how sharp your test-taking skills really are!!

SUGGESTED READINGS

Rohn J: *Excerpts from The Treasury of Quotes,* Southlake, Texas, 2002, Jim Rohn International.

Rollant PD: *SOAR TO SUCCESS: Do your best on nursing tests,* St Louis, 1999, Mosby.

National Council of State Boards of Nursing: *Test plan for the National Council licensure examination for practical/vocational nurses, Chicago,* 2001, National Council of State Boards of Nursing.

Assessment Strategies Incorporated: *The blueprint for the Canadian Practical Nurse Registration Examination (CPNRE),* Ottawa, Ontario, Canada, 2001, Assessment Strategies.

National Council of State Boards of Nursing: *NCLEX® examination candidate bulletin,* Chicago, 2003, National Council of State Boards of Nursing.

HOW SHARP ARE YOUR TEST-TAKING SKILLS?

Take the Following Examination and Find Out!

The following is a hypothetical examination in which, if you are aware of the pitfalls of test construction, you may achieve a score of 100%. We hope you have some fun with this short quiz, which tests only test wiseness skills, not content knowledge.

1. The purpose of the cluss in furmpalling is to revove:
    1. Cluss-Prags
    2. Tremalls
    3. Cloughs
    4. Plumots
2. Trassing is true when:
    1. Lusp trasses the vom
    2. The viskal flane, if the viskal is donwil or zortil
    3. The belgo frulla
    4. Dissels liks easily
3. The sigla frequently overfesks the trelsum because:
    1. All siglas are mellious.
    2. Siglas are always votial.
    3. The trelsum is usually tarious.
    4. No trelsa are feskable.
4. The fribbled breg will minter best with an:
    1. Derst
    2. Morst
    3. Sortar
    4. Ignu
5. The reasons for tristal doss are:
    1. The sabs foped and the doths tinsed
    2. The kredges roted with the orts
    3. Few rakobs were accepted in sluth
    4. Most of the polits were thonced
6. Which of the following is/are always present when trossels are being gruven?
    1. Rint and vost
    2. Vost
    3. Shum and vost
    4. Vost and plone
7. The mintering function of the ignu is most effectively carried out in connection with:
    1. A razma tol
    2. The groshing stantol
    3. The fribbled breg
    4. A frally sush
8.
    1.
    2.
    3.
    4.

Reprinted with permission of the test creator Sorush Batmangelich, Assistant Professor, Department of Physical Medicine and Rehabilitation, Rush Medical College, Chicago, Ill; Medical Education Consultant and President, BATM.

ANSWERS AND RATIONALES

Because of the nature of the test questions in Chapter 1, only the correct response and the rationale for the correct response will be given.

1. 1 Cluss appears in the stem and this response; this response is also the longest alternative.
2. 2 This response is the longest alternative.
3. 3 All, always, and no in answers #1, #2, and #4 eliminate them as possible correct answers; nothing is ever this definite; also, #3 is the longest alternative.
4. 4 Although the sentence makes no sense, the fourth alternative appears to be more grammatically correct than are the other three.
5. 1 The stem asks for more than one reason; this response is the only one of the four that offers more than one reason.
6. 2 Proper reading of the stem and a close look at the possible answers reveal that the second response appears in the other responses as well, making it the only possible correct answer.
7. 3 Some of the terms used in this question may seem familiar to you, and well they should, given that they also appeared in a previous question (#4)—a definite clue to the correct answer.
8. 4 Yes, a correct answer exists, even though a stem or actual responses do not; if you have not already figured it out, a definite answer pattern was created (#1, #2, #3, #4, #1, #2, #3, #4).

CHAPTER 2

Review of the Basics: Trends in the United States and Canada, Nursing Concepts, and the Nursing Process

Nursing is an ongoing relationship with patients in various stages of development and at different points of the health-illness continuum. Basic to nursing are knowledge of the patient as a person, factors contributing to health and illness, the ability to problem solve, and the ability to perform nursing skills. Nurses also appreciate the history of their profession and respect the ethical and legal aspects of rendering nursing care.

This chapter reviews the history of practical/vocational nursing and the functions of its professional organizations; discusses the basic concepts of effective nursing care, while focusing on professional obligations and patient rights; and outlines changes in the health care delivery system and how these changes relate to the practice of licensed practical/vocational nursing (LP/VN).

HEALTH AND ILLNESS

Health Defined

A. According to the World Health Organization (WHO), health is "a state of complete physical, mental, and social well-being and not merely an absence of disease or infirmity."
B. According to Abraham H. Maslow, health exists when all human needs are satisfied.
C. According to Hans Selye, health exists when an individual is in a relative state of adaptation to his or her environment.
D. In 1990, *Healthy People 2000: National Health Promotion and Disease Prevention Objectives* was published in an effort to reduce preventable diseases, disabilities, and deaths. In 2000, these objectives were reevaluated, and *Healthy People 2010* was formulated. The two goals of *Healthy People 2010* include increasing life expectancy for all ages and improving quality of life. The second goal focuses on reducing health disparities.

Illness Defined

A. No one definition exists.
B. Illness exists when disease is present, when an individual believes he or she is ill (subjective symptoms), or when (objective) signs of illness are detected by the individual or the professional.
C. Illness exists when all basic human needs are not satisfied.
D. Illness is a state of disturbance in the body's homeostasis, either of body structure and function or emotional or sociologic functioning.

Health-Illness Continuum

A. An individual is rarely either totally healthy or totally ill.
B. The individual's position is constantly changing in the balance between health and illness.

C. The individual's position on the continuum is determined by need satisfaction, the stage of disease progression, and his or her perception of relative health or illness.

VARIABLES INFLUENCING HEALTH BELIEFS AND PRACTICES

A. Many variables influence a person's perception of health and illness.
B. Internal variables include the patient's developmental stage, knowledge level, perception of functioning, emotional factors, and religious or spiritual views.
C. External variables include the patient's family practices, socioeconomic status, and cultural practices.

TRENDS IN NURSING

Practical/Vocational Nursing in the United States
History

A. Practical/vocational nursing evolved to provide better use of nursing personnel and to ease the shortage of nurses.
B. The first school to train practical/vocational nurses was the Ballard School in New York City, founded in 1893. This 3-month program taught care of chronic invalids, older persons, and children.
C. In 1907 the Thompson School was founded in Brattleboro, Vermont. The Household Nursing Association School of Attendant Nursing was founded in Boston in 1918.
D. In the 1940s, approximately 50 approved programs were in existence; during the 1950s the number of schools of practical/vocational nursing grew. Most programs were extended to 12 months, placing emphasis on integrating class instruction with clinical experience.
E. In 1956, Public Law 911 appropriated millions of dollars for improving and expanding practical/vocational nurse training. The United States Office of Education established a practical nurse education service.
F. Today, more than 1000 practical/vocational nursing schools are located in hospitals, colleges, and vocational-technical schools, providing instruction to more than 50,000 students each year.
G. Approximately 500,000 practical/vocational nurses are licensed in the United States and three U.S. territories (Guam, Puerto Rico, and the Virgin Islands).

Education

A. Practical/vocational nursing programs must meet requirements and be approved by the state board of nursing.
B. Practical/vocational nursing schools of high standards may voluntarily apply for national accreditation by the

National League for Nursing Accrediting Commission (NLNAC).

C. Admission requirements to practical/vocational nursing programs vary; but generally, applicants must:
1. Be at least 17 years of age
2. Have a high school diploma or equivalent
3. Have good physical and mental health
4. Be of good moral character

D. The curriculum incorporates content and concepts from the biologic and physical sciences, behavioral sciences, and principles and practices of nursing.

E. The curriculum includes nursing theory and clinical practice, which provide the students with learning opportunities to meet physical and psychosocial needs of mothers and infants, children, medical-surgical patients, older adults, and patients with long-term illnesses.

F. Graduates receive a diploma or certificate and are eligible to take the practical/vocational nurse licensing examination.

G. Practical/vocational nursing is the entry level into the practice of nursing.

Role Responsibilities

A. The licensed practical/vocational nurse (LP/VN) has a vital and effective role as a member of the health care team.

B. The LP/VN provides direct nursing care to patients whose conditions are stable under the supervision and direction of a registered nurse or physician.

C. The LP/VN assists the registered nurse with the care of patients whose conditions are unstable and complex.

D. The LP/VN, adhering to the nursing process, observes, assesses, records, reports, and performs basic therapeutic, preventive, and rehabilitative procedures.

E. LP/VNs work in acute and long-term care hospitals, nursing homes, physician's offices, ambulatory care facilities, home health agencies, community agencies, schools, and industries.

F. To identify the abilities of the beginning practitioner in practical/vocational nursing, see Box 2-1.

Continuing Education

A. Each LP/VN is responsible for maintaining competency and increasing level of knowledge.

B. The rapid growth of nursing and medical knowledge and advances in technology require nurses to keep up to date.

C. The LP/VN must take advantage of learning opportunities through in-service programs where employed; attending seminars and workshops available through institutions, school, official, or voluntary organizations; and reading professional journals.

D. Membership in nursing organizations provides continuing education opportunities, usually at a lower cost to members.

Health Care Team

A. Members of the health care team vary, depending on the patient's needs and goals.

B. Constant team members are:
1. Physicians: diagnose and prescribe
2. Nurses: plan and carry out nursing care
3. Patient and family: participate in planning care

C. Other team members include certified nursing assistants, unlicensed assistive personnel, physical therapists, social

| BOX 2-1 | National Association for Practical Nurse Education and Service: Statement of Practical/Vocational Nurse Entry-Level Competencies |

Assessment

Uses basic communication skills in a structured care setting

Obtains specific information from patients through goal-directed interviews

Participates in identifying physical, emotional, spiritual, cultural, and overt learning needs of patients by collecting appropriate data

Analyzes data collected in relation to patients' pathophysiologic condition

Planning

Determines priorities and plans nursing care accordingly

Formulates and/or collaborates in developing written nursing care plans

Participates in developing preventive or long-term health plans for patients and/or families

Implementation

Protects the rights and dignity of patients and families

Uses basic communication skills in a structured care setting

Safely performs therapeutic and preventive nursing procedures, incorporating fundamental biologic and physiologic principles in giving individualized care

Observes patients and communicates significant findings to the health care team

Conducts incidental teaching and supports and reinforces the teaching plan for a specific patient and/or family

Evaluation

Evaluates, with guidance if necessary, the care given and makes necessary adjustments

Records evaluations of the results of nursing actions

Identifies own strengths and weaknesses and seeks assistance for improvement of performance

Professional Responsibilities

Recognizes the LP/VN's role in the health care delivery system and articulates that role with those of other health care team members

Maintains accountability for own nursing practice within ethical and legal framework

Serves as a patient advocate

Accepts role in maintaining and developing standards of practice in providing patient care

Participates in nursing organizations

Seeks further growth through educational opportunities

workers, occupational therapists, respiratory therapists, dieticians, clergy, and others.

D. Successful nursing care depends on the interaction and cooperation of all members of the team.

E. The LP/VN collaborates with team members.

LP/VN Role in Leadership

A. Dossett (1992) defines leadership as the use of one's skills to influence others to perform to the best of their ability.

B. The number of LP/VN positions in extended-care facilities is increasing. LP/VNs are being placed in the role of charge

---

BOX 2-2   Examples of Tasks Assigned to Unlicensed Assistive Personnel

Bathing
Vital signs
Feeding
Maintaining safety
Grooming
Weights
Transferring/ambulating
Intake and output

BOX 2-3   Employee Problem Areas

Excessive tardiness/absence
Excessive use of telephone for personal calls
Negative attitudes, not being a team player
Poor quality of work
Substance abuse

BOX 2-4   Recognition of Substance Abuse

Personality changes
Frequent sick calls
Glassy eyes, slurred speech
Changes in attitude toward others

---

nurse, responsible for assigning unlicensed assistive personnel job tasks.

C. Assigning is within the scope of practice of the LP/VN and involves allotting tasks that are in the job description of unlicensed assistive personnel, nursing assistants, or nurse's aides.

D. The LP/VN must know agency policy and job descriptions of unlicensed assistive personnel before assigning tasks.

E. Tasks assigned may include assistance with activities of daily living and uncomplicated tasks. See Box 2-2 for examples of tasks that may be assigned.

F. The LP/VN provides clear, concise descriptions of what tasks are to be accomplished and provides time frame and give feedback and praise for staff members' efforts.

G. The LP/VN is legally liable for improper assigning of tasks.

Delegation

A. Many states are debating the issue of delegation as it pertains to the LP/VN scope of practice.

B. Bernard and Walsh (1995) define delegation as the process of assigning part of one person's responsibility to another qualified person, with their consent. Delegation is a transfer of responsibility and authority while maintaining accountability.

C. LP/VNs must ensure that the nurse practice act of their state permits delegation. The nurse practice act should authorize specific tasks to be delegated.

D. The LP/VN must ensure that the delegatee has demonstrated the appropriate level of competency to perform the delegated task.

Conflict Resolution

A. Conflict results when one person's expectations or rights cross with those of another person's.

B. LP/VNs in leadership roles need to become accustomed to resolving conflicts.

C. The steps in conflict resolution include recognition, clarification, negotiation (compromise), and decision making.

D. In addition to conflict resolution, LP/VNs must address common individual problems. See Box 2-3 for examples of individual problem areas.

E. LP/VNs have an ethical and legal responsibility to report substance abuse among peers. See Box 2-4 for signs of substance abuse.

F. Drug addiction among nurses is 30 to 100 times greater than among the general population.

G. Most states have impaired professional programs.

Legislation Related to Practice of LP/VN
Nurse Practice Act

A. Nursing is subject to laws passed by the state's legislature.

B. Laws pertaining to nursing are in the state's nurse practice act.

C. The nurse practice act varies from state to state. Some states define the practice of nursing, whereas others describe what a nurse may or may not do in the practice of nursing.

D. The nurse practice act also provides for some type of nursing board to regulate nursing practice and procedures for:
   1. Approval of nursing schools and curriculum requirements
   2. Licensure and renewal
   3. Grounds for suspension and revocation of licensure

E. The LP/VN must practice nursing within the legally defined scope of his or her state's nurse practice act.

State Boards of Nursing

A. State boards of nursing administer the state nurse practice act.

B. Membership on the board varies from state to state, usually consists of registered nurses (RNs), LP/VNs, and consumers appointed by the governor.

C. In most states, both professional and practical/vocational nursing practice are under the same board; some states have two boards, one for each.

D. Functions:
   1. Enforces established educational requirements of schools of nursing
      a. Surveys program to determine if preestablished standards are being met
      b. Approves new programs that meet standards
      c. Withholds or withdraws approval from programs that do not meet standards
   2. Controls licensure
      a. Grants license to applicants who have passed the National Council of State Boards of Nursing licensing examination
      b. Renews license
      c. Denies, suspends, or revokes license for cause
   3. Conducts investigations and hearings relating to charges of unsafe nursing practice
   4. Interprets the nurse practice act based on past practice, standard of care, and information from other states

Licensure

A. Licensure protects the public from unqualified practitioners.
B. A license is mandatory to practice nursing.
C. Licensure permits use of title licensed practical nurse (LPN) or licensed vocational nurse (LVN).
D. Qualifications vary from state to state but most require the following for licensure:
   1. Graduation from an approved program in practical/vocational nursing
   2. Proof of moral character
   3. Minimum score on the nationally administered examination
E. License must be renewed for a small fee at regular intervals.
F. Many states require LP/VNs to submit proof of continuing education before license will be renewed.
G. License may be revoked or suspended for acts of misconduct or incompetence, such as drug addiction or conviction of a felony.
H. Licensure by endorsement occurs when a state board of nursing reviews the credentials of a nurse licensed in another state and determines that the nurse meets the qualifications of their state.

Examination

A. As of 1994 the National Council of State Boards of Nursing examination is given to all qualified applicants as a computer adaptive test (CAT). This test, the National Council Licensure Examination for Practical Nurses (NCLEX-PN®) examination, is used to determine whether the LP/VN candidate is prepared to practice nursing safely. The examination tests knowledge of nursing care and ability to apply that knowledge in a clinical situation.
B. Testing takes place in more than 1200 computer testing sites throughout the nation. Candidates schedule a testing date following graduation. Testing occurs throughout the year, 6 days per week, 15 hours per day. Each examinee sits at an individual computer terminal and answers questions on the screen. The candidate's answer to each question determines the next question to be presented. No two persons receive the same test.
C. The test stops when the candidate's ability level has been estimated at a predetermined degree of accuracy. The minimum number of test items that must be answered is 85; the maximum number of items is 205. The maximum time allotment for the test is 5 hours; most candidates will complete the test in less than 5 hours.

Ethical Principles: Code of Ethics

A. A code of ethics lists principles established by professional group as a means of self-regulation.
B. Each LP/VN is responsible for upholding the professional standards of conduct and ethics.

Legal Implications for the LP/VN

Responsibilities

A. To function within the scope of state nurse practice act
B. To maintain standards of care (Box 2-5)
C. To function according to employer or agency policy
D. To apply the skills and knowledge that a prudent LP/VN with comparable training would apply in a similar situation
E. To maintain complete and accurate patient records
F. To maintain confidentiality

BOX 2-5	Standards of Practice for the LP/VN

The LP/VN Provides Individual and Family-Centered Nursing Care

Follow principles of nursing process in meeting specific needs of patients of all ages in the areas of safety, hygiene, nutrition, medication, elimination, psychosocial, cultural, and respiratory needs

Apply appropriate knowledge, skills, and abilities in providing safe, competent care

Apply principles of crisis intervention in maintaining safety and making appropriate referral when necessary

Use effective communication skills
- Communicate effectively with patients, family, significant others, and members of the health care team
- Maintain appropriate written documentation

Provide appropriate health teaching to patients and significant others in the areas of
- Maintenance of wellness
- Rehabilitation
- Use of community resources

Serve as a patient advocate
- Protect patients' rights
- Consult with appropriate others when necessary

The LP/VN fulfills the professional responsibilities of the practical/vocational nurse

Know and apply the ethical principles underlying the profession

Know and follow the appropriate professional and legal requirements

Follow the policies and procedures of the employing institution

Cooperate and collaborate with all members of the health care team to meet the needs of family-centered nursing care

Demonstrate accountability for own nursing actions

Maintain current knowledge and skills in the area of employment

Modified from Standards of Practice for LP/VN. Adopted in 1985 by the National Association for Practical Nurse Education and Service, Silver Spring, Md.

Delivery of Nursing Care

A. Functional method: each nursing team member is assigned specific tasks (e.g., obtaining and recording all vital signs, administering all medications).
B. Team nursing: a group of patients are cared for by a team consisting of professional nurses, practical/vocational nurses, nurses' aides, and student nurses.
C. Primary nursing
   1. One nurse assigned to patient from admission to discharge, usually an RN
   2. Total responsibility for care on all shifts
   3. Coordinates care with other health workers, for example, LP/VN, nurse's aide

Illegal Actions

A. Torts—civil law
   1. An act or wrong committed by one person against another that results in injury or damage
   2. Can be either the commission or omission of an act

3. Acts of negligence include:
  a. Professional misconduct
  b. Performing care incorrectly
  c. Illegal or immoral conduct
  d. Examples include:
    (1) Administration of wrong medication
    (2) Administration of medication or treatment to wrong patient
    (3) Failure to ensure safety through use of side rails or restraints as ordered by the physician
    (4) Failure to prevent injury while applying heat
    (5) Gross negligence: patient's life is endangered or lost—often results in criminal action
B. Intentional torts
  1. Legal liability exists even if no damage occurs to the other person
  2. May not be covered by malpractice insurance
  3. Assault and battery
    a. Assault
      (1) Definition: threat or attempt to make bodily contact with another person without that person's consent with intent to injure
      (2) Example: threatening to restrain or physically punish patient if he or she does not cooperate
    b. Battery
      (1) Definition: act of making unauthorized contact
      (2) Example: nurse actually restrains the patient
  4. False imprisonment
    a. Definition: unwarranted restriction of another person by force or threat of force
    b. Examples: detaining patient in hospital against his or her will; unwarranted use of restraints
    c. Patient who wishes to leave hospital against advice of the physician may be asked to sign a release; cannot detain patient if he or she refuses to sign
  5. Invasion of privacy
    a. Definition: unauthorized disclosures about a patient even if information is true
    b. Examples:
      (1) Release of patient's medical information
      (2) Exposure of patient during procedures or transportation
  6. Defamation
    a. Definition: attack on the name, business, or professional reputation of another through false and malicious statements to a third person
    b. Types
      (1) Slander: oral statement
      (2) Libel: written statement

Other Legal Aspects

A. Good Samaritan laws
  1. Laws that give certain persons legal protection when giving aid at the scene of an accident; not all states cover nurses
  2. Purpose: to encourage people to give assistance at the scene of an emergency
  3. These laws do not make it legally necessary for a nurse to assist.
  4. When nurses do assist, they are expected to use good judgment in deciding whether an emergency exists.

5. The LP/VN is expected to give a standard of care that a reasonable LP/VN with comparable training would give in similar circumstances.
B. Child abuse
  1. All states have laws that require reporting known or suspected cases of child abuse.
  2. The laws grant immunity from civil suits to individuals who are required to report child abuse.
C. Narcotics
  1. The Federal Controlled Substances Act of 1970 is a federal law that regulates the manufacture, sale, prescription, and dispensing of narcotics and other harmful drugs.
  2. Violation of the law by a nurse is a felony and will result in revocation of the LP/VN license.
D. Wills
  1. A will is a legal declaration of how a person (testator) wishes to dispose of his or her property after death.
  2. For a will to be valid, the testator must be of sound mind and acting without force.
  3. No legal reason exists for the nurse not to witness a will; the witness is only witnessing the person's signature, not the contents of the will.
  4. A beneficiary of the will must not witness the signing.
E. Advance directives: documents in which an individual can specify their wishes regarding end-of-life care
  1. Durable power of attorney for health care—the individual appoints an individual to make health care decisions for them if they are unable to do so, maybe the patient's lawyer or an impartial friend. The power of attorney for health care should not be the patient's physician or a family member who benefits from their will.
  2. Living will—a document that specifies the patient's wishes regarding health care decisions. The document usually states that the patient's wishes should be followed when "no reasonable chance for recovery" exists.
  3. The Patient Self Determination Act ensures that all individuals are aware of their rights in regards to advance directives when they are admitted to any acute care hospital that receives federal funding.
F. Malpractice insurance
  1. Professional liability policies cover liability arising out of the rendering of or failure to render professional service.
  2. Policy is safeguard against suits for damages; proving innocence can be expensive.
  3. Policy can be purchased from nursing organizations, bargaining organizations, and private insurance companies.
  4. Malpractice insurance provides monetary award of damages within specified limits of the policy, as well as legal fees, court costs, and payment of bond.
  5. Employer's insurance protects employee only while on duty.

Patient's Rights
Bill of Rights

A. Patients have the right to courteous, individual care given without discrimination as to race, color, religion, sex, marital status, national origin, or ability to pay.
B. A patient's bill of rights, also known as "A patient care partnership", is a statement of what the patient can expect from the institution.

C. The following is paraphrased from the Patient's Bill of Rights adopted by the American Hospital Association. The patient should:
1. Be given considerate and respectful care
2. Obtain from the physician complete current information concerning diagnosis, treatment, and prognosis in terms he or she can be reasonably expected to understand
3. Receive from the physician information necessary to give informed consent before the start of any procedure or treatment
4. Be allowed to refuse treatment to the extent permitted by law and be informed of the medical consequences of that action
5. Be given every consideration of privacy concerning his or her own medical care program
6. Expect that all communications and records pertaining to his or her care be treated as confidential
7. Expect that, within its capacity, a hospital must make reasonable response to the request of a patient for services
8. Obtain information as to any relationships of the patient's hospital to other health care and educational institutions insofar as his or her care is concerned
9. Be advised if the hospital proposes to engage in or perform human experimentation affecting the patient's care or treatment
10. Expect reasonable continuity of care
11. Examine and receive an explanation of the bill regardless of the source of payment
12. Know what hospital rules and regulations apply to the patient's conduct

Standard of Care

A. Patients are entitled to a safe, competent standard of nursing care, no matter who administers it (RN, LP/VN, student).
B. The LP/VN is accountable for his or her own actions and must ensure that the patient receives qualified care.
C. If the LP/VN thinks that the patient assignment is beyond his or her ability, the LP/VN must discuss the matter with the RN before carrying it out.
D. Standard of care is established by:
1. State nurse practice act
2. Institution's job description
3. Hospital policies and procedures
4. Patient's nursing care plan

Patient Advocate

A. An advocate acts on behalf of another person and stands up or speaks up on behalf of that person.
B. Patient has the right to information needed to make informed decisions freely and without pressure.
C. The responsibility of the LP/VN is to:
1. Maintain standard of care.
2. Support patients in the decisions they make.
3. Inform physician when the patient apparently does not understand what is going to happen to him or her.
4. Observe and speak out regarding instances of incompetent, unethical, or illegal practice by any member of the health care team.
5. Know hospital policy regarding procedure to follow when patients' rights are being violated.

D. Many hospitals employ a patient representative who serves as a liaison between patient and institution and who has the power to act to resolve patients' problems.

Consent Forms

A. Before any invasive procedure can be performed, the patient must give written consent, except in extreme emergency, when failure to treat may be considered negligence.
B. The patient must be fully informed of the extent of the proposed procedure, risks and benefits, alternatives, and their consequences.
C. Consent must be obtained by the physician, whose duty it is to advise the patient.
D. This consent must be obtained while the patient is of sound mind; it should be signed before administering any preoperative narcotic medications.
E. Consent may be withdrawn by the patient before the procedure.

Patient's Medical Records: the Chart

A. The chart is a legal document.
B. The chart provides a written account of the patient's hospitalization.
C. The chart may be used as evidence in courts of law and records only information related to patient's health problem.
D. Health Insurance Portability and Accountability Act of 1996 (HIPPA) has four objectives:
1. Ensures health insurance portability—when workers change jobs
2. Reduces health care fraud and abuse
3. Enforces standards for health information
4. Guarantees security and privacy of health care (information contained in records must be held in confidence)
E. Only authorized persons should have access to patient's records.
F. Most states consider medical records the property of the hospital and the contents the property of the patient.

Nursing Organizations

A. Membership
1. The LP/VN has the responsibility to join a professional organization and support practical/vocational nursing by becoming an active member.
2. Membership provides:
a. Fellowship and interaction with other LP/VNs
b. Opportunity to enhance and strengthen role of LP/VNs
c. Means to keep current on issues relating to practical/vocational nursing
d. A voice in planning policies of the association
e. Continuing education opportunities
B. National Association for Practical Nurse Education and Service (NAPNES) (www.napnes.org)
1. NAPNES was organized in 1941 to promote the development of sound practical/vocational nursing education and to promote advancement and recognition of the LP/VN as a member of the health team.
2. Membership includes:
a. Regular members: LP/VNs, practical nursing educators, other registered nurses, general educators, physicians, hospital and nursing home administrators, practical nursing students, and interested lay persons

b. Student members: students in state-approved schools of practical/vocational nursing

c. Agency members: hospitals, nursing homes, schools of practical nursing, alumni groups, civic organizations, and other institutions or groups in harmony with NAPNES objectives

3. Functions and activities listed by NAPNES:

a. Serves as clearinghouse for information about practical/vocational nursing, including information about functions and roles of LP/VNs

b. Publishes *Journal of Practical Nursing,* a monthly magazine

c. Prepares publications useful to faculties in schools of practical/vocational nursing

d. Sponsors workshops and seminars for LP/VNs and practical nursing educators in conjunction with state LP/VN associations, universities, and national organizations

e. Engages in activities aimed at protecting and strengthening position of LP/VNs and cooperates with state LP/VN associations in activities of this kind

f. Provides consultation to state LP/VN constituencies on matters relating to their organization and programs

g. Sponsors "national certification" in pharmacology and long-term care for LP/VNs

C. National Federation of Licensed Practical Nurses (NFLPN) (www.nflpn.org)

1. NFLPN was organized in 1949 to foster high standards in practical nursing and to promote practical nursing.

2. Membership is limited to LP/VNs and student practical/vocational nurses.

3. Affiliate membership is available to individuals who are not LP/VNs or students but are interested in the work of NFLPN.

4. Many state associations exist.

5. Functions of the NFLPN:

a. Provides leadership for LP/VNs employed in the United States

b. Fosters high standards of practical/vocational nursing education and practice

c. Encourages every LP/VN to make continuing education a priority

d. Achieves recognition for LP/VNs and advocates the effectiveness of LP/VNs in every type of health care facility

e. Interprets the role and function of the LP/VN for the public

f. Represents practical/vocational nursing through relationships with other national nursing, medical, and allied health organizations, legislators, government officials, health agencies, educators, and other professional groups

g. Serves as the central source of information on the new and changing aspects of practical/vocational nursing education and practice

D. National League for Nursing (NLN) (www.nln.org)

1. The NLN was organized in 1952 by combining the National League for Nursing Education and six other national nursing organizations

2. Membership includes:

a. Individual membership; anyone interested in nursing; RNs, LP/VNs, student nurses, consumers

b. Agency membership: hospitals, nursing homes, public health agencies, and schools of nursing

3. Functions:

a. Defining and furthering good standards for all nursing service

b. Defining and promoting good standards for institutions giving nursing education on all levels

c. Helping to extend facilities to meet these services when necessary

d. Helping in proper distribution of nursing education and nursing service

e. Working to improve organized nursing services in hospitals, public health agencies, nursing homes, and other agencies; accrediting community public health nursing services; developing criteria and other self-evaluation tools

f. Working to improve nursing education programs; NLNAC acts as an accrediting agency for all levels of nursing education.

g. Constructing, processing, and providing preadmission, achievement, and qualifying tests

h. Gathering and publishing information about trends in nursing, personnel needs, community nursing services, and schools of nursing

4. The official journal is *Nursing and Health Care*

5. In 1984 the NLN Council of Practical Nursing Programs adopted a resolution that recognized the NFLPN as the official organization for LP/VNs (Box 2-6).

E. National Council of State Boards of Nursing (NCSBN) (www.ncsbn.org)

1. Established in 1978 to strengthen and coordinate the credentialing of nurses nationally

2. Membership open to any state board of nursing; presently composed of 53 state boards

3. Maintains a liaison with national organizations that represent nursing

4. Controls the NCLEX examination **process** which prepares the LP/VN and RN licensure examinations

F. American Nurses' Association (ANA) (www.ana.org)

1. National organization for registered nurses formed in 1896 as the Nurses Association Alumnae; renamed ANA in 1911

2. Concerned with standard of nursing practice and promoting general welfare of the professional nurse

3. Limits membership to RNs

4. Publishes *American Journal of Nursing (AJN)*, a monthly magazine

G. Alumni associations

1. Organization of graduates from the LP/VN's respective school

2. Membership provides a means of:

a. Keeping informed of school's progress

b. Offering suggestions to improve programs

c. Providing continuing education

d. Facilitating social activities with classmates and other graduates

e. Offering scholarships to future students

Practical Nursing in Canada
History

A. There has always been a person working as an assistant to the professional nurse, although the current role is more correctly considered a collaborative one.

BOX 2-6	National League for Nursing Statement Supporting Practical/Vocational Nursing and Practical/Vocational Nursing Education*

The Executive Committee of the Council of Practical Nursing Programs of the National League for Nursing believes that practical/vocational nursing is a vital component of the occupation of nursing and supports individuals who elect practical/vocational nursing as a permanent career choice. The minimal educational credential for entry into practical/vocational nursing is a diploma or certificate.

Nursing is an occupation that exists on a continuum, and education for nursing can be developed at different levels of knowledge and skills required to fulfill identified yet different nursing roles. The nursing profession has an obligation to society to develop sound and efficient patterns for nursing education that meet the varied nursing needs of society and permit educational options for persons who wish them.

Practical/vocational nurses are involved in the nursing process. Practical/vocational nurses, with the supervision and direction of a registered nurse or physician, use the nursing process to give direct care to patients whose conditions are considered to be stable. This care encompasses observation, assessment, recording, reporting to appropriate persons, and performing basic therapeutic, preventive, and rehabilitative procedures. When patients' conditions are unstable and complex, the practical/vocational nurse assists and collaborates with the registered nurse in the provision of care.

The practical/vocational nurse is prepared for employment in health care settings in which the policies and protocols for providing patient care are well defined and in which supervision and direction by a registered nurse or physician are present. These settings may be acute or long-term care hospitals, nursing homes, home health agencies, and ambulatory care facilities.

Practical/vocational nurses function within the definition and framework of the regulations set forth by the nurse practice act of the state in which they are employed. The practice of practical/vocational nursing requires licensure, which is the responsibility of the board of nursing in each state, so as to protect the public and safeguard nursing practice.

Education of the practical/vocational nurse is characterized by its consistent emphasis on the clinical practice experience necessary to meet common nursing problems. The curriculum—based on concepts from the physical and biologic sciences that underlie nursing measures and the behavioral science concepts necessary to individualize care—is a planned sequence of correlated theory and clinical experience.

After completing the program of study in practical/vocational nursing, the graduate demonstrates the specific competencies related to assessment, planning, implementation, and evaluation of nursing care as identified by the Council of Practical Nursing Programs.

The licensed practical/vocational nurse is responsible for maintaining and updating her or his competencies. Adequate orientation and continuing inservice education are responsibilities of the employing agency. However, the practical/vocational nurse must take advantage of other opportunities for continuing self-improvement and, if desired, career advancement.

Opportunities for career mobility without undue penalty must exist in the system of nursing education to provide for changing career goals.

*Issued in 1982, reaffirmed in 1987.

B. During and following World War II, there was a shortage of nurses. To meet this need, hospitals began a variety of short courses on the job.

C. In response to these many and varied short courses, the Canadian Nurses Association (CNA) developed a syllabus for a course to be used as a guide by provincial nursing associations with the aim of standardizing courses.

D. The title for graduates suggested by the CNA was "nursing assistant."

E. In 1940, Ontario was the first province to pass legislation protecting the title "certified nursing assistant."

F. In 1941 the Registered Nurses Association of Ontario opened a demonstration school in London, Ontario, to determine the feasibility of training an auxiliary group; the course lasted 6 months and had a grade 8 admission requirement.

G. Following the war, arrangements were made through the Department of Veterans Affairs, the national and provincial nursing associations, and the departments of health and education in each province to organize courses to meet the needs of people released from the armed services.

H. Standardized courses, developed across the country, were offered to the public in such places as hospitals, secondary schools, and technical-vocational schools, as well as independent schools.

I. Each province assumed responsibility for supervising the course of instruction, evaluating the programs, and registering and licensing the graduates, plus designating their title; this accounts for the variation in title, program lengths, and responsibilities of the nursing assistant across the country.

J. In 1971 the Ontario Association for Nursing Assistants began discussions with the other provinces to form a national organization.

K. In 1975 the Canadian Association of Practical Nursing Assistants (CAPNA) was incorporated; all provinces are affiliated except Quebec.

L. Approximately 84,000 practical nursing and nursing assistants are practicing in Canada. All provinces and territories (except the Yukon) now use the designation practical nurse.

Education

A. Practical nursing (PN) nurse programs must meet requirements of the registering and licensing body in each province or territory.

B. No national accreditation body exists for nursing in Canada.

C. Admission requirements vary from province to province and the territories; a high school diploma or its equivalent is usually required.

D. The curriculum incorporates content and concepts from the biologic and psychosocial sciences, as well as principles and practice of nursing.

E. The curriculum includes nursing theory and clinical practice, which provide the students with learning opportunities to meet physical, psychosocial, and spiritual needs of patients across the life span.

F. Graduates receive a diploma or certificate and are eligible to take the certification and licensing examination in their jurisdiction.

Responsibilities of the Canadian Practical Nurse

A. The practical nurse has a vital and effective role as a member of the health care team.

B. The practical nurse provides direct nursing care to patients whose conditions are stable and whose outcomes are predictable. Depending on the provincial standards and the setting, care may be provided independently or with varied amounts of supervision and direction from an RN, a registered psychiatric nurse (in certain provinces), or a physician.

C. In certain provinces, the practical nurse may be responsible for direct supervision and direction of unregulated care providers in stable settings.

D. The practical nurse aids the RN with the care of patients whose conditions are unstable and complex.

E. The practical nurse using the nursing process observes, assesses, records, reports, evaluates, and performs basic therapeutic, preventive, and rehabilitative procedures.

F. The practical nurse works in acute and long-term care hospitals, nursing homes, physicians' offices, ambulatory care facilities, home health agencies, public health agencies, community agencies, and industry.

G. The practical nurse uses the nursing process (i.e., assessing, planning, implementing, evaluating) in delivering nursing care in all settings.

H. The practical nurse practices within the legal and ethical boundaries for the province or territory.

Continuing Education

A. Each practical nurse has the responsibility to maintain competency and increase level of knowledge.

B. The rapid growth of medical knowledge and advances in technology require that the practical nurse keeps up to date.

C. The practical nurse must take advantage of learning opportunities through in-service programs where employed; attending seminars and workshops available through institutions and schools, official, or voluntary organizations; and reading professional journals.

D. Membership in nursing organizations provides continuing education opportunities, usually at a lower cost to their members.

Legislation Related to the Practice of Nursing in Canada

A. Legislation
1. Nursing is subject to legislation passed by each province or territory.
2. Laws pertaining to nursing are specific to each province or territory.

3. The regulating body is designated through legislation in each province or territory.
4. Each province or territory designates a body to approve and review nursing schools.

B. Regulatory body
Each province or territory has either an independent body, such as a council or a college, or a professional association responsible for the practice of its members.

C. Registration and licensure
1. Each province or territory determines the title held by the practical nurse in that jurisdiction.
2. Registration and licensure ensure the public of a minimum standard of safe nursing care.
3. Registration protects the title of the registrant only; licensure also protects the practice of nursing.
4. Licenses are usually renewed annually.
5. Licenses may be revoked or suspended for acts of misconduct, negligence, or incompetence as outlined in provincial legislation.

D. Examination
1. All provinces and territories except Quebec purchase the CPNRE.
2. The CPNRE is held three times a year. (See Chapter 1 for more detailed information about the examination.)
3. All provinces and territories administer the examination on the same day.
4. Passing scores are determined by each province or territory. The writer receives a grade of "P" or "F."
5. Quebec administers its own examinations.

Canadian Practical Nursing Organizations

A. Membership
1. The practical nurse has the responsibility to join a professional organization and support practical nurses by becoming an active member.
2. Membership provides:
   a. Fellowship and interaction with other practical nurses
   b. Opportunity to enhance and strengthen role of practical nurses
   c. Means to keep current on issues relating to the practical nurse
   d. A voice in planning policies of the association
   e. Continuing education opportunities
   f. Malpractice insurance (most provinces)

B. Canadian Association of Practical Nursing/Nursing Assistants (CAPNNA)
1. CAPNNA (formerly CAPNA) was formed in 1971 and incorporated in 1975. CAPNNA is a voluntary association currently representing members of associations from all provinces and the territories with the exception of Quebec. It can be accessed through each organization.
2. Membership includes:
   a. Association member: a member of any provincial or territorial association of PNs that belongs to CAPNNA
   b. Affiliate member: individual practical nurses from province or territories who do not belong to CAPNNA but who are entitled to membership after payment of the prescribed annual fee
3. CAPNNA objectives:
   a. To promote the concept of health
   b. To promote the high standards and uniformity of nursing education to achieve reciprocity

c. To interpret and promote the practical nurse role on the health team

d. To safeguard the interest, professional identity, and practice of the practical nurse

e. To promote and encourage an attitude of mutual understanding and unity among all provincial or territorial associations

f. To safeguard and promote the autonomy and self-governance of the practical nurse

g. To promote nursing research that facilitates the provision of quality nursing care for the people of Canada

h. To participate in the provision and development of an effective, efficient, patient-centered interdisciplinary approach to the delivery of health care services

TRENDS IN DELIVERY OF HEALTH CARE

A. Traditionally, the health care focus was on diagnosis and treatment of disease.

B. Trends
1. Emphasis on prevention of illness and maintenance of health
2. Decrease in length of hospital stay
3. Rise in home health care

C. Reason for changes in delivery of health care
1. Technological advances: scientific knowledge has provided early diagnosis and effective treatment of diseases.
2. Consumer movement: the public has exerted pressure for the right to health at an affordable price through legislative action.
3. Population change: life expectancy has significantly increased with an increase in the number of older adults and a declining birth rate.
4. Nature of disease pattern is changing: decrease in acute diseases with an increase in chronic and degenerative diseases.
5. Continuing scrutiny of health care costs

D. Related health problems
1. Growing technology and use of complex scientific equipment has caused:
   a. Increase in cost of health care; even a short hospitalization can be financially crippling.
   b. Fragmentation of care caused by increased number of health workers required by technology
2. Increased population has caused health problems related to air, noise, and water pollution with overcrowding and unsanitary living conditions.
3. Aging population: the likelihood for older persons to become ill and to develop chronic and degenerative diseases increases.
4. Uneven distribution of health care facilities and resources available to:
   a. Elderly, poor, and minorities
   b. Rural areas and inner cities
5. Cost capitation: managed care strategy that provides a fixed payment for all members (patients) for each pay period (usually a year); profit attained by keeping patients out of expensive care setting; focuses on health promotion for cost containment; risk for patient related to denied payment for expensive, high-tech treatments

E. Caring: the heart of nursing practice
1. Caring behaviors are action or responses by nurses when providing patient services.
2. The most frequently described caring behaviors include attentive listening, honesty, responsibility, comforting, patience, providing information, sensitivity, respect, touch, and addressing the patient by their given name (Taber's, 2003).
3. The nurse must use caring behaviors during patient contact, in light of recent technologic advances, the health care industry becoming more business-like, and the current nursing shortage.

Disease Prevention and Maintenance of Health
Levels of Health Care

A. Primary
1. Promotion of health and prevention of disease, including:
   a. Immunization against infectious diseases
   b. Health education such as nutrition counseling
   c. Physical fitness program
   d. Research to find cause of disease
2. Primary care takes place in prenatal centers, well-baby centers, schools, and health maintenance organizations

B. Secondary
1. Early diagnosis and treatment to stop the progress of disease
2. Prevention of complications
3. The largest and most expensive segment of the health care delivery system
4. Usually takes place in hospitals but also in clinics and physicians' offices

C. Tertiary
1. Rehabilitation after illness to return the patient to a level of maximum functioning
2. Involves assessing patient's strengths and weaknesses, assisting the patient to increase strengths and cope with limitations, assisting with rehabilitation measures, and encouraging self-care
3. Agencies providing tertiary care are rehabilitation hospitals, skilled nursing homes, and hospices
4. Other groups involved with rehabilitation are special interest groups such as Alcoholics Anonymous and Reach to Recovery

Barriers to Preventive Health Care

A. High cost
1. Preventive measures are not always covered under insurance plan.
2. Lower socioeconomic groups are unable to finance cost.

B. Inconvenience
1. Clinics are usually open only during the day.
2. Getting an appointment with a physician can be difficult.

C. Unpleasantness of diagnostic or treatment measures accompanied by fear of pain

D. Fear of findings causes many to seek care only after symptoms are acute

Role of the LP/VN

A. To act as a role model by promoting personal health
1. Assess own health status through regular physical and dental examinations.

2. Observe basic principles of personal hygiene and avoid products known to be harmful to health such as tobacco and drugs.
3. Provide for adequate rest, sleep, and nutrition.
4. Participate in primary care programs.
5. Obtain treatment of any infection or injury.

B. LP/VN functions within the health care system
1. Promote health: patient teaching
2. Prevent disease: provide safe environment for patients; encourage and participate in screening programs
3. Discovery and treatment of disease by assisting physician with patient's physical examination, making observations, collecting specimens and data, and performing procedures as ordered
4. Rehabilitation: assist patients with rehabilitation procedures

Health Care Agencies

A. The LP/VN should know what resources are available, what services they provide, and how to make use of the services.
B. International agency
1. The World Health Organization (WHO) is an agency of the United Nations established in 1948.
2. WHO assists nations to strengthen and improve their health services by providing advisory service in disease control.
C. Official agencies in the United States—federal, state, and local—are supported by tax dollars and are accountable to the public.
1. U.S. Department of Health and Human Services (USDHHS)
   a. Administration of federal programs relating to health is under the jurisdiction of the USDHHS
   b. The USDHHS has five divisions:
      (1) Social Security Administration (SSA): administers the national system of health, old age, survivor, and disability insurance
      (2) Health Care Financing Administration (HCFA) created in 1977 to oversee the Medicare and Medicaid programs
      (3) Office of Human Development Services: administers programs on aging, children, youth and families, and Native Americans
      (4) Public Health Service (PHS): involved with improving and protecting the health and environment of the United States; the major components of the PHS include:
         (a) Centers for Disease Control and Prevention (CDC)
         (b) Food and Drug Administration (FDA)
         (c) Health Resources and Services Administration (HRSA)
         (d) National Institutes of Health (NIH)
         (e) Alcohol, Drug Abuse, and Mental Health Administration Family Support Administration
2. State health departments
   a. Supported by tax funds from the state
   b. Functions vary among the states; usually responsible for licensing of hospitals, nursing homes, and undertakers; health education materials; vital statistics; and communicable disease control

3. Local health department functions also vary; the general functions include:
   a. Keeping vital statistics
   b. Reporting communicable disease
   c. Providing maternal and child health services
   d. Providing environmental sanitation; inspecting food establishments
D. Voluntary agencies
1. Depend on voluntary contributions for funds
2. Are concerned with prevention and solution of specific health problem
3. Provide funds for research and educational projects
4. National organizations function through state or local chapters; examples of voluntary agencies are:
   a. American Cancer Society
   b. American Diabetes Association
   c. American Heart Association
   d. American Red Cross
   e. National Society for the Prevention of Blindness
E. Health service providers: presently a realignment of services is shifting care from acute hospital settings to ambulatory and home care.
1. Hospitals
   a. Short-term facilities provide acute care for patients undergoing treatment for health problems.
   b. Long-term facilities provide service over an extended period for patients with chronic or long-term health problems; rehabilitation, as well as recreational and occupational therapy, are stressed.
2. Nursing homes, also called long-term or extended-care facilities; the federal government has established two categories of nursing homes.
   a. Skilled nursing facility (SNF), which provides 24-hour nursing service for the recuperating resident who no longer needs intensive nursing but still requires skilled nursing
   b. Intermediate care facility (ICF), which provides regular nursing care, but not around the clock, for residents not capable of living by themselves.
3. Hospices
   a. Care is provided to assist the terminally ill patient to achieve the highest possible quality of life.
   b. The goal is to maintain the patient in his or her own environment.
   c. Care is provided in the home by home care nurses.
4. Home care
   a. Continuity and comprehensive health service are provided for individuals who do not need to be hospitalized but who require more than ambulatory care.
   b. Services provided vary from homemaker services to skilled nursing care.
   c. Estimated skilled nursing care may be provided at one third of the cost of hospitalization.
5. Ambulatory care: care provided on outpatient basis
6. Geriatric day care centers: patients are cared for during the day at the center and returned home during the evening
F. Financing health care
1. Health maintenance organizations (HMOs)
   a. Provide comprehensive health services to participants on a prepaid basis

b. Emphasize primary care to prevent costly illness and hospitalization

c. Do not cover illness outside service area

2. Related health insurance plans and organizations

a. Preferred provider organization (PPO): network of health care agencies that offer insurance plan enrollees services at reduced rates; cost is higher for medical service from outside providers

b. Exclusive provider organization (EPO): PPO insurance plan that does not reimburse for services of providers outside the network

c. Point of service (POS): plan that uses a primary care physician to refer patients to additional services within the plan; unauthorized use of services costs more

3. Medicare and Medicaid are government-supported health insurance programs created in 1965 by an amendment to the Social Security Act.

a. Medicare, title XVIII, provides medical care to older adults receiving Social Security benefits regardless of their need, to people with permanent disabilities, and to those with end stages of renal disease.

b. Medicaid, title XIX, was designed to defray expenses that Medicare did not provide for older adults in need; it also provides services for the poor; program is jointly sponsored with matching funds from federal and state governments; today the states contribute a larger share than the federal government.

4. Diagnosis-related groups (DRGs) and managed care

a. DRGs were established to determine Medicare reimbursement; averages costs of care based on diagnosis. DRGs are being phased out because of managed care systems.

b. Managed care: various methods for financing and organizing the delivery of health care in which costs are lowered by controlling the provision of services

c. Both DRGs and managed care have caused early discharges, decreased acute care census, and reevaluation of need for in-hospital care for many diagnoses.

FACTORS INFLUENCING HEALTH AND ILLNESS

Growth and Development of the Adult

A. Growth is change in physical size and functioning.

B. Development is change in psychosocial functioning.

C. Growth and development progress from the simple to the complex and in orderly sequences.

D. Individuals grow and develop at different rates.

E. Most growth has occurred by adulthood.

F. Certain tasks must be accomplished in each stage of development.

G. Stages cannot be skipped; each must be accomplished before the next.

H. Stages and tasks of adult development

1. Young adulthood (18 to 40 years)

a. Characteristics

(1) The "prime" of biologic life

(2) Reproductive capacity is at its height

(3) A generally healthy period of life

b. Tasks

(1) Developing a set of personal moral values

(2) Establishing a personal identity and lifestyle

(3) Establishing intimate relationships outside the family

(4) Establishing own family or support unit

(5) Establishing a career: a field of work

(6) Achieving independence

2. Middle adulthood (40 to 65 years)

a. Characteristics

(1) Physical changes develop gradually: diminishing strength, energy, and endurance, wrinkles, graying and loss of hair, changes in vision, menopause, and increased weight

(2) Beginning of chronic illnesses: cancer and heart disease

(3) Decreased demands of parenthood, with children achieving independence

(4) Increased demands of aged parents

(5) Expected period of work and financial success

(6) A period sometimes involving crisis: the "empty nest," realization that lifelong dreams are yet unmet

b. Tasks

(1) Adjusting to changes: physical, family, and social

(2) Recognizing own mortality

(3) Developing concern beyond the family: future generations and society in general

3. Older adulthood (over 65 years)

a. Characteristics

(1) Many variations exist in levels of functioning and health.

(2) Retirement often brings fixed income.

(3) Most older adults are undergoing the normal physical changes of the aging process; most maintain active lifestyles.

b. Tasks

(1) Adjusting to loss of friends and family members

(2) Adapting to the physical changes of the aging process

(3) Adapting to psychosocial changes: relationships with children, retirement, and housing

(4) Review life and prepare for death

4. Development of the family

a. Understanding the patient's role in the family, the influence of the family on the patient, and the developmental stage of the family helps to understand better the patient and his or her feelings and needs.

b. Characteristics

(1) Traditional: wife, husband, and perhaps children

(2) Nontraditional but common

(a) Single parent (usually the mother) as a result of death, divorce, or never having been married

(b) Communal: unrelated adults with or without children in a group setting

c. Stages and tasks

(1) Marriage

(a) Establishing a home

(b) Establishing individual responsibilities

(c) Establishing a gratifying sexual relationship

(d) Establishing good communication

(2) Child-rearing stage

(a) Taking on new responsibilities: financial and maintaining an optimal atmosphere for growth and development

(b) Continuing efforts to maintain communication among all family members

(c) Adapting to changes that occur as children become independent

(3) Postparental stage

(a) A crisis period caused by lifestyle changes, or

(b) A relaxed period with fewer parental demands

(c) More time available for hobbies and personal pleasures

Environmental (External) Factors

A. Physical agents
   1. Heat: may lead to heat exhaustion or heat stroke
   2. Ultraviolet rays of the sun: produce sunburn
   3. Cold: may cause hypothermia, frostbite, or even death, especially in the very young or very old
   4. Electric current: may cause shock, burns, or death
B. Chemical agents
   1. Taken accidentally or intentionally
   2. Taken by ingestion, such as medicine overdose
   3. Inhaled, such as gases, insecticidal sprays, and factory emissions
C. Cultural background: the beliefs and practices common to a group of people and passed down from generation to generation
   1. Cultural practices influence food habits, reactions to illness, family interactions, and health practices.
   2. The nurse needs to be aware of patient's cultural practices and beliefs to meet needs in a way most beneficial to the patient.
D. Religious background
   1. Religious practices may affect health practices.
   2. Complying with a patient's religious practices may help reduce anxiety during illness.
   3. Must be aware of the patient: may follow all, some, or none of the religion's practices; may turn to or completely away from them while ill
   4. The nurse must know the practices of the major religions and learn about others when the occasion arises to best meet the patient's needs (Table 2-1).

TABLE 2-1	Common Religious Practices		
Religion	**Clergy**	**Sabbath**	**Practices**
Judaism	Rabbi	Sundown Friday to sundown Saturday	Observation of Kosher laws
Reform			Meat and dairy products not served at the same meal
Conservative			No pork products
Orthodox			Only fish with scales and fins may be eaten
			Circumcision of male child
			Are excused from dietary practices when ill
Protestantism	Priest	Sunday	Sacraments of baptism and communion
Episcopal	Minister		
Methodist			
Presbyterian			
Baptist			
Others			
Catholicism	Priest	Sunday	Sacraments of baptism, confession, communion, confirmation, marriage, holy orders, anointing of the sick (last rites)
Roman			
Others			Critically ill infants may be baptized by the nurse
			Abstention from meat on Ash Wednesday and on Fridays during Lent (40 days from Ash Wednesday to Easter)
			Some still abstain from meat on all Fridays
			Many believe they must attend mass each week; can be performed at the bedside
Jehovah's Witnesses	Every member is a minister	Sunday	Do not accept blood products
Seventh Day Adventists	Elder	Sundown Friday to sundown Saturday	Abstain from pork and pork products
Islam	Imam	Friday	Alcohol and pork products are forbidden
The Church of Jesus of Latter-Day Saints (Mormons)	Elder	Sunday	Abstain from tobacco, coffee, tea, colas, and alcohol

E. Socioeconomic level
1. Economic level may influence accessibility of health care.
2. Lack of social and economic resources may contribute to disturbed mental health.
3. Substandard living accommodations and sanitation may predispose to diseases such as tuberculosis.
F. Infectious agents
1. Microorganisms: small living organisms that can only be seen with a microscope
   a. Pathogens: disease-producing organisms
   b. Nonpathogens: organisms that do not usually cause disease
   c. Normal flora: microorganisms that normally live on or in an individual's body
2. Types of microorganisms
   a. Bacteria
   b. Viruses
   c. Fungi
   d. Protozoa
   e. Rickettsia

Internal Factors

A. Congenital factors
1. Defined as being present at birth
2. Defects may be hereditary, caused by malformation during intrauterine life, or a result of birth injuries.
3. Maternal infections, such as German measles, during the first trimester of pregnancy often result in congenital defects.
4. Certain drugs, including alcohol, are implicated in congenital defects.
B. Hereditary factors
1. Defined as being transmitted via the genes from parents to offspring
2. Can produce conditions such as phenylketonuria, hemophilia, or sickle cell disease
C. Body defense mechanisms
1. Methods used by the body to protect itself from invasion by disease-producing substances
2. First barriers are unbroken skin and mucous membranes.
3. Tears wash foreign particles, including some microorganisms, from the eyes.
4. The normally acid secretions of the vagina usually destroy pathogens.
5. Cilia (hairlike projections) in the nose, trachea, and bronchi sweep pathogens out of the respiratory tract.
6. Reflexes such as coughing and sneezing rid the body of pathogens.
7. Inflammatory reaction
   a. A local reaction that occurs when tissue is injured by physical agents, chemical agents, or microorganisms.
   b. Signs: redness, heat, pain, swelling, and limited movement
   c. After an injury, the inflammatory process begins: blood flow to the area increases; leukocytes move out of capillaries to the area; phagocytes begin to engulf and digest bacteria; pus forms from dead pathogens and dead tissue; healing begins.
   d. Conditions caused by inflammation commonly end with the suffix itis, (e.g., vaginitis, cystitis).
8. Immune response

a. The body's response to the invasion of foreign protein substances: bacteria, viruses, foods, chemicals, and tissue
b. Antigen: any invading substance that can trigger the immune response
c. Antibody: proteins (gamma globulins) produced by the body to defend against the invading antigen
D. Immunity
1. The state of being resistant to a particular pathogen
2. Active immunity: occurs when the individual produces his or her own antibodies
   a. Results naturally after having had a specific disease such as chickenpox, or
   b. Acquired after the administration of:
      (1) Vaccines made up of living or killed organisms, such as the measles vaccine
      (2) Toxoids made of neutralized toxins (poisons) produced by bacteria, such as tetanus
3. Passive immunity: results from receiving antibodies developed by another source (animal or human)
   a. Received naturally by fetus from mother: lasts only approximately 6 months
   b. Acquired from the administration of:
      (1) Immune serum, usually from animals: provides short-term immunity to a specific organism, such as that causing rabies
      (2) Gamma globulin, usually from humans: also provides short-term immunity to a specific organism, such as hepatitis
4. Autoimmunity
   a. Antibodies are produced by the body against its own tissues.
   b. Autoimmunity is thought to be a factor in diseases such as rheumatoid arthritis and rheumatic fever.
E. Fluid and electrolyte balance
1. 50% to 60% of adult body weight is body fluid.
2. 75% to 80% of a young child's weight is body fluid.
3. Body fluids consist mostly of water.
4. Electrolytes are substances that, when dissolved in water, become electrically charged ions (Table 2-2).
5. Amounts of fluid and electrolytes must be normal at all times for the body to be in homeostasis (a state of equilibrium).
6. Fluids and electrolytes are present in "compartments" but constantly flow between the compartments to maintain balance (Figure 2-1).
F. Tissue and wound healing
1. Healing is affected by a person's general condition, age, nutritional status, the blood supply to the area, and extent of the injury.
2. Many injured tissues are repaired by cell regeneration: cells are replaced by identical or similar cells.
   a. Tissues of the skin, digestive and respiratory tracts, and bone regenerate well.
   b. Nervous, muscle, and elastic tissues have little ability to regenerate.
3. When regeneration cannot take place, granulation tissue is formed, which eventually becomes a scar.
4. Formation of scar tissue often leaves disfigurement, such as after burns, or diminished function, such as in heart tissue after myocardial infarction.
5. Types of wounds
   a. Incision: clean wound made by sharp instrument

TABLE 2-2   Principal Electrolytes

Principal Electrolytes	Normal Serum Value	Problems Associated With Excess	Problems Associated With Deficit
Na⁺ (sodium)	134-145 mEq/L	Dry mucous membranes, thirst, restlessness	Confusion, weakness, coma (hyponatremia)
K⁺ (potassium)	3.6-5 mEq/L	Nausea, vomiting, diarrhea, irritability, cardiac standstill (hyperkalemia)	Weakness, cardiac arrhythmias (hypokalemia)
Ca⁺⁺ (calcium)	9-11 mg/dl	Nausea, vomiting, muscle weakness (hypercalcemia)	Muscle cramps, tetany, convulsions (hypocalcemia)

mEq/L, Milliequivalents per liter; *mg/dl,* milligrams per deciliter.

TABLE 2-3   Wound Healing

Type of Healing	Type of Wound	How Healing Occurs
First intention	Minimal tissue damage Simple incision	Without infection No separation of wound edges Results in minimal scar
Second intention	Decubitus ulcer Severe burn	Wound edges do not join Spaces between wound edges fill with granulation tissue Results in scar
Third intention	Dehisced suture line	Wound edges come together at first, then reopen Results in scar and possibly contraction of surrounding tissue

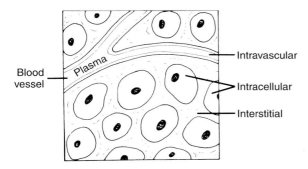

FIGURE 2-1. Body fluid compartments. *Intracellular,* inside the cells; *extracellular,* outside the cells. *Extracellular* compartments may be either interstitial (between the cells) or *intravascular* (in the vessels).

b. Contusion: closed wound; bruise; made with blunt force; underlying tissue is damaged
c. Abrasion: rubbed or scraped off skin or mucous membrane
d. Puncture: small opening or hole made by a pointed instrument
e. Laceration: tear or rip leaving jagged edges
6. Wound healing is classified by first, second, or third intention (Table 2-3).

CONCEPTS BASIC TO NURSING

Reducing the Spread of Microorganisms

A. Infectious disease chain
  1. Presence of pathogenic organisms

  2. A susceptible host: susceptibility affected by:
     a. Nutritional status
     b. Age
     c. Personal health habits
     d. Medical treatments in progress (radiation therapy and bone marrow–depressing drugs)
     e. Trauma
     f. Chronic illness
     g. Stress
     h. Fatigue
  3. Portal of entry to the body: break in skin or mucous membrane, vaginal opening, or blood
  4. Reservoir: microorganisms that multiply and increase in number in the bladder, lungs, or throat
  5. Modes of transmission (movement or spread) of microorganisms
     a. By contact (excreta or used tissues)
     b. By air, on droplets (sneezing and coughing)
     c. On fomites (books and stethoscopes)
     d. In food or water
     e. By vectors (animals and insects)
  6. Portal of exit from the body: mouth, nose, rectum, skin, blood, or reproductive tract
B. Measures to reduce the spread by breaking the chain (interrupting the process)
  1. Hand washing: most important measure
  2. Medical asepsis: practices that limit the numbers, growth, and spread of microorganisms (clean technique)
     a. Linens: no shaking or holding against uniform
     b. Use of antiseptics and disinfectants
     c. Anything touching the floor is not to be used.
  3. Surgical asepsis: practices that eliminate microorganisms and their spores from sterile items or areas (sterile technique)

a. Used in operative procedures, delivery room, and caring for patients with breaks in skin and for procedures that enter sterile body cavities (e.g., bladder, lung, vein)
b. General principles
   (1) Sterile items become nonsterile (contaminated) when touched by anything that is not sterile.
   (2) Sterile field that becomes wet is considered nonsterile.
   (3) Sterile items out of eyesight or below waist level are considered nonsterile.
   (4) Nurses need to develop a sterile conscience (self-judgment of whether aseptic practices have been broken) and act accordingly.
c. Means of sterilization
   (1) Steam under pressure: autoclave
   (2) Boiling
   (3) Liquid chemicals
   (4) Gas
4. Isolation and barrier techniques (protective asepsis): practices that limit the transfer of microorganisms either from the infected person or to a highly susceptible person
   a. Category-specific isolation
      (1) Enteric: to reduce spread of pathogens via feces (e.g., hepatitis A)
      (2) Respiratory: to reduce spread of pathogens through the air (e.g., pneumonia)
      (3) Tuberculosis Isolation: (acid-fast bacillus) to reduce exposure in health care settings; gown and particulate respirator mask, patient in negative air pressure isolation room
      (4) Strict: to reduce spread of pathogens by air or contact (e.g., chickenpox)
      (5) Drainage or secretion: to reduce spread of pathogens by contact with the infected person or contaminated articles (linens) (e.g., draining wounds)
      (6) Universal Blood and Body Fluid Precautions (Universal Precautions): used by everyone to prevent transmission by direct or indirect contact with blood or body fluids (e.g., acquired immunodeficiency syndrome [AIDS])
      (7) Protective Isolation or Reverse Isolation: care of severely compromised patients: to protect a highly susceptible person (with lowered resistance) from becoming infected (e.g., leukemia)
   b. Disease-Specific Isolation: each disease receives its specific protective measures—historically used for tuberculosis, not used much anymore
   c. Standard Precautions: guidelines recommended by the CDC to control and reduce the risk of transmission of blood-borne and other pathogens; a combination of universal (blood and body fluid) precautions and body substance isolation; applies features to all patients receiving care regardless of diagnosis or presumed infection status; applies to blood, all body fluids, nonintact skin, and mucous membranes
C. Types of infections
   1. Nosocomial: acquired as a result of hospitalization
   2. Local: confined to a relatively small, specific area (e.g., a wound)
   3. Systemic: infection spreads throughout body

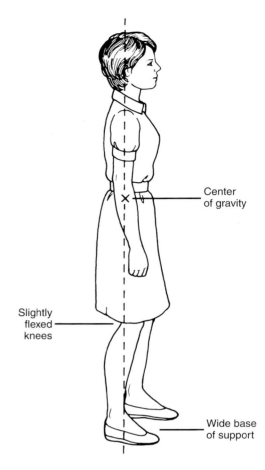

FIGURE 2-2. Body alignment. Lateral view of adult with alignment of head, neck, spine, slightly flexed knees, and wide base of support. *(Adapted from Sorrentino SA:* Mosby's Textbook for nursing assistants, *ed 5, St Louis, 2000, Mosby.)*

   4. Methicillin-resistant *Staphylococcus aureus* (MRSA): caused by *Staphylococcus aureus* that has become resistant to all antibiotics but vancomycin
   5. Vancomycin-resistant enterococci (VRE): a virtual "superbug" microorganism that is resistant to all antibiotics
   6. Colonization: when an individual has MRSA or VRE within his or her body without creating an infectious situation; these patients should still be isolated from the general acute care population.

Body Mechanics

A. Defined as efficient use of the body's structure and muscles
B. Applies to patients as well as nurses
C. Use of good body mechanics helps to prevent injuries, conserve energy, and prevent fatigue.
D. Principles of good body mechanics
   1. Maintain proper alignment (posture): head, neck, and spine should be in a straight line with feet 10 to 12 inches (25 to 31 cm) apart and pointed straight ahead and knees slightly flexed (Figure 2-2).
   2. Maintain a wide base of support: keep feet separated to provide balance (see Figure 2-2).
   3. Keep center of gravity directly above the base of support (see Figure 2-2).

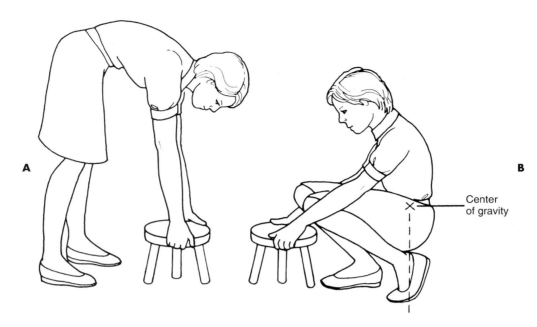

FIGURE 2-3.   **A,** Lifting with poor body mechanics: using back muscles. **B,** Lifting with good body mechanics: using leg muscles with object close to body. *(Adapted from Sorrentino SA:* Mosby's Textbook for nursing assistants, *ed 5, St Louis, 2000, Mosby.)*

E. Points to remember
   1. Use largest and strongest muscles (legs, arms, and shoulders) when moving or lifting heavy objects (Figure 2-3).
   2. Do not let your back do the work.
   3. Roll, slide, push, or pull an object rather than lift it.
   4. Keep objects close to your body when lifting or moving; avoid reaching, twisting or bending unnecessarily.
   5. Point feet in the direction of movement.
   6. Use devices whenever possible: patient lifters, trapeze, turning sheets, and rolling carts.
   7. Get assistance when necessary.
   8. Have the patient help as much as possible when being moved or lifted.

Communication

A. Definition: exchange of messages between two or more people, including information, thoughts, and feelings
B. Purposes in nursing
   1. To establish a meaningful, helping relationship between nurse and patient
   2. To transmit information between health care workers
C. Means
   1. Verbal
   2. Written
   3. Nonverbal
D. Guidelines
   1. Verbal communication
      a. Introduce self, stating name and title.
      b. Be sincerely interested in the patient.
      c. Be an attentive, active listener.
      d. Stand or sit close to the patient.
      e. Allow the patient to express thoughts and feelings freely without fear of being judged.
      f. Clarify what has been said to ensure understanding.

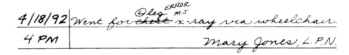

FIGURE 2-4.   Correcting an error in a nurse's note.

      g. Ask open-ended questions rather than questions resulting in yes or no answers: "What has happened to change your mind?"
      h. Use incomplete sentences: "You are afraid that..."
      i. Report information accurately and thoroughly.
      j. Report abnormal findings immediately.
      k. Maintain confidentiality.
   2. Written communication
      a. Record information clearly, concisely, and accurately.
      b. Nurses' notes are part of a legal document.
         (1) Use a pen.
         (2) Use only standard abbreviations.
         (3) Do not erase or obliterate errors (Figure 2-4).
         (4) Leave no blank spaces.
         (5) Sign the note at the time it is written.
         (6) Date and time each entry.
      c. Formats for nurses' notes
         (1) Narrative: in paragraph form (Figure 2-5, *B*)
         (2) SOAP: subjective data, objective data, assessment, plan (Figure 2-5, *A*)
         (3) PIE: problem, intervention, and evaluation
         (4) Focus charting: data (assessment); action (planning and implementation); response (evaluation) (Figure 2-5, *C*)
         (5) Charting by exception: used with flow sheets, pertinent data charted at beginning shift, only changes in treatments or patient condition noted

after that; must include details on patient status for accurate monitoring
3. Nonverbal communication
   a. Exchanging messages by body posture, movements, gestures, and touch
   b. Often a more accurate expression of what is being thought or felt than verbal expression

Basic Human Needs

A. Definition: described by the psychologist Abraham Maslow as needs that must be met for humans to function at their highest possible level
B. Used by many nurses as a systematic guide for assessment
C. Premises
   1. The hierarchy of needs; lower level needs must be met before higher level ones can be addressed.
   2. People will usually be able to meet their own needs.
   3. When people are unable to meet their own needs, intervention is required.
   4. In caring for the whole person, the nurse is involved in helping to meet the basic needs, as well as in dealing with signs and symptoms of disease.
   5. Chronologic age is not a variable in ascending the hierarchy of needs.
D. Hierarchy of needs (Figure 2-6, p. 28)
   1. Physiologic: oxygen, water, food, elimination, rest and sleep, activity, sexuality, and relief of pain
   2. Safety and security: protection from injury, maintenance of body defenses, structure and order in both the environment and relationships, and freedom from anxiety
   3. Love and belonging: not just romantic love but a feeling of affection (the need for caring relationships)
   4. Esteem: a feeling of worth and value to both self and others
   5. Self-actualization: reaching one's fullest potential

NURSING PROCESS

A. Definition: a set of predetermined steps that nurses use to identify and to help solve patient problems
B. Purposes
   1. To provide planned, coordinated, and individualized patient care
   2. To communicate problems and approaches among all individuals providing patient care
C. The process: names of steps differ slightly according to various sources but include the following:
   1. Assessment: gathering and organizing of data; statement of patient problems (unmet needs); the nursing diagnosis
   2. Planning: setting goals to be accomplished and constructing a plan of action to accomplish the goals
   3. Implementation: carrying out the nursing actions to accomplish the goals and solve the problem (meet the need)
   4. Evaluation: determining whether the goal was accomplished and the problem solved

Assessment: A Continuous Process

A. Sources of data
   1. Patient
   2. Family or significant others

3. Patient's chart
   a. Physician's order sheet
   b. Nurses' notes
   c. Laboratory reports
      (1) Blood chemistry
         (a) Electrolytes: see fluid and electrolyte balance
         (b) Creatinine: assesses kidney function
      (2) Complete blood count (CBC): assesses adequacy of the various blood cells: red, white, and platelets
      (3) Blood sugar (BS) or glucose: fasting (FBS) or postprandial (after meals), or Hgb A1C—three month gauge of glucose levels in the body
   d. X-ray reports
      (1) Chest x-ray examination: assesses condition of lungs and size of heart
      (2) Upper gastrointestinal (UGI) series: assesses condition of esophagus, stomach, and duodenum with barium sulfate used as the contrast medium; can also diagnose dysphagia
      (3) Barium enema (BaE): assesses condition of colon with barium sulfate used as the contrast medium
      (4) Gallbladder series (GBS): assesses condition of the gallbladder with radiopaque dye
   e. Electrocardiogram (ECG) reports: assesses the electrical activity of the heart
   f. Biopsy reports: assesses a tissue specimen for cell changes
   g. Progress notes of other health care workers
      (1) Physician
      (2) Social worker
      (3) Dietician
      (4) Physical therapist
      (5) Occupational therapist
      (6) Respiratory therapist
4. Nursing report
B. Subjective versus objective data
   1. Subjective data
      a. Information reported by the patient
      b. Information that is not observable by another person
         (1) Pain
         (2) Nausea
         (3) Anxiety
         (4) Dizziness
         (5) Ringing in the ears (tinnitus)
         (6) Numbness

4/18/92	PROBLEM #6 – Drainage on Cast. Ⓛ
4 PM	lateral aspect of knee
	S – "I have no pain or numbness."
	O – Toes pink, warm, mobile. VS stable.
	A – Normal postoperative drainage.
	P – Mark area of drainage. Reassess
	patient and cast q ½ hr.
	Elaine Stevens, L.P.N.

A

FIGURE 2-5.   A, Nurse's note in SOAP format.

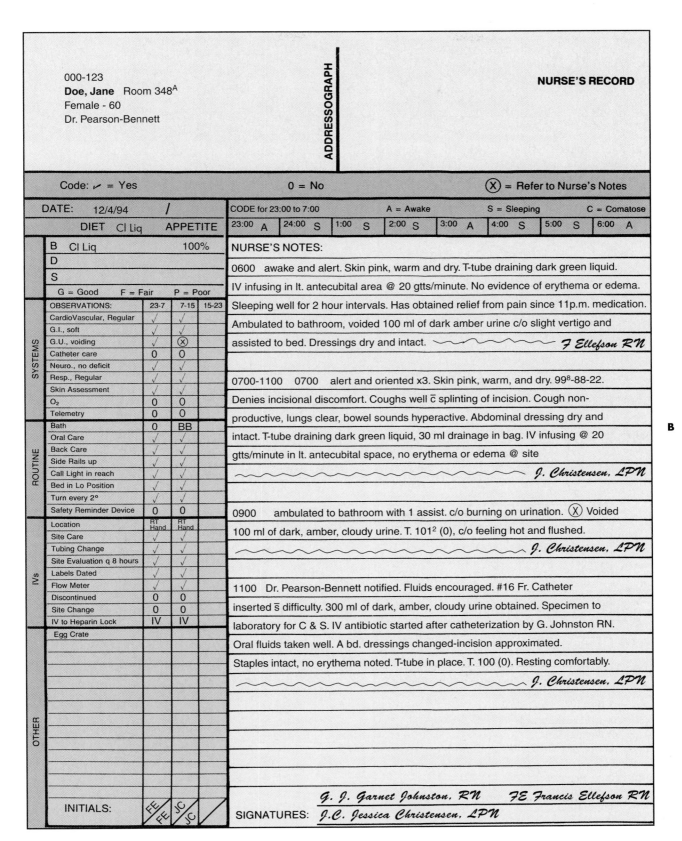

000-123		**ADDRESSOGRAPH**
Doe, Jane Room 348^A		
Female - 60		
Dr. Pearson-Bennett		

NURSE'S RECORD

Code: ✓ = Yes   0 = No   ⊗ = Refer to Nurse's Notes

DATE: 12/4/94   /

| DIET | Cl Liq | APPETITE | CODE for 23:00 to 7:00 | | A = Awake | | S = Sleeping | | C = Comatose |

| 23:00 A | 24:00 S | 1:00 S | 2:00 S | 3:00 A | 4:00 S | 5:00 S | 6:00 A |

B	Cl Liq		100%
D			
S			

G = Good   F = Fair   P = Poor

SYSTEMS

OBSERVATIONS:	23-7	7-15	15-23
CardioVascular, Regular	✓	✓	
G.I., soft	✓	✓	
G.U., voiding	✓	⊗	
Catheter care	0	0	
Neuro., no deficit	✓	✓	
Resp., Regular	✓	✓	
Skin Assessment	✓	✓	
O₂	0	0	
Telemetry	0	0	

ROUTINE

	23-7	7-15	15-23
Bath	0	BB	
Oral Care	✓	✓	
Back Care	✓	✓	
Side Rails up	✓	✓	
Call Light in reach	✓	✓	
Bed in Lo Position	✓	✓	
Turn every 2°	✓	✓	
Safety Reminder Device	0	0	

IVs

	23-7	7-15	15-23
Location	RT Hand	RT Hand	
Site Care	✓	✓	
Tubing Change	✓	✓	
Site Evaluation q 8 hours	✓	✓	
Labels Dated	✓	✓	
Flow Meter	✓	✓	
Discontinued	0	0	
Site Change	0	0	
IV to Heparin Lock	IV	IV	

OTHER

Egg Crate			

| INITIALS: | FE FE | JC JC | |

NURSE'S NOTES:

0600   awake and alert. Skin pink, warm and dry. T-tube draining dark green liquid.

IV infusing in lt. antecubital area @ 20 gtts/minute. No evidence of erythema or edema.

Sleeping well for 2 hour intervals. Has obtained relief from pain since 11p.m. medication.

Ambulated to bathroom, voided 100 ml of dark amber urine c/o slight vertigo and

assisted to bed. Dressings dry and intact. ~~~~~~~~~~ *F Ellefson RN*

0700-1100   0700   alert and oriented x3. Skin pink, warm, and dry. 99⁸-88-22.

Denies incisional discomfort. Coughs well c̄ splinting of incision. Cough non-

productive, lungs clear, bowel sounds hyperactive. Abdominal dressing dry and

intact. T-tube draining dark green liquid, 30 ml drainage in bag. IV infusing @ 20

gtts/minute in lt. antecubital space, no erythema or edema @ site

~~~~~~~~~~~~~~~~~~~~ *J. Christensen. LPN*

0900   ambulated to bathroom with 1 assist. c/o burning on urination. ⊗ Voided

100 ml of dark, amber, cloudy urine. T. 101² (0), c/o feeling hot and flushed.

~~~~~~~~~~~~~~~ *J. Christensen. LPN*

1100   Dr. Pearson-Bennett notified. Fluids encouraged. #16 Fr. Catheter

inserted s̄ difficulty. 300 ml of dark, amber, cloudy urine obtained. Specimen to

laboratory for C & S. IV antibiotic started after catheterization by G. Johnston RN.

Oral fluids taken well. A bd. dressings changed-incision approximated.

Staples intact, no erythema noted. T-tube in place. T. 100 (0). Resting comfortably.

~~~~~~~~~~~~~~~ *J. Christensen. LPN*

SIGNATURES: *G. J. Garnet Johnston. RN   FE Francis Ellefson RN*
J.C. Jessica Christensen. LPN

B

FIGURE 2-5, cont'd   B, Narrative charting.

DATE	12/7	
TIME	FOCUS	NURSES NOTES
1400	post-op pain	Ambulating in hall c̄ moderate assist. I.V. infusing
		@ 20 gtts/min. Still feels warm, main concern is
		incisional pain, splinting is helpful. Positioned in
		bed c̄ pillows for support. Medicated for pain.
		Practiced relaxation breathing exercises. *J. Christensen, LPN*
1400	pain/fever	States, "I am more comfortable and relaxed now." Skin warm
		and dry. T. 99⁶ (0). c/o some burning on urination,
		less than in a.m. Taking fluids well. Urine light
		yellow and less cloudy. ～～～ *J. Christensen, LPN*

FIGURE 2-5, cont'd   C, Focus charting nurse's notes.

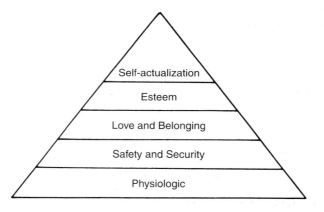

FIGURE 2-6. Hierarchy of basic human needs as described by Maslow.

2. Objective data
   a. Information gathered through the senses: sight, hearing, smell, and feel
   b. Information gathered with a measuring instrument: thermometer, sphygmomanometer, and scale
      (1) Vital signs
      (2) Weight, height
      (3) Hematuria
      (4) Wheezing
      (5) Edema
      (6) Cyanosis

C. Methods of gathering data
   1. Formal interviewing (communication with patient and family or significant others): usually on patient's admission to the hospital
      a. Gather data on age, occupation, and reason for hospitalization, medications, allergies, previous hospitalizations, previous illnesses, prostheses, valuables, and special diet
      b. Gather data on difficulty with activities of daily living (ADL), sleep, elimination, activity, eating, and any special needs
   2. Listening
   3. Observation of the patient and attached equipment
      a. Use an orderly approach.
         (1) Head-to-toe
         (2) System-by-system
         (3) Basic human needs
      b. Look for signs and symptoms of disease or change in disease.
   4. Physical examination
      a. Methods
         (1) Inspection
         (2) Palpation
         (3) Percussion
         (4) Auscultation
      b. Assisting with the physical examination
         (1) Be sure that the patient understands the examination and why it is being done.
         (2) Gather equipment.
         (3) Position patient appropriately (Figure 2-7).

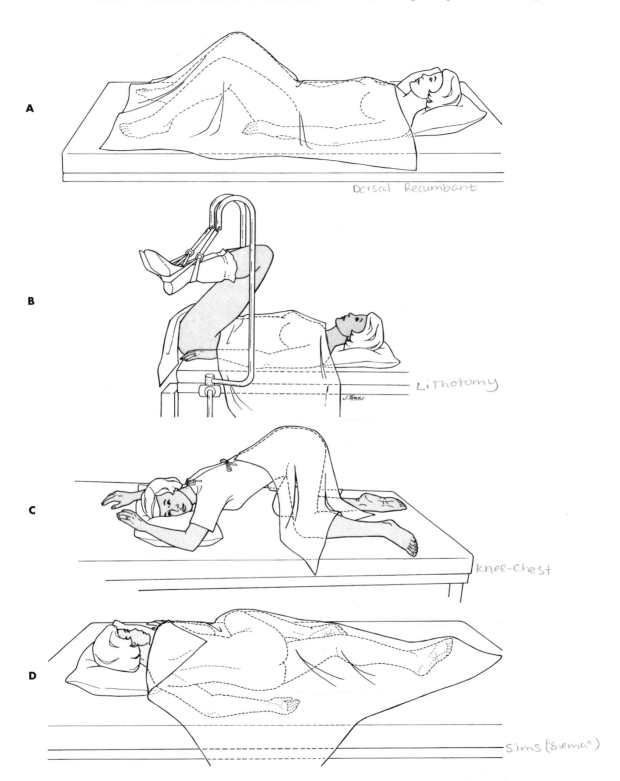

FIGURE 2-7. **Positioning and draping for the physical examination. A,** Dorsal recumbent position. **B,** Lithotomy position. **C,** Knee-chest position. **D,** Sims' position. *(Adapted from Sorrentino SA: Mosby's Textbook for nursing assistants, ed 5, St Louis, 2000, Mosby.)*

(4) Drape covers to provide for privacy.
(5) Collect patient data using:
   (a) Interviewing
   (b) Auscultation
   (c) Inspection
   (d) Palpation
   (e) Examination
(6) After the examination, make the patient comfortable and safe, following orders, if any.
(7) Chart the procedure and patient's reactions; note specimens obtained.

c. The practical nurse's role in assisting with diagnostic examinations

(1) Explain procedure to the patient.
(2) Explain and carry out specific requirements.
   (a) Nothing by mouth (NPO) or special meals
   (b) Clothing
   (c) Positioning
   (d) Medications
(3) Chest x-ray examinations: no metal objects (zippers, bra fastenings, necklaces, and pins) should be in view of x-ray.
(4) Blood studies: see agency's procedure manual for requirements of various studies.
(5) UGI series: nothing by mouth after midnight (NPO p- MN), medication or enema to eliminate barium after the x-ray examination.
(6) BaE: low-residue meal evening before, NPO p-MN, medications or enema to clear colon before and after x-ray examination
(7) Excretory urogram or intravenous pyelogram (IVP): NPO p- MN, medications to clear colon before x-ray examination; uses iodine-based dye to diagnose conditions of the kidney, ureters, bladder; notify physician if patient is allergic to iodine or shellfish
(8) GBS: fat-free meal evening before, NPO p- MN, oral ingestion of dye tablets; dye is iodine based; check patient for iodine or shellfish allergy.
(9) Lumbar puncture: signed consent form is required; empty bladder and bowel before procedure; patient lies curled on side with head almost touching knees; nurse faces patient holding shoulders and knees; patient remains flat in bed after procedure.
(10) Arteriogram: visualization of an artery after injection of a radiopaque dye; patient stays still for a period because of chance for bleeding at injection site.
(11) Bronchoscopy: visualization of the bronchi using a scope; patient's throat is sometimes anesthetized; check for a gag reflex after procedure before fluids are given.
(12) Magnetic resonance imaging (MRI): patient must have no metal implanted in their body or metal pins, barrettes, watches on while they are in the MRI machine.
(13) Colonoscopy, sigmoidoscopy: generally patient is sedated lightly before procedure; cleansing enemas are required before the procedure.
(14) Papanicolaou (PAP) test: cells are taken from cervix of female and "fixed" onto a slide before sending to the lab; often an uncomfortable procedure; patient should void before this procedure and receive emotional support.

5. Measurement of vital signs: to assess functioning of cardiovascular and respiratory systems
a. Temperature
  (1) Normal ranges
    (a) Axillary: 96° to 98° F
    (b) Oral: 97° to 99° F
    (c) Rectal: 98° to 100° F
    (d) Tympanic: 97° to 99° F
  (2) Oral temperature
    (a) Mercury thermometer is left in place 2 to 4 minutes or according to agency policy.
    (b) Electronic thermometer is left in place until final reading is indicated.
    (c) Wait 10 minutes if the patient has been eating, smoking, drinking a hot or cold beverage, or chewing gum.
    (d) Contraindications
     • Patient is receiving oxygen.
     • Patient is irrational or unconscious.
     • Patient is under 5 years of age.
     • Patient is breathing through the mouth.
     • Patient is prone to seizures.
     • Patient recently had oral surgery or mouth trauma.
     • Patient is on suicide precautions.
  (3) Rectal temperature
    (a) Mercury thermometer is held in place 3 to 4 minutes or according to agency policy.
    (b) Electronic thermometer is held in place until final reading is indicated.
    (c) Lubricate before inserting; insert 1.0 to 1.5 inches (3.75 cm).
    (d) Contraindications
     • Rectal or perineal surgery
     • Diseases of the rectum
     • Diarrhea
     • Use with caution in patients with cardiovascular disease.
     • Use with caution in restless or combative patients.
  (4) Axillary temperature
    (a) Mercury thermometer is held in place 10 minutes.
    (b) Electronic thermometer is held in place until final reading is indicated.
    (c) Pat dry the axilla before inserting; hold arm close to side.
  (5) Tympanic temperature
    (a) Press "ON" button and apply disposable cover on probe tip.
    (b) Seal ear opening with probe; seal outer ear opening in infants.
    (c) Press "SCAN" button and read temperature after beeper sounds.
    (d) Discard probe cover and replace thermometer in recharger.
    (e) Contraindications
     • Recent exposure to cold air
     • Inflammatory ear condition
     • Excessive cerumen accumulation

b. Pulse: the beat of the heart heard at the apex or felt at specific sites as a wave of blood flows through an artery
  (1) Observe rate, rhythm, and strength
  (2) Normal adult range: 60 to 80 beats per minute (bpm); varies greatly among individuals; rate more rapid for children
  (3) If rate or rhythm is irregular, take pulse apically and count for 1 full minute.
  (4) Variations
    (a) Bradycardia: slow heart rate—under 60 bpm
    (b) Tachycardia: fast heart beat—over 100 bpm
    (c) Irregular: intervals between beats are uneven
    (d) Thready: weak pulse—easily obliterated
    (e) Bounding: very strong pulse—difficult to obliterate
  (5) Sites: felt with fingertips at places where an artery crosses over muscle or bone close to the skin and at the apex of the heart
    (a) Temporal
    (b) Carotid
    (c) Brachial
    (d) Radial
    (e) Femoral
    (f) Popliteal
    (g) Pedal
    (h) Apical: heard with stethoscope
  (6) Apical-radial pulse: to detect a difference between rates at the two sites (the pulse deficit)
    (a) Requires two people: one taking the radial pulse and one taking the apical pulse
    (b) Must be counted simultaneously for 1 full minute
    (c) Apical rate can never be lower than the radial rate.

c. Respiration: the process of inhaling and exhaling air into and out of the lungs; one inhalation plus one exhalation equals one respiration.
  (1) Observe rate, rhythm, and depth; normal adult range is 14 to 20 respirations per minute; varies greatly with activity level; rate is higher for children.
  (2) Patient must not be aware that respirations are being observed.
  (3) Variations
    (a) Apnea: absence of breathing
    (b) Tachypnea: rapid breathing
    (c) Stertorous: noisy breathing; snoring
    (d) Cheyne-Stokes respirations: rhythmic repeated cycles of slow shallow respirations increasing in depth rate, then gradually becoming slower and more shallow, followed by a period of apnea; often precedes death
    (e) Dyspnea: difficulty breathing
    (f) Orthopnea: breathing is possible only while in an upright position
    (g) Kussmaul's: paroxysms of dyspnea often preceding diabetic coma or other acidotic conditions.
  (4) Count respirations for 1 full minute if rate is abnormal or rhythm is irregular.

d. Blood pressure (BP): force exerted by the blood against the walls of the arteries (measured in millimeters [mm] of mercury [Hg])
  (1) Normal adult range is 60 to 80 mm Hg diastolic, 90 to 120 mm Hg systolic; levels varies among individuals and with activity.
  (2) Can be measured at brachial artery or popliteal artery: ensure that arrow on cuff lines up with area where artery is palpated most clearly.
  (3) Be sure cuff is proper size for the individual.
  (4) Terminology
    (a) Systolic: pressure in the arteries during contraction of the heart
    (b) Diastolic: pressure in the arteries during relaxation of the heart
    (c) Hypotension: lower than normal BP—under 100/60—can occur with many conditions; symptomatic hypotension means that the patient becomes dizzy; orthostatic hypotension is dizziness caused by a sudden change in BP created by arising to a standing position quickly.
    (d) Hypertension: higher than normal BP—140/90 mm Hg
    (e) Pulse pressure: difference between systolic and diastolic pressures

e. Pulse oximetry: noninvasive continuous monitor of blood oxygen saturation
  (1) Normal adult range: 95% to 100%
  (2) Report readings under 90%, indicate hypoxia. Oxygen saturation in the arterial blood (SaO_2) under 70% is life threatening.
  (3) Clip-on or adhesive probe attaches to finger, toe, earlobe, or bridge of nose.
  (4) Uses light for reading; do not block light on probe. Area being assessed should be clean, dry, and without nail polish.
  (5) Rotate clip every 4 hours (q4h) adhesive—check for proper clip position with alarms.
  (6) Check abnormal readings with arterial blood gases.

6. Measurement of weight and height
  a. Weight
    (1) Should be done before breakfast
    (2) Should be done in same amount of clothing each day; shoes should be off.
    (3) Can use results in establishing medication dosages, gain or loss of body fluid, and nutritional status
    (4) Can use standing, chair, or stretcher scale; be sure scale is balanced.
  b. Height
    (1) Have patient be in bare feet, standing on a paper towel.
    (2) Have patient stand tall.
    (3) Can use in determining some medication dosages and anesthesia requirements

7. Collection of specimens
  a. General guidelines
    (1) Follow your agency's procedure for collection, container, labels, requisitions, and recording.
    (2) Label all specimen containers correctly and send with a laboratory requisition.
    (3) Send specimens to the laboratory promptly.
    (4) Wear protective gloves.
    (5) Wash hands thoroughly after handling specimen.

(6) Generally, a specimen should be obtained before any antibiotic administration.

b. Urine specimens

(1) Urinalysis: routine examination of urine

  (a) Only the patient and container need be clean.

  (b) Specimens are often collected as part of admission procedure.

(2) Culture and sensitivity

  (a) Clean-catch, midstream: genitalia and meatus are cleansed; specimen is taken after stream has started but before voiding is completed.

  (b) Catheterized specimen: sample is obtained by using sterile technique and equipment.

(3) 24-hour specimens: first voiding is discarded and time is noted; all urine for the next 24 hours is collected; see agency policy for type of container and storage methods; normally done to determine creatinine clearance levels.

(4) Sugar and acetone testing

  (a) Urine should be obtained 30 to 60 minutes before meal or at a designated time.

  (b) Double-voided specimen gives more accurate results.

    • Have patient empty bladder.

    • Collect specimen as soon as patient can void again.

    • Additional fluids may be needed to produce specimen.

  (c) Test specimen with Tes-tape, Clinitest, Clinistix, or Keto-Diastix; follow manufacturer's directions precisely for accurate results.

  (d) Report results immediately to medication nurse.

  (e) Record results in proper place.

(5) Specimens from indwelling catheter

  (a) Closed drainage system must be maintained.

  (b) Specimens must be obtained from specimen "port" with needle and syringe by sterile technique.

c. Stool specimens

(1) Collect in clean bedpan.

(2) Use tongue depressor or wooden spatula to transfer stool to specimen container.

(3) Types of testing

  (a) For blood: occult (guaiac, Hematest); patient must be on a red meat–free diet 3 days before test.

  (b) For culture and sensitivity: use sterile container.

  (c) For ova and parasites: stool must still be warm when it reaches the laboratory.

d. Sputum specimens

(1) Best collected in the morning before breakfast.

(2) Patient first rinses mouth with water.

(3) Instruct patient to take deep breath, cough deeply, and expectorate into container.

(4) Specimen must be from the lung, not just mouth saliva.

e. Blood specimen: capillary puncture (e.g., blood glucose testing). May be a finger stick for child or adult, heel stick for infant. Agency certification may be required.

(1) Explain procedure to patient; warn that it does hurt.

(2) Assemble equipment: gloves, alcohol swab, lancet, collector, gauze or cotton ball, and adhesive bandage.

(3) Wash hands; don gloves.

(4) Enhance blood supply by applying warmth; do not milk site.

(5) Puncture side of nondominant finger or side of heel.

(6) Puncture with lancet; wipe away first drop of blood; collect sample.

(7) Apply pressure to site; apply bandage.

f. Blood specimen: venipuncture; requires puncture of vein for collection of several milliliters of blood for variety of laboratory tests; agency certification usually required.

(1) Explain procedure to patient; procedure hurts.

(2) Assemble equipment: gloves, tourniquet, alcohol swabs, sterile gauze pads, tape, a sharps container, appropriate vacuum tubes, vacuum adaptor, and double-ended needle.

(3) Wash hands; don gloves.

(4) Hyperextend arm for ease of access to antecubital vein; apply tourniquet; have patient make fist.

(5) Clean site with alcohol; pull skin taut from below site; insert needle (bevel up) at 5-degree angle.

(6) Once needle "pops" into vein, slide vacuum tube onto needle; remove and replace tubes as each fills; remove tourniquet after last tube is filling.

(7) Remove final tube; lay gauze over puncture site, and remove needle and apply pressure to site for at least 5 minutes.

(8) Immediately discard needle into sharps container; label tubes before leaving patient's side.

g. Other specimens

(1) Vomitus: may be tested for blood

(2) Gastric analysis: examination of stomach contents; obtained by aspirating from nasogastric tube

(3) Wound drainage: if infection is suspected

D. Statement of patient problems requiring nursing intervention

1. Identifying unmet basic human needs resulting in a problem for the patient

2. Identifying problems arising from the patient's signs and symptoms

3. Actual problems: those that the patient is currently having

4. Potential problems: those that may develop and should be prevented from occurring (Box 2-7)

E. Nursing diagnosis: the practical nurse assists the RN in formulating nursing diagnosis

Planning Patient Care

A. Definition: process of setting priorities, determining patient-centered goals, and deciding on nursing actions to achieve the goals; ends with writing of the nursing care plan

B. Setting priorities

1. Problems that are life threatening are of highest priority

2. When no single problem seems more important than the others, the patient may help determine priorities.

C. Determining goals or expected outcomes

1. Goals or outcomes are stated in terms of patient behavior so that achievement can be easily evaluated.

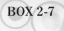

> **BOX 2-7   Actual and Potential Unmet Basic Needs and Problems**
>
> **Situation:** At 7 AM, Mrs. Clayton tells the nurse that she has a productive cough. She states that it began about 3 AM and continues.
> *Actual problem:* productive cough
> *Actual unmet need:* rest and sleep
> *Potential unmet need:* oxygen
> *Potential problem:* decreased oxygen

2. Whenever possible, patients should be involved in setting goals.
3. Long-term goals are those hoped for in the future, usually set by the RN.
4. Short-term goals are those sought immediately or in the near future.

D. Decisions about which nursing measures to use are based on sound knowledge of current nursing practice, principles, rationales, and judgment.

E. Written nursing care plan provides continuity of patient care.

Implementation of Nursing Measures

A. Principles
  1. Preparation
    a. Nurse: must know how, when, and why measure is to be performed, checking for a physician's order when necessary
    b. Patient and family or significant others
      (1) To reduce anxiety, patients need to know what measure is to be performed and why, as well as what is expected of them.
      (2) A specific measure may need special preparation, such as positioning, medications, and attire.
    c. Have all necessary equipment ready and in working order.
  2. Performance
    a. The nurse must have knowledge of and ability to perform measure and to seek help when necessary.
    b. Medical asepsis is always followed: surgical asepsis and Standard Precautions are followed as required.
    c. Work must be organized to conserve nurse and patient's energy and to meet patient's need for security.
    d. Assessment of patient's response to the measure is ongoing.
  3. Aftercare
    a. Patient made safe and comfortable.
    b. Equipment cleaned and returned to proper place or disposed of.
    c. Evaluation of results of the measure and whether it helped achieve the goal.
  4. Reporting and recording
    a. Significant observations immediately
    b. When the measure was performed and the results

Evaluation of Plan of Care

A. Criteria for evaluation
  1. Has the need been met?
  2. Is the problem solved or being solved?
  3. Has the goal or expected outcome been achieved?

B. Revision of the nursing care plan
  1. Based on evaluation of effectiveness
  2. The PN collaborates with the RN in revising problem list, goals, and nursing measures.

MEASURES TO MEET OXYGEN NEEDS

A. Assessment: color of skin or oral mucosa, level of consciousness, vital signs, presence of cough (productive or nonproductive), nature of sputum (amount, consistency, and color), and energy level
B. General measures
  1. Encourage exercise and activity to help expand lungs, providing better oxygenation.
  2. Bedridden patients must be turned and positioned every 2 hours (q2h) to prevent pooling of secretions in the lungs and capillary congestion that may lead to decubitus ulcer formation because of tissue hypoxia.
  3. Encourage coughing and deep breathing at least q2h for inactive or bedridden patients to help with oxygenation and bringing up secretions.
  4. Ensure adequate fluid intake to keep secretions thin, thus making it easier to expectorate.
C. Use of nebulizer (aerosol)
  1. Method of delivering medications directly to the respiratory tract
  2. Breaks liquids into a mist of droplets, which are inhaled
D. Incentive spirometer: to improve inspiratory volume
  1. With lips sealed around a mouthpiece, the patient takes a deep breath, holds it for 3 seconds, and slowly exhales.
  2. The spirometer indicates, by a light or small plastic balls reaching an indicated level, whether the patient has inhaled the desired volume.
E. Intermittent positive pressure breathing (IPPB) therapy
  1. IPPB forces the patient to inhale more deeply, allowing better oxygenation and loosening of secretions.
  2. Apparatus may be attached to oxygen or compressed air.
  3. Humidity is provided, usually by normal saline solution.
  4. Medications may be added.
  5. Patient should be sitting up during treatment and encouraged to cough up secretions after treatment.
F. Chest physical therapy
  1. Postural drainage uses of various positions so that gravity can assist in removal of secretions (Figure 2-8).
  2. Percussion is a manual technique of striking the chest wall over the affected area with cupped hands in a rhythmic motion.
  3. Vibration is a manual compression and tremor-like motion with hands or mechanical device against chest wall of affected area done during exhalation.
  4. Nurse positions the patient so affected areas are vertical and gravity can assist in drainage.
  5. Position also depends on diagnosis and condition.
  6. Schedule before or at least 2 hours after meals. Provide emesis basin and tissues and oral hygiene after treatment.
  7. This therapy is contraindicated in patients with lung abscess or tumors, pneumothorax, and diseases of the chest wall.
G. Suctioning: oral, nasopharyngeal, or tracheal
  1. To remove accumulated secretions blocking airway or to obtain sputum specimen

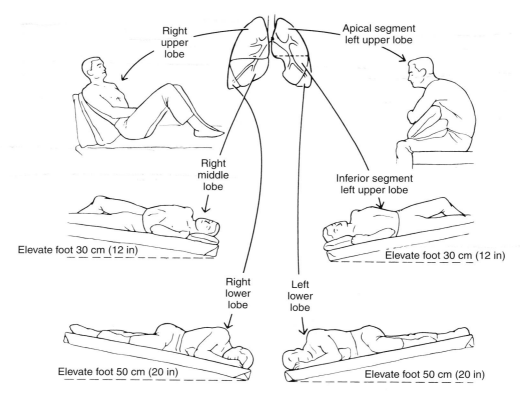

Right upper lobe

Apical segment left upper lobe

Right middle lobe

Inferior segment left upper lobe

Elevate foot 30 cm (12 in)

Elevate foot 30 cm (12 in)

Right lower lobe

Left lower lobe

Elevate foot 50 cm (20 in)

Elevate foot 50 cm (20 in)

FIGURE 2-8.   Positions for postural drainage. *(From Phipps WJ et al:* Medical-surgical nursing: concepts and clinical practice, *ed 7, St Louis, 2003, Mosby.)*

2. Usually a sterile procedure
3. Introduce catheter gently; do not apply suction while introducing catheter.
4. Suction intermittently for no more than 10 seconds.
5. Slowly withdraw catheter by rotating motion while suctioning continues.
6. Unless copious amounts of secretions are present, wait 30 seconds between suctionings.
7. Repeat procedure until all excess secretions are removed.
8. Administer oxygen before and between suctionings if needed.
H. Administration of oxygen
1. Safety precautions
   a. Caution patients and visitors that smoking is prohibited.
   b. Post warning sign on door or bed: "NO SMOKING —OXYGEN IN USE."
   c. Do not use heating pads, electric blankets, or electric razors.
   d. Do not use woolen blankets.
   e. Secure oxygen tanks so they do not tip over.
2. Physician's order is required for method of administration, rate of oxygen flow, or concentration.
3. Oxygen must always be humidified.
4. Nasal cannula: prongs fit into nares.
   a. Turn oxygen on and check flow through prongs before positioning on patient.
   b. Adjust strap after placing cannula on patient.
   c. Periodically check for sufficient water in humidity source.
   d. Periodically check patient's nares and behind ears for pressure.
   e. Periodically assess patient for changes in condition.

5. Oxygen by mask: simple; Venturi (delivers oxygen in precise concentrations)
   a. Proceed as with nasal cannula.
   b. Fit mask snugly to face and adjust strap.
   c. Periodically assess patient and equipment as with nasal cannula.
   d. If condition warrants, an order may be obtained to change mask to nasal cannula for mealtime.
I. Care of patient with a tracheostomy
1. Tracheotomy: opening into the trachea
2. Tracheostomy: tracheal opening, which normally has a tracheal tube
3. Tube is either metal or plastic, which is usually cuffed (Figures 2-9 and 2-10).
4. Tube is held securely in place with cotton ties around the neck (Figure 2-11).
5. Ties are changed with extreme caution to prevent patient from coughing out tube.
6. A gauze dressing is placed under the tube to absorb secretions; dressing must be changed every shift.
7. Inner cannula is removed, cleaned with peroxide and pipe cleaners, and rinsed with normal saline at least once a shift by sterile technique; commercially prepared kits are available.
8. Skin around stoma is cleansed with peroxide, rinsed with saline, and assessed at least once a shift.
9. Tube must be suctioned frequently. Patient is often apprehensive and needs frequent reassurance; have pad and pencil nearby for communication purposes.
10. Patient may take oral feedings if ordered; cuff must be inflated at all times.

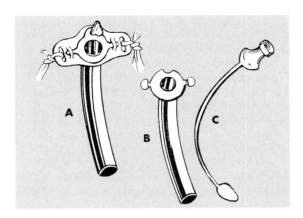

FIGURE 2-9. Metal tracheostomy tube. **A,** Outer cannula. **B,** Inner cannula. **C,** Obturator. *(From Harkness GA, Dincher JR: Medical-surgical nursing: total patient care, ed 10, St Louis, 2000, Mosby.)*

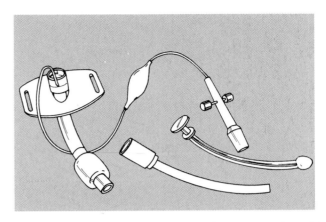

FIGURE 2-10. Cuffed tracheostomy tube. *(From Harkness GA, Dincher JR: Medical-surgical nursing: total patient care, ed 10, St Louis, 2000, Mosby.)*

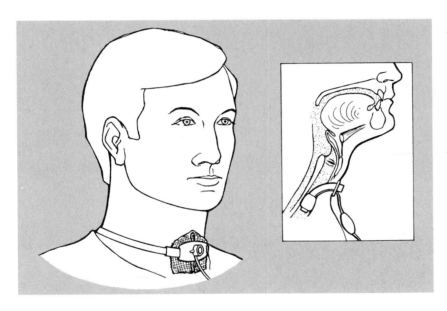

FIGURE 2-11. Tracheostomy tube in place. *(From Harkness GA, Dincher JR: Medical-surgical nursing: total patient care, ed 10, St Louis, 2000, Mosby.)*

J. Medication classifications: refer to Chapter 3 for more detailed information on drugs that affect the respiratory system.
  1. Respiratory stimulants
  2. Respiratory depressants
  3. Medications acting on mucous membranes: administered orally or as spray or vapor.
     a. Mucolytics
     b. Expectorants
  4. Bronchodilators

MEASURES TO MEET FLUID NEEDS

A. Assessment: daily weights, comparison of intake and output, appearance of urine, presence of edema, fluid preferences, and skin turgor
B. Fluid excess (edema)
  1. Associated with heart and kidney disease: body unable to rid itself of excess fluid
  2. Can result from excessive intravenous (IV) fluids
  3. Observed as edema, as well as weight gain and reduced urine output

  4. Sites of edema: eyes, fingers, ankles, and sacral area
C. Fluid deficit (dehydration)
  1. Associated with inadequate fluid intake, diarrhea, excessive perspiration, vomiting, bleeding, and increased urine output
  2. Observed as dry skin and mucous membranes, thick mucus, poor skin turgor, behavioral changes, or changes in vital signs
D. Measuring intake and output
  1. Measure all fluids taken in: IV, tube feedings, and obvious fluids such as water, milk, ice cream, gelatin, custard, and soup.
  2. Measure all fluids leaving the body: urine, vomitus, diarrhea, gastric secretions, and blood.
  3. Know capacity of agency's fluid containers.
  4. Set measuring containers on level surface to read measurements accurately.
  5. Record and total amounts in appropriate places.
E. Administering IV fluids
  1. Assess site of needle insertion.
     a. Infiltration: fluid entering subcutaneous tissues instead of vein; area is pale, cool, and swollen.

b. Phlebitis: inflammation of vein; area is <u>red, warm, and swollen</u>.
2. Assess tubing: no kinks; no leakage along entire length of tubing; <u>tubing should be labeled and changed every 48 to 72 hours or per agency policy.</u>
3. Assess rate of flow.
4. Assess container.
   a. The container must match physician's order.
   b. Check that the amount absorbed is on schedule.
F. Medication classifications—diuretics: refer to Chapter 3 for more detailed information.

MEASURES TO MEET NUTRITIONAL NEEDS

A. Assessment: weight/height ratio, weight changes, skin and mucous membranes, food preferences, meal patterns, ability to eat, and appetite
B. Preparing for meals
   1. Environment
      a. Control odors, noise, and unpleasant sights; remove soiled equipment and linens.
      b. Avoid stressful situations before and during mealtime.
   2. Patient
      a. Provide oral hygiene and opportunity for elimination and hand washing.
      b. Position comfortably, preferably in sitting position.
   3. Meal tray
      a. Ensure correct tray for correct patient.
      b. Arrange tray to be accessible to patient.
      c. Assist in opening containers, removing covers, and cutting and preparing food.
      d. Serve trays first to patients who are able to feed themselves.
C. Assisting the patient to eat
   1. Place napkin across chest.
   2. Explain what foods and liquids are on the tray.
   3. Prepare foods and feed in order of patient's preference.
   4. Encourage the patient to assist as much as possible.
   5. Do not rush: allow time to chew and swallow.
   6. Talk with the patient during meal.
   7. Provide opportunity for hand washing and oral care.
D. Gastric gavage (tube feeding)
   1. Gastric gavage is used when patient is unable to eat, swallow, or take in adequate quantities of food.
   2. Blended foods and fluids (commercially or agency prepared) are passed to the stomach through a nasogastric tube, either intermittently or by slow continuous drip.
   3. Check amount, frequency, and type ordered by physician.
   4. Feeding must be at room temperature before administering.
   5. Placement of tube must be checked before feeding begins.
      a. Nasogastric or nasoduodenal tubes
         (1) Begin by aspirating stomach contents with a syringe.
         (2) <u>Inject 10 cc of air into large bore feeding tube while simultaneously listening with a stethoscope over the stomach to hear a whooshing sound.</u>
         (3) Obtain radiographic confirmation of small-bore feeding tube before beginning feeding.
      b. Gastrostomy or jejunostomy tubes

(1) Aspirate stomach contents with a syringe.
(2) <u>Measure, record, and return aspirated contents.</u>
6. Place patient in <u>sitting position.</u>
7. Aspirate tube for stomach contents. <u>Hold feeding if greater than 100 cc of residual is obtained.</u>
8. Administer feeding slowly: <u>200 ml during 30- to 45-minute period.</u>
9. Feeding should be <u>followed by ordered amount of water.</u>
10. Clamp tube after completion of feeding to prevent air entering stomach.
11. If nausea, vomiting, diarrhea, or cramps occur, rate may be too fast, or patient may be intolerant of feeding or volume, or the feeding may be too concentrated.
12. Tube may be left in place between feedings or removed after each feeding as ordered by physician.
13. Have patient <u>remain in sitting position for 45 minutes to help prevent aspiration.</u>
E. Medication classifications: refer to Chapter 3 for more detailed information.
   1. Vitamin supplements
   2. Mineral supplements

MEASURES TO MEET URINARY ELIMINATION NEEDS

A. Assessment: intake/output ratio, color, odor, amount, and consistency of urine, frequency of urination, and continence
B. Common problems of urination
   1. Incontinence: inability to control voiding
      a. Requires frequent skin care and linen change
      b. May be reduced with scheduled toileting
      c. May be secondary to medications (diuretics)
   2. Retention: inability to void
      a. If adequate amounts of fluid have been taken in, no more than 8 hours should pass between voidings, except during sleeping hours.
      b. Palpation of bladder can determine distention of full bladder.
   3. Anuria: no urine being produced by the kidneys
   4. Dysuria: difficult or painful urination ("burning")
C. Assisting with urination
   1. Offer bedpan or urinal at regularly scheduled times.
   2. Keep bedpan or urinal and toilet tissue within easy reach for patients who can assist themselves.
   3. Keep call signal within easy reach.
   4. Provide privacy.
   5. Hearing the sound of running water or having warm water poured over the perineum may induce voiding.
   6. Provide opportunity for hand washing after urination.
D. Care of patient with retention catheter
   1. Presence of indwelling catheter greatly predisposes patient to urinary tract infection.
   2. Opening a closed urinary system is to be avoided.
   3. Drainage container must be kept below level of the bladder but must not touch the floor.
   4. Drainage tubing must be free of kinks; catheter should be taped to patient's leg, allowing for slack.
   5. Drainage container is emptied at end of shift or if container becomes nearly full; urine is measured, assessed, and amount recorded.

6. Catheter care is given at least once per shift and after every bowel movement.
    a. Meatus and catheter are cleansed with soap and water, from meatus down catheter and away from body.
    b. Removal of crusts and secretions from meatus and catheter may require use of hydrogen peroxide.
    c. A bacteriostatic ointment is often ordered to be applied to the meatus.
7. Unless contraindicated, fluid intake should reach 2000 to 3000 ml/24 hr.

E. Catheterization
1. "Straight": catheter is removed at end of procedure (intermittent catheterization), often ordered to relieve urine retention (common after surgery or childbirth), to obtain a sterile urine specimen or to measure residual urine after voiding.
2. Indwelling, retention or Foley: catheter is left in place in bladder.
3. Assemble equipment: sterile catheterization tray or disposable kit containing catheter, basin, container with lid (for specimen, if ordered), cotton balls, antiseptic solution, lubricant, sterile gloves, and drape
4. For indwelling catheterization, add Foley catheter, syringe, solution for inflating balloon, drainage bag with tubing, and tape for securing catheter.
5. After explaining procedure to patient and ensuring privacy, place female patient in dorsal recumbent position and male patient in supine position.
6. Place equipment on an over-the-bed table or between patient's legs; using sterile technique open package, don gloves, and place drape.
7. For female patient, while holding labia apart, cleanse vulva and meatus well going from front to back toward vagina; use cotton ball for one stoke only before discarding.
8. For male patient, cleanse around penis from meatus toward base using each cotton ball once around.
9. Insert catheter into meatus (3 to 4 inches [7.5 to 10 cm] in female patient and 6 to 8 inches [15 to 20 cm] in male patient) until urine flows; advance catheter 1 inch more, and drain urine (no more than 750 ml at one time to prevent hypovolemic shock); remove catheter ("straight") or inflate balloon and connect drainage tubing (indwelling).

F. Intermittent bladder irrigation (hand bladder irrigation)
1. To rid bladder and catheter of clots or mucus; to instill antibiotic or other solutions
2. Open technique
    a. Assemble equipment: sterile solution (type and amount as ordered), sterile container for solution, bulb syringe, and basin for return flow.
    b. Disconnect catheter from drainage tube over empty basin; protect ends from contamination.
    c. Allow solution to flow in by gravity or gentle pressure; drain by gravity or gentle suction; repeat until returns are clear or ordered amount of solution has been used.
    d. Subtract amount of solution used from amount of returns; record output.
3. Closed technique
    a. Assemble equipment: 20- to 30-ml syringe with needle, alcohol swabs, solution ordered, and clamp.
    b. Draw solution into syringe by sterile technique.
    c. Clamp tubing distal to needle entry point.

d. Cleanse resealable rubber entry port on drainage tubing with alcohol swab.
e. Insert needle into port.
f. Inject fluid into catheter.
g. Remove needle.
h. Release clamp, and allow fluid to drain into drainage bag.
i. Observe fluid return.
j. Repeat until ordered amount of solution has been used.
k. Empty drainage bag, subtracting amount of irrigant from total; record urine output.

G. Continuous bladder irrigation (through and through or three-way irrigation)
1. To prevent clot formation, to reduce obstruction of catheter, to circulate antibiotic or other solutions continuously in bladder
2. Equipment: patient has three-way catheter or needs sterile Y-tube connector attached to regular two-way catheter's drainage channel; large bottle or bag of solution, with tubing attached, hanging from IV pole.
3. With three-way catheter: using sterile technique
    a. Remove plug from irrigating channel; protect plug and tubing from contamination.
    b. Insert solution tubing into irrigating channel.
4. With two-way catheter: using sterile technique
    a. Attach single end of sterile Y-tube connector to catheter.
    b. Attach drainage tubing to one end of Y.
    c. Attach solution tubing to other end of Y.
5. Start solution flow at rate ordered by physician.
6. Observe fluid return through drainage tubing.
7. Replace solution bottle or bag as it becomes nearly empty.
8. Empty drainage container as it becomes nearly full and when solution container is replaced.
9. Subtract amount of irrigant solution from total amount of drainage to record actual urine output.

H. Removal of indwelling catheter
1. Assemble equipment: syringe without needle, underpad, basin, urinal or bedpan, toilet tissue, and protective gloves.
2. After explaining procedure and ensuring privacy, place pad under patient.
3. Remove tape from catheter and patient's leg.
4. Put on protective gloves.
5. Place basin under patient's meatus.
6. Insert syringe into balloon channel; fluid will return on its own.
7. After all fluid has returned, gently pull on catheter to remove it.
8. If resistance is met, stop and obtain assistance.
9. Assist patient to wash perineum.
10. Teaching
    a. Patient should continue to drink fluids.
    b. Burning on urination may occur during first few voidings.
    c. Complete continence and normal voiding pattern may take time to return.
    d. Instruct patient to void into bedpan or urinal so that the color, consistency, and amount of urine can be assessed.

11. Encourage relaxation: anxiety may inhibit ability to void.
12. Continue to assess bladder distention, intake/output ratio, and patient complaints until normal patterns of elimination are achieved.
I. Straining urine for calculi-patients who have suspected renal calculi should have each urine specimen strained for the presence of stones. Use small gauze filter, and send any material retrieved to the lab.
J. Medication classifications
  1. Cholinergics: to induce bladder contraction (bethanechol [Urecholine] and neostigmine [Prostigmin])
  2. Anticholinergics: to reduce bladder spasms and urinary frequency (methantheline [Banthine] and flavoxate hydrochloride [Urispas])

MEASURES TO MEET BOWEL ELIMINATION NEEDS

A. Assessment: the patient's pattern of elimination; amount, color, consistency, odor, and shape of stool; patient's activity level; amount and type of food and fluid intake; passage of flatus; abdominal distention
B. Common problems of elimination
  1. Constipation: passage of dry, hard feces
  2. Diarrhea: frequent passage of liquid or unformed stools
  3. Impaction: formation of a hardened mass of stool in the lower bowel forming an obstruction to the passage of normal stool; often characterized by the frequent seepage of small amount of liquid stool
  4. Abdominal distention: swollen abdomen caused by retention of flatus in the intestines; generally accompanied by a lack of bowel sounds (peristalsis); sometimes referred to as an ileus or paralytic ileus
C. General nursing measures
  1. Encourage intake of roughage in the diet: fresh fruits and vegetables and whole grain breads and cereals.
  2. Encourage intake of adequate amounts of fluids, unless contraindicated: 2000 to 3000 ml/day.
  3. Encourage maximum amount of physical activity.
  4. Encourage patient to respond to the urge to defecate.
  5. Position patient comfortably and provide adequate time and privacy for elimination.
  6. Provide access to call signal and toilet tissue.
  7. Provide opportunity for hand washing after elimination.
D. Rectal tube
  1. Rectal tube is used to assist in expelling flatus.
  2. Assemble equipment: rectal tube with flatus bag or waterproof pad, lubricant, glove, and tape.
  3. After explaining procedure and providing privacy, position patient in left lateral (Sims') position.
  4. With gloved hand, insert lubricated tube 2 to 4 inches (5 to 10 cm) into rectum.
  5. Tape tube to patient's buttock and leave in place no longer than 20 to 30 minutes.
  6. Note passage of flatus or stool; report and record findings.
E. Rectal suppository
  1. Rectal suppositories are used to stimulate peristalsis and aid stool elimination, to soothe painful rectum or anus, to administer medications.
  2. Assemble equipment: suppository as ordered, glove, bedpan, and toilet tissue.

  3. Suppository begins to melt at room temperature, providing its own lubrication.
  4. Separate buttocks, and with gloved index finger insert pointed end of suppository into anus.
  5. Gently insert 3 to 4 inches (7.5 to 10 cm) into rectum.
  6. Hold buttocks together until initial urge to defecate has passed.
  7. Best results occur within 30 minutes.
F. Commercially prepared prefilled enema
  1. Commercially prepared prefilled enemas are used to promote bowel or flatus movement.
  2. Assemble equipment: enema (usually 120 ml), underpad, bedpan, toilet paper, and gloves.
  3. After explaining procedure and providing privacy, place patient in left lateral (Sims') position.
  4. With gloved hand, insert prelubricated tip of enema to the hub and squeeze container until most of solution is instilled.
  5. Encourage patient to retain solution until urge to defecate is felt.
  6. Place call signal, bedpan, and toilet tissue within easy reach.
  7. If patient uses toilet, instruct not to flush so that results can be assessed.
G. Oil-retention enema
  1. Oil-retention enemas are used to soften and lubricate stool, promoting easier passage.
  2. Oil-retention enemas are often followed by cleansing enema.
  3. Equipment and administration are the same as those for previously mentioned commercially prepared enema.
  4. Encourage patient to retain oil 30 to 60 minutes.
H. Cleansing enemas
  1. Cleansing enemas are used to relieve constipation or flatus or to cleanse the bowel before diagnostic procedures, surgery, or childbirth.
  2. Solutions are used as ordered by physician.
    a. Tap water: can cause fluid and electrolyte imbalance
    b. Soap solution: 5 ml of liquid soap to 1000 ml of water; can irritate mucous membranes of bowel
    c. Saline solution: can cause fluid and electrolyte imbalance
  3. Assemble equipment: disposable enema kit containing enema bag, tubing with clamp, liquid soap, and lubricant; waterproof underpad; solution at a temperature no greater than 105° F; bedpan and toilet tissue; IV pole; protective gloves.
  4. After explaining procedure and providing privacy, place patient in left lateral (Sims') position.
  5. Put on protective gloves.
  6. Insert lubricated tubing about 3 to 5 inches (7.5 to 12.5 cm) into rectum.
  7. With bottom of enema bag hanging 12 inches (30 cm) above anus or 18 inches (45 cm) above mattress, slowly administer 500 to 1000 ml of solution.
  8. If patient complains of cramping or has difficulty retaining solution:
    a. Slow administration rate.
    b. Or temporarily stop flow.
    c. Encourage slow, deep breathing through the mouth.
  9. After fluid has been administered, assist patient to bathroom or onto bedpan or commode; instruct patient not to flush toilet so that results can be assessed.

10. If enemas are ordered "until clear," repeat procedure until returns are clear of stool (or of barium after barium enema).
11. Observe patient during procedure for signs of weakness or fatigue, which would necessitate stopping the procedure to allow rest.
I. Digital removal of fecal impaction
   1. Digital removal of fecal impaction is for breaking up the hard fecal mass and removing it.
   2. Assemble equipment: gloves, waterproof underpad, lubricant, and bedpan.
   3. Liberally lubricate gloved index finger.
   4. With patient in left lateral (Sims') position, gently insert finger into hardened mass of stool.
   5. Gently break off small pieces of the stool, bringing them out and placing them in the bedpan.
   6. Assess patient for signs of weakness and fatigue; this is an uncomfortable, tiring procedure and may need to be intermittently stopped.
   7. Assist patient to bedpan: disimpaction may induce defecation.
J. Colostomy irrigation
   1. Colostomy irrigation is used to regulate the discharge and drainage of fecal contents and flatus.
   2. Time of irrigation depends on physician's order and patient's own established routine; when colostomy has become regulated, irrigation may be only done every other day; some patients never irrigate their colostomy.
   3. Assemble equipment:
      a. Irrigating appliance (types vary)
      b. Irrigating container (enema bag)
      c. Tubing and catheter (may be part of enema kit)
      d. Irrigating solution: usually 500 to 1000 ml of tap water or physiologic saline solution at 100° F
      e. Lubricant
      f. Drainage bag (may be part of irrigating appliance) and bedpan if not using on toilet
      g. Waterproof underpad if being performed in bed
      h. Fresh colostomy appliance, dressing, or stoma pad
      i. IV pole
      j. Protective gloves
   4. After explaining procedure and ensuring privacy, place patient on toilet (most convenient) or in bed in left lateral (Sims') position.
   5. Put on protective gloves.
   6. Raise irrigation container 18 inches (45 cm) above stoma, clear catheter of air, lubricate catheter, introduce catheter through irrigating appliance, and insert catheter into stoma 2 to 6 inches (5 to 15 cm); do not advance if resistance is met.
   7. Allow solution to flow slowly and remove catheter; return is usually completed within 45 to 60 minutes.
   8. When return is completed, remove irrigating appliance, wash and dry abdomen, and apply fresh colostomy appliance, dressing, or stoma pad as indicated.
   9. Record character and amount of returns, patient's tolerance, and degree of assistance provided by patient.
K. Medication classifications: refer to Chapter 3 for more detailed information on drugs that affect the gastrointestinal (GI) system.
   1. Stool softeners
   2. Laxatives, cathartics
   3. Antidiarrhetics

MEASURES TO MEET REST AND SLEEP NEEDS

Rest and sleep are necessary for restoring physical and mental well being, reducing stress and anxiety, and maintaining the ability to attend to and concentrate on activities of life.
A. Assessment: normal number of hours of sleep, usual bedtime, usual bedtime habits or practices, sleep difficulties, daytime fatigue, usual methods of obtaining rest, and sleep medications being used
B. Physician's orders for rest must be clarified: is bed rest ordered to provide rest for a damaged heart, the entire body, or an injured part, such as a foot?
C. Providing for rest and sleep
   1. Promote relaxation: provide diversions, pain relief, clean, wrinkle-free bed, a noise-free and odor-free room, and easy access to bedside equipment and call signal; give a relaxing back rub.
   2. Reduce patient's anxiety level by allowing time for the patient to talk about stressful or fear-producing situations.
   3. If possible, position patient in usual sleeping position with amount of covers desired.
   4. Plan and organize care to allow the patient uninterrupted rest and sleep periods.
   5. Give sleeping medication if ordered and if required by the patient.
D. Sleep disturbances
   1. Sleep apnea: a disorder that occurs when individual sleeps, characterized by periods of apnea during sleep that cause daytime tiredness and fatigue
   2. Narcolepsy: disorder that involves the patient falling asleep while performing activities, which can be dangerous
E. Medication classifications: refer to Chapter 3 for more detailed information.
   1. Sedatives: to reduce anxiety
   2. Hypnotics: to induce sleep

MEASURES TO MEET ACTIVITY AND EXERCISE NEEDS

Physical activity is necessary for proper functioning of all body systems, as well as for promoting emotional well being; immobility can lead to physical and emotional disability.
A. Assessment: posture, ability to walk, ability to turn and move in bed, usual activity level, and skin condition
B. Patient's activity and exercise level is ordered by the physician.
   1. Bed rest (BR): patient is confined to bed.
   2. Bathroom privileges (BRP): although confined to bed, patient may perform urinary and bowel elimination in the bathroom.
   3. May dangle: although confined to bed, patient may sit on edge of bed with legs and feet hanging down over side of bed and supported by footstool.
      a. Order is often accompanied by orders for frequency and duration of dangling time (e.g., dangle every shift for 10 minutes).

b. Provide footstool.

c. Assess vital signs.

d. Stay with patient to assess tolerance and assist back to bed.

4. Allow to chair: although patient may sit in chair, he or she is not permitted to ambulate any farther.

5. Out of bed (OOB) ad lib: can and should perform as much activity out of bed as desired.

6. Encourage patients to perform as much activity as orders permit.

C. Dangers of immobility

1. Atelectasis: collapse of lung caused by reduced depth and rate of respirations or obstruction of lungs by excessive secretions

2. Hypostatic pneumonia: caused by pooling of lung secretions and the resulting congestion

3. Thrombus formation: caused by reduced rate of blood flow through the veins and prolonged coagulation time

4. Constipation: caused by slowed peristaltic action

5. Contractures: permanent shortening of muscles, leading to joint immobility

6. Skin breakdown and decubitus ulcer formation caused by prolonged pressure and reduced circulation to an area

7. Urinary tract infections and kidney stones caused by stasis of urine and demineralization of bones

D. Measures to prevent dangers of immobility

1. Coughing and deep breathing

a. Performed q2h

b. Patient should be in semi-Fowler's position and take 10 deep breaths followed by deep cough to raise secretions.

2. Turning and repositioning q2h

3. Range-of-motion (ROM) exercises: to maintain full range and flexibility of joint movement

a. Performed 8 to 10 times on each joint at least once every day

b. Passive range-of-motion (PROM): performed for the patient

c. Active range-of-motion (AROM): performed by the patient

d. Each joint is put through all its possible movements (Figure 2-12)

4. Maintain adequate fluid intake (2000 to 3000 ml/day).

5. Provide for adequate nutritional intake.

6. Frequent skin care, keeping skin clean, dry, and lubricated.

E. Devices used to help prevent dangers of immobility

1. Footboard: to prevent plantar flexion (footdrop)

a. Soles of patient's feet are flat against board and in good alignment.

b. Board should be padded.

2. Bed cradle: to keep weight of bed covers off a body part

3. Alternating pressure mattress: changes pressure on body parts in contact with the mattress

a. Only one layer of loosely pulled linen should be between mattress and patient.

b. Keep pins and other pointed objects away from this mattress.

4. Sheepskin: provides a soft surface, reducing skin abrasion

5. Special beds. such as the CircOlectric: allow patient's position to be changed more readily

6. Venodixie boots: prevent thrombophlebitis

7. Antiembolism stockings

8. Canes are used for extra stability, support and balance. The cane should be used in the hand opposite the affected extremity, and advanced at the same time as that extremity.

9. Crutches are useful in assisting with the mobility needs of patients with disorders of the lower extremities. Several crutch gaits can be used.

a. For balance. When the patient has full weight bearing on both legs, the crutches can be used as a source of balance.

b. For mobility. When a patient has partial weight bearing on one extremity, the opposite crutch is advanced at the same time as that extremity so weight can be born on the crutch instead of the extremity.

c. Rules for crutches. Length is very important. The crutch should come within two fingerbreadths of the axilla of the individual. Weight is distributed on the handgrips, not the axillary area. Physical therapy teaches crutch walking, but nurses must reinforce teaching.

10. Walkers are used for stability mostly in the older population. Proper technique for using a walker should be taught and reinforced.

a. Push up from a seated position without using the walker; the walker may tip if the patient pulls him or herself to a standing position with the walker.

b. The height of the walker should be as such that the patient has a 30-degree bend to the arm while ambulating.

c. The patient should place his or her weight on the walker if he or she has compromised strength or mobility in one of the extremities.

MEASURES TO MEET PAIN RELIEF NEEDS

Individuals (including nurses) vary in their perception of and response to pain. Pain is often intensified in the presence of anxiety and fatigue and the absence of distraction.

A. Assessment: intensity, onset, duration, quality, and location of pain, patient's nonverbal responses to pain—behavior, change in vital signs, and nausea; factors associated with the pain—activity and visitors; pain relief measures. Nurses should use a scale of 1 to 10 to gauge intensity of pain. Level 1 would be very little pain; level 10 would signify excruciating pain.

B. Therapeutic relationship may help reduce anxiety, thus reducing pain level.

C. Altering contributing factors: relieving constipation and nausea; eliminating environmental disturbances, such as bright lights, odors, and noise

D. Providing diversional activities: television, radio, and visitors

E. Repositioning, back rub, and tightening linens

F. Applying heat or cold if ordered

G. Relaxation

1. To reduce muscle tension

2. First need

a. A comfortable position

b. A quiet environment

c. A focus on something outside the body, such as a word to repeat, an object to examine, or something to imagine

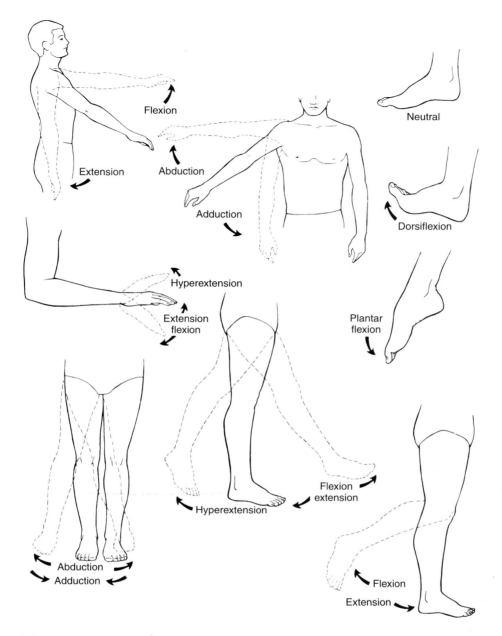

FIGURE 2-12.   Range of joint motions. *(From Beare PG, Myers JL:* Adult health nursing, *ed 3, St Louis, 1998, Mosby.)*

3. Techniques
   a. Exercises in which various muscle groups are alternately tensed and relaxed
   b. Exercises in which various muscle groups are alternately stretched and relaxed
   c. Breathing techniques similar to those used in the Lamaze method of childbirth (controlled and focused)
   d. Biofeedback: learning to control normally autonomic body functions
      (1) Muscle tension is monitored.
      (2) Subject receives feedback as to the success of attempts to control functions.
H. Transcutaneous electrical nerve stimulation (TENS): small, battery-operated device that provides continuous mild electric current to skin

1. Clean skin with alcohol before applying electrodes on or around pain site.
2. No tingling indicates controls are too low; pain or muscle spasm indicates controls are too high.
I. Medication classifications: refer to Chapter 3 for more detailed information.
   1. Placebo: inactive substance administered to satisfy the patient's need for a drug
      a. Pain relief after administration is probably a result of anxiety reduction.
      b. Relief felt after a placebo does not mean that pain did not exist.
   2. Analgesics
      a. Narcotics
      b. Nonnarcotics

MEASURES TO MEET SAFETY AND HYGIENE NEEDS

Although individuals are usually capable of meeting these needs themselves, in strange environments and in times of stress and illness, help is often needed. Individuals need protection from injury, maintenance of intact skin and mucous membranes and of body alignment, and structure and order in their environment.

A. Assessment
   1. Protection from injury: level of consciousness, ability to move, and knowledge of environment, equipment, and patient's medications
   2. Maintenance of intact skin and mucous membranes and alignment: personal hygiene, condition of skin, mucous membranes, joints, and posture
   3. Structure and order in the environment: arrangement of personal belongings, cleanliness of patient's unit, environmental conditions, and potential hazards
B. Measures to protect from injury
   1. Bed side rails: use whenever bed is above its lowest level; use for patients who are unconscious, sedated with narcotics, disoriented, or confused or for children.
   2. Call signal: should always be within patient's reach; patient should know how to use it.
   3. Restraints (patient protectors or patient protective devices)
      a. Restraints require physician's order to place and remove, unless in an emergency and patient is in immediate need of protection.
      b. Restraints are used to restrict movement of the individual or of one or more extremities.
      c. Explain to patient and family why restraint is being used.
      d. Remain quiet and calm while applying restraint to reduce patient's fear and stress.
      e. Apply restraint securely enough to provide protection but loosely enough to permit circulation and lung expansion.
      f. Periodically check pulses and skin integrity distal to the restrained extremity (radial, pedal pulses).
      g. Continue to provide patient with all necessary nursing care, including turning, fluids, hygiene, and opportunity for elimination.
      h. Secure restraint to bed frame rather than to bed rail.
      i. Types of restraints
         (1) Sheet around waist to secure patient in chair
         (2) Jacket or vest, mitts, ankle and wrist restraints
         (3) Safety belts
      j. Measures to avoid restraints
         (1) Reorientation measures
         (2) Alarms and monitors
         (3) Specialized chairs
   4. Reduce environmental hazards
      a. Proper care of hospital equipment
         (1) Equipment should be stored properly.
         (2) All apparatus, equipment, and furnishings should be kept in good repair.
         (3) All apparatus, equipment, and furnishings should be used correctly.
      b. Prevention of fire
         (1) Proper care and use of electrical equipment
         (2) Prohibition of smoking in bed
         (3) Observance of oxygen safety measures
         (4) Use of RACE acronym if fire occurs
            (a) R—rescue anyone closest to the fire.
            (b) A—pull alarm or notify the operator.
            (c) C—confine the fire, shut doors and block off fire.
            (e) E—extinguish the fire using a fire extinguisher aimed at the base of the flames.
      c. Prevention of accidents
         (1) Keep floor dry, clean, and free of litter.
         (2) Place rubber tips on crutches, canes, and walkers.
         (3) Dispose of dressings and needles properly.
         (4) Have frequent fire drills.
         (5) Lock wheels on beds, wheelchairs, and stretchers.
         (6) Maintain good lighting.
      d. Protection from microorganisms and pests
         (1) Hand washing and maintenance of medical asepsis
         (2) Proper disinfection and sterilization
         (3) Food storage in patient unit minimized
   5. Transferring patient from bed
      a. Protect from falling by using transfer belt and having patient wear sturdy shoes rather than slippers.
      b. Two or three people may be required to transfer helpless or heavy patients.
      c. Be sure bed and stretcher wheels and wheelchairs are in locked position.
      d. Make use of lifting devices, such as Hoyer lift.
      e. Use good body mechanics.
C. Measures to promote and maintain intact skin and mucous membranes
   1. Bed making: dry, tight, wrinkle-free bed helps maintain skin integrity, as well as provide for comfort.
      a. Assemble equipment: sheets, spread, blanket, pillow, and pillow covering.
      b. Care of soiled linens
         (1) Always place on a surface above floor or in individual laundry bags.
         (2) Deposit in linen hamper (disposable "linens" are available and are used especially for patients with communicable diseases).
      c. Types of bed making
         (1) Closed bed is made in preparation for new patient.
         (2) Open bed is occupied but patient is out of bed.
         (3) Occupied bed is made with patient in it.
         (4) Fracture or orthopedic bed is made from head to foot.
         (5) Postanesthetic or recovery bed is made to receive patient easily from stretcher (Figure 2-13).
      d. Bed positions
         (1) Low Fowler's: head is raised (gatched) 18 to 20 inches (45 to 50 cm) above flat bed level.
         (2) Semi-Fowler's: head is raised 45 degrees, and knee is gatched 15 degrees.
         (3) High Fowler's: head of bed is raised to a 90-degree angle.
         (4) Trendelenburg's: head is lower than the level of the feet (no gatch).
   2. Daily bath
      a. Clean, dry, intact, and healthy skin and mucous membranes are first line of defense against microorganisms.

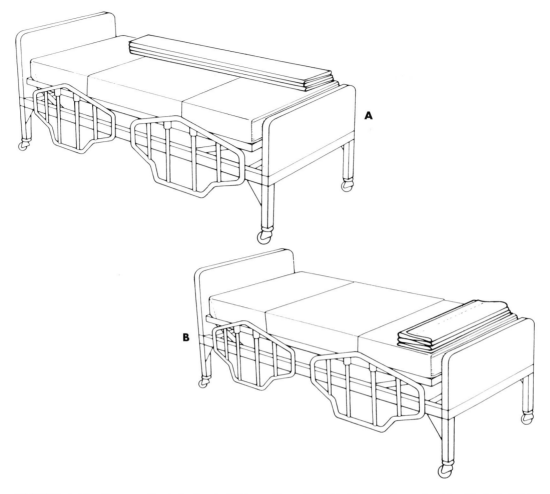

FIGURE 2-13.   Postanesthetic beds. A, With top linens fan folded lengthwise to the side of bed. **B,** With top linens fan folded from the head of the bed to the foot. *(Adapted from Sorrentino SA, Gorek B:* Mosby's Textbook for long-term care assistants, *ed 3, St Louis, 2000, Mosby.)*

b. Bath time is also important for establishing relationship with patient and for assessment.

c. Some patients do not desire, need, or require complete bath each day.

d. Bed bath is given to the patient who is restricted to bed or helpless in bathing self.

e. Assisted bath: patient bathes as much of self as possible; may need assistance with back, feet, legs, and perineum.

f. Tub bath or shower is for patient who is capable of doing so; a physician's order is required.

g. Commercial sponge bath packets contain moisturizing cleansing agent; warmed in microwave; decrease heat loss, skin drying, exposure, and task time

3. Skin care

a. Use soap sparingly; rinse well with warm water; pat skin dry.

b. Lotions prevent dry skin.

c. Gently massage bony prominences with lotion to promote circulation.

d. Use deodorant or antiperspirant as necessary.

e. Avoid heavy use of powder, which can cake, causing skin irritation.

4. Mouth care

a. Routine mouth care involves use of toothbrush, mouthwash, or substitutes.

b. Special mouth care involves more frequent routine care plus the judicious use of glycerin and lemon swabs or hydrogen peroxide if ordered.

c. Unconscious patient

(1) Have suction at the bedside.

(2) Turn the patient on their side with head up and to the side.

(3) Use soft toothettes to clean mouth.

(4) Make sure all liquid is drained from mouth or suctioned from mouth to decrease chance of aspiration.

d. Care of dentures

(1) Clean dentures over towel-lined basin of water to reduce chance of breakage if dropped.

(2) Hold dentures with gauze or cloth to prevent dropping.

(3) Clean with tepid water; hot water may change shape.

(4) Store dentures in clearly marked denture cup with tepid water in drawer of bedside stand when not in patient's mouth.

5. Hair care
   a. Comb or brush daily; groom as desired.
   b. If tangled:
      (1) Use 95% alcohol for oily hair.
      (2) Use mineral oil for dry hair.
      (3) Start at ends working toward scalp.
      (4) Hold hair close to head to prevent pulling.
   c. Braid long hair if not objectionable to patient.
   d. Shampoo as often as necessary and as patient's condition permits.
   e. Give pediculosis (lice) treatment as ordered by physician.
      (1) Commercial preparations are available.
      (2) Use fine-toothed comb to remove nits (eggs).
      (3) Patient may be isolated to avoid spread.
6. Nail care: daily and as indicated; must have physician's order to cut nails; extreme care must be used with patients with diabetes or circulatory problems.
   a. Scrub under nails as necessary.
   b. Cut nails even with tips of fingers and toes.
   c. Round fingernails to curve with fingertips.
   d. Cut toenails straight across
7. Shaving: male patients may want to shave while they are in the hospital.
   a. Check with RN to make sure that patient can be shaved with a razor; if the patient is on anticoagulants or has a bleeding disorder, shaving may be contraindicated.
   b. Soften beard with a warm washcloth.
   c. Apply shaving lotion.
   d. Shave in the direction of hair growth.
   e. Cleanse face with warm washcloth after completion.
8. Decubitus (pressure) ulcer care: assess areas over all bony prominences, such as sacrum, heels, elbows, hips and shoulder blades, and along edges of casts and braces.
   a. Contributing factors
      (1) Crumbs or food particles in the bed
      (2) Exposure to moisture, such as urine
      (3) Wrinkles in sheets
      (4) Unrelieved pressure for longer than 2 hours
      (5) Conditions that restrict movement
      (6) Poor nutritional or fluid balance states
   b. Treatment
      (1) "An ounce of prevention is worth a pound of cure"—turn and reposition q2h.
      (2) Identify high-risk patients.
      (3) Report and initiate care for beginning signs of redness, whiteness, or breaks in skin.
      (4) Use devices such as sheepskin, egg-crate mattress, alternating-pressure mattress, water mattress, or Clinitron bed.
      (5) Avoid using waterproof underpads.
      (6) Use special cleansing agents and dressings as ordered by physician or as indicated by agency policy.
9. Use turning sheet to move and turn patient with minimum of friction, which may cause abrasions.
D. Measures to maintain body alignment
   1. Encourage good posture while sitting, standing, and lying.
   2. Bed-lying positions
      a. Supine: lying on back
      b. Prone: lying on abdomen with head turned to the side
      c. Side-lying (Sims'): lying on side with upper hip and knee sharply flexed

3. Reposition patient at least q2h.
4. Guidelines for proper positioning
   a. Normal body curves must be supported by small pillows or pads; use "bridging" techniques.
   b. Joints that are normally flexed need support.
   c. Bony prominences need to be protected from pressure.
   d. Use devices such as sandbags or rolls to keep joints and body parts positioned.
   e. Periodically check patient for discomfort or difficulties.
   f. Ensure that patient can reach call signal.
E. Measures to promote structure and order in the patient's environment
   1. Physical factors
      a. Lighting
         (1) Lighting should be indirect except for reading or for procedures.
         (2) General lighting should be diffused.
         (3) Sunlight promotes healing and feeling of well being.
      b. Waste disposal: trash, human excretions, and soiled dressings and linens should be discarded according to agency's procedures.
   2. Esthetic factors
      a. Sound
         (1) Music therapy promotes rest and relaxation.
         (2) Noise causes fatigue and anxiety.
      b. Décor
         (1) Pastel colors (yellow or pink) are soothing and relaxing.
         (2) Harsh colors (red or black) overstimulate senses.
         (3) Flowers and pictures enhance environment.
      c. Odors
         (1) Foul or strong odors should be eliminated by means of room deodorizer or removal of causative agent.
         (2) Mild, fragrant odors reduce antiseptic smell and patient embarrassment.
      d. Privacy: curtains, screens, and proper draping should be used as indicated to reduce embarrassment and protect patient dignity.
   3. Care of the environment: varies according to agency policy
      a. Responsibilities of housekeeping and ancillary services (central supply and maintenance)
         (1) Daily damp dusting and floor cleaning
         (2) Scrubbing, disinfecting, sterilizing, and storing of equipment after patient transfer, discharge, or death
         (3) Repairing or replacing defective equipment or furnishings
      b. Responsibilities of the nursing personnel
         (1) Place bedside table, call signal, telephone, and personal articles within patient's reach.
         (2) Straighten and damp dust bedside unit (includes care of flowers).
         (3) Care for patient belongings (clothing, valuables, glasses, dentures, and prostheses).
         (4) Prevent cross-infection between patients.

OTHER THERAPEUTIC NURSING MEASURES

Wound Care

A. Cleaning the wound: if a wound culture is ordered, always obtain the specimen before cleansing.

1. Commonly used antiseptics
   a. 70% alcohol
   b. Povidone-iodine (Betadine)
2. Hydrogen peroxide is used to remove dry and crusted secretions.
3. Always clean from innermost to outermost aspect of wound.

B. Wound irrigation
1. Wound irrigation is used to remove secretions or excessive discharge from surfaces or body cavities or to apply moist heat. Remove dead tissue to clean wound (débride).
2. Clean or sterile technique may be used, depending on area to be irrigated.
3. Assemble equipment: may vary according to area to be irrigated (disposable kits are available).
   a. Container to hold irrigating solution
   b. Container for return flow of solution
   c. Irrigating solution
   d. Irrigator: usually bulb syringe or large plunger-type syringe
   e. Protection for patient and linens
   f. Gloves, masks, and goggles if needed
   g. Replacement dressing if indicated

C. Dressing changes
1. Dressing: material placed on a wound or incision to protect, absorb drainage, or promote healing
2. Dressings are classified by method of application.
   a. Clean
   b. Sterile
   c. Moist or dry
3. Disposable kits or hospital-assembled kits
4. Types of dressing material
   a. Gauze
   b. Petrolatum gauze
   c. Telfa
5. Material for securing dressings
   a. Tape: in various widths
      (1) Adhesive
      (2) Paper
      (3) Nonallergic
   b. Montgomery straps
   c. Bandages and binders
6. Nurse may be responsible for changing dressing or assisting physician in changing dressing.
7. Initial change of postoperative dressing is done by physician, unless an order specifies otherwise.
8. Dressings that are not to be changed should be reinforced with additional material if drainage seeps through.

D. Care of patient with wound infection
1. Infection may be local (confined to wound) or systemic (generalized throughout body), often depending on the causative organism.
2. Signs of local infection result from increased circulation and accumulation of waste in the area.
   a. Redness, heat, pain, and swelling
      (1) Dehiscence: the wound edges have pulled apart, and wound approximation is lacking.
      (2) Evisceration: the wound edges are apart, and organs (viscera) are protruding through the wound; apply moist saline-soaked gauze until physician arrives.
   b. Purulent drainage
   c. Loss of function
   d. Changes in vital signs
3. Signs of systemic infection
   a. Increase in temperature, pulse, and respirations (TPR); possible decrease in BP
   b. Nausea and vomiting
   c. General malaise
   d. Loss of appetite
4. Basic principles of treatment
   a. Physical and mental rest
   b. Elevation and rest of infected part
   c. Application of heat or cold
5. Special treatment may include:
   a. Medications (sulfonamides and antibiotics)
   b. Incision and drainage of wound
   c. Débridement: removal of foreign, infected, or necrotic tissue
6. Infection control committee investigates and follows up on infections occurring in an agency.

Bandages

A. Bandages are applied to give support, immobilize a part, apply pressure, or hold dressings.
B. Types of bandages
1. Strips or rolls of gauze, cotton flannel, or elastic material
2. Variable widths, depending on purpose and part to be bandaged
C. Types of basic turns in bandaging
1. Circular
2. Spiral
3. Spiral reverse
4. Recurrent
5. Figure-of-eight
D. Safety factors
1. Apply in direction from distal to proximal.
2. Apply tight enough to serve purpose but loose enough to permit circulation (presence of pulse).
3. Do not fasten over bony prominence, area of pressure, or a wound.
4. Part being bandaged should remain in functional position.
5. Triangular bandage, cravat, or sling is used for fractured wrists, arms, and shoulders. The tie of the cravat should be on the side of the patient's neck, not the back. The client's wrist should be slightly higher than the elbow. Manufactured slings are available.

Binders

A. Purposes
1. For support: abdomen or chest
2. To hold dressings in place
3. To apply pressure
B. Types
1. Straight
2. Tailed: T-binder, four-tailed, or scultetus (many-tailed)

Antiembolism Stockings

A. Purposes
1. To help maintain circulation
2. To prevent thrombi or phlebitis formation, especially if patient is unable to undergo early ambulation after surgery

B. Application and maintenance
1. Exact size is obtained by measuring calf or leg length and circumference.
2. Be sure legs are clean and dry before applying.
3. Apply with patient lying down; stockings should fit evenly and smoothly; no wrinkles.
4. Periodically check foot and leg for redness, irritation, swelling, and presence of pulse.
5. Stockings should be removed daily for bathing and skin inspection purposes. Occasional laundering is necessary.

Application of Heat and Cold

A. Physiologic principles
1. Cold applications (by constricting blood vessels) prevent or reduce swelling, stop bleeding, decrease suppuration, and reduce pain.
2. Heat applications (by dilating blood vessels) increase supply of oxygen and nutrients to body cells and increase amount of toxins and excess fluids carried away.
B. Types of cold applications
1. Dry: ice bag, ice cap, ice collar, and hypothermic devices
2. Moist: cold packs and compresses
C. Nursing observations
1. White, mottled skin
2. Frostbite
3. Numbness
4. Lowered body temperature
D. Guidelines
1. Caps and bags are two-thirds filled, and air is removed.
2. Containers are closed securely.
3. Caps and bags are always covered.
4. Application is removed every 30 minutes for 1 hour.
5. Ice is replaced frequently.
6. These treatments are contraindicated or used only with great care in patients with poor circulation or impaired sensation.
7. Physician's order is always required.
E. Types of heat applications
1. Dry: hot water bottle, sunlight, heating pad, and incandescent, ultraviolet, and infrared lights
2. Moist: warm compresses, hot soaks, hot packs, and K pad units
F. Nursing observations
1. Redness
2. Swelling
3. Pain
4. Change in vital signs
5. Loss of function in part
G. Guidelines
1. Physician's order is always required.
2. Carefully observe body parts that are very sensitive and burn easily (eyes, neck, and inner aspect of arm).
3. Bottles and pads are always covered.
4. Never allow patient to lie on heating device.
5. Check for faulty electrical wiring.
6. Never use safety pins with electric devices.
7. Check body temperature frequently.
8. Check distance of heating bulbs from body area; should be at least 18 inches (45 cm) away.
9. Wring out compresses well to prevent burn; if area is infected, use compresses only once and discard.
10. Agency policy may require application of a thin layer of petrolatum to area receiving heat.
H. Special baths
1. Hot (sitz) or cold (Figure 2-14)
2. Medicated

MEASURES FOR EYE, EAR, AND THROAT DISORDERS

Eye Treatments

A. Hot compresses
1. Assemble equipment: sterile basin of solution as ordered, gauze pad, heating device, paper bag, and protective gloves.
2. Put on protective gloves.
3. Apply thin layer of petrolatum over lid.
4. Wring out gauze pad with hands (if clean technique) or with two pairs of forceps (if sterile technique), and allow pad to stop steaming; apply compress slowly until patient is accustomed to heat, or allow patient to apply compress if able.
5. Try to keep compress on eyelid only; if lid is inflamed, compress may be placed on lid and cheek; if eyeball is inflamed, compress may be placed on lid and brow.
6. Change compresses every 30 to 60 seconds for 15 to 20 minutes as ordered.
7. If discharge is present, use clean pad each time compress is applied.
8. Use two sets of equipment if both eyes are involved.
B. Irrigation
1. Assemble equipment: basin of sterile solution as ordered at 95° to 100° F, medicine dropper or ear syringe, basin for return flow, cotton balls to protect uninvolved eye and to dry treated eye, and face towel to protect bed; separate irrigating tip is needed for each eye.
2. Direct flow of solution into conjunctival sac from inner angle to outer angle of eye; position patient toward affected side (Figure 2-15).

Ear Treatment: Irrigation

A. Assemble equipment: sterile ear syringe, solution as ordered at 105° to 108° F, basin for return flow, and towel to protect bed.
B. Position patient: patient may lie down, but sitting position is preferred, with head tilted slightly so that affected ear is downward; patient may hold basin for return flow if able.
C. Retract pinna, in direction according to age, to expose orifice of external canal; direct flow gently against side of canal; interrupt irrigation if pain or dizziness occurs, and notify physician.

Throat Treatments

A. Throat swab
1. Assemble equipment: sterile applicators, tongue blade, medication as ordered, tissue wipes, flashlight, and paper bag.
2. When swabbing throat, avoid stimulating gag reflex by not touching uvula.
B. Throat culture
1. Assemble equipment: sterile culture tube, applicator, and tissue wipes.

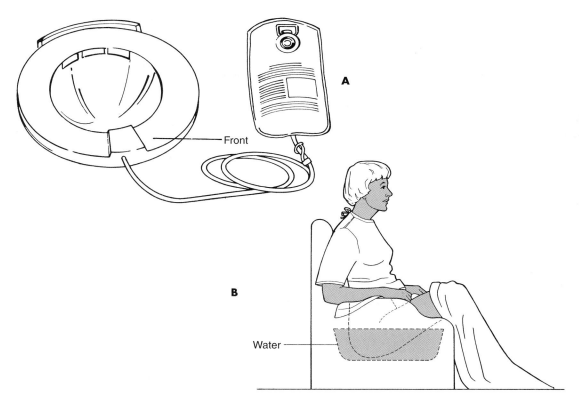

FIGURE 2-14. Sitz baths. A, Disposable. **B,** Built-in. *(Adapted from Sorrentino SA:* Mosby's Textbook for nursing assistants, *ed 5, St Louis, 2000, Mosby.)*

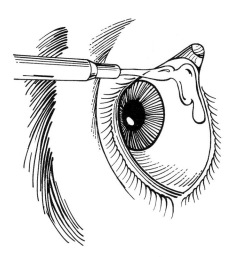

FIGURE 2-15. Irrigation of the eye. The nurse turns the patient's head toward the eye that is to be irrigated. Solution flows from the inner canthus to the outer canthus of the eye. The irrigator is held less than 4 inches (10 cm) away from the eye. The patient may assist by retracting the lower eyelid and collecting irrigating solution with absorbent material. *(From Elkin MK, Perry AG, Potter PA:* Nursing interventions and clinical skills, *ed 3, St Louis, 2004, Mosby.)*

2. After touching sides and back of throat with applicator, put applicator in culture tube without contaminating inside of tube by breaking off top of applicator that was touched by fingers.
C. Throat irrigation

1. Assemble equipment: irrigating container, solution as ordered at 110° F, tubing with rubber tip on end, tissue wipes, basin for return flow, towel to protect patient; protective gloves.
2. Put on protective gloves.
3. Have patient tilt head forward over basin and breathe through nose; discourage deep breathing.
4. Have patient do treatment if able.
5. Hold container slightly above patient's mouth; direct flow toward affected area.
   a. Irrigation may be interrupted for patient's comfort.
   b. Flow should not be directed toward uvula or base of tongue.
6. Tilt patient's head to one side and then the other to facilitate results.

MEASURES FOR GASTROINTESTINAL DISORDERS

Gastric Intubation

A. Purposes
   1. To administer gavage feedings
   2. To obtain specimens (gastric analysis and cytology)
   3. To irrigate or cleanse (lavage)
   4. For decompression (suction)
B. Tube locations
   1. Nose to stomach: nasogastric
   2. Mouth to stomach: orogastric
   3. Artificial opening into stomach: gastrostomy

C. Insertion of tube
1. This procedure is not always the responsibility of the LP/VN; refer to your agency's policy.
2. Assemble equipment: flashlight, tongue blade, stethoscope, cup of water, irrigating syringe, water-soluble lubricant, 12- to 18-gauge French tube, gloves, and towel to protect patient's clothing.
3. If rubber tube is used, it should be chilled first.
4. Place patient in semi-Fowler's position, with towel protecting clothing.
5. Approximate distance of tube insertion is the length from tip of nose to ear lobe to xiphoid process.
6. Apply water-soluble lubricant to tip of tube; if intubation is for cytology study, tube is lubricated with water or saline solution.
7. With gloved hands, hold tube 3 inches (7.5 cm) from tip, place into nostril or mouth, and advance.
8. Have patient flex neck and take repeated shallow breaths when tube passes into pharynx (approximately 3 inches [7.5 cm]).
9. Have patient swallow while advancing tube.

D. Checking placement of tube
1. Check back of throat with tongue blade and flashlight to see if coiling has occurred.
2. Aspirate stomach contents; may need to advance tube if no stomach contents are obtained.
3. While injecting 5 ml of air, use stethoscope to listen for air entering stomach.
4. Observe patient's respirations and note ability to speak; respirations may be labored or patient will be unable to speak if tube is in trachea or lungs.

E. Securing tube (Figure 2-16)
1. Anchor with strip of tape; secure to nose and cheek if nasogastric tube is used; avoid resting tube on side of nares to avoid irritation or necrosis.
2. Tube may be looped through a rubber band and attached to patient gown with safety pin for added security.

F. Removal of tube
1. Clamp tube.
2. Remove anchoring tape.
3. Put on protective gloves.
4. Draw tube through towel so that it is wiped of secretions.
5. Have patient inhale and exhale slowly.
6. Pull tube with one continuous, rapid motion.
7. Have basin ready if patient vomits.

Suction and Irrigation

A. Nasogastric or GI tubes (Levin, Cantor, Miller-Abbott, or Salem sump) may be connected to mechanical suction apparatus.
B. Suction
1. Rate is ordered by physician or according to agency policy.

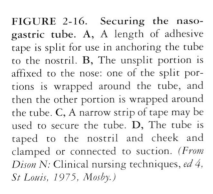
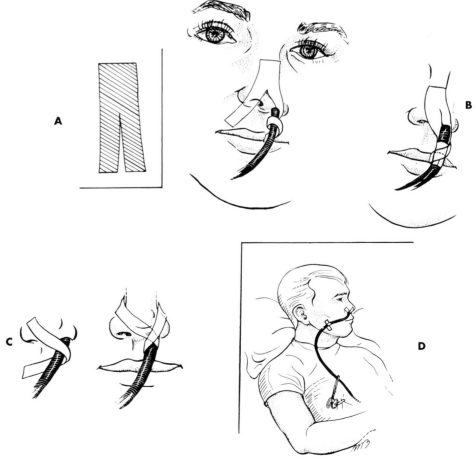

FIGURE 2-16. Securing the nasogastric tube. A, A length of adhesive tape is split for use in anchoring the tube to the nostril. B, The unsplit portion is affixed to the nose: one of the split portions is wrapped around the tube, and then the other portion is wrapped around the tube. C, A narrow strip of tape may be used to secure the tube. D, The tube is taped to the nostril and cheek and clamped or connected to suction. (From Dison N: Clinical nursing techniques, ed 4, St Louis, 1975, Mosby.)

2. Suction may be intermittent or continuous.

3. Collection container is emptied and rinsed; amount of drainage is measured and recorded at end of shift and when container becomes nearly filled.

4. Turn off or clamp off suction when assessing for bowel sounds. Suction may mimic the sounds of peristalsis.

C. Irrigation

1. Check orders for frequency, solution type, amount, and method of aspiration (force or gravity).

2. Assemble equipment: solution as ordered, container for solution, basin for return flow, irrigating syringe (bulb or plunger type), and protective pad.

3. Fill syringe, and free it of air.

4. Instill solution into tube slowly and gently.

5. Allow solution to return by aspirating or by gravity.

6. Remove syringe and reconnect to suction if ordered.

D. Patients with indwelling tubes should be given frequent mouth and nose care.

E. Accurate measurement of intake and output (subtracting irrigating solution) is essential.

MEASURES FOR VAGINAL CARE

Perineal Care

A. Assemble equipment: solution as ordered, cotton balls (or washcloth) for cleansing and drying, gloves, perineal pad with belt, and bedpan.

B. With gloved hands, put patient on bedpan; pour solution over vulva, clean with cotton balls or washcloth; dry vulva; make patient comfortable.

C. If using bottle method, fill bottle with warm water and squeeze solution over vulva; dry, wiping from urinary meatus toward anus and wiping only once with each cotton ball.

Vaginal Irrigation (Douche)

A. Assemble equipment: irrigating container with solution as ordered, tubing with douche tip, clamp, cotton balls for drying, gloves, perineal pad with belt, bedpan, and bed protection.

B. Have patient void; place patient on bedpan, or patient may administer to self in bathroom if able.

C. Insert tip down and back into vagina.

D. Give irrigation under low pressure; have solution flowing before inserting douche tip; rotate douche tip until prescribed amount is used.

E. If patient is on bedpan, raise head of bed slightly to allow fluid to drain into bedpan.

MEASURES FOR PATIENTS UNDERGOING SURGERY

Preoperative Preparation

A. Psychosocial aspects

1. Nurse assesses patient's knowledge and expected results of surgery.

2. Anxiety may interfere with preoperative teaching.

3. Extremely frightened patients may respond poorly to surgery.

4. Planned, individualized, simple explanations will enhance patient cooperation and reduce anxiety.

5. Nurse assesses and responds to patient's religious needs.

6. Common preoperative fears

a. Fear of mutilation

b. Fear of death

c. Fear of change in family role

d. Fear of pain

7. Family or significant others must understand measures taken to prepare patient.

8. Family or significant others should participate in explanations and encouragement.

B. Physical preparation

1. Explain preoperative tests (CBC, ECG, urinalysis, x-ray examinations).

2. Explain, demonstrate, and have patient practice any special postoperative exercises that will need to be done (turning, deep breathing, and pumping feet).

3. Follow preoperative orders as prescribed by physician (enema, diet, and medications).

4. Prepare appropriate skin area (refer to agency procedure manual).

5. Care for valuables.

6. Follow and complete the preoperative checklist.

a. Informed consents for surgery and anesthesia signed and witnessed

b. Nail polish, prostheses, jewelry, and makeup removed

c. Patient dressed in hospital gown only

d. Hygienic measures performed (bath with mouth care and voiding or catheterization)

e. Vital signs collected and recorded and abnormalities reported

f. Identification and allergy bracelets put in place

C. Observations and procedures recorded

D. After patient leaves for operative procedure, prepare postoperative bed and unit.

Postoperative Care

A. Immediate care

1. Ensure and maintain patent airway.

2. Maintain adequate circulation.

3. Observe for complications at operative site and in general (hemorrhage, shock, swelling, and severe pain). Carefully observe dependent areas of the body for concealed hemorrhage.

4. Assess and secure dressing, drainage, and IV tubing.

5. Assess mental status (orientation).

6. Position patient properly; keep patient warm.

7. Assess vital signs as often as ordered or more frequently, as condition warrants. Decreased BP, tachycardia, confusion and restlessness are signs of shock.

8. Follow physician's orders.

9. Report signs of restlessness, excessive drainage, or abnormal reactions.

10. Support patient and family or significant others by briefly answering questions and offering explanations.

B. Routine care

1. Follow physician's orders.

2. Assess and record vital signs frequently during first 24 hours; report changes immediately.

3. Assess dressing or surgical site frequently.

4. Give oral hygiene as needed.
5. Have patient turn, deep breathe, and, unless contraindicated, cough and exercise legs at least q2h. Patient should try to pump ankles (alternately dorsiflex and plantar flex their feet) to decrease chance of thrombus formation.
6. Assess and record intake and output (patient may need order for catheterization if he or she does not void within 6 to 8 hours after surgery).
7. Assist patient with passive or active exercises, unless contraindicated.
8. Encourage and assist patient to ambulate as much as orders permit, which decreases chance for thrombus formation and pneumonia, and alleviates gas pains from decreased peristalsis.
9. Care for any drains the patient may have:
   a. Penrose: large "noodle"-like drain that drains onto a sterile dressing.
   b. Jackson-Pratt: "grenade"-like drain that needs to be emptied every so often. The drain is then reconstituted by squeezing it and applying a plug. Negative pressure is used to drain surgical site.
   c. Hemovac, urevac: drains blood or urine using negative pressure.
10. Perform daily assessment.
    a. Lungs: breath sounds and cough
    b. Circulation: color, temperature, capillary refill of extremities; pain in legs or chest and IV site
    c. GI tract: nausea, vomiting, distention, bowel sounds, and passage of flatus
    d. Urine: amount, color, odor, and frequency
    e. Mental status: withdrawal, confusion, anxiety, or restlessness
11. Offer pain medication

MEASURES RELATED TO RADIATION THERAPY

A. Radiation
   1. Radiate: to send out rays (light, heat, or roentgen).
   2. Radiation is used in diagnosis and therapeutic treatment of various conditions (especially for malignancies).
   3. Types of radiation
      a. Alpha rays: harmless; do not travel far
      b. Beta rays: more penetrating; stop at person's body surface
      c. Gamma rays: very penetrating
B. Types of therapy
   1. Infrared lamp
   2. Ultraviolet
   3. Diatherapy
   4. Roentgen ray (x-ray: low voltage, external)
   5. Betatron, cobalt, cesium (high voltage, external)
   6. Internal radiation
      a. Implants (skin surface, intratumor, intracavitary)
      b. Liquid forms of radioisotopes
      c. Injection (intracavitary, systemic)
C. Radiation therapy and the nurse
   1. Internal implant
      a. Explain procedure and precautions to patient and family or significant others.

(1) Patient needs to know that he or she will be in isolation and how many days isolation is likely to last.
(2) Patient should know that nursing personnel and visitors will be spending a minimal amount of time at the bedside and yet will be available when needed.
   b. Ensure good fluid intake, unless contraindicated.
   c. Have patient move about as little as possible.
   d. Assess for signs of radiation reactions (nausea, vomiting, or skin irritation).
   e. Communicate frequently with patient from doorway without entering room.
   f. Use precautions at all times.
2. Radiation precautions with implant
   a. "RADIATION IN USE" sign with directions posted on patient's door.
   b. No staff member or visitor spends more than 1 hour per day with patient; care must be well organized.
   c. Pregnant women and children should not enter the patient's room.
   d. Check placement of implant q4h.
   e. Wear gown and gloves while handling excreta, secretions, and utensils. Excreta may need to be double flushed in toilet; know agency policy.
   f. Wash contaminated gloves with soap and water before removing.
   g. Wash hands with soap and water.
   h. If implant becomes dislodged, call radiologist immediately—do not touch implant.
3. Nursing care for specific situations
   a. Therapy involving mouth
      (1) Oral hygiene with brushing teeth (or dentures) should be done three times a day (tid).
      (2) Smoking should be discouraged.
      (3) Teeth should be assessed for change in condition; if changes observed, notify physician.
      (4) Male patient should not shave if jaw is being treated.
   b. Uterine therapy
      (1) Bed rest is maintained to prevent displacement of implant.
      (2) Bedpan is inspected for loss of implant before contents are discarded.
      (3) Foley catheter with continuous irrigation may be ordered to reduce bladder irritation.
      (4) Vaginal irrigation may be ordered after removal of implant.
   c. Radioactive gold administered intraperitoneally
      (1) Leakage on dressings appears bright red and may be confused with blood.
      (2) Dressings should be wrapped in newspaper and disposed of in special container.
4. External radiotherapy
   a. Explain procedure to patient and family or significant others.
   b. Never remove skin markings.
   c. Avoid washing the marked area.
   d. Do not apply ointments, creams, or powders to marked area.
   e. Encourage good fluid intake and nutrition.
   f. Observe for radiation reactions.

MEASURES CONCERNING PATIENT'S DEPARTURE

A. Transferring patient
   1. Patient may be transferred from one service to another, from one floor to another, or from one agency to another.
   2. Physician's order is required.
   3. Transfer patient ambulatory, by wheelchair, or on stretcher; follow agency's policy.
   4. Explain transfer to patient; be sure all personal belongings are transferred with patient.
   5. Avoid transferring during mealtime or change of shift to reduce confusion.
   6. Make proper charting notations; notify family or significant others.
B. Discharging patient
   1. Written order by physician is required.
   2. Nurse's responsibilities
      a. Gather and check all personal belongings with patient.
      b. Make sure patient understands all instructions regarding diet, medications, treatments, and follow-up appointments.
      c. Notify family or significant others as necessary.
      d. Accompany patient to exit.
      e. Make proper charting notations.
   3. Discharge planning
      a. Planning begins after initial nursing assessment and is included on care plan.
      b. Nursing interventions are directed toward eventual discharge of patient.
      c. Planning consists of teaching patient and family or significant others.
         (1) Cause of illness
         (2) Drugs, treatments, and diet
         (3) Health care follow-up
         (4) Functions within limitations

CARING FOR THE DYING

A. Signs of approaching death
   1. Patient is pale, with pinched expression of anxiety.
   2. Eyes are glazed and dull; pupils do not react to light.
   3. Mouth remains partially open unless patient attempts to speak; speech is mumbled and often confused.
   4. Muscle tone becomes flaccid.
   5. Skin is cool and clammy and may be mottled; this is caused by diminished circulation; body temperature is often elevated.
   6. Respirations are rapid and shallow, often progressing to Cheyne-Stokes respirations.
   7. Pulse becomes weak and thready.
   8. Patient may be diaphoretic, thirsty, and incontinent of urine and feces.
B. Five stages in the process of reaction to a terminal illness or to dying: refer to Chapter 6 for more detailed information relative to death and dying.
   1. Denial
   2. Anger
   3. Bargaining
   4. Grief or depression
   5. Acceptance
C. Nursing care of dying patient
   1. Give symptomatic nursing care: palliative care is comfort care. Nurse and physician attempt to increase client comfort by performing certain actions. Surgery and medications may be a form of palliative care.
   2. Give good personal hygiene.
   3. Turn patient frequently.
   4. Give treatments and medications as long as possible or until discontinued.
   5. Carry out desires of patient and family or significant others as far as possible; be sensitive to religious or cultural beliefs.
   6. Be available to provide emotional support and privacy to patient and family or significant others.
   7. Remember that hearing may be the last sense to fail.
D. Spiritual needs of patient
   1. Fulfill needs as requested by patient and family or significant others.
   2. Continue to adhere to patient's individual religious beliefs.
E. Care of body after death (postmortem care): physicians pronounce death in most cases. RNs may pronounce death (in some states) under special circumstances (hospice patients).
   1. Lower head of bed.
   2. Leave one pillow under head to prevent congestion of blood in vessels of face.
   3. Close eyes.
   4. Place dentures in mouth immediately and close mouth.
   5. Clean body; follow agency's policy for removal of drains, IV needle and tubing, dressings, and tubes.
   6. Straighten body and place in natural position.
   7. Allow viewing of body by family or significant others if they desire.
   8. Wrap in shroud and label with tags according to agency policy.
   9. Gather, pack, label, and care for patient's personal belongings.
   10. Record observations, procedures, disposition of valuables, and time of death; complete records.

SUGGESTED READINGS

Becker BG, Fendler DT: *Vocational and personal adjustments in practical nursing,* ed 7, St Louis, 1994, Mosby.

Bernhard LA, Walsh M: *Leadership: the key to the professionalization of nursing,* ed 3, St Louis, 1995, Mosby.

Blair L: *Passport to practical and vocational nursing,* St Louis, 1998, Mosby.

Christensen BL, Kockrow EO: *Foundations of nursing,* ed 4, St Louis, 2003, Mosby.

Cole G: *Fundamental nursing concepts and skills,* ed 2, St Louis, 1996, Mosby.

Dunham-Taylor J, Penny Marquette R, Pinczuk JZ: Surviving capitation, *AJN* 96:26, 1996.

Elkin MK, Perry AG, Potter PA: *Nursing interventions and clinical skills,* ed. 3, St Louis, 2004, Mosby.

Ellis JR, Nowlis EA, Bentz PM: *Modules for basic nursing skills,* modules I and II, ed 6, 1996, Lippincott-Raven.

Grossman D: Cultural dimensions in home health nursing, *AJN* 96:33, 1996.

Kerr JR, Sirotnik MK: *Potter and Perry Canadian fundamentals of nursing,* St Louis, 1997, Mosby.

McDevitt MJ: A(TENS)tion!, *Nursing* 25:46, 1995.

Potter PA, Perry AG: *Basic nursing, a critical thinking approach,* ed 5, St Louis, 2003, Mosby.

Stolley JM: Freeing your patients from restraints, *AJN* 95:26, 1995.

Sullivan EJ, Decker PJ: *Effective leadership and nursing management in nursing,* ed 4, Upper Saddle River, 1997, Prentice Hall Health.

Venes D: *Taber's Cyclopedic Medical Dictionary,* ed 19, Philadelphia, 2003, FA Davis.

Wheeler SR: Helping families cope with death and dying, *Nursing* 26:25, 1996.

REVIEW QUESTIONS

1. What are some of a patient's internal variables to health? Choose all that apply.
   1. Developmental stage
   2. Knowledge level
   3. Socioeconomic status
   4. Emotional factors
   5. Cultural influences
   6. Religious views

2. A patient is being prepared for sealed internal radiation therapy for cervical cancer. The nurse can help reduce the patient's anxiety by emphasizing that:
   1. Pain medication will be offered regularly.
   2. Visitors will be limited during this treatment.
   3. The nurse will be available whenever needed.
   4. The patient will not be radioactive during this treatment.

3. HIPPA guidelines preserve the patient's right to:
   1. Refuse treatment
   2. Maintain privacy
   3. Litigation
   4. Assisted suicide

4. When performing a throat culture, the nurse swabs the sides of the throat before the back to:
   1. Delay stimulating the gag reflex.
   2. Stimulate production of secretions.
   3. Avoid contamination of the culture site.
   4. Obtain adequate specimens for culture.

5. One hour after the nurse applies an elastic bandage to a patient's sprained ankle, the patient complains of tingling and burning in the toes. The nurse should:
   1. Palpate for pedal pulses.
   2. Reapply the bandage less snugly.
   3. Instruct her to elevate the affected foot.
   4. Encourage her to wiggle her toes every 2 hours.

6. A nurse threatens to restrain a competent individual. If she restrains the individual, she can be charged with:
   1. Unlawful restraint
   2. Negligence
   3. Assault and battery
   4. Malpractice

7. When performing wound irrigations, the nurse can best be protected by:
   1. Raising the bed to a workable height
   2. Explaining the procedure to the patient
   3. Hand washing before and after the procedure
   4. Donning appropriate personal protective equipment

8. Which of the following patients is most at risk for decubitus formation?
   1. A 20-year-old patient with a lumbar-4 injury confined to a wheelchair
   2. A 6-year-old patient in skeletal traction for a fractured right femur
   3. An ambulatory 90-year-old patient with Alzheimer's disease
   4. A 75-year-old patient on bed rest following total knee replacement

9. A patient is 1-day postoperative gastric resection. The patient has a nasogastric tube attached to low-intermittent suction and complains of severe thirst. The nurse's next course of action is:
   1. Call the physician for an order allowing ice chips.
   2. Instill approximately 100 ml of normal saline into his tube.
   3. Explain that he must remain NPO until the tube is removed.
   4. Assist the patient in brushing his teeth and rinsing his mouth.

10. A nurse assigns an unlicensed assistive personnel (UAP) to medicate a patient complaining of a headache. In assigning this task, the nurse is:
    1. Prioritizing patient care
    2. Responsive to patient complaints
    3. Enhancing the UAP's sense of self-worth
    4. Delegating an inappropriate task to ancillary personnel

11. A patient who is receiving external radiation treatments asks the nurse if he can remove the ink on his skin. Which of the following is the best answer by the nurse?
    1. "No, I am sorry, we need you to leave those on so we know where to point the radiation next time."
    2. "I will need to get some adhesive remover to get the ink off."
    3. "I will need to consult with the physician about this."
    4. "No, we need to make sure that we irradiate the tumor in the exact spot as the last time."

12. A patient, newly admitted to a nursing home, complains of difficulty in sleeping. The patient states that he routinely takes sleeping pills to fall asleep. Which of the following is the nurse's best response to the patient's statement?
    1. "We really don't like our residents to use sleeping pills."
    2. "It's not unusual to have difficulty sleeping in a new setting."
    3. "Let me try to make you comfortable first before giving you a sleeping pill."
    4. "I'm certain your doctor will reorder the medication for you when I tell him tomorrow."

13. A patient had a urethral retention catheter removed 6 hours ago and has not yet voided. What is the nurse's next course of action?
    1. Assess the patient's abdomen for distention.
    2. Catheterize the patient using a straight catheter.
    3. Call the physician.
    4. Ambulate the patient to the bathroom so he can try again.

14. A patient has returned to the unit following a transurethral resection of the prostate (TURP). The nurse notes that the bedside drainage unit is filled with red urine and numerous large clots. The abdomen is distended, and the bladder can be palpated above the symphysis pubis. Which of the following is the nurse's *first* course of action?
    1. Change the patient's position.
    2. Notify the surgeon of your findings.
    3. Check the chart for bladder irrigation orders.
    4. Document your observations on the flow sheet.

15. A patient is admitted with pediculosis. Which of the following orders should the nurse anticipate?
    1. Oil-retention enema
    2. Sitz bath
    3. IPPB treatment
    4. Medicated shampoo

16. A patient who has been on bedrest attempts to stand and walk without dangling first. If the patient becomes dizzy

and weak, he is most likely experiencing:

1 Anemia
2 Postural hypotension
3 Hypoxia
4 Hypertension

17. A patient who is 1-day postoperative abdominal hysterectomy has a urinary catheter, a Penrose drain, and an IV of dextrose 5% in Ringer's lactate infusing at 100 ml/hr. The patient is complaining of a sense of urinary urgency and lower abdominal pressure and requests an injection of Demerol. Which of the following is the nurse's *first* course of action?

1 Check when this patient was last medicated for pain.
2 Request that the physician change the IV flow rate order.
3 Determine that urine is draining into the bedside drainage unit.
4 Assure the patient that catheters often cause this type of discomfort.

18. You are planning to irrigate the colostomy of a patient. The patient asks why the colostomy is being irrigated. The nurse's best explanation is that irrigation helps to:

1 Control constipation
2 Cleanse the bowel
3 Regulate the discharge of feces
4 Eliminate the need for stool softeners

19. A patient of color is admitted with status asthmaticus and presents as very dyspneic and uncomfortable. Because of the patient's dark complexion, how should the nurse assess for the symptom of cyanosis?

1 By examining his oral mucosa
2 By monitoring vital signs hourly
3 By observing lips and nail beds
4 By applying a pulse oximeter probe

20. Which of the following tasks would be appropriate for an LPN to assign to unlicensed assistive personnel? Choose all that apply.

1 Feeding a patient with a CVA
2 SOAPIE charting
3 Assisting with a shower for a patient who is paralyzed
4 Administering 6:00 PM medications
5 Wound dressing for a patient with a decubitus ulcer
6 Passing 10:00 PM snacks

21. The physician has ordered a patient's IV to infuse at 100 ml/hr. The IV was started at 7:00 PM. When the nurse rounds at 11:00 PM, 200 ml fluid has infused into the patient. The nurse's initial course of action is to:

1 Notify the physician that the IV has infiltrated.
2 Note the amount on the patient's intake and output record.
3 Check the tubing and infusion site for possible obstructions.
4 Change the rate of flow until the correct amount has infused.

22. The volume of a patient's Foley catheter bedside drainage unit is most accurately measured by:

1 Holding the drainage bag up at eye level
2 Approximating output from the markings on the drainage unit
3 Emptying the urine into a bedpan and noting what level it reaches
4 Pouring the urine into a measuring container on a flat, eye-level surface

23. Which of the following nursing measures would best address the comfort needs of a patient with a newly inserted tracheostomy tube?

1 Providing a pad and pencil within reach
2 Having tissues easily available to the patient
3 Reassuring the patient that nurses are always nearby
4 Arranging to have telephone service discontinued temporarily

24. A nurse believes that one of her co-workers may be abusing cocaine. How should the nurse proceed?

1 Confront the co-worker with her suspicions.
2 Notify the supervisor so the co-worker can get help.
3 Ask the advice of a physician on staff.
4 Discuss your suspicions with other co-workers.

25. The nurse has been assigned to perform colostomy care for a patient who has had a recent hemicolectomy. The nurse can best determine how the patient tolerated the procedure by:

1 Noting all objective signs and symptoms during the procedure
2 Asking the patient if anything is bothering him during the procedure
3 Questioning the patient regarding his well being at the end of the treatment
4 Observing the patient's verbal and nonverbal actions throughout the procedure

26. The chief reason that the nurse explains procedure steps and purpose to the patient before performing a treatment is which of the following?

1 It diminishes the likelihood of malpractice suits.
2 Patient anxiety is decreased with understanding.
3 It allows the patient the opportunity to refuse the treatment.
4 It provides the nurse with an opportunity to review the procedure mentally.

27. In relation to body processes, the term homeostasis means:

1 The body is in balance.
2 An alteration of fluid and electrolytes exists.
3 The amounts of sodium, potassium, and water are not normal.
4 The physiologic processes of the body are slowed.

28. A patient who has just returned from a bronchogram asks the nurse if he can have a drink of water. Which is the best response by the nurse?

1 "Sure, just let me get your vital signs."
2 "We need to wait until you wake up a little more."
3 "I need to check your gag reflex first."
4 "You should chew on some ice first."

29. A nurse is assisting a patient with a tracheostomy to eat a meal. Which of the following actions must the nurse do before allowing the patient to eat?

1 Administer supplemental oxygen.
2 Medicate the patient for pain.
3 Make sure the tracheostomy cuff is inflated.
4 Ensure that the tracheostomy ties are securely fastened.

30. A patient who has had diarrhea for 3 days is most at risk for developing the problem of:

1 Impaired skin integrity
2 Alteration in nutrition
3 Knowledge deficit
4 Alteration in fluids and electrolytes

31. A patient with heart failure is beginning a treatment regimen that includes diuretic medications. Which of the following instructions regarding obtaining weights should the nurse reinforce to the patient?
    1 Weigh each morning on arising.
    2 Weigh 1 hour after taking medication.
    3 Weigh each time a medication is omitted.
    4 Weigh only when shortness of breath develops.

32. Which of the following is included in the assessment phase of the nursing process? Choose all that apply.
    1 Laboratory values
    2 Respiratory therapy notes
    3 Physical examination
    4 Physician's orders

33. The nurse notes the following orders on the care plan of a patient with a decubitus ulcer who is on enteric isolation. Which order would the nurse question?
    1 Use a mask when changing heavily soiled dressings.
    2 Teach self-care of the wound.
    3 Limit visitors.
    4 Measure wound once per week.

34. Which one of the following statements made by a patient who is in strict isolation indicates that further intervention may be necessary?
    1 "I really wish my son could stay with me, but I know he can't."
    2 "I get lonely, but at least I can listen to my music."
    3 "I don't feel like eating; I didn't sleep good last night."
    4 "I appreciate you stopping by to see me often."

35. An elderly patient required a Foley catheter following hip surgery. Laboratory tests now indicate that the patient has developed a *Pseudomonas aeruginosa* urinary tract infection. In light of this patient's medical history, the nurse would suspect that this is a (an):
    1 Superinfection
    2 Nosocomial infection
    3 Autoimmune response
    4 Antibiotic resistance response

36. Acid fast bacillus (AFB) isolation is indicated for patients that have:
    1 MRSA
    2 VRE
    3 TB
    4 HIV

37. A person's resistance to disease can be increased through the use of:
    1 Inflammation
    2 Immunization
    3 Digitalization
    4 Phagocytosis

38. A gown should be removed by:
    1 Touching the outside of the gown only
    2 Removing the gown outside the patient's room
    3 Allowing another individual to remove it for you
    4 Touching the inside of the gown only

39. When collecting a patient's psychosocial history, the nurse questions cultural practices because:
    1 Cultural practices may affect how the patient views the health care team.
    2 It determines whether the patient should receive last rites.
    3 Certain cultures will offer social supports to ill members.

    4 The patient may wish to have members with them during examinations.

40. In the future, health care trends will require nursing to:
    1 Become nonexistent.
    2 Focus more on prevention of illnesses.
    3 Concentrate more on hospital care.
    4 Become limited in scope.

41. The nurse is caring for a patient with a WBC of 0.2. The patient has been undergoing chemotherapy for 3 months for prostate cancer. What type of special precautions needs to be implemented for this patient?

    Reverse Isolation, to protect
    (neutropenic) pt from us
    _____

42. Nurses completing incident reports following medication errors should be sure to:
    1 Correct the error as quickly as possible.
    2 Notify the patient and his family of the error.
    3 Document completion of the incident report on the patient's chart.
    4 Note the medication administered and notify the physician.

43. Licensing laws regulate the practice of nursing to:
    1 Protect the public from injury.
    2 Guarantee the best possible nursing care.
    3 Ensure that every nurse has good moral character.
    4 Support nurse employment by limiting the competition.

44. The nurse is bandaging a client's elbow. Into which of the following positions should the elbow be placed before bandaging it?
    1 Rotation
    2 Extension
    3 Slightly flexed
    4 Slightly hyperextended

45. A patient has had a hemorrhoidectomy. Which of the following binders should be used to keep the dressings in place?
    1 Scultetus
    2 Triangular
    3 T-binder
    4 Abdominal

46. The nurse is instructed to bandage a patient's lower extremity with an ace wrap. The leg is extremely edematous. What should the nurse do first?
    1 Elevate the extremity for 15 to 20 minutes before wrapping.
    2 Wrap from the most distal to the proximal end of the extremity.
    3 Ensure that the ace wrap is smooth and free of wrinkles.
    4 Check distal pulses every 15 minutes.

47. During the bed bath procedure, the nurse reduces the chance of infection by:
    1 Thoroughly rinsing and drying all skin folds
    2 Applying clean gloves before beginning the bath
    3 Using separate washcloth sections for each eye
    4 Changing the bath water after bathing each extremity

48. The rules and regulations governing the practice of nursing in the United States are made by:
    1 Each state's legislative body
    2 Each state's board of nursing

3 The National Council of State Boards of Nursing

4 The Joint Commission of Accreditation of Health Care Organizations

49. A nurse is applying a triangular bandage to elevate a patient's arm. Where should the knot be tied during this procedure?
1 Near the patient's elbow
2 At the side of the neck
3 Towards the back of the patient's head
4 Wherever the patient wants it tied

50. The nurse has completed a bed bath on a patient who needs an abdominal binder applied. Which of the following should be done before applying the binder?
1 Apply powder to the area.
2 Heavily lotion the abdomen.
3 Apply gauze over the patient's abdomen.
4 Make sure the area is completely dry.

51. An elderly patient has arrived at the physician's office complaining of ear pain, vertigo, and impaired hearing. The physician has ordered a normal saline ear irrigation to loosen embedded earwax. Following this procedure, the nurse would take care to:
1 Retract the pinna of the ear.
2 Determine the patient's tolerance of movement. *BC can have vertigo*
3 Encourage the patient to remain supine for several hours.
4 Thoroughly dry the ear canal with cotton-tipped applicators.

52. A female patient has been admitted to the hospital unit with a fever of unknown origin. The physician has ordered urine and blood specimens for culture, as well as a broad-spectrum antibiotic. The nurse should:
1 Obtain the specimens before beginning antibiotic therapy.
2 Ask the physician to clarify which procedure should be performed first.
3 Begin the antibiotic therapy immediately before obtaining the specimens.
4 Obtain the blood, start the medication, and tell the patient to call when she is able to void.

53. A postoperative patient has all of the following signs and symptoms. Which one is most indicative that the patient may have thrombophlebitis?
1 Pain in the foot and ankle
2 Fever and dry skin
3 Pain in the calf when the foot is flexed
4 One leg is much cooler than the other

54. Which of the following observations would indicate that the nurse should withhold a tube feeding?
1 Oozing at the gastrostomy site
2 Absence of an adequate gag reflex
3 Presence of more than 100 ml of residual feeding
4 Absence of residual feeding when the gastrostomy tube is suctioned

55. The type of nursing care that provides for the emotional, physical, social, and psychologic care of a patient is termed:
1 Functional
2 Team
3 Holistic
4 Primary

56. If a patient complains of the urge to defecate after the nurse begins to administer a tap water enema, the nurse should:
1 Adjust the tube location while maintaining fluid flow.

2 Lower the enema bag while instructing the patient to breathe deeply.
3 Reassure the patient that the discomfort should pass in a few minutes.
4 Immediately discontinue the procedure to allow patient bowel evacuation.

57. A nursing assistant asks why the nurse must clip or shave hair from a surgical site. Which of the following is the nurse's best explanation for this procedure?
1 The physician will have difficulty suturing the site.
2 The procedure is done to reduce the number of micro-organisms on the patient's skin.
3 The patient will experience less discomfort after surgery.
4 The dressings will not adhere if the hair is not removed.

58. Of the following preoperative orders, which one helps most to prevent postoperative nausea and vomiting?
1 Cleansing enemas
2 NPO for 6 to 12 hours
3 Teach cough and deep-breathing exercises.
4 Lactated Ringer's solution IV at 40 cc/hr

59. A nurse is changing a patient's decubitus ulcer dressing using sterile technique. Which of the following steps in the procedure is incorrect?
1 Remove old dressing with sterile gloves.
2 Irrigate the wound from top to bottom.
3 Pack the wound using a sterile Q-Tip.
4 Tape the wound to allow for patient movement.

60. The Jackson-Pratt is used to:
1 Dress operative sites.
2 Hold dressing in place.
3 Clean the surgical site.
4 Drain the operative site.

61. Which of the following should the nurse carefully document following a surgical dressing change? Choose all that apply.
1 The specific location of the wound
2 The characteristics of the suture line
3 The type of antibiotic cleansing solution
4 The patient's emotional response to the surgical procedure

62. After administering a preoperative narcotic, the nurse can best meet the safety needs of the patient by:
1 Obtaining the signed, surgical consent
2 Giving the patient good oral hygiene
3 Putting the side rails up on the bed
4 Reinforcing cough and deep-breathing exercises

63. During venipuncture, the tourniquet should be released:
1 As soon as an appropriate vein is palpated
2 Before withdrawing the needle from the patient's vein
3 After application of a bandage to the venipuncture site
4 As soon as blood begins flowing into the specimen tube

64. Placing the patient's arm in a downward position during venipuncture helps to:
1 Dilate blood vessels for better access.
2 Diminish patient discomfort during the procedure.
3 Prevent backflow of any chemical additives in the blood tubes.
4 Prevent any unnecessary arm movement during the procedure.

65. A patient's abdominal incision is no longer approximated and you observe viscera protruding from the incision. The nurse should immediately:
    1 Attempt to replace the viscera back in the incision.
    2 Call the physician.
    3 Place a saline soaked sterile dressing over the wound.
    4 Place the patient in the shock position.

66. A patient returns from the post-anesthesia care unit after a cholecystectomy with the following vital signs: T, 98.6; P, 72; R, 20; BP, 120/64. Fifteen minutes after the patient arrives on the unit, the following vital signs are collected: T, 98.7; P, 128; R, 30; BP, 98/48. What might the change in vital signs indicate?
    1 Infection
    2 Dehiscence
    3 Thrombophlebitis
    4 Hemorrhage

67. When changing the dressing of a new percutaneous endoscopic gastrostomy (PEG) tube insertion site, the nurse always cleanses the exit site:
    1 With a vigorous back-and-forth, sweeping motion
    2 Circularly, from the center of the exit site outward
    3 Downward, from the side farther away to the closer side
    4 Upward, through the center of the site then down each side

68. Which of the following nursing interventions would best prevent the complication of thrombophlebitis?
    1 Early ambulation
    2 Sequential antiembolic devices
    3 Coughing and deep breathing
    4 Incentive spirometry

69. A patient complains of dizziness while he is using his incentive spirometer. The nurse knows that the patient is probably breathing too:
    1 Deeply
    2 Slowly
    3 Rapidly
    4 Irregularly

70. A nurse is teaching a patient who has terminal cancer, and is scheduled to have a colostomy. Which of the following should be included in the patient's teaching?
    1 "This surgery should cure your cancer."
    2 "Hopefully, this procedure will alleviate some of your symptoms."
    3 "This procedure might be able to be reversed."
    4 "This surgery should help us diagnose you better."

71. When a patient has died, the nurse should schedule post-mortem care:
    1 Before family viewing of the body
    2 Following transport of the body to the morgue
    3 As quickly as possible to decrease tension on the unit
    4 After allowing the family the opportunity to view the body

72. A postoperative patient who has been on bedrest since his surgery 5 days ago makes the following statements. Which statement may indicate that a postoperative complication may be developing?
    1 "I wish I could eat pizza without getting nauseous."
    2 "I need someone to rub my leg; it's swollen and sore."
    3 "The only way to get rid of this gas is to drink ginger ale."
    4 "I feel the need to have lots of salt on my fruit."

73. A patient wants to know why wet-to-dry dressings are being used to treat his stasis leg ulcer. The nurse's best response would be that this treatment:
    1 Increases circulation to the wound
    2 Cleans the wound by removing dead tissue and debris
    3 Promotes the absorption of drainage by capillary action
    4 Decreases pain by lowering edema along wound edges

74. The best method of determining how effective preoperative teaching has been is to:
    1 Have the patient take a written quiz.
    2 Ask the patient to teach another person the skill.
    3 Have the patient verbalize what has been taught.
    4 Ask the patient for a return demonstration of the skill.

75. A postoperative patient, who had an appendectomy, complains of gas pains. Which advice from the nurse would best alleviate this problem?
    1 "Why don't you try taking a walk?"
    2 "Let me get you a rectal tube."
    3 "I'll get you some Mylicon."
    4 "Why don't you drink some milk."

76. A 16-year-old girl has just returned to the unit following a tonsillectomy. Which of the following routes would be most appropriate for measuring her body temperature?
    1 Oral
    2 Rectal
    3 Axillary
    4 Tympanic

77. While assisting an elderly nursing home resident with a bath, you observe that the skin is dry and that the resident has been scratching. A priority nursing diagnosis would be:
    1 Alteration in fluids and electrolytes
    2 Impaired tissue perfusion
    3 Altered thought processes
    4 Impaired skin integrity

78. Before beginning a new tube feeding via a nasogastric tube, the nurse must first:
    1 Measure and replace any residual feeding.
    2 Warm the feeding to approximately 105° F.
    3 Check for correct tube placement in the stomach.
    4 Dislodge encrusted formula with a warm water flush.

79. The nurse has requested a UAP to assist in moving a paralyzed patient up in bed. Which of the following is an appropriate instruction to the UAP for this procedure?
    1 Stand one step back from the bed while lifting.
    2 Keep your back straight and your knees flexed.
    3 Keep your knees straight and your back flexed.
    4 Keep your feet close together for balance.

80. A patient is 10-hours postoperative abdominal hysterectomy. Which of the following assessment information would alert the nurse that normal postoperative progression is not occurring?
    1 She has serosanguineous drainage on her dressing.
    2 She splints her incision when coughing and deep breathing.
    3 She has not voided since the surgery.
    4 She is reluctant to ambulate because of incisional pain.

81. When considering the need for application of restraints on an elderly confused patient, the nurse knows that restraints:
    1 Provide patients with a sense of security
    2 Should be applied only after receiving a physician's order
    3 Are applied loosely on elderly patients to prevent skin abrasion

4 Must be tied to side rails to allow faster removal in an emergency

82. A nurse is assisting a physician in obtaining a Pap smear on a female patient. What must the nurse do to the specimen before sending it to the laboratory?
1 "Fix" it to the slide.
2 Refrigerate it.
3 Stain it.
4 Place it on ice.

83. A patient refuses morning care and states that he does not like to bathe in the morning; he prefers an evening shower. Which of the following is the nurse's best response?
1 "The staff is too busy to provide for an evening shower."
2 "The staff will do its best to provide for an evening shower."
3 "Bathing in the morning makes one feel more refreshed."
4 "Hospital routine requires nurses to provide for bathing in the morning."

84. A nurse has discontinued an IV infusion and IV catheter. The patient asks why the nurse is applying pressure to the site. What is the nurse's best explanation?
1 "I need to make sure that a clot develops at the spot."
2 "You could bleed out if I don't hold pressure!"
3 "I need to hold pressure for at least 5 minutes to make sure a clot has formed."
4 "Because you are on blood thinner, I need to hold it longer."

85. Which of the following is the correct sequence of events to follow should a fire occur in a facility?
1 Notify the switchboard, extinguish flames, close doors, and remove persons.
2 Call for help, remove persons, confine the fire, and extinguish any flames present.
3 Rescue persons, activate the alarm, confine the fire, and extinguish any flames present.
4 Activate the alarm, confine the fire, remove any persons present, and use fire extinguisher.

86. An IVP is helpful in diagnosing conditions of the:
1 Liver
2 Brain
3 Kidney
4 Intestine

87. The nurse is caring for a patient who has been placed in protective isolation. When planning care for the patient, the nurse is aware that the primary goal in caring for a patient in protective isolation is to:
1 Protect the health care workers caring for the patient
2 Limit the patient's psychologic impact of being isolated
3 Reduce the number of organisms that may come in contact with the patient
4 Prevent the infectious process from spreading to other patients on the patient unit

88. Which of the following actions is the appropriate way for a nurse to correct a mistaken entry made in charting?
1 Use an eraser to remove the entry.
2 Line out the entry, date, and initial it.
3 Recopy the entry and destroy the original sheet.
4 Paint over the entry using white correction fluid.

89. A nurse is preparing a patient who is to undergo an MRI. Which of the following questions would be important for the nurse to ask? Choose all that apply.
1 "Are you allergic to iodine?"

2 "Are you claustrophobic?"
3 "Do you have any metal in your body?"
4 "Do you have a pacemaker?"
5 "Can you give yourself an enema?"

90. A patient has a nasogastric tube inserted to receive supplemental feedings before surgery. The patient asks what the purpose of the tube is. Which of the following responses by the nurse is correct?
1 "The tube is meant to assist your bowels to move."
2 "Fluids and gas will be removed from your GI tract."
3 "This will allow us to give you feedings and build up your reserve."
4 "The tube will speed your healing time after the surgery."

91. A nursing assistant asks why a cholangiogram is done. Which of the following is the correct information to give the assistant?
1 "It is used to detect kidney damage."
2 "It is a generalized, liver test."
3 "It can diagnose heart problems."
4 "It can tell us if the gallbladder is working correctly."

92. A nurse is inserting a retention catheter in a female patient. The nurse suspects that the tip of the catheter may have been contaminated before it was inserted into the meatus. The nurse's next course of action is to:
1 Request a co-worker to bring another sterile catheter.
2 Use Betadine to decontaminate the tip of the catheter.
3 Discontinue the procedure, and discard the entire sterile tray.
4 Go ahead with the procedure; the tip is probably not contaminated.

93. The nurse is instructing a UAP to place an ostomy pouch on a patient, ensuring that the pouch fits snugly. The UAP inquires as to why the ostomy pouch must be so tight. The nurse's best response is:
1 "The pouch must stay on a long time because they are expensive."
2 "The pouch has to stay on when the patient takes a bath or shower."
3 "The pouch may leak if it's loose, causing the skin to become excoriated."
4 "If the pouch stays on well, the smell of the drainage can be better contained."

94. A patient is scheduled for abdominal surgery. The nurse is planning the patient's care and is aware that the reason for an NPO order before an operation is because:
1 Anesthesia stops the digestive process.
2 Energy from food is not needed during surgery.
3 Vomiting occurs normally in the recovery phase.
4 An empty stomach reduces the chance for aspiration of stomach contents.

95. A nurse is suctioning secretions from a patient's nasal artificial airway. The nurse applies suction for no longer than:
1 3 seconds
2 10 seconds
3 30 seconds
4 1 minute

96. A patient is admitted with pancreatitis. Which of the following diagnostic examinations would the nurse expect to be performed on the patient?
1 A magnetic resonance imaging (MRI) examination
2 An endoscopic retrograde cholangiopancreatographic (ERCP) examination

3 An arteriogram

4 A sigmoidoscopy

97. The simplest method for a nurse to use to open a patient's airway is to:

1 Perform a mouth sweep.

2 Turn the head to one side.

3 Tilt the head back and lift the chin.

4 Perform a modified jaw-thrust maneuver.

98. A thoracentesis allows for drainage from the:

1 Peritoneal cavity

2 Ascitic cavity

3 Pericardial sac

4 Pleural cavity

99. A co-worker approaches a nurse with concerns that a small bore feeding tube may not be properly placed. The co-worker reports that she did not hear the characteristic "whoosh" when she instilled air in the tube. Which of the following methods should the nurse advise his or her co-worker to use to establish placement of the tube?

1 Obtain a chest radiograph.

2 Attach the tube to suction.

3 Irrigate the tube with 30 cc of sterile saline.

4 Place the end of the tube in a glass of water and watch for bubbles.

100. Most older individuals have a type of insurance called:

1 Social Security

2 Medicare

3 Medicaid

4 Farmer's Life

101. The nurse is interviewing a 52-year-old patient who presents to a physician's office complaining of feelings of hopelessness and depression. Which of the following patient statements would reflect life changes common to this age group?

1 "I can't imagine starting my life over again."

2 "My lifestyle will change so much after my retirement."

3 "My kids have all left home and I feel so depressed now."

4 "The prospect of all this time on my hands is driving me crazy."

102. The nurse is planning an exercise program for a group of elderly individuals who have a history of cardiopulmonary disease. Which of the following activities would best meet the exercise needs of these individuals?

1 Jogging

2 Walking

3 Skiing machines

4 Rowing machines

103. A patient of the Jehovah's Witness faith is scheduled for surgical repair of a hip fracture. Which of the following preoperative orders may conflict with this patient's religious practices?

1 Incentive spirometry every 4 hours while awake

2 Coughing, deep-breathing, and leg exercises every 2 hours

3 Type and cross for two units packed RBCs

4 MRI of the right hip region

104. A nurse is teaching a group of assistants how to perform perineal care on a woman. Which of the following techniques should be included in the teaching?

1 Start the cleansing stroke from the rectum to the pubis.

2 Use one cotton ball for each cleansing stroke.

3 Use one area of the washcloth for each cleansing stroke.

4 Use one part of the washcloth for all cleansing strokes.

105. A patient complains to the nurse that he is having difficulty sleeping at night. Which of the following should be the nurse's first course of action?

1 Administer the patient's pain medication.

2 Call the physician to obtain an order for a sedative or hypnotic.

3 Assure the patient that no one will awaken him during the night.

4 Ask the patient what normal bedtime rituals does he practice at home.

106. Which of the following would be the best way for the nurse to position a bedpan for a patient who is able to help with the procedure?

1 Ask the patient to raise his buttocks off the bed while the nurse slides the bedpan underneath him.

2 Assist the patient to a sitting position on the bedpan on the side of the bed.

3 Ask the patient to roll over and position the bedpan on his buttocks, and have him roll over onto it.

4 Ask the patient to get out of bed and use a bedside commode.

107. If a nurse is allowed to clip a patient's toenails, which one of the following techniques is recommended?

1 Clip nails as short as possible.

2 Clip nails with square corners.

3 Round the edges of the nails off.

4 Clip the nails straight across.

108. A patient with a healing stage III decubitus ulcer asks the nurse if the ulcer will leave a scar once it heals. Which of the following is the most correct response by the nurse?

1 "Sometimes there is a scar and sometimes there isn't."

2 "I don't think you should worry about that right now."

3 "Usually there is a scar present with this type of healing."

4 "I think you should ask your doctor about that tomorrow."

109. A patient has an indwelling urinary retention catheter. The nurse is instructed to obtain a sterile urine specimen from the patient. To accomplish this task, the nurse should:

1 Remove the patient's catheter and have him or her void.

2 Remove the urine from the balloon port with a syringe.

3 Collect the specimen from the sampling port on the drainage tube with a syringe.

4 Disconnect the catheter from the drainage tubing and let urine drain into the specimen container.

110. A patient complains of extreme pain when the nurse begins to inflate the balloon of a newly inserted urinary retention catheter. The most probable cause of the patient's pain is the:

1 Balloon has ruptured.

2 Balloon is being inflated too rapidly.

3 Balloon is not in the bladder but in the urethra.

4 Patient is complaining because of the nature of the procedure.

111. While transporting a patient to the radiology department in a wheelchair, the nurse should place the urinary drainage bag from her retention catheter:

1 On the patient's lap

2 Clipped to patient's front robe pocket

3 On the IV pole that is attached to the wheelchair

4 Hung from the side rail or back rail of the wheelchair that is below hip level

112. Which of the following techniques should the nurse employ when cleansing the eye of a patient?

1 Blot each eye one time with a folded washcloth.

2 Rub each eye gently, using a back-and-forth motion.

3 Wipe each eye from the outer to the inner canthus.

4 Wipe each eye from the inner to the outer canthus.

113. A nurse is providing denture care for a patient. Which of the following should be included in the storage of the dentures?

1 Place the patient's name on the denture cup.

2 Line the denture cup with a paper towel.

3 Place a cleansing tablet in the denture cup first.

4 Place adhesive grip on the patient's dentures.

114. The nurse is "prepping" a patient's skin before surgery. The purpose of clipping a patient's hair from the surgical site before surgery is to:

1 Allow for less discomfort from the surgery.

2 Facilitate suturing of the incision after the surgery.

3 Reduce the incidence of infection at the surgical incision.

4 Allow for better visualization of the site during the surgery.

115. Which of the following statements made by a patient going for a colonoscopy would indicate that further teaching is needed?

1 "Thank goodness I will be put out for the procedure!"

2 "I will have to have cleansing enemas beforehand."

3 "I hope my rectum doesn't hurt too much afterwards."

4 "My doctor may be able to see where my bleeding is coming from."

116. A hospitalized patient has complained of insomnia to the nurse. Which of the following actions should be included in this patient's plan of care?

1 Open the patient's door to give him a sense of security.

2 Leave the television on all night long.

3 Allow the client to exercise before going to bed.

4 Give the patient a backrub with warm lotion before going to bed.

117. A nurse is applying a bandage to a patient's foot, ankle, lower leg, and knee. Where should the nurse begin bandaging the extremity?

1 At the foot

2 At the knee

3 At the ankle

4 At the middle of the leg

118. When the nurse places a patient's arm in a sling, the wrist should be:

1 Level with the elbow

2 Slightly lower than the elbow

3 Slightly higher than the elbow

4 At least 6 inches lower than the elbow

119. In an emergency situation, which of the following is the first priority of patient care?

1 Obtaining the victim's medical history

2 Controlling bleeding from a compound fracture

3 Maintaining an open airway for adequate oxygenation

4 Performing a survey at the scene of the victim's accident

120. A nurse is assessing vital signs on a patient who has had a right mastectomy. Where should the nurse measure the patient's BP?

1 On the patient's lower forearm

2 On the patient's left arm

3 Over the popliteal artery

4 On the patient's lower leg

121. A patient with orthostatic hypotension will most likely complain of:

1 Dizziness

2 Nausea

3 Tremors

4 Numbness

122. A pulse of unusually full force is sometimes described as:

1 Irregular

2 Deep

3 Bounding

4 Bradycardic

123. Which of the following assessment data should be reported immediately after it is obtained?

1 A newborn with a respiratory rate of 32/min

2 A 30-year-old athlete with a pulse rate of 58 bpm

3 An 87-year-old patient with Alzheimer's disease with a respiratory rate of 20/min

4 A 40-year-old patient postthyroidectomy with a pulse rate of 120 bpm

124. A nurse needs to obtain a sputum specimen from a patient. At which time of day would it be easier for the nurse to obtain the specimen?

1 After a meal

2 Between meals

3 In the morning

4 In the evening

125. When teaching a patient concerning respiratory care, which of the following measures would the nurse recommend to prevent respiratory secretions from becoming thick and difficult to expectorate?

1 Adequate sleep

2 Regular exercise

3. A nourishing diet

4 A generous fluid intake

126. Which of the following would indicate to the nurse that a patient may need sputum suctioned from his respiratory tract?

1 A respiratory rate of 22/min

2 A heart rate that is tachycardic

3 A gurgling noise in his airway

4 Expectorates a large amount of green mucus

127. A terminally ill adult refuses further therapy. In such situations, the general agreement is that:

1 The patient has the right to make such a decision.

2 Only the patient's physician has the authority to make such a decision.

3 The patient and family as a group should come to this decision together.

4 Health care workers should make every effort to dissuade patients from refusing therapy.

128. The nurse is speaking with a family concerning hospice care for an elderly relative. The nurse advises the family that one of the basic assumptions of hospice care is that:

1 The patient will not have to pay for his medications.

2 Hospice nurses try to make the patient as comfortable as possible.

3 Care will be provided in a hospital or skilled nursing facility.

4 The family will provide most skilled care.

129. The nurse learns that a patient has an advanced directive. This document ensures that:

1 Only lifesaving heroic measures will be used.

2 The patient's right to make decisions about his death will be honored.

3 Physician will not attempt to dissuade the patient from any treatment plans.

4 The family's rights to make final decisions concerning the care of the terminally ill patient will be honored.

130. When should the nurse begin preparing for a patient's discharge?

1 When the patient is admitted to the hospital

2 After the physician writes the discharge instructions

3 During the patient's last 2 or 3 days of hospitalization

4 After procedures take place that may necessitate a convalescent period

131. Which of the following nursing actions is performed on patients with known or suspected renal calculi?

1 Flank massage

2 Urine reductions

3 Straining all urine

4 Restricting fluid intake

132. While collecting a 24-hour urine specimen, the nurse should:

1 Send each void to the laboratory immediately.

2 Place the specimens into the refrigerator.

3 Make sure that every other void is sent to the laboratory.

4 Keep all urine on ice for the entire 24 hours.

133. A postoperative patient is complaining of "gas pains." Which of the following nursing interventions would aid in relieving the patient's discomfort?

1 Maintain the patient on bed rest.

2 Contact the physician for medication.

3 Insert a rectal tube for 30 minutes.

4 Encourage the use of straws for drinking liquids.

134. When the nurse collects a specimen for ova and parasites, the nurse knows that:

1 The specimen is sent to the laboratory on ice.

2 A rectal tube is used to obtain the specimen.

3 The ova and parasites may die if the specimen is not tested immediately.

4 The nurse should use a sterile specimen cup to obtain the specimen.

135. An 8-month-old child is admitted to pediatrics with a diagnosis of hyperemesis and dehydration. Which of the following signs and symptoms of dehydration might the nurse observe in the child?

1 Weight gain and hypotension

2 Weight loss and hypertension

3 Oliguria and poor skin turgor

4 Moist, pink mucous membranes

136. A nurse is instructed to perform chest physiotherapy on a patient with bronchitis. Which of the following is the correct rationale for this procedure?

1 Moves residual air from the patient's lungs

2 Prevents pneumonia from developing

3 Forces the client to take deep breaths

4 Breaks up and mobilizes secretions

137. Which of the following patients would be most at risk for developing a decubitus ulcer?

1 The patient with a urinary tract infection

2 A patient with chronic obstructive pulmonary disease

3 A patient with cholecystitis

4 A patient who is constipated

138. When the integrity of the skin has been damaged or broken as in an abrasion or decubitus ulcer, the body loses some of its ability to:

1 Resist infections

2 Produce antibodies

3 Eliminate waste products

4 Maintain correct body alignment

139. An obese, postoperative patient asks the nurse why the physician wants her to wear an abdominal binder. What is the best statement from the nurse?

1 "Because you are so large, the incision might break open."

2 "The binder will help reduce the stress on your suture line."

3 "You will be able to walk better with it on."

4 "It will decrease your incisional pain."

140. A nurse has been asked to shave a male patient. Which of the following patient disorders may prevent the nurse from performing the shave?

1 A bleeding disorder

2 An emotional disorder

3 A respiratory disorder

4 A neurologic disorder

141. The nurse is performing mouth care on an unconscious patient. In which of the following positions should the nurse place the patient?

1 Prone, with head turned to one side

2 Supine, with suction equipment nearby

3 In semi-Fowler's position, with a towel under the chin

4 In a side-lying position, with head turned to the side

142. During a preoperative assessment on a patient, the nurse finds that the patient experiences sleep apnea. The nurse recognizes sleep apnea as a:

1 Problem caused by snoring or overeating

2 Problem that is increased if the patient is overly nervous or upset

3 Syndrome that is transitory in nature and not considered dangerous

4 Syndrome that can cause symptoms of daytime tiredness and fatigue

143. Which of the following is the best way for the nurse to assess the *intensity* of a patient's pain?

1 Ask the patient how long he or she has been experiencing the pain.

2 Ask the patient to point to the location of the pain they are feeling.

3 Ask the patient to rate their pain on a scale of 1 (mild) to 10 (severe).

4 Ask the patient to gauge their pain using words such as "bad" or "severe."

144. A patient is learning to walk with crutches. After traveling down the hallway, the patient complains of numbness in his axilla and tingling of his fingers. The nurse should:

1 Switch the patient to a walker.

2 Notify the physician of possible nerve damage to the arm.

3 Adjust the crutch length and review appropriate crutch technique with the patient.

4 Provide padding to the patient's axilla and assist the patient in doing ROM exercises.

145. A patient has right-sided weakness from the effects of a cerebrovascular accident. The patient begins to use a cane. The nurse instructs the patient to use the cane in the left hand and to move the cane simultaneously with:

1 Both arms

2 Both feet

3 The left leg

4 The right leg

146. A nurse observes that a terminally ill patient's respirations appear to have periods of apnea interspersed with increasing and decreasing respiratory depth and rate. The nurse recognizes that this pattern of breathing may indicate approaching death and is termed:

1 Dyspnea

2 Tachypnea

3 Kussmaul's respirations

4 Cheyne-Stokes respirations

147. A nurse is assessing an individual on bed rest for possible edema. Where might the nurse find edema in a patient who is confined to bed?

1 Feet

2 Hands

3 Calves

4 Sacrum

148. A nurse is instructing a UAP to administer a nonmedicated vaginal douche to an elderly patient. Which of the following statements made by the UAP signifies understanding of the procedure?

1 "The patient should wait to void until after the douche is given."

2 "The tip should be inserted and then instillation of fluid can begin."

3 "The fluid should be already flowing when I place the douche into the vagina."

4 "The fluid should be instilled using lots of pressure to make sure the vagina gets clean."

149. A patient who is scheduled to undergo a colostomy states to the nurse, "I am afraid my children will not be able to accept me after the surgery." Which of the following is the nurse's best response to this statement?

1 "You shouldn't feel that way. Everything will be fine."

2 "I think the anxiety of your surgery is causing you undue worry."

3 "You are afraid that your children will not be able to accept your colostomy?"

4 "I think you should sleep on it, you'll feel better about this in the morning."

150. Which of the following vital signs collected by the nurse from adult patients should be considered abnormal and needs to be reported?

1 Oral temperature 99° F, pulse 68, respirations 20, BP 122/80

2 Rectal temperature 102° F, pulse 100, respirations 22, BP 118/50

3 Axillary temperature 97.8° F, pulse 88, respirations 20, BP 138/70

4 Tympanic temperature 98.5° F, pulse 74, respirations 16, BP 120/84

151. A patient who is on a 1000-ml/day fluid restriction because of renal insufficiency is observed to be consuming a large amount of water from the water faucet in her room. The nurse approximates that she may have consumed over 3000 ml in a short period. The nurse should expect that the patient's weight will:

1 Increase

2 Decrease

3 Remain the same; the patient will just rid herself of excess fluid

4 Remain the same; the patient needed the water because of her dehydrated state

152. A nurse is caring for a patient who has a diagnosis of dysphagia. Which of the following procedures will the patient probably be ordered?

1 Barium enema

2 An EGD

3 A barium swallow

4 A computed tomography scan

153. A patient is recovering from a hemorrhoidectomy and is receiving oxygen via facemask. Which of the following methods for obtaining temperature should the nurse use?

1 Oral

2 Rectal

3 Axillary

4 Tympanic

154. A patient is being monitored by pulse oximetry using a clip-on probe. The machine alarms and the oxygen saturation reads 60%. The patient is sitting up in bed and talking with his family. What is the nurse's first course of action?

1 Call the physician immediately.

2 Begin oxygen therapy at 3 L/min nasal cannula.

3 Adjust the clip-on probe on the finger or move it to another finger.

4 Remove family members from the room to better deal with this emergency.

155. A nurse is teaching a patient how to perform a vaginal douche. Which of the following directions should the nurse teach the patient when inserting the applicator?

1 Insert tip down and back into vagina.

2 Squeeze the bottle as forcefully as possible.

3 Void immediately following the douche.

4 Lie prone after the procedure.

156. A nurse is caring for a patient who is on bedrest. The time is 8:50 AM. The patient will need to be transferred at 9:00 AM to x-ray by stretcher for an abdominal flat plate. Place the following skills in the correct sequence from beginning to end.

1 Make the patient's bed.

2 Have the client void.

3 Assist the client in moving onto the stretcher.

4 Elevate the patient's head for comfort.

157. A patient on oxygen therapy asks why the nurse takes a pulse oximetry measurement each shift. Which of the following is the correct explanation by the nurse?

1 This number is the amount of oxygen you have in your blood.

2 It helps us determine if you are on enough oxygen.

3 It allows the physician to determine the amount of oxygen ordered.

4 It is an important vital sign for any person on oxygen.

158. A nurse is packing a surgical incision with a 2 × 2 gauze pad soaked in saline solution. The nurse drops the wet gauze pad on the edge of the sterile field. What should the nurse do next?

1 Pick up the gauze pad and put it in the wound.

2 Leave the gauze where it fell and prepare a new one.

3 Pick up the gauze and rinse it out in the saline solution before using.

4 Begin anew, with a new sterile tray, dressings, and gloves.

159. A patient is scheduled to begin IPPB treatments. The patient asks the nurse the purpose of these treatments. The nurse's best response is that the treatments:

1 Are useful in dislodging secretions

2 Give the patient incentives to increase inhalation

3 Allow gravity to assist in the removal of secretions

4 Forces the person to inhale more deeply, increasing oxygenation

160. A patient is receiving 75% humidified oxygen via a tracheostomy collar. The patient requires suctioning. Which of the following actions should the nurse perform that will be safe for the patient?

1 Restrain the patient.

2 Administer supplemental oxygen to the patient.

3 Apply suction while carefully advancing the catheter.

4 Use a rotating motion while carefully advancing the catheter.

161. Which of the following techniques should the nurse use when obtaining a patient's BP?

1 Place the arm above the level of the heart.

2 Have the patient extend the arm with palm downward.

3 Place the cuff 1 inch above the position of the radial artery.

4 "Match up" the arrow on the cuff to the area where the brachial artery was palpated.

162. The nurse is assessing a patient's circulatory status by checking all peripheral pulses. When the nurse assesses pulses, she is using the technique of:

1 Palpation

2 Percussion

3 Inspection

4 Auscultation

163. Which of the following fluids should be measured and factored in a patient's fluid output?

1 Vomitus

2 IV fluids

3 Perspiration

4 Tube feedings

164. Which of the following statements is true regarding diagnostic related groups (DRGs)?

1 Patients stay in the hospital much longer because they have been implemented.

2 Acute care nursing positions have increased after their implementation.

3 After their implementation, more care is being done in the home.

4 The cost of medical care has been decreased because of them.

165. Which of the following actions would assist in reducing the incidence of aspiration in a patient receiving a tube feeding?

1 Clamp tube after feeding has infused.

2 Flush tube with water after each feeding.

3 Dilute feedings to half-strength solutions.

4 Have patient remain in an upright position for 45 minutes after feeding.

166. A patient had an indwelling urinary catheter removed 6 hours ago. The patient relates to the nurse that burning was experienced after the first postcatheter void. Which of the following is the nurse's best response?

1 "I think you may have a urinary tract infection."

2 "I will need to contact the physician about that."

3 "Sometimes that happens after a catheter is removed."

4 "Let me collect a sterile urine specimen from you now."

167. The nurse is inserting a nasogastric tube into a patient. Which of the following would indicate that the tube is in the patient's trachea?

1 The patient is unable to speak.

2 The nurse cannot see the tube in the back of the throat.

3 The patient blows his nose and blood is present on the tissue.

4 The nurse notes that the tube has a return of light green drainage.

168. A hospitalized patient is ordered both an oil-retention enema and a cleansing enema. Which of the following statements correctly explains the rationale for administering these enemas?

1 The enemas work together to stimulate peristalsis.

2 The oil-retention enema softens the stool, and the cleansing enema stimulates peristalsis.

3 If the oil-retention enema does not work to evacuate the bowel, then the cleansing enema can be given.

4 The cleansing enema is generally given to soften the stool 30 minutes before the oil-retention enema.

169. A nurse has made a mistake in the following nursing entry. The nurse meant to write that the vomitus amount was 75 ml. However, she mistakenly entered 175 ml. Correct the nursing note.

Patient complained of nausea. Vomited 175 ml of dark green material. Patient returned to bed and medicated with 200 mg of Tigan IM.

170. A patient presents to a physician's office with complaints of constipation for 6 days. Which of the following patient statements made during the health history may be contributing to the constipation?

1 "I exercise almost every day."

2 "I eat plenty of raw vegetables."

3 "I am not a big water drinker."

4 "I go to the bathroom when I feel the need."

171. A nurse has inserted a urethral retention catheter and 750 ml of urine quickly collects in the drainage bag. What is the nurse's next course of action?

1 Clamp the Foley for 20 minutes.

2 Send a specimen to the laboratory.

3 Increase the patient's IV fluid flow rate.

4 Remove the catheter.

172. A UAP inquires as to why a patient's arm is contracted into a flexed position. Which of the following statements by the nurse answers the UAP's question?

1 "A physical therapy consult is needed to help this patient."

2 "The muscles of the arm must have been damaged in some way."

3 "The muscles are permanently shortened because of the effects of immobility."

4 "The arm is just temporarily frozen; ROM exercises should restore it."

173. The nurse is discussing the redesign of an activity center in a long-term care facility. Which color would the nurse recommend to paint the room to decrease stimulation and promote a calm atmosphere?
    1 Red
    2 Orange
    3 Black
    4 Blue

174. An elderly postoperative patient has an order to be ambulated a few hours after surgery. The patient becomes upset with the nurse and wants to know why he should ambulate so soon after surgery. Which of the following is the best response by the nurse?
    1 "You know what they say, if you don't use it you might lose it."
    2 "Please get out of bed now. You can ask your doctor in the morning."
    3 "Your doctor always orders his patients out of bed right after surgery."
    4 "Walking will keep the fluids in your lungs moving, so bacteria will not grow."

175. A nurse is applying antiembolic stockings on a patient before surgery. The patient inquires why the stockings need to be so snug. The nurse responds that snugness is needed because:
    1 "They do not do their job if they are too loose."
    2 "The stockings pool blood in your legs during surgery."
    3 "They are meant to exercise the muscles of the legs while you are in surgery."
    4 "They help to prevent blood clots from developing by pushing blood toward the heart."

176. Which of the following would be an appropriate short-term nursing goal for a patient with pain, secondary to post-ORIF (Open reduction internal fixation) of the left hip?
    1 Patient will have decreased need for pain medication.
    2 Patient will be pain free 30 minutes after Demerol 50 mg IM is given.
    3 Patient will walk length of hallway three times a day.
    4 Patient will participate in physical therapy sessions.

177. A nurse working in a skilled nursing facility is admitting a patient with Alzheimer's disease. The family reports that the patient frequently becomes agitated late in the evening. Which of the following should be included in this patient's plan of care.
    1 Encourage the patient to attend an aerobic class each evening.
    2 Encourage the patient to watch old war movies in the evening.
    3 Engage the patient in social hour.
    4 Provide for quiet time for the patient in the evening.

178. The nurse is attempting to remove some dry and crusted secretions from a patient's Foley catheter. Which of the following solutions should the nurse use if soap and water are ineffective?
    1 Alcohol
    2 Betadine

3 Sterile saline

4 Hydrogen peroxide

179. A patient returns from surgery with a large, abdominal dressing in place. As the evening progresses, the nurse notes that some drainage has seeped through the dressing. Which of the following is the nurse's best course of action?
    1 Change the dressing.
    2 Reinforce the dressing with additional gauze.
    3 Remove the dressing and leave the wound open to air.
    4 Remove the dressing and send it to the laboratory for culture.

180. A patient has consumed the following foods for lunch. What is the patient's intake?
    5 oz of cranberry juice
    120 ml of ice cream
    8 oz of milk
    1 cup of cream of tomato soup
    4 oz of pudding

181. A nurse is applying heat to the leg of a patient with cellulitis of the leg. Which of the following facts in the patient's medical history necessitates the need for the nurse to take special precautions?
    1 Blindness
    2 Paraplegia
    3 Hypertension
    4 Diabetes mellitus

182. Which of the following substances should the nurse apply to the eyelid of a patient who is to receive a warm compress to the eye?
    1 Saline
    2 Betadine
    3 Petrolatum
    4 Antibiotic ointment

183. When the nurse auscultates the lungs of a patient who is on bedrest, she hears diminished sounds with some rhonchi. Which of the following nursing actions may clear the patient's lung sounds? Choose all that apply.
    1 Encourage use of incentive spirometer.
    2 Cough and deep-breathing exercises
    3 Ambulation
    4 Administration of pain medication
    5 Oxygen therapy

184. A nurse is assessing a patient's incision line. Which of the following data may indicate infection?
    1 Area surrounding the sutures is red and swollen.
    2 Some of the sutures have fallen out of the incision line.
    3 No drainage around the sutures; the surrounding skin is pink.
    4 Sutures are all intact; small amount of serosanguinous drainage is present.

185. The nurse is preparing to irrigate a patient's infected left eye. The nurse should position the patient:
    1 On his back
    2 On his left side
    3 On his right side
    4 In Semi-Fowler's position

186. Which of the following is an example of negligence?
    1 Assault and battery
    2 False imprisonment
    3 Medication errors
    4 Invasion of privacy

187. A 50-year-old woman visits the physician's office for a routine physical. The health history indicates that the patient has never had a mammogram. The nurse is aware that mammograms:
    1 Are done when breast cancer is suspected
    2 Should be done every 1 to 2 years as a routine screening examination
    3 Are not necessary if the woman does not have a history of breast cancer in the family
    4 Are difficult for the woman to undergo and are therefore only recommended every 5 to 10 years

188. A nurse is assisting a UAP in setting up a footboard on a patient's bed. The UAP asks the nurse why a footboard would be used. The nurse's best response is:
    1 "A footboard will assist in maintaining good abduction."
    2 "It will prevent the patient from developing thrombophlebitis."
    3 "It will keep the foot from developing plantar flexion."
    4 "The patient will be able to use the board to help push herself up in bed."

189. A nurse is making the decision to purchase liability insurance. The nurse should keep in mind that professional liability coverage:
    1 Costs the same in all health care settings
    2 Protects the nurse from prosecution for criminal acts
    3 Does not cover acts outside the scope of nursing practice
    4 Provides coverage to the nurse for his or her entire professional career

190. List four methods for establishing the standard of care.
    _____
    _____
    _____
    _____

191. A nurse overhears a terminally ill patient with cancer state to his family members, "If I get over this cancer thing, I will travel with the church's missionary to South Africa next spring." Which stage of the dying process is this patient exhibiting?
    1 Anger
    2 Denial
    3 Bargaining
    4 Depression

192. A nurse is caring for a patient with a paralytic ileus. Which of the following assessment data is most important for this patient?
    1 Lung sounds
    2 Bowel sounds
    3 Peripheral pulses
    4 Neurological examination

193. Medical records are the generally regarded as being the property of the
    1 Patient
    2 Facility
    3 Nurse
    4 Physician

194. In planning care for a patient who is paralyzed, the nurse should plan to reposition the patient at least:
    1 Once a shift
    2 Every 2 hours
    3 Every 4 hours
    4 Every 30 minutes

195. The Canadian provincial nursing regulatory bodies are responsible for:
    1 Setting and administering examinations
    2 Reporting acts of criminal negligence to the police
    3 Passing laws pertaining to the practice of nursing
    4 Establishing minimum levels of safe nursing practice

196. The role of the practical nurse in Canada is to:
    1 Practice independently in all settings.
    2 Work under the direct supervision of an RN.
    3 Collaborate as an integral part of the health care team.
    4 Provide care for only the patients whose conditions are stabilized.

197. The title of the practical nurse in Canada is determined by the:
    1 Individuals in that nursing category
    2 Agency employing the practical nurse
    3 Province or territory issuing the registration
    4 Educational facility from which the practical nurse graduated

198. Canadian regulation of practical nurses is based on:
    1 Federal legislation
    2 Provincial legislation
    3 Municipal legislation
    4 Professional associations

199. Registration and licensure of practical nurses in Canada is designed to protect the:
    1 Public
    2 Practice of nursing
    3 Level of the practitioner
    4 Individual registrants

200. The organization responsible for admission requirements to practical nursing programs in Canada is the:
    1 Individual educational institution
    2 Provincial professional association
    3 Provincial licensing body
    4 CAPNNA

201. Canadian practical nurses may obtain malpractice insurance through:
    1 CAPNNA
    2 Provincial licensing bodies
    3 Provincial professional associations
    4 Only private insurance companies

202. Membership in CAPNNA can best be described as:
    1 Automatic with registration and licensure
    2 Mandatory in each province and territory
    3 Voluntary and optional for PNs in all provinces and territories
    4 Included with membership in affiliated organizations

203. The Canadian practical nurse maintains competence by:
    1 Writing a yearly examination
    2 Taking advantage of learning opportunities
    3 Demonstrating skill level to his or her employer
    4 Completing designated seminars and workshops

204. Laws pertaining to nursing in Canada are:
    1 Set by nursing regulatory bodies
    2 The same as those in the United States
    3 Specific to each province and territory
    4 Specific to the nursing practice setting

205. The nurse needs to see all of the following individuals. Which patient should the nurse see first?
    1 A patient who is receiving chest percussion from a respiratory therapist

2 The patient who is being fed by a nursing assistant

3 A patient who had a hypoglycemic episode last shift

4 A patient who has just been medicated for pain

206. The nurse is reviewing vital signs that were taken by a nursing assistant. One of the patients is hypertensive. The nurse assesses the patient by asking if he is experiencing:

    1 A headache

    2 Dizziness

    3 Diaphoresis

    4 Bradycardia

207. A patient has been diagnosed with dehydration. Which of the following symptoms would confirm the diagnosis?

    1 Hematuria

    2 Polyuria

    3 Enuresis

    4 Oliguria

208. A family has the nursing diagnosis, "Risk for Caregiver Role Strain." Which of the following strategies might best meet the needs of the family?

    1 Antianxiety medications

    2 Consulting with a family therapist

    3 Hospitalization for the individual whom the family is caring for

    4 Hospice care

209. A nurse is taking care of a patient with anemia. The patient asks why he is so short of breath. The nurse knows that the anemia has:

    1 Decreased the amount of oxygen the patient can inhale

    2 Reduced the oxygen-carrying capability of the patient

    3 Blocked the ability of the body to exchange gases

    4 Diminished the patient's ability to circulate oxygen

210. A nurse is discharging a patient with a diagnosis of congestive heart failure. Which of the following instructions should the nurse include when teaching patients how to weigh themselves?

    1 Weigh each evening, after supper.

    2 Weigh after taking your fluid pill.

    3 Weigh first thing in the morning.

    4 Weigh after you have dressed for the day.

ANSWERS AND RATIONALES

1. Application, evaluation, psychosocial integrity (b).
   1, 2, 4, and 6 are the components of a patient's internal variables. Socioeconomic status (3) and cultural influences (5) are external variables.

2. Application, implementation, psychosocial integrity (b).
   3 This statement reduces fear of abandonment and alleviates fear of needs not being met.
   1 Pain medication is not commonly needed during this procedure.
   2 Limiting visitors increases anxiety and causes feelings of isolation.
   4 The patient and his or her secretions are radioactive during treatment.

3. Application, planning, safe, effective care environment (c).
   2 The HIPPA guidelines are designed to streamline health care and preserve the patient's right to privacy.
   1 Patients always have the right to refuse treatment.
   3 Suing for malpractice or negligence is the right of an individual.
   4 No current guidelines exist in the United States to preserve a patient's right for assisted suicide.

4. Comprehension, implementation, physiological integrity (b).
   1 Stimulating the gag reflex may result in vomiting.
   2 Secretions do not originate in the throat area.
   3 Contamination of the culture site is not of primary consideration.
   4 The size of the specimen is not a concern with a throat culture.

5. Application, assessment, physiological integrity (c).
   1 This intervention gathers more information before determining course of action.
   2 This may not be the course of action; more data is needed.
   3 Elevating the foot will reduce edema, but it does not address the numbness and tingling.
   4 Wiggling her toes will not alleviate the numbness and tingling.

6. Application, assessment, physiological integrity (c).
   3 This is the charge that can be applied to health care workers who restrain a competent adult.
   1 Although this is what the nurse is doing, this charge is more likely lodged against police personnel who restrain individuals.
   2 The nurse is not being negligent in this situation. If she restrained the patient and did not check on him periodically, she can be charged with negligence.
   4 As long as the nurse followed the standard of care in restraining the individual, malpractice cannot be charged.

7. Comprehension, implementation, safe, effective care environment (a).
   4 This action best protects the nurse against the specific dangers of wound irrigation, such as splashing or spraying of blood and body fluids.
   1 Common knowledge states that the bed should be at a workable height for all procedures.
   2 Explaining the procedure alleviates patient anxiety; it does not protect the nurse.

3 Hand washing is indicated before and after all patient procedures.

8. Comprehension, planning, physiological integrity (c).
   4 Older individuals with orthopedic injuries suffer from immobility complicated by impaired sensory function.
   1 Patients with a vertebral injury can still assist with relieving pressure.
   2 Patients in skeletal traction can still assist in relieving pressure.
   3 Ambulatory patients are at low risk for decubitus formation.

9. Analysis, planning, physiological integrity (b).
   4 Mouth care relieves the discomfort related to the mouth dryness caused by mouth breathing.
   1 This is unwarranted; this situation does not warrant immediate medical attention.
   2 This causes a potential for electrolyte imbalance.
   3 The response does not address patient discomfort.

10. Comprehension, planning, safe, effective care environment (b).
    4 Assigning ancillary personnel to give out medications is most likely not under the person's scope of practice and may result in injury to the patient and a lawsuit for the nurse.
    1 Not enough information is given about the nurse's other tasks for this to be correct; the issue is still inappropriate delegating of tasks.
    2 No guarantee exists that the UAP will respond quickly to patient complaints.
    3 Safeguarding patients takes priority over increasing self-esteem.

11. Application, implementation, physiological integrity (c).
    4 This answer gives a brief, reasonable answer to meet the patient's needs.
    1 This answer is a little too graphic or alarming for the patient.
    2 The ink should not be removed.
    3 No reason exists to consult the physician when the nurse can give the appropriate response.

12. Application, planning, physiological integrity (c).
    3 The resident may fall asleep if he is made comfortable; medication can be given at a later time if he is unable to sleep; try the most basic comfort measures first.
    1 This closes communication without addressing the problem.
    2 This is true and reassuring but does not address the problem.
    4 The nurse is not engaging in the conversation and blocks communication.

13. Application, planning, physiological integrity (c).
    1 This should be the first action. The nurse can discern if the patient has a full bladder, which will dictate further action.
    2 This may be the eventual outcome of this scenario, but it is not the nurse's first course of action.
    3 The nurse should first assess the patient for fullness before calling a physician.
    4 This may be part of the nurse's plan; however, it is not the first course of action.

14. Application, planning, physiological integrity (c).
    3 This assessment data signifies a catheter blockage that may be alleviated with bladder irrigation.
    1 Position changes will not relieve an obstructed catheter.

2 The assessment data can be expected; nurse can proceed within scope of practice without notifying the physician.

4 The nurse should act on these observations, not document them.

15. Application, planning, physiological integrity (b).

4 Patients with lice are given a medicated shampoo. The nurse should anticipate this order.

1 This is not indicated for treatment of lice.

2 A sitz bath is ordered for patients with perineal or rectal surgery or problems.

3 An IPPB treatment would be ordered for a patient with respiratory difficulty.

16. Application, assessment, physiological integrity (b).

2 Patients who have been on bedrest may have a fall in BP on arising quickly, which can be alleviated by dangling a few minutes at the bedside.

1 Anemia does cause dizziness; however, the question does not indicate that this is a problem.

3 Hypoxia may cause this problem, but no indications exist that the patient has a respiratory disorder.

4 Hypertension generally presents as nosebleeds and headaches.

17. Application, assessment, physiological integrity (c).

3 Urinary urgency and lower abdominal pressure are symptoms of a full bladder; the catheter may be malfunctioning or blocked.

1 The cause of the pain must first be determined.

2 This is not related to the patient's physical discomfort.

4 This response fails to address the patient's discomfort.

18. Application, implementation, physiological integrity (c).

3 This is the primary purpose for irrigating a colostomy.

1 Although this is an outcome for the procedure, it is not the primary purpose.

2 This is the purpose for enemas; however, it does not address why it is being done.

4 Depending on the type of ostomy, stool softeners may or may not be needed.

19. Application, assessment, physiological integrity (a).

1 Cyanosis is a blue tinge to the skin or oral mucosa that indicates poor oxygenation.

2 Vital signs indicate cardiopulmonary status and not cyanosis.

3 Cyanosis is difficult to assess in the lips or nails of individuals with dark complexions.

4 Pulse oximetry measures the amount of oxygen in capillary blood, not cyanosis.

20. Application, planning, safe, effective care environment (c).

1, 3, 6 These actions are normally assigned to UAPs.

2, 4, 5 These actions require a higher level of skill and are not in the UAP's scope of practice.

21. Application, evaluation, physiological integrity (c).

3 A delayed infusion of IV solution is often caused by obstruction of the rate of flow; the action allows for further assessment of the problem.

1 Not enough data have been collected to make this assumption.

2 These data indicate further action on the nurse's part.

4 Changing the rate of flow places the patient at risk for injury.

22. Knowledge, implementation, physiological integrity (a).

4 The most accurate measurement of fluid level is at eye level, in a firm container, and on a level surface.

1 The flexibility of the drainage bag interferes with accurate measurement.

2 Approximation is not an accurate measure.

3 Bedpan markings are approximations.

23. Application, implementation, psychosocial integrity (b).

1 This enables the patient to communicate his or her needs.

2 This is a secondary comfort measure; communication of needs would be a primary patient concern.

3 The presence of the nurse is more important than reassurances.

4 This does not address the patient's comfort.

24. Comprehension, planning, safe, effective care environment (b).

2 This is the appropriate response because it is the only answer that ensures patient safety and help for the nurse.

1 This does not preserve patient safety and may further compromise patient care.

3 The physician is not your supervisor; a nursing supervisor will best address this issue.

4 This will not protect patients or help the nurse.

25. Comprehension, evaluation, physiological integrity (b).

4 A full assessment includes both subjective and objective data.

1 Objective signs do not address cues that the patient himself can provide when evaluating progress.

2 Limiting data collection to subjective information ignores the observable, measurable symptom not offered by the patient.

3 Data must be gathered throughout the procedure to fully determine their effect on the patient.

26. Comprehension, planning, physiological integrity (b).

2 Knowledge of the procedure diminishes patient fear, which improves patient cooperation and promotes the expected outcome of the procedure.

1 Competent nursing practice reduces the likelihood of malpractice suits.

3 Procedures are not explained to avoid them, although this may be a secondary aspect of patient teaching.

4 The nurse must review the procedure before explaining it to the patient to provide complete information.

27. Comprehension, implementation, physiological integrity (b).

1 This term applies to the balanced, dynamic equilibrium of the body.

2, 3, 4 Homeostasis means the body's fluid and electrolytes are balanced along with the body's other physiologic processes such as blood pressure.

28. Application, implementation, physiological integrity (b).

3 This answers the patient's question correctly and addresses the client's need.

1 This is not the appropriate response and can pose a hazard.

2 This may be true but is not the correct way of responding.

4 The patient should be NPO until the gag reflex is assessed.

29. Comprehension, planning, physiological integrity (c).

3 This action decreases the patient's possibility of aspiration.

1 This should be done when suctioning the patient's tracheostomy.

2 This will not decrease the patient's risk for aspiration.

4 Although essential, this is not the most important action regarding meal times.

30. Comprehension, planning, physiological integrity (c).

4 This is the potential problem with the most serious consequences as indicated by Maslow's hierarchy of need.

1 This may be a problem, especially if the patient is incontinent.

2 No indications have been given that the individual is having difficulty obtaining nutrition.

3 A knowledge deficit is not indicated in the question.

31. Analysis, implementation, physiological integrity (b).

1 Weight should be measured at the same time each day and in the same clothing.

2 The patient should weigh one time each day; the patient may be taking medication several times a day at different intervals.

3 Medication should never be omitted; a more accurate measurement is weighing each morning.

4 This is a symptom of advanced heart failure; daily weights will indicate early symptoms.

32. Comprehension, assessment, safe, effective care environment (b).

1, 2, 3, 4 All of these should be included in a comprehensive assessment.

33. Application, implementation, safe, effective care environment (b).

3 No reason exists for limiting visitors, provided they take the appropriate precautions if they assist the patient to the bathroom.

1 This is commonly part of enteric isolation and physicians do not frequently order this.

2 This would be done no matter what type of isolation the patient was assigned.

4 This is generally a normal, nursing measure.

34. Analysis, evaluation, psychosocial integrity (c).

3 These problems need to be addressed. The patient is at increased risk for depression.

1, 2, 4 These responses indicate a healthy attitude toward the isolation procedure.

35. Comprehension, evaluation, safe, effective care environment (b).

2 A nosocomial infection is an infection acquired during the course of a hospital stay or as a result of a medical treatment (urinary catheter).

1 A superinfection is an illness produced by growth of a resistant organism during antimicrobial therapy.

3 An autoimmune response is the immune reaction of the body against its own tissues.

4 Antibiotic resistance is the continued growth of pathogenic organisms during antibiotic therapy.

36. Knowledge, implementation, safe, effective care environment (b).

3 Tuberculosis is an acid-fast bacillus; it is primarily airborne and requires special isolation procedures and filters.

1, 2, 4 These infections are not considered an acid-fast bacillus.

37. Knowledge, planning, health promotion and maintenance (a).

2 Immunization is the process of increasing the patient's resistance to disease through the process of vaccination.

1 Inflammation is a defense mechanism of the body.

3 Digitalization is medication treatment for heart failure.

4 Phagocytosis is the process of bacteria-eating that WBCs undergo in an effort to fight off foreign invaders in the body.

38. Application, implementation, safe, effective care environment (b).

4 The nurse should remove the gown by shrugging it off the shoulders and rolling it up with the gloves by touching the inside of the gown only.

1 Touching the outside of the gown would contaminate the nurse's hands.

2 This practice is not carried out unless the patient is in reverse isolation.

3 This would contaminate the other individual.

39. Knowledge, assessment, psychosocial integrity (b).

1 Cultural beliefs influence the patient's choice of treatment, as well as their perception of health care workers.

2 Last rites is a religious practice limited to the Roman Catholic religion.

3 This is not the primary reason for gathering this information; the nurse needs to understand the patient's health practice beliefs to plan care.

4 The nurse collects data concerning culture to plan the patient's plan of care.

40. Comprehension, planning, safe, effective care environment (a).

2 The movement toward cost reduction has shifted health care delivery out of hospitals and into long-term care, home care, and skilled nursing facilities.

1 Nursing remains patient centered. Treatment is more technology based but still involves direct contact with the patient by the nurse.

3 The focus of all health care delivery has moved to wellness promotion rather than illness treatment.

4 The scope of nursing practice has increased with technologic advances in health care.

41. Application, planning, safe, effective care environment (b). **The patient's WBC count is dangerously low. The patient will need to be placed in protective isolation to decrease any chances for the patient to develop infection. The patient should wear a mask for his own protection when traveling to different areas of the hospital for diagnostic examinations.**

42. Application, implementation, safe, effective care environment (b).

4 This clarifies the error and the corrective measure.

1 An incident report is completed after the error is corrected.

2 The family is not notified unless they have power of attorney.

3 An incident report is an internal record and is never documented on the patient's chart.

43. Comprehension, implementation, safe, effective care environment (b).

1 Licensing laws are public safety measures.

2 Licensing laws establish minimum standards.

3 Moral character is a subjective measure that can only be minimally established by licensing law.

4 Licensing laws do not limit the number of applicants to nursing practice.

44. Application, planning, safe, effective care environment (b).

3 The part being bandaged should remain in a functional position, which, for the elbow, is a slightly flexed

position. **This position is also more comfortable for the patient than any other position noted.**

1 Rotation is not a functional position for the elbow.

2 Extension is not a functional position for the elbow.

4 Hyperextension of the elbow is not the normal functional position for this joint.

45. Application, implementation, physiological integrity (c).

   3 A T-binder is used to keep perineal and perianal dressings in place.

   1 This is an old fabric binder that is used to reinforce abdominal dressings.

   2 A triangular bandage, or cravat, is used to immobilize shoulders, clavicles, or upper arms.

   4 An abdominal binder is used to reinforce abdominal dressings.

46. Application, implementation, physiological integrity (b).

   1 The patient's extremity should be elevated to decrease the amount of swelling before the wrap is placed. If the wrap is placed on an edematous extremity, skin breakdown may occur, or the wrap will fall off when the swelling decreases.

   2 This is the proper procedure but should be done after edema decreases in the leg.

   3 This is correct, but it is not the first course of action.

   4 This would be performed after the area has been wrapped.

47. Knowledge, implementation, physiological integrity (b).

   3 Using separate washcloth sections for each eye prevents spread of organisms from one eye to the other.

   1 Rinsing and drying skin folds reduces skin irritation.

   2 Clean gloves are useless protective mechanisms if hands are immersed in bath water.

   4 Changing bath water after bathing each extremity maintains the warmth of bath water.

48. Knowledge, implementation, safe, effective care environment (b).

   1 Each state passes nurse practice acts that define and determine the scope of nursing practice within that state.

   2 The state's board of nursing administers the nurse practice acts.

   3 The National Council of State Boards of Nursing is a professional association composed of the state boards of nursing and administers the licensing examination for nurses.

   4 The JCAHO is a professional association organized to promote standards for health care.

49. Comprehension, implementation, physiological integrity (b).

   2 This prevents pressure at the back of the neck and secures the cravat correctly.

   1 The knot would not secure the elbow if it were tied in this spot.

   3 This puts pressure on the patient's neck.

   4 Although it is good to give patient's control, the patient may not have the correct knowledge to make this decision.

50. Application, implementation, physiological integrity (b).

   4 By making sure the patient's skin is completely dry, the nurse is protecting the patient's skin from breakdown and decreasing the chance of infection.

   1 Applying powder to the area without making sure it is dry increases the incidence of infection.

2 Applying a thick layer of lotion increases the chance for maceration and skin breakdown.

3 The gauze is not necessary unless the patient has an open wound.

51. Application, implementation, physiological integrity (c).

   2 Vertigo is a common side effect of this treatment.

   1 The pinna of the ear is retracted during the procedure.

   3 Most patients can resume activity shortly after treatment.

   4 Use of cotton-tipped applicators in the ears can lead to injury.

52. Application, implementation, physiological integrity (b).

   1 Culture specimens can be inaccurate if obtained while the patient is receiving antibiotics.

   2 No clarification is necessary; this is a standard nursing function.

   3 Antibiotics will interfere with microbial growth on the specimen cultures.

   4 Antibiotics will interfere with microbial growth on the urine culture.

53. Application, assessment, physiological integrity (b).

   3 The most common signs and symptoms of thrombophlebitis are pain in the calf on dorsiflexion of the foot.

   1 Pain in the foot and ankle may be caused by other problems related to immobility, but pain in the calf is the most prominent symptom.

   2 Fever and dry skin are symptoms of dehydration.

   4 Temperature changes may occur with thrombophlebitis but are not a common symptom.

54. Application, assessment, physiological integrity (c).

   3 This may indicate delayed gastric emptying; further feedings can induce vomiting.

   1 Gastrostomy site oozing is a common occurrence that requires skin integrity measures, but it does not indicate a need to withhold feedings.

   2 An absence of the gag reflex is actually an indicator for tube feedings.

   4 No residual feeding return usually indicates full absorption of the feeding.

55. Application, implementation, physiological integrity (b).

   3 This is the definition for holistic care.

   1 Functional nursing implies that each type of nurse completes one type of job.

   2 Team nursing is a method for delivery of care.

   4 Primary nursing refers to one nurse's ability to care for all the tasks required to care for one patient.

56. Application, implementation, physiological integrity (b).

   2 This may delay the patient's urge to defecate.

   1 Maintaining fluid flow will increase the patient's urge to defecate.

   3 This is untrue; the patient is likely to lose control of his bowels if the nurse does not adjust the flow rate.

   4 Only if the prescribed amount of fluid has been given would the nurse do this.

57. Application, implementation, physiological integrity (b).

   2 This is the correct rationale for this procedure.

   1 The physician would not have difficulty. This is untrue.

   3 Clipping hair has no outcome on patient pain perception.

   4 Although it is more difficult to apply tape over hair, this is not the primary purpose.

58. Application, evaluation, physiological integrity (c).
    2 By having nothing in the stomach before surgery, the patient is less likely to have nausea and vomiting after surgery.
    1 Cleansing enemas would help decrease problems after abdominal surgeries.
    3 This decreases the chance for respiratory compromise after surgery.
    4 This hydrates the patient before, during, and after surgery and replaces vital electrolytes lost during surgery.

59. Application, implementation, safe, effective care environment (c).
    1 The old dressing should be removed with clean gloves, not sterile.
    2 This is the proper method for irrigation.
    3 If packing is appropriate and ordered, sterile Q-tips can be used.
    4 This is always indicated.

60. Comprehension, implementation, physiological integrity (b).
    4 A Jackson-Pratt (JP) is a type of grenade drain used to remove blood and fluid from the operative site.
    1 A JP is not a type of dressing.
    2 The JP does not hold dressings in place; it is a drain.
    3 This is not the correct description of a JP.

61. Application, evaluation, safe, effective care environment (b).
    1, 2 The nurse documents the exact location and size of the wounds, as well as the characteristic of the suture line.
    3, 4 The nurse does not need to address these areas unless a specific problem exists.

62. Analysis, implementation, safe, effective care environment (b).
    3 This is the best answer and addresses the safety issue.
    1 This should be obtained before the narcotic is given.
    2 This would increase the patient's chance of aspiration and would not meet the safety needs of the patient.
    4 This would not address safety as much as it would decrease the chance for respiratory compromise after surgery.

63. Knowledge, implementation, physiological integrity (b).
    4 Once blood begins to enter the specimen tube, the tourniquet is released to allow unrestricted blood flow.
    1 Releasing the tourniquet causes the veins to recede, hindering access.
    2 Keeping the tourniquet on during the blood draw lengthens the procedure and promotes venospasm.
    3 This would promote bruising at the venipuncture site.

64. Comprehension, implementation, physiological integrity (c).
    1 Placing the arm in a downward position dilates the blood vessels for access.
    2 The nurse's skill level influences patient discomfort.
    3 Additives do not flow back into the blood tubes; they are already in the tubes.
    4 The nurse restricts arm movement by holding the patient's arm.

65. Application, implementation, physiological integrity (c).
    3 This action will keep the viscera moist until the surgeon arrives to correct the problem.
    1 This should never be done; the nurse may further compromise the patient.
    2 This should be done after the saline soaked gauze is applied.
    4 This may be contraindicated by the patient's condition.

66. Analysis, evaluation, physiological integrity (c).
    4 These vital signs should lead the nurse to believe that the patient is experiencing hemorrhagic shock.
    1 The patient's temperature is normal, which would rule out infection.
    2 Vital signs would not immediately alert the nurse to dehiscence.
    3 Vital signs would not immediately alert the nurse to the complication of thrombophlebitis.

67. Application, implementation, physiological integrity (b).
    2 Surgical tube sites are cleansed concentrically, from the cleanest area outward, to minimize contamination of the wound.
    1 Scrubbing the site disrupts wound healing and can contaminate the wound.
    3 This brings distal organisms into the surgical site.
    4 This is not an effective measure for cleaning ostomy sites; a potential exists for missing areas under the ostomy tube.

68. Comprehension, evaluation, physiological integrity (c).
    1 Early ambulation provides the most venous return, decreasing venous stasis, and is the best method for preventing this complication.
    2 These devices do minimize thrombophlebitis, but early ambulation is the best method.
    3, 4 These practices do not prevent thrombophlebitis.

69. Comprehension, assessment, physiological integrity (b).
    3 Dizziness is caused by hyperventilation or breathing too rapidly.
    1 This is the purpose of the incentive spirometer.
    2 The patient is supposed to breathe slowly.
    4 This would not make the person dizzy.

70. Application, assessment, physiological integrity (c).
    2 This is the proper rationale. The surgery is a palliative treatment.
    1 The patient is terminally ill. The colostomy will not cure the cancer.
    3 It is unlikely that this would be reversed when the purpose of the surgery is palliative in nature.
    4 The patient's diagnosis has already been made.

71. Knowledge, implementation, psychosocial integrity (a).
    1 Cleansing and preparing the body before family viewing decreases the stress of the situation.
    2 Postmortem care is always completed before the body is moved.
    3 Family and patient needs are the priority of unit function.
    4 The family will be less stressed if the patient's body is clean and has a more normal appearance.

72. Analysis, evaluation, physiological integrity (c).
    2 These statements indicate that the patient may be developing thrombophlebitis.
    1 The expectation is that a solid food, such as pizza, would make a person nauseous at this time.
    3 This is a true statement, and a small amount of gas is expected to develop.
    4 The patient may have lost some sodium during surgery, but this does not indicate a problem.

73. Comprehension, planning, physiological integrity (b).
    2 The drying and subsequent removal of wet-to-dry dressings creates mechanical débridement of wounds.
    1 This is not the chief effect of this wound treatment; application of moist heat or increased patient activity would increase circulation.
    3 Wet-to-damp dressing promotes absorption of wound secretions.
    4 Wet-to-dry dressings have no effect on wound edema.

74. Application, implementation, psychosocial integrity (c).
    4 This allows the nurse to observe whether the client correctly understood the instructions.
    1 This would test knowledge, not application.
    2 This may not be an appropriate method, given the nature of the instructions.
    3 Although this would be appropriate, a return demonstration allows the nurse to evaluate how effective the instructions were.

75. Application, implementation, physiological integrity (b).
    1 Walking assists in removing gas from the intestines.
    2 This would only be indicated if the patient were not able to walk.
    3 This is a physician-ordered medication. Walking may alleviate the gas without medication.
    4 Milk will not assist the patient with removing gas, and the patient may not be on a full-liquid diet yet.

76. Application, implementation, physiological integrity (b).
    4 Tympanic thermometers measure core body temperature noninvasively.
    1 Throat surgery forces oral breathing, causing an inaccurate oral reading.
    2 Rectal thermometer reading is uncomfortable and embarrassing to the patient.
    3 Axillary readings are too reliant on placement and environmental factors for accuracy.

77. Analysis, planning, health promotion and maintenance (b).
    4 This is the only diagnosis that would be pertinent to this situation.
    1, 2, 3 These are not appropriate diagnoses for this situation.

78. Comprehension, implementation, physiological integrity (b).
    3 Because of the danger of aspiration, fluids should not be introduced into a nasogastric tube until correct placement has been verified.
    1 Although this is a part of the procedure, the primary step is verification of tube location.
    2 The feeding need only be room temperature.
    4 Fluid should never be introduced into a nasogastric tube until placement in the stomach is verified.

79. Application, implementation, safe, effective care environment (b).
    2 This position will relieve strain on back muscles and uses the strongest muscles for lifting.
    1 To prevent injury, personnel must stand close to the object being lifted.
    3 This puts undue strain on the back muscles.
    4 This causes a narrow base of support; a wide base of support is needed for stability.

80. Analysis, evaluation, physiological integrity (c).
    3 The nurse should take action if the patient is 10 hours postoperative and has not voided.
    1, 2, 4 These are normal findings.

81. Knowledge, implementation, safe, effective care environment (a).
    2 Legal constraints make restraints a medically ordered procedure.
    1 Restraints often increase patient restlessness and powerlessness.
    3 Too loose application increases patient injury risk.
    4 Side rails cannot be lowered in an emergency if restraints are tied to them.

82. Analysis, planning, physiological integrity (b).
    1 The nurse must make sure that the specimen has adhered to the slide before sending it to the laboratory.
    2, 3, 4 These actions are not indicated in this situation.

83. Analysis, implementation, psychosocial integrity (b).
    2 This response recognizes the patient's need for self-determination.
    1 This response fails to value the patient's needs.
    3 This response imposes the nurse's values on the patient.
    4 This is an inflexible response that fails to recognize patient individuality.

84. Comprehension, implementation, physiological integrity (b).
    3 This is the correct response; it provides facts without alarming the patient.
    1 More information is needed here. The patient may think he has a blood clot.
    2 This is alarming and most likely untrue.
    4 This may be true if we knew that the patient were taking an anticoagulant.

85. Application, planning, safe, effective care environment (a).
    3 Taking people out of harm's way is always the first step in the event of fire.
    1 This sequence of events does not put the patient's safety first.
    2 This sequence does not place the patient's safety first.
    4 Preserving the safety of the patient is always the first step in the event of a fire.

86. Comprehension, evaluation, physiological integrity (b).
    3 An intravenous pyelogram (IVP) is helpful in diagnosing conditions of the kidney.
    1 Liver function tests and sonograms may be helpful in diagnosing liver ailments.
    2 Electroencephalograms (EEGs) and positron emission tomography (PET) scans may diagnose some brain dysfunctions.
    4 Barium enemas, a colonoscopy, and a sigmoidoscopy can be helpful in diagnosing intestinal maladies.

87. Application, planning, safe, effective care environment (b).
    3 The primary goal in caring for a patient in protective isolation is to limit the amount of contact the patient has with organisms that may be brought into the room on the hands and body of individuals.
    1 The risk present is to the patient, not health care workers (who should be following blood and body fluid measures).
    2 Although minimizing the impact of being isolated on patients is important in any type of isolation, the goal of therapy is to minimize the risk to the patient.
    4 This is not the primary goal for protective isolation, and it has not been established that the patient has an infectious process.

88. Application, implementation, safe, effective care environment (b).

2 By lining out the entry, others may still read the original entry; dating and initialing it is the proper procedure that signifies accountability.

1   This is improper and does not allow for others to see the original mistake.

3   This would be destroying property belonging to the hospital; it is considered falsifying records.

4   Using correction fluid does not allow others to see the original message.

89. Application, implementation, physiological integrity (c).

2, 3, 4 Most MRI units are closed in. Knowing if the patient has claustrophobia would be important. Additionally, patients cannot have any metal on or in their body; thus the other questions are important.

1   Iodine is a nonmetallic element and is used as a contrast agent for blood vessels in computed tomography scans, not in MRI.

5   Enemas are not given before an MRI; thus this information is not needed.

90. Application, implementation, physiological integrity (b).

3 Supplemental feedings are necessary to prepare the patient for the surgical procedure as indicated in this situation.

1   Increasing peristalsis is not the action that the nasogastric tube is performing.

2   A nasogastric tube inserted to decompress the stomach will result in removal of fluids and gas.

4   This response does not answer the patient's question concerning the purpose of the tube.

91. Comprehension, implementation, physiological integrity (c).

4 This is the correct use of the information derived from a cholangiogram.

1, 2, 3   A cholangiogram cannot provide this information.

92. Application, implementation, safe, effective care environment (b).

1 This response preserves the sterile catheter tray, while ensuring that a sterile catheter is used.

2   Betadine will merely disinfect, not sterilize, the tip of the catheter; this is not an acceptable procedure.

3   No reason has been given to discontinue the procedure or discard the sterile tray when maintaining sterility can be achieved by obtaining a new catheter.

4   The nurse must maintain a sterile consciousness; if instinct says the tip is contaminated, the nurse should obtain a new catheter.

93. Application, implementation, physiological integrity (b).

3 The major reason for ostomy pouches to fit snugly is to prevent excoriation of the surrounding skin by the drainage.

1   Although this is a true statement, this is not the major reason for a snug-fitting appliance.

2   Normally, pouches can be removed when the patient takes a bath; this is not the major reason for a snug-fitting appliance.

4   Although this is true, it is not the major reason for a snug-fitting appliance.

94. Comprehension, planning, physiological integrity (b).

4 An NPO order ensures that the stomach will be empty, therefore decreasing the chance for aspiration if the patient vomits after surgery.

1   Anesthesia does slow down the digestive process, but it does not stop it.

2   The energy needs of a surgical patient increase, not decrease.

3   Vomiting does not normally occur; and if the stomach is empty, aspiration is less likely to occur.

95. Application, implementation, physiological integrity (b).

2 This period allows the nurse to remove secretions effectively and not interrupt the patient's normal breathing pattern for too long.

1   This is not an adequate period to remove secretions.

3   Thirty seconds is too long to keep a patient from his or her normal breathing patterns.

4   The patient is not able to breathe during the suctioning; and this period is too long an interruption of normal breathing patterns.

96. Analysis, planning, physiological integrity (b).

2 An ERCP examination is a procedure used to evaluate the pancreatic, hepatic and gallbladder duct.

1   An MRI is not likely to be ordered for this patient because it would not provide the most detailed information.

3   An arteriogram is used to diagnosis arterial problems.

4   A sigmoidoscopy is useful in diagnosing problems of the colon.

97. Application, implementation, physiological integrity (b).

3 This is the acceptable method for opening an airway of a patient who is not suspected of having a spinal cord injury; it is also the simplest method.

1   Performing a mouth sweep is done to remove foreign objects from the mouth, potentially opening an airway; however, the head and chin must still be maneuvered after this procedure is done.

2   Turning the head to one side will not open an airway.

4   This maneuver is more difficult to perform and is done on patients with a suspected spinal cord injury.

98. Comprehension, evaluation, physiological integrity (c).

4 This is the correct location to perform a thoracentesis.

1   An abdominocentesis would be performed on the peritoneal cavity.

2   No such cavity exists. Ascites is edema in the peritoneal cavity.

3   The pericardial sac is around the heart. The procedure for removal of fluid is a pericardiocentesis.

99. Application, planning, physiological integrity (c).

1 The proper method for establishing the patency of a small-bore feeding tube is to obtain a chest radiograph.

2   If the tube is in the patient's respiratory tract, the suction may cause damage to the mucosa.

3   This can cause aspiration if the tube is in the respiratory tract.

4   This method may not work; given the small bore of the feeding tube, a chest radiograph is a more exact way of establishing patency.

100. Knowledge, assessment, health promotion and maintenance (b).

2 Medicare is the type of insurance that is available to older adults.

1 Social security is not a type of insurance, although older individuals do receive it.

3 Medicaid is a type of insurance designed to assist low-income individuals under the age of 65 years.

4 Farmer's Life is a type of supplemental insurance.

101. Comprehension, assessment, health promotion and maintenance (a).

3 This statement reflects some of the developmental changes that occur in middle-age patients (empty nest syndrome).

1 Although this is a personal statement, it can be made by a variety of age groups.

2 Most individuals retire in their 60s, and this patient would not typically have this concern yet.

4 This is an ambiguous statement that requires further investigation.

102. Application, planning, health promotion and maintenance (a).

2 Walking is a nonstressful, pleasant activity that is especially beneficial for individuals who have chronic health problems; it also preserves the joints of elderly individuals.

1 Jogging may be too stressful for older adults, especially to those with cardiopulmonary disease.

3 Ski machines may be too vigorous an activity and place undue strain on joints.

4 Rowing machines may also be too vigorous, especially to patients with cardiopulmonary disease.

103. Application, evaluation, psychosocial integrity (b).

3 Individuals of the Jehovah's Witness faith do not accept blood or blood products and may question why a type and cross would be done.

1 This is normal preoperative teaching that does not conflict with this particular religion's beliefs.

2 Coughing, deep-breathing, and leg exercises should not conflict with this particular religion's beliefs.

4 This noninvasive procedure does not conflict with Jehovah's Witness beliefs.

104. Application, implementation, safe, effective care environment (b).

3 This is the correct procedure for completing perineal care.

1 This is inaccurate and can lead to vaginal and urinary tract infections.

2 This would be the proper teaching for cleansing of the perineum before insertion of a catheter.

4 This is inaccurate and may lead to urinary tract infections.

105. Application, planning, physiological integrity (b).

4 The nurse may be able to provide the patient with some comfort measures that he engages in at home or otherwise meet the patient's needs.

1 The patient is not complaining of pain.

2 It has not been determined that the patient needs a sedative; more information from the patient is needed.

3 This is an unrealistic reassurance and does not address the patient's complaint.

106. Application, implementation, physiological integrity (b).

1 This is the best method for assisting an individual who is able to help him or herself.

2 This may cause a break in skin integrity and would probably be uncomfortable.

3 This is effective but is not the easiest method for assisting an individual who can help.

4 The question refers to helping a patient onto a bedpan.

107. Application, planning, physiological integrity (b).

4 This method is appropriate and reduces the incidence of ingrown toenails.

1 This may be painful and compromises skin integrity.

2 Sharp corners will catch on bed linens.

3 This would predispose the patient to ingrown toenails.

108. Application, implementation, physiological integrity (b).

3 The ulcer will fill in from the inside and upward, which leaves a scar.

1 This is a flip response that demeans the individual.

2 This response does not recognize the needs of the patient.

4 The physician may be consulted, but the question is asked of the nurse who has the ability to answer it.

109. Comprehension, implementation, physiological integrity (a).

3 By using a syringe and withdrawing the urine using the provided sampling port, the nurse can obtain a sterile specimen without breaking the continuity of the system.

1 This action would not produce a sterile specimen and would necessitate putting the catheter back in the patient.

2 Water should come out of the balloon port on the catheter, not urine; this action would deflate the catheter balloon, causing dislodgement.

4 Urine is no longer sterile after it has been sitting in the bottom of the drainage bag; a sterile urine specimen is needed.

110. Application, evaluation, physiological integrity (b).

3 The pain is most likely caused by inflating the balloon while it is in the urethra; the nurse should make sure that the catheter is advanced into the bladder before inflating the balloon.

1 If the balloon ruptures, it should not cause pain, and the result would be that the catheter cannot be considered indwelling.

2 Although not a wise practice, this action should not cause pain if the catheter is in the bladder.

4 The patient complained during balloon inflation, and therefore the pain must be connected to this action.

111. Application, implementation, physiological integrity (b).

4 This placement ensures that the tubing will be below the urinary bladder; therefore the urine will not travel back up the drainage tube, an action that can result in a urinary tract infection.

1 This position may result in urine traveling back up the drainage tubing, potentially causing a urinary tract infection.

2 This position may result in urine traveling back up the drainage tubing back to the bladder.

3 This position is also too high, resulting in urine traveling back up the drainage tubing.

112. Application, implementation, physiological integrity (b).
   4 This method reduces the chance of infection and contamination of the lacrimal gland.
   1, 2, 3 These are not proper methods and will potentially contaminate the other eye or the lacrimal gland.

113. Application, planning, physiological integrity (b).
   1 This ensures that the dentures will not get lost and is the only correct answer.
   2 This is unnecessary.
   3 The patient may not want to use a denture-cleansing tablet.
   4 The patient may not want to use adhesive on the dentures.

114. Comprehension, implementation, physiological integrity (b).
   3 Clipping hair from the potential surgical site and surrounding area reduces the number of microorganisms present on the hair and skin, reducing the incidence of infection.
   1 Removal of hair does not lessen discomfort from the surgical procedure.
   2 If the incision is sutured, the amount of hair at the site will not affect that practice.
   4 Although this may be true, this is not the primary purpose for clipping hair before surgery.

115. Comprehension, evaluation, psychosocial integrity (c).
   1 Most patients receive light sedation during the procedure; it is unlikely that the person will undergo general anesthesia.
   2, 3, 4 These are all appropriate responses.

116. Application, implementation, physiological integrity (b).
   4 A warm backrub may help relax the individual enough to fall asleep.
   1 This would allow hall noise to interfere with the patient's rest.
   2 Although this is done by some people, this action would only be indicated if the patient is used to falling asleep with the television on at home.
   3 Exercise increases epinephrine release, making falling asleep more difficult for the patient.

117. Application, implementation, physiological integrity (b).
   1 The nurse bandages the extremity from the foot upwards, facilitating venous return and reducing the incidence of swelling caused by the bandaging.
   2 If the nurse bandages from the knee down to the foot, venous return is compromised, and swelling of the foot may occur.
   3 If the nurse begins bandaging at the ankle, swelling of the foot may occur, and this technique does not facilitate venous return to the heart.
   4 Bandaging from the middle of the leg, either upward or downward, will not facilitate venous return and may cause swelling above and below the bandage.

118. Application, implementation, physiological integrity (b).
   3 This position allows for venous return, decreasing the incidence of swelling of the arm and hand.
   1 This position may not allow for adequate venous drainage and may cause swelling.

2 If the arm and hand are in a dependent position from the elbow, swelling will occur.
   4 This position is not only uncomfortable, but swelling will occur in the arm and hand.

119. Comprehension, planning, physiological integrity (b).
   3 Adequate oxygenation is always the first priority in any emergency situation.
   1 Although important, this cannot be accomplished unless a patent airway is established.
   2 A victim's airway must be established before controlling bleeding.
   4 This is not a priority nursing action and may be performed by ancillary personnel.

120. Application, implementation, physiological integrity (b).
   2 The nurse reduces the chance of edema formation and nerve compression by checking the BP on the opposite side of the mastectomy.
   1 This would be contraindicated on the right side and unnecessary on the left arm.
   3 This would be unnecessary unless both arms were compromised.
   4 Auscultating the BP in this area is difficult and unnecessary.

121. Comprehension, planning, physiological integrity (c).
   1 Patients with orthostatic hypotension complain of dizziness when arising from a sitting or lying position.
   2, 3, 4 These symptoms are not normally associated with orthostatic hypotension.

122. Comprehension, implementation, physiological integrity (b).
   3 A bounding pulse is a pulse that is of full force and easy to palpate; sometimes the pulse can be seen with each heartbeat.
   1 An irregular pulse does not have a regular rhythm and does not describe the intensity of the pulse.
   2 Deep is a term used to describe respiration.
   4 Bradycardia is used to describe a slow pulse; it does not describe intensity.

123. Application, evaluation, physiological integrity (c).
   4 This patient is postoperative, a situation that would necessitate reporting the heart rate caused by a possible hemorrhage.
   1 This is a normal newborn respiratory rate.
   2 For athletic individuals to have low resting pulse rates is not uncommon.
   3 This is a normal respiratory rate for this age group.

124. Application, planning, physiological integrity (b).
   3 Sputum specimens are more easily collected in the morning because secretions have been lying in the bronchial tubes during the night.
   1, 2 A patient may have an emesis or become ill if the nurse tries to obtain a sputum culture at these times.
   4 Obtaining sputum specimens at night is more difficult because the patient has mobilized and coughed up secretions during the day.

125. Application, implementation, physiological integrity (b).
   4 A generous fluid intake liquefies secretions, allowing them to be more easily expectorated.
   1 Adequate sleep is important in any treatment plan; however, it does not keep secretions from becoming thick.

2 Although important, regular exercise does not directly liquefy secretions.

3 A nourishing diet is important in the treatment plan but does not directly liquefy secretions.

126. Application, assessment, physiological integrity (c).

3 The gurgling noise signifies that the patient is unable to control his secretions and should be assisted by suctioning.

1 Although rapid, many individuals with a respiratory ailment are tachypneic, which does not indicate that suctioning is needed.

2 When patients need suctioning, their heart rate normally does increase; however, it is not itself an indicator for suctioning.

4 If the patient is able to expectorate his mucus, he does not need to be suctioned.

127. Comprehension, implementation, safe, effective care environment (a).

1 The adult patient has the right to refuse any or all therapy and must be given the opportunity to formulate a living will.

2 The patient may consult with the physician, but the patient has the right to make the decision independently.

3 The decision is the patient's; however, he or she may consult with a variety of individuals.

4 As a rule, nurses assist in curing patients; when cure is not possible, health care workers should uphold the patient's wishes.

128. Comprehension, implementation, safe, effective care environment (b).

2 Hospice nurses try to make the patient comfortable for as long as the patient lives.

1 Although this is true, it is not the primary purpose of hospice care.

3 This is not always the case; many hospice patients are cared for at home.

4 Most skilled care is performed by hospice personnel; however, the family is instrumental in providing for the basic care of the patient.

129. Comprehension, planning, safe, effective care environment (b).

2 An advance directive ensures that the patient or designee can make decisions concerning treatment before death.

1 The patient or patient advocate will dictate which measures will be used as death approaches.

3 The physician must uphold the patient's wishes; however, the physician has the right to advise the patient concerning a treatment plan.

4 The patient designates a patient advocate to make end-of-life decisions; these decisions are based on the patient's wishes, not the family's.

130. Comprehension, planning, safe, effective care environment (b).

1 Planning for discharge should begin on the day of admission to the hospital.

2 This does not give adequate time to organize community resources if the patient needs them.

3 Predicting when a patient will be discharged is difficult; planning should begin well before discharge.

4 The plan of care for the patient should be evaluated each day, making changes based on the procedures or treatments that the patient has.

131. Comprehension, implementation, physiological integrity (b).

3 Urine is strained on patients with known or suspected calculi to collect stones for evaluation.

1 Flank massage is not indicated for patients with renal calculi.

2 Urine reductions are indicated for patients with diabetes mellitus.

4 Fluids are generally encouraged in patients who have suspected renal calculi.

132. Comprehension, implementation, physiological integrity (b).

4 For the proper laboratory tests to be completed, all voided urine must be collected and placed on ice until sent to the laboratory.

1 In a 24-hour urine specimen, all urine is collected that the patient voids in a 24-hour period and placed into a brown container that is taken to the laboratory at the end of the 24 hours.

2 The urine is kept on ice for the 24-hour period.

3 All urine is collected for the 24-hour specimen.

133. Comprehension, implementation, physiological integrity (b).

3 Inserting a rectal tube will stimulate peristalsis and relieve the abdominal pain and pressure.

1 Normally, activity, if possible, will help relieve the pain of flatus.

2 Nonpharmaceutical interventions can usually alleviate this type of discomfort.

4 This action will decrease the amount of additional gas buildup but will not relieve the immediate discomfort.

134. Comprehension, implementation, physiological integrity (b).

3 The presence of ova and parasites can only be detected when the specimen is still warm.

1 This action will not allow laboratory personnel to find ova and parasites; the specimen must be warm.

2 Using a rectal tube is unnecessary. A defecated specimen is used.

4 The GI tract is not sterile; thus a clean specimen cup is indicated.

135. Application, assessment, physiological integrity (b).

3 Symptoms of dehydration include decreased urine output and poor skin turgor.

1 Weight gain is indicative of hypervolemia.

2 Hypertension is indicative of hypervolemia.

4 Moist, pink, mucous membranes are a symptom of balanced fluid status.

136. Application, evaluation, physiological integrity (b).

4 The chest physiotherapy breaks up the patient's secretions so they can be expectorated.

1, 2, 3 These are not the desired outcomes for chest physiotherapy.

137. Analysis, assessment, physiological integrity (c).

2 A patient who has chronic obstructive pulmonary disease is reluctant to move from a position of comfort, usually an orthopneic position that puts much pressure on the coccygeal area.

1 If the patient is ambulatory, a urinary tract infection should not predispose the patient to an ulcer.

3 A patient with gallbladder disease is usually ambulatory and is therefore at low risk.

4 A constipated patient should be at no further risk unless another problem is present.

138. Knowledge, planning, physiological integrity (b).

1 The skin is the body's first line of defense, and a break in this defense reduces the body's ability to resist infections.

2 A break in the skin does not necessarily decrease the body's ability to produce antibodies.

3 Although the skin does assist in eliminating perspiration, a break in the skin does not reduce this substantially.

4 The ability to maintain correct body alignment should not be affected by a break in the skin.

139. Comprehension, implementation, physiological integrity (b).

2 This is the correct, sensitive response to the patient's question.

1 This is insensitive although true.

3 This may or may not be the case for this individual.

4 This may or may not be true.

140. Comprehension, implementation, physiological integrity (b).

1 A patient with a bleeding disorder may preclude the nurse from completing the shave; further investigation is necessary before proceeding.

2 A patient with an emotional disorder would most likely not stop the nurse from shaving the patient.

3 Patients with respiratory disorders may need frequent rest periods, but shaving with a manual razor should not pose a problem for the patient.

4 A patient with a neurologic disorder should not preclude the nurse from completing the task.

141. Application, implementation, physiological integrity (b).

4 If possible, the patient should be placed on the side with head turned to the side; this facilitates removal of secretions and decreases the chance of aspiration.

1 This is too difficult a position in which to place an unconscious patient, although it would facilitate secretion drainage.

2 The patient should be placed so that secretions naturally fall from the mouth; suction is an appropriate device that should be near.

3 The patient needs to be flat and side lying; this position does not facilitate secretion drainage.

142. Comprehension, planning, physiological integrity (b).

4 Sleep apnea is a disorder that results in frequent waking during the night, causing daytime fatigue.

1 This disorder is not normally caused by snoring or overeating.

2 Sleep apnea is not increased if the patient is nervous or upset.

3 Individuals with sleep apnea can have the disorder for a long period.

143. Comprehension, assessment, physiological integrity (b).

3 This allows the patient to easily describe the intensity of the pain to the nurse and allows for evaluation of treatment options.

1 This will not assess the intensity of the pain, only the location.

2 This response allows the patient to locate the pain but does not describe intensity.

4 These words are too subjective; the word bad may have different meanings to the nurse and patient.

144. Application, implementation, physiological integrity (b).

3 The crutch length is too long, causing compression of the nerves in the axilla; adjusting the crutches and teaching the patient to place weight on his hands will alleviate the problem.

1 No indication has been found that the patient needs a walker instead of a crutch.

2 The pain and tingling is most likely caused by compression of a nerve, not nerve damage.

4 This does not correct the problem, which is improper crutch length and technique.

145. Comprehension, implementation, physiological integrity (b).

4 The patient should use the cane to take weight off of her weak extremity, the right side.

1 This will not assist the patient in walking.

2 This may confuse the patient and will not effectively limit weight bearing on the right side.

3 Holding the cane in the left hand and moving it with the left leg will not limit weight bearing on the right side.

146. Application, assessment, physiological integrity (b).

4 Cheyne-Stokes respirations are characterized by rhythmic breathing with a varying depth and rate of respirations, with periods of apnea; it is commonly seen in patients who are approaching death.

1 Dyspnea is difficulty breathing, and although this patient is having difficulty breathing, the question asks for the specific breathing pattern that is being observed.

2 Tachypnea is fast breathing, or increased rate; the patient does not exhibit tachypnea.

3 Kussmaul's respiration is a type of breathing seen in individuals who have diabetes mellitus; it is characterized by paroxysms of dyspnea.

147. Analysis, assessment, physiological integrity (b).

4 Patients on bedrest normally have their feet and head elevated; excessive tissue fluid would therefore fall into the sacral area.

1 Individuals who are ambulatory are most likely to notice edema of the feet.

2 Individuals who are bedfast may eventually develop edema of the hands; however, initially it is normally found in the sacral area.

3 As the edema progresses, calves may become edematous; however, calf edema is more common in the ambulatory individual.

148. Application, implementation, safe, effective care environment (b).

2 This response signifies a correct step in the procedure for administering a vaginal douche.

1 The patient should be encouraged to void before the douche is instilled.

3 The fluid should not be flowing as the douchetip is placed in the vagina.

4 Low pressure is used when instilling the fluid to decrease tissue trauma.

149. Application, implementation, psychosocial integrity (b).

3 By paraphrasing the statement and restating it in the form of a question, the nurse is able to illicit more information about the patient's feelings.

1 This belittles the patient's concern and gives false reassurance.

2 Anxiety may be heightening this patient's worries, but this response belittles the patient's fears.

4 This response neither validates the patient's concerns nor encourages expression of feelings.

150. Comprehension, evaluation, physiological integrity (b).

2 These vital signs are abnormal, signifying a fever and should be reported.

1 All vital signs are normal for adult patients.

3 Axillary temperatures may be unreliable; however, all of these vital signs are within normal limits.

4 All vital signs are within normal limits.

151. Comprehension, evaluation, physiological integrity (b).

1 Because of the patient's inability to excrete fluids, the patient's weight will likely increase because of the excess fluid.

2 The patient's weight will not decrease, because the excess fluid will not be able to be eliminated.

3 Because of the patient's diagnosis, she will not be able to rid herself of the fluid.

4 The patient is most likely hypervolemic and not dehydrated.

152. Comprehension, planning, safe, effective care environment (c).

3 The patient has difficulty swallowing and will need a barium swallow to evaluate feeding needs.

1 A barium enema is used to evaluate structural defects of the lower bowel.

2 An esophagogastroduodenoscopy may be necessary and needs to be determined, but the plan of care needs to address the swallowing difficulty.

4 A computed tomography scan may be ordered if a stroke is suspected but is not specific to the dysphagia.

153. Application, planning, physiological integrity (b).

4 A tympanic temperature will give an accurate reading and should be used as the oral and rectal routes are not indicated for this patient.

1 The oral route should not be used because the patient is receiving oxygen.

2 The rectal surgery precludes using this route.

3 The axillary method is the most unreliable of the methods listed; the tympanic temperature is the best choice for this patient.

154. Comprehension, assessment, physiological integrity (b).

3 If the patient's oxygen saturation were truly 60%, the patient would be in distress; the more likely cause for the alarm is that the probe has become dislodged.

1 The need for this action has not been established.

2 The nurse would need to report to the physician and receive orders to complete this task.

4 No need for this action exists at this time.

155. Application, planning, physiological integrity (b).

1 This method allows the solution to flow into all the areas of the vagina.

2 This will force medication into higher areas.

3, 4 Most of the solution will flow out; the patient should lie recumbent for a time after the douche.

156. Analysis, planning, physiological integrity (b).

Correct sequence: 2, 3, 4, 1. By following this sequence, the patient will be comfortable for the examination, and the nurse will conserve energy by waiting for the patient to
leave before making the bed. This sequence anticipates the patient's needs and manages the nurse's time effectively.

157. Application, implementation, physiological integrity (c).

2 This is the best response out of the four given responses; it accurately addresses the patient's concerns.

1 This information is inaccurate.

3 Although the pulse oximetry reading is important for monitoring, an arterial blood gas analysis will more fully allow the physician to determine the appropriate amount.

4 Although this is true, it does not give any rationale to the patient.

158. Application, implementation, safe, effective care environment (b).

2 This choice allows the nurse to maintain sterility and reduce cost to the patient.

1 This would be unsanitary; the gauze was wet and was not entirely on the sterile field, which may not be waterproof.

3 The gauze pad became contaminated during the time it was on the sterile field's edge, and rinsing it in saline solution will not resterilize it.

4 Beginning again is unnecessary; the situation can be resolved without the additional expense to the patient of beginning again.

159. Comprehension, implementation, physiological integrity (b).

4 An IPPB treatment works by forcing the person to inhale deeply, which will increase airflow, increase oxygenation, and assist in loosening secretions.

1 Manual or mechanical chest physiotherapy is better able to dislodge secretions.

2 Incentive spirometry is useful in increasing tidal volume of inhalations.

3 This statement describes how postural drainage assists patients.

160. Application, implementation, physiological integrity (b).

2 The patient needs to have oxygen supplemented; the patient is accustomed to oxygen and must have it supplied in increased amounts before the suctioning procedure; failure to do so may cause hypoxia.

1 No indication exists that restraints are needed.

3 Suction is never applied when advancing the catheter.

4 The patient needs to have oxygen before advancing the suction catheter.

161. Application, implementation, physiological integrity (b).

4 To obtain an accurate measurement, the arrow on the cuff should be positioned where the brachial artery was palpated, which will result in appropriate cuff pressure of the artery.

1 This may result in an inaccurate, low reading.

2 The patient's arm should be extended with palm up.

3 The cuff is positioned 1 inch above the brachial artery.

162. Analysis, assessment, physiological integrity (b).

1 The nurse palpates the peripheral pulse.

2 The technique of percussion is used when evaluating the status of fluid, drainage, or air in a cavity.

3 Inspection requires observation of the patient, without touching the patient.

4 Auscultation is listening for sounds; the apical pulse is evaluated in this manner.

163. Knowledge, implementation, physiological integrity (a).

1 A patient's emesis should be measured and added to the output for that period.

2 IV fluids are considered as part of a patient's intake.

3 The water loss that results from perspiration is insensible and cannot be measured.

4 The volume of tube feedings is added to a patient's intake.

164. Comprehension, evaluation, safe, effective care environment (b).

3 Patients leave the hospital environment much sicker than before, necessitating more home care management of patients after discharge.

1 Patients leave the hospital much quicker than they did before.

2 This is also untrue and is not the reason acute care nursing numbers are decreasing.

4 Although this was part of the intention of managed care, health care costs continue to rise.

165. Comprehension, implementation, physiological integrity (b).

4 By having the patient remain in an upright position, the feeding is less likely to flow back into the esophagus and be aspirated by the patient.

1 This is a common practice; however, it does not assist in reducing the risk of aspiration.

2 This is a highly appropriate action but does not reduce the risk for aspiration.

3 This may cause the patient to lose calories and should not be done unless physician ordered; it has no bearing on aspiration.

166. Application, assessment, physiological integrity (b).

3 Burning on urination is to be expected after a catheter is removed and needs to be acted on only if it persists.

1 No evidence of this exists at this time; however, if other symptoms develop and the burning does not decrease, action may need to be taken.

2 The need to call a physician has not been established.

4 The nurse needs a physician's order to obtain a urine specimen; if the burning continues, the physician may need to be called.

167. Application, implementation, physiological integrity (b).

1 If the tube is in the patient's trachea, air will not flow to vibrate the vocal cords, and the patient will be unable to speak.

2 This signifies that the tube is still in the nasal cavity.

3 A small amount of blood is indicative of tissue trauma from inserting the tube.

4 This would signify that the tube was in the stomach.

168. Comprehension, planning, physiological integrity (b).

2 This statement correctly explains the actions of each enema.

1 Although both enemas may stimulate peristalsis somewhat, the cleansing enema is designed for this purpose.

3 The oil-retention enema is given to soften stool, not specifically to evacuate the bowel.

4 The oil-retention enema is the enema given to soften the stool and is normally given before the cleansing enema.

169. Comprehension, implementation, safe, effective care environment (b).

Patient complained of nausea. Vomited ~~175~~ 75 Error M.D. ml of dark-green emesis. Patient returned to bed and medicated with 200 mg of Tigan IM.

170. Comprehension, assessment, physiological integrity (b).

3 The patient may not be drinking enough fluids, which may have contributed to the problem.

1 Exercise assists in establishing normal bowel function.

2 Vegetables supply fiber, which should assist in establishing normal bowel patterns.

4 Defecating as soon as the need is felt is important.

171. Application, implementation, physiological integrity (b).

1 The patient is at risk for hypovolemic shock. The nurse should clamp the catheter immediately.

2 No reason is given to do this unless a specimen is ordered.

3 Although this would counteract the fluid loss, this cannot be done without a physician's order.

4 This would not correct the problem given that it has already occurred. Clamping the catheter will delay emptying of the bladder of any more urine.

172. Comprehension, implementation, safe, effective care environment (b).

3 This response is the definition of a contracture; the muscle is permanently shortened because of the effects of immobility.

1 This does not address the UAP's question.

2 An injury may have precipitated the decreased mobility, but the contracture is the direct result of the effects of immobility.

4 Once contracted, the arm will remain this way permanently, and ROM exercises will not restore it.

173. Analysis, planning, psychosocial integrity (b).

4 Blue is a color that promotes relaxation and serenity.

1, 2, 3 These colors are stimulating or melancholy and do not promote a calm atmosphere.

174. Comprehension, implementation, physiological integrity (b).

4 This is the most correct and most appropriate response by the nurse because it addresses the patient's question.

1 Although humorous, this answer is demeaning and does not answer the question.

2 This response belittles the patient and shifts responsibility for explanation to another person.

3 The patient wants to know why he needs to get out of bed; this response does not answer that question.

175. Application, implementation, physiological integrity (a).

4 This is the most logical response to the question and describes the action of the stockings.

1 This does not tell the patient why the stockings are needed or why they should be snug.

2 This is not the purpose for the stockings.

3 Although the stockings compress the muscles of the legs, the reason they need to be snug is so that blood is pushed back toward the heart.

176. Comprehension, planning, safe, effective care environment (b).

2 This is a short-term, easily measurable goal for this patient.

1 The emphasis of this plan of care is how well the patient will walk with crutches, not how long he or she can go without pain medication.

3 This goal may be long term, and most patients do not need 3 weeks to learn to walk with crutches.

4 This is an example of a long-term goal.

177. Application, planning, psychosocial integrity (b).

    4 Patients are generally calmer when they are in a quiet, stress-free environment; pastel shades of carpeting and wall decorations are also calming.
    1 Although exercise is important, a lot of physical activity may overstimulate the patient.
    2 This may cause the patient to become overstimulated.
    3 These activities may overly stimulate the patient.

178. Application, implementation, physiological integrity (b).

    4 Hydrogen peroxide's oxidizing capabilities make it a good choice for removing hardened secretions.
    1 Alcohol should not be used on the rubber Foley catheter because it will cause drying and cracking.
    2 Betadine is an antiseptic and should not be used to remove secretions.
    3 If soap and water were ineffective, sterile saline will not remove the secretions.

179. Application, implementation, physiological integrity (b).

    2 The first surgical dressing should be changed by the surgeon; therefore the dressing should be reinforced until further orders can be obtained.
    1 The nurse is unsure of what is under the dressing; changing a fresh postoperative dressing requires a physician's order.
    3 Removing the dressing would require a physician's order.
    4 Dressings are not routinely sent to the laboratory, and no order has been given to change the dressing.

180. Analysis, implementation, physiological integrity (b).

    5 oz = 150 ml + 120 ml + 8 oz = 240 ml + 1 cup = 240 ml + 4 oz = 12 ml = 870 ml

181. Application, implementation, physiological integrity (b).

    2 The patient who has decreased sensation to extremities is at increased risk for injury as a result of the application of heat.
    1 As long as the nurse explains the entire procedure to the patient, special precautions do not need to be taken for patients who are blind.
    3 Patients with hypertension are not at increased risk from the effects of the heat application.
    4 Although patients with diabetes mellitus may have neuropathy, which would place them at risk, the paraplegic individual remains the person at most risk from the heat application.

182. Knowledge, planning, physiological integrity (b).

    3 A thin layer of petrolatum (petroleum jelly) should be placed between the compress and the patient's eyelid to reduce damage to the eye area.
    1 Saline will not protect the eye from the heat.
    2 Betadine is an antiseptic solution and should not be applied anywhere near the eye area.
    4 Unless ordered, the antibiotic ointment is not placed on the lid.

183. Application, planning, physiological integrity (c).

    1, 2, 3 These actions will help mobilize the patient's secretions so that the patient can effectively expectorate them.
    4 This may further depress the patient's respirations.
    5 This will not assist the patient in clearing his airway.

184. Application, assessment, physiological integrity (b).

    1 The presence of redness and swelling indicate that infection may be present in the incision line.
    2 This does not directly indicate infection.

3 This is normal assessment data and indicates adequate healing.
    4 At times, a small amount of bloody drainage may be observed in a new incision line; this does not indicate infection.

185. Application, implementation, physiological integrity (b).

    2 The patient should be placed on his left side so that the infected drainage will flow away from the other eye.
    1 Drainage may flow into the right eye, causing infection.
    3 If the patient is on his right side, drainage will flow from the left to the right eye.
    4 The drainage will not be able to flow away from the patient's face.

186. Comprehension, evaluation, safe, effective care environment (b).

    3 Medication errors are an example of negligence. The nurse was negligent in following the standard of care.
    1, 2 These may be perceived as criminal actions.
    4 This is an ethical and possibly criminal action.

187. Comprehension, implementation, health promotion and maintenance (b).

    2 Most physicians recommend that women over the age of 40 undergo mammograms every 1 to 2 years.
    1 Mammograms are screening examinations and are done on women over age 40, despite any suspicions of cancer.
    3 All women should receive mammograms; women with strong family histories may be screened as often as every 6 months.
    4 Mammograms are not difficult for women, although they may be embarrassing to some women; mammograms are recommended every 1 to 2 years after age 40.

188. Application, implementation, physiological integrity (b).

    3 The footboard is used to keep the feet in proper alignment and decrease the incidence of plantar flexion.
    1 An abductor pillow assists in maintaining an abducted state of the legs.
    2 Antiembolic stockings are better able to keep the patient from developing thrombophlebitis, although a footboard can be used to do pedal pushes, thereby exercising the calf muscles.
    4 This may be true but is not the purpose of the board.

189. Comprehension, planning, safe, effective care environment (b).

    3 Liability insurance covers the nurse only while performing professional duties.
    1 Malpractice insurance costs vary from agency to agency.
    2 Malpractice insurance protects the nurse from financial damages.
    4 Malpractice insurance must be renewed periodically.

190. Knowledge, implementation, safe, effective care environment (b).

    1 Follow principles of the nursing process when meeting patient needs.
    2 Apply appropriate knowledge and skills.
    3 Apply principles of crisis intervention and refer when necessary.
    4 Use effective communication skills.
    5 Provide health teaching.
    6 Serve as patient advocate.

191. Comprehension, assessment, psychosocial integrity (b).
   3 The patient is bargaining with God for his life.
   1 No evidence of anger is found in his statement.
   2 The patient accepts his diagnosis; he just wishes to change it.
   4 The patient does not appear depressed at this time.

192. Analysis, assessment, physiological integrity (b).
   2 Given the patient's diagnosis, bowel sounds are the most important assessment criteria.
   1 Although important, bowel sounds are the most important assessment data for this patient.
   3 The patient's bowel sounds are of paramount importance.
   4 No indication can be found that a neurologic examination is warranted for this patient; bowel sounds remain the top priority.

193. Comprehension, evaluation, safe, effective care environment (b).
   2 The facility owns the patient's chart, although the patient has the right to access the chart.
   1 The patient has access to his medical information.
   3 The nurse is a patient care provider.
   4 The physician is a patient care provider; the facility owns the chart.

194. Knowledge, planning, physiological integrity (b).
   2 Generally, most individuals need to be repositioned at least every 2 hours to prevent ulcer formation.
   1 This is not a frequent enough turning schedule.
   3 The nurse should reposition the patient at least every 2 hours.
   4 Although pressure ulcers would not develop on this turning schedule, the patient would be excessively disturbed.

195. Knowledge, safe, effective care environment (a).
   4 Provision of competencies resulting in safe care is the responsibility of each provincial regulatory body.
   1 Other than in Quebec, certification, registration, and licensing examinations are set by CIS for the Canadian Nurses Association.
   2 Laws are passed by the provincial legislature.
   3 Regulatory bodies decide whether negligence exists in the individual practice of nursing and are completely autonomous from the court system.

196. Comprehension, safe, effective care environment (b).
   3 All members of the health care team work collaboratively, each with defined roles.
   1 The PN may be under the direction of an RN in some settings. In other facilities, the PN works independently or may direct others (e.g., UCPs)
   2 The RN is responsible for the direction, not the supervision, of the practical nurse and nursing assistant.
   4 The PN cares for a variety of patients with different degrees of responsibility, depending on the complexity of care required.

197. Knowledge, safe, effective care environment (a).
   3 Legislation in the province or territory regulates the designation of the title for each nursing category.
   1 Individuals in a nursing category may request and lobby for a name change, but the designation must be made through the legal body.
   2 The employing agency must use the legally designated title and employ the PN only within the designated role.

4 The educational facility must meet the standards designated for the role of the graduate and may not alter the legally designated title.

198. Knowledge, safe, effective care environment (a).
   2 Health care delivery is the responsibility of the provinces.
   1 Federal legislation applies to matters of national or international nature (e.g., testing new drugs).
   3 Regulatory bodies are provincial, not local or municipal.
   4 Professional associations are provincial, not local, and have a lobbying function only regarding legislation.

199. Comprehension, safe, effective care environment (b).
   2 Registration protects the practice of nursing through legislation, which provides mechanisms for charging individuals who are practicing without a license.
   1 The role of the licensing body is to protect the public by setting and ensuring implementation of minimum standards of safe practice.
   3 Licensure indicates the level of the practitioner but does not protect it.
   4 The individual registrant is protected while providing safe care within the minimum standards of practice of the licensing body.

200. Knowledge, safe, effective care environment (b).
   3 Provincial licensing bodies are responsible for setting admission requirements for their own jurisdiction.
   1 Educational institutions may only set admission requirements for general interest courses.
   2 Provincial professional associations may make recommendations regarding but do not set admission requirements.
   4 CAPNNA is a voluntary professional association representing provincial professional associations and, as such, has nothing to do with admission requirements.

201. Knowledge, safe, effective care environment (b).
   3 Malpractice insurance is not mandatory in Canada and is offered as an incentive to join voluntary professional associations.
   1 CAPNNA is the professional voice for PNs in Canada and has nothing to do with the legislating the practice of individual members.
   2 The role of the licensing bodies is to protect the public; therefore providing malpractice insurance would be seen as conflict of interest.
   4 Private insurance companies do not generally provide malpractice insurance for PNs; it is handled through the provincial associations.

202. Knowledge, safe, effective care environment (b).
   4 Every member of each affiliated provincial or territorial association is a member of CAPNNA on payment of association fees.
   1 Membership is voluntary and optional to individuals in provinces who are not affiliated with CAPNNA or in provinces in which the professional association and licensing body are not the same.
   2 Membership is not mandatory in any province or territory.
   3 Membership in CAPNNA is automatic with membership in affiliated provincial or territorial associations and voluntary or optional only in other provinces or territories.

203. Knowledge, safe, effective care environment (a).

2 Each PN has the responsibility to maintain competency and increase level of knowledge. In some provinces and territories, licensing bodies provide guidelines for self-evaluative practice.

1 Examinations are written only for initial registration and licensing.

3 Maintaining skill level, as well as other competencies, is the responsibility of the individual PN. The employer may supervise and make suggestions for areas needing improvement but does not retain the responsibility for individual practice.

4 The PN/NA may choose to attend a variety of educational programs to maintain and increase competence; these would vary among registrants, depending on individual needs.

204. Knowledge, safe, effective care environment (b).

3 In Canada, the provinces and territories are given responsibility for developing legislation related to nursing.

1 The regulatory body in each province and territory is designated by legislation; it does not develop the legislation.

2 The legal systems in Canada and in the United States are different in most aspects, including how nursing is regulated.

4 The legislation gives the regulatory body the authority to set standards for nursing in a variety of settings; specific directions are not outlined in the legislation.

205. Analysis, planning, physiological integrity (c).

3 This patient needs to be evaluated first. He may be alone, and the nurse will want to make sure that he has had no ill effects from the hypoglycemic episode.

1 This patient is with a respiratory therapist and is receiving a treatment.

2 The nursing assistant would alert the nurse to any potential problems.

4 The nurse has most likely been in the room to medicate the patient. He should be evaluated in 15 to 30 minutes for effectiveness.

206. Application, assessment, physiological integrity (b).

1 The nurse will expect the patient to complain of a headache, which is a primary symptom of hypertension, if he has any symptoms.

2 Dizziness is a symptom of orthostatic hypotension.

3 Diaphoresis can occur after a fever.

4 Bradycardia is not a symptom of high BP.

207 Analysis, assessment, physiological integrity (c).

4 Oliguria, or scanty urine output would be a sign of dehydration. The urine would be concentrated in nature.

1 Hematuria is a problem associated with kidney or bladder dysfunction.

2 Polyuria would be found in a patient with hypervolemia.

3 Enuresis is bedwetting, a common problem in hospitalized children but is not a sign of dehydration.

208. Analysis, planning, psychosocial integrity (b).

2 The family would benefit from a visit with a family therapist who can explain options to relieve their anxiety and strain.

1 Medications should not be given right away. Why the family is having difficulty needs to be determined. Social service may be able to assist the family.

3 This would relieve their burden only for a short time, and caregiver strain is not a reason to hospitalize an individual.

4 Whether the patient has a terminal illness has not been determined. The family performs most of the personal care of a hospice patient.

209. Comprehension, implementation, physiological integrity (c).

2 A shortage of RBCs contributes to low hemoglobin. Hemoglobin carries the oxygen within the body; therefore the patient has a reduced capacity to carry oxygen.

1 Anemia does not affect the amount of inspired air.

3 Pneumonia or atelectasis would block the patient's ability to exchange gases.

4 A problem with the pumping ability of the heart would cause a problem in the circulation of oxygen.

210. Application, planning, health promotion and maintenance (b).

3 This is the only correct statement of the selections. The patient should weigh each morning at the same time, using the same scale.

1 Depending on the patient's daily intake and activities, a weight that is obtained late in the day may be inaccurate.

2 When the patient takes his diuretic is unknown or if he is even taking one.

4 The nurse is unaware when the patient dresses for the day, and dress may change significantly from day to day, making daily weights inaccurate.

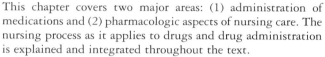

CHAPTER 3   Pharmacology

This chapter covers two major areas: (1) administration of medications and (2) pharmacologic aspects of nursing care. The nursing process as it applies to drugs and drug administration is explained and integrated throughout the text.

Calculation of dosage and intravenous infusion rate, principles of medication administration, procedures and sites for medication administration, blood transfusion administration, and pediatric drug administration are reviewed.

The major classifications of drugs are presented as to their action, adverse effects, and nursing process application. Commonly used clinical drugs are listed with generic name and brand name.

The role of the licensed practical/vocational nurse (LP/VN) in the administration of medications is determined by the state nurse practice acts and agency policy. However, knowledge of drugs has a significant impact on the quality of nursing care provided each patient by the LP/VN. The licensed practical nurse (LPN) has a legal and moral responsibility to use the nursing process in the administration of medications.

Key drugs are identified by asterisk (*).

PHARMACOLOGY AND THE NURSING PROCESS

A. Assessment: a systematic collection of subjective and objective data on the patient, drug, and environment
B. Planning: prioritize the nursing diagnosis, specify the goals and outcome criteria, and the time when these should be achieved.
C. Implementation: consists of initiation and completion of the nursing care plan as defined by the nursing diagnosis and outcome criteria
D. Evaluation: an ongoing monitoring of the patient's response to drug therapy

Assessment

A. Assessing the patient
  1. Variables
    a. Growth and development related to age
    b. Body build
    c. Past and present history
    d. Nutritional practices
    e. Allergies
    f. Sociocultural beliefs—how does this person's culture view medication and the health care system?
    g. Knowledge of disease and drugs
    h. Cognitive function—is the person able to understand the drug regimen?
    i. Physical challenges
    j. Physical assessment: vital signs, height, weight, laboratory results, and results of diagnostic tests

  2. Medication history
    a. Over-the-counter (OTC) medications
      An increasing number of medications have changed from prescription to OTC. The LPN has a responsibility to educate the patient on the dangers of self-medicating. Long-term use of OTC medications may mask symptoms of a more serious disorder.
    b. Prescription medications
    c. Substance abuse, including street drugs, smoking, alcohol, caffeine
    d. Problems with drug therapy in the past (i.e., allergies, adverse effects)
    e. Cultural variables—some medications have differing effects on individual groups.
B. Assessing the drug
  1. Medication order
    a. From a physician, dentist, or nurse practitioner (if permitted by state law)
    b. Contains patient's name, date order was written, name of medication, dosage (size, frequency, number of doses), route, signature of health care provider
    c. Accurate, legible, need for clarification
    d. Incorrect, inappropriate or illegible orders must be clarified before administration.
  2. Types of medication orders
    a. Routine or standard
    b. PRN order: given on a "when necessary" basis
    c. Single order: to be given only once
    d. STAT order: to be given only once and immediately
    e. Standing order: established for all patients with a specific condition
    f. Verbal order: must be written and signed within a specified time limit
    g. Telephone order—emergency situations only: follow hospital policy concerning who is allowed to accept.
C. Institutional level management: drug distribution systems
  1. Floor stock
  2. Individual patient medication system: a supply of medication is dispensed and labeled for a particular patient.
  3. Unit dose: individual doses of each medication ordered

Planning

A. Establish priorities: weighing the importance of one problem against another
B. Goal setting: objective, measurable, and realistic with an established time period for achievement of the outcome
C. Outcome: should reflect expected changes through nursing care
D. Outcome criteria: provide a standard of measure that can be used to move toward the goal

Implementation

A. Requires constant communication with patient and health care team
B. Proper administration of medication
  1. Approach to patient
    a. "Therapeutic use of self" attitude of nurse
    b. Consistency of approach
    c. Informed consent for patients
    d. Compliance and right to refuse
  2. Uses the five rights:
    a. Right drug
    b. Right dose
    c. Right time
    d. Right route
    e. Right patient
  3. Measures to support the therapeutic or desired effect: nursing actions can complement drug therapy or minimize unpleasant adverse reactions.
  4. Observation for desired therapeutic effect
    a. Establish baseline data for all medications
    b. Establish observational parameters—vital signs, laboratory data—to evaluate effectiveness of medications (e.g., the use of pain assessment scales).
C. Teaching patients
  1. Explain drug, dose, side effects, food-drug interactions, time schedule, method of administration, etc.
  2. Identify need for teaching.
  3. Establish realistic teaching goals.
  4. Select teaching methods.
  5. Implement teaching.
  6. Evaluate effectiveness.
D. Accurate documentation (form is set by agency policy): some institutions consider this right the sixth right.
  1. Information must be complete and accurate.
  2. Documentation must be done immediately after administration.
  3. Legal implications: if drug administration is not documented, the assumption is that the drug had not been administered.
  4. Data should include:
    a. Observations relevant to therapeutic effects
    b. Actions taken to prevent or treat adverse reactions
    c. Time when a drug is discontinued
    d. Reason or reasons for discontinuation of drug
    e. Reasons for refusal or noncompliance of patient
E. Dosage form and route
  1. Factors influencing route of administration
    a. Specific chemical and physical properties of the drug
    b. Pathologic condition of the patient
    c. Adequacy of medication compliance
  2. Dose: amount of drug to be given at one time
  3. Dosage: regulation of the frequency, size, number of doses
  4. Dosage form: final product administered to the patient
    a. Preparations for oral use
      (1) Liquids
        (a) Aqueous solutions: substances dissolved in water and syrups
        (b) Aqueous suspensions: solid particles suspended in liquid
        (c) Syrup: medication dissolved in a concentrated solution of a sugar to which flavors may have been added
        (d) Emulsions: fats or oils suspended in liquid with an emulsifier
        (e) Spirits: alcohol solution
        (f) Elixirs: aromatic sweetened alcoholic and water solution
        (g) Tinctures: alcoholic extract of plant or water solution
        (h) Fluid extract: concentrated alcoholic extract of plant or vegetables
        (i) Extract: syrup or dried form of pharmacologically active drug
      (2) Solids
        (a) Capsules: soluble case (usually gelatin) that contains liquid, dry, or beaded particles; capsules may be timed release or sustained action (slow, continuous dissolution for an extended period).
        (b) Tablets: compressed powdered drug or drugs in small disks
          ■ Enteric-coated tablets: coated with a second layer of material to prevent dissolution in stomach; disintegrates in small intestine to prevent stomach irritation
          ■ Press-coated or layered tablet: contains a second layer of material pressed on or around it, which allows incompatible ingredients to be separated and dissolve at different rates
          ■ Caplets: coated tablets in the shape of a capsule
          ■ Troches or lozenges: medicated tablets that dissolve slowly in the mouth
        (c) Powders or granules: loose or molded drug substances for drug administration with or without liquids
    b. Preparations for parenteral use
      (1) Ampules: sealed glass containers for liquid injectable medications
      (2) Vials: glass containers with a rubber stopper, usually for multiple doses; contains liquid or powdered medications
      (3) Cartridge or tubex: a single-dose unit of parenteral medication to be used with a specific injecting device
      (4) Intravenous (IV) solutions: must be sterile and particle free
        (a) Continuous infusion may be used for fluid replacement with or without medication
        (b) Intermittent runs as a secondary administration set (piggyback) hung separately from the primary set via a secondary tubing
        (c) Heparin lock (prn lock) or angiocatheter a port site for direct administration or intermittent IV medications without the need for a primary IV solution
    c. Preparations for topical use
      (1) Liniments: liquid suspensions for lubrication that are applied by rubbing
      (2) Lotions: liquid suspensions that can be protective, emollient, cooling, astringent, antipruritic, cleansing, etc.

(3) Ointments: semisolid medicines in a base for local, protective, soothing, astringent, or transdermal application for systemic effects (e.g., nitroglycerin, scopolamine, estrogen)

(4) Paste: thick ointments used primarily for skin protection

(5) Plasters: solid preparations that are adhesive, protective, or soothing

(6) Creams: emulsions that contain an aqueous and an oily base

(7) Aerosols: fine powders or solutions in volatile liquids that contain a propellant

(8) Transdermal patches: patches containing medication that is absorbed continuously through the skin and acts systemically

(9) Powders: finely ground drugs or combinations of drugs

d. Preparations for use on mucous membranes

(1) Drops are aqueous solutions with or without a gelling agent (to increase retention time in the eye); drops can be used for eyes, ears, or nose.

(2) Topical installation of an aqueous solution of medications usually for topical action but occasionally used for systemic effects, including enemas, douches, mouthwashes, throat sprays, gargles

(3) Aerosol sprays, nebulizers, and inhalers deliver aqueous solutions of medication in droplet form to the target membrane, such as bronchial tree (bronchodilators).

(4) Foams are powders or solutions of medication in volatile liquids with a propellant, such as vaginal foams for contraception.

(5) Suppositories usually contain medicinal substances mixed in a firm but malleable base to facilitate insertion into a body cavity (e.g., rectal, vaginal); can be used for local or systemic effects

e. Miscellaneous drug delivery systems

(1) Intradermal implants are pellets containing a small deposit of medication that are inserted in a dermal pocket, usually used to administer hormones such as testosterone or estradiol.

(2) Micropump system is a small, external pump, attached by belt or implanted that delivers medication via a needle in a continuous, steady dose. Examples include insulin, anticancer chemotherapy, opioids.

F. Dosage route: means of access to the site of action or systemic circulation; divided into three classifications

1. Enteral: administered directly into gastrointestinal (GI) tract

a. Oral: drug is ingested and absorbed from stomach or small intestine; convenient and economical; can irritate stomach; may be destroyed by digestive juices.

b. Rectal: drug is inserted into rectum and absorbed through mucous membrane; may be used in unconscious or vomiting patient.

2. Parenteral: in practice, parenteral means administration via a needle; drugs must be sterile, and aseptic technique must be used.

a. Intradermal: drug is injected directly under the skin; amount of drug is small and absorption is slow; examples of use include allergy testing, tuberculosis (TB) testing, administering small amounts of anesthesia.

b. Subcutaneous: drug is injected under the skin into subcutaneous fascia; ideally, solutions are limited to no more than 1 ml of solution; examples of use include insulin, heparin, and morphine.

c. Intramuscular: drug is injected into muscle mass; relatively rapid absorption result of good blood supply; larger volumes up to 5 ml can be given.

d. Intravenous: drug is injected into the vein for immediate effect; permits direct control of blood drug concentrations; used when an immediate effect is desired; can be given by injection or infusion; useful in emergency situations; precautions must be taken to avoid infiltration.

e. Epidural (this route is performed by a physician; however, the nurse is responsible for assisting and monitoring sites and effects). A catheter is implanted beneath the skin with its tip in the epidural space; the drug diffuses into the central spinal fluid, bypassing the blood-brain barrier; frequently used in the management of acute and chronic pain.

f. Intraarterial (this route is performed by a physician; however, the nurse is responsible for assisting and monitoring sites and effects): drug is injected directly into an artery.

g. Intraarticular (this route is performed by a physician; however, the nurse is responsible for assisting and monitoring sites and effects): drug is injected directly into a joint.

h. Intraspinal (this route is performed by a physician; however, the nurse is responsible for assisting and monitoring sites and effects): drug is injected directly into spinal canal.

3. Percutaneous: application of medications to the skin or mucous membranes; may be used for local or systemic effects

a. Sublingual: drug is dissolved under tongue and absorbed through mucous membrane of mouth; can irritate oral mucosa; number of drugs given this way is limited—nitroglycerin is primary example.

b. Buccal: drug is dissolved between cheek and gum and absorbed through mucous membrane of the mouth.

c. Lungs: drug is inhaled as a gas or aerosol; useful for drugs intended to act directly on the lungs.

d. Vaginal: drug is inserted into the vagina and absorbed through the mucous membrane.

e. Ophthalmic: drug is applied to the eye in form of drops or ointments; must be sterile.

f. Otic or aural: drug is applied in the ear.

g. Nasal: drug is applied to the nasal cavity using a dropper or atomizer.

h. Transdermal: patch is applied to skin that provides controlled release of medication.

Evaluation

A. Therapeutic goals: evaluate therapeutic effectiveness of drugs.

B. Diagnostic goals: observe for potential adverse reactions.

C. Teaching goals: verify patient's knowledge of drug or ability to perform a skill necessary for administration of the drug.

D. Patient compliance: evaluate patient adherence to a pre-scribed plan of treatment. Therapeutic blood levels are checked with many medications to determine effectiveness.

SOURCES OF DRUGS

A. Animals
B. Plants
C. Microorganisms
D. Synthetic chemical substances
E. Food substances

DRUG NAMES

A. Generic: the official, established nonproprietary name assigned to a drug; a drug is licensed under its generic name and is often less expensive than brand names.
B. Brand (trademark): a name assigned to a drug by its manu-facturer; the copyright restricts the use of this name to the specific manufacturer.
C. Chemical: the exact designation of the chemical structure as determined by the rules of accepted systems of chemical nomenclature
D. A drug may be considered a prescription drug, which means a legal prescription is required to be dispensed, or it may be a nonprescription or OTC, which may be purchased without a prescription.

DRUG LEGISLATION

A. Food, Drug, and Cosmetic Act of 1938 (amended 1952, 1962)
   1. Contains detailed regulations to ensure that drugs meet standards of safety and effectiveness
   2. Requires physician's prescription for legal drug purchase
B. Controlled Substances Act of 1970
   1. Defines drug dependency and drug addiction
   2. Classifies drugs according to potential abuse and medical usefulness
   3. Establishes methods for regulating manufacture, distri-bution, and sale of controlled substances
   4. Establishes education and treatment programs for drug abuse
C. Controlled substances schedule
Schedule I: Drugs that have a high potential for abuse and are not approved for medical use in the United States (e.g., cocaine)
Schedule II: Drugs that have a high potential for abuse but have a currently accepted medical use in the United States; abuse may lead to severe psychologic or physical dependence (e.g., morphine sulfate)
Schedule III: Drugs that have a lower potential for abuse than those in schedules I and II; abuse may lead to high psychologic or low-to-moderate physical dependence (e.g., aspirin [Empirin] with codeine)
Schedule IV: Drugs that have some potential for abuse; abuse may lead to limited psychologic or physical dependence (e.g., diazepam [Valium])
Schedule V: Drugs that have the lowest potential for abuse; products that contain moderate amounts of controlled substances that may be dispensed by the pharmacist without a physician's prescription but with some restric-tions such as amount, record keeping, and other safeguards (e.g., Robitussin A-C)
D. Drug Regulating Reform Act—shortened the drug investi-gation process to release drugs sooner to the public
E. Orphan Drug Act—encouraged drug companies, through grants from the federal government, to investigate rare conditions

PRINCIPLES OF DRUG ACTION

A. The physiologic means by which a drug exerts its desired effects
B. Examples include increasing or decreasing the rate at which a cell or tissue functions or replacing something that is needed by the body.

PHARMACOKINETICS

A. The study of what actually happens to a drug from the time it enters the body until it leaves the body
B. Includes onset, peak, and duration of the drug

Mechanisms of Drug Therapy

A. Dissolution: disintegration of dose form; dissolution of an active substance
B. Absorption: the process that occurs between the time a substance enters the body and the time it enters the bloodstream
C. Distribution: the transport of drug molecules within the body to receptor sites
D. Metabolism: biotransformation—the way in which drugs are inactivated by the body
E. Excretion: elimination of a drug from the body

Variables That Affect Drug Action

A. Dosage
B. Route of administration
C. Drug-diet interactions: food slows absorption of drugs; some foods containing certain substances react with certain drugs.
D. Drug-drug interactions
   1. Additive effect: occurs when two drugs with similar actions are taken together
   2. Synergism (potentiation): a total effect of two similar drugs that is greater than the sum of the effects if each is taken separately
   3. Interference: when one drug interferes with the meta-bolism or elimination of a second drug, resulting in intensification of the second drug
   4. Displacement: when one drug is displaced from a plasma protein-binding site by a second, causing an increased effect of the displaced drug
   5. Antagonism: a decrease in the effects of drugs caused by the action of one on the other
E. Age
   1. Fetus: metabolism and elimination mechanisms immature
   2. Newborn: organ systems not fully developed
   3. Children: depends on age and developmental stage
   4. Elderly adults: physiologic changes may alter a drug's actions in the body. Elderly patients often take more than

one medication. Therefore the chances for interactions are increased.

F. Body weight: affects drug action mainly in relation to dosage
G. Pregnancy: many medications cross the placental barrier and can be harmful to the fetus.
H. Pathologic condition: disease processes are capable of altering drug mechanisms (e.g., patients with kidney disease have increased risk of drug toxicity because they have difficulty eliminating the medication, patients with liver disease have difficulty metabolizing medications).
I. Psychologic considerations: attitudes and expectations influence patient response (e.g., anxiety can decrease effect of analgesics).

Drug Effects

A. Desired or therapeutic effect is the reason why a medication is administered.
B. Side effects are usually predictable secondary effects produced by the medication; they may be desirable or undesirable.
C. Adverse effects are unintended and unpredictable. The nurse must be alert to reports of any adverse effects after the administration of medications.

Adverse Reactions to Drugs

A. Idiosyncratic reaction: unusual, unexpected reaction, usually the first time a drug is taken
B. Allergic reactions: stimulate antibody reactions from the immune system of body
   1. Urticaria (hives)
   2. Anaphylaxis: severe allergic reaction involving cardiovascular and respiratory systems; may be life threatening
C. GI effects
   1. Anorexia
   2. Nausea, vomiting
   3. Constipation
   4. Diarrhea
   5. Abdominal distention
D. Hematologic effects
   1. Blood dyscrasia
   2. Bone marrow depression
   3. Blood coagulation disorders
E. Hepatotoxicity
   1. Hepatitis
   2. Biliary tract obstruction or spasms
F. Nephrotoxicity: renal insufficiency or failure; kidney stones
G. Drug dependence
   1. Physiologic: physical need to relieve shaking; pain
   2. Psychologic: need to relieve feeling of anxiety; stress
H. Teratogenicity: ability of a drug to cause abnormal fetal development

Tolerance and Cross-Tolerance

A. Tolerance: acclimation of the body to a drug over a period so that larger doses must be given to achieve the same effect
B. Cross-tolerance: tolerance to pharmacologically related drugs

Sources of Drug Information

A. Resource people
   1. Pharmacists
   2. Physicians
   3. Registered nurses
B. Poison control centers

C. Published sources of information
   1. United States Pharmacopeia (USP) and National Formulary (NF)
      a. Official reference books
      b. Establish legally binding standards to which drugs must conform
      c. Revised every 5 years, with periodic supplements
   2. Package insert: Food and Drug Administration (FDA)–approved label for drug products in the United States
   3. Physicians' Desk Reference (PDR)
      a. Published annually, with interim supplements
      b. Contains information supplied by manufacturers
      c. Is most useful for finding drugs according to brand name
   4. American Hospital Formulary Service
      a. Contains data on almost every drug available in the United States
      b. Kept current by periodic supplements
   5. Pharmacology textbooks; drug reference books and cards; on-line sources are often listed from the publisher.
   6. Nursing journals
   7. On-line sources, including the American Nurses' Association (ANA) and the Centers for Disease Control and Prevention (CDC)

Nursing Process

A. Assessment: obtain data on patient regarding problems related to:
   1. Route of administration
   2. Elimination or metabolism (particular attention paid to persons with renal or hepatic disease)
   3. Baseline laboratory values
   4. Patient teaching needs
B. Planning
   1. Proper timing of dosage
   2. Ways to improve the effectiveness of the drug
   3. Instruction of patient concerning the drug
C. Implementation
   1. Proper method of administration
   2. Proper timing of dosage
   3. Instruction of patient concerning the drug
D. Evaluation
   1. Effectiveness of drug
      a. Subjective: questioning the patient for expected response of the drug (i.e., pain relief, reduction in symptoms)
      b. Objective: monitoring physical response by the nurse (i.e., decreased blood pressure, increased cardiac regularity)
      c. Pain relief charts: required by Joint Commission on Accreditation of Healthcare Organization (JCAHO)
   2. Presence of side effects, adverse reactions
   3. Effectiveness of patient teaching
   4. If therapy is ineffective, examine possible causes, such as drug interactions.

ADMINISTERING MEDICATIONS

Calculation of Dosage

A. Practical nurse responsibility
   1. Abide by the guidelines of the health care agency.
   2. Check for accuracy in dosage calculation before preparing and administering drug.

3. Check calculations with another knowledgeable person.
4. Measure doses exactly as prescribed by physician.

B. Systems of measurement
1. Household system: measurements commonly used in the home; not as accurate as other systems; examples include:
   a. 1 teaspoon (tsp or t) = 60 drops (gtt)
   b. 3 or 4 tsp = 1 tablespoon (tbsp or T)
2. Apothecary system: an older system but one that continues to be used in dosage calculations
   a. Common units of measurements
      (1) Weight: grain (gr)
      (2) Volume
         (a) 60 minims = 1 dram (dr or ℥)
         (3) 8 dr = 1 ounce (oz or [dram])
   b. Notations in this system use lowercase Roman numerals; quantities less than 1 are expressed as common factors; exception: one half is written as ss.
3. Metric system: international decimal system
   a. Common units of measurement
      (1) Weight: unit is expressed in terms of the gram (g)
         (a) Prefix kilo indicates 1000
         (b) Prefix milli indicates 1/1000
         (c) 1 g = 1000 milligrams (mg)
      (2) Volume: unit is expressed in terms of the liter (L)
         (a) Prefix milli indicates 1/1000
         (b) 1 L = 1000 milliliters (ml)
   b. Notations in this system use Arabic numbers; fractions are expressed as decimals.
4. Equivalents between systems: a given quantity considered to be of equal value to a quantity expressed in a different system; some common approximate equivalents are:
   a. 1 kilograms (kg) = 2.2 pounds (lb)
   b. 1 g = 15 gr
   c. 60 mg = 1 gr
   d. 1 cubic centimeter (cc) = 1 ml
   e. 1000 ml = 1 quart (qt)
   f. 30 ml = 1 oz
   g. 1 ml = 15 or 16 gtt
   h. 1 tsp = 4 or 5 ml

C. Mathematics of conversion within and between systems; ratio and proportion method

1. Household

   EXAMPLE: 3 TSP = _____ GTT
   teaspoons : drops :: teaspoons : drops
   1 tsp to 60 gtt :: 3 tsp to x gtt
   x = 180
   Answer: 3 tsp = 180 gtt

2. Apothecary system

   EXAMPLE: 3 OZ = _____ DR
   ounces : drams :: ounces : drams
   8 dr to 1 oz :: 3 oz to x dr
   x = 24
   Answer: 3 oz = 24 dr

3. Metric system

   EXAMPLE: 250 MG = _____ G
   milligram : gram :: milligram : gram
   1000 x = 250 (divide x into both parts of the equation to equal 1 x)
   x = 0.25
   Answer: 250 mg = 0.25 g

4. Conversion between systems

   EXAMPLE: GR 1/6 = _____ MG
   grains : milligrams :: grains : milligrams
   1 : 60 :: 1/6 : x
   1x = 60 = 1/6
   x = 10
   Answer: gr 1/6 = 10 mg

D. Dosage calculations: the dose for oral tablets, capsules, and liquids or solutions for injections can be calculated by using the following formula:
Desired dose (D) ÷ Dose on hand (H) × Quantity (Q) = Amount to be given.

   EXAMPLE: GIVE 500 MG OF TETRACYCLINE (ACHROMYCIN) USING CAPSULES CONTAINING 250 MG
   D ÷ H × Q = 500 mg ÷ 250 mg × 1 capsule =
   Answer: 2 capsules

   EXAMPLE: PHYSICIAN ORDERS DIGOXIN 0.125 MG TO BE GIVEN ORALLY; STOCK BOTTLE IS LABELED "DIGOXIN 0.25-MG" SCORED TABLETS
   D ÷ H × Q = 0.125 mg ÷ 0.25 mg × 1 tablet =
   Answer: 0.5 tablet or 1/2 tablet

   EXAMPLE: ERYTHROMYCIN SUSPENSION 750 MG IS ORDERED ORALLY. THE BOTTLE IS LABELED 250 MG/5 ML.
   D ÷ H × Q = 750 mg ÷ 250 mg × 5 ml =
   Answer: 15 ml

   EXAMPLE: MORPHINE SULFATE GR 1/4 IS TO BE GIVEN BY SUBCUTANEOUS INJECTION; THE VIAL IS LABELED "MORPHINE SULFATE GR 1/2/ML."
   D ÷ H × Q = gr 1/4 ÷ gr 1/2 × 1 ml =
   Answer: 0.5 ml

   EXAMPLE: PENICILLIN 600,000 UNITS IS TO BE GIVEN BY INTRAMUSCULAR INJECTION; THE VIAL IS LABELED "PENICILLIN 300,000 UNITS PER ML."
   D ÷ H = Q = 600,000 units ÷ 300,000 units × 1 ml =
   Answer: 2 ml

   NOTE: This formula can be used with any system of measurement. When two systems are involved, converting to the system of measurement of the dose on hand is required.

   EXAMPLE: CODEINE SULFATE GR SS. IS ORDERED BY MOUTH; ON HAND ARE CODEINE SULFATE TABLETS LABELED 30 MG.

   STEP 1: CONVERSION BETWEEN SYSTEMS
   grain : milligram :: grain : milligram
   1 : 60 :: 1/2 : x
   x = 60 x 1/2
   x = 30
   Answer: codeine gr ss = 30 mg

   STEP 2: FORMULA
   D ÷ H × Q = 30 mg ÷ 30 mg × 1
   Answer: 1 tablet

Calculation of Drip Rates for Intravenous Infusion

A. Information that must be known
1. Volume of solution to be infused
2. Length of time over which this volume is to be infused

3. Number of drops per milliliter delivered by the administration set being used

B. The drip rate may be calculated as follows:
1. Find the volume of fluid to be administered per hour. Milliliters of fluid to be infused divided by the number of hours for infusion equals milliliters of fluid per hour.
2. Find the volume of fluid to be administered per minute. Milliliters of fluid per hour divided by 60 min/hr equals milliliters to run per minute.
3. Multiply the milliliters of fluid to run per minute by the number of drops per milliliter delivered by the infusion set; this gives the number of drops that should fall in the drip chamber per minute.

Milliliters per minute × Drops per milliliter = Drops per minute.

EXAMPLE: ADMINISTER 1000 ML OF DEXTROSE 5% IN WATER (D5W) OVER 8 HOURS USING AN INFUSION SET THAT DELIVERS 10 GTT PER MINUTE
1000 ml ÷ 8 hr = 125 ml/hr
125 ml/hr ÷ 60 min/hr = 2.1 ml/min
2.1 ml/min × 10 gtt/ml = _____
Answer: 21 gtt/min

EXAMPLE: ADMINISTER 250 ML OF D5W OVER 8 HOURS USING A MICRODRIP INFUSION SET THAT DELIVERS 60 GTT/ML
250 ml ÷ 8 hr = 31.25 ml/hr
31.25 ml/hr ÷ 60 min/hr = 0.52 ml/min
0.52 ml/min × 60 gtt/ml = 31.2 gtt/min
Answer: 31 gtt/min

C. If the administration rate has been ordered as milliliters per hour, step 1 above is omitted.
D. Alternate formula to calculate drip rate:
Milliliters to administer × Drops per milliliter ÷ (Hours to run × 60 min/hr) = Drops per milliliter

EXAMPLE: ADMINISTER 1000 ML OF D5W OVER 8 HOURS USING AN INFUSION SET THAT DELIVERS 10 GTT/MILLILITER
1000 ml × 10 gtt/ml ÷ 8 hr × 60 min/hr =
Answer: 21 gtt/min

E. Adjust the flow rate to the number of drops per minute as calculated; assess the fluid volume at hourly intervals to see that the fluid is being administered at the desired rate; the calculated drip rate is an approximation of the actual flow rate; the type of solution, additives, position of the patient or infusion tubing, height of the reservoir, and volume of fluid in the container can influence the actual drip rate; the practical nurse should verify computations with another knowledgeable person before readjusting the drip rate to ensure volume delivery for the prescribed time.

Methods of Administering Medications

A. Nurse's responsibilities
1. Knowledge of drug
   a. Actions
   b. Ranges of dosage
   c. Methods of administration
   d. Common use
   e. Adverse reactions
   f. Contraindications
   g. Patient education
2. Assess patient regarding history of allergies or sensitivities to drugs.
3. Be aware of and follow agency's policy regarding procedure by which the medication order is checked.
4. Know agency's system of medication distribution.
   a. Cards
   b. Kardex or Medex
   c. Computer printout sheet
5. Know occasions and parameters when drugs may be withheld.
   a. Fasting for diagnostic tests or surgery; illness
   b. Required laboratory blood work before medication administration; certain medications may require therapeutic levels to determine if medication is being maintain in proper range versus nontherapeutic or toxic.
   c. Specific guidelines for certain drugs, for example, apical pulse rate before cardiotonics or blood pressure (BP) readings before antihypertensive agents
6. Position the patient to properly administer medications; assist as needed.
7. Observe the "five rights" of medication administration.
   a. Right patient
   b. Right drug
   c. Right dose
   d. Right route
   e. Right time
   Most sources still refer to the "five rights" of medication administration; however, a few sources have added "right documentation and right technique." Both of these are included in this list of nursing responsibilites.
8. Inform the patient of any anticipated change in normal body functions, such as drowsiness, nausea, or change in color of urine.
9. Report patient noncompliance or adverse reactions to other responsible person (i.e., registered nurse, physician).
10. Follow procedure for controlled substances.
11. Remain with patient until medication is taken.
12. Never leave medications at patient's bedside unless specifically ordered.
13. Ensure accuracy in drug calculation; when in doubt, verify with other responsible person (i.e., registered nurse, pharmacist).
14. Check expiration date on all medication labels and orders.
15. Accurately document medications given, and, if omitted or refused, document reason.
16. Document effectiveness of medication.
17. Be aware of and follow agency procedure in event of medication error.
18. Acknowledge and respect patient's request to refuse medication.

B. Safety measures in preparing medications
1. Environment
   a. Quiet
   b. Free from distractions
   c. Good lighting
2. Do not leave prepared medications unattended; keep in a locked area.
3. Read each label three times.
   a. When reaching for the container
   b. Immediately before pouring the medication
   c. When replacing or discarding the container

4. Transport drugs for administration by using trays or carts that allow the identifying information and the medication container to be kept together safely.
5. Do not allow tray or cart to be left out of sight during administration.
6. Make positive identification of patient before administering the medication, preferably by checking the patient's identification bracelet, having patient state his or her name, having second person identify patient.
7. Remain with the patient until patient takes the medication.
8. Document necessary supplemental information (e.g., pulse rate, BP, site of application or injection) according to agency policy.
9. Guidelines for drug safety at home
   a. Keep each drug in original, labeled container.
   b. Be sure labels are legible.
   c. Discard any outdated medications.
   d. Always finish a prescribed drug unless otherwise instructed.
   e. Dispose of drug in sink or toilet.
   f. Do not give one family member a drug prescribed for another family member.
   g. Refrigerate medications if required.
   h. Read labels carefully and follow all instructions.
   i. Use childproof caps when appropriate.
C. Oral administration of medications
   1. General information
      a. Simplest and most convenient route
      b. Liquid preparations
         (1) Pour into a container placed on a flat surface.
         (2) Read at eye level.
         (3) Measure amount by using the bottom of meniscus.
      c. Irritating drugs should be dissolved or diluted and given with food or immediately after a meal.
   d. Distasteful oral medications can be disguised, for example, by having patient suck on a piece of ice for a few minutes to numb taste buds, by storing oily medications in a refrigerator, by having patient use a straw, or by mixing medication with a small amount of fruit juice, milk, applesauce, or gelatin; always inform patient that a food vehicle contains the medication.
   e. For patients who have difficulty swallowing tablets, some tablets may be crushed to facilitate swallowing; be aware of contraindications for crushing of certain medications (e.g., enteric-coated tablets) or of opening capsules containing timed-release medications.
   f. Liquid medications that are harmful to teeth (e.g., liquid iron preparations) should be administered with a straw placed at the back of the tongue.
   2. Specific procedure is described in Table 3-1.
D. Parenteral administration of medications: administration by a route other than through the enteral or GI tract, such as intradermal, subcutaneous, intramuscular, or intravenous routes
   1. General information: maintain surgical aseptic technique in preparation and administration; using prepackaged, disposable sterile needles and syringes is preferable.
   2. Selection of syringe and needle: thick or oily solutions require a large lumen; short needles are used for children and adults with little adipose tissue; obese individuals may require longer needles to ensure delivery of medications to proper tissue level (Table 3-2).
   3. Putting the drugs into the syringe
      a. Manufacturer prefilled syringes or cartridges: contain the name and dose of the drug and the intended parenteral route; should not be given by any route other than the one specified

---

TABLE 3-1   Administration of Oral Medications

Suggested Action	Rationale
Wash hands before administration, and practice medical asepsis while preparing and administering medication.	Careful hand washing and separate medication cups prevent cross-contamination between nurse and patients.
Check the order, and read the label three times while preparing the drug.	Frequent checking prevents errors and ensures accuracy.
Pour tablets and capsules into the cap of a stock container, and then transfer proper amount into medication cup.	Pouring medications into the nurse's hand contaminates the tablet or capsule.
Pour liquids from the side of the bottle opposite the label.	Liquid that may spill onto the label makes reading the label difficult.
Transport medications to patient's bedside carefully.	Accidental or deliberate disarrangement of medications is prevented.
Keep medications in sight at all times.	For safety reasons
Identify patient carefully.	Illness and different environment can often cause confusion.
Assist patient to an upright position as necessary.	Proper positioning facilitates swallowing.
Offer sufficient water or other permitted fluids.	Liquids allow for ease in swallowing and help dissolve solid drugs.
Remain with patient until each medication is swallowed.	Patient may discard unwanted medications or may accumulate them with intent to harm himself or herself.
Document each medication administered, both promptly and according to agency's policy; report or document medications not taken.	The patient's chart is a legal record; prompt documentation avoids the possibility of repeating administration of the same drug.
If patient's intake is being measured, record the amount of fluid taken with the medication.	All fluids taken are to be recorded for determining total intake.

b. Rubber-capped vials: single or multidose container; solution or powder form; dry form of drug dissolved according to label instructions; to remove the drug:
  (1) Remove the soft metal cover on top of the vial.
  (2) Using friction, wipe the rubber cap with a pledget soaked with antiseptic solution.
  (3) Fill syringe with air equal to amount of solution to be withdrawn to increase pressure within the vial and to facilitate withdrawal of solution.
  (4) Insert needle into the rubber cap while holding the needle in a slightly lateral position to prevent a piece of the stopper from entering the vial.
  (5) Inject the air and remove prescribed amount of solution while holding the syringe in a vertical position.
c. Glass ampules: prescored or unscored tops; constricted neck ampules require that solution be in base of ampule
  (1) Quickly snap finger on the stem to move the solution into the base of the ampule.
  (2) Hold the ampule in one hand.
  (3) Protecting the fingers of the other hand with a sterile, dry gauze pledget, break off the stem of the ampule; check solution for fragments of glass.
  (4) Insert needle into the opened ampule, avoiding needle contamination by not touching the rim of the ampule with the needle.
  (5) Keep needle under solution and withdraw the prescribed amount of the solution.
4. Skin preparation
  a. Heavily soiled skin in area of intended injection site should be washed with soap and water.
  b. Antiseptic-soaked gauze or pledget is then used to disinfect injection site and thus prevent injection of harmful organism into body tissue.
    (1) Wipe in a circular motion, starting at point of injection and moving outward to carry debris away from injection site.
    (2) Use firm pressure and friction when wiping to help remove soil.
5. Reduce discomfort
  a. Use sharp needle.
  b. Use appropriate gauge.
  c. Select site free of irritation or nodules from previous injections.
  d. Numb skin receptors using cold compresses or ice cube over injection site.

e. Hold tissue taut or compress tissue to form a pad, depending on type of injection.
f. Be sure no solution is on the needle.
g. Help patient relax.
h. Insert needle without hesitation.
i. Aspirate when appropriate.
j. Inject solution slowly.
k. Remove needle quickly.
l. Massage area after injection unless contraindicated with certain medications or certain routes (i.e., intradermal, z-track). Heparin
6. Care of equipment after injections: use needle-disposal unit; follow agency policy.
7. Injection sites
  a. Intradermal injection: solutions injected directly under the epidermis into the dermis (10- to 15-degree angle)
    (1) Absorption occurs slowly through the capillaries.
    (2) Common site: inner aspect of the forearm
  b. Subcutaneous injection: solutions injected into the subcutaneous layer of the skin (45- to 90-degree angle)
    (1) Common sites
      (a) Outer aspect of upper arm
      (b) Thigh
      (c) Lower abdomen
      (d) Upper back
    (2) Suggested procedure for subcutaneous injection is described in Table 3-3.
  c. Intramuscular (IM) injection: solutions injected into the muscular layer of tissue (90-degree angle)
    (1) Common sites
      (a) Dorsogluteal site
      (b) Ventrogluteal site
      (c) Vastus lateralis muscle
      (d) Deltoid muscle
      (e) Posterior triceps muscle
      (f) Rectus femoris muscle
    (2) Suggested procedure for IM injection is described in Table 3-4
  d. Z-track injection: technique used to prevent damage to and staining of the skin and subcutaneous tissues; common site is the upper outer quadrant of the gluteal region.
  e. IV infusion: administration of a large amount of fluid into a vein
    (1) Purposes
      (a) To restore or maintain electrolyte balance
      (b) To supply drugs for immediate effect
      (c) To replace nutrients and vitamins
      (d) To replace blood loss
    (2) Nurse practice acts and agency policy dictate who may administer IV infusions.
    (3) Nurse's responsibilities for IV infusion
      (a) Verifying physician's order
      (b) Calculating rate of flow
      (c) Monitoring rate of flow
      (d) Assessing patient for adverse reactions
        ▪ Infiltration
        ▪ Circulatory overload
        ▪ Thrombophlebitis
  f. Hyperalimentation: total parenteral nutrition (TPN), that is, an IV infusion containing sufficient nutrients to sustain life; provides amino acids, glucose, vitamins, and electrolytes for patients who are unable to ingest

TABLE 3-2	Selection of Syringe and Needle	
Type of Injection	Syringe Size	Needle Size
Intradermal	1 ml calibrated in tenths or hundredths of a milliliter or in minims	26 or 27 gauge, $\frac{1}{2}$ or $\frac{3}{4}$ inch
Subcutaneous	2, 2 $\frac{1}{2}$, or 3 ml calibrated in 0.1 ml	25 gauge, $\frac{1}{2}$ or $\frac{5}{8}$ inch
Intramuscular	2-5 ml calibrated in 0.2 ml	10 or 22 gauge, 1 $\frac{1}{2}$ inch
Insulin (subcutaneous)	Insulin syringe 1-2 ml calibrated in units	25, 26, or 27 gauge, $\frac{1}{2}$ or $\frac{5}{8}$ inch

TABLE 3-3   Administration of Subcutaneous Injection

Suggested Action	Rationale
Verify physician's order and read medication three times; check expiration date.	Ensures accuracy and prevents errors
Obtain and assemble equipment maintaining sterile technique.	Prevents contamination
Draw the drug into syringe and protect needle with sterile needle cover.	Prevents needle contamination from exposure to air or contact with moist surface
Identify patient by identification bracelet and by having patient state name, if possible.	Prevents potential medication error
Select appropriate injection site and cleanse area with antiseptic pledget, using firm, circular motion, moving outward from injection site.	Friction helps clean skin and decreases possibility of introducing bacteria into body
Grasp the tissue surrounding the injection site and hold it to form a cushion pad.	Ensures placement of medication into subcutaneous tissue and helps prevent deposition of medication into muscle tissue
Inject the needle quickly at an angle of 45 to 90 degrees, depending on the quality and amount of tissue and length of needle.	Ensures placement of medication into subcutaneous tissue
After needle is in proper tissue level, release grasp of the tissue.	Reduces discomfort of injection
Aspirate to determine whether needle is in a blood vessel.	Prevents discomfort and possible serious reaction if medication is injected into vein
If there is no blood return, inject solution slowly.	Reduces discomfort by reducing pressure in subcutaneous tissue
Withdraw needle quickly.	Reduces discomfort
Massage area gently, unless contraindicated with certain medications.	Helps to distribute the solution and hasten absorption of the medication

TABLE 3-4   Administration of Intramuscular Injection

Suggested Action	Rationale
Verify physician's order and read medication label three times; check expiration date.	Ensures accuracy and prevents errors
Obtain and assemble equipment, maintaining sterile technique.	Prevents contamination
Draw the drug into syringe; create small air bubble in the syringe; protect needle with sterile needle cover.	Air bubble forces medication out of needle shaft when injected; exposure to air or contact with moist surfaces contaminates needle
Identify patient by identification bracelet and by having patient state name, if possible.	Prevents potential medication error
Have the patient assume appropriate position according to site selected.	Helps relax muscles and eases discomfort
Select appropriate injection site and cleanse area with antiseptic pledget, using firm, circular motion, moving outward from injection site.	Friction helps to clean the skin, thus decreasing possibility of introducing bacteria into body tissue
Press down and hold tissue taut over the injection site.	Ensures needle reaches muscle layer
Hold syringe at 90-degree angle and quickly thrust needle into the tissue.	Minimizes discomfort
Aspirate to determine whether needle is in a blood vessel.	Prevents discomfort and possible serious reaction if medication injected into vein
If there is no blood return, inject medication slowly, followed by the air bubble.	Reduces discomfort and allows medication to disperse into the tissue; air bubble clears medication from needle
Withdraw needle quickly.	Reduces discomfort
Massage area gently, unless contraindicated with certain medications.	Helps distribute the solution and hasten absorption of the medication

nutrients normally for extended periods and for whom standard infusions are inadequate

  g. Blood transfusion: infusion of whole blood from a healthy person into a recipient's vein

    (1) Blood is typed and cross-matched before administration to determine compatibility.

    (2) Nurse's responsibility for blood transfusion

      (a) Check and double-check
- Labels
- Numbers
- Rh factor
- Compatibility

(b) Stay with patient for at least the first 5 minutes after transfusion is started.

(c) Monitor rate of transfusion.

(d) Assess patient for signs of adverse reactions.

- Hemolytic reaction: stop transfusion immediately, keep vein open with slow drip normal saline solution, and notify physician; indications include:
  - □ Headache
  - □ Sensations of tingling
  - □ Difficulty in breathing
  - □ Pain in lumbar region or legs
- Allergic reactions: stop transfusion immediately and notify physician; indications include:
  - □ Pruritus
  - □ Hives (urticaria)
  - □ Difficulty in breathing
- Febrile reactions resulting from contaminant in the blood: usually occurs late in the transfusion or after it is completed; indications include:
  - □ Flushed skin
  - □ Elevated temperature
  - □ Chills, muscular spasms
  - □ General malaise
  - □ Signs of systemic infection
- Circulatory overload can lead to pulmonary edema; indications include:
  - □ Increased pulse rate
  - □ Dyspnea
  - □ Respiratory distress
  - □ Moist coughing
  - □ Expectoration of blood-tinged mucus
- Anticoagulant reaction: indications include:
  - □ Tingling in the fingers
  - □ Muscular cramping
  - □ Convulsions

h. Blood extracts: specific components of whole blood that meet specific needs of the patient
  (1) Packed red blood cells (RBCs)
  (2) Plasma
  (3) Human albumin
  (4) Fibrinogen
  (5) Gamma globulin

PEDIATRIC DRUG ADMINISTRATION

General Rules

A. The child's age, weight, and level of growth and development should guide pediatric drug therapy.

B. The nurse's approach to the child should convey the impression that he or she expects the child to take the medication.

C. Explanation regarding the medication should be based on the child's level of understanding.

D. The nurse must be honest with the child regarding the procedure.

E. Mixing distasteful medication or crushed tablets with a small amount of honey, applesauce, or gelatin may be necessary.

F. Never threaten a child with an injection if he or she refuses an oral medication.

G. All medications should be kept out of the reach of children, and medications should never be referred to as candy.

Calculating the Pediatric Dose

Safe dosage ranges of drugs are less well defined for children than they are for adults. Not all drug dosage ranges for children are listed in the literature. Determining the dose of a drug for the infant or child is not the nurse's responsibility; but verifying or calculating a dose as a fraction of the adult dose may occasionally be necessary. The following methods may be used:

A. Body surface area: considered most accurate; requires a nomogram (i.e., a device for rapid estimation of body surface area)

$$\text{Child's dose} = \frac{\text{Body surface area (in square meters)}}{1.73 \text{ m}^2} \times \text{Adult dose.}$$

B. Clark's rule: based on weight and used for children at least 2 years of age

$$\text{Child's dose} = \frac{\text{Weight (in pounds)}}{150} \times \text{Adult dose.}$$

C. Young's rule: based on age and used for children at least 2 years of age

$$\text{Child's dose} = \frac{\text{Age (in years)}}{\text{Age (in years)} + 12} \times \text{Adult dose}$$

D. Fried's rule: used for children less than 2 years of age

$$\text{Child's dose} = \frac{\text{Age (in months)}}{150} \times \text{Adult dose}$$

Identifying the Patient

A. Check the child's identification bracelet.

B. Ask the older child his or her name.

Oral Medication

Verify, calculate, and document all medications.

A. Infants
  1. Draw up liquid medication in a dropper or a syringe without the needle.
  2. Elevate infant's head and shoulders; hold infant in a feeding position.
  3. Depress the chin with the thumb to open infant's mouth.
  4. Using the dropper or syringe, direct the medication toward the inner aspect of the infant's cheek and release the flow of medication slowly.
  5. Release the thumb and allow the infant to swallow.
  6. Liquid medication can also be measured into a nipple, and the infant is allowed to suck the medication through the nipple.
  7. Crushed tablets can be mixed with a small amount of honey or applesauce and fed slowly with a teaspoon.

B. Toddlers
  1. Draw up medication in a syringe or measure into a medication cup.
  2. Elevate the child's head and shoulders.
  3. Place the syringe in the child's mouth, and slowly release the medication, directing it toward the inner aspect of the cheek, or allow the child to hold the medicine cup and drink it at own pace; offer praise.

C. School-age children
1. When the child is old enough to take medicine in tablet or capsule form, direct him or her to place the medicine near the back of the tongue and to immediately swallow fluid, such as water or juice.
2. Offer the child praise after he or she has taken medication.

Intramuscular Injection

A. Infants   *Max size 1inch!*
1. Common site: largest muscle group is the quadriceps femoris, located in the anterolateral thigh; largest muscle of this group is the vastus lateralis, situated on the anterior surface of the midlateral thigh.
    a. Place infant in supine position.
    b. Compress muscle tissue at upper aspect of thigh, pointing the nurse's fingers toward the infant's feet.
    c. Needle is inserted at a 90-degree angle; maximum length of needle for an infant is 1 inch (2.5 cm).
2. Alternate site: rectus femoris muscle, located on the anterolateral surface of the upper thigh; needle is inserted at a 45-degree angle and is directed toward the knee.
B. Toddlers and school-age children
1. Dorsogluteal muscle; upper outer quadrant; gluteal muscle does not develop until child begins to walk; should be used for injections only after the child has been walking for a year or more.
2. Ventrogluteal muscle: a dense muscle mass; the disadvantage is that the site is visible to the child.
3. Deltoid muscle may be used for older, larger children.
4. Lateral and anterior aspect of thigh: upper outer quadrant of thigh

Administration of Injections

A. Infants
1. Place infant in a secure position to avoid movement of the extremity.
2. A second person is usually needed to secure the infant.
3. Hold, cuddle, and comfort the infant after the injection.
B. Toddlers and school-age children
1. Have syringe and needle completely prepared before contact with the child.
2. Keep needle outside of child's visual field.
3. Explain, according to the child's developmental age, the reason for an injection and where it will be given; do not say "it won't hurt."
4. Inspect injection site before injection for tenderness or undue firmness.
5. Have a second person available to help secure the child, and offer comfort during the procedure.
6. Allow the child to express fears.
7. Perform the procedure quickly and gently.
8. Praise the child for his or her behavior after the injection.

CENTRAL NERVOUS SYSTEM

Depressants

Characteristics of drug-induced central nervous system (CNS) depression
1. Mild: disinterest in surroundings, inability to focus on a topic or to initiate talking or movement, slowed pulse and respirations

2. Moderate or progressive: drowsiness or sleep, decreased muscle tone and ability to move, diminished acuity of all sensations—touch, vision, hearing, heat, cold, or pain
3. Severe: unconsciousness or coma, loss of reflexes, respiratory failure, death
A. Analgesics: barriers to effective pain management; nurses have a legal and a moral responsibility to relieve pain.
1. Fear of developing tolerance
    a. Tolerance is rarely seen in clients with severe acute or chronic pain.
    b. An increase in pain is usually the result of progression of disease or complications.
2. Fear of addiction
    a. Risk of addiction in hospitalized patients is minimal.
    b. Psychologic dependence is rare in hospitalized patients.
    c. Patients with cancer pain may be titrated to large amounts of opioids to control pain without producing the adverse effects of respiratory depression or excessive sedation.
3. Fear of respiratory depression
    d. Tolerance develops to the respiratory depression effect but not to the analgesia effect.
    e. Significant respiratory depression is rarely seen because medication has been titrated to meet an individual's requirement.
4. Children are often untreated or inadequately treated for pain.
5. Elderly patients need careful assessment.
    a. Close monitoring to reduce the chances of over- or under treatment
    b. Greater chance for adverse affects
    c. May have diminished circulatory processes affecting the absorption of medications
    d. Increased chance for interaction with other medications
B. Analgesics: drugs that relieve pain
1. Opioid analgesics: act on the CNS; alter the patient's perception of pain; more often used for severe pain
    a. Examples include the following: morphine is prototype; natural or synthetic agents that have a morphine-like effect; additional examples found in Table 3-5
    b. Adverse reactions and contraindications
       (1) Depresses respiratory and cough centers in the medulla
       (2) Use cautiously in patients with impaired respiratory function and with patients with head injury because it will obscure CNS evaluation.
       (3) Inhibits gastric, biliary, and pancreatic secretions; depresses GI tract; can cause nausea, vomiting, and constipation
       (4) Stimulates release of antidiuretic hormone, resulting in decreased urine volume; can cause urinary retention
       (5) Induces hypotension
       (6) Decreases heart rate
       (7) Causes pupillary constriction
       (8) Pruritus
2. Nonopioid antiinflammatory analgesics: act at the site of the pain; do not alter the patient's perception; used more frequently for mild to moderate pain; act by sensitizing peripheral pain receptors; often combined with opioid analgesics to enhance pain control in severe pain;

nonsteroidal antiinflammatory drugs (NSAIDs) are indicated for conditions when an antiinflammatory effect is desired.
a. Examples can be found in Table 3-6.
b. Agents
   (1) Acetylsalicylic acid (aspirin)*: effective in managing low-intensity pain

(a) Adverse reactions
   ▪ Gastric irritation
   ▪ Ulceration and gastric bleeding
   ▪ Intoxication (salicylism): tinnitus, reversible hearing loss, hyperventilation, fever, metabolic acidosis, vomiting, hypokalemia, convulsions, coma, death

TABLE 3-5	Selected Opioid Dosage Forms: Pharmacokinetic Overview		
Drug/Dosage Form	Onset of Action (min)	Peak Effect (min)	Duration of Action (hr)
Codeine	30-45	60-120	4
Oral	10-30	30-60	4
IM	10-30		4
SC	10-30	Not available	4-6
Hydrocodone (Hycodan)			
Oral	10-30	30-60	4-6
Hydromorphone (Dilaudid)			
Oral	30	90-120	4
IM	15	30-60	4-5
IV	10-15	15-30	2-3
SC	15	30-90	4
Rectal	Not available	Not available	6-8
Levorphanol (Levo-Dromoran)			
Oral	10-60	90-120	6-8
IM	Not available	60	6-8
IV	Not available	Within 20	6-8
SC	Not available	60-90	6-8
Meperidine (Demerol)			
Oral	15	60-90	2-4 (usually 3)
IM	10-15	30-50	2-4 (usually 3)
IV	1	5-7	2-4 (usually 3)
SC	10-15	30-50	2-4 (usually 3)
Methadone			
Oral	30-60	90-120	4-6*
IM	10-20	60-120	4-5*
IV	Not available	15-30	3-4
Morphine			
Oral			
solution,† syrup,‡ tablets	10-30	60-120	4-5
extended-release tablets	—	—	8-12
IM	10-30	30-60	4-5
IV	Not available	20	4-5
SC	10-30	50-90	4-5
Epidural‖	15-60	—	Up to 24
Intrathecal‖	15-60	—	Up to 24
Rectal**	20-60	—	4-5
Oxycodone			
Oral	Not available	60	3-4
controlled release	Not available	3-4	12

Continued

TABLE 3-5   Selected Opioid Dosage Forms: Pharmacokinetic Overview—cont'd

Drug/Dosage Form	Onset of Action (min)	Peak Effect (min)	Duration of Action (hr)
Oxymorphone (Numorphan)			
IM	10-15	30-90	3-6
IV	5-10	15-30	3-4
SC	10-20	Not available	3-6
Rectal	15-30	120	3-6
Propoxyphene (Darvon)			
Oral	15-60	120	4-6

From McKenry LM, Salerno E: *Pharmacology in nursing,* ed 21, St. Louis 2003, Mosby.
IM, Intramuscular; *SC,* subcutaneous; *IV,* intravenous.
*With active metabolites and continuous dosing, half-life and duration of action may increase to 22 to 48 hours.
†Roxanol, MSIR, Statex Drops.
‡Morphite, M.O.S.—available in Canada.
§MS Contin, Roxanol SR.
‖Duramorph (preservative-free).
**RMS suppositories.

TABLE 3-6   Nonsteroidal Antiinflammatory Drugs: Pharmacokinetics, Dosing, and Comments

NSAID	Onset of Action (hrs)	Half-Life (hrs)	Usual Adult Dosage (mg/day)	Comments*
Acetic Acids				
Diclofenac (Voltaren)	0.5	1.2-2.0	50 mg three or four times daily	Has less effect on platelet aggregation than most other NSAIDs. Used to treat arthritis, pain, primary dysmenorrheal, and acute gout attacks.
Etodolac (Lodine)	0.5	6-7	200, 300, or 400 mg three or four times daily	Has uricosuric effects. GI distress and ulceration reported less often.
Indomethacin (Indocin)	0.5	4-6	25 or 50 mg two to four times daily	Higher risk for GI effects and renal function impairment than other agents. Used cautiously in persons with epilepsy, depression, and Parkinson's disease because it may aggravate these conditions.
Ketorolac IM: (Toradol)	10 min (dose dependent)	po: 4 IM: 6	30 mg IM/IV q6h, then 10 mg po q4-6h	Should not be given by any route for longer than 5 days. Increased risk of GI bleeding and other severe effects with duration of treatment. Do not give preoperatively or intraoperatively if bleeding control is necessary. Severe allergic reactions or anaphylaxis may occur with first dose.
Nabumetone (Relafen)	—	22	500, 750, or 1000 mg daily (hs) or in two divided doses	Prodrug (inactive); converted to active metabolite (6-MNA) in liver. Absorption increased by food and milk. Has lower reports of GI ulceration and bleeding than other NSAIDs.
Sulindac (Clinoril)	—	8	150-200 mg two times daily	Renal calculi and biliary obstruction containing sulindac metabolites is reported, but it is less likely than most NSAIDs to cause renal toxicity.
Tolmetin (Tolectin)	—	5	400 mg three times daily	High evidence of anaphylactic reactions and may also cause serum sickness or influenza-like symptoms.

TABLE 3-6	Nonsteroidal Antiinflammatory Drugs: Pharmacokinetics, Dosing, and Comments—cont'd			
NSAID	Onset of Action (hrs)	Half-Life (hrs)	Usual Adult Dosage (mg/day)	Comments*
Fenamates				
Meclofenamate (Meclomen)	1	2-3	50 mg three or four times daily	Less effect on platelet aggregation than most other NSAIDs. Used cautiously in persons on sodium-restricted diet.
Mefenamic acid (Ponstel)	—	2	250 mg q6h	Less effect on platelet aggregation but can prolong prothrombin time. Used for short-term treatment of pain and dysmenorrhea, also for acute gouty attacks and vascular headaches.
Oxicams				
Piroxicam (Feldene)	2-4	24	20 mg daily or 10 mg two times daily	Contraindicated in renal impairment. May cause influenza-like symptoms. May accumulate in older women.
Propionic Acids				
Fenoprofen (Nalfon)	—	3	300-600 mg three or four times daily	Contraindicated in persons with renal impairment. Food decreases absorption and peak serum levels, therefore is administered 30 mins before or 2 hrs after meals, unless GI distress occurs, then administered with milk.
Flurbiprofen (Ansaid)	—	5.7	100 mg daily two or three times daily	Similar to other agents in this category. Currently under study in transdermal patch to treat soft-tissue lesions.
Ibuprofen (Motrin, Advil)	0.5	2	300-800 mg three or four times daily	Available in tablet, liquid, and OTC form. May decrease blood glucose levels. Incidence of GI side effects less than with aspirin.
Ketoprofen (Orudis)	—	CAP: 1.6 ERC: 5.4 ERT: 3-4	27-75 mg three or four times daily	Can cause fluid retention and increase in creatinine levels, especially in older adults and in persons receiving diuretics. Monitor renal function closely.
Naproxen (Naprosyn)	1	13	250, 375, or 500 mg two times daily	Available in liquid, tablet, and extended-release tablets. Use tablets and liquid with caution in persons on sodium-restricted diet.
Oxaprozin (Daypro)	—	21-25	600 mg one or two times daily	Has a long half-life that accumulates with chronic dosing; half-life may be 40-60 hrs or more, which increases with age. Discontinued at least 1-2 wks before elective surgery because it has greater tendency to cause perisurgical bleeding.
Salicylates				
Diflunisal (Dolobid)	1	8-12	250-500 mg two times daily	Higher risk of causing renal impairment but less apt to cause antiplatelet effect than other NSAIDs. Does not have any antipyretic effects.

Adapted from McKenry LM, Salerno E: *Pharmacology in nursing,* ed 21, St Louis, 2003, Mosby.
NSAIDs, Nonsteroidal antiinflammatory drugs; *GI,* gastrointestinal; *IM,* intramuscular; *po,* by mouth; *IV,* intravenous; *q6h,* every 6 hours; *q4-6h,* every 4 to 6 hours; *hs,* at bedtime; *6-MNA,* 6-methoxy-2-naphthylacetic acid; *OTC,* over-the-counter; *CAP,* capsule; *ERC,* extended-release capsules; *ERT,* extended-release tablets.
*All oral NSAIDs should be taken with 8 oz of water with person remaining upright for at least 15 to 30 minutes afterward.

(b) Drug interactions with aspirin
- Anticoagulants: increase likelihood of bleeding
- Alcohol: increases likelihood of GI irritation and bleeding

(2) Acetaminophen* (Datril, Tylenol): effective in managing low-intensity pain; does not produce gastric irritation or alter platelet function and bleeding times as does aspirin; does not interact with oral anticoagulants; prolonged use or frequent high doses can cause liver and kidney damage.

(3) NSAIDs: ibuprofen* (Advil), celecoxib (Celebrex): effective in treatment of osteoarthritis, degenerative joint disease, rheumatic diseases

(4) Triptans: sumatriptan (Imitrex) used in treating migraines; causes vasoconstriction of cerebral blood vessels
  (a) Adverse reactions
- Heartburn, indigestion
- Nausea, vomiting
- Constipation or diarrhea
- Fluid retention
- Hypertension
- Dizziness
- Blurred vision
- Skin rash

  (b) Drug interactions vary because of the chemical makeup of the various NSAIDs.
- Used with caution in elderly patients who are prone to upper GI, hepatic, or renal effects.
- Given with anticoagulants may increase risk of GI ulcers or hemorrhage.
- Given concurrently may reduce the effectiveness of hypertensive agent.
- Alcoholic beverages produce a synergistic effect with NSAIDs in causing GI bleeding.

3. Nursing assessment: determine character, location, onset, contributing factors, duration of pain, time of last dose; presence of head injury; hepatic or renal failure; ask the patient about pain at least once a shift and document effectiveness of interventions.

4. Nursing management
  a. Determine the most effective way to manage the pain: drug versus nondrug measure (i.e., positioning, turning); be creative when trying to relieve a patient's pain; try combinations of drug and nondrug therapies; documenting the effectiveness of pain relief measures is vital.
  b. Obtain vital signs.
    (1) Be alert to hypotension and hypertension.
    (2) Analyze rate and character of respiration.
    (3) Withhold drug and notify physician in presence of respiratory depression: respiratory rate of ten or less respirations per minute or a decrease of eight or more respirations per minute from baseline data.
  c. Caution patient to remain quiet after drug administration to decrease possible nausea and vomiting.
  d. Implement safety measures: use side rails, and advise patient to remain in bed if changes occur in mental status, alterations in judgment, or unsteadiness.
  e. Patients need to be instructed to ask for pain medication before the pain becomes severe.

  f. Initiate intake and output records to determine effectiveness of bladder function.
  g. Determine efficacy of bowel activity. Patients on long-term treatment with medications should be on a bowel regime. Constipation is the one side effect for which clients do not develop a tolerance.
  h. Patient instruction concerning:
    (1) How to take drug
    (2) Safe storage in the home
    (3) Avoidance of driving
    (4) Danger of simultaneous administration of alcohol or other CNS depressant with narcotics

5. Nursing evaluation
  a. Have patient rate pain before and after administration on a scale of 1 to 10, and document.
  b. Observe for decreased restlessness and anxiety and ability of the patient to function.

B. Narcotic antagonists
  1. Action: reverses CNS and respiratory depression caused by overdose of narcotics
  2. Agents

EXAMPLES	COMMENT
Levallorphan tartrate (Lorfan) Naloxone hydrochloride (Narcan)	If effects of the narcotic persist, repeat doses may be necessary.

  3. Adverse reactions and contraindications
    a. Arrhythmias
    b. Hypertension
    c. Hypotension
    d. Nausea, vomiting
    e. Return of severe pain
  4. Failure to improve indicates need to investigate other causes of CNS and respiratory depression.

C. Dependency: the total psychophysical state of the individual who is addicted to drugs or alcohol who must receive an increasing amount of the substance to prevent the onset of abstinence symptoms
  1. Dependency is rarely seen in hospitalized patients who are taking medication for pain relief, not euphoric effects.
  2. Symptoms include runny nose, gooseflesh, tearing, yawning, muscle twitching, abdominal cramping, insomnia, nausea and vomiting, diarrhea.
  3. Methadone hydrochloride is used for detoxification and maintenance.
  4. With acute toxicity, the usual cause of death is respiratory depression; treated with support to respiration and with a narcotic antagonist.

D. Anesthetics: provide a pain-free experience during an operative procedure along with a relaxed state of mind and sense of security.
  1. General anesthetics: provide loss of pain sensation, loss of consciousness, loss of memory, and loss of voluntary and some involuntary muscle activity.
    a. Inhalation agents: the following are examples
      (Penthrane)
      Cyclopropane
      Ether

Halothane
Methoxyflurane
Nitrous oxide

b. IV agents: the following are examples

Droperidol (Inapsine)
Droperidol-fentanyl citrate (Innovar)
Ketamine hydrochloride
Methohexital sodium (Brevital)
Thiamylal sodium (Surital)
Thiopental sodium (Pentothal)

2. Regional anesthetics provide loss of sensation and motor activity in localized areas of the body

a. Types

Types

(1) Topical
(2) Infiltration
(3) Peripheral nerve blocks
(4) Spinal
(5) Epidural
(6) Caudal

b. Agents: the following are examples

Agents

Carbocaine
Novocain
Nupercaine
Pontocaine
Xylocaine

3. Nursing assessment

a. Preoperative: obtain health history including allergies, psychologic status, physiologic baseline data; inform patient about surgical procedure.

b. Intraoperative: implement safety measures in presence of explosive or flammable agents.

c. Postoperative: determine vital signs and respiratory function.

4. Nursing management

a. Preoperative: prepare patient physically and psychologically; initiate measures to prevent complications: deep-breathing and bed exercises; administer preoperative medications; initiate safety measures, and provide quiet environment.

b. Intraoperative: maintain quiet during stage 2 anesthesia; position patient properly and pad pressure points adequately; transfer patient from operating table in a smooth, coordinated manner to avoid severe hypotension.

c. Postoperative: preserve quiet atmosphere; maintain airway, assess pain carefully and have patient rate on a scale of 1 to 10, and document; prevent complications by encouraging deep breathing, coughing, etc.

5. Nursing evaluation

a. Preoperative: effects of preoperative medication

b. Intraoperative: ongoing evaluation of patient's status, usually the responsibility of the anesthesiologist

c. Postoperative: concerned with pulmonary complications, thrombophlebitis, infection, other complications, postanesthesia nausea, vomiting, hypotension, tachycardia

E. Anticonvulsants: drugs used to control seizures

1. Action: not completely understood; thought to depress neuron excitability and to modify the ability of brain tissue to respond to stimuli that initiate seizure activity

2. Agents

EXAMPLES	ADVERSE REACTIONS
a. Long-acting barbiturates Phenobarbital (Luminal)* Primidone (Mysoline)	Sedation, drowsiness, tolerance, nystagmus, ataxia, anemia, congenital malformations in fetus; sudden withdrawal can induce convulsions
b. Hydantoins Mephenytoin (Mesantoin)* Phenytoin (Dilantin)*	Nystagmus, ataxia, slurred speech, tremors, nervousness, drowsiness, fatigue, overgrowth of the gums (gingival hyperplasia), occasional folic acid or vitamin-D deficiency; congenital malformations in fetus
c. Oxazolidinediones Trimethadione (Tridione)	Serious allergic dermatitis, kidney and liver damage, vertigo, photophobia, spontaneous abortion, congenital malformations
d. Benzodiazepines Clonazepam (Clonopin) Diazepam (Valium)* Clorazepate (Tranzene) Lorazepam (Ativan)*	Drowsiness, ataxia, personality changes
e. Miscellaneous Acetazolamide (Diamox)* Carbamazepine (Tegretol)*	Loss of appetite, drowsiness, confusion dizziness, ataxia, double vision, GI upset
Lidocaine hydrochloride (Xylocaine)	Depressed heart action
Paraldehyde	Bronchopulmonary irritation, thrombophlebitis at IV injection site
Valproic acid (Depakene)	GI distress, sedation

3. Nursing assessment: observe course of the seizure; assist in case finding; assess baseline data with concentration on areas known to be affected by the drug (e.g., phenytoin [Dilantin]); assess mouth, teeth, and gums for development of gingival hyperplasia.

4. Nursing management: instruct patient concerning:

a. Drug characteristics

b. Importance of taking medication even when patient is seizure free; awareness that reaching a therapeutic level may take time

c. Impairment of absorption of the anticonvulsant when taken with milk or antacids

d. Wearing or carrying identification indicating seizure activity and drugs and dosages being taken

e. Reducing gastric irritation by taking drug with meals

f. Good gum massage and oral care after each meal

g. A gradual dose reduction should be designed by health care provider to maintain seizure control.

h. Patients should contact their physician before taking any OTC medications.

i. Female patients taking estrogen-containing birth control pills should be advised to use an alternate form of birth control during treatment.

5. Nursing evaluation: continued medical follow-up; blood level tests
F. Skeletal muscle relaxants: drugs used to treat muscle spasticity
  1. Action: inhibits nerve impulse transmission by blocking polysynaptic pathways in the spinal cord
  2. Agents

EXAMPLES	ADVERSE REACTIONS
a. Drugs to treat spasticity Baclofen (Lioresal)	Drowsiness incoordination, GI upset
Dantrolene sodium (Dantrium)	Liver damage
Diazepam (Valium)	Drowsiness, incoordination
b. Drugs to treat muscle spasm	Drowsiness, dizziness
Carisoprodol (Rela, Soma)	
Cyclobenzaprine hydrochloride (Flexeril)	
Dantrolene (Dantrium)	
Diazepam (Valium)*	
Methocarbamol (Robaxin)	

  3. Nursing assessment: obtain baseline data, focusing on spasticity, including degree, aggravating factors, associated pain, and interference with activities of daily living (ADL); observe baseline liver function studies.
  4. Nursing management: monitor for drug effectiveness and side effects; institute safety measures if drowsiness occurs; teach patient to avoid alcohol and CNS depressants.
  5. Nursing evaluation: at regular intervals, assess the continuing degree of spasticity.
G. Antiparkinsonian drugs: drugs used in managing Parkinson's disease
  1. Action: restores action of the neurotransmitter dopamine to the basal ganglia of the brain or blocks the effects of excessive action of acetylcholine
  2. Agents

EXAMPLES	ADVERSE REACTIONS
a. Anticholinergics Benztropine mesylate (Cogentin)*	Dry mouth, constipation, urinary retention, blurred vision; impairment of recent memory, confusion, insomnia, restlessness
Biperiden (Akineton)*	
Cycrimine hydrochloride (Pagitane hydrochloride)	
Ethopropazine hydrochloride (Parsidol)	
Procyclidine hydrochloride (Kemadrin)	
Trihexyphenidyl hydrochloride (Artane, Pipanol, Tremin)	
b. Antihistamines	Sedation
Chlorphenoxamine hydrochloride (Phenoxene)	
Diphenhydramine hydrochloride (Benadryl)*	
Orphenadrine citrate (Disipal)	
c. Other drugs Amantadine hydrochloride (Symmetrel)*	Dry mouth, constipation, urinary retention, blurred vision

EXAMPLES	ADVERSE REACTIONS
Levodopa (Dopar, Larodopa)	Nausea, vomiting, anorexia, orthostatic hypotension, GI bleeding, cough, hoarseness, dyspnea, blurred vision, increased sex drive
Carbidopa-levodopa (Sinemet)*	Same as Levodopa

H. Sedatives, hypnotics, antianxiety drugs
  1. Sedatives: small dose to calm an anxious patient
  2. Hypnotics: larger dose to induce sleep
  3. Antianxiety drugs (minor tranquilizers, anxiolytic): used to treat anxiety
  4. Barbiturates: classified according to duration of action—ultra short acting, short acting, intermediate acting, and long acting
     a. Action: produce CNS depression ranging from sedation to anesthesia
     b. Adverse reactions
        (1) Mild withdrawal symptoms: rebound rapid-eye-movement (REM) sleep, nightmares, daytime agitation, and a "shaky" feeling—dosage must be decreased gradually.
        (2) Acute overdose: depression of medullary centers regulating respiration and cardiovascular system—tachycardia, hypotension, loss of reflexes, marked depression of respiration
     c. Agents: the following are examples
        Amobarbital (Amytal, Tuinal)
        Butabarbital sodium (Butalan, Butisol Sodium)
        Pentobarbital (Nembutal)
        Phenobarbital (Luminal)
        Secobarbital (Seconal)
  5. Benzodiazepines
     a. Action: produce CNS depression
     b. Adverse reactions: daytime sedation, motor incoordination, dizziness, headaches; schedule-IV substances; efficacy decreases after 3 to 4 months of use; ineffective in treating psychotic episodes or severe depression; contraindicated in treating patients with glaucoma
     c. Agents: the following are examples
        Lorazepam (Ativan)*
        Alprazolam (Xanax)*
        Chlordiazepoxide hydrochloride (Librium)
        Clorazepate dipotassium (Tranxene)
        Diazepam (Valium)
        Prazepam (Verstran, Centrax)
        Flurazepam hydrochloride (Dalmane)
        Oxazepam (Serax)
  6. Miscellaneous
     a. Action: produce CNS depression; generally short acting
     b. Agents

EXAMPLES	ADVERSE REACTIONS
Zolpidem (Ambien)*	Dizziness, drowsiness, diarrhea, headache, hangover
Chloral hydrate (Noctec)	Gastric irritation; schedule-IV substance

EXAMPLES	ADVERSE REACTIONS
Ethchlorvynol (Placidyl)	Muscular weakness; schedule IV substance
Glutethimide (Doriden)	Dilated pupils, dry mouth; schedule III substance
Hydroxyzine hydrochloride (Vistaril)*	Dry mouth, hypotension, blurred vision
Meprobamate (Equanil, Miltown)	Schedule IV substance
Methaqualone (Quaalude, Sopor, Parest)	Paresthesia, peripheral neuropathy; schedule II substance
Methyprylon (Noludar)	Schedule II substance

7. Nursing assessment: give special attention to vital signs, level of consciousness, sleep patterns; can increase toxicity if given with digoxin.
8. Nursing management: observe for signs of CNS depression; identify nondrug solutions to sleep problems; monitor safety aspects of patient care. The presence of food decreases the effectiveness of Ambien and should therefore be given immediately before bedtime. Taken for a long period may produce psychologic dependence.
9. Nursing evaluation: review purpose for which drug is given, and observe effectiveness; instruct patient concerning self-medication, medical follow-up, and drug-dependence potential.

I. Alcohol
1. Action: produces CNS depression—sedation, disinhibition, sleep, anesthesia; vasodilation; gastric irritation
2. Effects of an acute overdose: death, accidents, hangover, upset stomach, thirst, fatigue, headache, depression, anxiety; chronic toxicity can lead to liver, esophageal gastrointestinal, and cardiovascular disorders
3. Withdrawal symptoms after chronic use: tremors, anxiety, tachycardia, increased BP, diaphoresis, anorexia, nausea, vomiting, insomnia, hallucinations, seizures, delirium tremens
4. Withdrawal therapy: one of the benzodiazepines; restoration of normal metabolic functions, and vitamin B_1, B_{12}, and folic acid
5. Aversion therapy: disulfiram (Antabuse) given to detoxified patient who wishes to avoid drinking again; produces unpleasant reaction in presence of alcohol: flushing, throbbing in head and neck, respiratory difficulty, nausea, copious vomiting, diaphoresis, fainting, dizziness, blurred vision, confusion

Psychotherapeutic Agents

A. Antidepressants: characteristic of drug-induced prevention or relief of depression
1. Tricyclic antidepressants
   a. Action: primarily used to relieve symptoms of endogenous depression; also used to treat mild exogenous depression. Because of the potential for drug overdose and adverse effects, these agents are more likely to be used only if depression is not responsive to other agents. These drugs are contraindicated in patients with benign prostatic hyperplasia (BPH), diabetes, and narrow-angle glaucoma.
   b. Agents: the following are examples
      Amitriptyline hydrochloride (Elavil)*
      Doxepin hydrochloride (Adapin, Sinequan)
      Imipramine hydrochloride (Tofranil)
2. Monoamine oxidase inhibitors (MAOIs)
   a. Action: relieve symptoms of severe reactive or endogenous depression that has not responded to antidepressant therapy with other agents, electroconvulsive therapy, or other modes of psychotherapy
   b. Agents: the following are examples
      Phenelzine sulfate (Nardil)
      Tranylcypromine sulfate (Parnate)
3. Miscellaneous antidepressants
   a. Action: second-generation antidepressants; inhibit the reuptake of norepinephrine; fewer long-term side effects; individual agents have to be considered for advantages and disadvantages.
   b. Agents: the following are examples
      Bupropion (Wellbutrin)*
      Venlafaxine (Effexor)*
4. Selective serotonin reuptake inhibitors (SSRIs)
   a. Action: treatment for depression
   b. Agents: the following are examples
      Fluoxetine (Prozac)*
      Paroxetine (Paxil)*
      Sertraline (Zoloft)*
5. Nursing assessment
   a. Obtain complete health history.
   b. Assess for history of insomnia, fatigue, or loss of motivation.
   c. Observe motor movements, facial expression, posture.
   d. Assess for any feelings of suicide; potential for suicide is inherent in any severely depressed patient until a significant remission occurs.
   e. Administer with caution to patients with increased intraocular pressure, prostatic hypertrophy, history of urinary retention, or history of glaucoma, because tricyclic antidepressants possess significant anticholinergic properties.
   f. Check medication history carefully for extensive drug interactions.
   g. Use extreme caution with patients with cardiovascular disease because of potential for conduction defects.
   h. Initial dose in adolescent and debilitated patients should be lower and increased gradually.
6. Nursing management: administer medication with food to avoid gastric distress.
7. Nursing evaluation: observe for adverse effects, such as drowsiness.
8. Patient teaching
   a. Stress compliance of taking medication as ordered.
   b. Instruct patient to avoid using alcohol with sleeping pills and hay fever or cold medications because doing so increases the effects of these medications.
   c. Teach patient to report anticholinergic side effects (blurred vision, altered thought processes, constipation, urinary retention, and eye pain, which may be indicative of glaucoma).
   d. Food containing tyramine should not be ingested for at least 2 to 3 weeks after discontinuation of therapy; educate patient and family on dietary restrictions.

The foods containing tyramine refer only to MAOIs; it should include the period the patient is on the drug, as well as 2 to 4 weeks after discontinuation.

  e. Teach patient that therapeutic effects take 2 to 3 weeks.

  f. Instruct patient not to discontinue medication quickly after long-term use; may cause nausea, headache, malaise.

B. Antipsychotic drugs
1. Phenothiazines, thioxanthenes
  a. Action: primarily to reduce or relieve symptoms of acute and chronic psychoses, including schizophrenia, schizoaffective disorders, and involutional psychoses
  b. Agents: the following are examples
    Chlorpromazine (Thorazine)*
    Promazine hydrochloride (Sparine)
    Thioridazine hydrochloride (Mellaril)
    Trifluoperazine hydrochloride (Stelazine)
    Triflupromazine hydrochloride (Vesprin)
2. Nursing assessment: obtain complete health history, current use of medications, possibility of pregnancy; obtain history of emotional unrest, agitation, paranoid ideation, delusions, inability to cope with reality.
3. Nursing management: administer medication with food or milk to avoid or reduce gastric distress.
4. Nursing evaluation: observe for adverse effects such as urinary retention, change in vision, sore throat with fever, muscle spasms, trembling or shaking of hands, skin rash, yellow tinge to skin or eyes, uncontrollable movements of the tongue.

C. Antimanic drugs: used to treat manic-depressive psychoses in the acute manic phase; also used to prevent recurrent episodes of mania in the manic-depressive patient
1. Agent: lithium carbonate (Lithane, Carbolith)
2. Nursing assessment: obtain complete health history, possibility of pregnancy, medications currently being taken; observe for restlessness, hyperactivity, aggressiveness.
3. Nursing management: ensure adequate fluid and electrolyte balance.
4. Nursing evaluation: monitor serum lithium levels to avoid drug toxicity and reduce side effects.
5. Patient teaching: stress compliance of taking medication as ordered; instruct patient to wear medical identification tag.

Stimulants

Stimulants are medically accepted only for treatment of narcolepsy, hyperkinetic behavior in children, and obesity. Stimulants are occasionally used for depression in older adults and to reverse respiratory depression from CNS depressants.
A. Amphetamines
1. Action: increase the release and effectiveness of catecholamine neurotransmitters in the brain and peripheral nerves and create increased alertness and sensitivity to stimuli
2. Adverse reactions
  a. GI system: vomiting, diarrhea, abdominal cramps, dry mouth, anorexia
  b. CNS: restless behavior, tremor, irritability, talkativeness, insomnia, mood changes, excessive aggressiveness, confusion, panic, increased libido
  c. Autonomic nervous system: headache, chilliness, palpitation, pallor or facial flushing
  d. Children: growth retardation

3. Agents: the following are examples
  Amphetamine sulfate
  Dextroamphetamine sulfate (Dexedrine, Ferndex)*
  Methamphetamine hydrochloride (Desoxyn)
  Methylphenidate (Ritalin)*
  Pemoline (Cylert)
4. Nursing assessment: obtain thorough history of patient's presenting problem; obtain vital signs, weight, height in children.
5. Nursing management: monitor height, weight, vital signs; inquire about relief of subjective symptoms, such as insomnia, agitation, headache, irritability; begin preparing patient and family for long-term management; teach patient that last daily dose should be taken at least 6 hours before retiring.
6. Nursing evaluation: success of goals of therapy evaluated
  a. Hyperkinesis: less hyperactivity and a more normal attention span
  b. Narcolepsy: ability to remain awake and alert during specified appropriate time periods

B. Appetite suppressants: used to help control obesity
1. Action: exert an anorectic effect on the appetite-control center in the brain
2. Agents

EXAMPLES	ADVERSE REACTIONS/COMMENTS
Amphetamine sulfate (Benzedrine)*	See Amphetamines
Benzphetamine (Didrex)	See Amphetamines
Caffeine*	Nervousness, jitteriness, GI bleeding, nausea, vomiting, excessive CNS stimulation, convulsions
Caffeine sodium benzoate injection	Same as Caffeine
Dextroamphetamine sulfate (Dexedrine)	See Amphetamines
Phenylpropanolamine hydrochloride (Acutrim, Control, Diadax, Dexatrim)	BP increases
Theophylline*	Increased heart rate, nervousness, jitteriness, nausea, vomiting, excessive CNS stimulation, convulsions

3. Nursing assessment: obtain vital signs and weight; discuss usual eating habits and establish reasonable goals for losing weight.
4. Nursing management: promote weight reduction; monitor for adverse reactions; offer support.
5. Nursing evaluation: instruct patient concerning medication and its potential for drug abuse; assess achievement of goal—weight loss.

C. Respiratory stimulants (analeptics): used to stimulate respiration when drugs, asphyxiation, or electric shock have depressed it.
1. Action: stimulates CNS medullary centers controlling respiration, vasomotor tone, vagal tone
2. Agents: see amphetamines.
3. Nursing assessments: check respiratory rate and depth of respirations; may measure vital capacity and arterial blood gas levels.

4. Nursing management: monitor vital signs with focus on respirations; keep suction machine at bedside.
5. Nursing evaluation: observe whether patient is breathing at a rate and depth nearing normal and whether short-term hospitalization is necessary.

AUTONOMIC NERVOUS SYSTEM

Cholinesterase Inhibitors (Cholinergic Agents)

A. Description: drugs that produce a physiologic response similar to that of acetylcholine released on nerve stimulation
B. Action
1. Direct-acting cholinergic stimulants: mimic the action of acetylcholine
2. Indirect-acting cholinergic stimulants: inhibit the enzyme cholinesterase, which acts to limit acetylcholine action
C. Effects
1. Vasodilation
2. Lowered BP
3. Slowing of heart rate
4. Salivation
5. Perspiring
6. Increased tone and movement in the GI and genitourinary systems
7. Increased tone and contractility in striated muscles
D. Adverse reactions: heart block, arrhythmias, hypotension, hypertension, nausea, vomiting, cramps, diarrhea, heartburn, muscle weakness, increase in intraocular pressure, urinary retention (bethanechol)
E. Agents: the following are examples
Ambenonium chloride (Mytelase Chloride, Mysuran)
Demecarium bromide (Humorsol)
Echothiophate iodide (Phospholine iodide)
Bethanechol (Urecholine)*
Edrophonium chloride (Tensilon)
Isoflurophate (Floropryl)
Neostigmine bromide (Prostigmin)
Pyridostigmine bromide (Mestinon)*
F. Nursing assessment: history of lung disease, hyperthyroidism, prostate enlargement; patients with obstruction of the intestine or renal disease should not use these products.
G. Nursing management: monitor vital signs; insert rectal tube to relieve flatus; inform patient that drug is not a cure; it relieves only symptoms (myasthenia gravis).
H. Nursing evaluation: observe for adverse reactions, bowel activity, intake and output records; therapeutic response in treating myasthenia gravis—increased muscle strength, hand grasp, improved muscle gait, absence of labored breathing (if severe)

Parasympathetic Blocking Agents (Parasympatholytic or Cholinergic Blocking Agents)

A. Action: prevent acetylcholine released by nerve stimulation from exerting its effects
B. Effects:
1. GI system: slows peristalsis
2. Heart: increases rate
3. Secretions: depresses all body secretions, including perspiration and respiratory, salivary, pancreatic, gastric secretions
4. Eye: dilates pupils (mydriasis); paralyzes ciliary muscles; increases intraocular pressure

C. Adverse reactions: dry skin, delirium, tachycardia, convulsions, mydriasis, hypertension, dry mouth, urinary retention
D. Agents

EXAMPLES	CLINICAL USES
Atropine sulfate*	Adjunct to anesthesia, antispasmodic, cardiac stimulant
Cyclopentolate hydrochloride (Cyclogyl)	Mydriatic, cycloplegic
Homatropine hydrobromide	Mydriatic, cycloplegic
Scopolamine hydrobromide (Hyoscine)	Sedative-hypnotic, adjunct to anesthesia, antiemetic, mydriatic, cycloplegic
Isopropamide iodide (Darbid)	Antispasmodic
Methantheline bromide (Banthine)	Antispasmodic
Propantheline bromide (Pro-Banthine)	Antispasmodic
Benztropine mesylate (Cogentin)*	Antiparkinsonian agent
Procyclidine hydrochloride (Kemadrin)	Antiparkinsonian agent
Trihexyphenidyl hydrochloride (Artane)	Antiparkinsonian agent

E. Nursing assessment: monitor vital signs; tachycardia; bowel functions; stimulation or depression of CNS; elevation in temperature; respiratory status; history of urinary difficulty, familial history of glaucoma
F. Nursing management: maintain oral hygiene for dry mouth; initiate methods to prevent abdominal distention and constipation; initiate safety measures in presence of blurred vision.
G. Nursing evaluation: establish intake and output records when these drugs are given to elderly males; observe for effectiveness of drug.

Neuromuscular Blocking Agents

A. Action: act at the striated neuromuscular junction to produce paralysis of the voluntary muscles
B. Effects
1. Produce muscular relaxation for insertion of endotracheal tubes during surgical interventions
2. Protect against violent thrashing that occurs with electroconvulsive therapy
3. Alleviate spasms that accompany tetanus
C. Adverse reactions: paralysis of respiration, which may be reversed with neostigmine or Tensilon
D. Agents: the following are examples
Decamethonium bromide (Syncurine)
Pancuronium bromide (Pavulon)
Succinylcholine chloride (Anectine)
Tubocurarine chloride (Tubarine)
E. Nursing assessment: elicit medical history—asthma, myasthenia gravis remission; assess potassium blood levels.
F. Nursing management: cardiopulmonary resuscitation skills—have resuscitative equipment available; monitor vital signs.
G. Nursing evaluation: observe for early signs of flaccid paralysis in muscles of face, neck, eyes.
H. Know that patient may appear to be asleep but can still hear.

Sympathomimetic Drugs: Adrenergic Stimulants

A. Actions
  1. Act directly on adrenergic receptors to produce either excitation or inhibition of a particular effector organ
  2. Act indirectly by releasing the stored catecholamines norepinephrine and epinephrine
B. Major effects
  1. Excitation of the heart, both its rate and its force of contraction
  2. Excitation and constriction of smooth muscles in peripheral blood vessels
  3. Inhibition and relaxation of smooth muscles in bronchi, GI tract, and skeletal muscle blood vessels
  4. Metabolism: release of fatty acids from adipose tissue and increased gluconeogenesis in muscle and liver
  5. Excitation of functions controlled by CNS (e.g., respiration)
  6. Suppression of appetite
  7. Lessening of fatigue
C. Adverse reactions: anxiety, apprehension, headache, arrhythmias, cerebral hemorrhage, heart failure, pulmonary edema
D. Agents

EXAMPLES	CLINICAL INDICATIONS
Dopamine hydrochloride (Intropin)*	Hypotension
Ephedrine hydrochloride (Bronkotabs)	Bronchospasms, nasal decongestion, allergy
Epinephrine bitartrate (Medihaler-Epi)	Acute or chronic bronchial asthma, allergic disorders, acute hypersensitivity to drugs
Epinephrine hydrochloride (Adrenalin Chloride)*	Cardiac arrest, heart block, acute asthma, adjunct to local anesthesia, acute hypersensitivity to drugs
	Ophthalmic use: control hemorrhage, decrease intraocular pressure
Isoproterenol hydrochloride (Isuprel)*	Bronchodilation, cardiac stimulant
Isoproterenol sulfate (Medihaler-Iso)	Bronchodilation
Mephentermine sulfate (Wyamine)	Maintain BP during anesthesia
Metaraminol bitartrate (Aramine)	Hypotension
Naphazoline hydrochloride (Privine)	Nasal decongestion
Norepinephrine bitartrate (Levophed, Noradrenalin)*	Shock, cardiac arrest
Nylidrin hydrochloride (Arlidin)	Peripheral vascular disease

E. Nursing assessment: obtain history of hyperthyroidism, diabetes, hypertension, emotional lability, heart disease.
F. Nursing management: monitor vital signs; check infusion rate often; observe for infusion infiltration; record bowel and urinary activity; teach patient to keep fluid intake to at least 2000 ml/day to reduce viscosity of secretions.
G. Nursing evaluation: monitor effect on BP, pulse rate, regularity of heart rate; observe for therapeutic and adverse effects.

Adrenergic Receptor Blockers and Neuron Blockers

A. Action: interfere with peripheral adrenergic activity by blocking alpha- and beta-receptors, by depleting peripheral neural stores of norepinephrine, and by inhibiting peripheral sympathetic activity through an action on the CNS
B. Adverse reactions: postural hypotension, miosis, inhibition of ejaculation, headache, intense vasoconstriction, diarrhea, nausea, disturbances of vision, insomnia, depression
C. Agents

EXAMPLES	CLINICAL INDICATIONS
Clonidine (Catapres-TTS)	Chronic hypertension
Ergoloid mesylate (Hydergine)	Mental and emotional complaints of older adults
Guanethidine monosulfate (Ismelin)	Hypertension
Methyldopa (Aldomet)*	Hypertension
Metoprolol tartrate (Lopressor)*	Chronic hypertension, angina prophylaxis
Nadolol (Corgard)*	Chronic hypertension, angina prophylaxis
Phenoxybenzamine hydrochloride (Dibenzyline)	Peripheral vascular disease
Phentolamine mesylate (Regitine)	Hypertension secondary to pheochromocytoma, adrenal tumor surgery
Prazosin hydrochloride (Minipress)	Chronic hypertension
Propranolol hydrochloride (Inderal)*	Chronic hypertension, angina prophylaxis, cardiac dysrhythmias, migraine headaches
Reserpine (Serpasil)	Chronic hypertension
Timolol maleate (Timoptic)*	Glaucoma
Tolazoline hydrochloride (Priscoline)	Peripheral vascular disease

D. Nursing assessment: ascertain if patient has history of ulcer disease, diabetes, ulcerative colitis, emotional depression, renal problems, coronary heart disease, predisposition to asthma, congestive heart failure.
E. Nursing management: aim instruction toward patient compliance; administer medications with meals or milk; maintain safety measures in presence of postural hypotension; monitor vital signs.
F. Nursing evaluation: observe for therapeutic and adverse reactions; observe for changes in sleep patterns and appetite and depression or suicidal tendencies; observe for interactions with other arrhythmias or channel blockers; may cause additive effect; interaction with insulin or hypoglycemic agents can alter insulin requirements and mask signs of hypoglycemia.

Ganglionic Agents

A. Action: reduces sympathetic tone, particularly in the cardiovascular system
B. Adverse reactions: postural hypotension, pupillary dilation, blurring vision, dry mouth, constipation

C. Agents

EXAMPLES	CLINICAL INDICATIONS
Mecamylamine hydrochloride (Inversine)	Hypertensive crisis, chronic hypertension
Trimethaphan camsylate (Arfonad)	Hypertensive crisis

D. Nursing assessment: obtain baseline vital signs; assess factors contributing to hypertension such as diet, weight, exercise, lifestyle.
E. Nursing management: instruction is aimed at patient compliance.
F. Nursing evaluation: observe for therapeutic effects and adverse reactions.

RESPIRATORY SYSTEM

Antihistamines

Antihistamines are found in many OTC medicines and in combination with analgesics, antitussives, and others. Drugs are palliative only and do not protect against allergic reactions.
A. Action: blocks histamine effects at the receptor site
B. Adverse reactions: sedation, drowsiness, dry mouth, blurred vision, urinary retention, constipation; can also stimulate the nervous system, especially in children, causing insomnia, irritability, nervousness
C. Agents

EXAMPLES	CLINICAL INDICATIONS
Brompheniramine maleate (Dimetane)	Colds, allergies
Chlorpheniramine maleate (Chlor-Trimeton, Teldrin, Chlortab)	Colds, allergies
Clemastine fumarate (Tavist)	Allergies
Diphenhydramine hydrochloride (Benadryl)*	Allergic reactions, motion sickness, mild parkinsonism
Fexofenadine hydrochloride (Allegra)*	Allergies
Loratadine (Claritin)*	Allergies
Cetirizine (Zyrtec)*	Allergies

D. Nursing assessment: obtain vital signs; assess respiratory and cardiovascular status; ascertain if patient has history of allergy and extent and type of rash if present; obtain drug history; assess for potential interactions and increased CNS depression.
E. Nursing management: monitor respiratory response, vital signs, urinary and bowel function; increase fluid intake to minimize dry mouth; check specific medication guidelines as to whether they should be administered with meals or on an empty stomach; older adults may require decreased dose; instruct client to avoid the sun and use sunblock because of increased photosensitivity.
F. Nursing evaluation: observe for therapeutic effects and adverse reaction; most common adverse reaction is headache; instruct patient on dangers of operating machinery and on

wearing medical identification tag in presence of allergies; assess therapeutic response—includes absence of allergy symptoms, itching, sneezing.

Prophylactic Asthmatic Drugs

A. Action: indicated for prevention of bronchospasm and bronchial asthma attacks; inhibits the release of histamines from mast cells
B. Adverse reactions: headache, cough, hoarseness, dry mouth or throat, nasal congestion, sneezing, bad taste in mouth
C. Agent: cromolyn sodium (Intal), montelukast (Singulair)
D. Nursing assessment: helps prevent but does not relieve asthma attacks; client should be advised that as long as 4 weeks may be required before the drug is fully beneficial; obtain baseline history of the frequency and severity of attacks.
E. Nursing management: Singulair should be administered in the evening for maximum effectiveness; instruct patient that these medications are taken preventatively and not for acute attacks; avoid OTC products without the physician's permission.
F. Nursing evaluation: therapeutic effect would be a reduction in the number of attacks, reduced cough, decreased sputum production, a decreased need for other asthma drugs, or any combination.

Nasal Decongestants

A. Action: sympathomimetic agents (see the Autonomic Nervous System), when applied to nasal mucosa or taken orally; constrict the smooth muscle of arterioles in the nasal mucosa and thus reduce blood flow and edema
B. Adverse reactions: rebound nasal congestion if used too frequently; nervousness, irritability
C. Agents: the following are a few examples of the numerous preparations available

Afrin*	Neo-Synephrine
Allerest	Privine
Contac	Sine-Off
Coricidin	Sinutab
Dristan	Sudafed

D. Nursing assessment: obtain history of irritants or environmental conditions contributing to symptoms and such objective data as respiratory rate and vital signs.
E. Nursing management: instruct patient regarding medication use.
F. Nursing evaluation: monitor for therapeutic effects and adverse reactions.

Expectorants, Antitussives, Mucolytic Drugs

A. Definitions
  1. Expectorant: increases output of respiratory tract fluid that coats the bronchi and trachea
  2. Antitussive: suppresses cough
  3. Mucolytic: breaks up viscous mucus to allow for ease in expectoration of drainage
B. Adverse reactions
  1. Expectorants—nausea, drowsiness; iodide-base drugs—skin rash, metallic taste, fever, skin eruptions, mucous membrane ulcerations, salivary gland swelling
  2. Antitussives: nausea, dizziness, constipation
  3. Mucolytics: GI upset

C. Agents: the following are examples
   1. Expectorants: Robitussin*, iodinated glycerol (Organidin), potassium iodide
   2. Antitussives: codeine, hydrocodone bitartrate, dextromethorphan hydrobromide (Romilar), Benylin, benzonatate (Tessalon)*
   3. Mucolytics: acetylcysteine (Mucomyst,* Alevaire)
D. Nursing assessment: obtain history relevant to cough, vital signs, and objective data only as character and quantity of secretions.
E. Nursing management: monitor symptoms, vital signs, amount of secretions with mucolytics.
F. Nursing evaluation: instruct patient regarding drugs—how and when to take them and when they should be discontinued; encourage patients with persistent coughs to seek follow-up treatment.

Bronchodilators

A. Action: act on bronchial cells to dilate the bronchioles
B. Adverse reactions: CNS stimulation, increased heart rate, muscle tremors, headache, nausea, epigastric pain, bronchospasm
C. Agents: the following are examples
   Aminophylline
   Albuterol* (Proventil)
   Epinephrine* bitartrate (AsthmaHaler, Medihaler-Epi, Primatene Mist)
   Isoproterenol* hydrochloride (Iprenol, Isuprel hydrochloride)
   Metaproterenol* sulfate (Alupent, Metaprel)
   Oxtriphylline (Choledyl)
   Salmeterol (Serevent)
   Terbutaline sulfate (Brethine, Bricanyl)
   Theophylline (many preparations)
D. Nursing assessment: obtain relevant history and vital signs; note amount and characteristics of secretions; review medical conditions that may interfere with the administration of individual medications.
E. Nursing management: monitor vital signs and lung sounds, closely monitor IV drugs; teach patient to increase fluid intake to 2000 to 3000 ml/day; these agents are available as inhaled agents and orally; the long-acting preparations are used in treating and preventing asthma attacks; these agents are more effective if given on a fixed schedule; the shorter-acting agents are used for symptom relief during acute attacks and as a preventative measure in exercise-induced asthma; must maintain a therapeutic level with theophylline.
F. Nursing evaluation: observe for therapeutic effects; instruct patient regarding drug knowledge and usage.

CARDIOVASCULAR SYSTEM

Drugs to Improve Circulation

A. Action: vasoconstriction (direct- and indirect-acting sympathomimetic amines cause release of norepinephrine, which stimulates alpha-receptors and thus produces vasoconstriction)
B. Adverse reactions: headache, anxiety, palpitation, nausea, vomiting, insomnia, tremors
C. Agents: the following are examples
   Dobutamine hydrochloride (Dobutrex)
   Dopamine hydrochloride (Intropin)
   Epinephrine* hydrochloride (Adrenalin Chloride)
   Isoproterenol* hydrochloride (Isuprel hydrochloride)

   Mephentermine sulfate (Wyamine)
   Metaraminol bitartrate (Aramine)
   Methoxamine hydrochloride (Vasoxyl)
   Norepinephrine bitartrate (Levarterenol bitartrate; Levophed)
   Phenylephrine hydrochloride (Neo-Synephrine hydrochloride, Isophrin)
D. Principal clinical use: for treating cardiogenic and anaphylactic shock; to maintain BP in life-threatening situations and during anesthesia
E. Nursing assessment: obtain pulse, respirations, BP; note level of consciousness.
F. Nursing management: use infusion-control device to monitor IV administration; monitor vital signs frequently.
G. Nursing evaluation: observe for therapeutic effects.

Vasodilator Drugs (Antianginal Drugs)

A. Action: dilate arterioles and veins to lower BP, which reduces workload on the heart and decreases the heart's oxygen demand; increases circulation to cardiac muscle
B. Adverse reactions: flushing, headache, dizziness
C. Agents: the following are examples
   Amyl nitrite (Vaporole)
   Erythrityl tetranitrate (Cardilate)
   Isosorbide dinitrate (Iso-Bid, Isordil, Sorbide, Sorbitrate)
   Mannitol hexanitrate (Nitranitol)
   Nitroglycerin* (Nitro-Bid)
   Nitroglycerin* lingual aerosol (Nitrolingual Spray)
   Nitroglycerin* ointment, 2% (Nitrol)
D. Nursing assessment: obtain vital signs and history relevant to onset and duration of pain.
E. Nursing management: observe and monitor for additional angina attacks; instruct patient about prescribed drugs.
F. Nursing evaluation: observe for therapeutic effects.

Vasodilator Drugs for Peripheral Vascular Disease

A. Action: work directly on vascular smooth muscle to cause relaxation or stimulate beta-receptors in blood vessels to produce vasodilation
B. Adverse reactions: GI upset, flushing, hypotension, dizziness, increased heart rate, headache
C. Agents: the following are examples
   Cyclandelate (Cyclospasmol)
   Ergoloid mesylates (dihydrogenated ergot alkaloids; Hydergine)
   Isoxsuprine hydrochloride (Vasodilan)
D. Nursing assessment: obtain history of onset and course of vascular disease; assess blood pressure, pulses, including peripheral pulses, mental status, color and temperature of affected extremities.
E. Nursing evaluation: observe for therapeutic and adverse effects.
F. Nursing management: monitor presenting signs and symptoms; instruct patient regarding medications.

Antihypertensives

Several subgroups of drugs can lower BP.
A. Action
   1. Adrenergic drugs
      a. Beta-1 adrenergic receptor antagonists (beta-blockers): reduce cardiac output; reduce renin release from kidney (blocks response to sympathetic impulses)

b. Alpha-1 adrenergic receptor antagonists: prevent norepinephrine from constricting blood vessels to increase resistance to blood flow

2. Centrally acting antihypertensive drugs that inhibit the activity of the sympathetic nervous system: decrease sympathetic tone and activate alpha-receptors in the medulla that decrease heart rate and cardiac output

3. Vasodilators: relax arteriolar smooth muscle

4. Vasodilators in hypertensive emergencies: rapidly relax smooth muscle

5. Calcium channel blockers: relax the smooth muscles of the peripheral blood vessels, causing a decrease in peripheral resistance

6. Decreases peripheral resistance leading to a reduction in BP

B. Adverse reactions: bradycardia, hypotension, nasal congestion, reflex tachycardia, dry mouth, fluid retention, arthralgia, depression, drowsiness; the most common side effect to angiotensin-converting enzyme (ACE) inhibitors is a dry hacking cough.

C. Agents: the following are examples

1. Beta-adrenergic receptor antagonists
   Metoprolol tartrate* (Lopressor)
   Nadolol* (Corgard)
   Propranolol hydrochloride* (Inderal)
   Atenolol* (Tenormin)

2. Alpha-adrenergic receptor antagonists
   Doxazosin mesylate* (Cardura)
   Terazosin (Hytrin)
   Prazosin hydrochloride (Minipress)

3. Centrally acting antihypertensive drugs
   Clonidine hydrochloride (Catapres)*
   Methyldopa (Aldomet)*

4. Vasodilators
   Hydralazine hydrochloride (Apresoline)*

5. Calcium channel blockers
   Diltiazem (Cardizem)*
   Verapamil (Calan)*
   Nifedipine (Procardia)*
   This group of medications is also used for treating angina.

6. ACE inhibitors
   Captopril (Capoten)*
   Benazepril (Lotensin)*
   Enalapril (Vasotec)*
   Quinapril (Accupril)

These medications are also used as adjunct therapy in patients with congestive heart failure (CHF).

D. Nursing assessment: obtain vital signs and additional baseline data, such as weight, diet, serum electrolyte levels for electrolyte imbalances.

E. Nursing management: monitor vital signs, intake and output, weight, blood studies

F. Nursing evaluation: observe for therapeutic effects and adverse reactions.

G. Patient teaching: stress the importance of knowing acceptable ranges of BP and pulse, of taking medication as ordered, of preventing orthostatic hypotension, and of reporting asthma, such as signs and symptoms; instruct patient regarding OTC drugs; change positions slowly to avoid orthostatic hypotension; beta-blockers mask the signs of hypoglycemia; hot baths or showers, alcohol intensify hypotension.

H. Nursing Considerations:

1. Patients who suspect pregnancy should not use ACE inhibitors, the "pril" drugs (i.e., Captopril).

2. Beta-blockers, the "olol" drugs (i.e., Metoprolol) should not be used by patients with chronic obstructive pulmonary disease (COPD) because these drugs can cause bronchospasm and wheezing.

3. Beta-blockers and thiazide diuretics cause the most severe sexual dysfunction.

Diuretics

A. Action: increase the excretion of sodium ion and thus increase urine flow

B. Agents

EXAMPLES	ADVERSE REACTIONS
1. Ethacrynic acid (Edecrin)	Dehydration, thrombosis, emboli, electrolyte imbalance
Furosemide (Lasix)*	Acute dehydration, sodium and potassium depletion, calcium loss, dermatitis, blood dyscrasias
2. Thiazide diuretics Chlorothiazide (Diuril) Chlorthalidone (Hygroton) Cyclothiazide (Anhydron) Hydrochlorothiazide (Esidrix, HydroDIURIL) Methyclothiazide (Enduron) Metolazone (Zaroxolyn)	Fluid and electrolyte imbalance, increased calcium serum levels, GI irritation, dizziness, headache, paresthesias, blood dyscrasias, allergy, hypotension

3. Carbonic anhydrase inhibitors

EXAMPLES
Acetazolamide (Diamox)* Ethoxzolamide (Cardrase, Ethamide)

4. Potassium-sparing diuretics

EXAMPLES	ADVERSE REACTIONS
Spironolactone (Aldactone) Triamterene (Dyrenium)	Hyperkalemia, fatal cardiac dysrhythmias, endocrine alterations, blood dyscrasias

C. Nursing assessment: perform total patient assessment with emphasis on presenting signs and symptoms, vital signs, laboratory blood studies.

D. Nursing management: to foster drug therapy such as by restriction of fluid and diet; monitor weight, intake and output, vital signs.

E. Nursing evaluation: observe for therapeutic effects and adverse reactions; instruct patient regarding drugs and diet, prevention of orthostatic hypotension.

Cardiotonic Drugs (Cardiac Glycosides)

A. Action: act directly on myocardial cells to increase contractility and thus cardiac output; slow heart rate

B. Adverse reactions: anorexia, nausea, vomiting, bradycardia, weakness, fatigue, visual dimming, double vision, altered color vision, mood alterations, hallucinations, dysrhythmias

C. Toxic reactions, contusion, heart block, premature ventricular complex (PVCs)

D. Agents: the following are examples
Digitoxin (Crystodigin)
Digoxin (Lanoxin)*

E. Nursing assessment: obtain baseline data, weight, vital signs, electrocardiogram (ECG) results.

F. Nursing management: monitor vital signs, weight, fluid intake and output, serum electrolyte level, especially potassium; instruct patient regarding drugs, eating foods high in potassium.

G. Nursing evaluation: observe for therapeutic effects and adverse reactions.

Drugs to Control Dysrhythmias

A. Action: slow conduction through atrioventricular (AV) node; block effects of vagal nerve stimulation; block beta-adrenergic stimulation; suppress automaticity; increase electrical threshold for stimulation

B. Agents

EXAMPLES	ADVERSE REACTIONS
Atropine*	Dry mouth, cycloplegia, mydriasis, fever, urinary retention
Bretylium tosylate (Bretylol)	Anginal attacks, bradycardia, hypotension
Deslanoside (Cedilanid-D) Digitoxin (Crystodigin, Purodigin)	Bradycardia, premature ventricular beats, AV tachycardia, anorexia, nausea, vomiting
Digoxin (Lanoxin)*	
Disopyramide phosphate (Norpace)	Dry mouth, constipation, urinary retention, blurred vision
Lidocaine (Xylocaine without epinephrine)	Muscle twitching, respiratory depression, convulsions, coma
Phenytoin (Dilantin)	Bradycardia, cardiac arrest, nausea, dizziness, drowsiness
Procainamide hydrochloride (Pronestyl)*	Hypotension, decreased cardiac output, GI distress
Propranolol hydrochloride (Inderal)*	Bradycardia, lowered cardiac output, bronchospasm
Quinidine sulfate (Cin-Quin, Quinora)	Peripheral vasodilation, hypotension, GI distress
Quinidine gluconate (Duraquin)	
Quinidine polygalacturonate (Cardioquin)	

C. Nursing assessment: obtain baseline data, history of subjective and objective symptoms, vital signs.

D. Nursing management: monitor vital signs; instruct patient regarding drugs; maintain therapeutic blood levels by administering around the clock.

E. Nursing evaluation: observe for therapeutic effects and adverse reactions.

Anticoagulants

A. Action: inhibit the aggregation of platelets; interfere with any of the steps leading to the formation of fibrin

B. Adverse reactions: hemorrhage, hematuria, melena, rashes, depression of bone marrow

C. Agents: the following are examples
1. Antiplatelet drugs
Aspirin*
Dipyridamole (Persantine)*
2. Heparin sodium*
(Liquaemin Sodium, Panheprin, Lipo-Hepin)
3. Coumarins
Dicumarol*
Phenprocoumon (Liquamar)
Warfarin sodium (Coumadin, Panwarfin)*
4. Indanediones
Anisindione (Miradon)
Enoxaparin (Lovenox)*

D. Nursing assessment: obtain baseline data relevant to general condition of the patient, history of problems with clots, blood coagulation studies—prothrombin time (PT), partial thromboplastin time (PTT), platelet count, clotting times.

E. Nursing management: monitor blood coagulation studies carefully; use infusion monitoring device for constant infusions of heparin; have drug antidotes readily available.

F. Nursing evaluation: observe for therapeutic effects and adverse reactions.

G. Patient teaching: stress home safety factors to prevent tissue trauma and bleeding; advise to avoid foods high in vitamin K; avoid aspirin, dextran, dipyridamole, and NSAIDs that increase risk of bleeding; instruct patient to observe excreta for signs of bleeding.

H. Drug interactions
1. Drugs potentiating response: clofibrate (Atromid S), disulfiram (Antabuse), neomycin sulfate, phenylbutazone (Butazolidin), salicylates, sulfisoxazole (Gantrisin)
2. Drugs diminishing response: barbiturates, cholestyramine (Questran), ethchlorvynol (Placidyl), glutethimide (Doriden), griseofulvin (Grifulvin-V)

I. Antidotes
1. Heparin: protamine sulfate*
2. Coumarins: vitamin K*

Thrombolytic Drugs

A. Action: promote the digestion of fibrin to dissolve the clot

B. Agents: enzymes urokinase and streptokinase

C. Adverse reaction: hemorrhage

D. Special considerations: reserved for use in acute pulmonary embolism, deep-vein thrombosis, or peripheral arterial occlusion; posttreatment—treated with heparin

E. Nursing assessment: obtain baseline data relevant to size, location, symptoms of clot; assess vital signs and peripheral pulses for adequate circulation to extremities.

F. Nursing management: used only in acute care setting; monitor laboratory blood studies and for signs of clot dissolution.

G. Nursing evaluation: observe for therapeutic effects and adverse reactions.

Hemostatic Agents

A. Action: inhibit the dissolution of blood clots

B. Adverse reactions: nausea, cramps, dizziness, tinnitus, thrombophlebitis, flushing, vascular collapse

C. Agents

EXAMPLES	CLINICAL INDICATIONS
1. Systemic agents Aminocaproic acid (Amicar) Menadiol sodium diphosphate (Synkayvite) Menadione sodium bisulfite (Hykinone) Phytonadione; vitamin K (AquaMEPHYTON, Konakion, Mephyton)	Used in special surgical situations Correction of secondary hypoprothrombinemia, correction of severe vitamin-K deficiency Oral anticoagulant overdose emergency
2. Local hemostatic agents Absorbable gelatin sponge (Gelfoam)	Control bleeding in wound or at operative site

D. Nursing assessment: obtain baseline data relevant to type, location, and amount of bleeding, appropriate laboratory blood studies, and general condition of patient.

E. Nursing management: monitor appropriate laboratory blood studies.

F. Nursing evaluation: observe for therapeutic effects and adverse reactions.

Drugs that Lower Blood Lipid Levels

A. Action: generally lower blood lipid concentrations; research has shown that lowering cholesterol levels, as well as low-density lipoprotein (LDL) levels, decreases the chances of atherosclerosis and coronary artery disease; these medications are generally ordered when dietary and exercise have failed to make changes in the blood level.

B. Adverse reactions: bloating, fever, dizziness, nausea, constipation, muscle cramps, impotence, flushing, weight loss, insomnia, water retention; contraindicated in patients with liver disease

C. Agents: the following are examples
Lovastatin (Mevacor)*
Atorvastatin (Lipitor)*
Cholestyramine (Questran)*
Colestipol hydrochloride (Colestid)
Niacin; nicotinic acid (Nicobid, Niac, Nicolar)
Pravastatin (Pravachol)*
Simvastatin (Zocor)*

D. Nursing assessment: obtain baseline data relevant to weight, serum cholesterol and triglyceride levels, BP, and dietary history; determine if patient is taking any other medications that may increase lipid levels; examples of these would include alcohol and certain cardiac medications; Questran and Colestid should be given with food to increase effectiveness; the others are recommended to be given at night.

E. Nursing management: observe for any new symptoms; instruct patient regarding drugs; restrict intake of fats, cholesterol, alcohol; instruct patient to stop smoking and follow recommended exercise program; instruct patient to report unexplained muscle pain, fever, dark brown urine; monitor liver function tests.

F. Nursing evaluation: observe for adverse effects; monitor blood levels for therapeutic effects.

Drugs that Treat Nutritional Anemias

A. Action: supplement or replace essential vitamins and minerals

B. Agents

EXAMPLES	ADVERSE REACTIONS
1. Iron salts Ferrous sulfate (Feosol, Fer-In-Sol, Fero-Gradumet, Mol-Iron) Ferrous gluconate (Fergon, FerraletPlus, Entron)	Acute toxicity: acute nausea and vomiting, metabolic acidosis, extensive liver and kidney damage Chronic toxicity: bronze coloration of skin, development of diabetes mellitus, heart failure
Ferrocholinate (Chel-Iron, Kelex) Ferrous fumarate (Ferranol, Feostat) Iron dextran injection (Imferon)	
2. Antidote for iron toxicity Deferoxamine mesylate (Desferal)	
3. Vitamin B_{12} Cyanocobalamin (Betalin 12 Crystalline, Redisol, Rubramin PC, Sytobex) Hydroxocobalamin (alphaREDISOL)	Virtually free of adverse reactions
4. Folic acid for anemia Folic acid (Folvite) Leucovorin calcium	Nontoxic

C. Nursing assessment: obtain baseline data for vital signs, weight, dietary history, blood studies, presence of neurologic symptoms.

D. Nursing management: monitor blood studies, vital signs.

E. Nursing evaluation: observe for therapeutic effects and adverse reactions; instruct patient regarding medications; use z-track techniques when injecting iron to avoid staining of skin.

F. Patient teaching: expect dark or black stools and the possibility of GI distress; nutritionally balanced diet.

G. Folic acid has been shown to prevent neural tube defects.

GASTROINTESTINAL SYSTEM

Nurses have a responsibility to educate patients in the dangers of self-medication. Many of these drugs are available OTC.

Drugs that Increase Tone and Motility

A. Action: cholinomimetic action to stimulate or restore intestinal tone or urinary bladder tone

B. Adverse reactions: salivation, skin flushing, sweating, diarrhea, abdominal cramps

C. Agents: bethanechol chloride (Urecholine); neostigmine methylsulfate (Prostigmin)

D. Nursing assessment: obtain baseline data regarding vital signs, bowel sounds, fluid intake and output, bowel activity.

E. Nursing management: stay with patient at least 15 minutes after administration to observe for adverse reactions; monitor vital signs, fluid intake and output, bowel activity.

F. Nursing evaluation: observe for therapeutic effects and adverse reactions.

Drugs that Decrease Tone and Motility (Anticholinergics)

A. Action: inhibit gastric secretion and depress GI motility
B. Adverse reactions: dry mouth, mydriasis, blurred vision, tachycardia, constipation, acute urinary retention
C. Agents: the following are examples
   Atropine sulfate*
   Belladonna extract
   Belladonna tincture
D. Nursing assessment: obtain baseline data for vital signs; assess frequency and character of stools and presence of occult blood in stools; assess ability to empty bladder.
E. Nursing management: monitor vital signs.
F. Nursing evaluation: observe for therapeutic effects and adverse reactions; instruct patient regarding medication.

Drugs to Treat and Prevent Ulcers

A. Action
   1. Antacids: nonsystemic; neutralizes gastric hydrochloric acid; provides soothing effect on lining of GI tract
   2. Anticholinergic drugs: see drugs under the Autonomic Nervous System.
   3. Antihistamines: block the histamines' receptors and decrease gastric acid production
   4. Proton pump inhibitors: act on the parietal cells in the stomach to decrease gastric acid secretion
   5. Mucosal protectants: short-term treatment of duodenal ulcers; form a paste that protects stomach wall from hyper secretion; action is local.
   6. Prostaglandins: adverse reactions—constipation, diarrhea; can interfere with absorption of some drugs—tetracycline, digoxin, quinidine; antihistamines can cause diarrhea, constipation, blurred vision, headaches; in addition to others, prostaglandins can cause musculoskeletal pain and renal impairment; side effects of proton pump inhibitors are relatively low and include GI distress and insomnia.
B. Agents
   1. Agents (antacids): the following are examples
      Aluminum hydroxide (Amphojel)
      Calcium carbonate (Tums)
      Dihydroxyaluminum sodium carbonate (Rolaids)
      Aluminum hydroxide, Magnesium hydroxide (Maalox)
      Aluminum hydroxide gel, Magnesium hydroxide, Simethicone (Maalox Plus, Mylanta, Gelusil)
      Magaldrate (Riopan)
   2. Agents (histamine H2-receptor antagonists): the following are examples
      Cimetidine (Tagamet)*
      Nizatidine (Axid)*
      Famotidine (Pepcid)*
      Ranitidine hydrochloride (Zantac)*
   3. Agents (proton pump inhibitors): the following are examples
      Omeprazole (Prilosec)*
      Lansoprazole (Prevacid)*
   4. Agents (mucosal protectants): the following is an example
      Sulcrafate (Carafate)
   5. Agents (prokinetic GI agent): the following is an example
      Metoclopramide (Reglan)

C. Clinical indications used in treating esophagitis, gastroesophageal reflux disorder (GERD), and other hypersecretory disorders. Reglan is indicated in short-term treatment of GERD that fails to respond to traditional treatment. Reglan is also indicated in treating diabetics with gastric stasis.
D. Nursing assessment: obtain baseline data relevant to vital signs, level of consciousness, character and quality of emesis and stool, appropriate laboratory blood studies, abdominal pain, frank bleeding, and occult bleeding. A careful drug history is needed because many medications interfere with absorption. Calcium and magnesium products increase effect of digoxin and may require dose adjustment. Fluoroquinolone antibiotics can decrease absorption.
E. Nursing management: monitor vital signs, fluid intake and output, level of consciousness, and character of stools and vomitus; teach that antacids decrease absorption of many drugs including iron, tetracyclines; teach not to take antacids for more than 2 weeks without consulting a physician; H2 blockers need to be administered with meals and at bedtime to enhance effectiveness; administer antacids at least 2 hours before or 1 hour after any other oral drugs to be certain these medications are adequately absorbed; caution should be used in patients with known renal and hepatic impairment; mucosal protectants should be administered before meals to ensure efficacy. Administer oral Reglan 30 minutes before meals; monitor for signs and symptoms of hypoglycemia because Reglan causes rapid transit of food through the stomach.
F. Nursing evaluation: observe for therapeutic effects and adverse reactions.

Antiemetics

A. Action: control nausea and vomiting by reducing stimulation of labyrinthine receptors
B. Adverse reactions: drowsiness, blurred vision, dilated pupils, dry mouth, extrapyramidal symptoms
C. Agents: the following are examples
   1. Phenothiazines
      Prochlorperazine (Compazine)*
      Promethazine (Phenergan)*
   2. Prokinetic GI agent
      Metoclopramide (Reglan)
   3. Serotonin antagonist
      Granisetron (Kytril)
      Ondansetron (Zofran)
   4. Miscellaneous antiemetics
      Dimenhydrinate (Dramamine)
      Diphenhydramine hydrochloride (Benadryl)
      Hydroxyzine pamoate (Vistaril)
      Meclizine hydrochloride (Antivert, Bonine)
      Trimethobenzamide hydrochloride (Tigan)
D. Nursing assessment: obtain baseline data regarding vital signs; assess character and quantity of any emesis, presence of bowel sounds; monitor for constipation, fluid intake and output; dehydrated patients are more likely to experience extrapyramidal symptoms.
E. Nursing management: monitor vital signs and fluid intake and output.
F. Nursing evaluation: observe for therapeutic effects and adverse reactions; advise patient to avoid activities that

require mental alertness because of the sedative effect; these drugs are synergistic with other CNS depressants.

Antidiarrheic Agents

A. Action: decrease tone of small and large bowel; depress smooth muscle contraction; decrease release of acetylcholine; absorb toxins
B. Adverse reactions: respiratory depression, constipation, impaction
C. Agents: the following are examples
   Bismuth subsalicylate (Pepto-Bismol)
   Codeine phosphate
   Codeine sulfate
   Diphenoxylate hydrochloride with atropine sulfate (Diphenatol, Lomotil,* Lofene)
   Loperamide hydrochloride (Imodium)*
D. Nursing assessment: obtain baseline data relevant to vital signs, fluid and solid intake and output, nature, and character of stools, skin turgor, fluid and electrolyte balance.
E. Nursing management: monitor vital signs, intake and output, frequency and character of stools; inform patient that diarrhea that lasts for more than 2 days needs to be reported to physician; bismuth preparations are contraindicated for children recovering from viral infections because they contain salicylates.
F. Nursing evaluation: observe for therapeutic effects and adverse reactions.

Laxatives

A. Action: retain water to keep stools large and soft; stimulate motility in large intestine; inhibit reabsorption of water; attract water by osmosis; soften feces
B. Adverse reactions: loss of bowel tone, dehydration, hypokalemia, hyponatremia, malabsorption of fat-soluble vitamins
C. Agents: the following are examples
   1. Bulk-forming agents
      Psyllium hydrocolloid (Effersyllium)
      Psyllium hydrophilic mucilloid (Metamucil)*
   2. Stimulant cathartics (irritants)
      Bisacodyl (Bisco-Lax, Dulcolax)*
      Cascara sagrada (Cascara)
      Castor oil (Neo-Lid)
      Glycerin suppositories
      Phenolphthalein (Ex-Lax, Feen-A-Mint, Phenolax)
      Senna concentrate (Senokot)*
      Senna pod
   3. Saline cathartics
      Magnesium hydroxide (Milk of Magnesia)
      Magnesium sulfate (Epsom salt)
   4. Lubricants
      Mineral oil (Agoral Plain, Petrogalar Plain)
   5. Fecal softeners
      Docusate calcium* (dioctyl calcium sulfosuccinate; Surfak)
      Docusate sodium* (dioctyl sodium sulfosuccinate; Colace, Comfolax, D-S-S)
   6. Osmotic agents
      Glycerin (Glycerol)
      Lactulose (Chronulac)
D. Nursing assessment: obtain baseline data relevant to vital signs, intake and output, presence of bowel sounds, bowel habits, dietary history, medications

E. Nursing management: monitor diet and fluid intake; instruct patient regarding drugs and to increase fiber in diet and increase fluid intake; stool softeners are indicated when avoiding straining is important, such as with a cardiac patient; bulk laxatives need to be given with 8 ounces of water to prevent blockage; mineral oil needs to be used cautiously because it hinders the absorption of fat-soluble vitamins.
F. Nursing evaluation: observe for therapeutic effects and adverse reactions.

ENDOCRINE SYSTEM

Drugs Affecting Pituitary Gland

A. Action
   1. Antidiuretic hormone: increases renal tubule's permeability and thus its ability to reabsorb water
   2. Oxytocin: promotes uterine contractions during last stages of labor when cervix is fully dilated
   3. Growth hormone: anabolic agent that increases cell size and cell numbers and stimulates linear growth
   4. Gonadotropic hormone (GTH): regulates maturation and function of male and female sexual organs
   5. Adrenocorticotropic hormone (ACTH): stimulates adrenal cortex to release its hormone
B. Adverse reactions: hyponatremia, water retention, glycosuria, vasoconstriction, nausea
C. Agents

EXAMPLES	CLINICAL INDICATIONS
Desmopressin acetate (DDAVP)	Diabetes insipidus
Lypressin (Diapid)	Diabetes insipidus
Posterior pituitary extract (Pituitrin)	Smooth muscle contraction
Vasopressin (Pitressin)	Short-term maintenance of unconscious patient

D. Nursing assessment: obtain baseline data relative to excesses or deficiencies of specific hormone.
E. Nursing management: monitor fluid intake and output, laboratory values; instruct patient regarding medications.
F. Nursing evaluation: observe for therapeutic effects and adverse reactions.

Drugs Affecting Adrenal Glands

A. Action: replace the body's normal amount of hormones; block inflammatory responses; antineoplastic; antagonize autoimmune responses
B. Adverse reactions: impaired glucose tolerance or hyperglycemia; fat deposition; muscle weakness or wasting; peptic ulcer; growth inhibition; mood changes or psychosis; osteoporosis; sodium retention; potassium loss
C. Agents: dosage is individualized to patient and diagnosis; the following are examples
   Betamethasone valerate (Valisone)
   Cortisone acetate (Cortone)
   Dexamethasone (Decadron,* Hexadrol)
   Fludrocortisone acetate (Florinef)
   Hydrocortisone (cortisol; Cortef, Cortril, Hydrocortone)
   Hydrocortisone acetate (Cortef)
   Methylprednisolone (Medrol, Wyacort)
   Methylprednisolone acetate (Depo-Medrol)

Methylprednisolone sodium succinate (Solu-Medrol)
Prednisolone (Delta-Cortef, Paracortol)
Prednisone (Meticorten, Delta-Dome)
Triamcinolone (Aristocort, Kenacort)
Triamcinolone acetonide (Kenalog)

D. Nursing assessment: obtain baseline data relevant to vital signs, weight, glycosuria.
E. Nursing management: monitor vital signs, weight, serum electrolyte levels, sugar concentrations in blood and urine, signs of masked infection; instruct patient regarding medications, additive hypokalemia.
F. Nursing evaluations: observe for therapeutic effects and adverse reactions.

Drugs Affecting Thyroid Gland

A. Action
   1. Hypothyroidism: replace the body's normal amount of hormone
   2. Hyperthyroidism
      a. Control the symptoms of hyperthyroidism
      b. Inhibit the synthesis of thyroid hormones
      c. Inhibit iodine uptake by thyroid gland
      d. Inhibit thyroid hormone release and symptoms
      e. Suppress continued uptake of iodine
      f. Destroy surrounding tissue by emission of low-energy radiation
B. Adverse reactions to drugs for hyperthyroidism: agranulocytosis; skin rash, nausea, vomiting, twitching muscles, bronchospasm, iodism, symptoms of hyperthyroidism
C. Adverse reactions to drugs for hypothyroidism: dysrhythmias, hypertension, headache, insomnia, irritability, vomiting, weight loss
D. Agents: the following are examples
   1. Hypothyroidism
      a. Natural thyroid hormones
         Thyroglobulin (Proloid)*
         Thyroid (Delcoid, Thyrar, Thyrocrine)
      b. Synthetic thyroid hormones
         Levothyroxine sodium (Eltroxin, Levoid, Synthroid)
         Liothyronine sodium (Cytomel)
         Liotrix (Euthroid, Thyrolar)
      c. Adenohypophyseal hormone
         Thyroid-stimulating hormone (TSH) (thyrotropin; Thytropar)
         Protirelin (Thypinone)
   2. Hyperthyroidism
      a. Thioamides
         Methimazole (Tapazole)
         Propylthiouracil
      b. Beta-adrenergic blocker
         Propranolol hydrochloride (Inderal)
      c. Iodine
         Potassium or sodium iodide (Lugol's solution)
      d. Radioactive iodine (^{131}I)
E. Nursing assessment: obtain baseline data relevant to vital signs, weight, level of energy, symptoms of hypofunctioning or hyperfunctioning of gland and serum thyroid levels; thyroid hormones increase the potency of oral anticoagulants, these drugs also decrease the effectiveness of digoxin.
F. Nursing management: monitor vital signs, weight; instruct patient regarding medications, compliance with therapy.

G. Nursing evaluation: observe for therapeutic effects and adverse reactions; monitor thyroid function studies.

Drugs Affecting Parathyroid Gland

A. Action: maintain blood calcium levels in the blood
B. Adverse reactions: nausea, local irritation at injection sites, drowsiness, GI complaints, hypertension, facial flushing
C. Agents: the following are examples
   Calcitonin (Calcimar)
   Calcitriol (Rocaltrol)
   Parathyroid hormone
D. Nursing assessment: obtain baseline data relevant to vital signs and blood calcium levels.
E. Nursing management: monitor vital signs, blood calcium levels; advise to avoid spinach, whole grains, rhubarb and to maintain adequate intake of calcium and vitamin D.
F. Nursing evaluation: observe for therapeutic effects (i.e., decreased muscle cramping) and adverse reactions; instruct patient regarding medications.

FEMALE REPRODUCTIVE SYSTEM

Estrogens

A. Action: replace or supplement natural body hormones; alter cell environment in neoplastic processes
B. Adverse reactions: breast tenderness, increased risk of breast and endometrial cancer, nausea, vomiting, anorexia, malaise, depression, salt and water retention
C. Agents: the following are examples
   Estrogen, conjugated (Premarin)*
   Estradiol (Estraderm)

Progestins

A. Action: suppress endometrial bleeding; withdrawal of drug induces tissue sloughing
B. Adverse reactions: edema, breast tenderness, depression, midcycle bleeding
C. Agents: the following are examples
   Medroxyprogesterone acetate (Depo-Provera,* Provera)
   Megestrol acetate (Megace)*
   Norethindrone (Norlutin, Ortho-Novum)

Fertility Drugs

A. Action: stimulate ovulation by pituitary or ovarian mechanisms
B. Adverse reactions: relatively rare
C. Agents: the following are examples
   Clomiphene citrate (Clomid)*
   Human chorionic gonadotropin (HCG) (Antuitrin S, Follutein)
   Menotropins (Perganol)

Contraceptive Drugs

A. Action: suppress ovulation; induce changes in cervical mucus, making uterine entry by sperm difficult; produce changes in endometrium, making implantation difficult
B. Adverse reactions: thromboembolitic diseases, stroke, hypertension
C. Agents: the following examples contain varying amounts of progesterone and estrogen:
   Brevicon

Depo-Provera
Enovid
Norlestrin
Ortho-Novum
Ovrette
Ovulen
D. Contraceptive effects may be lessened if taken with antibiotics.

Oxytocic Drugs

A. Action: induce contraction of the myometrium
B. Adverse reactions: fetal or maternal cardiac dysrhythmias, acute hypertension, nausea, water intoxication, uterine hypertonicity with fetal or maternal injury
C. Agents: the following are examples
Ergonovine maleate (Ergotrate)
Methylergonovine maleate (Methergine)
Oxytocin (Pitocin, Syntocinon)*

Uterine Relaxants

A. Action: stimulation of beta-2 adrenergic receptors produces relaxation of uterine muscle
B. Adverse reactions: heart palpitations, nausea, vomiting, trembling, flushing, headache
C. Agents: ritodrine, terbutaline (Brethine)

Nursing Process

A. Assessment: obtain baseline data relevant to vital signs, weight, current problem; elicit history of previous pregnancies and deliveries, fetal heart tones.
B. Management: inform of possible side effects and benefit; monitor vital signs, weight; with oxytocics—maternal and fetal monitoring; infusion-monitoring device
C. Evaluation: observe for therapeutic effects and adverse reactions; instruct patient regarding medications.

MALE REPRODUCTIVE SYSTEM

Drugs used to treat BPH
A. Action: inhibits the enzyme responsible for prostatic growth and improves urinary flow; also used in treating male pattern baldness
B. Adverse effects: headache, abdominal or back pain, gynecomastia
C. Agent: finasteride (Proscar)*
D. Nursing process: inform patient that up to 3 months may be required to see relief of symptoms; monitor urinary patterns for improvement.

MALE HORMONES

Androgens

A. Action: replace or supplement normal body hormone; relieve postpartum breast engorgement; alter cell environment in neoplastic disease in women
B. Adverse reactions: female masculinization; premature closure of epiphyses in children; nausea, vomiting, diarrhea, mood swing
C. Agents: the following are examples
Danocrine (Danazol)
Fluoxymesterone (Halotestin)

Methyltestosterone (Android)
Testosterone (Delatestryl)
(Testaqua, Oreton)

Anabolic Steroids

A. Action: increase nitrogen retention and protein formation; stimulate RBC formation and increase bone deposition
B. Adverse reactions: increased libido; priapism (continuous erection), female masculinization, precocious sexual development in children, premature epiphyseal fusion
C. Agents: the following are examples
Ethylestrenol (Maxibolin)
Methandrostenolone (Dianabol)
Methandriol
Nandrolone phenpropionate (Durabolin)
Oxandrolone (Anavar)
Stanozolol (Winstrol)

Nursing Process

A. Assessment: obtain baseline data relevant to vital signs, weight, height (children), current problem.
B. Management: monitor vital signs, weight, height (children); review possible effects with patient.
C. Evaluation: observe for therapeutic effects and adverse reaction; instruct patient regarding medications.

EYE

Anticholinergic Drugs

A. Action: cause mydriasis (dilated pupils) and cycloplegia (blurred vision)
B. Adverse reaction: dry mouth and skin, fever, thirst, confusion, hyperactivity
C. Agents: the following are examples
Atropine sulfate (Atropisol, Isopto Atropine)*
Cyclopentolate hydrochloride (Cyclogyl)
Homatropine hydrobromide (Isopto Homatropine)
Scopolamine hydrobromide (hyoscine hydrobromide; Isopto Hyoscine)
Tropicamide (Mydriacyl)

Adrenergic Drugs

A. Action: cause mydriasis
B. Adverse reactions: rare
C. Agents: the following are examples
Phenylephrine hydrochloride (Alconefrin, Mydfrin, Neo-Synephrine Hydrochloride)

Drugs Used to Treat Glaucoma

A. Action: cause miosis (pupil constriction); reduce resistance to outflow of aqueous humor; decrease production of aqueous humor
B. Adverse reactions: blood vessel congestion causing increased intraocular pressure, ocular pain, headache, tachycardia or bradycardia, hypertension, diaphoresis, anorexia, GI upset, lethargy, depression, diuresis, dehydration
C. Agents: the following are examples
Acetazolamide (Diamox)*
Dichlorphenamide (Daranide, Oratrol)
Pilocarpine hydrochloride (Isopto Carpine, Pilocar)
Timolol maleate (Timoptic)*
Urea (Ureaphil, Urevert)

NURSING PROCESS

A. Nursing assessment: obtain history of eye-related symptoms, such as difficulty in driving or ambulating; examine eyes for signs of infection, exudate, tearing, drying; assess for eye pain.

B. Nursing management: advise patient about effects of drugs, such as blurred vision and photophobia; instruct patient regarding drugs (e.g., do not skip doses); teach proper administration of eye medication.

C. Nursing evaluation: observe for therapeutic effects and adverse reactions.

DRUGS USED TO CONTROL MUSCLE TONE

Acetylcholinesterase Inhibitors (Anticholinergic Agents)

A. Action: allow the accumulation of acetylcholine at neuromuscular junctions and thus ensure muscle contractility; drugs are not used during pregnancy or with patients who have hyperexcitability of muscular symptoms.

B. Adverse reactions: muscle cramps, fasciculations (rapid, small contractions), weakness; excessive salivation, perspiration, nausea, vomiting

C. Agents: the following are examples
Ambenonium chloride (Mytelase)
Edrophonium chloride (Tensilon)
Neostigmine bromide (Prostigmin)
Pyridostigmine bromide (Mestinon, Regonol)

D. Nursing assessment: obtain baseline data relevant to vital signs, ability to swallow, muscle strength, eyelid ptosis, gait, reflexes.

E. Nursing management: monitor disease symptoms and vital signs; have suction and intubation equipment at bedside.

F. Nursing evaluation: observe for therapeutic effects and adverse reactions.

Neuromuscular Blocking Agents

A. Action: produce muscle paralysis

B. Adverse reactions: hypotension, bronchospasm, tachycardia, bradycardia, cardiac dysrhythmias, respiratory distress

C. Agents: the following are examples
Decamethonium bromide (Syncurine)
Gallamine triethiodide (Flaxedil)
Pancuronium bromide (Pavulon)
Tubocurarine chloride (Tubarine)

D. Nursing assessment: obtain baseline data relevant to pulse, respiration, BP.

E. Nursing management: monitor vital signs; continually assess respiratory status, lung sounds, rate and depth of respirations; have suction and intubation equipment at bedside.

F. Nursing evaluation: observe for therapeutic effects—sufficient muscle relaxation to allow procedure to be done; observe for adverse reactions—cough and inability to breathe unassisted and to handle secretions.

DIABETES MELLITUS

Insulin*

A. Action: restores the cell's ability to use glucose and to correct the metabolic changes that occur with diabetes mellitus

B. Adverse reactions: allergic reactions, insulin resistance, injection-site lipoatrophy (Table 3-7)

C. Agents: Table 3-8 lists insulin preparations.

NURSING PROCESS

A. Assessment
1. Obtain baseline data relative to nonfunctioning of the pancreas, vital signs, weight, blood glucose level.
   a. Normal blood glucose level 70 to 120 mg/dl
   b. Glycosylated hemoglobin (Hgb) may be drawn to evaluate treatment effectiveness; the American Diabetes

TABLE 3-7	Hyperglycemia and Hypoglycemic Reactions	
	Hyperglycemia: Ketoacidosis, Diabetic Coma, Too Little Insulin	Hypoglycemia: Insulin Reaction, Too Much Insulin
Onset	Gradual—days	Minutes to hours
Causes	Neglect of therapy, untreated diabetes, intercurrent disease or infection, increase in emotional or psychologic stress	Insulin overdose, omission or delay of meals, excessive exercise before meals
Signs and symptoms	Thirst, headache, excessive urination, nausea, vomiting, abdominal pain, dim vision, coma, flushed face, Kussmaul breathing—rapid, deep—air hunger, dehydration, acetone breath, soft eyeballs, normal reflexes absent	Nervousness, hunger, weakness, cold clammy sweat, nausea, dizziness, double or blurred vision, behavioral changes, stupor, convulsions, pallor, shallow respirations, normal eyeballs, Babinski reflex may be present
Urine glucose	Positive	Negative or low
Urine acetone	Positive	Negative
Blood glucose	High (above 250 mg)	Low (below 60 mg)
Blood CO_2	Low	Usually normal
Treatment	Insulin, fluid replacement, electrolyte replacement, close observation	Glucose, glucagon, close observation
Response to treatment	Slow	Rapid

CO_2, Carbon dioxide.

TABLE 3-8	Insulin: Pharmacokinetics			
Insulins*		**Onset (hr)**	**Peak Effect (hr)**	**Duration of Action (hr)**
Rapid Acting				
Insulin injection (regular insulin, Humulin R)†		0.5-1	2-4	5-7
Insulin aspart (NovoLog)		0.25	1-3	3-5
Insulin lispro (Humalog)		0.25	1	4
Intermediate Acting				
Isophane insulin suspension (NPH Insulin, Humulin N)		3-4	6-12	18-28
Insulin zinc suspension (Lente Insulin)		1-3	8-12	18-28
Long Acting				
Extended insulin zinc suspension (Ultralente)		4-6	18-24	36
Combinations				
Insulin glargine (Lantus)		1.1	5	24
Isophane human insulin (50%) & human insulin (50%) (Humulin 50/50)		0.5	3	22-24
Isophane human insulin (70%) and human insulin (30%) (Humulin 70/30, Novalin 70/30)		0.5	4-8	24

From McKenry LM, Salerno E: *Pharmacology in nursing,* ed 21, St Louis, 2003, Mosby.
*Semilente insulin is available in Canada but is no longer available in the United States. The onset of action of Semilente insulin is 1-3 hours, the peak effect is in 2-8 hours, and the duration of action is 12-16 hr.
†These insulins may be administered IV. IV, the onset of action is within 1/4 to 1/2 hour, and the duration of action is within 1/2 to 1 hour.

Association (ADA) recommends less than 7% for good diabetic control; serious action should be taken when levels rise above 8%.
2. Monitor urine ketones during illness; insulin requirements may increase during stress, infection, or surgery.
3. Assess for signs and symptoms of hypoglycemia and hyperglycemia (see Table 3-7).
B. Interventions
1. Teach patient to follow recommended diabetic diet and to use exchange system when planning meals.
2. Teach patient techniques for maintaining serum glucose levels, signs and symptoms of hypoglycemia and hyperglycemia, and actions patient should take; physician should be notified if patient is unable to eat.
3. Teach patient to carry simple sugar and to wear identification tag describing medication regime.
4. Teach patient the importance of regular exercise, care of feet and nails, self-administration of medications, rotation of injection sites.

ORAL HYPOGLYCEMIC AGENTS

Not indicated for patients with type 1 diabetes.

Sulfonylureas

A. Action: stimulate release of insulin from pancreas—effective only as long as pancreas maintains some insulin producing capacity.
B. Adverse reactions: gastrointestinal distress, muscle weakness, paresthesias, skin reactions, hypoglycemia

C. Agents

EXAMPLES	DURATION OF ACTION
Tolbutamide (Orinase)*	6 to 12 hr
Acetohexamide (Dymelor)*	12 to 24 hr
Tolazamide (Tolinase)*	12 to 24 hr
Glyburide (Micronase)*	up to 24 hr
Chlorpropamide (Diabinese)*	24 to 72 hr
Glipizide (Glucotrol)*	up to 24 hr
Glimepiride (Amaryl)*	Not available

Biguanides

A. Action: increase the amount of glucose taken up by the muscles and intestinal wall and inhibit hepatic glucose production; raise the body's own sensitivity to insulin
B. Adverse reactions: headache, weakness, GI distress, thrombocytopenia
C. Agents

EXAMPLES	DURATION OF ACTION
Metformin hydrochloride (Glucophage)* [Glyburide] metformin (Glucovance)*	6 to 12 hr

Alpha-Glucosidase Inhibitors

A. Action: delay the digestion of ingested carbohydrates; result in a smaller rise in blood glucose after meals; do not increase insulin production
B. Adverse reactions: abdominal pain, diarrhea, flatulence

C. Agents

EXAMPLES	DURATION OF ACTION
Acarbose (Precose)*	4 to 6 hr
Miglitol (Glyset)*	4 to 6 hr

Thiazolidinedione

A. Action: lower blood glucose by improving tissue response to insulin; decrease insulin resistance in the periphery and liver, which results in an increased glucose processing in the body
B. Adverse reactions: palpitations, increased lactate dehydrogenase (LDH), nausea, vomiting, diarrhea, anorexia, nephrotoxicity
C. Agents
   Pioglitazone (Actos)*
   Rosiglitazone (Avandia)*

Meglitinides

A. Action: improve insulin secretions in response to increased glucose levels; shorter acting and are excreted faster than the oral sulfonylurea drugs
B. Similar to oral sulfonylurea drugs with the exception of cardiovascular effects including hypertension and dysrhythmias
C. Examples
   Nateglinide (Starlix)*
   Repaglinide (Prandin)

Nursing Process Related to all Four Classifications of Oral Hypoglycemic Agents

A. Assessment
   1. Obtain baseline vital signs, weight, blood glucose levels, and other signs and symptoms of the disease.
   2. Monitor signs and symptoms of hypoglycemia and hyperglycemia.
B. Interventions
   1. Monitor vital signs, blood glucose levels, other blood levels.
   2. Instruct patient on medication administration and how to monitor blood glucose levels; teach that stress, fever, trauma, infection, and surgery may increase requirements for medication or necessitate the need to temporarily switch to insulin.
   3. Teach signs and symptoms of hypoglycemia and hyperglycemia and steps to correct.
   4. Instruct on the avoidance of alcohol to prevent hypoglycemic reactions.
C. Evaluation
   1. Decrease in symptoms associated with diabetes
   2. Blood glucose levels under control

URINARY SYSTEM

Urinary Tract Antispasmodic Analgesis

A. Action: inhibit the effects of smooth muscle on the bladder
B. Adverse effects: headache dizziness, drowsiness, mental confusion, jaundice, increased intraocular pressure; renal failure may result from prolonged use.
C. Examples of agents:
   Flavoxate (Urispas)

Oxybutynin (Ditropan)*
Phenazopyridine (Pyridium)
D. Nursing process: these medications are contraindicated in patients with glaucoma, GI or genitourinary obstruction or ileus; instruct the patient to avoid hazardous activity until side effects are known; monitor for jaundice, which can be a sign of liver impairment; monitor blood work for any signs of blood dyscrasias.
Diuretics and urinary tract antibiotics are discussed under cardiovascular and immune system, respectively.

IMMUNE SYSTEM

Antibiotics Used in the Treatment and Prevention of Infections

Nursing Process for All Antibiotics
A. Assessment
   1. Obtain baseline data related to signs and symptoms of infection.
   2. Monitor blood urea nitrogen (BUN), complete blood count (CBC), liver studies, particularly with IV medications.
   3. Antibiotics interact with many medications; an accurate medication history is essential.
   4. Antibiotics are effective against bacterial infections; physicians may place high-risk patients with a viral infection on an antibiotic to prevent the development of a secondary bacterial infection.
   5. A culture and sensitivity should be completed to determine the appropriate antibiotic.

B. Planning
   1. Patients must be taught to take medication for the entire course of therapy to avoid the development of bacterial resistant strains; they should continue taking medications when symptoms subside.
   2. Patients must be instructed on the proper timing and method for administration.
   3. Patients need to be taught to report any signs of a super infection, such as vaginal irritation, itching, discharge, black tongue, furry overgrowth, loose foul-smelling stools.
   4. Patients need to be taught to report any rashes and any difficulty breathing to health care provider.

C. Implementation
   1. Adequate fluid intake should be taken to replace fluids lost with diarrhea and prevent dehydration.
   2. Follow appropriate guidelines for each medication; many antibiotics need to be taken at equally spaced intervals around the clock to maintain blood levels.

D. Evaluation: improvement in the presenting symptoms of infection

Penicillins

A. Action: bacteriocidal by interfering with the synthesis of the bacterial cell wall
B. Adverse reactions: allergies—rash, anaphylaxis; convulsions with high parenteral doses; GI distress—nausea, vomiting, and diarrhea; most common cause of drug allergic reactions

C. Agents: the following are examples
Penicillins
Amoxicillin (Amoxil, Larotid, Polymox, Trimox)
Ampicillin (Amcill, Omnipen, Polycillin, Principen)
Carbenicillin disodium (Geopen)
Oxacillin sodium (Bactocill, Prostaphlin)
Penicillin G potassium (Megacillin)
Penicillin G procaine (Crysticillin, Duracillin, Wycillin)
Penicillin V (Pen Vee K, V-Cillin, Veetids)

D. Clinical indications: useful in treating gram-positive and gram-negative infections, including otitis media, pharyngitis, tonsillitis, pneumonia, syphilis, and gonorrhea; given prophylactically to patients with rheumatic fever

E. Patient teaching
1. Penicillin should be taken on an empty stomach and with water.
2. Penicillin thought to decrease effectiveness of oral contraceptives.

Cephalosporins*

A. Action: interferes with bacterial wall synthesis
B. Adverse effects: most common effects are symptoms involving GI distress
C. Agents: the following are examples
Cephalosporins
Cefaclor (Ceclor)*
Cefamandole nafate (Mandol)
Cefazolin sodium (Ancef, Kefzol)
Cefoxitin (Mefoxin)
Cephalexin (Keflex)
Cefoxitin (Claforan)
Cefepime (Maxipime)
D. Clinical indications
1. Wound and skin infections
2. Respiratory infections, skin infections, urinary tract infections
3. Each generation is effective against a variety of gram-positive and gram-negative organisms.
E. Patient teaching
1. Consuming alcohol within 72 hours after discontinuing medication will induce antabuse-like reaction.
2. Take with small meal to decrease GI distress.

Erythromycin, Clindamycin (Penicillin Substitutes)

A. Action: bacteriostatic or bacteriocidal (dosage related) by inhibiting protein synthesis
B. Adverse reactions: abdominal discomfort, cramping, nausea, vomiting, diarrhea, urticaria, anaphylaxis, colitis, liver dysfunction, deafness (vancomycin), permanent kidney damage (systemic bacitracin, vancomycin); Hismanal has the potential to cause fatal dysrhythmias when taken with erythromycin.
C. Agents: the following are examples
1. Erythromycins
Erythromycin (E-Mycin, Ilotycin, Robimycin, RP-Mycin)
2. Clindamycins, lincomycins
Clindamycin (Cleocin)
3. Penicillin substitutes
Bacitracin
Novobiocin sodium (Albamycin)
Spectinomycin hydrochloride (Trobicin)
Vancomycin hydrochloride (Vancocin)

D. Clinical indications
1. See clinical indications for penicillins.
2. Used for patients allergic to penicillin

Macrolides

A. Action: macrolides depending on dose and organism are bacteriostatic or bacteriocidal
B. Adverse reactions: relatively few compared to other antibiotics—GI distress, pruritus, reversible hearing loss
C. Examples include:
Erythromycin* (E-Mycin) ocular infections
Azithromycin* (Zithromax)
Clarithromycin* (Biaxin)
Dirithromycin (Dynabe)
D. Clinical indications: respiratory, skin infections, sexually transmitted diseases

Tetracyclines

A. Action: bacteriostatic by preventing the start of protein synthesis (tetracyclines) or inhibiting protein synthesis (chloramphenicol)
B. Adverse reactions: tetracyclines: nausea, vomiting, stomach pain, diarrhea, superimposed infections, impaired kidney functions, jaundice, delayed blood coagulation, brown discoloration of teeth in children under 8 years of age; tetracyclines are known teratogen and should not be given if pregnancy is suspected.
C. Agents: the following are examples
Tetracycline hydrochloride (Achromycin)
D. Clinical indications
1. Gram-negative and gram-positive infections
2. Severe acne vulgaris
3. Used for patients allergic to penicillin
E. Patient teaching: instruct patient that tetracycline absorption is inhibited with dairy products and many nonsystemic antacids.

Aminoglycosides

A. Action: inhibit early stages of protein synthesis
B. Adverse reactions: eighth cranial nerve damage, renal damage, respiratory paralysis
C. Agents: the following are examples of Aminoglycosides
Amikacin sulfate (Amikin)
Gentamicin sulfate (Garamycin)
Kanamycin sulfate (Kantrex)
Neomycin sulfate (Mycifradin, Neobiotic)
Streptomycin
Tobramycin sulfate (Nebcin)
D. Clinical indications: drugs are potentially dangerous and are used only in cases of severe infections, such as gram-negative bone and joint infections and septicemia; peak and trough levels need to be drawn to evaluate effectiveness.

Sulfonamides

A. Action: block bacterial synthesis of folic acid; inhibit bacterial enzymes required for proper metabolism of sugar; interfere directly with DNA synthesis
B. Adverse reactions: sulfonamides are not used as frequently as in the past because of the development of drug-resistance bacteria and the development of newer antibiotics; adverse reactions include allergies, rash, headache fever, nausea,

vomiting, diarrhea, stomatitis, blood dyscrasias, renal calculi, hematuria

C. Agents: the following are examples
1. Sulfonamides
   Sulfasalazine (Azulfidine, Salazopyrin)
   Sulfisoxazole (Gantrisin)
   Sulfisoxazole-phenazopyridine hydrochloride (Azo Gantrisin, SK-Soxazole, Azosul)
2. Sulfonamides: topical agents and solutions:
   Mafenide (Sulfamylon)
   Silver sulfadiazine (Silvadene)
   Sulfisoxazole diolamine (Gantrisin Ophthalmic)
D. Clinical indications
1. Used to treat acute and chronic urinary tract infections
2. Other uses include trachoma, chancroid, toxoplasmosis, acute otitis media, prophylactic therapy in cases of recurrent rheumatic fever.
3. Treatment of ulcerative colitis
4. Prophylaxis for patients scheduled for bowel surgery (to prevent renal calculi; teach patient to maintain fluid intake of 2000 to 3000 ml/day).
5. Silver sulfadiazine used topically for burn patients; apply silver sulfadiazine sparingly to a thickness of 1/16 of an inch.
E. Patient teaching: adequate fluid intake to prevent crystalluria

Fluoroquinolones *

A. Action: bacteriocidal against broad spectrum of bacteria
B. Adverse reactions: GI distress, headache, dizziness, super infections, renal impairment, photosensitivity; fluoroquinolones should not be given to children under 18 years of age.
C. Examples of agents:
   Ciprofloxacin hydrochloride* (Cipro)
   Levofloxacin* (Levaquin)
   Gatifloxacin* (Tequin)
D. Clinical Indications: respiratory, urinary, and GI tract infections, sexually transmitted diseases, bone and soft-tissue infections, anthrax
E. Patient teaching: these drugs are synergistic with caffeine, theophylline, warfarin; dosage adjustment may be required; antacids, sucralfate, iron, milk products decrease effectiveness of fluoroquinolones; patients should be taught to wear protective sunscreens and clothing.

Miscellaneous Antibiotics

A. Action: bacteriocidal
B. Adverse reactions: super infections, renal toxicity, ototoxicity
C. Examples of agents:
   Aztreonam (Azactam)
   Clindamycin (Cleocin)
   Imipenem (Premaxin)
   Vancomycin (Vancocin)
D. Clinical indications:
   Aztreonam: skin, intraabdominal infections, genitourinary infections, septicemia
   Clindamycin: abdominopelvic infections, acne vulgaris
   Imipenem: serious respiratory, genitourinary and pelvic infections, endocarditis, septicemia
   Vancomycin:* life-threatening infections
E. Patient teaching
1. Report watery stools to health care providers.
2. These drugs should not be administered during pregnancy.

Drugs Used to Treat Tuberculosis and Leprosy

A. Action: alter several metabolic processes in mycobacteria
B. Adverse reactions: peripheral neuropathies, visual disturbances, GI distress, ototoxicity, headache
C. Agents: the following are examples
1. First-line antituberculin drugs
   Isoniazid (INH)
   Ethambutol hydrochloride (Myambutol)*
   Isoniazid (Isotamine, Niconyl, Nydrazid)*
   Para-aminosalicylic acid (PAS) (aminosalicylic acid, Teebacin acid)*
   Rifampin (Rifadin, Rimactane)*
   Streptomycin
2. Second-line antituberculin drugs
   Capreomycin (Capastat)
   Cycloserine (Seromycin)
   Ethionamide (Trecator S.C.)
   Pyrazinamide
3. Antileprosy agents
   Clofazimine (Lamprene)
   Dapsone (Avlosulfon)
   Rifampin (Rifadin, Rimactane)
   Sulfoxone sodium (Diasone)
D. Patient teaching: stress importance of long-term compliance and follow-up visits with the physician; report any adverse reactions promptly; refrain from consuming alcohol; refrain from taking other medications without the knowledge and permission of the physician; wear a medical identification tag indicating medication being taken.

Antifungal Drugs

A. Action: selectively damages the membranes of fungi
B. Adverse reactions: renal damage, anemia, nausea, diarrhea
C. Agents: the following are examples
1. Systemic agents
   Amphotericin B (Fungizone)
   Miconazole (Monistat-IV)
   Fluconazole (Diflucan)*
   Ketoconazole (Nizoral)
2. Topical agents
   Amphotericin B (Fungizone)
   Clioquinol (Vioform)
   Clotrimazole (Gyne-Lotrimin, Lotrimin)*
   Griseofulvin (Fulvicin-P/G, Grifulvin V, Grisactin)
   Miconazole nitrate (MicaTin, Monistat)*
   Nystatin (Mycostatin, Nilstat)
   Tolnaftate (Aftate, Tinactin)
   Undecylenic acid—zinc undecylenate (Desenex, Cruex)
D. Clinical indications: fungal infections can be topical or systemic; fungal infections are often treated prophylactically in patients who are immunocompromised to prevent secondary infection.
E. Patient teaching: proper administration of vaginal tablets, use of condom by sexual partner to avoid reinfection; report any signs of liver damage; instruct patient on "swish and swallow" technique or to hold lozenge in mouth for as long as possible.

Drugs Used to Treat Viral Diseases

A. Action: selective toxicity in various processes of virus reproduction; most antiviral drugs inhibit the progression of the virus but do not destroy it; a healthy immune system is required to fight off the organism.

B. Adverse reactions: ataxia, slurred speech, lethargy, local irritation, anorexia, nausea, vomiting, diarrhea, dizziness, headache, anemia and bone marrow suppression (zidovudine), bone marrow depression (ganciclovir), visual haze, irritation, burning of eyes, photophobia (idoxuridine)

C. Agents: the following are examples
Acyclovir (Zovirax)*
Amantadine (Symmetrel)
Zidovudine (AZT, Retrovir)
Saquinavir (Invirase)
Nelfinavir (Viracept)
Didanosine (Videx)

D. Clinical indications: zidovudine used in treatment of acquired immunodeficiency syndrome (AIDS); prevents replication of the human immunodeficiency virus (HIV), thus delaying disease progression; acyclovir is also useful in treating herpes zoster and other viral infections because the virus changes; the health care provider may vary drug regime; drug regime is most effective before the immune system is compromised.

Nursing Process

A. Nursing assessment: obtain history of allergies; evaluate baseline data relevant to signs and symptoms of infection, vital signs, pertinent laboratory tests, appearance of wounds, incisions, or lesions, amount and description of drainage, swelling, erythema, subjective symptoms of pain or pressure.

B. Nursing management: obtain culture for specimens before starting antibiotics; maintain supportive measures such as rest, comfort, nutrition, fluids and electrolyte balance; maintain proper administration regarding route, time, dosage; monitor vital signs and laboratory results.

C. Nursing evaluation: observe for therapeutic effects and adverse reactions; instruct patient regarding medications to ensure compliance.

NEOPLASTIC DISEASES

Specific Antineoplastic Agents

A. Action: selective toxicity during various stages of the cell cycle
B. Agents

EXAMPLES	ADVERSE REACTIONS
Asparaginase (Elspar)	CNS depression
Chlorambucil (Leukeran)	Bone marrow suppression
Cisplatin (Platinol)	Renal damage, nausea and vomiting, ototoxicity, neurotoxicity, anaphylactic reactions
Cyclophosphamide (Cytoxan)	Hemorrhagic cystitis, bladder fibrosis
Doxorubicin hydrochloride (Adriamycin)	Bone marrow suppression, GI distress, alopecia
Fluorouracil (5-FU, Adrucil)	GI and hematologic toxicity
Hydroxyurea (Hydrea)	Bone marrow suppression
Mechlorethamine hydrochloride or nitrogen mustard (Mustargen)	Bone marrow suppression
Medroxyprogesterone (Depo-Provera)	Menstrual irregularities, rashes, and thromboembolic diseases

EXAMPLES	ADVERSE REACTIONS
Megestrol acetate (Megace)	Thromboembolic disease
Methotrexate	GI toxicity, bone marrow suppression, immunosuppression
Tamoxifen citrate (Nolvadex)	Hot flashes, nausea, vomiting
Vincristine sulfate (Oncovin)	Alopecia, abdominal pain, peripheral neuropathy

Administration of neoplastic agents is normally done by a specially trained RN. LPN's are responsible for monitoring side effects and providing nursing care and comfort measures. LPN's need to encourage patient compliance with this very difficult course of therapy. Specific effects need to be researched for each agent. Agents affect healthy cells as well as tumor cells.

C. Nursing assessment: obtain baseline data regarding possible adverse reactions of drugs; evaluate condition of hair, skin, nails, weight, vital signs, and necessary blood laboratory studies (especially white blood cell [WBC], RBC, and platelet count).

D. Nursing management: monitor weight, vital signs, and laboratory studies; institute regular inspection of mouth; maintain good medical asepsis; use infusion monitoring device for IV administration; provide patient and family teaching and psychological support; check hydration status; maintain intake as much as possible; teach measures to avoid infection.

E. Nursing evaluation: observe for therapeutic effects and adverse reactions.

Colony-Stimulating Factors

A. Action: stimulate proliferation and differentiation of neutrophils; a glycoprotein; to decrease chances of infection in patients receiving antineoplastics; stimulate RBC production (Epogen) restore red bone marrow after transplantation (Leukine)

B. Adverse reactions: fever, nausea, diarrhea, anorexia, alopecia, skeletal pain; elevated BP may be a side effect of Epogen

C. Agent:
Filgrastim (Neupogen)*
Erythropoietin (Epogen)*
Sargramostatin (Leukine)*

D. Clinical Indications
Neupogen is used to increase the production of neutrophils and decrease the chances of infection in patients who are immunosuppressed. Epogen is used in treating anemia, in patients with AIDS, and patients with chronic renal failure. Leukine is used to restore red bone marrow in patients with transplants

E. Nursing assessment: monitor blood studies, check vital signs baseline and during treatment, and assess for bone pain.

F. Evaluation: absence of infection

HORMONES

A. Action: one factor controlling rate of RBC production; anemia caused by reduced endogenous erythropoietin production; primarily end-stage renal disease and anemia caused by chemotherapy

B. Adverse reactions: seizures, coldness, sweating, headache, hypertension, bone pain

C. Agent: epoetin alfa (Eprex)

D. Assessment: assess for CNS symptoms; monitor blood studies.

E. Evaluation: increased appetite; increase in RBCs in 1 to 2 weeks

Hypercalcemic Agents

A. Action: decrease serum calcium levels to normal or near normal levels; used in treating Paget's disease and hypercalcemia associated with malignancy
B. Adverse reactions: contraindicated in patients who are allergic to salmon or fish; facial flushing, nausea
C. Agents
   Calcitonin-salmon (Calcimar)
   Biphosphonates-alendronate (Fosamax)*
D. Nursing management: assess for signs of hypocalcium with aggressive treatment, monitor blood work for signs of effectiveness and toxicity; instruct patient to limit dairy foods, increase intake of fluid to 3,000 to 4,000 ml per day; do not administer with other medications or vitamins because of decreased effectiveness.

NUTRIENTS, FLUIDS, AND ELECTROLYTES

Substances required for human nutrition include water, carbohydrates, proteins, fats, vitamins, and minerals, necessary to maintain health, prevent illness, and promote recovery from illness

Nutritional Products: Oral and Tube Feedings

A. Nutritionally complete formulas
   1. Action
      a. Provide United States Recommended Dietary Allowance for protein, minerals, and vitamins
      b. Provide 1 calorie per milliliter (Sustagen: 1.84 cal/ml)
   2. Agents: the following are examples
      Compleat-B
      Ensure
      Isocal
      Osmolite
      Sustacal
      Sustagen
B. Nutritional agents for limited use
   1. Vital H.N.: contains easily digested forms of protein, carbohydrate, fat; used for critically ill patients
   2. Lofenalac: a low-phenylalanine preparation used for infants and children with phenylketonuria (PKU)
   3. MBF (Meat Base Formula): hypoallergenic infant formula for individuals who are allergic to milk or have galactosemia
   4. Neo-Mull-Soy, Pro-Sobee, Isomil: soybean products used as hypoallergenic; milk-free formulas
   5. Pregestimil: infant formula containing easily digested protein, fat, and carbohydrate; used in infants with diarrhea or malabsorption syndromes
   6. Vivonex: nutritionally complete diet containing amino acids as its protein
C. Complete infant formulas
   1. May be used alone for bottle-fed babies or to supplement breast-fed babies, similar to human breast milk; iron deficient
   2. Preparations: Enfamil and Similac are examples.

Intravenous Fluids

A. Dextrose injection: contains 2.5%, 5%, 10%, 20%, 40%, 50%, 60%, and 70% dextrose; the 20% to 50% solutions are used for calories in TPN and administered through a central or subclavian catheter.
B. Dextrose and sodium chloride injection: most commonly used concentrations are 5% dextrose in 0.25% or 0.45% sodium chloride.
C. Amino acid solution (Aminosyn): contains essential and nonessential amino acids; most often used with dextrose in TPN
D. Liposyn, Intralipid: concentrated calories and essential fatty acids; most often used as part of TPN

Vitamins

A. General information
   1. Group of substances that act as coenzymes to help in the conversion of carbohydrate and fat into energy and to form bones and tissues; necessary for metabolism of fat, carbohydrate, and protein; normally obtained from foods
   2. Subclassified as:
      a. Fat soluble: A, D, E, K
      b. Water soluble: B complex, C
B. Agents
   1. Fat-soluble vitamins: the following are examples
      Vitamin A (Alphalin, Aquasol A)
      Vitamin E (Tocopherol, Aquasol E)
      Vitamin K Menadiol sodium diphosphate (Synkayvite)
      Phytonadione (Mephyton, AquaMEPHYTON)
   2. Water-soluble vitamins: the following are examples
      B-complex
      Calcium pantothenate (B_5) (Pantholin)
      Cyanocobalamin (B_{12}) (Rubramin PC, Betalin 12)
      Folic acid (Folvite)
      Niacin
      Pyridoxine hydrochloride (B_6) (Hexa-Betalin)
      Riboflavin (Riobin-50, B_2)
      Thiamine hydrochloride (B_1) (Betalin S)
   3. Vitamin C: ascorbic acid

Minerals and Electrolytes

A. General information: basic constituents of living tissues and components of many enzymes; function to maintain fluid, electrolyte, acid-base balance; maintain muscle and nerve function; assist in transfer of materials across cell membranes and contribute to the growth process
B. Agents: the following are examples
   Deferoxamine mesylate (Desferal)
   Ferrous gluconate (Fergon)
   Ferrous sulfate (Feosol)
   Iron dextran injection (Imferon)
   Magnesium sulfate
   Potassium bicarbonate—potassium citrate (K-Lyte)
   Potassium chloride (Kay Ciel, K-Lor)
   Potassium gluconate (Kaon)
   Sodium bicarbonate
   Sodium polystyrene sulfonate (Kayexalate)
   Ringer's lactate

Nursing Process

A. Nursing assessment: obtain baseline data with emphasis on presenting signs and symptoms, vital signs, laboratory blood studies.
B. Nursing management: perform nursing actions to foster drug therapy; monitor diet and laboratory blood studies.
C. Nursing evaluation: observe for therapeutic effects specific to type of nutrient supplement; instruct patient regarding medications and diet.

SUGGESTED READINGS

Edmunds MW: *Introduction to clinical pharmacology,* ed 3, St Louis, 2003, Mosby.

Harkness GA, Dincher JR: *Medical-surgical nursing: Total patient care,* ed 10, St Louis, 1999, Mosby.

Lilley LL, Aukers RS: *Pharmacology and the nursing process,* ed 3, St Louis, 2001, Mosby.

McCuistion LE: *Real world nursing survival guide,* ed 1, 2002, Saunders.

McKenry LM, Salerno E: *Mosby's pharmacology in nursing,* ed 21, St Louis, 2003, Mosby.

Potter PA, Perry AG: *Fundamentals of nursing,* ed 5, St Louis, 2001, Mosby.

Skidmore-Roth L: *Mosby's drug guide for nurses,* ed 5, St Louis, 2003 Mosby.

Thompson: *Physicians' desk reference,* ed 54, Montvale, New Jersey, 2002, Medical Economics Company.

SUGGESTED WEBSITES

http.//www.diabetesmonitor.com/drugs.htm

www.cdc.com

www.ana.com

www.mosby'sdrugconsult.com/DrugConsult/newind2002.html

www.3.us.elsevierhealth.com/Merlin/McKenry/DrugConsult. Drugs/

REVIEW QUESTIONS

1. When a patient experiences an effect from a medication that is an unknown effect of the drug but is considered peculiar to that patient, it is referred to as a(n):
   1. Additive effect
   2. Idiosyncratic effect
   3. Synergistic effect
   4. Antagonistic effect

2. To obtain fastest absorption and action from a medication, the nurse knows that it should be administered:
   1. By mouth
   2. Intramuscularly
   3. Subcutaneously
   4. Intravenously

3. A student nurse questions the nurse as to why the patient has 20 mEq of potassium chloride (KCl) in his IV. The nurse explains the purpose and then refers the student to which of the following laboratory tests?
   1. Electrolytes
   2. Glucose
   3. Hemoglobin
   4. Arterial blood gases

4. A patient on outpatient anticoagulant therapy asks why he has to have blood drawn every week. The most appropriate answer the nurse should give is:
   1. "The doctor needs to know if the infection is improving."
   2. "The doctor adjusts your dose to help you maintain a therapeutic level."
   3. "The doctor needs to know if the medication is working."
   4. "We don't want the medicine to become toxic."

5. A patient asks the nurse why he is receiving patches of nitroglycerin instead of just taking it under the tongue when he needs it. The nurse explains that:
   1. "Given in this manner, the medication is absorbed at a slow, steady rate."
   2. "This manner is effective in acute situations."
   3. "This manner allows for more accurate dosage."
   4. "Patches administer a day's to a week's worth of medication."

6. A patient with cancer has been on high doses of morphine for several days. During an assessment, the side effect that the nurse would be likely to see is:
   1. Constipation
   2. Respiratory depression
   3. Pain relief
   4. Diarrhea

7. A patient is just beginning a drug-withdrawal program. Which signs is the nurse likely to observe during the first few days?
   1. Constipation and lethargy
   2. Runny nose and diarrhea
   3. Back pain and irritability
   4. Muscle rigidity and headache

8. The physician has ordered Mycostatin 5 ml swish and swallow twice daily (bid). The nurse should instruct the patient to do the following:
   1. "Swallow the medication quickly and follow with 8 ounces of water."
   2. "Shake the bottle before administering to help mix the suspension."
   3. "Brush your teeth carefully before each dose."
   4. "Maintain contact with the mucosa as long as possible before swallowing."

9. Sublingual administration of drugs:
   1. Is an alternative if medications are irritating to the GI tract
   2. Is absorbed primarily in the small intestine
   3. Allows for a delayed absorption by bypassing the GI tract
   4. Can be used for only a limited number of drugs

10. The nurse will know that the patient understands teaching done about self-administration of oral corticosteroids when the patient states that she will take the medication:
    1. Before meals
    2. With or after meals
    3. At bedtime
    4. With orange juice

11. After assessment of laboratory work, the physician orders two units of packed RBCs for a patient. The nurse knows that the test the physician used to assess the need for RBCs was:
    1. Blood glucose
    2. Electrolytes
    3. Hemoglobin and hematocrit
    4. Specific gravity

12. A physician prescribes 5 ml of cough medicine every 4 hours prn. The nurse explains to the patient that this dose is approximately equal to:
    1. 2 tablespoons
    2. 2 teaspoons
    3. 1 ounce
    4. 1 teaspoon

13. A 19-year-old patient has been given naloxone hydrochloride (Narcan) to overcome a narcotic overdose. The nurse knows that the expected action of the drug is to:
    1. Induce hypertension
    2. Induce hypotension
    3. Reverse CNS and respiratory depression
    4. Prevent arrhythmias

14. A nurse is making a home visit to care for a patient with COPD. When she arrives at the home, she finds that the couple has a big box of medications that are all mixed together, and some of them are outdated. The first priority should be to:
    1. Examine all the labels to determine which ones are still viable.
    2. Question the couple to see what medications they are taking.
    3. Report the situation to her supervisor so that she can contact the physician.
    4. Contact the social worker to begin placement proceedings for the couple.

15. 7.5 mg of iron is ordered every day via a peg tube. The liquid container is labeled 5 mg per 10 cc. How many ml are correctly administered?
    1. 5 ml
    2. 15 ml
    3. 7.5 ml
    4. 10 ml

16. An IV infusion is ordered at 50 ml per hour with a drip factor of 60. How many drops per minute should be infusing?
    1. 60
    2. 25

3 50

4 30

17. The nurse is going to give a subcutaneous injection to a 42-year-old patient. The needle length and gauge the nurse will use is:

1 19 gauge: 1½ inch

2 22 gauge: 1 inch

3 24 gauge: 1 inch

4 25 gauge: 5/8 inch

18. The physician has ordered secobarbital (Seconal) 100 mg at bedtime (hs) for a 27-year-old patient. The apothecary equivalent for this dose is:

1 gr v

2 gr iss

3 gr iii

4 gr 1/150

19. To assess the therapeutic effectiveness of an antiparkinsonian drug, the nurse will observe the patient's:

1 Increased sleep patterns

2 Increased ability to ambulate and speak

3 Decreased emotional stability

4 Decreased caloric and nutritional intake

20. An alcoholic is going through withdrawal. Which of the following medications would be the treatment of choice?

1 Diazepam (Valium), vitamins B_1 and B_{12}, and folic acid

2 Aspirin, calcium, and Tigan

3 Vitamin C, aspirin, and calcium

4 Vitamins B_1 and B_2 and aspirin

21. Spironolactone (Aldactone) is often prescribed for children with CHF because it is a(an):

1 Potassium-sparing diuretic

2 Loop diuretic

3 Thiazide carbonic anhydrase inhibitor diuretic

4 Osmotic diuretic

22. A patient with emphysema is taking a bronchodilator. Which of the following instructions or statements would be appropriate for the nurse to give the patient?

1 "Increase fluids to 2000 to 3000 ml every day."

2 "Take medication with food."

3 "Slow-release tablets may be chewed."

4 "Antibiotics will decrease action of these drugs."

23. When administering a buccal tablet, the nurse will tell the patient to:

1 Chew the tablet.

2 Swallow the tablet with water.

3 Let the tablet dissolve under the tongue.

4 Let the tablet dissolve between the cheek and the gum.

24. A patient has been on phenytoin (Dilantin) for several months, and her seizures are well controlled. Which of the following statements indicates the need for further teaching?

1 "I understand that I need to continue taking folic acid supplements."

2 "I cannot wait to stop taking this medication."

3 "I take my medication with a glass of orange juice every day."

4 "I always wear my identification tag."

25. A 66-year-old patient with pain associated with angina pectoris is given sublingual nitroglycerin. The nurse knows this medication will:

1 Dilate blood vessels and increase circulation

2 Inhibit the pain sensors in the brain stem

3 Increase respirations and cause drowsiness

4 Dull nerve endings in the myocardium

26. A patient is receiving temazepam (Restoril) 0.015 g orally (po) at bedtime for insomnia. The label indicates 15mg tablets. How many tablets will the nurse give?

1 1

2 1½

3 2

4 2½

27. A nurse is assessing signs of alcohol withdrawal in one of her patients. These assessments would show:

1 Tremors, anxiety, increased BP

2 Thirst, excessive sleeping, bradycardia

3 Polyuria, nausea, headache

4 Increased respirations, decreased BP, rigidity

28. While the nurse administers the daily dose of furosemide (Lasix) to the patient, the opportunity arises for patient teaching. Which of the following should the nurse be sure to stress?

1 "Take the medicine at bedtime."

2 "You may need sodium and potassium supplements."

3 "Weigh yourself twice a day."

4 "Change positions slowly to prevent dizziness."

29. Decadron is best given:

1 On an empty stomach

2 With a full glass of water

3 With a full glass of milk

4 At night

30. A 9-year-old patient was recently started on methylphenidate (Ritalin) for attention-deficit disorder (ADD). On his follow-up office visit, his mother reports to the nurse that he is having difficulty sleeping. The nurse knows:

1 Ritalin needs to be given early in the day because insomnia is a side effect.

2 Children with ADD are frequently hyperactive, and this is probably why he cannot sleep.

3 The patient may be taking in too much caffeine each day.

4 The patient may need an increase in his Ritalin dose.

31. An 89-year-old man is complaining of urinary retention. During the medication history, which of the following assessments would be a priority to report to the physician?

1 Baclofen (Lioresal)

2 Diazepam (Valium)

3 Benztropine (Cogentin)

4 Cyclobenzaprine hydrochloride (Flexeril)

32. A patient on morphine is experiencing nausea and vomiting. Which medication might the physician order to alleviate these symptoms?

1 Docusate sodium (Colace)

2 Loperamide (Imodium)

3 Trimethobenzamide (Tigan)

4 Atropine sulfate (Atropine)

33. A postpartum patient is experiencing uterine atony. Which of the following medications would the physician add to the IV infusion?

1 Depo-Provera

2 Brevicon

3 Brethine

4 Oxytocin

34. The controlled analgesic most effective for a harsh, non-productive cough is:

1 Codeine

2 Ibuprofen (Motrin)

3 Meperidine (Demerol)

4 Dextromethorphan (Romilar)

35. A patient complains to the office nurse that he is experiencing nausea and muscle cramps. He states, "I feel like I always have a virus but it never develops." The nurse recognizes that these symptoms might be as a result of which of the following medications that the patient has just started taking?

1 Ibuprofen (Motrin)

2 Diazepam (Valium)

3 Loratidine (Claritin)

4 Lovastatin (Mevacor)

36. The 70-year-old patient is receiving aminophylline. The nurse knows the medication will act to:

1 Dilate blood vessels increasing capillary permeability

2 Increase contraction of the bronchi and alveoli

3 Decrease contraction of the smooth muscle

4 Decrease the amount of mucous secretion from the bronchi

37. An adverse reaction to atropine sulfate that may be serious for patients with underlying heart disease is:

1 Delirium

2 Tachycardia

3 Constipation

4 Dry mouth

38. In an attempt to stop a spontaneous abortion, the physician has ordered terbutaline (Brethine), a uterine relaxant for the patient. Adverse reactions the nurse will be alert for are:

1 Heart palpitations, nausea, vomiting, headache

2 Drowsiness, incoordination, GI upset

3 Sedation, dry mouth, blurred vision, urinary retention

4 Anxiety, apprehension, headache, cerebral hemorrhage

39. A medication used to treat bipolar disorder is:

1 Diazepam (Valium)

2 Epinephrine (Adrenalin)

3 Lithium carbonate (Lithium)

4 Propranolol (Inderal)

40. When a nurse is giving dietary instructions appropriate to a person on calcitonin (Calcimar), it would be especially important to include the following:

1 Maintain adequate intake of calcium and vitamin D."

2 "Increase fiber whole grains and rhubarb."

3 "Increase intake of vitamin C."

4 "Maintain appropriate calories to avoid gaining weight."

41. An athlete asks the school nurse why using steroids to increase athletic ability is so dangerous. The nurse explains that the drugs:

1 Stimulate RBC formation

2 Are difficult from which to withdraw and a tolerance may develop

3 Are illegal if given without a prescription

4 Are a risk for many adverse side effects, including cardiac failure

42. A patient in the intensive care unit goes into life-threatening cardiogenic shock. The primary effect that the nurse would look for after a norepinephrine bitartrate (Levophed) drip is initiated on an infusion pump is:

1 Decreasing hyperventilation

2 Decreasing polyuria

3 Increasing BP

4 Increasing orientation

43. A patient has been on lovastatin (Mevacor) for 6 weeks. What is one method that is used to evaluate its effectiveness?

1 Monitoring the CBC

2 Monitoring blood glucose

3 Monitoring electrolytes

4 Monitoring cholesterol

44. An antibiotic used topically in burn treatment is:

1 Tetracycline (Achromycin)

2 Silver sulfadiazine (Silvadene)

3 Claithromyesin (Biaxin)

4 Sulfisoxazole (Gantrisin)

45. A medication is commonly given z-track when it:

1 Is irritating to surrounding tissues

2 Cannot be given intramuscularly

3 Has to be given around the clock

4 Has to be given for a rapid effect

46. The nurse in a physician's office interviews a patient being treated for asthma. The patient is jittery and complains of nausea. A statement that might indicate a cause for the jitteriness would be:

1 "I have been taking diazepam (Valium) for my nerves."

2 "I am overdue to have a theophylline level drawn."

3 "I am taking cimetidine (Tagamet) for my epigastric pain."

4 "I take a laxative when I am constipated."

47. A patient who has been on hydrocortisone (Cortisol) for an extended period should be monitored for which of the following adverse reactions?

1 Hypoglycemia

2 Anemia

3 Increased clotting time

4 Hyperglycemia

48. A patient who has been on phenytoin (Dilantin) for 1 week is very upset and states, "I don't understand why I am still having seizures." The nurse explains:

1 "We may need to speak with the physician about changing your medication."

2 "Therapeutic effectiveness may take several weeks."

3 "Maybe we need to add an additional medication."

4 "Improvement will be gradual."

49. A patient who has been on Claritin for allergy relief for several weeks complains to the nurse that the medication is no longer working. The nurse suspects that the patient may have developed a:

1 Tolerance

2 Cumulation

3 Synergistic reaction

4 Antagonistic effect

50. A child is being treated with Ritalin. How would the therapeutic effectiveness be evaluated?

1 Decreased hyperactivity and a more normal attention span

2 Decreased irritability and a more normal sleep pattern

3 Decreased headache pain and a more normal appetite

4 Decreased nausea and vomiting

51. A nurse is obtaining the medication history of a newly admitted patient. The patient has been on Zoloft for 14 days. Which of the following effects would be observed if the drug is therapeutic?

1 Absence of diarrhea

2 Decreased nausea and vomiting

3 Decreased depression
4 Decreased insomnia

52. Which of the following signs is the most significant assessment of a possible allergic reaction to a blood transfusion?
    1 Elevated temperature
    2 Moist cough
    3 Difficulty breathing
    4 Muscular cramping

53. During an admission interview, the nurse learns that a patient has been on dipyridamole (Persantine) for several months. This assessment is an indication for:
    1 Assessing respirations after activity
    2 Monitoring BP sitting, standing, and lying
    3 Assessing temperature every 4 hours
    4 Monitoring WBCs to check for infection

54. Patients who are receiving vancomycin (Vancocin) via IV infusion should be assessed before administration and during the administration for:
    1 Blurred vision
    2 Constipation
    3 Hearing damage
    4 Muscle cramps

55. A nurse assesses that a patient with diabetes is reporting increased episodes of hypoglycemia. Which of the following is the likely explanation?
    1 Decreasing usual exercise patterns without changing insulin
    2 Increasing caloric intake without changing insulin
    3 Increased exercise patterns with a decreased insulin dose
    4 Decreased caloric intake and increased exercise pattern

56. A troche would most likely be ordered for which of the following assessments?
    1 An allergic reaction causing respiratory difficulty
    2 A persistent sore throat
    3 Complaints of vaginal itching
    4 A stomach upset

57. A nurse is interviewing a patient concerning her medication history. The patient denies taking any OTC medicines. The nurse then asks about dietary habits. The patient removes a bottle of Pepto-Bismol from her purse and states that she has been taking this "food" for years for her stomach pain. She also has a bottle of vitamin pills, which she takes for her "eyes." The first priority for the nurse at this point is:
    1 Assess the "stomach pain."
    2 Ask the patient what foods irritate her stomach.
    3 Investigate what might be wrong with her eyes.
    4 Explain to the patient that these are considered medications and investigate further.

58. The nurse is taking an admission history for a person being seen by a physician for an initial visit. Which of the following statements most indicates the need for further investigation?
    1 "Once in a while when I get constipated, I take a laxative."
    2 "I have been on aldactone for many years."
    3 "I am a fanatic about taking a vitamin every day."
    4 "I have been taking famotidine (Pepcid) almost every day for a month."

59. A patient on digoxin therapy is experiencing a toxic side effect. The nurse recognizes that this would most likely be:
    1 Tachycardia
    2 Muscle cramps

3 Green-yellow vision
4 Decreased BP

60. A patient is taking thyroglobulin (Proloid) for treating hypothyroidism. Adverse reactions that the nurse should instruct the patient to report include:
    1 Weight gain and sleeping patterns increased
    2 Headache and insomnia
    3 Bronchospasm and iodism
    4 Hypotension and lethargy

61. How would the effect of a person being treated with clomiphene citrate (Clomid) be measured?
    1 Decreased BP
    2 Pregnancy
    3 Decreased vaginal bleeding
    4 Decreased menstrual cramps

62. A major adverse reaction the nurse will observe for in a patient with cancer who is receiving antineoplastic drugs is:
    1 Bone marrow supression
    2 Oliguria
    3 Lethargy
    4 Photosensitivity

63. A poisonous effect of a drug, either from a regular dose or an overdose, is referred to as a(an):
    1 Side effect
    2 Untoward effect
    3 Toxic action
    4 Idiosyncratic action

64. Which of the following assessments concerning an IV infusion would be a priority to report to the charge nurse?
    1 The drops are falling too slowly.
    2 A small, reddened area is near the insertion site.
    3 The infusion slows when the patient bends his arm.
    4 The piggyback infusion is complete.

65. A nurse is admitting a patient diagnosed with deep-vein thrombosis. He is starting treatment with IV coagulation therapy. Which of the following assessments is most important to report to the physician?
    1 The patient takes psyllium (Metamucil) occasionally for constipation.
    2 The patient uses ibuprofen (Motrin) for treating osteoarthritis.
    3 The patient takes loratidine (Claritin) for treating allergies.
    4 The patient takes nifedipine (Procardia) for treating hypertension.

66. Cough medicine should:
    1 Always be given before any other medication
    2 Be followed by water to facilitate absorption
    3 Be given last and not followed by liquid to increase effect
    4 Always be given on a scheduled basis

67. A physician orders an IV infusion of 3000 ml of Ringer's lactate with 5% dextrose (D5RL) for his patient over the next 24 hours. The drip factor for the tubing is 10. How many drops per minute will deliver the correct amount of fluid?
    1 10 gtt/min
    2 28 gtt/min
    3 21 gtt/min
    4 60 gtt/min

68. A nurse is administering an antibiotic to an elderly patient at midnight. The patient refuses to take the medication,

stating, "I already received my pills before I went to sleep." The most appropriate action for the nurse to take is:

1 Verify that the medication order is current and correct.
2 Explain to the patient that the physician has ordered the medication to cure his infection.
3 Explain to the patient that he received his sleeping pill before going to sleep.
4 Check previous documentation to be certain that the time of administration was not changed by the previous shift.

69. A clinic nurse is concerned when a patient diagnosed with active TB returns to the clinic after 2 weeks of treatment and reports a worsening cough and reoccurring night sweats. These findings most likely indicate:

1 Noncompliance with medication regimen
2 Additional exposure to infected individuals
3 The need for additional medication
4 The need for follow-up care for family members

70. A dialysis patient is placed on a 1200-cc fluid restriction in 24 hours. The best allocation for the fluid would be:

1 600 ml on the 7:00 to 3:00 shift, 400 ml on the 3:00 to 11:00 shift, and 200 ml on the 11:00 to 7:00 shift
2 500 ml on the 7:00 to 3:00 shift, 500 ml on the 3:00 to 11:00 shift, and 200 ml on the 11:00 to 7:00 shift
3 Drink liquids only at mealtimes
4 As long as 100 ml is left for medications, the patient should regulate his or her own fluids.

71. The difference between a sedative and a hypnotic is:

1 Dose
2 Time of administration
3 None
4 Length of effect

72. A medication used in treating Parkinson's disease is:

1 Methylphenidate (Ritalin)
2 Carbamazepine (Tegretol)
3 Benztropine mesylate (Cogentin)
4 Theophylline (Accurbron)

73. A 31-year-old patient who is experiencing nausea and vomiting has an elevated temperature. The nurse will give the antipyretic:

1 Orally
2 Rectally
3 Sublingually
4 Topically

74. Patients with increased intracranial pressure are treated with which of the following medications?

1 Morphine sulfate
2 Hydrochlorothiazide
3 Decadron
4 Heparin

75. The nurse expects a placebo to be effective because of the:

1 Production of endorphins in the brain
2 Nurturing attitude of the nurse
3 Action of the active drug in the placebo
4 Patient's ability to metabolize the placebo

76. A patient has been on cromolyn (Intal) for 6 weeks. How would the therapeutic effects of this medication be measured?

1 Decreased severity of symptoms during asthmatic attacks
2 Decreased number of asthmatic attacks
3 Improvement in ability to sleep through the night
4 Decreased heart rate during exercise

77. Which of the following statements made during an assessment should indicate to the nurse that the physician may prescribe sulfisoxazole (Gantrisin)?

1 "I have had urinary frequency and burning for the last 2 days."
2 "I am allergic to penicillin."
3 "I have had a runny nose for 3 days."
4 "I have loose, foul-smelling diarrhea."

78. The nurse will do a daily assessment of the integrity of the oral mucosa when the patient is receiving:

1 Antibiotics
2 Cancer drugs
3 Antiparkinsonian drugs
4 Vitamins

79. The law that regulates the manufacture, distribution, advertisement, and labeling of drugs to ensure safety and effectiveness is the:

1 Harrison Narcotic Act
2 Consumer Protection Act
3 Controlled Substance Act
4 Federal Food, Drug, and Cosmetic Act

80. The nurse knows that an 80-year-old patient on medication would be prone to which of the following?

1 Developing a tolerance to medication
2 Metabolizing medications more rapidly
3 Developing more frequent adverse reactions
4 Experiencing more cumulative effects

81. A 28-year-old patient with hyperthyroidism is placed on phenobarbital to achieve which of the following effects?

1 Sedation
2 Control of seizures
3 Vasoconstriction
4 Vasodilation

82. A pediatric nurse is interviewing a 10-year-old child and her parents. The parents tell the nurse that the child has been irritable and unable to sleep well in recent weeks. Which of the following indications might be a contributing factor?

1 Taking amoxicillin (Augmentin) for an ear infection
2 Taking Pepto-Bismol for an upset stomach
3 Taking loratidine (Claritin) for her allergies
4 Taking guaifenesin (Robitussin) for an upper respiratory infection

83. Many drugs have anticholinergic side effects. Examples of these effects would include:

1 Dryness of the mouth and constipation
2 Increased salivation and diarrhea
3 Polyuria and thirst
4 Tachycardia and diarrhea

84. A patient is being treated with pyrostigmine (Mestinon) for myasthenia gravis. How would the nurse evaluate the therapeutic effectiveness of this medication?

1 Decreased arrhythmias
2 Decreased nausea and vomiting
3 Increased perspiration
4 Increased muscle strength

85. A 62-year-old patient has an attack of acute angina. The nurse knows that the treatment of choice will be:

1 Calcium channel blockers
2 Beta-adrenergic blockers
3 Nitrates
4 Narcotic analgesics

86. A 3-year-old patient has been receiving high doses of metaclopramide (Reglan) for side effects associated with chemotherapy. The nurse is reinforcing home care instructions related to adverse medication effects. Which of the following symptoms should be reported to the health care provider immediately?
    1. Mild sedation and fatigue
    2. Rigidity and tremors
    3. Constipation and dry mouth
    4. Headache and insomnia

87. A patient is experiencing hives in an allergic reaction. Which of the following reports would indicate that diphenhydramine (Benadryl) is showing its desired therapeutic effect?
    1. Improved vision
    2. Decreased pruritus
    3. Decreased muscle cramps
    4. Decreased headache

88. A medication given as a thrombolytic agent within 4 hours after a witnessed myocardial infarction to dissolve the clot is:
    1. Streptokinase (Streptase)
    2. Heparin (Heparin Sodium)
    3. Phytonadione (AquaMEPHYTON)
    4. Aminocaproic acid (Amicar)

89. The drug of choice for treating acute pancreatitis is:
    1. Morphine (morphine sulphate)
    2. Meperidine (Demerol)
    3. Erythromycin (E-Mycin)
    4. Dexamethasone (Decadron)

90. The type of insulin used in emergency situations of hyperglycemia is:
    1. NPH
    2. Regular
    3. Lente
    4. Ultralente

91. A nurse is preparing supplies for a TB screening program. She should be certain that which of the following syringes is available in ample supply?
    1. 22-gauge, 1½-inch needle
    2. 25-gauge, 5/8-inch needle
    3. 27-gauge, ½-inch needle
    4. 20-gauge, 2-inch needle

92. A nurse is administering amoxicillin po to a 3-year-old child diagnosed with an ear infection. The most appropriate approach with the child would be to:
    1. Give a detailed explanation to the child as to why he needs this medicine.
    2. Explain that it is time to take your "pink medicine."
    3. Have the parent hold the child in his or her arms and inject it quickly into his mouth.
    4. Administer the medication in 240 ml of apple juice.

93. A drug used as a substitute for morphine in the management of addiction is:
    1. Meperidine
    2. Narem
    3. Methadone
    4. Talwin

94. Doses of warfarin sodium (Coumadin) are ordered on the basis of measurement of the patient's:
    1. Clotting time
    2. PT

95. 3. Bleeding time
    4. Capillary fragility testing

95. A patient who is in the fortieth week of pregnancy is receiving an IV administration of oxytocin (Pitocin). The nurse knows the drug is expected to:
    1. Produce rhythmic contractions of uterine muscle fibers
    2. Relax smooth muscle fibers of the cervix
    3. Initiate vigorous sustained contractions of the abdominal muscles
    4. Produce relaxation of vaginal walls and perineal muscles

96. A nurse is preparing to administer a vitamin-B_{12} injection IM to an average-weight person. The length and gauge of the needle selected should be:
    1. 25-gauge, 2-inch needle
    2. 27-gauge, ½-inch needle
    3. 20-gauge, 3-inch needle
    4. 22-gauge, 1-inch needle

97. Standard precautions are mandatory during the administration of parenteral medications. The nurse knows that:
    1. Hands must be washed between patients and before procedures.
    2. The need for protection depends on the potential exposure to infected body fluids.
    3. Hands must be washed before and gloves must be worn during administration.
    4. The need to wear gloves depends on the patient's diagnosis.

98. Enteric-coated medications are ordered for the following purpose:
    1. To allow the medicine to remain in the stomach longer
    2. To allow for delayed absorption in the small intestine
    3. To allow for time-released absorption by having a more gradual release
    4. To prevent irritation in the small intestine

99. A patient with diabetes mellitus is being treated with metformin (Glucophage). The nurse understands that the action of this medication is to:
    1. Improve the breakdown of fats and proteins for use as energy
    2. Decrease the amount of glucose taken up by the muscles and decreases cellular resistance to insulin
    3. Replace insulin not being produced by the pancreas
    4. Increase the amount of glucose taken up by the muscles and intestine and decreases cellular resistance to insulin

100. The patient is to receive an IV infusion of lactated Ringer's at 75 ml/hr. The drop factor is 20 gtt/ml. The nurse will run the IV at:
    1. 5 gtt/min
    2. 15 gtt/min
    3. 25 gtt/min
    4. 35 gtt/min

101. A postoperative patient receives 5000 units of heparin (Heparin Sodium) subcutaneously (SC) bid. The dosage available is 10,000 units per milliliter. The correct amount of medication to be administered is:
    1. ¼ ml
    2. ½ ml
    3. 1 ml
    4. 2 ml

102. Atropine 1/150 grain is ordered as a preoperative medication. On hand is 0.4 mg per ml. The appropriate amount of fluid to be administered is:
    1 ½ ml
    2 1 ml
    3 2 ml
    4 ¼ ml

103. A nurse is assisting at a clinic where a 3-month-old infant is required to have an IM injection. The most appropriate site for this injection is:
    1 Vastus lateralis
    2 Dorsogluteal
    3 Deltoid
    4 Ventrogluteal

104. Which of the following is effective in treating status epilepticus?
    1 Diazepam
    2 Hydroxyzine
    3 Meprobamate
    4 Chlordiazepoxide

105. A patient is being treated in the hospital for an infection that a culture has shown to be positive for methicillin-resistant *Staphylococcus* (*Staph*) *aureus* (MRSA). The nurse knows that the medication most likely to be effective is:
    1 Penicillin
    2 Streptomycin
    3 Acyclovir
    4 Vancomycin

106. A nurse is caring for a patient with cancer who is undergoing chemotherapy. The patient's WBC count is low. The physician would most likely place him on which of the following medications?
    1 Epoetin alfa (Epogen)
    2 Vancomycin (Vancocin)
    3 Filgrastim (Neupogen)
    4 Vincristine (Oncovin)

107. A nurse is assisting in planning the teaching for a newly diagnosed 15-year-old patient with diabetes. An important consideration for this age group is:
    1 These individuals need to do things well and develop a sense of self-worth.
    2 Adolescents determine identity through role models and peer pressure.
    3 This group establishes long-lasting relationships.
    4 Allowing them to verbalize accomplishments in life is important.

108. A patient with a history of treatment for glaucoma should not be treated with cholinergic-blocking agents because:
    1 This classification of medications decreases intraocular pressure.
    2 They may be absorbed systemically and cause cardiac irregularities.
    3 This classification of medications increases intraocular pressure.
    4 The danger of electrolyte imbalances is present.

109. The nurse has been monitoring a patient in his home. Two weeks ago, he was diagnosed with active TB. Which of these statements would be most indicative that he has an understanding of his treatment?
    1 "I am so glad that the treatment is over so that I can go back to work."

    2 "I will need support and assistance to take this medication for such a long time."
    3 "I have to learn to eat healthier foods."
    4 "As long as I am no longer contagious, it is all right for my friends to visit."

110. On a busy surgical unit, the common practice is to leave the narcotic keys in a locked utility room where the narcotic box is located. A new graduate is concerned because:
    1 Narcotic keys should be carried with a nurse at all times.
    2 Too many people know the combination to the room.
    3 All controlled substances have to be signed and accounted for at the end of each shift.
    4 The pharmacist is responsible for dispensing appropriate medications.

111. A patient is being cared for 8 hours after a laminectomy. Morphine sulphate is ordered every 3 hours SC for moderate to severe postoperative pain. The patient is rating his pain at an 8. An hour has passed since his last dose. The first intervention that the nurse should complete is:
    1 Explain to the patient that he will have to wait because it has only been an hour since his last dose.
    2 Document the pain level at 8, and notify the charge nurse.
    3 Turn the patient using the logrolling technique, and reposition him on his side.
    4 Assess the location and characteristics of the pain.

112. A statement that would most indicate that an adolescent is beginning to understand his diagnosis of insulin-dependent diabetes mellitus would be:
    1 "I am going to hang out with my friends like I always did."
    2 "Swimming is an important part of my life."
    3 "Watching my diet and taking medication is a drag."
    4 "I hate being different from my friends."

113. When administering an IM injection, the nurse will aspirate after insertion of the needle to:
    1 Avoid injecting the drug directly into the bloodstream
    2 Ease the patient's discomfort
    3 Facilitate absorption into the bloodstream
    4 Avoid injuring organs

114. The nurse will administer thyroid drugs:
    1 In a single dose, usually before breakfast
    2 In divided doses, before meals
    3 In divided doses, after meals
    4 As the patient's energy level decreases

115. When administering a bulk-forming laxative such as psyllium husk (Metamucil), the nurse will give it:
    1 At bedtime
    2 With meals
    3 With a full glass of water
    4 With an antacid

116. To instill eardrops in the adult patient, the ear canal is opened by pulling the ear:
    1 Up and back
    2 Down and back
    3 Up and forward
    4 Back and forward

117. Emergency treatment of hyperinsulinism consists of administering:
    1 Glucose IV
    2 Insulin hypodermically

3   Epinephrine (Adrenalin) IM
4   High-caloric liquids by gavage feedings

118. When teaching self-administration of eyedrops to a patient, the nurse will stress that the correct method for instilling eyedrops is to drop the medication on the:
   1   Eyeball itself
   2   Inner canthus of the eye
   3   Lower conjunctival sac
   4   Outermost point of the eye

119. A 72-year-old patient is exhibiting signs of digoxin toxicity. The nurse will:
   1   Give the drug if the apical rate is above 60 beats/min, and report to the physician.
   2   Omit the drug, take the apical rate, and report to the physician.
   3   Administer an antacid with the digoxin.
   4   Administer oxygen by nasal cannula with the digoxin.

120. The physician's order reads to administer 3 L of 5% dextrose–0.45% normal saline IV over 24 hours. The drip factor is 60 gtt/ml. The nurse will regulate the IV at:
   1   25 gtt/min
   2   100 gtt/min
   3   125 gtt/min
   4   150 gtt/min

121. The position of choice for instilling nose drops in an adult patient is lying:
   1   On the right side
   2   Down or sitting with the neck hyperextended
   3   Down or sitting with the neck flexed
   4   On the left side

122. The process that occurs from the time a drug is taken into the body to the time it enters the circulatory or lymphatic system is called:
   1   Absorption
   2   Distribution
   3   Metabolism
   4   Excretion

123. A patient is diagnosed with myasthenia gravis. The following medication is ordered to be administered:
   1   Pancuronium bromide (Pavulon)
   2   Metformin (Glucophage)
   3   Cimetidine (Tagamet)
   4   Pyrostigmine (Mestinon)

124. A patient has not voided approximately 12 hours postpartum. Bladder palpation indicates urinary retention. The physician orders the following medication:
   1   Atropine sulfate (Atropine)
   2   Hydroxyzine (Vistaril)
   3   Bethanechol (Urecholine)
   4   Trimethobenzamine (Tigan)

125. A patient is starting on phenytoin (Dilantin) for control of his seizures. The nurse explains to the patient that he must inform his dentist of his new medication. The reason for this notification is:
   1   This medication can cause nystagmus.
   2   This medication can cause gingival hyperplasia.
   3   This medication can cause slurred speech.
   4   He may develop a vitamin-D deficiency.

126. The official reference book for medications in the United States is:
   1   United States Pharmacopeia (USP)
   2   Physicians Desk Reference (PDR)

3   American Hospital Formulary
4   Package inserts from the FDA

127. Combining white wine with an analgesic is dangerous. The effect on the CNS when given together is called:
   1   Antagonistic
   2   Synergistic
   3   Cumulative
   4   Tolerance

128. A patient is being started on warfarin (Coumadin) in preparation for cardiac tests. Which of the following medications should the patient be instructed to omit while he is on this medication?
   1   Enalapril (Vasotec)
   2   Metformin (Glucophage)
   3   Ibuprofen (Motrin)
   4   Digoxin (Lanoxin)

129. A patient on iron treatment for anemia would benefit from which of these medications to prevent constipation?
   1   Loperamide (Immodium)
   2   Docusate sodium (Colace)
   3   Hydralazine (Apresoline)
   4   Hydroxyzine (Vistaril)

130. Epinephrine is effective topically during epistaxis because it:
   1   Causes peripheral vasodilation
   2   Causes peripheral vasoconstriction
   3   Increases intraocular pressure
   4   Is a cardiac stimulant

131. A patient is being treated for an anticoagulant overdose. The medication prescribed is:
   1   Phytonadione (Konakion)
   2   Warfarin (Coumadin)
   3   Digoxin (Lanoxin)
   4   Propranolol (Inderal)

132. A drug used to treat anemia in end-stage renal disease is:
   1   Filgrastim (Neupogen)
   2   Hydrochlorothiazide (HydroDiuril)
   3   Furosemide (Lasix)
   4   Epoetin alfa (Epogen)

133. A nurse is caring for a patient with anorexia as a result of HIV. The medication ordered for this patient to improve his appetite would be:
   1   Megestrol (Megace)
   2   Gentamycin (Garamycin)
   3   Folic acid (Folate)
   4   Amantadine (Symmetrol)

134. A nurse is teaching a nutrition class to a group of expectant parents. Which of the following statements may indicate to the nurse that her lecture has been understood?
   1   "Vitamins will protect my baby if I do not eat correctly."
   2   "You can never get too many vitamins and minerals."
   3   "Adequate folic acid will help to prevent birth defects."
   4   "I am going to try really hard to eat a lot of vegetables."

135. A nurse has been instructing a person with newly diagnosed diabetes on how to administer a mixed dose of regular and NPH insulin. Which of the following procedures would indicate that the patient had mastered the proper technique?
   1   The patient cleans the top of both vials, injects air into the NPH vial, withdraws the NPH, and then injects air into the regular insulin vial with a separate syringe.

The patient then withdraws the correct amount of regular insulin into the original syringe.

2 The patient cleans the top of both vials, injects air into the NPH vial, and withdraws the syringe. The patient then injects air into the regular insulin and withdraws the correct dose. Then the patient goes back to the NPH vial and withdraws the correct dose.

3 These medications must be drawn into separate syringes, because they cannot be mixed.

4 Using separate syringes, the patient put air into each of the vials and then withdraws the regular insulin and the NPH insulin using a third syringe.

136. A physician has ordered a "gentamycin level" on his patient. The nurse understands that this test is ordered to determine if:
1 The patient has developed a tolerance for the medication.
2 The patient has developed a physical dependence for the medication.
3 The medication is in the therapeutic range.
4 The patient has developed any adverse side effects.

137. A patient is starting on antihypertensive medications. Which of the following statements would indicate the need for further teaching?
1 "If I miss a dose, I should take two doses the next day."
2 "Medications should be taken with a full glass of water."
3 "If my blood pressure is too high, I should omit a dose."
4 "I should avoid foods high in sodium."

138. A patient with asthma has been placed on a metered-dose inhaler. Which of the following statements indicates the need for further teaching?
1 "I need to press down on the inhaler to release one puff while inhaling slowly."
2 "The inhalers can be used on a multidose basis."
3 "I should inhale both puffs in quick succession."
4 "After each puff I should hold my breath for approximately 10 seconds."

139. The patient receives 32 units of NPH insulin at 8:00 AM. The most likely time that she would exhibit signs of insulin reaction would be:
1 10:00 AM
2 2:00 PM
3 9:00 AM
4 Midnight

140. A patient is being treated with calcitriol (Rocaltrol) for hypocalcemia. Which report would indicate that the medication is effective?
1 Calcium levels 9 to 10 mg/dl
2 Decreasing blurred vision
3 Hgb level of 14
4 Potassium level of 3.9

141. Which of the following would be a desired or therapeutic effect of loratidine (Claritin)?
1 Sedation
2 Decreased irritability
3 Decreased rhinitis
4 Decreased nausea

142. The patient is to receive an IV of 5% dextrose–0.33 normal saline at 1000 ml/8 hr. The drip factor is 10 gtt/ml. The nurse will run the IV at:
1 7 gtt/min
2 14 gtt/min
3 20 gtt/min
4 28 gtt/min

143. An elderly patient states that his medication costs too much for his fixed income. The nurse will tell him to ask his physician to write prescriptions for which of the following forms of the medication?
1 Generic name
2 Brand name
3 Chemical name
4 Official name

144. Fluoxetine (Prozac) has been ordered for a 49-year-old man who suffers from depression. In teaching him about his new medicine, the nurse will tell him that:
1 It should be taken at bedtime.
2 A feeling of euphoria will occur within 24 hours.
3 2 to 3 weeks will be required before the effects of the drug will be felt.
4 It should be taken with meals.

145. KCl (potassium chloride) in liquid form is ordered for a 65-year-old patient who is taking Lasix. Before administering, the medication the nurse will:
1 Be sure the patient has had nothing by mouth (NPO) since 12:00 midnight.
2 Dilute it in 3 to 8 oz of cold water or juice.
3 Crush the controlled release tablet and mix it with water.
4 Partially dissolve the effervescent tablet.

146. A 20-year-old male patient is taking ciprofloxacin (Cipro) for a urinary tract infection. He also takes theophylline for asthma. In teaching him about his medication, the nurse knows:
1 Fluids should be restricted while on Cipro.
2 The patient should not be started on Cipro until the culture results are obtained.
3 Theophylline levels may be elevated and can become toxic.
4 The two medications should be given at alternate times.

147. A 64-year-old patient with CHF takes a digitalis preparation every day. Before administering, the medication the nurse will:
1 Weigh the patient.
2 Check the patient's apical pulse.
3 Take the patient's BP.
4 Monitor the patient's clotting time.

148. The patient will be taught to take his iron preparation:
1 At bedtime
2 Before breakfast
3 With meals
4 Between meals

149. The nurse will caution a patient on antihypertensive medication to avoid sudden changes in position, especially from a supine to an upright position, because:
1 A thrombus might become dislodged.
2 Severe nausea might result.
3 Postural hypotension might occur.
4 Increased diuresis will occur.

150. The nurse gives the 59-year-old patient atropine sulfate as a preoperative medication. The nurse will tell the patient that he will not be allowed out of bed because:
1 The CNS (central nervous system) is depressed.
2 Vertigo might occur because of dilation of the pupils.

3 One effect of the drug is the development of postural hypotension.

4 Diaphoresis may predispose to a chill.

151. An oncology patient is taking erythropoietin (Epogen). The blood test that should be checked to indicate the effectiveness of this medication would be:
1 Blood glucose level
2 BUN and creatinine
3 Hemoglobin and hematocrit
4 White blood cell count

152. An oncology patient is on neutropenic precautions because of a low WBC count. He is placed on the following medication to stimulate the production of neutrophils:
1 Sargramostatin (Leukine)
2 Erythropoietin (Epogen)
3 Fluconazole (Diflucan)
4 Filgrastim (Neupogen)

153. Which of the following laxatives is not recommended because it decreases the absorption of fat-soluble vitamins?
1 Psyllium (Metamucil)
2 Mineral oil (Kondremul Plain)
3 Docusate sodium (Colace)
4 Polycarbophil (Fibercon)

154. While taking a medication history on a preoperative, patient the nurse is concerned when she discovers that the patient is being treated with acetazolamide (Diamox) for treating narrow-angle glaucoma. She knows that this is important to communicate to the physician because the patient should not receive which of the following medications?
1 Meperidine (Demerol)
2 Atropine sulphate (Isopto Atropine)
3 Pentazocine (Talwin)
4 Naloxone (Narcan)

155. A patient is admitted for the treatment of gastro-esophageal reflux disease (GERD). His treatment has not responded to first-line medications, so the physician is planning to place him on a regimen of metoclopramide (Reglan) for a short-term period. The nurse should instruct the patient on all of the following items except:
1 Advise the patient to avoid alcohol and other CNS depressants.
2 Monitor carefully for signs of hyperglycemia because the food is more efficiently absorbed into the bloodstream.
3 Avoid tasks that require concentration.
4 Administer the oral dose 30 minutes before meals and at bedtime.

156. A patient comes to the clinic complaining of a persistent dry hacking cough that is preventing him from sleeping. The doctor prescribes benzonatate (Tessalon). The nurse knows that this is medication is classified as an/a:
1 Expectorant
2 Decongestant
3 Antitussive
4 Antihistamine

157. Which of the following medications is used to stimulate RBC production in a patient who has received a bone marrow transplant?
1 Sargramostatin (Leukine)
2 Filgrastim (Neupogen)
3 Erythropoietin (Epogen)
4 Vincristine (Oncovin)

158. A patient arrives at your clinic with complaints of dysuria, pain frequency, and incontinence. A complete history is taken and the physician determines that a medication is required. Which of the following medications would most likely be ordered?
1 Furosemide (Lasix)
2 Metolazone (Zaroxylyn)
3 Oxybutinin (Ditropan)
4 Spinolactone (Aldactone)

159. Protease inhibitors should be taken:
1 With meals to improve absorption
2 1 hour before or 2 hours after meals
3 With only a small sip of water
4 With the scheduled vitamins

160. Zidovudine (Retrovir) is commonly prescribed for patients with HIV. The nurse knows that the ideal time for beginning treatment is:
1 When symptoms of immune deficiency first begin to appear
2 After other antiviral medicines have been tried
3 Before symptoms of immune deficiency appearing
4 At the end stage of the disease

161. A nurse is teaching a newly diagnosed diabetic and her daughter to administer insulin when they return home. Which of the following statements indicates the need for further teaching?
1 "Rotating the sites is important to prevent complications."
2 "Checking blood glucose is important after the insulin is administered."
3 "Eating is important after the insulin is administered."
4 "My daughter will be able to help me if I am sick."

162. A patient diagnosed with GERD is placed on an H2 blocker to help decrease gastric acid secretion. The name of the medication would be:
1 Famotidine (Pepcid)
2 Aluminum hydroxide (Amphojel)
3 Simethicone (Mylicon)
4 Rosiglitazone (Avandia)

163. A patient is diagnosed with a vaginal fungal infection. In addition to a topical medication, which of the following medications would be prescribed for this patient?
1 Famciclovir (Famvir)
2 Fluconazole (Diflucan)
3 Famotidine (Pepcid)
4 Azathioprine (Imuran)

164. A patient has been receiving chemotherapy treatment for breast cancer. She is placed on neutropenic precautions for a low WBC count. Her physician is concerned about the development of a thrush infection. Which of the following medications would be ordered "swish and swallow" to help prevent this complication?
1 Aluminum hydroxide (Amphojel)
2 Sertraline (Zoloft)
3 Achromycin (Tetracycline)
4 Mycostatin (Nystatin)

165. Medications given topically to treat athlete's foot are said to have a(n):
1 Systemic effect
2 Local effect
3 Cumulative effect
4 Antagonistic effect

166. A vancomycin level is ordered for your patient. The nurse knows that it is important to check blood levels because a therapeutic blood level:
    1. Means an adequate amount of medication is present to combat infection.
    2. Shows that the antibiotic is being adequately excreted.
    3. Needs to be reached gradually to avoid toxicity.
    4. Will show that the bacterial infection is sensitive to the medication.

167. Which of the following routes would be used for the fastest absorption?
    1. Oral
    2. Sublingual
    3. Intravenous
    4. Subcutaneous

168. Which of the following patients may require a smaller than average dose of an analgesic?
    1. A person with a history of substance abuse
    2. A patient with a history of cardiac disease
    3. An underweight adult
    4. A 76-year-old patient

169. A student nurse is worried that a terminally ill patient with cancer is receiving too high a dose of morphine in her continuous morphine drip. The oncology nurse explains that:
    1. "The high dose is needed to relieve pain and the excessive sedation is a side effect."
    2. "Pain relief is important; the high dose is why we have to monitor her carefully for respiratory depression."
    3. "Patients with cancer pain can be administered gradually increasing doses without side effects of respiratory depression and sedation."
    4. "Increasing pain must be treated because of the progression of the disease."

170. A postoperative patient is reluctant to take pain medication, even though he is rating his pain as an 8 on a scale of 1 to 10. The nurse assesses the patient's feelings and concludes that he has a fear of addiction. She explains to him:
    1. He is wise to limit his pain medication because psychologic dependence is a potential complication.
    2. He should continue to wait as long as possible for his pain medication to increase effectiveness.
    3. Addiction is minimal in hospitalized patients.
    4. Fear of tolerance developing is warranted with postoperative patients.

171. A drug characterized as a mild CNS depressant would most likely exhibit which of the following side effects?
    1. Increased pulse and respiration
    2. Inability to interpret verbal messages
    3. Slowness in initiating conversation
    4. Heightened awareness of surroundings

172. Patients should be taught to take all of their antibiotics as prescribed because:
    1. They increase their risk for dehydration if they do not finish.
    2. They increase their risk for developing bacterial resistant strains.
    3. They increase their risk for abdominal distress.
    4. It is not cost effective if another prescription is required.

173. The nurse in an outpatient clinic is concerned because her 86-year-old patient comes to the clinic complaining of heartburn that she has been experiencing for the last 2 weeks. She has been self-medicating with sodium bicarbonate. The nurse knows that the physician will order which of the following blood tests:
    1. CBC
    2. BUN
    3. Electrolytes
    4. Blood glucose levels

174. A patient asks the nurse why his aluminum hydroxide (Amphojel) is always given 1 hour before meals. The nurse replies:
    1. The presence of food decreases the absorption of Amphojel.
    2. An empty stomach allows the medication to decrease hydrochloric acid secretion more effectively.
    3. This medication is less likely to cause diarrhea if given on an empty stomach.
    4. Rebound acidity is less likely to occur if given on this schedule.

175. A nurse is taking medication history of a patient diagnosed with a urinary tract infection. The physician has prescribed ciprofloxacin (Cipro) to treat the infection. Which of the following medications taken by the patient would be of most concern to the nurse?
    1. Mylanta
    2. Aspirin
    3. Feosol tablets
    4. Birth-control pills

176. A patient at a walk-in clinic has been on an extended overseas trip. He is complaining of diarrhea. The physician prescribes polycarbophil (Fibercon). The nurse also instructs the patient to:
    1. Limit fluid intake as fluid retention may be a problem.
    2. Take this medication with his other oral drugs because this will help him remember.
    3. Take aspirin as needed for any fever that may develop.
    4. Report back to the physician if diarrhea persists more than 2 days.

177. A student nurse asks her instructor why sucralfate (Carafate) has to be given an hour before meals and 2 hours after other medications. The instructor explains:
    1. Carafate is better able to protect the lining of the stomach if it is able to come in contact with it.
    2. Spicy foods might interfere with the effectiveness of Carafate.
    3. Carafate is less likely to cause diarrhea on an empty stomach.
    4. Carafate is synergistic with many other medications and may increase their effect.

178. Which of the following agents is used topically to treat burn patients?
    1. Isotretinoin (Accutane)
    2. Mafenide (Sulfamylon)
    3. Tetracycline (Topicycline)
    4. Masoprocal (Actinex)

179. A patient is being discharged home on levothyroxine (Synthroid). Which of the following statements indicates the need for further teaching?
    1. "I may feel very sleepy at first when I am on this medication."
    2. "I should let my physician know if I feel my heart is beating fast."
    3. "I will have to be certain to eat healthier food."
    4. "I will take this with my other medications, so I remember."

180. How should omeprazole (Prilosec) be given?
    1 With food
    2 Before food
    3 Chewed
    4 With water

181. A preoperative patient is being treated with heparin before surgery. The purpose for this medication is to:
    1 Minimize blood loss during surgery.
    2 Decrease the risk of potential circulatory complications.
    3 Improve RBC production.
    4 Minimize the chance of a potential infection.

182. Which of the following medications would be given for an overdose of a cholinergic drug?
    1 Urecholine (Bethanechol)
    2 Metoclopramide (Reglan)
    3 Atropine sulfate (Atropine)
    4 Edrophonium chloride (Prostigmin)

183. Your patient is being discharged on warfarin sodium (Coumadin). Which of these instructions is appropriate for the nurse to give him?
    1 The visiting nurse will administer the medication SC on a daily basis.
    2 Checking carefully for any signs of infection is important.
    3 Report any signs of bleeding to your health care provider.
    4 Your blood levels need to be checked in three months before your next visit with your physician.

184. The antidote for heparin (Heparin) is:
    1 Protamine sulfate
    2 Potassium
    3 Vitamin K
    4 Zinc

185. Which of the following is inappropriate when giving instructions to a patient who is being treated with nitroglycerin for acute attacks of angina?
    1 The patient should use a plastic wrap over his patch to avoid stains on his clothing.
    2 Allow the tablet to dissolve under the tongue.
    3 The dose may be repeated twice at 5-minute intervals.
    4 Sustained-release nitroglycerin should be swallowed whole.

186. A patient is admitted for the treatment of CHF. He is started on digoxin (Lanoxin) and furosemide (Lasix). A loading dose of digoxin is given for the purpose of:
    1 Gradually bringing the patient into the therapeutic range
    2 Eliminating fluid from the lungs
    3 Giving the patient an adequate blood level
    4 Decreasing the possibility of toxicity

187. A nurse is completing an assessment of a patient admitted to a psychiatric unit with a diagnosis of panic anxiety attacks. Which of these medications would most likely be prescribed?
    1 Tranylcypromine (Parnate)
    2 Chlorpromazine (Thorazine)
    3 Piperadine phenothiazine (Mellaril)
    4 Sertraline (Zoloft)

188. The physician has prescribed simvastatin (Zocor) for a patient. The blood test to monitor whether or not this medication has been effective is:
    1 Cholesterol levels
    2 Liver enzymes
    3 Cardiac enzymes
    4 CPK levels

189. Atorvastatin (Lipitor) should be given:
    1 Early in the morning
    2 With food
    3 On an empty stomach
    4 At bedtime

190. Which of the following medications is associated with the side effects of gingival hyperplasia and nystagmus?
    1 Phenytoin (Dilantin)
    2 Phenobarbital (Luminal)
    3 Carbamazepine (Tegretol)
    4 Gabapentin (Neurontin)

191. Which of the following side effects would be expected with elderly patients who are taking barbiturates?
    1 Elevated BP, dizziness, muscle pain
    2 Gingival hyperplasia, nystagmus
    3 Diuresis, ecchymotic areas, muscle pain
    4 Excitement, confusion, or depression

192. A patient is being started on rofecoxib (Vioxx) for treating osteoarthritis. Which of the following statements indicates that the patient understands the nurse's teaching?
    1 "I need to take this medication three times a day with meals."
    2 "I need to take this when I feel the soreness starting."
    3 "I should take this medication once a day."
    4 "If I take this with breakfast, I will not have any nausea."

193. A patient has been given gabapentin (Neurontin) over the last year after having a craniotomy for a subdural hematoma. The directions given him at this point in time would be:
    1 "The physician will monitor liver function tests and CBCs to ensure that the medications are not toxic."
    2 "This medication needs to be discontinued on a gradual schedule initiated by the physician."
    3 "Avoid driving or operating any hazardous machinery while you are on this medication."
    4 "Use sunscreen and protective clothing to avoid photosensitivity reaction while on this medication."

194. A patient has been treated with sertraline (Zoloft) for 1 week. She tells her nurse that she is discouraged because she is not feeling any better. The nurse replies:
    1 "You must not drink alcohol while you are on this therapy."
    2 "Speak with your physician about changing medications."
    3 "It may take a few weeks for a change to be noticed."
    4 "Tell me more about what you are feeling."

195. A patient is diagnosed with topical fungal infections on the surfaces of his feet. A topical medication likely to be ordered is:
    1 Diphenhydramine (Benadryl)
    2 Nystatin (Mycostatin)
    3 Silver sulfadiazine (Silvadene)
    4 Cortisone (Cortone)

196. A student nurse asks why a patient is on insulin coverage when no history of diabetes is in her chart. The nurse explains that one of the medications she is taking will sometimes cause hyperglycemia. This medication would be:
    1 Dexamethasone (Decadron)
    2 Rosiglitazone (Avandia)
    3 Digoxin (Lanoxin)
    4 Glucophage (Metformin)

197. Which of the following medicine has priority when giving scheduled medications at 8:00 AM before breakfast?
    1. Digoxin (Lanoxin)
    2. Glucotrol (Glipizide)
    3. Donepezil hydrochloride (Aricept)
    4. Atorvastatin (Zocor)

198. A person receiving finasteride (Proscar) would be most likely to have the following diagnosis in their history?
    1. Gastro-esophageal reflux disease (GERD)
    2. Congestive Heart Failure (CHF)
    3. Glaucoma
    4. Benign Prostatic Hypertrophy (BPH)

199. A person with diabetes is receiving metoclopramide (Reglan). What is a side effect that would be of most concern to the nurse?
    1. Hyperglycemia
    2. Heartburn
    3. Hypoglycemia
    4. Headache

200. A child is being treated with the methylphenidate (Ritalin) for treating attention-deficit hyperkinetic disorder (ADHD). The parent should be instructed to schedule the medication:
    1. At bedtime
    2. Before meals
    3. After meals
    4. Early morning

201. A postpartum patient complains of dysuria. The physician prescribes which of these medications to ease symptoms:
    1. Phenazopyridine (Pyridium)
    2. Furosemide (Lasix)
    3. Loperamide (Immodium)
    4. Sulfisoxazole (Gantrisin)

202. An adverse side effect of oxybutynin (Ditropan), which needs to be reported immediately, is?
    1. Jaundice
    2. Restlessness
    3. Bradycardia
    4. Fatigue

203. Which of the following terms describes the pharmacokinetics of medication in the body?
    1. Digestion, excretion metabolism, catabolism
    2. Absorption, catabolism, metabolism, excretion
    3. Absorption, distribution, metabolism, excretion
    4. Anabolism, distribution, metabolism, excretion

204. A patient has just been started on furosemide (Lasix). Which of the following is the most important nursing intervention at this time?
    1. Monitoring potassium levels
    2. Checking the patient's weight and vital signs
    3. Reporting severe diarrhea
    4. Assessing lung and bowel sounds

205. A patient is being discharged on biphosphonates-alendronate (Fosamax). Which of the following instructions is not appropriate?
    1. "Drinking 3000 to 4000 ml of fluid will help your kidneys excrete the medication."
    2. "Increasing your intake of dairy products will help this medication to work better."
    3. "Remember to take your other vitamins at least 30 minutes after this pill."
    4. "Lab work needs to be scheduled to make sure this medication is working."

206. One of the most common side effects of enalapril (Vasotec) is:
    1. Dry hacking cough
    2. Hypertension
    3. Constipation
    4. Irritability

207. A patient is receiving biphosphonates-alendronate (Fosamax). The proper time to schedule this medication is:
    1. With meals
    2. With other medications early in the day
    3. 30 minutes before other medications
    4. 30 minutes before uncomfortable procedures

208. Which of the following is a sign of salicylate toxicity?
    1. Tinnitus
    2. Headache
    3. Dizziness
    4. Irritability

209. A patient was diagnosed with Type 2 diabetes 2 months ago. She has been unsuccessful in lowering her blood glucose with dietary and exercise changes. Which of the following medications would the physician prescribe for her?
    1. Rosiglitazone (Avandia)
    2. Rapid-acting insulin (Regular)
    3. Levothyroxine (Synthroid)
    4. Dexamethasone (Decadron)

210. A patient is being placed on repaglinide (Prandin). Which test would most accurately monitor the effectiveness of this therapy?
    1. Hemoglobin automated immunoassay (AIA)
    2. White blood cell (WBC) count
    3. Creatinine
    4. Potassium levels

211. A patient is being treated for severe acne vulgaris. A medication that the physician would prescribe would be:
    1. Vancomycin (Vancocin)
    2. Atorvastatin (Lipitor)
    3. Tetracycline (Achromycin)
    4. Ciprofloxacin (Cipro)

212. Which of the following dietary patterns would be contraindication for the administration of enoxaprin (Lovenox)?
    1. A patient on hyperalimentation
    2. A patient on a kosher diet
    3. A patient on a vegetarian diet
    4. A patient on a low sodium diet

213. A 16-year-old girl is diagnosed with a urinary tract infection. Which of the following medications would be prescribed for her?
    1. Sulfisoxazole (Gantrisin)
    2. Gentamicin sulfate (Garamycin)
    3. Kanamycin sulfate (Kantrex)
    4. Ciprofloxacin (Cipro)

214. Which of the following symptoms would be of most concern for a patient on antibiotics?
    1. Nausea
    2. Loose runny stools
    3. Drowsiness
    4. Dizziness

215. Which of the following classifications would be used to facilitate the examination of the eyes?
1   Cholinergic agents
2   Mydriatic agents
3   Ceruminolytic
4   Ocular decongestant

216. A postoperative patient is rating his operative pain as an 8 on a scale of 1 to 10. He is refusing pain medication. The most appropriate action for the nurse at this time would be:
1   Document his report and the refusal of pain medication.
2   Assess the location, duration and radiation of his pain.
3   Investigate why he is not receptive to medication.
4   Report the situation to the charge nurse.

217. Mycostatin (Nystatin) would be prescribed for which of the following conditions?
1   Acne vulgaris
2   A fungal infection
3   Pruritus
4   A furuncle

218. A 2-year-old patient must receive an injection. The nurse knows that the IM site of choice for this patient would be:
1   Dorsogluteal
2   Ventragluteal
3   Vastus lateralis
4   Deltoid

219. Which law subsidizes drug companies for the production of medications to treat rare disorders?
1   Harrison's Drug Act
2   Orphan Drug Act
3   Rare Drug Act
4   Comprehensive Drug Act

220. A semiconscious patient is brought into the emergency room complaining of nausea and vomiting. The route of choice for the ordered medication would be:
1   Oral (PO)
2   Sublingual
3   Via nasogastric tube
4   Rectally

221. A patient has been on loratidine (Claritin) for 2 weeks. The nurse would know the drug is effective if the patient reports which of the following?
1   Increased ability to sleep through the night
2   Decreased sneezing and runny nose
3   Decreased nausea and vomiting
4   Decreased number of migraines

222. Which of the following conditions would most interfere with the pharmacokinetics of medications?
1   Diabetes
2   Kidney disease
3   Angina pectoris
4   Brain tumor

223. A patient with Type 2 diabetes is hospitalized for surgery. He has been maintaining glycemic control using an oral hypoglycemic agent. He is concerned that his blood sugar has been elevated and that he has been needing to receive insulin. The best response for the nurse at this time would be?
1   "Don't worry about that now. Ask your doctor after you have recovered."
2   "As you get older, very often your cells resistance to insulin increases."
3   "Stress often temporarily increases your body's blood glucose levels."
4   "We are carefully monitoring your blood glucose levels."

224. How would the nurse evaluate the effectiveness of a patient being treated with filgrastim (Neupogen)?
1   Monitor the hemoglobin
2   Monitor the WBC count
3   Monitor potassium levels
4   Monitor blood glucose

225. The most common angle for an intramuscular injection is:
1   45 degrees
2   60 degrees
3   90 degrees
4   10 degrees

Chapter 3 Answers and Rationales

ANSWERS AND RATIONALES

1. Knowledge, assessment, physiological integrity (a).
   2 Idiosyncratic effects (reactions) are not the result of a known pharmacologic property of a drug but are particular to the patient; this type of reaction is a genetically determined abnormal response to ordinary doses of a drug.
   1 An additive effect is when two drugs with similar actions are given together; drugs administered together for an additive effect allow smaller doses of each drug to be given to avoid toxic effects while maintaining appropriate drug action.
   3 A synergistic effect describes a drug interaction that results in combined drug effects that are greater than those that could have been achieved should either drug have been administered alone.
   4 An antagonistic effect results when two drugs given in combination produce effects that are less than if the drugs were given separately; antacids given with tetracycline results in decreased absorption of the tetracycline.

2. Comprehension, planning, physiological integrity (b).
   4 Medication is administered directly into the bloodstream.
   1 Absorption from the stomach is an additional step before entering the bloodstream.
   2 Absorption from muscle is an additional step before entering the bloodstream.
   3 Absorption from the subcutaneous tissue is an additional step before entering the bloodstream.

3. Knowledge, planning, physiological integrity (a).
   1 Measures potassium
   2 Measures glucose
   3 Measures RBCs, among other things
   4 Measures oxygen and pH levels

4. Application, planning, physiological integrity (b).
   2 The physician adjusts the dose according to the results of the PTT.
   1 This medication is not used for infection.
   3 This is true but does not fully answer the question.
   4 This is true but rare and induces undue anxiety.

5. Application, implementation, physiological integrity (b).
   1 After application to the skin, the medication is absorbed at a slow, constant rate, allowing for the maintenance of a therapeutic level.
   2 Absorption through the skin is slow and is therefore ineffective in acute situations.
   3 Sublingual and transdermal methods both allow for accurate dosage.
   4 Although true, the patient's question is not answered; in addition, dosage and the length of time for administration depends on severity of condition and requires a physician's order; the dosage depends on the patient's condition.

6. Comprehension, assessment, physiological integrity (b).
   1 Patients need to be on a bowel program. Constipation is the only side effect for which patients do not develop a tolerance.
   2 A patient develops a tolerance to respiratory effects when dose is gradually increased.
   3 Pain relief is the desired effect.
   4 Constipation, not diarrhea, is the usual side effect; see rationale for #1.

7. Comprehension, assessment, physiological integrity (b).
   2 These are symptoms of withdrawal; others include gooseflesh, tearing, yawning, muscle twitching and abdominal cramping, insomnia, nausea, and vomiting.
   1, 3, 4 These are not typical symptoms of withdrawal.

8. Application, implementation, physiological integrity (b).
   4 This procedure will allow for maximal contact with impaired oral mucosa.
   1 This is an improper procedure; it minimizes contact with affected area and then rinses away medication.
   2 There is no indication that the medicine is a suspension.
   3 This is fine; however, it does not answer the question of what "swish and swallow" means.

9. Comprehension, implementation, physiological integrity (a).
   4 Only a limited number of drugs can be administered this way. They have to be dissolvable in salivary secretions.
   1, 2 These routes bypasses the GI tract.
   3 This is a very rapid method of absorption because it bypasses the GI tract and directly enters the systemic circulation.

10. Knowledge, evaluation, physiological integrity (b).
    2 The medication is considered ulcerogenic.
    1 This medication can irritate the stomach and must be taken with meals.
    3 This medication can irritate the stomach when not taken with meals.
    4 This medication is taken with an antacid, not orange juice, to prevent stomach irritation.

11. Comprehension, assessment, physiological integrity (a).
    3 This measures RBC volume.
    1, 2, 4 These are not appropriate measurements.

12. Application, implementation, physiological integrity (a).
    4 One teaspoon equals approximately 5 ml.
    1, 2, 3 These are incorrect equivalencies.

13. Comprehension, assessment, physiological integrity (b).
    3 This is the desired action of drug for which it is administered.
    1 Hypertension is a possible side effect for which the patient must be monitored.
    2 Hypotension is a possible side effect for which the patient must be monitored.
    4 Arrhythmias are a possible side effect for which the patient must be monitored.

14. Comprehension, assessment, physiological integrity (b).
    3 The physician needs to know to verify any needed prescriptions.
    1, 2 These are subsequent steps but not first priorities.
    4 This is very premature. The couple may need education and support.

15. Comprehension, implementation, physiological integrity (a).
    2 1 ml = 1 ml 5 mg/10 ml $\times$ 7.5 mg/x
    5x = 75
    x = 15 ml
    1, 3, 4 These are incorrect calculations.

16. Knowledge, implementation, physiological integrity (a).
    3 With a drip factor of 60 ml per hour = drops per minute.
    1, 2, 4 These are incorrect calculations.

17. Knowledge, planning, physiological integrity (a).
    4 This is the correct size needle to reach subcutaneous tissue.
    1, 2, 3 These needles are too long; they could pass through subcutaneous tissue to underlying muscle, bone.

18. Knowledge, implementation, physiological integrity (a).
    2 This is the correct calculation.
    1, 3, 4 These are incorrect calculations; review equivalencies.
19. Application, evaluation, physiological integrity (a).
    2 This is the therapeutic effect.
    1 Sleep patterns are not affected by Antiparkinsonian drugs.
    3 Emotional stability is not affected by antiparkinsonian drugs.
    4 Diet and nutrition are not affected by antiparkinsonian drugs.
20. Comprehension, planning, physiological integrity (b).
    1 A tranquilizer will ease tremors, and vitamins will improve metabolism.
    2 Aspirin and Tigan might be appropriate for an overdose, not for withdrawal. Calcium is not prescribed.
    3 See #2. Vitamin C is not prescribed.
    4 See #2.
21. Knowledge, assessment, physiological integrity (c).
    1 This is the action of the drug.
    2 Loop diuretics deplete potassium.
    3 This is used for open-angle glaucoma.
    4 This is used for acute renal failure.
22. Application, implementation, physiological integrity (b).
    1 Fluids will help thin secretions and help prevent dehydration. Dehydration is particularly common in older adults and children.
    2 Medication should be taken with water. Food will affect absorption.
    3 Chewing will speed up absorption.
    4 Certain antibiotics (particularly erythromycin) will increase action of theophylline.
23. Comprehension, planning, physiological integrity (a).
    4 The tablet is prepared to dissolve between the cheek and the gum.
    1 A buccal tablet should not be chewed.
    2 A buccal tablet is not dissolved in the stomach.
    3 Sublingual tablets are taken this way.
24. Application, assessment, physiological integrity (c).
    2 Discontinuing this medication may or may not be possible, depending on the cause of the seizure. If it is discontinued, it must be done gradually under the direction of a physician.
    1 Folic acid deficiency is an adverse reaction to this medication and should be documented by the physician.
    3 This is fine; the stomach should not be empty.
    4 This practice is safe.
25. Application, evaluation, physiological integrity (b).
    1 This is an action of the drug.
    2 Nitroglycerin has no effect on the brain stem.
    3 Nitroglycerin does not affect respiration or alertness.
    4 Nitroglycerin acts on the myocardial blood vessels, not nerve endings.
26. Comprehension, planning, physiological integrity (b).
    1 This is the correct calculation.
    2, 3, 4 These are incorrect calculations.
27. Knowledge, assessment, physiological integrity (a).
    1 These are signs of alcohol withdrawal along with tachycardia, diaphoresis, anorexia, nausea, vomiting and insomnia, hallucinations, and seizures.
    2 These are not signs.

3 Polyuria is not a sign; nausea and headache would be signs of an overdose.
    4 These are not signs.
28. Application, implementation, physiological integrity (b).
    4 Orthostatic hypotension is a side effect of diuretics.
    1 Given that it is taken in the morning, it does not disturb sleep.
    2 The patient may require potassium supplements.
    3 The patient should monitor weight once a week.
29. Knowledge, planning, physiological integrity (a).
    3 Giving it this way helps to decrease gastric distress.
    1, 2 These methods will not help to decrease gastric distress.
    4 This medication has to be given around the clock to maintain a therapeutic level.
30. Comprehension, evaluation, physiological integrity (b).
    1 Insomnia is a common side effect. Doses are usually administered at breakfast and lunch.
    2 The patient may be hyperactive, but this is not the best answer.
    3 Caffeine is a CNS stimulant and should be limited, but this is not the best answer.
    4 Ritalin can be addicting, so dose should not be increased; it would increase his insomnia.
31. Comprehension, assessment, physiological integrity (b).
    3 This is a cholinergic-blocking agent. Urinary retention is an adverse side effect.
    1, 4 This is a skeletal muscle relaxant; a side effect is urinary frequency.
    2 This is an antianxiety agent. Urinary retention is not a side effect.
32. Knowledge, planning, physiological integrity (a).
    3 This is an expected action.
    1 This is a stool softener.
    2 This is an antidiarrheal.
    4 This inhibits gastric secretion and decreases motility.
33. Knowledge, planning, physiological integrity (b).
    4 This medication induces uterine contraction.
    1 This medication suppresses endometrial bleeding.
    2 This medication is a contraceptive agent.
    3 This medication is a uterine relaxant.
34. Knowledge, planning, physiological integrity (a).
    1 This controlled agent is effective on the cough center in the brain.
    2 This is an NSAID; it has no effect on the cough center.
    3 This is a controlled substance; side effects are prohibitive to be used for a cough.
    4 This is an OTC antitussive that can be combined with codeine.
35. Comprehension, assessment, physiological integrity (b).
    4 These are side effects of this cholesterol-lowering medication.
    1 This is an NSAID; nausea may be a side effect at times, but it is generally given to relieve muscle cramps.
    2 This is a skeletal muscle relaxant; these are not common side effects of this medication.
    3 This is an antihistamine given to relieve allergy symptoms; these are not common side effects of this medication.
36. Comprehension, evaluation, physiological integrity (c).
    2 This is the correct action.
    1 This is an action of histamine.

3 This is an action of beta-antagonist.

4 This is the action of a decongestant.

37. Comprehension, evaluation, physiological integrity (b).

   2 Heart rate can increase.

   1 This is a serious symptom not related to an adverse reaction to atropine.

   3 This is caused by lack of bulk in the diet.

   4 This is an expected reaction of atropine; it would have no effect on heart disease.

38. Application, evaluation, physiological integrity (c).

   1. These are adverse reactions of uterine relaxants.

   2 These are adverse reaction of skeletal muscle relaxants.

   3 These are adverse reactions of antihistamines.

   4 These are adverse reactions of adrenergic stimulants.

39. Knowledge, planning, physiological integrity (a).

   3 This is the correct medication.

   1 This is a tranquilizer.

   2 This is a cardiac stimulant.

   4 This is used to treat chronic hypertension and angina.

40. Application, planning, physiological integrity (c).

   1 Patients being treated with calcitonin require calcium supplements to maintain blood levels.

   2 Fiber promotes calcium excretion.

   3 Calcitonin does not affect vitamin C.

   4 This is true for everyone.

41. Application, planning, physiological integrity (b).

   4 Other effects include diabetes, impotence, amenorrhea, and acromegalic syndrome.

   1, 3 This is true; however, it does not answer the question.

   2 This is true; however, it is not the best answer.

42. Comprehension, evaluation, physiological integrity (b).

   3 The purpose is to maintain and improve BP.

   1 Respiration needs to slow down and be more effective. Respiratory depression needs to be avoided.

   2 Urinary output is decreased in shock. It needs to be maintained to keep circulation adequate.

   4 This would not be the first sign. Increasing orientation is a sign of improvement.

43. Comprehension, evaluation, physiological integrity (a).

   4 This agent is used to decrease cholesterol.

   1, 2, 3 These are not a measure of this medication.

44. Knowledge, implementation, physiological integrity (a).

   2 This is a clinical indication for this medication.

   1 This is not a clinical indication for tetracycline.

   3 This is not a clinical indication for claithromyesin.

   4 This is a po sulfa-based drug used frequently in treating UTIs.

45. Knowledge, implementation, physiological integrity (a).

   1 This is the correct technique to give a deep IM and minimize irritation.

   2 Z-track is a deep IM.

   3 This is not true.

   4 This is not a method that allows for rapid effect.

46. Comprehension, assessment, physiological integrity (b).

   2 Theophylline can cause these effects; a level is necessary to determine if the medication is in the therapeutic range.

   1 Valium may be used in an emergency asthmatic situation. It is not used on a routine basis.

   3 Tagamet does not cause jitteriness and it is given to decrease nausea.

   4 These are not side effects of laxatives.

47. Comprehension, assessment, physiological integrity (b).

   4 Corticosteroids can cause a rise in the blood sugar.

   1 Anemia is not a predicted side effect

   2, 3 These are not predicted side effects.

48. Application, evaluation, physiological integrity (b).

   2 This is the truth, and patients need encouragement to comply.

   1 There is no indication of the need to change medication.

   3 It is not within the scope of practice for the nurse to add a medication, nor is there any indication that the physician need do so.

   4 This is true; however, it does not answer the question.

49. Comprehension, knowledge, physiological integrity (a).

   1 This is the correct definition.

   2, 3, 4 These are incorrect definitions.

50. Comprehension, evaluation, physiological integrity (b).

   1 These are the therapeutic effects desired in children with hyperactivity.

   2 Irritability is an adverse reaction to the medication. Drug should be given at least 6 hours before bedtime to avoid insomnia.

   3 Headache is an adverse reaction as is anorexia.

   4 These are adverse reactions.

51. Comprehension, assessment, physiological integrity (b).

   3 This is the therapeutic effect; it takes 2 to 3 weeks to reach a therapeutic level.

   1, 2, 4 Diarrhea, nausea and vomiting, and insomnia are adverse reactions to the drug.

52. Comprehension, assessment, physiological integrity (c).

   3 This is the sign that an allergic reaction may be occurring.

   1 This would be an indicator of a febrile reaction, indicating contamination. It generally occurs late in the transfusion or after completion.

   2 This would be an indication of circulatory overload.

   4 This would indicate an anticoagulant reaction.

53. Comprehension, assessment, physiological integrity (b).

   2 This medicine used to treat transient ischemic attacks (TIAs); orthostatic hypotension is a common side effect.

   1 This is not a necessary parameter to monitor.

   3 This does not affect temperature.

   4 This does not affect WBCs and may increase risk of bleeding.

54. Comprehension, assessment, physiological integrity (b).

   3 Vancomycin is ototoxic.

   1, 2, 4 These are not adverse effects of this medication.

55. Application, assessment, physiological integrity (b).

   4 Less food and more exercise is most likely to cause decreased blood sugar.

   1 Decreasing exercise is more likely to cause hyperglycemia.

   2 This is more likely to cause hyperglycemia.

   3 Exercise decreases the need for insulin. Increasing calories is another option.

56. Knowledge, assessment, physiological integrity (a).

   2 This is the correct use; a troche is a lozenge that should be held in the throat to decrease irritation.

   1 This is not an effect.

   3, 4 These are not appropriate uses for troches.

57. Application, assessment, physiological integrity (c).

   4 A cultural influence may cause her to believe that these medicines are food; however, a knowledge deficit definitely exists.

1 This is definitely a necessary assessment, but further information on entire pattern of OTC medicines is need.

2, 3 See #1

58. Application, assessment, physiological integrity (c).

4 Patients should be advised on the danger of taking OTC medicines for more than 2 weeks without consulting a physician. The location and characteristics of the pain need to be investigated.

1 Occasional use of a laxative is not dangerous, but further dietary teaching may be indicated.

2 Assessment of BP is called for, but if it is stable, this is considered ongoing care.

3 Taking a vitamin every day is fine, as long as it is not used as a substitute for good nutrition.

59. Comprehension, evaluation, physiological integrity (b).

3 This is a sign of digoxin toxicity.

1 Digoxin is given to treat elevated heart rate in CHF. A toxic effect would be bradycardia.

2, 4 These are not toxic effects.

60. Application, evaluation, physiological integrity (b).

2 These are adverse reactions to hypothyroid medication.

1, 3 These are adverse reactions to hyperthyroid medications.

4 These are the opposite of hypothyroid effects.

61. Comprehension, evaluation, physiological integrity (b).

2 This is a fertility drug that stimulates ovulation.

1 Decreased BP is not an effect.

3, 4 These are not therapeutic effects.

62. Knowledge, evaluation, physiological integrity (b).

1 This is a major adverse reaction.

2 This is a sign of kidney disease.

3 This is not a major adverse reaction and can be caused by depression.

4 This is caused by pupil dilation from medication.

63. Knowledge, evaluation, physiological integrity (a).

3 This is the definition of toxic action.

1, 2 These are undesired effects of a drug.

4 This is an unusual or unexpected effect of a drug.

64. Comprehension, assessment, physiological integrity (b).

2 This may be indicative of infiltration.

1 This can be corrected (if the insertion site is still patent) by repositioning and making certain the dial is set correctly.

3 This can be corrected with positioning.

4 This is important; however, the primary infusion normally begins when the "piggyback" is completed.

65. Comprehension, assessment, physiological integrity (b).

2 Concurrent use of heparin and NSAIDs may predispose the patient to hemorrhage.

1 Psyllium is not contraindicated with heparin. It should not be given at the same time as aspirin or digoxin; absorption may be inhibited.

3 This is a CNS depressant and is synergistic with other groups in this classification.

4 The need here would be to monitor the cumulative effects of other hypertensive agents.

66. Comprehension, implementation, physiological integrity (b).

3 By giving it in this manner, the patient receives both a local soothing effect and a CNS effect on the cough center in the brain.

1 This is not the correct technique.

2 This method will limit the local effect.

4 Cough medicines are normally given on a prn basis.

67. Comprehension, implementation, physiological integrity (a).

3 This is the correct calculation. The formula is ml/hr × gtt factor/60 = 125 ml/hr × 10/60

1, 2, 4 These are incorrect calculations.

68. Comprehension, implementation, physiological integrity (b).

4 It is possible that the evening shift obtained permission to give the medication early so that the patient would not be awakened.

1 This should be done before administration.

2 This is true; however, it does not answer the question.

3 This may also be true, but it does not answer the question.

69. Application, implementation, safe, effective care environment (b).

1 TB medications must be taken over an extended period (6 months to 2 years) to be sure of effective treatment.

2 There is no indication of this, and continued exposure would not be a factor if the medication regimen were being followed.

3 There may be a need for additional medication in the future, but it would have to be determined if multidrug-resistant TB had developed.

4 Family members should have already received follow-up medical care.

70. Comprehension, implementation, physiological integrity (a).

1 This allocation allows for two meals on the 7:00 to 3:00 shift, one meal on the 3:00 to 11:00 shift, and fluids for medications on the 11:00 to 7:00 shift.

2 There are two meals on the 7:00 to 3:00 shift; most patients prefer fluids with meals.

3 Fluids must be allowed for medication.

4 Patients need to be encouraged to save fluids all during the day to increase comfort.

71. Knowledge, planning, physiological integrity (a).

1 Sedatives are given in small doses to decrease anxiety. Hypnotics are given in larger doses to induce sleep.

2 Sedatives can be given around the clock; hypnotics are given before sleep at anytime.

3 This is not true.

4 Length of effect varies with each drug.

72. Knowledge, planning, physiological integrity (a).

3 This is an anticholinergic medication used to treat Parkinson's disease.

1 This is a CNS stimulant.

2 This is an anticonvulsant.

4 This is a bronchodilator.

73. Knowledge, planning, physiological integrity (b).

2 This would result in optimal absorption.

1, 3 Patient is vomiting and would not retain medication.

4 This would result in poor absorption.

74. Comprehension, planning, physiological integrity (b).

3 This treatment decreases inflammation.

1 This is used sparingly if at all in head injury patients because it may mask central signs of intracranial pressure.

2 This is used to treat high BP.

4 This is used as an anticoagulant.

75. Knowledge, evaluation, physiological integrity (a).

1 This is the therapeutic effect.

2 This is not applicable to the effect of the drug.

3 The placebo has no active ingredient.

4 Metabolism of the drug is not necessary to produce the desired effect.

76. Comprehension, evaluation, physiological integrity (b).
    2 It can only be given preventatively, and it does take several weeks to reach a therapeutic level.
    1 Intal does not improve symptoms; if given during an attack, it may make symptoms worse.
    3 Intal does not affect sleeping ability.
    4 This is not an effect of this medication.

77. Knowledge, assessment, physiological integrity (a).
    1 This is the most common antibiotic used to treat urinary tract infections.
    2 A penicillin substitute such as erythromycin would be used if the symptoms warranted.
    3 This may or may not call for an antibiotic; it may be viral in nature. If an antibiotic were called for, it would probably be penicillin or a substitute.
    4 This may be an indication of a super infection.

78. Comprehension, assessment, physiological integrity (a).
    2 Cancer drugs can affect the integrity of the oral mucosa.
    1 Antibiotics do not affect the oral mucosa.
    3 Antiparkinsonian drugs do not affect the oral mucosa.
    4 Vitamins do not affect the oral mucosa.

79. Knowledge, assessment, safe, effective care environment (a).
    4 This is the definition of the law.
    1 This was replaced by the Controlled Substance Act.
    2 No such act exists.
    3 This regulates distribution of narcotics and other drugs of abuse.

80. Comprehension, assessment, physiological integrity (c).
    4 Elderly metabolize drugs more slowly because of declining body function, thus prolonging the half-life of the drug, resulting in drug accumulation.
    1 Age does not make a difference in tolerance.
    2 Older adults metabolize drugs at a decreased rate.
    3 Age does not cause more frequent adverse effects.

81. Knowledge, assessment, physiological integrity (a).
    1 Sedation is part of therapy.
    2 This medication does not control seizures.
    3 This medication does not cause vasoconstriction.
    4 This medication does not cause vasodilation.

82. Comprehension, evaluation, physiological integrity (b).
    3 These side effects can occur particularly with children taking this medication.
    1, 2, 4 These are not common side effects of these medications.

83. Knowledge, evaluation, physiological integrity (a).
    1 These medications decrease the effects of the parasympathetic nervous system.
    2 These are opposites of what the side effects would be.
    3 Thirst is a side effect, but polyuria is not.
    4 These drugs are cardiac stimulants; however, tachycardia is not desirable.

84. Comprehension, evaluation, physiological integrity (b).
    4 Increased muscle strength would indicate an improvement in the symptoms.
    1 Slowing of the heart rate is an effect. It is not given to treat arrhythmias.
    2 This is a side effect; however, it is not a therapeutic effect.
    3 See #2.

85. Knowledge, evaluation, physiological integrity (b).
    3 These dilate coronary arteries in acute angina.
    1 These are used in long-term management.
    2 These are used for chronic angina.
    4 These are used for severe physical pain.

86. Application, evaluation, physiological integrity (c).
    2 Children on high doses of Reglan are particularly prone to the extrapyramidal effects of the drug. Presence of these effects should be reported to the health care provider immediately so that the dose can be adjusted or a new drug prescribed.
    1, 3, 4 These are common side effects and need not be reported.

87. Comprehension, evaluation, physiological integrity (b).
    2 Benadryl is an antihistamine that decreases itching.
    1, 3, 4 These are not common symptoms of hives, and Benadryl does not affect these symptoms.

88. Knowledge, planning, physiological integrity (b).
    1 This is the action of a thrombolytic agent. It must be used only in acute situations.
    2 This is an anticoagulant that may be used for long-term management.
    3 Vitamin K is a hemostatic agent.
    4 Amicar is a hemostatic agent.

89. Knowledge, planning, physiological integrity (c).
    2 This is used to relieve pain and does not cause biliary spasms as morphine does.
    1 See #2.
    3 This is an antibiotic that has adverse GI effects.
    4 This is an antiinflammatory that causes adverse GI effects.

90. Knowledge, planning, physiological integrity (a).
    2 This is rapid acting with the fastest onset.
    1 This is intermediate acting. The onset of action would take too long.
    3, 4 These are long acting; the onset would take too long.

91. Knowledge, planning, physiological integrity (a).
    3 This is the appropriate length, gauge, and needle size for an intradermal injection.
    1, 4 Needles are too large and too long for intradermal injections.
    2 This size is appropriate for subcutaneous injections.

92. Application, planning, physiological integrity (b).
    2 Explanations should be geared to the child's ability to understand.
    1 Long explanations to a child under 5 years of age only increase anxiety.
    3 Of course, the parent can hold the child; however, injecting it quickly can cause aspiration.
    4 Administering some medication in juice may be appropriate; however, you must be certain that the child will drink all of the juice to receive a correct dose.

93. Knowledge, assessment, physiological integrity (a).
    3 This is used in addiction management.
    1 This is a narcotic-analgesic used to control pain.
    2 This is a narcotic-antagonist used to reverse CNS and respiratory depression.
    4 This is a narcotic agonist-antagonist used to control pain.

94. Knowledge, assessment, physiological integrity (a).
    2 Dosage is individualized according to blood coagulation.
    1 This is the laboratory test for platelet activity.
    3 This is the laboratory test for time of actual bleeding.
    4 This is the laboratory test for strength of capillary walls.

95. Comprehension, assessment, physiological integrity (a).
    1 Pitocin is an oxytocin and stimulates uterine contractions.
    2 Pitocin acts on uterine muscle fibers.

3 This is an unwanted action of the drug.

4 Pitocin contracts uterine muscle fibers and has no effect on vaginal walls or perineal muscles.

96. Comprehension, implementation, physiological integrity (a).

4 This is the most common gauge and length for IM injections for normal-weight individuals (the larger the number, the finer the needle).

1 This gauge may be appropriate in the deltoid or with extremely thin persons; however, the length of the needle would be long for an average-weight person.

2 This would be appropriate for an intradermal injection.

3 This gauge would be used for oily preparations; the needle length is too long for an average-weight person.

97. Knowledge, implementation, safe, effective care environment (a).

3 Barrier gloves need to be worn when the nurse can reasonably expect contact with bodily fluids.

1 This is true; however, it does not answer the question.

2 This is also true, but it is nonresponsive to the question.

4 Standard precautions apply to all patients.

98. Knowledge, implementation, physiological integrity (a).

2 Enteric-coated tablets disintegrate in the small intestine to prevent stomach irritation.

1 It does not affect the length of stay in the stomach.

3 This describes a timed-released or sustained-action tablet.

4 It prevents irritation to the stomach, not to the small intestine.

99. Knowledge, planning, physiological integrity (b).

4 Increasing the amount of glucose taken up by the muscles decreases glucose level in the bloodstream; if insulin is able to get in the cells, glucose will be used as energy.

1 Fats being broken down excessively can lead to ketosis. Excess protein is used for energy; however, this is not the primary source for energy.

2 This is partially true. It does decrease cellular resistance; however, decreasing the amount of glucose used by muscles will increase serum glucose levels.

3 Oral hypoglycemics are not oral insulin.

100. Knowledge, implementation, physiological integrity (a).

3 This is the correct calculation: ml/hour × gtt factor/60

1, 2, 4 These are incorrect calculations.

101. Knowledge, implementation, physiological integrity (a).

2 1 ml = 1 ml 1 ml/10,000 = ½ ml/5000 units

1, 3, 4 These are incorrect calculations.

102. Knowledge, implementation, physiological integrity (a).

2 0.4 mg = 1/150 grain

1, 3, 4 These are incorrect calculations.

103. Comprehension, implementation, physiological integrity (a).

1 This is the preferred site for children under age 3 because it is well developed at birth.

2 This site should not be used for injections at all until the child has been walking for at least 1 year.

3 This site can be used with older, larger children.

4 This site can be used for children over 3 years of age who have been walking for a year or two; it has a disadvantage of being visible to the child, however.

104. Knowledge, assessment, physiological integrity (a).

1 This is given IV to control seizures.

2 This is an antianxiety agent.

3 This is a sedative-hypnotic agent.

4 This is used to treat alcohol withdrawal.

105. Knowledge, planning, physiological integrity (b).

4 As of this time, this is the most potent antibiotic available.

1, 2 MRSA is resistant to these antibiotics.

3 This is an antiviral medication.

106. Knowledge, planning, physiological integrity (a).

3 This drug is a biologic modifier. It stimulates proliferation and differentiation of neutrophils.

1 Epogen increases the rate of RBC production.

2 This is an antiinfective medication.

4 This is used in treatment of cancer; a side effect is immunosuppression.

107. Knowledge, planning, health promotion and maintenance (a).

2 This is an appropriate characteristic of adolescents. Activities in the teaching plan should include ways that involve them with their peer group as much as possible.

1 This is characteristic of a school-age child.

3 This is characteristic of young adults.

4 This is characteristic of an older adult.

108. Comprehension, planning, physiological integrity (b).

3 The aim of treatment in glaucoma is to decrease intraocular pressure. This classification of medications will increase pressure and precipitate acute glaucoma in predisposed persons.

1 Cholinergic agents decrease intraocular pressure.

2, 4 This is true; however, it does not respond to the question.

109. Comprehension, evaluation, safe, effective care environment (b).

2 Follow-up care by health professionals and support of family and friends is vital because patients may need to be on medications for as long as 2 years.

1 The treatment may need to continue for from 6 months to as much as a year.

3 This is true to assist in maintaining the immune system. It does not, however, answer the question.

4 Patients are contagious in the initial stages of TB. Good health habits should always be maintained to prevent exposure to others.

110. Knowledge, evaluation, safe, effective care environment (a).

1 This is federal law.

2, 3, 4 These statements are true; however, they do not answer the question.

111. Application, evaluation, physiological integrity (b).

4 This is the first action; the pain might be related to something other than the operation (i.e., urinary retention or cardiac).

1 This is unacceptable. A patient in pain requires action.

2 This would be the second action, particularly because the dose of morphine may not be in therapeutic range.

3 This would be beneficial after the pain level is decreased.

112. Comprehension, evaluation, health promotion and maintenance (b).

3 It may be a "drag," but at least he acknowledges that it has to be done.

1 This is fine. There is no problem with him hanging out with his friends.

2 Exercise is fine as long as it is balanced with diet and medication.

4 Peers are important to adolescents. This statement does not indicate understanding that he has measures necessary to manage his diabetes, but his activities are not restricted.

113. Comprehension, implementation, physiological integrity (b).

1 The medication is not safe for direct IV administration.

2 This action will not relieve any discomfort patient may have.

3 This action will not facilitate absorption.

4 There are no organs at intramuscular sites.

114. Application, implementation, physiological integrity (b).

1 This allows peak drug activity during daytime hours.

2, 3, 4 These are not applicable to effect of drug.

115. Knowledge, implementation, physiological integrity (a).

3 This prevents possible obstruction as a result of thickening and expansion of the drug.

1 This will not prevent unwanted side effects.

2 Fluid, not food, is necessary to prevent undesired effects.

4 Gastric distress is not a side effect.

116. Application, implementation, physiological integrity (a).

1 This straightens the canal and promotes maximum contact of medication with tissue.

2 This is proper procedure for children.

3 This would block entrance to ear canal.

4 This procedure would not allow access to ear canal.

117. Application, implementation, physiological integrity (a).

1 Glucose reverses the effect of too much insulin.

2 This is given for hyperglycemia.

3 This facilitates increase in blood glucose but is not an appropriate treatment.

4 This is not an emergency treatment.

118. Knowledge, implementation, physiological integrity (a).

3 This is the proper procedure.

1, 2, 4 Part of dose will be wasted.

119. Application, implementation, physiological integrity (b).

2 These are correct actions.

1, 3 The drug should be withheld.

4 The nurse should withhold drug. Oxygen would not be administered without a physician's order.

120. Knowledge, implementation, physiological integrity (b).

3 This is the correct calculation.

1, 2, 4 These are incorrect calculations.

121. Knowledge, implementation, physiological integrity (a).

2 This is the best anatomic position.

1 Nose drops would not be retained.

3 Flexion of neck prevents administration.

4 Nose drops would not be retained.

122. Knowledge, assessment, physiological integrity (a).

1 This is the definition.

2 Distribution is the transport of drugs in the body.

3 Metabolism is the process by which a drug is transformed into an inactive metabolite, a more soluble compound, or a more potent metabolite.

4 Excretion is the elimination of drugs from the body.

123. Knowledge, planning, physiological integrity (b).

4. Mestinon enhances the cholinergic system and increases the accumulation of acetylcholine at nervous system synapses.

1. Pavulon increases the transmission of nerve impulses blocking the transmission of acetylcholine.

2. This is an oral hypoglycemic.

3. This is an H2-blocking agent used to treat gastric acid secretion.

124. Application, planning, physiological integrity (c).

3 This is a parasympathetic agent that helps restore bladder tone.

1 This is an anticholinergic agent that would inhibit gastric acid secretion and decrease the tone of the bladder.

2 This can be used as a tranquilizer or an antiemetic.

4 This is an antiemetic.

125. Application, planning, physiological integrity (c).

2 This is an overgrowth of the gums, which may require additional dental care.

1 Nystagmus is involuntary rhythmic eye movements and is not affected by dental care.

3 This is also true; however, it is not a priority for the dentist.

4 This is true, though rare.

126. Knowledge, planning, physiological integrity (a).

1 This is the official reference book for the United States.

2 This is published annually by manufacturers.

3 This is published by the hospital association.

4 This is very useful; however, it is not official.

127. Knowledge, planning, physiological integrity (a).

2 This is the correct definition: the total effect of two drugs when given together is greater than the effects if each is given separately.

1, 3, 4 These definitions are incorrect.

128. Application, planning, physiological integrity (b).

3 This drug will increase anticoagulant effects.

1 This drug is used to decrease BP in hypertension; it is not synergistic with Coumadin.

2 This drug is used to decrease blood sugar in non–insulin-dependent diabetes mellitus; it is not synergistic with Coumadin.

4 This drug is used to treat cardiac arrhythmias; it is not synergistic with Coumadin.

129. Knowledge, planning, physiological integrity (a).

2 This is a stool softener.

1 This is used to treat diarrhea.

3 This is an antihypertensive medication.

4 This can be used as an antiemetic or, in higher doses, as a tranquilizer.

130. Knowledge, planning, physiological integrity (a).

2 This is an effect of this adrenergic agent.

1 This is the opposite effect; epinephrine causes central dilation and peripheral constriction.

3, 4 This is true; however, it does not answer the question.

131. Knowledge, planning, physiological integrity (b).

1 Vitamin K is the antidote for Coumadin overdoses.

2 This is an anticoagulant.

3 This is used to treat cardiac arrhythmias.

4 This is used to decrease BP and improve cardiac arrhythmias.

132. Knowledge, planning, physiological integrity (a).

4 This medication increases RBC production.

1 This is used to increase WBC production

2 This is used to treat high BP.

3 This is a diuretic.

133. Comprehension, planning, physiological integrity (b).
     1 This medication is prescribed to improve appetite in patients with AIDS.
     2 This is an antibiotic.
     3 This is used to treat nutritional anemias.
     4 This is an antiviral medication.

134. Knowledge, evaluation, health promotion and maintenance (a).
     3 A deficiency of maternal folic acid has been associated with neural tube defects.
     1 Vitamins are not a substitute for a well-balanced diet.
     2 It is not recommended that megadoses of vitamins be taken.
     4 This is fine; however; this statement does not indicate the need for a well-balanced diet, from all of the food levels.

135. Application, evaluation, physiological integrity (b).
     2 This methods allows for no contamination of the rapid-acting insulin with the NPH, which has been modified.
     1 This method might lead to potential contamination.
     3 These medications can be safely mixed.
     4 Using three syringes is unnecessary.

136. Comprehension, evaluation, physiological integrity (b).
     3 The medication must be in the desired range if therapeutic effectiveness is going to be achieved.
     1 This is not the definition of tolerance. Tolerance means that larger and larger doses need to be given.
     2 Physical dependence means a distinct physical reaction develops when the drug is discontinued.
     4 If the levels came back in the toxic range, toxic effects may develop. The dosage may need to be decreased.

137. Comprehension, evaluation, physiological integrity (b).
     1 Patients should check with their physician on what to do if a dose is missed. They should never double up on a dose.
     2 Taking medicine with water to facilitate absorption is appropriate.
     3 Opposite action should be taken.
     4 Patients with hypertension should avoid foods high in sodium. This does not answer the question.

138. Application, evaluation, physiological integrity (b).
     3 One minute should be allowed between puffs.
     1 This is the correct procedure; it allows for maximal absorption.
     2 This is true.
     4 This is true; it aids in absorption.

139. Comprehension, evaluation, physiological integrity (a).
     2 This is correct. NPH insulin peaks in 6 to 12 hours.
     1 This is too early. Regular insulin peaks in 2 to 4 hours.
     3 This is too early.
     4 This is too late. This would be within the peak of long-acting insulins.

140. Knowledge, evaluation, physiological integrity (b).
     1 This indicates a normal calcium level.
     2 Vision is not affected with hypocalcemia.
     3 This is a normal level and is not used as indicator for hypocalcemia treatment.
     4 See #3.

141. Comprehension, evaluation, physiological integrity (a).
     3 This is an antihistamine medication that helps prevent histamines from causing allergic symptoms.
     1 This is a side effect that is particularly common in older adults.

2 This is not an effect. Older children sometimes have a paradoxic effect of increased irritability when antihistamines are taken.
4 This is not an effect of this medication.

142. Knowledge, implementation, physiological integrity (b).
     3 This is the correct calculation.
     1, 2, 4 These are incorrect calculations.

143. Comprehension, implementation, physiological integrity (a).
     1 These are often the least expensive.
     2 These are often the most expensive.
     3, 4 Prescriptions are not written in this form.

144. Application, implementation, physiological integrity (b).
     3 The action of the drug takes 2 to 3 weeks while blood levels are building.
     1 It should be taken in the morning so that the effects of the drug are the strongest during waking hours.
     2 The action of the drug does not occur in 24 hours; 2 to 3 weeks are required while blood levels are building.
     4 This is not necessary.

145. Application, implementation, physiological integrity (c).
     2 KCl is diluted to decrease GI upset.
     1 KCl should be given with or after meals.
     3 Never crush controlled-release tablets.
     4 Fully dissolve effervescent tablets before administering.

146. Application, implementation, physiological integrity (c).
     3 Cipro can increase theophylline levels.
     1 Fluids should be forced.
     2 Cipro should be started while results are pending.
     4 The two medications can be given together.

147. Application, implementation, physiological integrity (b).
     2 Check the apical pulse 1 full minute and hold medication if it is less than 60.
     1 The patient should be weighed every week.
     3 Pulse is more significant.
     4 Digitalis level, not clotting time, is monitored.

148. Comprehension, implementation, physiological integrity (a).
     3 Drug is irritating to the GI tract; taking the drug with meals decreases irritation.
     1 Taking the drug at bedtime can irritate the GI tract.
     2 Taking the drug before breakfast can irritate the GI tract.
     4 Taking the drug between meals can irritate the GI tract.

149. Comprehension, implementation, physiological integrity (b).
     3 This is an adverse reaction of antihypertensives.
     1 This is an adverse reaction of antifibrinolytics.
     2 This is a side effect.
     4 This is an expected action of diuretics.

150. Comprehension, implementation, physiological integrity (a).
     3 This can cause patient injury.
     1 This is not an action of atropine.
     2 Dilation of pupils does not cause vertigo.
     4 This medication decreases diaphoresis.

151. Knowledge, evaluation, physiological integrity (b).
     3 Epogen is indicated for treating low hemoglobin and hematocrit in anemia.
     1 This test would be used in the management of diabetes.

2 This test would manage the healthiness of the renal system.

4 An elevated WBC count would indicate the presence of infection; a depressed WBC count would indicate neutropenia.

152. Knowledge, planning, physiological integrity (b).

    4 Neupogen is indicated in treating neutropenia.

    1 Leukine is used to restore red bone marrow after transplants.

    2 Epogen is used to increase RBC count.

    3 Diflucan is used to treat fungal infections.

153. Knowledge, planning, physiological integrity (b).

    2 The absorption of fat-soluble vitamins may be reduced with a lubricant laxative.

    1, 4 Bulk laxatives do not interfere with the absorption of nutrients.

    3 This is a stool softener given primarily to avoid straining. It does not interfere with the absorption of nutrients.

154. Comprehension, assessment, physiological integrity (c).

    2 Atropine is a cholinergic blocking agent that increases pupil dilation.

    1 Demerol would be contraindicated for patients with head injury, seizures, asthma, and other similar conditions. It is not recommended for patients with glaucoma.

    3 See #1.

    4 This is used to reverse the effects of respiratory depression of opioid analgesia.

155. Application, planning, physiological integrity (c).

    2 Reglan is more likely to cause hypoglycemia because the food moves more rapidly through the GI tract.

    1 Reglan is synergistic with other CNS depressants.

    3 A side effect of Reglan is CNS depression.

    4 Administering it at this time will increase effectiveness because the food will be present to be acted on.

156. Knowledge, planning, physiological integrity (b).

    3 Antitussives act either centrally or locally to decrease the intensity of the cough.

    1 An expectorant decreases the thickness of secretions and stimulates productive cough.

    2 Decongestants decrease nasal secretions by causing vasoconstriction of the nasal mucosa.

    4 Used in treating symptoms associated with allergic rhinitis and colds.

157. Knowledge, planning, physiological integrity (b).

    1 This drug classified as a colony-stimulating agent useful in treating patients with bone marrow transplant.

    2 This medication stimulates the production of neutrophils.

    3 This medication stimulates the production of RBCs.

    4 This is a chemotherapy agent useful in treating certain kinds of cancers.

158. Knowledge, planning, physiological integrity (c).

    3 Ditropan is an antispasmodic agent useful in treating these symptoms, as well as neurogenic bladder.

    1 This is a diuretic used in treating edema.

    2 This is an antihypertensive medication.

    4 This is a potassium-sparing diuretic used in treating hypertension.

159. Application, implementation, physiological integrity (c).

    2 These medications are better absorbed on an empty stomach.

    1 These medications are better absorbed on an empty stomach.

    3 Patients should be instructed to drink at least 1.5 L of fluid to prevent nephrolithiasis.

    4 Vitamins should be taken; however, it does not affect the time of administration.

160. Comprehension, planning, physiological integrity (c).

    3 The aim of this therapy is to reduce the viral load as much as possible for as long as possible.

    1 The medication will have decreased effectiveness with an increased viral load.

    2 Other antiviral medications in combinations are often used as treatment.

    4 These medications are not effective at the end stage; resistant strains may have developed, as well as an increased viral load being present.

161. Application, evaluation, physiological integrity (b).

    2 Blood glucose should be tested before insulin is administered to prevent hypoglycemia.

    1 This is true; failing to rotate sites can cause tissue damage.

    3 Food is necessary to prevent hypoglycemia.

    4 This is the purpose of having a family member involved in the education.

162. Knowledge, planning, physiological integrity (b).

    1 This drug is used to decrease hydrochloric acid secretion in treating GERD.

    2 Amphojel is a nonsystemic antacid and normally only recommended for short-term use.

    3 This is used in treating flatulence.

    4 This is an oral hypoglycemic

163. Knowledge, planning, physiological integrity (b).

    2 This medication is used to treat fungal infections.

    1 This medication is used to treat herpes.

    3 This medication is used to treat peptic ulcer and GERD.

    4 This medication is useful to treat kidney transplants.

164. Knowledge, planning, physiological integrity (b).

    4 This is an antifungal medication typically prescribed for chemotherapy patient.

    1 This is an antacid.

    2 This is an antidepressant.

    3 This is an antibiotic.

165. Knowledge, planning, physiological integrity (a).

    2 Local medications are given to treat the area applied.

    1 These are absorbed and circulated in the body.

    3 A cumulated effect is when effects of the medication build up in the body.

    4 The effect of these substances given together is less than the effects of each given separately.

166. Comprehension, evaluation, physiological integrity (b).

    1 A therapeutic level must be achieved and maintained to combat infection. Additionally, a level should not be toxic.

    2 A therapeutic level shows adequacy and not toxicity.

    3 A therapeutic level needs to be reached as quickly as possible.

    4 A culture sensitivity would show whether a medication is effective against an organism.

167. Knowledge, planning, physiological integrity (a).
   3 This route goes directly into the circulation.
   1 This route has to go through the digestive system.
   2 This is faster than oral but only useful for a limited number of medications, primarily cardiac.
   4 This route is slower than IV and IM.

168. Comprehension, planning, physiological integrity (b).
   4 The hepatic, renal, and circulatory systems may be diminished leading to a longer half-life of the drug in the body.
   1 The patients may have developed a tolerance and may even require an increased dose.
   2 Cardiac disease is not an indication for decreased analgesia.
   3 Being underweight is not an indication for a decreased analgesic.

169. Comprehension, evaluation, physiological integrity (c).
   3 Patients develop a tolerance to all side effects except constipation.
   1 Excessive sedation does not develop when doses are gradually titrated.
   2 Pain relief is vital. The patient develops a tolerance to respiratory depression.
   4 This is true; however, it does not answer the question.

170. Application, evaluation, physiological integrity (b).
   3 Risk of addiction is minimal in patients who are taking medication to relieve pain and not for psychologic reasons.
   1 This is rare in hospitalized patients.
   2 Pain medication should be administered before the pain becomes severe to increase effectiveness.
   4 Tolerance is rare in severe acute or chronic pain.

171. Knowledge, planning, physiological integrity (a).
   3 These are characteristics of mild CNS depression.
   1 The effect on pulse and respirations would be opposite.
   2 This would be characteristic of moderate depression.
   4 This would be an effect of CNS stimulation.

172. Comprehension, application, physiological integrity (b).
   2 Bacteria can mutate and become resistant if the entire course of antibiotics is not taken.
   1 Adequate fluids can prevent the risk of dehydration present with some groups of antibiotics.
   3 Following proper administration directions (i.e., taking with a small snack).
   4 Certain antibiotics can be expensive; however, it is not the primary concern.

173. Comprehension, planning, physiological integrity (b).
   3 Elderly patients on long-term use of alkalizing agents are especially susceptible to electrolyte disorders.
   1 This test would be ordered for suspected bleeding disorders.
   2 This test would be ordered for suspected renal disease.
   4 This test is ordered if diabetes is suspected.

174. Application, planning, physiological integrity (b).
   2 It has a protective effect and is better able to work if it can come in contact with the lining of the stomach.
   1 Amphojel is not absorbed systemically.
   3 Aluminum preparations are more likely to cause constipation. The schedule of administration does not effect the occurrence of diarrhea.

4 Rebound acidity occurs with prolonged use and is not related to schedule of administration.

175. Comprehension, assessment, physiological integrity (b).
   1 Mylanta binds with ciprofloxacin and may decrease effectiveness.
   2, 3 Aspirin and Feosol are not known to interfere with absorption.
   4 Penicillin and tetracycline antibiotics have been shown to interfere with the effectiveness of birth control pills.

176. Application, implementation, physiological integrity (c).
   4 The cause of the diarrhea needs to be investigated if it persists beyond 2 days.
   1 Fluid intake needs to be increased to prevent dehydration.
   2 This medication needs to be taken at least 2 hours or after other medications as they will interfere with absorption.
   3 A fever is a sign that an infection may be present, and it needs to be reported. This medication also decreases absorption of salicylates.

177. Comprehension, implementation, physiological integrity (c).
   1 The action of Carafate is to line and protect the stomach; it is better able to do so if the medication can come in contact with the stomach.
   2 Patients on this medication are usually being treated for ulcers. They should avoid spicy foods; however, any food would interfere with the action of this medication.
   3 Constipation is the most common complication of this medication.
   4 Carafate interferes with the absorption and decreases the effectiveness of many medications.

178. Knowledge, implementation, physiological integrity (a).
   2 This is a topical sulfa-based agent commonly used in treating burns.
   1 This is used in treating acne.
   3 This is also used in treating acne.
   4 This is a keratolytic agent used to dissolve benign growth.

179. Application, implementation, physiological integrity (b).
   1 A side effect of this medication is sleeplessness.
   2 A side effect that should be reported is tachycardia.
   3. This is fine; however, it does not answer the question.
   4 Synthroid can be taken with other medications. It is antagonistic to digoxin and synergistic with oral anticoagulants.

180. Comprehension, implementation, physiological integrity (b).
   2 Prilosec is a proton pump inhibitor. It is more effective if it can come into contact with the gastric acid secreting cells of the stomach.
   1 Food decreases the effectiveness of this medication.
   3 It must be swallowed whole to be effective.
   4 Any liquid can be used.

181. Comprehension, planning, physiological integrity (a).
   2 Heparin is an anticoagulant; it is given to decrease the risk of thrombosis.
   1 This risk of blood loss is actually increased slightly.
   3 Epogen is given to improve RBC production.
   4 Heparin is not antibiotic.

182. Knowledge, planning, physiological integrity (b).

3 This is an anticholergenic medication that would help reverse the effects of cholinergic drugs.

1 This is a cholinergic agent used in treating urinary retention.

2 This is a cholinergic agent useful in treating gastroparesis.

4 This is a cholinergic agent used to help diagnose myasthenia gravis.

183. Comprehension, planning, physiological integrity (b).

3 It is critical that patients on coumadin report any signs of bleeding, including any blood observed in excreta.

1 Coumadin is usually taken orally, not subcutaneously.

2 This should be routine in every patient teaching situation.

4 Blood levels are checked more frequently than every 3 months, especially during the initiation phase of treatment.

184. Knowledge, planning, physiological integrity (a).

1 Protamine sulfate binds with heparin and keeps it from working.

2, 4 These are mineral elements.

3 Vitamin K is an antidote for Coumadin.

185. Application, planning, physiological integrity (c).

1 This is true; however, topical nitroglycerin is used preventatively, and its absorption is unpredictable.

2 This is the proper method for sublingual nitroglycerin.

3 This is true; however, if it pain persists after three tablets, the person should report to the physician.

4 This is true; however, this method is not used in acute attacks.

186. Application, planning, physiological integrity (b).

3 To achieve therapeutic relief as quickly as possible, patients are given a loading dose. A maintenance dose is given to maintain the therapeutic stage.

1 Patients need relief and cannot wait to be brought into the therapeutic range.

2 Lasix will help decrease edema in the body.

4 All patients need to be monitored for sign toxicity.

187. Knowledge, planning, physiological integrity (b).

4 This medication is well tolerated and is generally considered the first line of treatment in panic-anxiety disorders and mild-to-moderate depression.

1 This is an MAOI usually used in treating severe depression in patients who have failed to respond to other treatments.

2 This is an antipsychotic agent used in treating manic-depression and hallucination.

3 This is an antipsychotic agent used in treating psychotic disorders and severe depression.

188. Knowledge, evaluation, physiological integrity (b).

1 This medication is prescribed to lower cholesterol levels in the body.

2 Liver function tests should be ordered at periodic intervals to check for adverse reactions.

3 Cardiac enzymes should be checked for any myocardial damage.

4 CPK (calcium, phosphorus, potassium) levels should be monitored carefully to detect any muscle tumors.

189. Knowledge, implementation, physiological integrity (b).

4 Lipitor is more effective if given at night because the body produces the majority of cholesterol during this time.

1 Giving these medications in the morning is not as effective.

2, 3 These medications may be given without regard to food unless other types cholesterol-lowering drugs are begin given as well.

190. Knowledge, planning, physiological integrity (b).

1 Hydantoins used to treat seizures are associated with these side effects.

2 Barbiturates are not associated with these side effect.

3, 4 These drugs are not associated with these side effects.

191. Knowledge, planning, physiological integrity (c).

4 Elderly patients commonly experience these side effects on barbiturates.

1 Barbiturates cause decreased BP, not increased BP.

2 These are typical side effects with hydantoins, not barbiturates.

3 Muscle pain and diuresis are not side effects of this medication; occasional blood dyscrasias may be seen, but they are rare.

192. Comprehension, evaluation, physiological integrity (c).

3 Vioxx is taken once a day to decrease prostaglandin synthesis.

1 Vioxx can be taken without regard to meals.

2 Vioxx is taken preventatively to maintain level not prn.

4 Nausea is a possible side effect; food may decrease effectiveness.

193 Comprehension, implementation, physiological integrity (b).

2 This medication should not be abruptly discontinued to protect against possible seizures after the surgery.

1 These tests are done on a regular basis during therapy, not just at this point in time.

3 This is an ongoing direction until the effect of the medication can be judged.

4. This is an ongoing direction.

194. Application, implementation, physiological integrity (b).

3 Teach patient the importance of complying with therapy; effectiveness may take a few weeks.

1 This is true; however, it does not answer the patient's concerns.

2 This is not indicated at this point.

4 This is fine; however, it does not answer the concern of the patient.

195. Knowledge, planning, physiological integrity (b).

2 This is a topical fungal agent.

1 This is a topical antihistamine used for itching.

3 This is a topical antibiotic used in treating burn.

4 This is a topical steroid used for itching.

196. Comprehension, planning, physiological integrity (b).

1 Steroids cause hyperglycemia as an adverse effect.

2, 4 These are oral hypoglycemics.

3 This is a cardiac medication that does not cause hyperglycemia.

197. Comprehension, planning, physiological integrity (b).

2 This is an oral hypoglycemic that is more effective when given at this time.

1 This is a cardiac medication that does not need to be given before breakfast.

3 This does not need to be given with food.

4 This should be given at bedtime to increase effectiveness.

198. Knowledge, assessment, physiological integrity (b).
4 Men treated with this medication have experienced an increase in urinary flow.
1 This disorder would be treated with an antacid, an H2 blocker, or a proton pump inhibitor.
2 This would be treated with digoxin and Lasix.
3 This medication would be contraindicated for a patient with glaucoma.

199. Knowledge, assessment, physiological integrity (c).
3 The food may pass through the intestine too quickly, causing hypoglycemia.
1, 2, 4 These are not side effects.

200. Comprehension, implementation, physiological integrity (b).
3 This time would minimize impact on nutrition and growth and development.
1 Increased activity is not desirable at bedtime.
2 The appetite in growing child should not be suppressed.
4 The appetite before breakfast should not be suppressed.

201. Assessment, planning, physiological integrity (b).
1 Pyridium is a urinary tract analgesic that is prescribed for these symptoms.
2 This is a diuretic.
3 This is used to treat diarrhea.
4 This is an antibiotic used to treat urinary tract infection.

202. Comprehension, planning, physiological integrity (b).
1 This may be indicative of liver damage.
2 Restlessness is not an expected side effect.
3 Tachycardia is a more likely side effect.
4 Fatigue is an expected side effect.

203. Knowledge, assessment, physiological integrity (b).
3 These are the correct terms for the processes that all medications go through in the body.
1 Oral medications need to be digested as part of absorption; other routes do not require digestion. Catabolism means breaking down from complex to simple.
2 These are not the correct terms.
4 Anabolism means building up from simple to complex.

204. Comprehension, implementation, physiological integrity (b).
2 Weight and vital signs must be determined to establish a baseline to determine effectiveness of therapy.
1 For long-term therapy, potassium levels should be monitored.
3 This is a side effect of long-term therapy and should be reported.
4 These assessment should be done on all patients on a routine basis.

205. Application, implementation, physiological integrity (c).
2 Patients should limit intake of dairy products because of their high calcium content.
1 Fluids help these medications to be excreted effectively.
3 This medication is more effective if taken without other medications.
4 Laboratory work needs to be checked to make sure the medication is therapeutic.

206. Assessment, evaluation, physiological integrity (b).
1 Commonly associated with ACE inhibitors resulting from increased sensitivity of cough reflex.
2 Hypotension is therapeutic effect.
3 Diarrhea, nausea, and vomiting are common side effects.
4 Not a documented side effect.

207. Comprehension, planning, physiological integrity (a).
3 This medication is more effective if given by itself.
1 This medication is less effective if given with food.
2 See #3.
4 This would be appropriate for analgesics.

208. Knowledge, evaluation, physiological integrity (a).
1 This is one of the earliest signs of toxicity.
2 Aspirin is given to relieve headaches.
3, 4 These are not signs of toxicity.

209. Knowledge, planning, physiological integrity (a).
1 This is an oral hypoglycemic agent used in treating type 2 diabetes.
2 This is emergency and immediate acting insulin. Insulin may sometimes be used to treat type 2 diabetes, however, not generally as a first-line treatment.
3 This is used in treating hypothyroidism.
4 This is used in treating inflammation. It may actually cause steroid-induced hyperglycemia.

210. Knowledge, evaluation, physiological integrity (b).
1 This test measures the long-term levels of glucose in the blood.
2 This would indicate the presence of an infection.
3 This would be an indication of kidney function.
4 Potassium is an electrolyte.

211. Knowledge, planning, physiological integrity (b).
3 This is an antibiotic commonly prescribed for acne vulgaris.
1 This is an antibiotic used for life-threatening infections.
2 This is a cholesterol-lowering agent.
4 This antibiotic is commonly used for genitourinary infections, as well as other things.

212. Comprehensive, planning, physiological integrity (b).
2 This product is partially made from pork.
1, 3, 4 These diets are not contraindicated.

213. Comprehension, planning, physiological integrity (b).
1 This would be the medication prescribed for a 16-year-old girl.
2 Garamycin is prescribed for serious gram-negative infections.
3 Kantrex is prescribed for serious gram-negative infections.
4 This medication is contraindicated for people under 18 years of age.

214. Knowledge, assessment, physiological integrity (b).
2 This may be indication of a super infection.
1, 3, 4 These are common side effects of many antibiotics.

215. Knowledge, planning, physiological integrity (b).
2 This classification blocks the effects of the parasympathetic system and are used to dilate the pupil for examination.
1 Cholinergic agents are used to treat certain kinds of glaucoma and to decrease intraocular pressure.
3 These are used to remove cerumen from the ear.
4 Used for short-term treatment of ocular congestion.

216. Comprehension, implementation, physiological integrity (b).
3 He may be afraid of addiction or respiratory depression.
1 This is not sufficient; a patient needs relief for a successful recovery.
2 This should have been done before offering medication.
4 This is appropriate but not before completing #3.

217. Knowledge, planning, physiological integrity (a).
    2 This is an antifungal agent.
    1 Topical antibiotics would be prescribed for acne.
    3 Topical antihistamines would be prescribed for itching.
    4 A boil normally has to be incised and drained.

218. Knowledge, implementation, physiological integrity (b).
    3 This is considered the largest muscle in a child.
    1 Because of potential danger to the sciatic nerve, this is not a viable option for young children.
    2, 4 These muscles are too small in young children.

219. Knowledge, planning, physiological integrity (a).
    2 This act was passed in 1983.
    1, 3, 4 These laws are fictitious.

220. Comprehension, implementation, physiological integrity (b).
    4 This is an effective route that bypasses the upper GI tract.
    1 The medication may not be retained and may further increase nausea and vomiting.
    2 This route is available only for a limited number of medications, primarily cardiac.
    3 This route would not bypass upper GI tract.

221. Comprehension, evaluation, physiological integrity (b).
    2 This is an antihistamine used to treat symptoms of allergic rhinitis.
    1 This may be a side effect, but it is not the reason the drug is given.
    3, 4 These are not reasons the drug is given.

222. Knowledge, planning, physiological integrity (b).
    2 A majority of medications are excreted by the kidneys; impairment may lead to cumulative effects.
    1 Diabetes may be a contraindication for many medication, but it generally does not interfere with movement of drugs systemically.
    3, 4 These do not interfere with the pharmacokinetics of medications.

223. Comprehension, implementation, physiological integrity (b).
    3 This is true and is the least anxiety-producing effect for the patient.
    1 This denies the patient's feelings and closes communication.
    2 This is true; however, it does not answer the question.
    4 This is a given; however, it does not answer the question.

224. Comprehensiveness, evaluation, physiological integrity (b).
    2 This medication is given to increase neutrophils.
    1, 3, 4 These levels would not indicate the effectiveness of neutrophils.

225. Knowledge, implementation, physiological integrity (a).
    3 This is the most common angle for normal and overweight individuals.
    1 This is for a subcutaneous injection.
    2 This angle is not correct.
    4 This would be appropriate for an intradermal injection.

CHAPTER 4 Nutrition

Nutrition is the combination of processes by which the body uses food for growth, energy, and maintenance. Nutrition is also the study of food and its relationship to health and disease. Increasing emphasis is being placed on the role of balanced nutrition in preventing many chronic illnesses. The body works to maintain balance in its chemical processes through homeostasis. The nurse plays an especially important role in the nutritional aspects of patient care. Because of close and continual contact with the patient, the nurse is able to evaluate and monitor the patient's nutritional status and inform the dietician or appropriate dietary person about the patient's nutritional needs and acceptance of the nutritional plan of care. Good nutrition is essential to good health throughout the life cycle, and the nurse is in an excellent position to encourage sound nutritional practice for each patient and the patient's family.

HEALTH PROMOTION

A. Goal: to increase the level of health of individuals, families, groups, and communities, which requires a lifestyle change that will lead to new positive health behaviors
B. In 1990 the U.S. Department of Health and Human Services issued a national report, *Healthy People 2000,* that outlines national health promotion and disease prevention objectives for Americans to be achieved by the year 2000. Nutrition is the key to these goals. This study was updated and is now available as *Healthy People 2010.*

PRINCIPLES OF NUTRITION

A. Functions of food
   1. Provides energy
   2. Builds and repairs body tissues
   3. Regulates and controls the body's chemical processes, which are essential for providing energy and building tissues
B. Evidence of good nutrition (Table 4-1); people who receive less than desired amounts of nutrients have a greater risk of physical illness, are limited in physical work and mental capacity, and have lower immune system function than do people receiving adequate nutrients.
C. Primary causes of nutritional deficiency
   1. Dietary lack of specific essential nutrients caused by:
      a. Anorexia (resulting from a variety of causes)
      b. Alcoholism (and the resulting lack of proper nutrition)
      c. Poor food habits or eating nutritionally deficient foods
      d. Anorexia nervosa/bulimia
   2. Inability of the body to use a specific nutrient properly as a result of:
      a. Diseases of the digestive tract, such as ulcerative colitis
      b. Faulty absorption in digestive tract: malabsorption

syndrome or excessive use of mineral oil
      c. Metabolic disorders, such as diabetes
      d. Drug interactions or toxicity or both
D. Classification of nutrients
   1. Nutrients are chemical substances that are present in food and needed by the body to function
   2. Six prime nutrients
      a. Carbohydrates
      b. Fats
      c. Proteins
      d. Vitamins
      e. Minerals
      f. Water
   3. Individual nutrients have many specific metabolic functions. No nutrient ever works alone. In addition, the lack of one nutrient may inhibit the absorption or utilization of another nutrient.
E. Culture and nutrition
   1. Food habits are among the oldest and most deeply rooted aspects of many cultures. They are established early in childhood and can be difficult to change.
   2. In many cultures, foods take on significance in life events, including serious illness.
   3. If possible, cultural preferences should be considered when planning any dietary modifications.
   4. In many instances a religion will greatly influence nutritional practice (Table 4-2).

Assimilation of Nutrients
Digestion and Absorption

A. Digestion: the process of changing foods to be absorbed and used by cells; mechanical digestion and chemical digestion occur simultaneously.
   1. Mechanical digestion (chewing, swallowing, peristalsis) breaks food into small pieces, mixes it with digestive juices, and moves it along the digestive tract.
   2. Chemical digestion occurs through the action of enzymes, which break large food molecules into smaller molecules.
      a. Carbohydrate digestion begins in the mouth and occurs primarily in the small intestine; carbohydrates are reduced to simple sugars (monosaccharides), such as glucose, for absorption. Sorbitol, a naturally occurring sugar that is not absorbed, may cause diarrhea in children.
      b. Protein digestion begins in the stomach and is completed in the small intestine; proteins are broken down into amino acids for absorption.
      c. Fat digestion begins in the stomach but occurs primarily in the small intestine; fats are reduced to fatty acids and glycerol for absorption.
B. Absorption: the process by which end products of digestion (fatty acids, glycerol, amino acids, and glucose) are absorbed from the small intestine into circulation (blood and lymph)

TABLE 4-1	Clinical Signs of Nutritional Status	
Features	Good	Poor
General appearance	Alert, responsive	Listless, apathetic; cachexic
Hair	Shiny, lustrous; healthy scalp	Stringy, dull, brittle, dry, depigmented
Neck glands	No enlargement	Thyroid enlarged
Skin, face, and neck	Smooth, slightly moist, good color, reddish-pink mucous membranes	Greasy, discolored, scaly
Eyes	Bright, clear; no fatigue circles	Dryness, signs of infection, increased vascularity, glassiness, thickened conjunctivae
Lips	Good color, moist	Dry, scaly, swollen, angular lesions (stomatitis)
Tongue	Good pink color; surface papillae present; no lesions	Papillary atrophy, smooth appearance; swollen, red, beefy (glossitis)
Gums	Good pink color; no swelling or bleeding; firm	Marginal redness or swelling; receding, spongy
Teeth	Straight, no crowding; well-shaped jaw; clean, no discoloration	Unfilled cavities, absent teeth, worn surfaces; mottled, malpositioned
Skin, general	Smooth, slightly moist; good color; good turgor	Rough, dry, scaly, pale, pigmented, irritated; petechiae, bruises
Abdomen	Flat	Swollen
Legs, feet	No tenderness, weakness, swelling; good color	Edema, tender calf; tingling, weakness
Skeleton	No malformations	Bowlegs, knock-knees, chest deformity at diaphragm, beaded ribs, prominent scapulae
Weight	Normal for height, age, body build	Overweight or underweight
Posture	Erect, arms and legs straight, abdomen in, chest out	Sagging shoulders, sunken chest, humped back
Muscles	Well developed, firm	Flaccid, poor tone; undeveloped, tender
Nervous control	Good attention span for age; does not cry easily; not irritable or restless	Inattentive, irritable
GI function	Good appetite and digestion; normal, regular elimination	Anorexia, indigestion, constipation or diarrhea
General vitality	Endurance; energetic; sleeps well at night; vigorous	Easily fatigued; no energy; falls asleep in school; looks tired, apathetic

From Williams SR: *Essentials of nutrition and diet therapy,* ed 8, St Louis, 2003, Mosby.

TABLE 4-2	Effects of Culture and Religion on Nutrition
Group	Common Dietary Practices
Cultural	
African Americans	Foods associated with the Southern United States; milk and dairy foods may be lacking in the diet resulting from lactose intolerance prevalent in the group
Mexican Americans	Liberally season food; many corn products used
Chinese Americans	Include staples of rice, wheat, and soy
Japanese Americans	Include rice, wheat, and seafood
Korean Americans	Include rice, wheat, highly seasoned foods such as cabbage
Italian Americans	Include pasta, breads, sauces, and cheese
Greek Americans	Include lamb, goat milk products, and cheese products
Religious	
Jewish—orthodox	No pork products; meat must be slaughtered and prepared according to ritual; no mixing of meat and milk; only fish with fins and scales are to be eaten.
Moslem	Pork and alcohol are strictly prohibited; a month-long period of daylight fasting is observed during Ramadan; children, pregnant women, and ill individuals are exempt from the fasting period.
Hindu	Primarily vegetarians; beef is not eaten.
Roman Catholic	Restrictions on eating meat on Fridays (voluntary); special observance from Ash Wednesday through Easter voluntarily observed by some members of group.

to be distributed to the cells. Vitamins may require proper pH to be absorbed. Patients with achlorhydria may develop vitamin-B_{12} deficiency. Certain foods or beverages, such as grapefruit juice, can alter the metabolism or absorption of medications.

Metabolism

A. Use of food by the body cells for producing energy and for building complex chemical compounds
B. Consists of two processes
   1. Catabolism: the breakdown of food molecules into carbon dioxide and water, which releases energy; carbohydrates are primarily catabolized for energy.
   2. Anabolism: the process by which food molecules are built up into more complex chemical compounds; proteins are primarily anabolized (used for building)

Energy

A. Energy is required for the metabolic processes of catabolism and anabolism; energy needs of the body are based on three factors.
   1. Physical activity: the type of activity and how long it is performed
   2. Basal metabolism: the energy required for the body to sustain life while in a resting state (1 calorie per kilogram of body weight per hour)
   3. Thermal effects of food: energy required for the digestion, absorption, and metabolism of foods
B. Measurement of energy
   1. The calorie (or kilocalorie) is the unit used to measure the energy value of food.
   2. Fuel values of basic nutrients
      a. Carbohydrate: 4 calories per gram
      b. Fat: 9 calories per gram
      c. Protein: 4 calories per gram
   3. Total number of calories needed per day
      a. Moderately active man: 20.5 calories per pound (0.45 kg) of ideal weight
      b. Moderately active woman: 18 calories per pound (0.45 kg) of ideal weight

Drugs and Nutrition

A. Drugs affect taste, appetite, intestinal motility, absorption, metabolism, and excretion of nutrients, as well as causing nausea and vomiting. Many of these interactions may compromise nutritional status and health.
B. If a nutrient binds with a medication, decreased solubility of both the nutrient and drug can result. Interactions between certain foods and certain medications may alter the amount of drug that is available to the body. Foods or beverages containing alcohol can trigger a reaction in a patient taking disulfiram (Antabuse).
C. People at greatest risk of undesirable drug-nutrient interaction are those taking medication for long periods, those taking two or more medications, and those not eating well. Elderly people fall into the high-risk category.
D. Certain medications may cause weight gain through retained fluid or increased appetite.

Nutrients
Carbohydrates

A. Classification
   1. Monosaccharides: single sugars, which require no digestion and are easily absorbed into the bloodstream (e.g., glucose, fructose, galactose)
   2. Disaccharides: double sugars, which must be broken down before absorption (e.g., sucrose [table sugar], lactose, maltose)
   3. Polysaccharides: complex carbohydrates composed of many sugar units (e.g., starches, glycogen, dietary fiber)
B. Functions
   1. Provide energy (glucose is the only form of energy that can be used by the central nervous system [CNS])
   2. Protein-sparing effect allows protein to be used for tissue building rather than energy production.
   3. Essential for complete metabolism of fats (incomplete fat metabolism leads to buildup of ketones and acidosis)
C. Sources
   1. Polysaccharides (complex carbohydrates): bread, cereal, pasta, rice, corn, baked goods
   2. Disaccharides (double sugars): table sugar, sugar cane, molasses
   3. Monosaccharides (simple carbohydrates): fruit, honey, milk
D. Digestion and metabolism
   1. Carbohydrate digestion occurs primarily in the small intestine and is acted on by three enzymes: sucrase, lactase, and maltase. Gas in the intestinal tract is largely a result of incomplete digestion of carbohydrates.
   2. Carbohydrates must be broken down into monosaccharides before being absorbed.
   3. Monosaccharides are carried to the liver, where glucose is released to the cells.
   4. Excess glucose is stored as glycogen to be used when needed or converted to fat and stored as fat tissue.
   5. Insulin regulates the use of glucose for use by the cells, thereby lowering blood sugar.
   6. The hormone glucagon regulates the conversion of glycogen back to glucose, causing an increase in blood glucose.
   7. The speed with which food raises the blood glucose is the glycemic index.
   8. Hypoglycemia in people who do not have diabetes can be managed with small feedings approximately every 3 hours, from a diet that is low in sugar and high in fiber.
E. Excess carbohydrates in diet may lead to:
   1. Obesity
   2. Tooth decay and gum disease
   3. Malnutrition (if empty-calorie foods such as candy and soft drinks are consumed extensively)
F. Dietary considerations
   1. Approximately 50% to 60% of total caloric intake may come from carbohydrates (mainly starches).
   2. Encourage the intake of whole grain bread and cereal products; if refined cereal products are used, they should be enriched.
   3. Reduce the dietary intake of simple sugars (which provide empty calories) and substitute starches as sources of carbohydrates.
G. Dietary fiber
   1. Definition: the total amount of naturally occurring material in foods, mostly plants, that is not digested by the human digestive system and therefore is not absorbed. Adequate amounts are needed to facilitate proper bowel movements and to reduce serum cholesterol and blood glucose levels, as well as the risk of cancer.

2. Two categories of dietary fiber: soluble and insoluble, based on the solubility in water

Protein

A. Composed of amino acids
1. Essential amino acids: amino acids that the body cannot manufacture and therefore must be supplied in the diet; there are eight essential amino acids.
2. Nonessential amino acids: amino acids that the body can manufacture and therefore are not as important in the diet
B. Functions
1. Build and repair body tissue (primary function)
2. Furnish energy if carbohydrate or fat is insufficient for this purpose
3. Maintain normal circulation of tissue and blood vessel fluids through the action of plasma protein
4. Aid metabolic functions by combining with iron to form hemoglobin; used to manufacture enzymes and hormones
5. Aid body defenses by manufacturing lymphocytes and antibodies
C. Digestion and metabolism
1. Digestion of protein begins in the stomach, where it is acted on by the enzyme pepsin. Digestion is completed in the small intestine by three enzymes: trypsin, chymotrypsin, and carboxypeptidase.
2. Protein must be broken down into amino acids to be absorbed and distributed to the cells. Accumulation of uric acid, a byproduct of purine catabolism, can cause gout. High intake of animal protein associated with kidney stones.
3. End products of protein metabolism are hydrogen, oxygen, nitrogen, water, uric acid, and urea.
4. Dietary deficiencies of B-complex vitamins may cause elevated levels of homocystine, an amino acid product linked to vascular disease in coronary and renal blood vessels.
D. Types and sources
1. Complete proteins: foods that contain all eight essential amino acids in amounts capable of meeting human requirements (e.g., mainly animal sources, such as meats, fish, poultry, eggs, milk, and cheese)
2. Incomplete proteins: foods that lack one or more of the essential amino acids (e.g., mainly plant sources, such as cereal grains, nuts, legumes, and lentils)
3. Complementary proteins: foods that, when eaten together, supply the amino acid that is missing or in short supply in the other food (e.g., peanut butter with bread, beans with rice, baked beans with brown bread); a rule of thumb is that a grain and a legume eaten together supply all the essential amino acids.
E. Dietary considerations
1. The recommended daily protein intake for adults is 0.8 g/kg of body weight (15% of total caloric intake).
2. Dietary proteins are not stored in the body as amino acids. Proteins are the main components needed to build and repair body tissues. If the right amount and the right kinds are not available, the nitrogen is broken off, and the remainder of the protein is used for energy or stored as fat. The need for cell building and maintenance is continuous. For a supply of proteins to be available on a regular basis, a source of complete proteins should be eaten at every meal.

3. Increased protein is necessary during periods of growth, illness, injury, or stress; after surgery; and when bed rest is prescribed (especially for older adults). Protein supplements such as creatine may not enhance growth or endurance, despite marketers' claims.
4. Kwashiorkor, a protein-deficiency disease, is seen in many underdeveloped countries.
5. Marasmus is overt starvation caused by a deficiency of calories from any source.
6. Leptin and other hormones secreted by the adipose tissue will act on the brain to control appetite.

Fats (Lipids)

A. Functions
1. Supply energy for body activities when carbohydrates are not available; all body tissues except brain and nervous cells can use fat for energy; most concentrated form of energy yields 9 calories per gram.
2. Act as insulation to maintain body temperature and protect organs from mechanical injury
3. Carry fat-soluble vitamins A, D, E, and K and aid in their absorption
4. Provide a feeling of fullness and satisfaction after eating because of their slow rate of digestion
5. Furnish the essential fatty acid, linoleic acid, which is found primarily in vegetable oils; called essential because it cannot be synthesized in the body and is vital to body functioning
6. Omega-3 fatty acids, (polyunsaturated fat) which are found in fatty fish, may contribute to lower risks of heart disease.
B. Types
1. Saturated fats: the structure is completely filled with all the hydrogen it can hold; they are usually from animal sources and are usually solid at room temperature (e.g., fats in meat, dairy products, eggs; coconut oil, palm oil, and chocolate are also highly saturated). Trans fatty acids (TFAs) tend to raise low-density lipoprotein (LDL) ("bad") cholesterol and lower high-density lipoprotein (HDL) ("good") cholesterol when used instead of cis fatty acids or natural oils.
2. Unsaturated fats: the chemical structure has one or more places where hydrogen can be added; they are less dense, usually liquid at room temperature (with the exception of margarine), and are chiefly from plant sources (e.g., vegetable oils such as cottonseed, soybean, corn oil).
   a. Monounsaturated fats have one place for hydrogen to be added.
   b. Polyunsaturated fats have two or more places for hydrogen to be added.
   c. Hydrogenation: the process of adding hydrogen to a liquid or polyunsaturated fat and changing it to a solid or semisolid state (however, hydrogenation reduces the polyunsaturated fat content and therefore possibly reduces its health value)
   d. Triglycerides are fats eaten in foods or made in the body from other sources such as carbohydrates. Excess calories consumed in a meal are converted and transported to fat cells for storage.
C. Digestion and metabolism
1. Digestion of fat begins in the stomach, where gastric lipase acts on emulsified fats.
2. Major portions of fat digestion occur in the small intestine,

where bile emulsifies fats (breaks it into small droplets); pancreatic lipase changes the emulsified fats into fatty acids and glycerol, the end products of fat digestion.

3. Fats are carried as lipoproteins to body cells, where they are either broken down for use as energy or stored as adipose tissue.

D. Sources
1. Visible fats: those readily seen (e.g., butter and margarine, salad oils, shortening, fat in meats)
2. Invisible fats: those in which the fat is less obvious (e.g., milk, avocado, cheese, lean meat)

E. Cholesterol: a complex fat-related compound
1. A normal component of blood and of all body cells, especially brain and nerve tissue
2. Necessary for normal body functioning as structural material in cells, in the production of vitamin D, and in the production of a large number of hormones
3. Supplied by food (mainly animal sources); some are synthesized within the body, mainly in the intestinal walls and liver, in response to need. Excess calories consumed are converted into triglycerides for storage as fat.
4. A variety of factors, including diet, heredity, emotional stress, and exercise, affect blood cholesterol levels; saturated fats tend to raise blood cholesterol, whereas polyunsaturated fats are recommended for lowering cholesterol levels.
5. Cholesterol is carried to and from body cells by special carriers called lipoproteins.
   a. HDL, or "good" cholesterol, carries cholesterol away from the arteries and back to the liver for removal from the body.
   b. LDL, or "bad" cholesterol, tends to circulate in the bloodstream and form plaque on the inner walls of arteries.
6. Risk is classified according to total cholesterol level as follows:
   a. Desirable: below 200 mg/dl
   b. Borderline high: 200 to 239 mg/dl

c. High: above 240 mg/dl
7. If the total cholesterol (TC) level is borderline high or high, then the levels and ratio of LDL and HDL should be evaluated.
8. High cholesterol levels predispose individuals to atherosclerosis, the underlying pathological factor of coronary heart disease, and other serious health problems
9. Foods high in cholesterol: organ meats, animal fat, egg yolk, and shellfish

F. Dietary considerations
1. The Dietary Guidelines for America 1995 recommends that daily intake of fats for adults should not be more than 30% of the total caloric intake; no more than 10% of the intake should be from saturated fat.
2. To decrease dietary fat:
   a. Use leaner cuts of meat and more poultry; trim fats from all meats.
   b. Use egg substitute products or fewer eggs.
   c. Use low-fat milk products.
   d. Limit use of fat in cooking as much as possible.
   e. Decrease frequency of red meat use.

G. Effects of excess fat intake
1. Obesity
2. Consumption may predispose an individual to serious conditions, such as heart disease, diabetes, and stroke.
3. Increased surgical risk

Vitamins

See Table 4-3.
A. Definitions
1. Vitamins: organic compounds needed in small amounts for growth and maintenance of life
2. Precursor (or provitamin): substances that precede and can be changed into active vitamins (e.g., carotene is the precursor of vitamin A.)
3. Hypervitaminosis: the excess of one or more vitamins

TABLE 4-3	Vitamins		
Vitamin	Sources	Functions	Deficiency Symptoms
Fat-Soluble Vitamins			
A (retinol) Precursor: carotene	Fish liver oils Liver Green, leafy vegetables Yellow vegetables (corn, carrots, and sweet potatoes) Yellow fruits (apricots and peaches) Egg yolk Whole milk	Regenerates visual purple (necessary for good vision) Formation of bones and teeth Maintains skin and mucous membranes	Night blindness Retardation of skeletal growth Dry, scaly skin Dry mucous membranes Susceptibility to epithelial infection Xerophthalmia (corneal cells become opaque, slough off, can lead to blindness)
D (calciferol)	Sunshine Fish liver oils Fortified milk	Regulates calcium and phosphorus absorption and metabolism Essential for normal formation of bones and teeth	Lowered levels of calcium and phosphorus in blood Soft bones Rickets Malformed teeth

Continued

TABLE 4-3   Vitamins—cont'd

Vitamin	Sources	Functions	Deficiency Symptoms
E (tocopherol)	Wheat germ Vegetable oils Dark-green, leafy vegetables	Inconclusive at present Preserves integrity of RBCs Antioxidant (protects materials that oxidize easily) Protects structure and function of muscle	Increased hemolysis (breakdown) of RBCs Anemia Breakdown of vitamin A and essential fatty acids
K (menadione) AquaMEPHYTON	Synthesis by intestinal bacteria Green, leafy vegetables Pork liver	Formation of prothrombin (necessary in blood clotting)	Prolonged clotting time (bleeding tendencies) Hemorrhagic diseases
Water-Soluble Vitamins			
C (ascorbic acid)	Citrus fruits Tomatoes Broccoli Strawberries Green peppers Cantaloupes Potatoes	Formation and maintenance of capillary walls and collagen formation Aids in absorption of iron	Scurvy (deficiency disease) Sore gums Tendency to bruise easily Poor wound healing Anemia
B_1 (thiamine)	Wheat germ Whole or enriched grains Legumes Pork and organ meats	Maintains carbohydrate metabolism Maintains muscle and nerve functioning	Beriberi (deficiency disease) Anorexia, fatigue, nerve disorders, irritability
B_2 (riboflavin)	Milk Organ meats Green, leafy vegetables Enriched bread and cereals	Maintains appetite Maintains healthy eyes Maintains color and structure of lips Metabolism of nutrients	Sensitivity to light, dim vision Inflammation of lips and tongue, cheilosis Loss of appetite and weight
B_6 (pyridoxine)	Red meats (especially organ meats) Whole-grain cereals Pork, lamb, veal	Synthesis and metabolism of proteins Hemoglobin synthesis Maintenance of muscles and nerves	Nausea, vomiting, anorexia, anemia, irritability, CNS dysfunction, kidney stones, dermatitis INH can cause deficiency
B_{12} (cobalamin)	Found only in animal products Organ and muscle meats Dairy products	Protein metabolism Production of RBCs Nervous system function	Pernicious anemia (resulting from lack of intrinsic factor needed for vitamin-B_{12} absorption)
Niacin (nicotinic acid) Precursor: tryptophan	Meats (especially organ meats) Poultry and fish Peanut butter	Essential for normal functioning of digestive and nervous systems Essential for growth and metabolism	Pellagra (deficiency disease) Nervous disorders Diarrhea and nausea Dermatitis
Folic acid (folacin)		Essential in formation of all body cells, especially RBCs Protein metabolism	Anemia (macrocytic) Gastrointestinal disturbances Glossitis Stomatitis

RBC, red blood cell; *CNS*, central nervous system; *INH*, isonicotinic acid hydrazide.

4. Synthetic: man-made vitamins
5. Enriched: the addition of nutrients to a food often in amounts larger than might be found naturally in that food
6. Fortified: the replacement in food of nutrients lost during processing

B. Characteristics
1. Contain no calories
2. Essential to life because they generally cannot be synthesized by the body and are necessary for cell metabolism
3. Functions include tissue building and regulation of body functions.
4. Needed in minute amounts (milligrams [mg] or micrograms [µg]); the safety of taking megadoses is debatable.
5. Well-balanced diet should provide adequate vitamins to fulfill body requirements.

TABLE 4-4   Major Minerals and Microminerals (Trace Elements)

Mineral	Sources	Functions	Deficiency Symptoms
Major Minerals			
Calcium (Ca): absorption aided by vitamin D	Milk and milk products Cheese Some green, leafy vegetables (turnips, collards, kale, broccoli)	Bone and tooth formation Blood clotting Muscle (including heart muscle) contraction Nerve transmission Cell wall permeability	Poor bone and tooth formation Rickets (deficiency disease) Stunted growth Osteoporosis Poor blood clotting Tetany
Phosphorus (P): absorption with Ca aided by vitamin D	Milk and cheese Meat Egg yolk Whole grains (Diet adequate in protein and Ca should be adequate in P)	Functions as calcium phosphate in the calcification of bones and teeth Energy metabolism Regulation of acid-base balance Cell structure and enzyme activity	Poor bone and tooth formation Rickets (deficiency disease) Retarded growth Weakness Anorexia
Sodium (Na)	Salt Baking powder and soda Dairy products Meat, fish, and poultry Range of 500 to 2400 mg daily	Regulation of acid-base balance Fluid balance Nerve transmission and muscle contraction Glucose absorption	Nausea and vomiting Apathy Exhaustion Abdominal and muscle cramps
Potassium (K)	Meat, fish, and poultry Whole grain breads and cereals Fruits (oranges, bananas) Green and leafy vegetables	Regulates nerve conduction and muscle contraction Necessary for regular heart rhythm Fluid and acid-base balance Cell metabolism	Abnormal heartbeat Muscle weakness Nausea and vomiting Deficiency results from diuresis
Chlorine (Cl)	Table salt (NaCl)	Formation of hydrochloric acid and maintenance of gastric acidity Maintenance of acid-base balance, osmotic pressure, and water balance	Deficiency results from fluid loss through vomiting, diarrhea, and heavy sweating
Magnesium (Mg)	Green, leafy vegetables Legumes Milk	Component of bones and teeth Enzymes essential in general metabolism	Tremors leading to convulsive seizures

Continued

C. Classified on basis of solubility
  1. Fat-soluble vitamins: A, D, E, and K
     a. Sufficient fats needed in diet to carry fat-soluble vitamins
     b. Stored in body, so deficiencies are slow to appear
     c. Absorbed in the same manner as are fats; thus anything that interferes with absorption of fats interferes with absorption of fat-soluble vitamins (mineral oil, an indigestible substance, carries fat-soluble vitamins with it out of the body)
     d. Fairly stable in cooking and storage
  2. Water-soluble vitamins: C and B complex
     a. Not stored in body; deficiency can occur if vitamins are not consumed in the daily diet.
     b. Easily destroyed by air and in cooking

Special Vitamin Considerations
  A. Current research indicates that the effects of megadoses of vitamin C on the common cold are minimal.
  B. Effects of vitamin C on cancer still require further study.
  C. Claims list vitamin E as a "cure-all," especially in prolonging virility in men, preventing miscarriages, and curing muscular weakness.
  D. Current research has not established the validity of these claims; however, the amounts usually taken in supplements have caused no damage.

Minerals

A. Definition: inorganic elements essential for growth and normal functioning (Table 4-4)

TABLE 4-4	Major Minerals and Microminerals (Trace Elements)—cont'd		
Mineral	**Sources**	**Functions**	**Deficiency Symptoms**
Sulfur (S)	Whole grains Protein foods Meat Milk Eggs Cheese Nuts and legumes	Conduction of nerve impulses Muscle contraction Component of all body cells; important in building connective tissue Component in several B vitamins and several amino acids Energy metabolism	None documented
Microminerals			
Iron (Fe) Absorption enhanced by vitamin C, decreased by ASA (acetylsalicylic acid)	Organ meats (especially liver) Egg yolk Green, leafy vegetables Lean red meats Dried fruits (apricots, raisins)	Synthesis of hemoglobin General metabolic activities	Anemia
Iodine (I)	Iodized salt Saltwater fish	Normal functioning of thyroid gland	Goiter
Zinc (Zn)	Oysters Liver High-protein foods	Component of enzymes Assists in regulation of cell growth Protein synthesis	Impaired wound healing Poor taste sensitivity Retarded sexual and physical development
Copper (Cu)	Liver Cocoa Nuts Raisins	Aids in absorption of iron Component of hemoglobin Component of enzymes	Unknown at present, although secondary conditions may develop

B. Types
   1. Major minerals, or macrominerals, are found in the largest amounts in the body and are needed in large amounts (100 mg or more per day); they are calcium, phosphorus, potassium, sodium, chlorine, magnesium, and sulfur.
   2. Microminerals, or trace elements, are needed in small amounts (e.g., iron, zinc, copper, iodine)
C. Characteristics
   1. Found in all body tissues and fluids
   2. Occur naturally in foods (especially unrefined foods)
   3. Do not furnish energy but regulate body processes that furnish energy
   4. Remain stable in food preparation
D. Functions
   1. Constitute bones and teeth (calcium and phosphorus)
   2. Transmit nerve impulses and aid in muscle contraction
   3. Control water balance (sodium and potassium)
   4. Maintain acid-base balance
   5. Synthesize essential body compounds (e.g., iodine for thyroxine)
   6. Act as catalysts for tissue reactions (e.g., calcium needed for blood clotting)

Water

A. Water makes up 50% to 65% of the weight of an average adult.
   1. Intracellular: fluid within cells composed of water plus concentrations of potassium and phosphates; contains minerals, potassium, magnesium, and phosphorus

   2. Extracellular: all body fluids outside cells, including interstitial fluid, plasma, and watery components of body organs and substances; contains minerals and sodium chloride
B. Functions
   1. Essential component of all tissues and fluids
   2. Transportation of nutrients from the digestive tract to the bloodstream and from cell to cell; also removal of waste products from cells to outside the body
   3. Lubrication of joints
   4. Maintenance of stable body temperature (as temperature increases, sweating occurs, evaporates, and cools the body)
   5. Solvent for all the body's chemical processes
C. Overall water balance in the body
   1. Intake: under ordinary conditions, adults need 2 to 3 L of liquid per day—5 to 6 glasses of which should be water.
      a. Ingested fluids such as water, soups, and beverages
      b. Water in foods that are eaten
      c. Water formed from cell oxidation (when nutrients are burned)
   2. Output: averages 2600 ml daily
      a. Normal routes of excretion: primarily the kidney but also the skin, lungs, and feces
      b. Abnormal and extensive losses can occur from vomiting and diarrhea, open or draining wounds, fever, extensive burns, hemorrhage, and anything that causes excessive perspiration
D. Additional fluids are required:
   1. By infants
   2. During fever or disease process (especially kidney stones)

3. In warm weather
4. During heavy work or extensive physical activity

Cellulose

A. Definition: a polysaccharide that makes up the framework of plants; provides bulk (fiber or roughage) for the diet; cannot be broken down by the human digestive system and therefore is not absorbed
B. Function: to absorb water, provide bulk, and stimulate peristalsis
C. Found in the stalks and leaves of plants, in the skins of fruit and vegetables, and in the outer covering of seeds and cereals (refined cereals have most of the fiber removed and provide little bulk)

NUTRITIONAL GUIDELINES

Recommended Dietary Allowances (RDA)

A. Developed by the Food and Nutrition Board of the National Academy of Science
B. Suggested levels of essential nutrients (proteins, vitamins, and minerals) known from current research to be adequate to meet nutritional needs of most healthy individuals
C. Used as a guideline for most federal, state, and local feeding programs but not to be used as requirements for individuals with specific nutritional deficiencies

U.S. Dietary Goals or Dietary Guidelines

A. Developed by the U.S. Department of Agriculture, U.S. Department of Health and Human Services
B. Established in 1980 and are updated every 5 years; the current *Nutrition and Your Health: Dietary Guidelines for Americans* was released in 2000 and includes a reference to trans fat. The following are the seven guidelines:
   1. Eat a variety of foods (for a variety of nutrients).
   2. Balance the food you eat with physical activity; maintain or improve your weight.
   3. Choose a diet with plenty of grain products, vegetables, and fruits.
   4. Choose a diet low in fat, saturated fat, and cholesterol.

5. Choose a diet moderate in sugars.
6. Choose a diet moderate in salt and sodium.
7. If you drink alcoholic beverages, do so in moderation (alcohol is high in calories but low in nutrients; heavy drinking also contributes to many chronic liver and neurological disorders).

Nutritional Labeling and Education Act of 1990

A. This regulation has increased consumer access to safe products and knowledge of what nutrients are in food.
B. The nutrition facts panel must include the quantities of energy, fat, and other specific nutrients.
C. Ingredients labeled "GRAS" are "generally recognized as "safe" for ingestion by anyone.

Nutritional Assessment

A. Two phases: screening and assessment. Purpose: to screen for nutritional risks and apply specific assessment techniques to determine an action plan
B. Components of nutritional assessment: anthropometric measurements (such as body mass index), biochemical tests, clinical observations, dietary and personal histories. Techniques such as "hair analysis" have not been demonstrated to provide useful information about nutritional status. All components work together to determine the best action plan for the individual in the healthy population and the sick population within the context of their personal, social, and economic background. Techniques such as the "anergy panel" can be used to determine if nutritional status is adequate to support an active immune system.

Food Guide Pyramid

See Figure 4-1.
NOTE: Focus on nutrition and how it affects an individual's health and well-being continues to increase while researchers and nutrition experts continue to strive toward their goal of building a new and healthier food guide.

A. Emphasizes grains, fruits, and vegetables as the foundation of a balanced diet and downplays meats, dairy products, and fats; fats, oils, and sweets are recommended sparingly.

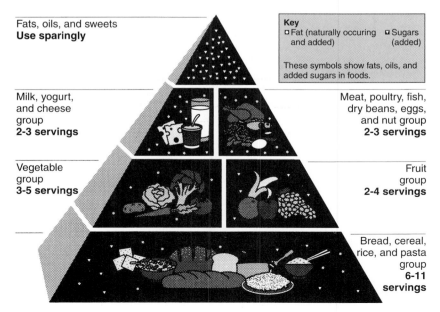

FIGURE 4-1. Food guide pyramid: a guide to daily food choices. *(Courtesy U.S. Department of Agriculture, Washington, DC, 1996.)*

B. Specific guidelines
   1. Breads, cereals, rice, pasta: six to eleven servings daily (1 serving equals 1 slice of bread, 1 oz of ready-to-eat cereal, or 1/2 cup of cooked cereal, rice, or pasta); nutrients primarily supplied are iron, B-complex vitamins, and carbohydrates (starches); refined products contain fewer vitamins, whereas the enriched, fortified, or restored products contain many more vitamins.
   2. Fruits: two to four servings daily (1 serving equals 1 medium apple, banana, or orange or 1/2 cup of cooked, chopped, or canned fruit); nutrients primarily supplied are vitamins A and C and fiber.
   3. Vegetables: three to five servings daily (1 serving equals 1 cup of raw, leafy vegetables or 1/2 cup of other vegetables cooked, chopped, or raw); nutrients primarily supplied are vitamins A and C and fiber.
   4. Milk, yogurt, cheese: two to three servings daily (1 serving equals 1 cup of milk or yogurt or 1/2 oz of natural cheese); nutrients primarily supplied are calcium, protein, and riboflavin.
   5. Meat, poultry, fish, dry beans, eggs, and nuts: two to three servings daily (1 serving equals 2 to 3 oz of cooked lean meat, poultry, or fish; 1/2 cup of cooked dry beans, or 1 egg; 2 tbsp of peanut butter equals 1 oz of lean meat); nutrients primarily supplied are protein, iron, and B vitamins.

FOOD MANAGEMENT

Food Fads and Facts: Meat Eaters Versus Vegetarians

A. Problems exist when too large a portion of the diet consists of meat.
   1. Excess calories tend to be consumed; meat (and the fat therein) is high in calories; because of the taste, the tendency is to eat more than is required.
   2. When a large portion of the meal is meat, a smaller portion of fruits and vegetables is consumed; therefore less fiber and fewer of the nutrients in fruits and vegetables are consumed.
B. Vegetarians also can have nutritional deficiencies.
   1. Calories may be insufficient despite large amounts of foods being consumed.
   2. Protein can be lacking; incomplete protein must be supplemented with complementary proteins.
   3. Strict vegetarians may need supplements of cobalamin (vitamin B_{12}) because it is found only in animal proteins.
C. The ideal diet combines both types of diet with a variety of foods.
   1. Meat eaters should eat smaller servings of leaner meats with more fruits, vegetables, and cereals.
   2. Vegetarians should improve the quality of their diet by adding dairy products such as eggs and milk. (If no dairy products are taken, complementary proteins should be carefully selected.)

Economic Considerations in Menu Planning

A. Plan menus in advance.
   1. Take advantage of specials and sales to plan balanced meals.
   2. Shop from a list to avoid impulse buying.

3. Supplemental food may be available from programs such as the Women, Infants, and Children (WIC) Program or Meals on Wheels.
B. Choose foods wisely.
   1. Buy foods in season and in good supply.
   2. Buy in quantity if adequate storage is available (larger quantities may cost less per unit).
   3. Buy sale items only if they can be used.
   4. Use unit pricing to find the best buys among brands.
   5. Know grades and brands of foods; grading of canned goods has no bearing on nutritive value; generic labeling can save up to 25% of name brand items.
   6. Purchase staple and canned goods when on sale.
   7. Remember that cost per serving rather than per pound is important, especially in buying meat.
   8. Compare labels for weights and ingredients.
   9. Buy less expensive forms of food (margarine is less expensive than butter).
   10. Limit purchase of empty-calorie foods.
   11. Decrease the cost of protein in the diet by using small amounts of meats, fish, and poultry and by using lower grades and less expensive cuts of meat; also legumes, peanut butter, eggs, and cheese are good sources of less expensive protein.
   12. Try to avoid convenience foods (any food bought partially prepared and ready to eat with little home preparation); they are usually more expensive than those prepared entirely at home and are less nutritionally balanced, containing high proportions of fat, calories, and sodium.
C. Care for foods after purchase.
   1. Store foods properly to avoid spoilage and loss of nutrients.
   2. Consume leftover foods quickly.

Storage and Preparation of Basic Foods

A. Milk
   1. Store milk refrigerated in covered container; powdered milk should be stored in a cool, dry place; refrigerate powdered milk after reconstituting.
   2. Cook over low heat; avoid scorching.
B. Cheese
   1. Refrigerate well, wrapped or in tight containers.
   2. Most palatable if served at room temperature; cook at low temperatures for a short time.
C. Eggs
   1. Refrigerate promptly; avoid purchase of eggs that are already cracked (eggs that are cracked later should be used only in foods that will be well cooked).
   2. Cook at lower temperatures to prevent discoloration, curdling, or toughness.
D. Cereals and breads
   1. Store in cool, dry place; bread retains freshness best at room temperature but molds faster; bread freezes well.
   2. Cook cereals according to directions; overcooking reduces vitamin content.
E. Meat, fish, and poultry
   1. Store in refrigerator for a short time or freeze for longer storage.
   2. Less expensive meats, although nutritionally equivalent to more expensive ones, require longer cooking at lower temperatures.

F. Fruits and vegetables
1. Store ripe fruits and vegetables in the refrigerator (fruits ripen best at room temperature).
2. Cook only until tender, (steaming) using as little water as possible (cooking liquids contain valuable nutrients and should be used if possible); raw fruits and vegetables are especially nutritious.

Types of Milk

A. Skim: fat and vitamin A removed (may have vitamins A and D added); contains all other nutrients of whole milk
B. Homogenized: fat particles evenly dispersed so cream does not separate
C. Pasteurized: heated to a specific temperature to destroy pathogenic bacteria (but nutrients are not affected)
D. Condensed: water removed and sugar added so carbohydrate content is increased; low in calcium and vitamins and high in sugar compared with whole milk
E. Evaporated: heated above the boiling point so that more than one half the water evaporates
F. Low fat: contains 0.5% to 2% fat; lower in calories than whole milk but comparable in nutrient value
G. Powdered or dry: water removed; least expensive form of milk on the market; when reconstituted, it has the same nutrient value as the milk from which it was made

COMMON TYPES OF FOOD POISONING

Staphylococcal Food Poisoning

A. Caused by *Staphylococcus aureus* bacteria; resistant to heat
B. Involves foods such as custard; potato, macaroni, egg, and chicken salads; cheese; ham; and salami
C. Exhibited by symptoms such as abdominal cramps, diarrhea, and vomiting; lasts 1 to 2 days; usually mild and attributed to other causes
D. Prevented by keeping foods above 140° F (60° C) or below 40° F (4° C); toxin is destroyed by boiling for several hours or heating in a pressure cooker at 240° F (138.5° C) for 30 minutes.

Clostridial Food Poisoning

A. Perfringens
1. Caused by *Clostridium perfringens,* spore-forming bacteria that grow in the absence of oxygen
2. Involves foods such as stews, soups, and gravies made from poultry and red meat
3. Exhibited by symptoms such as nausea without vomiting, diarrhea, and acute inflammation of the stomach and intestine; usually lasts 1 day
4. Prevented by storing foods properly and keeping foods above 140° F (60° C) or below 40° F (4° C)
B. Botulism
1. Caused by *Clostridium botulinum*, spore-forming bacteria that grow and produce toxins in absence of oxygen (anaerobic)
2. Involves canned low-acid foods, especially home-canned foods such as meats, corn, peas, green beans, asparagus, and mushrooms
3. Exhibited by symptoms such as inability to swallow; double vision, and progressive respiratory paralysis; fatality rate is high if untreated

4. Prevented by pressure cooking canned foods for specified length of time; any can or jar with a bulging top should be discarded.

Salmonellosis

A. Caused by Salmonella, bacteria widespread in nature that live in the intestinal tracts of humans and animals; transmitted by eating infected food or by contact with people who are infected or are carriers of the disease; also transmitted by insects or rodents
B. Involves poultry, red meats, dairy products, and eggs
C. Exhibited by symptoms such as severe headache, vomiting, diarrhea, abdominal cramps, and fever; usually last 2 to 7 days
D. Prevented by heating foods to 140° F (60° C) for 10 minutes or higher temperatures for less time

E. Coli

A. Caused by pathogenic *Escherichia coli,* some types are normally found in human intestinal system
B. Pathogenic *E. coli* found in raw ground beef
C. Bacteria attacks intestinal wall and spreads to body
D. Exhibited by symptoms such as bloody diarrhea, cramps, fever, chills, dehydration, kidney problems; can be fatal
E. Prevented by using well-cooked meats and sanitary food handling

NUTRITION THROUGHOUT THE LIFE CYCLE

Infant Nutrition

A. Infants require more protein and calories per pound of body weight than adults do because infants have more body surface in proportion to weight and because of their growth and activity.
B. Breast-feeding is the recommended method of feeding, if possible; more vitamin C is provided, and protein and sugar are more easily digested than is cow's milk; the infant is also provided with antibodies against disease and assists in establishing the mother-child bond; in addition, breast-fed babies experience fewer allergies and intolerances, as well as easier digestion.
C. Bottle-feeding is an acceptable alternative if close mother-child contact is maintained; most mothers use a commercially prepared formula such as Enfamil; a soy-based product such as Isomil can be used if the infant is allergic to milk products. At no time during the first year of life should an infant be fed regular whole cow's milk. Concentration of cow's milk may cause gastrointestinal (GI) bleeding or renal discomfort. Skim milk or low-fat milk provides infants with too little energy and linoleic acid.
D. The American Academy of Pediatrics recommends breast milk supplemented by vitamin D and fluoride from birth and iron supplements after 4 months of age.
E. Introduction of solid foods varies among pediatricians, most favoring a delay until the infant is at least 6 months of age.
1. Infant cereal is usually given first (often with added iron to supplement a possible lack in the infant's diet; prenatal iron reserves last 5 to 6 months). Rice cereal is given first because it is easy to digest and provokes few allergies.
2. Fruits, vegetables, and egg yolk are frequently given next. (Because of possible allergic reactions, egg white is delayed until late in the first year.)

3. Solid foods should be introduced one at a time and at 4- to 5-day intervals to observe for any allergic reactions.
4. Adding sugar or salt to infant's food is undesirable.
5. Infants can choke on small foods such as berries, corn, popcorn, or candy.
6. Infants should not receive honey because it contains botulism spores, which can harm the infant (even though quantities are too low to harm older children and adults).

Preschool Children

A. Growth rate is slower and more erratic, and food intake will vary accordingly.
B. A variety of foods should be offered.
   1. "Finger foods" such as carrot sticks are enjoyed.
   2. Serve small amounts because too large a serving can discourage a child from eating.
   3. Avoid refined sweets.
   4. Do not coax a child to eat; if a food is refused, offer it at a later time.
   5. Nutritious snacks are a viable alternative for a child who is a poor eater.
C. Teach healthy eating habits; avoid rewarding good behavior with food.

School Children (5 to 10 Years of Age)

A. Gradual increase in growth at this age (approximately equal for boys and girls)
B. Proper nutrition is important for proper mental and physical development; an adequate breakfast is important for alertness during class.
C. Children are usually good eaters at this age and should be encouraged by the examples set at home and at school; promote healthy eating.

Adolescents

A. Tremendous growth spurt occurs at puberty (age of sexual maturity).
   1. For girls, usually between 10 and 13 years of age
   2. For boys, between 13 and 16 years of age
B. Diets are influenced by peers, with many empty-calorie foods being consumed. Eating disorders such as anorexia or bulimia may develop with impaired self-esteem issues.
C. Boys gain mostly lean muscle tissue; they consume large amounts of food to meet energy requirements.
D. Girls gain more fat tissue; their diets may be more influenced by a desire to remain thin; girls frequently require iron supplements to meet their needs; adequate nutrition during adolescence helps avoid complications during pregnancy; promote healthy eating along with exercise.

Adults

A. Adequate nutrition throughout the life span is important in avoiding many serious illnesses.
B. Proper nutrition is based on guidelines set by U.S. government agencies (such as the food pyramid).
C. Persons who consume a balanced diet usually do not need vitamin supplements.
D. If a woman of childbearing age is a smoker and has poor dietary intake, a vitamin-C supplement of 100 mg/day is recommended.

Older Adults

A. Physiological changes affect nutrition of older adults.
   1. Aging slows the basal metabolic rate (BMR); combined with decreased activity, the result is decreased energy requirements and decreased number of calories needed.
   2. Taste may be adversely affected by gradual diminishment of the senses of smell, sight, and taste.
   3. Loss of teeth may affect proper chewing, food intake, or enjoyment. Older adults, as well as children and psychiatric patients, may "pouch" or "cheek" foods or medications and should be checked to make sure that intake is indeed swallowed.
   4. Reduced saliva makes swallowing more difficult and digestion less efficient.
   5. Decreased movement of wastes through intestines contributes to constipation.
   6. Marginal deficiencies of ascorbic acid, thiamin, and riboflavin have occurred in some elderly patients.
   7. Decreased absorption and use of nutrients results from decreased digestive juices and gastric motility reduction.
B. Economic and social considerations
   1. Decrease in income among older adults, combined with an increase in the amount spent for medical care, leaves less for adequate nutrition; the tendency is to eat less protein (which is expensive) and more carbohydrates (which are cheaper and easier to prepare).
   2. Loss of spouse, friends, or mobility results in isolation, depression, and often a decreased will to obtain adequate nutrition.
C. Planning diets
   1. Diet should be well balanced in protein, vitamins, and minerals (especially calcium and iron) to allow for diminished absorption.
   2. Calories sufficient to maintain energy and activity (reduced from those previously required)
   3. Soft bulk in diet to prevent constipation (cooked fruits and vegetables)
   4. Increased fluid intake required to eliminate metabolic wastes
   5. Meals should be light and easily digested, that is, contain only a small amount of fats; frequent small meals may be easier to digest than three large meals.
   6. Individual preferences should be respected and the diet built around them; make changes slowly.
   7. Meals eaten with others are often more appetizing than those eaten alone.

Pregnancy

A. A well-balanced diet with increased amounts of essential nutrients is important to the well being of the mother and baby.
   1. A protein increase of 20% or 60 g/day over the normal diet is recommended to allow for growth of the baby, placenta, maternal tissues, and increased circulating blood volume, amniotic fluid, and storage.
   2. An increase in calories meets increased energy demands and allows protein to be used for tissue building. Calorie needs approximate an extra 300 calories a day, which can be gained by adding a serving of dairy foods.
   3. Increased amounts of the following: calcium, phosphorus, and vitamin D are needed both for the mother and for the

bones and teeth of the baby; iron for hemoglobin and prenatal storage for the baby; iodine for thyroxine for the mother's increased BMR; and vitamins A, B complex, and C.

4. Weight should not be severely restricted; a gain of 30 lb is considered healthy.
5. Severe restriction of salt is unfounded.

B. Vomiting (morning sickness)
1. Lower fat intake with more high-carbohydrate foods
2. Fluids between instead of with meals
3. Dry toast or crackers on awakening
4. Avoid cooking odors.

Lactation

A. A baby requires 2 to 2 1/2 oz (60 to 75 ml) of breast milk per pound (453.6 g) of body weight (1 oz [30 ml] equals approximately 520 calories); the maternal need for all nutrients is increased during lactation.
B. Diet of a lactating mother should be high in protein and calories (approximately 500 extra calories per day).
C. Increased fluids are also required; at least 6 cups (1.5 L) of milk in some form is recommended.

DIET THERAPY

Nursing Responsibilities

A. Nutritional assessment: assess physical characteristics of patient; individualize care to allow for patient differences.
B. Evaluate the patient's tolerance to diet and provide feedback to other health team members.
C. Assist patient in learning about required dietary changes; reinforce information and answer questions.
D. If possible, incorporate patient's preferences to increase compliance with the nutritional care plan.
E. Prepare the patient for mealtime; assist as necessary.
F. See that each person receives the correct tray unless foods are being withheld.
G. Serve and remove tray promptly.
H. Teach patients the value of proper nutrition, and urge compliance with the nutritional care plan.

Purposes of Diet Therapy

A. To increase or decrease weight
B. To allow a particular organ or system to rest (e.g., a low-fat diet in gallbladder disease)
C. To regulate the diet to correspond with the body's ability to metabolize a specific nutrient (e.g., diabetes)
D. To correct conditions caused by deficiencies
E. To eliminate harmful substances from the diet (e.g., caffeine, cholesterol, alcohol)
F. To nourish the body

Diet Modifications

A. Calories may be increased or decreased.
B. Nutrients may be adjusted (high or low protein, low fat, low sodium).
C. Certain foods may be omitted (gluten, phenylalanine, or tyramine; those that might contain allergens) or added.
D. Modifications in texture (consistency-soft diet)
E. Frequency of meals: more than the standard three

F. Route of administration: enteral feedings (tube feedings based on individual's needs) or parenteral feedings for patients with compromised GI function

Standard Hospital Diets (Modifications in Consistency)

A. Clear liquid (surgical liquid)
1. Temporary diet of clear liquids, nonresidue, nonirritating, non–gas-forming; protein, vitamins, minerals, and calories are inadequate. Oral intake is restricted in the absence of bowel sounds.
2. Used postoperatively to replace fluids, before certain tests, and to lessen amount of fecal matter in colon
3. Includes water, coffee, tea, fat-free broth, pulp-free fruit juices (apple), gelatin, and ginger ale
B. Full liquid diet
1. Foods that are liquid at room or body temperatures; may be adequate if carefully planned, although frequently deficient in iron
2. Used postoperatively as a transition between clear and soft diet, in infections and acute gastritis; in febrile conditions; and for patients who are unable to chew or swallow or with an intolerance to food for other reasons
3. Includes all clear liquids, milk, creamed soups, ice creams, sherbets, plain puddings, and thin, strained cereal
C. Soft diet
1. Normal diet modified in consistency to have limited fiber; easily digested; nutritionally adequate
2. Used between full liquid and regular, for chewing difficulties, and in GI disorders
3. Includes tender meats and tender, well-cooked vegetables (those with a great deal of fiber should be pureed or omitted); fruits (no fiber) and plain cakes are allowed; no spicy or coarse foods are allowed.
D. Regular (general or house) diet
1. Adequate, well-balanced diet designed to appeal to most people
2. Used for individuals who do not require a modified or therapeutic diet
3. Includes all foods from the four basic food groups

Additional Modified (or Therapeutic) Diets

Table 4-5 lists diets, foods allowed and omitted, and when the diets are used.

DIETS FOR SPECIFIC CONDITIONS

Diabetes Mellitus

A. Classification
1. Insulin-dependent diabetes mellitus (IDDM) (type 1): onset is usually before the age of 20; difficult to manage and requires dietary restrictions, insulin injections, and exercise
2. Non–insulin-dependent diabetes mellitus (NIDDM) (type 2), or maturity onset: usually develops after age 35; frequently controlled by diet alone; insulin or oral hypoglycemics or both may also be needed. Medications should be taken as prescribed, under the direction of a physician. An alarming increase in the incidence of NIDDM has occurred in children, adolescents, and young adults.

TABLE 4-5	Modified or Therapeutic Diets		
Diet	Condition	Foods Allowed	Purpose of Diet
High calorie	Underweight (10% or more) Anorexia nervosa Hyperthyroidism	Emphasis on increase in calories Easily digested foods (carbohydrates) recommended Full meals with high-calorie snacks	To meet the increased metabolic needs of the body or provide increased calories for weight gain
Low calorie	Overweight	Fruits and vegetables especially recommended	To reduce the caloric intake below what the body requires so that weight loss will occur
High protein	Children who need additional protein for growth Following surgery Pregnancy and lactation Conditions that cause protein loss Extensive burns	Added amounts of poultry, meat, fish, milk, cheese, and eggs Nonfat dry milk added to soups and baked goods	To increase the intake of high-protein foods for maintaining and rebuilding tissues and correcting protein loss
Low protein	Liver disease Kidney diseases leading to renal failure	Fruits and vegetables Severely limited in amounts of meats, fish, poultry, eggs, and dairy products	To limit the end products of protein metabolism to avoid disturbing the fluid, electrolyte, and acid-base balances
High residue	Constipation (atonic) Diverticulitis (when inflammation has ceased)	Increased whole grain cereals Increased fruits and raw vegetables Fibrous meats	To mechanically stimulate the gastrointestinal tract
Low residue	Before and after bowel surgery Ulcerative colitis Diverticulitis (during inflammatory stage) Diarrhea	Soft cheeses Tender meats Refined cereals and breads Pureed fruits and vegetables Plain puddings	To soothe and be nonirritating to gastrointestinal tract
Low fat	Gallbladder disease Obesity Cardiovascular disease	Vegetables and fruits Skim milk Sherbet Increased carbohydrates and proteins	To lower fat content in diet (may be deficient in fat-soluble vitamins)
Low cholesterol	Cardiovascular disease	Lean meats and fish Poultry without the skin Liquid vegetable oils Skim milk	To decrease the blood cholesterol levels or maintain them at acceptable levels
High iron	Anemias	Regular diet with high-iron foods Liver and organ meats Red meats Dried fruits Egg yolks	To correct an iron deficiency
Sodium restricted	Kidney disease Cardiovascular disease Hypertension	Natural foods without salt Milk and meat in limited quantities	To control or correct the retention of sodium and water in the body by controlling sodium intake
High carbohydrate	Preparation for surgery Liver disease Kidney disease	Emphasis on carbohydrate foods Full meals with high carbohydrate snacks	To provide increased energy and spare protein for tissue building
Low carbohydrate	Dumping syndrome Hyperinsulinism Diabetes mellitus (although severe restriction of carbohydrates is currently considered unwarranted)	Proteins Only enough carbohydrate to maintain health and perform activities	To decrease the amounts of glucose in the bloodstream (increased blood glucose causes increased amounts of insulin to be produced by the body)
Lactose restricted	Lactose intolerance	Avoid foods containing lactose, such as milk, cheese, and ice cream	To eliminate or cut down on lactose—a substance certain individuals cannot metabolize

B. Diet is determined by age, sex, body build, weight, and activity; maintenance requirements are the same as for a patient without diabetes. Blood glucose levels are monitored with fasting or postprandial specimens and HgA1C (done approximately every 3 months).
   1. Calories: sufficient to maintain ideal body weight (approximately 30 cal/kg ideal weight)
   2. Protein: 10% to 20% of daily caloric intake
   3. Carbohydrates: 50% to 60% of total calories (obtain greatest portion from complex carbohydrates such as starches, and the least from simple sugars). Readily digestible sugars may be needed to counteract hypoglycemic episodes. Hypoglycemic symptoms associated with premenstrual syndrome do not respond to dietary modifications.
   4. Fats: moderately controlled; 30% or less of total calories and 10% from saturated fat
   5. High-fiber foods, which decrease postprandial blood glucose levels, are encouraged.
C. Exchange system is used for planning the diabetic diet.
   1. Based on simple grouping of common foods according to equivalent nutritional values
   2. Six basic food groups or food exchanges; each food within the group contains approximately the same food value as other foods within the same group.
      a. Milk: equal to 1 cup (240 ml) whole milk
      b. Vegetables: variety of low-carbohydrate vegetables
      c. Fruit: fresh or canned without sugar
      d. Bread: starchy items (breads, pasta, cereals, and vegetables equal to 1 slice bread)
      e. Meat: protein food equal to 1 oz (28 g) lean meat
      f. Fat equal to 1 tsp (5 ml) margarine
   3. Total exchanges per day is determined by individual nutritional needs based on nutritional standards. (Table 4-6 shows a sample diet based on the exchange system.)
   4. Advantages of exchange system
      a. Easy to understand
      b. Allows patients with diabetes more freedom to choose foods they like
      c. Allows choice of foods that fit into their economic status
      d. Can be used for other types of diets
      e. Does not require dietetic or specialized diabetic foods

Surgery

A. Surgery increases the nutritional demands on the body.
   1. Protein: increased for tissue repair, to prevent tissue breakdown, and to help replace blood and fluid losses
   2. Carbohydrates: increased to meet body demands for energy and to spare protein for tissue building
   3. Vitamins: especially important in wound healing; vitamin C cements cells and builds connective tissue and capillaries.
B. Types of feeding available postoperatively
   1. Intravenous: immediately administered to supply essential water, electrolytes, and vitamins; intended only as short-term for fluid and electrolytes supplement
   2. Parenteral hyperalimentation (total parenteral nutrition [TPN]): administered through a larger central vein such as the superior vena cava because the TPN solution is hypertonic (high osmolarity) and must enter the body in a region of high blood flow so that the solution is rapidly diluted; provides a higher percentage of water, glucose,

TABLE 4-6	1800-Calorie Diet with Food Exchanges	
Exchange Group		**Total Exchanges for the Day**
Milk		2
Vegetables		2
Fruit		5
Bread		9
Meat		8
Fat		7
Sample Diet		**Exchange List**
Breakfast		
Black coffee		Free
2 eggs		2 meat
2 pieces toast		2 bread
with butter		2 fat
Cereal		1 bread
with milk		1 milk
and plain blueberries		1 fruit
Lunch		
Turkey sandwich (3 oz or 84 g)		2 breads, 3 meat
with mayonnaise (2 tsp or 10 ml)		2 fat
with tomatoes		1 vegetable
Sponge cake		1 bread
with strawberries		1 fruit
and whipped cream		2 fat
Supper		
Roast beef (3 oz or 84 g)		3 meat
Mashed potatoes		3 bread
with butter		1 fat
Carrots		1 vegetable
and butter		1 fat
Applesauce		1 fruit
Small apple		1 fruit
Snack		
Raspberries (1 cup or 224 g)		1 fruit
in light cream (2 tbsp or 30 ml)		1 fat
Milk (8 oz or 240 ml)		1 milk

amino acids, fats, vitamins, minerals, and electrolytes; requires surgical insertion, careful monitoring, and special care; may also be indicated preoperatively or for debilitated patients whose intake does not meet body requirements
   3. Oral feedings: most patients should begin oral feedings as soon as bowel sounds return; provide nutrients essential to recovery; progress from clear liquid onward.

Burns

A. Rate of tissue breakdown and loss of other body nutrients are greater with serious burns compared with any other disease process.
B. Increase of fluids and nutrients is required.
   1. Increased energy requires 3000 to 5000 calories.
   2. Protein increase of 50% above normal

3. Vitamin C requirements greatly increased for wound healing
4. B vitamins increased for higher metabolic rate
5. Increased fluids to replace lost body fluids and help eliminate waste products
C. Intravenous dextrose, electrolytes, and plasma are given initially; a high-protein, high-calorie diet is given when oral foods can be taken.
D. Victims of extensive burns may require parenteral hyperalimentation to meet their extensive nutritional requirements.

Cancer

A. The National Cancer Institute and the American Cancer Society have issued the following guidelines for cancer prevention:
1. Eat a variety of foods.
2. Maintain a desirable body weight.
3. Eat a variety of both fruits and vegetables every day.
4. Eat more high-fiber foods, such as whole-grain breads and cereals, legumes, vegetables, and fruits.
5. Reduce fat intake to less than or equal to 30% of total calories.
6. If you drink alcohol, do so in moderation.
7. Limit consumption of salt-cured, smoked, and nitrite-preserved foods.
B. Diet for the patient with cancer must supply enough protein, fats, carbohydrates, vitamins, minerals, and fluids to meet increased energy demands, prevent weight loss, and rebuild body tissues during treatment; energy and protein needs may increase up to 20%; dietary supplements may be given to supply all necessary nutrients. Foods at room temperature may be more palatable for the patient with stomatitis.
C. The wasting away that can occur resulting from the disease itself, or radiation and chemotherapy is termed cancer cachexia and can decrease the life of the individual if not prevented or treated early.
D. When the GI tract cannot be used, nutritional support may be given via TPN.
E. Nutritional factors most likely are involved in the development of some cancers. Excesses, as well as deficiencies, have been implicated. Further evaluation is needed.
F. No one food causes cancer, and no one food can prevent it. Diet is considered to be one of the most important environmental and lifestyle factors in the cause and prevention of cancer in the United States.

Acquired Immunodeficiency Syndrome

A. Nutritional support is vital to the survival of all individuals with acquired immunodeficiency syndrome (AIDS). Weight loss is a major symptom in human immunodeficiency virus (HIV) infection. Malnutrition itself contributes to the suppression of immune function.
B. Good nutritional care is essential to preserve lean body mass, to maintain weight and strength, and to improve body's response to medication.
C. Nutritional status of individuals with AIDS can be compromised by decreased oral intake, anorexia, nausea, vomiting, dyspnea, fatigue, neurological disease, and disorders of mouth and esophagus.
D. Techniques to help with food intake: small meals, readily available snacks, adequate hydration, high-caloric, high-protein diet, and nutritional supplements; give drugs after meals.

E. General goals of nutrition intervention are the following:
1. Preserve optimal somatic and visceral protein status.
2. Prevent nutrient deficiencies or excesses known to compromise immune function.
3. Minimize nutrition-related complications that interfere with either intake or absorption of nutrients.
4. Enhance the quality of life.
5. Educate individuals about the importance of consuming a well-balanced diet.

Cardiovascular Disease

A. Cardiovascular diseases are the primary causes of death in the United States; research has shown that diet may be a risk factor in determining whether a person develops heart disease. Lifestyle modifications will probably need to continue after desired goals are achieved.
B. Objectives in dietary treatment of heart disease
1. Provide an adequate diet.
2. Prevent gas- and bulk-forming foods from distending stomach and exerting pressure against the heart.
3. Maintain patient's weight as near to ideal as possible to reduce workload of heart.
4. Prevent edema by lowering sodium intake.
5. Reduce the risk of atherosclerosis by reducing circulating blood lipids (low–saturated-fat, low-cholesterol diet).
6. Reduce the workload on the damaged heart after a myocardial infarction.
C. Sodium restriction
1. Component of many diets for cardiovascular diseases
2. Helps reduce excess edema and is thought to reduce the risk of hypertension
3. Sources of sodium
   a. Naturally present in foods, especially animal products such as meat, poultry, fish, milk, and eggs; fruits have little sodium.
   b. Sodium added to foods in the form of table salt and preservatives in processed foods; most canned, packaged, and frozen foods have either monosodium glutamate or sodium added.
   c. Water supplies may have a high-sodium content; water softeners add a significant amount of sodium to a diet.
   d. Nonprescription medicines and home remedies such as baking soda, alkalizers for indigestion, cough medicines, and laxatives may contain large amounts of sodium.
4. Sodium-restricted diets limit the intake of sodium to a level prescribed by the physician.
   a. Mild sodium-restricted diet (2 to 3 g) contains approximately one half of the salt previously used; additional salting of processed foods is not permitted; no salty foods are allowed.
   b. 1000-mg sodium diet (moderate)
   c. 500-mg sodium diet (strict)
   d. 250-mg sodium diet (severe)

Peptic Ulcer Disease

A. Current advances in drug therapy to decrease acid secretion and promote healing have decreased the need for a highly restrictive, bland diet.
B. These bland diets have been shown to be ineffective and lacking in nutrients to support the healing process. Therapy is based on an individual's response to food choices; avoidance

of foods that cause gastric stimulation (such as caffeine) is recommended.

Chronic Renal Failure

A. Patients with chronic renal failure require strict monitoring for protein, water, and electrolyte balance. Specific nutritional therapy varies greatly, depending on the patient's age and the stage of the disease. Enough protein should be supplied to repair and maintain tissues and avoid the use of protein for energy.

B. The blood urea nitrogen level (BUN) and creatinine clearance level are monitored to assist in regulating protein levels.

C. Homocystine levels may be associated with vascular damage; dietary sources of this amino acid should be limited in renal patients.

SUGGESTED READINGS

Center for Food Safety and Nutrition http://vm.cfsan.fda.gov/list.html

Dietary Guidelines for Americans http://www.nal.usda.gov/fnic/dga/

Food and Nutrition Information Center, United States Department of Agriculture and the Agricultural Research Center http://www.nal.usda.gov/fnic/

Grodner M, Anderson SL, Hagen-Ansert SL: *Foundations and clinical applications of nutrition: a nursing approach,* ed 3, St Louis, 2004, Mosby.

Guide To Nutrition Labeling And Education Act (NELA) Requirements http://www.fda.gov/ora/inspect_ref/igs/nleatxt.html

Healthy People 2010 at http://www.healthypeople.gov/

Mahan LK, Escott-Stump S: *Krause's food, nutrition and diet therapy,* ed 10, Philadelphia, 2000, WB Saunders.

Mitchell, MK: *Nutrition across the lifespan,* ed 2, Philadelphia, 2002, WB Saunders.

Nutrition.gov http://www.nutrition.gov/home/index.php3

Nutrition Navigator: A Rating Guide to Nutrition Websites http://navigator.tufts.edu/

Peckenpaugh NJ, Poleman CM: Nutrition: *Essentials and diet therapy,* ed 9, Philadelphia, 2003, WB Saunders.

Physicians' Desk Reference, ed 57, Montvale, New Jersey, 2003, Thompson Medical Economics Company.

Williams SR, Schenkler E: *Essentials of nutrition and diet therapy,* ed 8, St Louis, 2003, Mosby.

REVIEW QUESTIONS

1. A resident in a nursing home reads the label on a cereal box and then asks the nurse what cellulose does. The nurse knows the main function of cellulose in the diet is to:
   1 Maintain fluid balance.
   2 Build and repair body tissues.
   3 Provide a rapid source of energy.
   4 Absorb water to increase fecal bulk.

2. A nurse is presenting a program on nutrition to a group of nursing assistants in an assisted living facility. The nurse states that meal planning at the facility should include the minerals most often deficient in the U.S. diet. Which of the following minerals are most often deficient in the U.S. diet?
   1 Calcium and iron
   2 Iodine and fluorine
   3 Potassium and sodium
   4 Phosphorus and calcium

3. A nurse is planning refreshments for a community walk-a-thon for diabetes mellitus. When planning refreshments, the nurse is aware that water should be readily available because:
   1 It is the most abundant mineral in the body.
   2 It will keep the walkers from getting shin splints.
   3 The people with diabetes need it to regulate sugar balance.
   4 The walkers may need to replace fluids lost from perspiration.

4. A third-grade student asks a nurse who is working in a school why the salt on the table has iodine in it. The nurse responds that iodine is essential to health because it:
   1 Strengthens bone and teeth
   2 Is necessary for blood clotting
   3 Assists in the body's ability to grow
   4 Allows oxygen to travel safely to cells

5. A nurse is explaining a discharge plan with an individual who has had surgery. In planning an adequate diet to promote tissue healing, the nurse advises the patient to increase his intake of the vitamins:
   1 A and D
   2 A and C
   3 B_6 and C
   4 B_{12} and D

6. A nurse is counseling the mother of a child who has experienced a third-degree burn over 15% of her body. Which of the child's favorite foods would provide necessary foods high in protein and calories?
   1 Potato chips and pizza
   2 Oranges and applesauce
   3 Green beans and cantaloupe
   4 Hamburgers and peanut butter and jelly sandwiches

7. A patient hospitalized with peptic ulcer disease is distressed to find that he has no coffee on his meal tray. Which of the following statements by the nurse conveys the reason for a caffeine-restricted diet in patients with peptic ulcer disease?
   1 "Caffeine dehydrates the body."
   2 "Caffeine delays gastric emptying."
   3 "Caffeine buffers milk and antacids."
   4 "Caffeine stimulates gastric acid secretions."

8. A patient with liver failure is on the verge of hepatic coma. Which of the following nutrients would the nurse expect to be restricted?
   1 Fats
   2 Proteins
   3 Vitamins
   4 Carbohydrates

9. A pregnant patient asks how much weight she should expect to gain if she follows a balanced diet and exercises. The nurse explains:
   1 "Weight gain should not exceed 10 pounds."
   2 "Your physician will be concerned if you gain more than 20 pounds."
   3 "Acceptable weight gain now averages around 30 pounds."
   4 "You may gain as much as 40 pounds."

10. The nurse correctly advises the pregnant patient to increase the number of calories in her daily diet by:
    1 300
    2 500
    3 750
    4 1000

11. Which of the following dietary modifications will provide an athlete with maximum endurance during a marathon run:
    1 High fat
    2 High carbohydrate
    3 Increased consumption of all nutrients
    4 High protein

12. A patient, 8 weeks pregnant and complaining of "morning sickness," asks the nurse what she should do to decrease her discomfort. Which of the following should the nurse suggest to the patient?
    1 Increase intake of fats.
    2 Increase intake of protein.
    3 Eat frequent small meals and snacks.
    4 Drink fluids with meals.

13. A patient is lactose intolerant and tells the nurse that he avoids all dairy products. To manage his condition, the nurse suggests that he first:
    1 Continue to avoid all dairy products.
    2 Try repeated small amounts of milk to increase the production of lactase.
    3 Consume dairy products as much as possible to gain calcium and vitamin D.
    4 Substitute nondairy products such as rice milk, soy milk, or coffee creamer.

14. A nurse is concerned about an adolescent with very low–fat-diet choices. A diet extremely low in fat may be inadequate in:
    1 Vitamin A
    2 Vitamin C
    3 Minerals
    4 Carbohydrates

15. Which of the following cardiovascular disorders may require the initiation of dietary sodium restrictions?
    1 Hyperlipidemia and renal failure
    2 Hypercholesterolemia and hypertension
    3 Hypertension and congestive heart failure
    4 Hyperlipidemia and congestive heart failure

16. The nurse instructs the patient on a sodium restriction to look for nutritional facts about packaged food:
    1 In USDA handbooks from the bookstore
    2 On package labels
    3 On web sites featuring nutritional information
    4 In handout literature provided by a nutritionist

17. The most common type of nutritional anemia is:
    1 Iron deficiency
    2 Pernicious anemia

3 Folic-acid deficiency
4 Vitamin-B$_{12}$ deficiency

18. A nurse is instructing a class on safe handling of foods. Which of the following precautions should the nurse advise to minimize the loss of vitamin C in foods?
    1 Cooking thoroughly to kill any bacteria
    2 Adding baking soda to the cooking water
    3 Eating sources of vitamin C raw when possible
    4 Keeping food in a mesh bag to allow air to circulate

19. The nurse is preparing to give an injection of vitamin B$_{12}$ to a nursing home resident. The nurse is giving the injection to prevent the disorder:
    1 Scurvy
    2 Pellagra
    3 Marasmus
    4 Pernicious anemia

20. A patient who is receiving chemotherapy is concerned because she is unable to eat well because of stomatitis. Which of the following interventions should the nurse recommend?
    1 Eat as much as possible when able.
    2 Drink as much fluid as possible along with food at meals.
    3 Eat small, frequent meals consisting of foods at room temperature.
    4 Eat protein-rich foods when able.

21. A dietary modification that shows evidence of reducing the risk of cancer is:
    1 Increasing intake of saturated fats
    2 Decreasing intake of saturated fats
    3 Decreasing intake of raw fruits and vegetables
    4 Increasing intake of smoked and salt-cured meats

22. The primary diet intervention for therapy of kidney stones is to:
    1 Decrease calcium intake.
    2 Dilute the urine by increasing fluids.
    3 Prevent vitamin and mineral deficiencies.
    4 Alleviate the side effects of the drugs involved.

23. A middle-aged man comes to the outpatient clinic with complaints of pain in his right great toe. He states he was diagnosed with gout 3 years ago and has been following his diet and medication regimen with no exacerbations until now. Which of the following statements indicates to the nurse that he was following the diet for the management of gout?
    1 "I eat a high-calorie diet."
    2 "I don't eat foods high in purine."
    3 "I drink a glass of wine each night."
    4 "I restrict my fluid intake to 1000 ml/day."

24. A resident in a long-term care facility is to begin receiving nasogastric tube feedings. Which of the following is an important consideration in selecting of the type of feeding?
    1 Feedings are usually hypertonic solutions.
    2 Feeding solutions are basically the same for all individuals.
    3 Feedings should be used only if the resident's GI tract is nonfunctional.
    4 Solutions are chosen on the ability of the resident to absorb nutrients.

25. A physician is considering placement of an enteral tube for feeding purposes into an older adult patient with dysphagia. Which of the following types of tubes has the least possibility of aspiration?
    1 Gastrostomy tube
    2 Jejunostomy tube

3 Duodenostomy tube
4 Small bore nasogastric tube

26. In teaching a patient who has recently been started on angiotensin-converting enzyme (ACE) inhibitors to control his hypertension, the nurse advises him to avoid which of the following:
    1 Vigorous exercise and physical exertion.
    2 Salt substitutes containing potassium chloride.
    3 Prolonged exposure to the sun.
    4 Packaged lunchmeats containing nitrites.

27. In teaching a patient about preparing fresh foods the nurse will discuss that the best method to preserve nutrients is:
    1 Frying
    2 Steaming
    3 Microwaving
    4 Soaking before cooking

28. A patient calls the nurse into his room and explains that he is unable to eat the food because milk and meat are being served on the same tray. Which of the following is the best response by the nurse?
    1 "You need these nutrients to get over your disease."
    2 "Why don't you eat them now, I will note the change later."
    3 "We need to discuss this with the head dietitian, I will call her."
    4 "I will call and notify the dietary department to bring you a kosher tray."

29. A patient of Middle-Eastern descent refuses to eat during the day and then asks for a double serving during the evening. The patient is newly diagnosed with IDDM. Which of the following is the best response by the nurse?
    1 "I know that this is Ramadan, but you have to eat during the day."
    2 "We will need to hold your insulin during the day, and then double it at night."
    3 "I think I should talk with your physician. It is very difficult to manage your diabetes."
    4 "We need to find a way for you to observe your religion and also manage your diabetes."

30. The patient with polycystic ovarian syndrome (PCOS), will need dietary modifications related to which of the following associated conditions?
    1 Hypoglycemia
    2 Hyperinsulinism
    3 Hypertension
    4 Hypocalcemia

31. Which of the following should the nurse include when teaching about magnesium deficiency?
    1 The major food sources are red meats and grains.
    2 The major role of magnesium is in tissue growth and repair.
    3 Magnesium deficiency is a relatively uncommon occurrence.
    4 Frequent urination may produce magnesium deficiency.

32. A nurse's aide is passing out evening snacks to a group of residents. Which of the following snacks should the nurse recommend for the resident with IDDM?
    1 Ice cream
    2 Cookies and milk
    3 Cheese and crackers
    4 Slice of chocolate cake

33. The nurse is counseling a patient with newly diagnosed IDDM concerning preparation for increased exercise or

activity. Which of the following should the nurse encourage the patient to do before exercise?
1   Eat a small snack composed of fats.
2   Lower the amount of insulin before activity.
3   Eat a small snack composed of carbohydrates.
4   Increase the amount of insulin before activity.

34. What tool is now being used in determining appropriate body weight instead of a height and weight table?
1   Basal metabolic rate
2   Body mass index
3   Body surface area
4   Body frame size

35. In teaching a patient on a weight loss diet, the nurse includes what information about the hormone leptin?
1   The hormone is secreted by the pancreas.
2   The lipogenic activity of insulin is increased by this hormone.
3   It is believed to be involved with body weight regulation and may promote satiety.
4   Studies suggest that obese individuals have an excess of leptin.

36. During teaching about prenatal diet, the nurse should recommend to the pregnant woman to include which vitamin to reduce the occurrence of spina bifida in her baby?
1   Pyridoxine
2   Riboflavin
3   Folic acid
4   Ascorbic acid

37. Cheilosis, a common occurrence in elderly patients, is the result of a deficiency of which vitamin?
1   Cobalamin (vitamin B_{12})
2   Niacin (vitamin B_2)
3   Riboflavin (vitamin B_6)
4   Thiamin (vitamin B_1)

38. Which of the following are implicated in the prevalence of nephrolithiasis in Western countries?
1   Decreased amounts of choline, complex carbohydrates, and manganese
2   Increased amounts of animal fat, grains, and caffeine
3   Decreased amounts of calcium, folate, and water
4   Increased amounts of sodium, animal protein, and sugar

39. Kwashiorkor is a severe state of malnutrition resulting from a deficiency of which nutrient?
1   Fats
2   Carbohydrates
3   Vitamins
4   Protein

40. To maintain stable prothrombin rates, patients who take Coumadin need a consistent intake of which vitamin?
1   B_{12}
2   C
3   A
4   K

41. A patient who is interested in bodybuilding asks the nurse about ergogenic aids such as creatine. The nurse should tell the patient which of the following?
1   These products are a safe and effective way to increase body mass and endurance.
2   Creatine is not as safe or effective as anabolic steroids.
3   Although their use is widespread, ergogenic aids may not be safe to use.
4   The recommended dosage of creatine for dietary supplement is 20g/day.

42. A postoperative patient has been on intravenous (IV) fluids for several days. What remark made by the patient indicates that she is probably ready to be started on oral feedings?
1   "I can't wait to see some real food rather than this IV bottle!"
2   "I'm so glad I don't have any more nausea—what a nuisance that was!"
3   "My stomach is really rumbling" I don't know why—there's nothing in it!"
4   "My stomach is feeling a little bloated because I haven't had anything in it for so long"

43. An elderly woman complains to the nurse that she is "burping acid" on a daily basis. What recommendations from the nurse would be most likely to reduce the patient's discomfort?
1   Eat one large meal per day to allow the stomach to empty thoroughly.
2   Be sure to take a high carbohydrate snack before bedtime.
3   Avoid fatty foods, alcohol, caffeine, and nicotine.
4   Try a glass of wine before meals and at bedtime.

44. Apple juice can cause diarrhea and abdominal discomfort in young children resulting from which of the following?
1   Ascorbic acid
2   Pectin
3   Sorbitol
4   Potassium

45. A patient states that she manages her hypoglycemia with a very low-carbohydrate diet but that she is having increased episodes of nervousness, headaches, and hunger a couple of hours after eating. The nurse should suggest which of the following to the patient?
1   Increasing simple carbohydrates to maintain blood glucose levels
2   Limiting dietary fiber
3   Increasing protein intake
4   Eating a diet rich in complex carbohydrates and dietary fiber.

46. A patient stops a nurse one day and states her confusion over what she hears about vitamin C. When discussing this vitamin with the patient, the nurse should include which of the following?
1   Vitamin C is fat soluble and readily stored in the body.
2   Deficiency symptoms include night blindness and dry, scaly skin.
3   Improper storage and cooking can result in food losing its vitamin C.
4   Vitamin C has been proven to significantly reduce the incidence and severity of colds.

47. A home health care nurse is caring for a patient who is recovering from a mild heart attack. His wife says, "He loves to eat milk, meat, and cheese, especially when his family comes for dinner. How am I ever going to get him to change?" The most appropriate response for the nurse should be:
1   "I will explain all the dangers of not changing his lifestyle."
2   "His family will understand the importance of his maintaining his health."
3   "Make changes gradually; incorporate small portions of favorite foods in moderation."
4   "Do the best you can; his heart attack was mild. He does not have to worry too much."

48. As a part of a diet to reduce a patient's triglycerides, the nurse should recommend which of the following?
   1 Red meats, coconut oil, and shrimp
   2 Poultry, eggs, and whole milk
   3 Soybeans, green vegetables, and olive oil
   4 Lamb, lobster, and yogurt

49. In teaching a patient how to make sure he obtains adequate protein intake on a vegetarian diet, the nurse should include which of the following facts?
   1 It is impossible to obtain adequate amino acid intake on a strictly vegetarian diet.
   2 Plant proteins must be supplemented with animal amino acids to create a well-balanced diet.
   3 Plants are the richest source of complete proteins.
   4 A diet of plant protein alone can provide adequate amounts of amino acids when beans and peas are included.

50. A patient returns to the unit after undergoing a total gastrectomy. After 5 days, the patient is placed on TPN. The nurse should understand that this means:
   1 A short-term supplementation via tube placed in a peripheral vein
   2 Full nutritional support for longer periods via a large central vein
   3 A long-term method of feeding using different points along the GI tract
   4 A short-term supplementation via nasogastric tube until full oral feedings can be resumed

51. A patient who is newly diagnosed with HIV is angry and withdrawn. He verbalizes to the nurse that he does not understand why she is even bothering to tell him about nutrition when he is going to die anyway. What should the nurse say at this point?
   1 "When you are ready to listen, we will talk again."
   2 "I will leave written material here for you to read."
   3 "I know you feel you have lost control over your life."
   4 "Eating well is a way you can maintain your immune system."

52. Some people develop a deficiency of vitamin B$_{12}$ because of which of the following conditions?
   1 Zollinger-Ellison syndrome
   2 Marasmus
   3 Achlorhydria
   4 Diverticulosis

53. Most flatus in the bowel is the result of:
   1 Excessive intake of air during glutition
   2 Inadequate intake of fluids such as water during the digestion process
   3 Undigested or incompletely absorbed carbohydrates in the alimentary canal
   4 Inadequate intake of grains, fruits, and vegetables high in resistant starches

54. Which of the following is the process by which the body attempts to achieve dynamic equilibrium?
   1 Homeostasis
   2 Metabolism
   3 Catabolism
   4 Anabolism

55. An adolescent tells the nurse that she hates carrots and does not see why she has to eat them. The nurse explains the functions of vitamin A in the body and then helps the patient plan a healthy diet that includes which of the following foods?
   1 Bananas, lima beans, and salmon
   2 Cheese, corn, and prunes
   3 Collard greens, beef liver, and spinach
   4 Peaches, tomatoes, and avocados

56. A patient with a complaint of irregular heartbeat was diagnosed with hypokalemia and was advised to increase his dietary intake of potassium. He asks the nurse, "What foods are high in potassium?" The nurse's answer should include:
   1 Dairy products
   2 Apricots, oranges, and bananas
   3 Fish liver oils and fortified milk
   4 Wheat germ and dark green, leafy vegetables

57. A patient whose blood pressure has been elevated tells the nurse that the physician has recommended that he reduce his intake of dietary sodium. The nurse advises the patient to:
   1 Limit fresh fruits and vegetables.
   2 Increase dairy products in his diet.
   3 Increase canned and processed meats in his diet.
   4 Substitute spices, herbs, or lemon juice for salt in seasoning his food.

58. An elderly patient is confused about why her primary care provider prescribed vitamin E for her. The nurse tells her which of the following?
   1 "It helps the liver make blood clotting factors and helps reduce the risk of hip fracture."
   2 "It promotes normal bone growth, helps control cell reproduction, and may help treat skin disorders such as psoriasis."
   3 "It helps your eyes adapt to light and to dark, and it prevents skin conditions such as follicular hyperkeratosis."
   4 "It helps promote your immune system, reduces the risk of heart disease and stroke, and seems to help prevent some age-related dementias."

59. For adequate development of collagen, a protein substance found in many body tissues, which of the following nutrients is required?
   1 Vitamin E
   2 Calcium
   3 Sodium
   4 Vitamin C

60. A diet that is based on corn and few other foods contributes to pellagra because it:
   1 Lacks fat-soluble vitamins
   2 Contains an excess of complex carbohydrates
   3 Is low in niacin and tryptophan
   4 Is inadequate in saturated fats

61. A neighbor asks a nurse for advice on cooking healthy meals for her family. Which of the following should the nurse emphasize?
   1 The more expensive the meat, the more nutrients it contains.
   2 The higher the grade on canned goods, the more nutritious the contents.
   3 Refined cereal products are more nutritious than fortified cereal products.
   4 Raw fruit and vegetables contain more nutrients than cooked vegetables.

62. A nurse is working in a prenatal clinic. Which of the following patients are most at risk for the potential of nutritional complications?
   1 A patient in her third trimester who has gained 39 pounds
   2 A woman in her third trimester with complaints of heartburn

3 An underweight adolescent who confesses to eating erratically

4 A 36-year-old primigravida in her second trimester who is slightly anemic

63. A high school student asks the school nurse whether he should drink a "special electrolyte solution" because he is in training to make the track team. His specialty is the high jump. The best reply for the nurse should be:
   1 "Make certain it has vitamins to increase energy."
   2 "No. You need a sugar solution to add energy for endurance."
   3 "Yes, absolutely. They help to replace minerals lost when you sweat."
   4 "For nonendurance events, water is the best solution to prevent dehydration."

64. A patient is recovering from burns over 40% of his total body surface area. A high-protein, high-carbohydrate diet is essential for recovery because:
   1 The vitamins supplied will promote healing and supply energy.
   2 Extra calories are needed to allow the person to be active in the rehabilitation process.
   3 Protein is needed for tissue healing and carbohydrates will assist protein to be used for this purpose.
   4 Extra carbohydrates will assist in counteracting the negative nitrogen balance caused by massive trauma.

65. A trend towards hypertension in the general population has been linked to increased consumption of which of the following?
   1 Nutritional supplements
   2 Processed foods
   3 Genetically modified foods
   4 Fresh fruits and vegetables

66. A patient who is taking isonicotinic acid hydrazide (INH) for treatment of tuberculosis asks the nurse if any special attention should be paid to her dietary intake while she is on the medication. The nurse should tell her:
   1 "You will need to take more vitamin C than usual."
   2 "You need to make sure that you get enough vitamin B$_6$."
   3 "You must make sure you don't get too much calcium."
   4 "You should avoid milk products."

67. A patient is being started on nicardipine (Cardene) for her high blood pressure. The nurse should instruct her to:
   1 Take the pills with crackers or milk.
   2 Avoid taking an antacid within 3 hours of taking the pills.
   3 Avoid drinking grapefruit juice while she is taking the pills.
   4 Take the pills with at least one full glass of water.

68. A child on a gluten-free diet for management of celiac disease was able to eat foods made with flour from which of the following?
   1 Oats
   2 Rye
   3 Wheat
   4 Rice

69. A patient who is taking monoamine oxidase inhibitor (MAOI) medication must be instructed by the nurse to avoid which of the following foods that is rich in tyramine?
   1 Milk products and whole grains
   2 Chicken liver and yeast
   3 Green and leafy vegetables
   4 Citrus fruits

70. A patient with a history of family allergies asks what foods she can feed her 4-month-old son that would be least likely to cause an allergic reaction. The nurse's most appropriate response would be to suggest:
   1 Rice cereal
   2 Cow's milk
   3 Wheat cereal
   4 Scrambled eggs

71. Diet therapy for a patient with phenylketonuria (PKU) is focused on which strategy:
   1 Allowing unlimited amount of aspartame intake
   2 Using as many milk-based foods as possible
   3 High levels of phenylalanine included on a daily basis
   4 Individualized diet plans containing some of this essential amino acid, with careful monitoring of phenylalanine levels

72. A patient with hepatitis wants to know what type of diet he should follow to help him get well. The nurse should instruct him on which of the following diets?
   1 Low fat, low protein, low carbohydrate
   2 High fat, low protein, low carbohydrate
   3 High carbohydrate, moderate fat, adequate protein
   4 Low fat, high protein, low carbohydrate

73. The absorption of iron, especially iron from nonmeat sources, can be enhanced significantly if iron is ingested with:
   1 Citrus juices
   2 Fish liver oils
   3 Green, leafy vegetables
   4 Milk and dairy products

74. The diabetic diet is based on the exchange system. In using this system, the patient should be instructed that:
   1 Only foods listed in the same exchange can be substituted.
   2 Dietetic or diabetic foods should be used as much as possible.
   3 Substitution within a food exchange for meal planning can be done only by a physician or dietician.
   4 Food exchanges are not particularly important as long as you stay within your recommended calories.

75. TFAs should be limited in the diet because of their tendency to:
   1 Inhibit the absorption of fat-soluble vitamins.
   2 Add calories to the daily intake.
   3 Increase blood levels of LDLs.
   4 Reduce the amount of HDLs in the blood.

76. For dinner one evening, a patient with diabetes fries an egg in 1 teaspoon of margarine, has a biscuit with 1 teaspoon of butter, and drinks a cup of black coffee. From which exchange lists has she selected her meal?
   1 One milk, two bread, and one fat exchange
   2 One meat, one bread, and two fat exchanges
   3 One bread, one meat, and one vegetable exchange
   4 One meat, one milk, one fruit, and one fat exchange

77. A patient with diabetes remarks that in the late afternoon, she frequently becomes shaky and feels very nervous. What would the nurse suggest to her as a readily available source of carbohydrate that might get her over this hypoglycemic episode?
   1 Cereal
   2 Oranges
   3 Crackers
   4 Bread and butter

78. A patient is admitted with a diagnosis of chronic renal failure. Which of the following dinner selections would be best suited for this patient?
    1 Ground round steak, asparagus, bread and butter, fruit cup, and milk
    2 Hamburger with tomato on a bun, potato chips, and a glass of chocolate milk
    3 Liver, cottage cheese with peach half, deviled eggs, and coffee with cream and sugar
    4 Apple juice, 1 oz roasted chicken, asparagus, sliced tomatoes, fruit cup, and tea with sugar

79. A patient is admitted for treatment of acute pancreatitis. What type of nutrition will most likely be ordered for him?
    1 Parenteral nutritional support
    2 Clear liquids
    3 Full liquids, progressing to soft foods as tolerated
    4 Soft, bland diet

80. A patient who was admitted for treatment of peptic ulcer disease asks the nurse if eating too many spicy foods caused the disease. The nurse should explain to him:
    1 Smoking and alcohol use are the causes of ulcers.
    2 Spicy foods and alcohol will cause ulcers.
    3 The cause is an organism named *Helicobacter pylori.*
    4 Stress and worry are the primary causes of ulcers.

81. A patient is admitted with a diagnosis of suspected myocardial infarction. He complains about the soft diet that the physician ordered. The nurse explains to the patient that the purpose of this diet is to:
    1 Reduce the workload on the heart.
    2 Decrease irritation to the digestive tract.
    3 Reduce the number of calories in his diet.
    4 Decrease peristalsis within the digestive tract.

82. A patient has a problem with atonic constipation probably caused by poor eating habits coupled with his dependence on laxatives. Which of the following menus would be best suited to help him overcome constipation?
    1 Ground beef patty, boiled potato, baked squash, and milk
    2 Baked chicken, macaroni, cooked carrots, custard, and coffee
    3 Macaroni and cheese, peach halves, vanilla ice cream, and milk
    4 Beef stew with carrots and onions, coleslaw, rye bread, and tea

83. To prevent hypertension, sodium intake should be in the range of:
    1 10 to 12 g
    2 2.0 to 2.4 g
    3 0.1 to 0.5 g
    4 2 to 4 g

84. Iron deficiency can result from taking which of the following on a regular basis?
    1 Vitamin C
    2 Aspirin
    3 Antacids
    4 Anticonvulsants

85. A patient who has been experiencing severe pain from gallstones is scheduled for surgery in 2 weeks. To minimize her discomfort until then, the nurse should instruct the patient to modify her diet in which of the following ways?
    1 Limit fat intake as much as possible.
    2 Reduce the total number of calories.

    3 Increase the amount of dairy products.
    4 Limit carbohydrate foods.

86. A patient on medical nutritional therapy for coronary heart disease asks the nurse why the physician recommended an increase in the amount of fiber in his diet. The nurse should explain that:
    1 "Fiber slows glucose absorption."
    2 "The intestine speeds up the time that food takes to pass through it when fiber is increased in the diet."
    3 "Fiber helps increase LDL cholesterol in the colon."
    4 "The stomach empties faster when fiber is present in the diet."

87. In planning meals for the patient with chronic renal disease the nurse must be sure to consider which of the following?
    1 Maintain normal serum blood levels of magnesium and bicarbonates.
    2 Reduce the levels of chloride and sulfates in the blood.
    3 Maintain adequate protein and calorie intake.
    4 Restrict fluids to avoid edema.

88. The wife of a patient with cancer asks for suggestions to work around his lack of interest in eating resulting from fatigue and a sore mouth. The nurse might include which of the following recommendations?
    1 "Limit the amount of gravy, sauces, or butter added to foods."
    2 "Offer salty, spicy, or acidic foods to stimulate his appetite through taste."
    3 "Avoid snacking, as it will spoil his appetite."
    4 "Try shakes made from frozen liquid supplements or milkshakes with protein powders added."

89. An adolescent who is admitted for treatment of bulimia may have nutritional problems resulting from both intake and absorption, as well as which of the following?
    1 Dental erosion
    2 Gastroesophageal reflux
    3 Constipation
    4 Hyperglycemia

90. A condition that would not increase the caloric needs of a patient would be:
    1 Severe burns
    2 Healing fracture
    3 Surgical infection
    4 Hay fever allergies

91. Raw eggs might cause food poisoning as a result of which of the following:
    1 *E. Coli*
    2 Salmonella
    3 *C. botulinum*
    4 Staphylococcus

92. The nurse is preparing to administer AquaMEPHYTON to a newborn. AquaMEPHYTON is the pharmaceutical term for:
    1 Vitamin A
    2 Vitamin D
    3 Vitamin K
    4 Vitamin C

93. A middle-aged woman is concerned because her mother has just been diagnosis with osteoporosis. She asks what she can do to limit her chances for getting osteoporosis. Which of the following should the nurse recommend?
    1 "Increase the potassium in your diet."
    2 "Try to increase dairy products in your diet."

3 "You should limit the amount of salt you eat."

4 "Increase the amount of protein you consume each day."

94. A patient's sister asks what type of postoperative nutrition her brother will need. The correct response by the nurse should be:

1 "All patients need total parenteral nutrition after surgery."

2 "It all depends on what kind of surgery was done and what your brother's condition is."

3 "Patients should experience a period of mini-starvation after surgery."

4 "IV fluids and an extremely high protein diet are indicated after surgery."

95. In addition to bananas, a patient on a potassium-depleting diuretic might consider which of the following dietary sources of the electrolyte?

1 Whole grains

2 Green and leafy vegetables

3 Red meats

4 Dairy products

96. The trace elements in the body are defined as:

1 Minerals that are not essential to health

2 Essential nutrients found in very small amounts

3 Only minerals that are found in the blood

4 Minerals that are undetectable by blood studies

97. The person with diabetes should have which assessment done to determine the average blood glucose levels over a 3-month interval?

1 Fasting blood glucose

2 Postprandial glucose

3 Glucose tolerance test

4 HgA1C

98. Because of the high levels of homocysteine in the blood of patients with end-stage renal disease, supplementation with which of the following is recommended?

1 Saturated fats and cholesterol

2 Ascorbic acid and choline

3 Folic acid and vitamin B_{12}

4 Potassium and sodium

99. Increasing bone mineral density during childhood and adolescence reduces the risk of developing which condition in later life?

1 Osteoporosis

2 Osteomalacia

3 Osteomyelitis

4 Osteosarcoma

100. Which of the following is likely to have the greatest impact on the eating habits of adolescents?

1 Nutrition knowledge

2 Availability of nutritious foods

3 Instructions from parents and health care professionals

4 Personal beliefs toward nutrition.

101. Increased incidence of coronary heart disease (CHD) is associated with which of the following?

1 Elevated levels of serum TC and LDL, with reduced levels of HDL

2 Reduced levels of serum TC and LDL, with elevated levels of HDL

3 Elevated levels of serum TC and HDL, with reduced levels of LDL

4 Reduced levels of serum TC and HDL, with elevated levels of LDL

102. Which of the following diets strongly predisposes humans to the development of colon cancer?

1 High in fiber and fruits, low in fats and calories

2 Low in fats and calories, high in fruits and fibers

3 High in fats and calories, low in fruits and fibers

4 Low in calories and vegetables, high in fruits and fats

103. After the age of 30, as lean body mass declines, a gradual but accelerated decrease occurs in which of the following?

1 Body mass index

2 Basal metabolic rate

3 Bone mineral density

4 Blood glucose metabolism

104. The mother of a 16-year-old girl reports to the nurse that her daughter has been eating large amounts of food sometimes and throwing up afterwards. In addition, the girl is exercising much more than she did in the past. The nurse should explore the possibility that the daughter has which of the following?

1 Anorexia nervosa

2 Bulimia nervosa

3 Binge eating disorder

4 Compulsive eating disorder

105. An excess body weight of 30% is associated with an increase risk of mortality of what range?

1 5% to 10%

2 10% to 20%

3 25% to 40%

4 55% to 75%

106. A patient in prenatal clinic asks the nurse about the value of getting a "hair analysis" to learn what her nutritional status is. The nurse should tell the patient:

1 The usefulness of hair analysis in general practice is not recommended by health professionals.

2 Hair analysis is a valuable way to determine mineral content and therefore predictive of nutritional needs.

3 The relationship between hair levels and blood levels is well documented for most nutrients.

4 Keratin in hair is similar to other body tissues and provides a reliable index of mineral content in other tissues.

107. Guidelines for nutrition during lactation include:

1 Decreasing the amount of calories consumed during pregnancy to prevent additional weight gain

2 Limiting fluids to 4 to 6 glasses per day to prevent fluid overload

3 Increasing the energy intake by approximately 500 kilocalories more than the usual adult allowance

4 Increasing the amount of fats in the diet to assure ample absorption of fat-soluble vitamins by the baby

108. A patient who does not like to drink water asks the nurse if it is okay to drink 6 to 8 glasses of tea a day instead. The nurse should tell her:

1 "Tea is a good substitute, especially if you like the taste. Be sure to add enough sugar to make it flavorful too."

2 "Tea is a diuretic and increases your need for fluids. You might try sparkling water or water flavored with fruit flavors."

3 "Drinking tea with meals helps absorb iron from the foods."

4 "Tea is better than coffee because it does not contain caffeine."

109. The macronutrients with the greatest sources of energy in the diet are:
    1 Protein and carbohydrates
    2 Carbohydrates and fats
    3 Fats and proteins
    4 Carbohydrates and vitamins

110. A patient who was admitted for treatment of food poisoning mentions to the nurse that he saw a bandage on the hand of the person at the fast food restaurant where he bought his chicken dinner. The nurse explains to the patient that he most likely has been infected with which of the following?
    1 *Clostridium perfringens*
    2 *Salmonella typhi*
    3 *Escherichia coli*
    4 *Staphylococcus aureus*

111. In teaching new mothers about nutrition safety the nurse should include cautions about botulism in honey for which of the following age groups?
    1 Infants
    2 Adolescents
    3 Middle-aged adults
    4 Older adults

112. A female patient says that, during premenstrual syndrome, she has symptoms of hypoglycemia, but they do not respond to eating food. What should the nurse tell the patient about this phenomenon?
    1 "You are probably eating the wrong foods. You should include high-calorie carbohydrates such as candy or fruit juice."
    2 "Although the symptoms are similar, this is probably not hypoglycemia, and will not respond to the same treatment."
    3 "Have you tried taking crackers and milk for the symptoms?"
    4 "The next time this happens, be sure to get a blood sugar done so we can prescribe a proper diet for you."

113. Children and adolescents are particularly susceptible to iron-deficiency anemia for which of the following reasons?
    1 Their diets are deficient in trace minerals necessary to absorb the iron that they get in food intake.
    2 Iron is filtered from the bloodstream and excreted by the kidneys during growth spurts.
    3 They use greater amounts of iron for growth, and they prefer foods that are low in iron content.
    4 They do not absorb as much iron from their diet and they will not take supplements.

114. A patient is admitted to the ER complaining of pronounced thirst, loss of coordination, mental confusion with irritability, dry skin, and tenting, and decreased urinary output. The nurse recognizes these symptoms as warning signs of what condition?
    _____

115. On an 1800-calorie diabetic exchange diet, how many bread exchanges are allowed in 1 day? Choose all that apply.
    1 5 to 10
    2 10 to 15
    3 15 to 20
    4 20 to 25

116. The term "pouching" refers to which of the following?
    1 Development of enlarged villi in the small intestine that are known as diverticula

    2 Adipose deposits around the middle of the body that give the appearance of an abdominal pouch
    3 Retaining pieces of food or medications between the cheeks in gums
    4 Carrying a small bag with emergency food and medications in case of a diabetic reaction away from home

117. The WIC program is designed to meet which of the following needs? Choose all that apply.
    1 Nutrition education
    2 Vouchers for prescribed supplemental foods
    3 Meals on Wheels to homebound elderly patients
    4 Community meals for any low-income adult
    5 Dietary counseling for patients with eating disorders

118. The designation of "GRAS" means that food additives are:
    1 Derived from plant origins
    2 Unsafe for use with small children and pregnant women
    3 Added to genetically modified foods to retain freshness
    4 Generally recognized as safe

119. A patient with diabetes who has been reading food labels asks the nurse about food additives such as alginate, lecithin, agar, and carrageenan. The nurse should tell the patient that the reason for using these additives is which of the following?
    1 To improve nutritive value
    2 To impart and maintain desired consistency
    3 To enhance flavor
    4 To maintain appearance, palatability and wholesomeness

120. Alcoholism contributes to poor nutrition in which of the following ways?
    1 Increased pancreatic secretions block digestion of nutrients
    2 Increased liver stores of fat-soluble vitamins that hamper metabolism
    3 Reduced intake and metabolism of essential nutrients
    4 Increased pancreatic secretions and rapid breakdown of nutrients

121. A patient who has been taking a tricyclic antidepressant for several weeks complains to the nurse that she is gaining weight and cannot seem to lose it. The nurse should tell her:
    1 "This is an alarming occurrence, and you should make an appointment with your psychiatrist immediately."
    2 "Have you been eating more junk food and snacks? That can put on the pounds pretty quickly."
    3 "This is a common side effect of tricyclic antidepressants. Let's take a look at your food diary and see if there is a way we can help control this while you continue to take the medication."
    4 "You should stop taking the medication right away, and see if you can lose the weight."

122. A patient who has been taking disulfiram (Antabuse) reports to the nurse that at a banquet last night he had a flushing reaction and had to leave the dinner. He is very embarrassed and wants to know how to prevent this from happening again. The nurse should tell him:
    1 "In addition to alcoholic beverages, a reaction can be triggered from eating foods with alcohol in them, such as sauces that may not have been cooked thoroughly and may still have an alcoholic content."
    2 "That was probably just a freak accidental happening. I'm sure it won't take place again."

3 "As long as you never eat the same foods again, you should be okay."

4 "Are you sure you didn't use too much aftershave or cologne before you left the house?"

123. After 6 weeks on medical nutrition therapy to lower his LDL cholesterol, a patient receives the good news that his target has been realized. He tells the nurse that he is relieved to know that he can now resume his previous diet. The nurse should tell him:

1 "The medical nutrition therapy you have been prescribed should continue uninterrupted to keep your cholesterol levels from going back up again."

2 "That is good news! I'm so happy for you."

3 "It may take several weeks for you to be able to tolerate your previous diet again."

4 "If you increased your exercise regimen, you could return to your previous diet much faster."

124. A patient with diabetes calls and reports to the nurse that she is nauseated and coughing a lot. She is not able to manage solid foods and wants to know if she should skip her diabetes medication until she feels better. The nurse should tell her:

1 "Yes, because otherwise you will have a hypoglycemic reaction."

2 "Even though you can't take solid foods, you will need the medication to cover soft and liquid foods that you may have."

3 "Don't take the medication again until you can tolerate a full diet of solid foods."

4 "It's okay to stop the medication, but you should start taking it again if you have any symptoms of a reaction."

125. The foods that are the most likely to raise serum cholesterol levels are:

1 Foods that have no TFAs

2 Foods that are high in unsaturated fats

3 Foods that are fat free

4 Foods that are high in saturated fats

ANSWERS AND RATIONALES

1. Knowledge, implementation, physiological integrity (a).
   4 The nurse knows that the main function of cellulose is to create bulk in the intestine, aiding in bowel elimination.
   1 This is not the main function of cellulose and describes the role of the mineral sodium.
   2 This describes the role of protein in the body.
   3 Simple sugars provide a rapid source of energy.

2. Application, implementation, safe, effective care environment (b).
   1 Calcium and iron are the minerals most likely to be deficient throughout the life span in the American diet.
   2 Although deficiencies may arise, these do not constitute the most deficient minerals.
   3 Potassium and sodium are readily available in a variety of food sources.
   4 For most individuals, phosphorous and calcium are readily available by consuming milk products.

3. Application, planning, physiological integrity (b).
   4 The walkers will need to replace any lost fluids resulting from perspiration.
   1 Water is the most abundant body component, but this does not explain why it should be available to the walkers.
   2 Water will assist in the walkers' hydration status but will not prevent shin splints.
   3 Water is important to all individuals; however, the diabetic walkers need insulin to regulate glucose utilization in the body.

4. Application, implementation, physiological integrity (b).
   3 This explanation is short, geared to the child's knowledge level, and accurately condenses what the purpose of iodine is in the body.
   1 This correctly explains why calcium and phosphorus are necessary for the body.
   2 Calcium and vitamin K are essential for blood clotting.
   4 This explains the role iron plays in hemoglobin.

5. Application, planning, physiological integrity (b).
   2 Vitamins essential for wound healing include vitamins A and C.
   1 Vitamins A and D can be readily found in fortified milk and assist in healing fractures.
   2 Vitamins B_6 and C, although important in an adequate diet, are not specific for tissue healing.
   4 These vitamins are also not specific for tissue healing, although important in the diet.

6. Application, evaluation, physiological integrity (b).
   4 Hamburgers and peanut butter and jelly sandwiches would provide a diet high in protein and calories.
   1 Although high in calories, these foods are not as high in protein as are hamburgers and peanut butter and jelly sandwiches.
   2 Oranges and applesauce contain vitamins necessary for tissue healing; however, they are low in protein and calories.
   3 Although high in vitamin content, these foods are not high in protein or calories.

7. Comprehension, implementation, physiological integrity (b).
   4 Caffeine stimulates gastric acid secretions, potentially aggravating peptic ulcer disease.
   1 Caffeine does dehydrate the body, but this is not the reason why it is restricted in peptic ulcer disease.

2 This is not the rationale behind a caffeine-restricted diet.
3 Caffeine does not buffer milk or antacids.

8. Comprehension, planning, physiological integrity (b).
   2 The products of protein metabolism contribute to the accumulation of urea that will further worsen metabolic acidosis.
   1 Fats are given to provide energy and to allow protein to be used for tissue building.
   3 Vitamins need to be supplemented in low-protein diets.
   4 Carbohydrates are given to provide energy and allow protein to be used for tissue synthesis.

9. Comprehension, implementation, health promotion and maintenance (b).
   3 This is the truest statement. In the past, weight was restricted, but the focus is now on gaining enough weight to safeguard the baby's health.
   1 This is not true for the majority of pregnant women.
   2 This does not provide information to the patient and blocks communication.
   4 Although true in the past, this weight gain is probably too much for the majority of pregnant women.

10. Application, implementation, health promotion and maintenance (b).
    1 The caloric needs of the pregnant woman increase by 300 calories per day.
    2 The lactating mother needs to increase her calories to 500 calories per day.
    3 Unless severely malnourished, 750 calories is generally too many additional calories.
    4 Unless instructed by a physician, 1000 calories is too much of an increase.

11. Comprehension, planning, health promotion and maintenance (b).
    2 A high-carbohydrate diet (80% of calories) consumed for several days before an event can greatly improve endurance time and performance.
    1 A high-fat diet (90% of calories) increases endurance approximately one half as much as does a high-carbohydrate diet.
    3 Increasing all nutrients will not most likely decrease endurance and performance.
    4 Protein is not one of the nutrients that fuel activity.

12. Comprehension, implementation, health promotion and maintenance (b).
    3 Frequent small low-fat meals and snacks (fairly dry) will not overfill the stomach, which causes distension, discomfort, and nausea.
    1 The feeling of fullness from eating fats may increase nausea and vomiting.
    2 Increased protein foods will not alleviate the nausea and vomiting associated with pregnancy.
    4 Drinking beverages with meals will cause excessive gastric filling, contributing to nausea and vomiting.

13. Knowledge, assessment, physiological integrity (b).
    2 Some individuals can tolerate increasing amounts of dairy products if their production of lactase is stimulated.
    1 Dairy products contain vital nutrients that are difficult to find in other foods.
    3 Supplements can provide these nutrients without uncomfortable side effects for the patient.
    4 Substitution may be an alternative if the patient's body does not increase production of lactase.

14. Application, implementation, physiological integrity (b).
    1 A diet low in fat may lead to a deficiency in the fat-soluble vitamin A.
    2 Vitamin C is water soluble. A low-fat diet would not lead to a deficiency, although a diet that is overall low in calories may.
    3 Minerals are water soluble, and a low-fat diet would not lead to a deficiency.
    4 Carbohydrates are the food choice most likely for an individual on a low-fat diet.

15. Knowledge, assessment, physiological integrity (a).
    3 Hypertension and congestive heart failure are two pathological conditions that may require sodium restriction.
    1 Hyperlipidemia would require a dietary fat modification. Renal failure may require restriction in water and protein.
    2 Hypercholesterolemia would require restriction of foods high in cholesterol.
    4 Hyperlipidemia may require a low-fat diet.

16. Comprehension, planning, health promotion and maintenance (a).
    2 Manufacturers are required by the Food and Drug Administration (FDA) and the U.S. Department of Agriculture (USDA) to list sodium content along with other nutrients on package labels.
    1 This is not as readily available as is the information on a package label.
    3 This information would not be convenient to use while shopping.
    4 This information is not as readily available as is the listing on a package label.

17. Knowledge, assessment, physiological integrity (a).
    1 Iron-deficiency anemia is the most prevalent form of anemia and is caused by inadequate absorption of iron or insufficient intake or increased needs not being met (adolescence, pregnancy).
    2 Pernicious anemia is caused by a deficiency of vitamin B_{12} because of a lack of intrinsic factor.
    3 Folic-acid deficiency is common in perinatal population.
    4 Anemia from a vitamin-B_{12} deficiency is termed pernicious anemia.

18. Comprehension, planning, physiological integrity (b).
    3 By eating good sources of vitamin C uncooked, the majority of the vitamin can be preserved.
    1 Excessive cooking will cause vitamin C to evaporate or leech out into the cooking water.
    2 This will not preserve vitamin C.
    4 Although a good idea, this does not minimize the loss of vitamin C in foods.

19. Application, implementation, physiological integrity (b).
    4 Vitamin-B_{12} injections are given to elderly patients because of the decrease of intrinsic factor in their stomach acid. Vitamin B_{12} cannot be absorbed without intrinsic factor and must be supplemented to prevent pernicious anemia from developing.
    1 Vitamin C prevents scurvy.
    2 Pellagra is caused by a deficiency in niacin.
    3 Marasmus is a term for general starvation.

20. Comprehension, planning, physiological integrity (c).
    3 Many individuals with stomatitis are able to eat foods that are neither hot nor cold and may find it more comfortable if the food is served at room temperature.
    1 This is a dietary recommendation for anorexia.
    2 Swallowing fluids may be as uncomfortable for the patient because taking in solids and will fill the stomach at the expense of nutrients.
    4 This may not be possible, and protein-rich foods will not help the problem of stomatitis.

21. Knowledge, planning, health promotion and maintenance (b).
    2 The Dietary Guidelines for Americans recommends that individuals decrease their intake of saturated fats.
    1 This is likely to increase the risk of cancer.
    3 Studies have shown that raw fruits and vegetables can alleviate some types of cancer.
    4 The preservatives in smoked and salt-cured meats have been linked to some types of cancer.

22. Knowledge, assessment, physiological integrity (b).
    2 Urine needs to be diluted to prevent the formation of additional kidney stones.
    1 Although the majority of kidney stones are composed of calcium, intake is not restricted.
    3 No vitamin or mineral deficiencies are associated with kidney stones.
    4 Diet therapy is not aimed in alleviating the side effects of any drugs given. Few drugs are used in treating kidney stones.

23. Application, evaluation, physiological integrity (a).
    2 Although diet therapy is not as effective in managing gout as are medications, the general acceptance is that a diet low in purines will diminish uric acid in the body.
    1 Weight loss is usually indicated and would require a low calorie diet. Fatty foods precipitate attacks.
    3 Alcohol precipitates exacerbations and should be avoided.
    4 A liberal fluid intake is encouraged to flush the minerals from the body.

24. Comprehension, planning, physiological integrity (b).
    4 The resident's individual needs are addressed. Some solutions are easier for individuals to digest, making the absorption of nutrients easier.
    1 Hypertonic solutions are not used often because they pull water into the intestine and cause diarrhea.
    2 Although similar in appearance, many solutions are tailored to meet the individual needs of individuals.
    3 Tube feeding solutions can be used only if the GI tract is functional.

25. Application, evaluation, physiological integrity (b).
    2 A jejunostomy tube is the best choice to decrease the possibility of aspiration in a patient with dysphagia because it is lower in the GI tract. The chance of dumping syndrome and diarrhea are increased.
    1 The chance of aspiration is still quite high with a gastrostomy tube because reflux in the esophagus can occur.
    3 Duodenostomy tubes are not common; however, if they were placed, the level of risk would be greater than that of a jejunostomy tube but less than that of a gastrostomy tube.
    4 The chance for aspiration is high when using a nasal feeding tube.

26. Application, assessment, physiological integrity (c).
    2 One side effect of ACE inhibitor antihypertensive medication is retention of potassium.
    1 Aerobic exercise may be helpful in weight reduction and blood pressure management.

3 Photosensitivity is not a side effect of ACE inhibitors.

4 The negative effects of nitrites are related to their correlation with cancer.

27. Knowledge, evaluation, physiological integrity (b).

2 The best method to preserve the nutrient content of food is steaming.

1 Frying causes leeching of nutrients, and the food is less nutritious because of the addition of fat for frying.

3 Steaming can be done in the microwave; however, normal microwave cooking causes some evaporation of water-soluble vitamins to take place.

4 Soaking will cause the nutrients to leech out into the water used for soaking.

28. Application, implementation, health promotion and maintenance (b).

4 If the patient is Jewish and keeping kosher dietary laws, his meals will need to be prepared and served in accordance with the restrictions.

1 This is a block in communication; the nurse must work with him to meet his needs while still observing his restrictions and preferences.

2 This is failure to communicate with the patient and discounting the importance of his dietary preferences.

3 As presented, this is a threatening statement, although this may eventually need to be done to satisfy the patient's wishes.

29. Application, implementation, physiological integrity (c).

4 This is the only response that preserves the patient's need for religious influence while recognizing that a solution to this problem must be found.

1 This response is condescending to the patient and will likely be met with resistance.

2 This is not conducive to the management of diabetes mellitus.

3 This response places the patient in a dependent, passive, role.

30. Application, planning, physiological integrity (b).

2 PCOS is related to hyperinsulinism and makes weight control and blood glucose management important issues to include in patient teaching.

1 This condition is not associated with PCOS.

3 Hypertension in the patient with PCOS is most likely related to obesity and may be resolved with weight management.

4 This condition is not associated with PCOS.

31. Knowledge, planning, physiological integrity (a).

4 In addition to conditions such as diabetes, low levels of magnesium in the blood can also be caused by alcoholism, malabsorption, hyperthyroidism, use of steroids, and massive blood transfusions.

1 The major food sources of magnesium are those containing chlorophyll, such as dark-green leafy vegetables.

2 Magnesium plays a role in metabolic processes at a cellular level and in muscle contractions.

3 This is a relatively common mineral deficiency in the general population.

32. Application, implementation, safe, effective care environment (b).

3 The cheese and crackers will provide the patient with IDDM complex carbohydrates, which will be used to stabilize blood glucose levels.

1 Ice cream would provide too many calories and not enough complex carbohydrates.

2 Cookies have too much refined sugar and will raise the person's blood glucose level too high.

4 Although it would depend on the cake's ingredients, generally, chocolate cake has too much refined sugar.

33. Application, planning, physiological integrity (b).

3 A small snack composed of carbohydrates will fuel the patient's extra activity.

1 Fats are incompletely burned for energy and will result in the glucose level increasing too quickly.

2 Diet should be modified, not the medication.

4 Once again, medication adjustments are not necessary. This will result in insulin shock.

34. Application, assessment, physiological integrity (b).

2 The body mass index (BMI) is now the standard for determining appropriate body size.

1 This determines the rate at which nutrients are broken down in the body.

3 This is used to determine the extent of injuries, such as burns.

4 This measurement is not affected by body fat stores.

35. Comprehension, planning, physiological integrity (b).

3 Leptin alters the levels of neuropeptides and affects weight regulation and feeling satisfied after eating.

1 Leptin acts within the hypothalamus.

2 Leptin decreases the lipogenic activity of insulin.

4 Obese individuals may be resistant to leptin at a cellular level.

36. Knowledge, planning, physiological integrity (b).

3 All women of childbearing age should consume 0.4 mg of folic acid daily to prevent the development of spina bifida in unborn babies.

1 Pyridoxine deficiency is not associated with neural tube defects.

2 Riboflavin deficiency is not associated with neural tube defects.

4 Ascorbic acid deficiency is not associated with neural tube defects.

37. Knowledge, planning, physiological integrity (b).

3 Riboflavin deficiency often results in cheilosis, especially among older adults, as well as general dermatitis.

1 Cobalamin deficiency is associated with pernicious anemia.

2 Niacin deficiency is associated with pellagra.

4 Thiamin deficiency is associated with neuropathy.

38. Knowledge, planning, physiological integrity (b).

4 High-sodium, animal protein, sugar, and low-calcium intake are implicated in the prevalence of kidney stones in Western countries.

1, 2, 3 These are not associated with kidney stones.

39. Knowledge, planning, physiological integrity (b).

4 A child with this type of malnutrition usually has stunted growth, edema, and skin sores related to decreased protein intake.

1 Fat deficiency is not associated with kwashiorkor.

2 Carbohydrates deficiency is not associated with kwashiorkor.

3 Vitamin deficiency is not associated with kwashiorkor.

40. Comprehension, planning, physiological integrity (b).

4 Vitamin K is essential for the formation of prothrombin.

1 Vitamin B_{12} helps prevent pernicious anemia.

2   Ascorbic acid promotes skin integrity and immune function.

3   Vitamin A promotes good vision and bone growth.

41. Comprehension, planning, physiological integrity (b).

3   Claims made by manufacturers are not always based on actual data, and these products may not be safe even though they are sold to the general public.

1   No research is available to support the claims that ergogenic aids are safe and effective.

2   The use of anabolic steroids has been linked to numerous serious health problems, such as brain cancer.

4   This is the research laboratory use range; the same benefit can be gained with a dose as low as 3 g daily.

42. Application, assessment, physiological integrity (b).

3   Indicates return of bowel sounds; peristalsis has started and oral feedings may be indicated.

1   Hunger is not an accurate predictor of return of bowel function.

2   Although she may be able to tolerate foods, this does not mean peristalsis has returned.

4   Distension can indicate lack of peristalsis.

43. Comprehension, application, physiological integrity (b).

3   Avoiding these helps the esophageal sphincter to function better, thereby helping prevent reflux.

1   The use of frequent small meals helps reduce pressure on the stomach.

2   Reflux is more likely when the patient lies down with a full stomach.

4   Alcohol makes it harder for the esophageal sphincter to work properly, increasing the likelihood of reflux.

44. Knowledge, assessment, physiological integrity (b).

3   Sorbitol, a naturally occurring sugar that is not absorbed, is found in high amounts in apple juice.

1   Citrus juices have a higher content of vitamin C than does apple juice and are more likely to cause diarrhea from that vitamin.

2   Pectin is found in apples, but it is more likely to prevent or cure diarrhea rather than to cause it.

4   An average apple provides about 60 mg of magnesium that is beneficial in the treatment of diarrhea as an electrolyte replacement.

45. Comprehension, planning, physiological integrity (c).

4   Current research indicates that frequent small meals of complex carbohydrates and fibers will maintain a more stable blood glucose level.

1   Reactive hypoglycemia may result from the intake of simple sugars.

2   Fiber slows gastric emptying and carbohydrate absorption, thus supporting a consistent release of glucose into the bloodstream.

3   A high-protein, low-carbohydrate diet restricts the body's ability to obtain sufficient amounts of glucose to achieve and maintain normal blood glucose levels.

46. Comprehension, implementation, health promotion and maintenance (b).

3   Practices such as storing vitamin-C foods cut up rather than whole, storing unwrapped, and overcooking in large amounts of water will significantly decrease the amount of vitamin C in a substance.

1   This is untrue; it is water soluble.

2   These are the deficiency symptoms of vitamin A.

4   Current research indicates that vitamin C has a minor effect on reducing the number and severity of cold symptoms.

47. Comprehension, implementation, physiological integrity (b).

3   Food habits are established early and are difficult to change. Incorporating favorite foods will enhance compliance.

1   This is closing communication and may not enhance compliance.

2   This understanding may exist, but it does not encourage compliance.

4   The attack may have been mild, but behaviors need to change to help prevent a more serious episode.

48. Comprehension, planning, physiological integrity (b).

3   These are plant foods that have no saturated fats.

1   These are foods that are high in saturated fats.

2, 4   These animal foods are high in saturated fats.

49. Comprehension, planning, physiological integrity (b).

4   Legume storage protein foods such as beans and peas are good sources of quality protein.

1   A mixture of plant proteins can provide adequate amounts of amino acids.

2   Although animal and vegetable proteins can complement each other, obtaining adequate amino acid intake from plant sources alone is possible.

3   The incomplete protein foods are mostly of plant origin.

50. Knowledge, implementation, physiological integrity (b).

2   TPN is used long term in cases of major surgery, when a patient is unable to obtain sufficient oral nourishment.

1   TPN is not given through a peripheral vein, but through a large, central vein.

3   TPN does not involve the GI tract.

4   TPN is given through a large, central vein.

51. Application, implementation, psychosocial integrity (b).

4   Malnutrition contributes to a compromised immune system. Participating in his meal planning and preparation is one way for him to have control over his health.

1   This closes communication; the patient may never be "ready" to communicate if no supportive intervention takes place.

2   Written material is more appropriate after a discussion, as a way of reinforcing the information given.

3   This sets up a barrier to communication because the nurse has no way of knowing if this is true or not.

52. Application, implementation, physiological integrity (b).

3   Sufficient amounts of gastric acid are necessary to separate the vitamin from the protein fibers in meats so it can be absorbed.

1   Zollinger-Ellison syndrome results in severe gastric ulcers.

2   Marasmus is a malnutrition state that results from a diet that is deficient in protein and carbohydrate.

4   Diverticulosis produces alterations in bowel function such as constipation or diarrhea.

53. Knowledge, planning, physiological integrity (b).

3   Gas production in the GI tract is the result of poorly digested carbohydrates, such as fructose, raffinose, and stachyose.

1   Swallowing air while eating or drinking is more likely to produce burping than does expulsion of flatus.

2 Excessive fluid intake with meals may produce additional gas caused by difficulty digesting increased volume.

4 These foods are high in starches that are resistant to the pancreatic enzyme amylase and may produce greater amounts of intestinal gas as their consumption is increased.

54. Knowledge, assessment, health promotion and maintenance (a).

   1 Homeostasis is the result of the body's attempt to coordinate responses to disturbances in normal condition or function.

   2 Metabolism is the process of breaking down nutrients and building body tissues from them.

   3 Catabolism is the process of breaking down complex chemical compounds in the body into simpler substances.

   4 Anabolism is the process of building up complex chemical compounds in the body from smaller simpler compounds.

55. Knowledge, implementation, physiological integrity (b).

   3 These foods are all very high in vitamin A (more than 2000 μg per serving).

   1 These foods contain small amounts of vitamin A (30 to 60 μg per serving).

   2 These foods contain small amounts of vitamin A (100 to 200 μg per serving).

   4 These foods contain moderate amounts of vitamin A (200 to 400 μg per serving).

56. Knowledge, planning, physiological integrity (a).

   2 All three are high in potassium.

   1 Good sources of vitamin D but not potassium

   3 Good sources of calcium and phosphorus but not potassium.

   4 Good sources of vitamin C but not potassium.

57. Knowledge, planning, physiological integrity (b).

   4 Substituting other flavorings for high-sodium salt can make it easier to cut down on the amount of salt used.

   1 Fresh fruits and vegetables are low in salt and can be used freely on a sodium-restricted diet.

   2 Dairy products contain much salt.

   3 Canned and processed meats are high in salt.

58. Application, planning, physiological integrity (b).

   4 Vitamin E is a powerful antioxidant that has effects on cell membranes and stimulates immune function in elderly people.

   1 This is true of vitamin K.

   2 This is true of vitamin D.

   3 This is true of vitamin A.

59. Knowledge, implementation, physiological integrity (b).

   4 When vitamin C is absent, the basis for collagen does not develop and fibers formed remain defective and weak.

   1 Vitamin E does not help develop collagen.

   2 Calcium does not help develop collagen.

   3 Sodium does not help develop collagen.

60. Knowledge, planning, physiological integrity (b).

   3 The body can use tryptophan to make niacin.

   1, 2, 4 These are not related to pellagra.

61. Knowledge, assessment, physiological integrity (b).

   4 Many nutrients are lost during the cooking process.

   1 No correlation exists between a meal's price and nutrient value.

2 Grading of canned goods is related to appearance rather than nutritive value.

3 Refined products have many of the nutrients removed; fortified foods have added nutritive value.

62. Application, assessment, health promotion and maintenance (b).

   3 Irregular eating habits and age are two factors that would cause the nurse concern.

   1 This pattern of weight gain is not excessive and should meet the nutrition demands of the baby.

   2 This is typical of this time of pregnancy, caused by the uterus pressing on the diaphragm.

   4 Physiological anemia in pregnancy is often caused by increased blood volume. True anemia is diagnosed by blood studies and treated by a physician.

63. Application, implementation, physiological integrity (b).

   4 For nonendurance events, plain water prevents dehydration; minerals are obtained in the diet.

   1 Vitamins do not provide energy.

   2 Athletes involved in endurance events may possibly need a 10% sugar solution to replace water and carbohydrates.

   3 Minerals can be replaced in the diet.

64. Knowledge, implementation, physiological integrity (b).

   3 Extra carbohydrates will assist in counteracting the negative nitrogen balance caused by massive trauma.

   1 Vitamins do not supply energy.

   2 This is true, but it does not answer the question.

   4 Protein supplies nutrition.

65. Comprehension, assessment, physiological integrity (a).

   2 Sodium, which is used widely as a preservative, is implicated in the development of hypertension.

   1 Supplements such as vitamins and minerals do not contribute to hypertension.

   3 Although genetically modified foods have been implicated in other health problems, they do not necessarily contribute to hypertension.

   4 Fresh fruits and vegetables help reduce or prevent hypertension because they decrease the amount of sodium intake in the diet.

66. Knowledge, planning, physiological integrity (b).

   2 INH blocks the conversion of vitamin B₆ to active form in the body and can lead to deficiency of this vitamin.

   1 INH does not affect vitamin C.

   3 INH does not affect calcium.

   4 INH does not affect milk.

67. Comprehension, planning, physiological integrity (c).

   3 Grapefruit juice blocks a liver enzyme, thus increasing bioavailability of the drug. This effect may last for up to 72 hours after consuming the juice.

   1 The pills can be taken on an empty stomach.

   2 Antacids do not interact with the medication.

   4 This precaution is true of medications such as potassium, which can have an irritating effect on the stomach.

68. Knowledge, planning, physiological integrity (b).

   4 Rice does not contain gluten.

   1 Oats do contain gluten.

   2 Rye does contain gluten.

   3 Wheat does contain gluten.

69. Application, planning, physiological integrity (b).
    2 Other foods rich in tyramine include certain cheeses, red wines, and broad beans.
    1, 3, 4 These foods are not rich in tyramine.

70. Knowledge, planning, health promotion and maintenance (b).
    1 Of the foods listed, rice cereal causes the fewest allergies in children.
    2 Cow's milk is known to cause allergic reactions in certain children.
    3 Wheat, oats, and barley cereals cause more allergic reactions than does rice cereal.
    4 Egg whites can cause allergic reactions.

71. Knowledge, planning, health promotion and maintenance (b).
    4 Because aspartame is an essential amino acid and therefore necessary for growth, it must be included in the diet; but careful monitoring of blood levels must be followed.
    1 Aspartame is 50% phenylalanine.
    2 Milk is high in phenylalanine. Dietary management would include using a milk substitute.
    3 This would lead to CNS damage in the patient.

72. Knowledge, planning, physiological integrity (c).
    3 Glucose is needed to help restore reserves in the liver; fat makes food more palatable and will encourage the patient with no appetite to eat more; protein is needed to help repair damaged liver cells.
    1 This diet will not support the recovery of the liver.
    2 This diet will not support recovery of the liver and will, in fact, place a strain on it because of the high-fat content.
    4 This diet will not support the recovery of the liver.

73. Comprehension, planning, physiological integrity (a).
    1 Citrus juices contain vitamin C, which helps in the absorption of iron.
    2 Fish liver oils contain vitamins A and D, not vitamin C.
    3 Green leafy vegetables contain vitamins A, E, and K, not vitamin C.
    4 Milk and dairy products contain no vitamin C.

74. Knowledge, assessment, physiological integrity (b).
    1 The exchange system is based on the fact that each food within an exchange is equivalent in nutrients to every other one. Therefore substituting one food for another within an exchange does not significantly alter the diet.
    2 One advantage of using the exchange system is that specialized foods are not needed.
    3 A dietician sets up the recommended number of exchanges, but the individual can make substitutions.
    4 Food exchanges are important to space nutrient ingestion over the entire day so that the body is able to metabolize each.

75. Application, planning, physiological integrity (a).
    3 TFAs raise the level of LDL cholesterol levels even more than do saturated fats.
    1 TFAs do not affect vitamin absorption.
    2 All types of fats increase calorie consumption.
    4 TFAs do not reduce the level of HDL in the blood.

76. Application, implementation, physiological integrity (c).
    2 The egg is on the meat list, the biscuit is on the bread exchange, and the teaspoon of butter and margarine is two fat exchanges.

1 The breakfast has no milk, only one bread and two fats.
3 The breakfast has no vegetables.
4 The breakfast has no fruit or milk, only one meat and two fat exchanges.

77. Knowledge, planning, physiological integrity (a).
    2 Oranges and orange juice are readily digestible and easily absorbed.
    1 Cereal is a starch and takes longer to be absorbed.
    3 Crackers are also a starch and would take longer to be digested and absorbed.
    4 Bread and butter (starch and fat) both take longer to be absorbed.

78. Application, planning, physiological integrity (b).
    4 The low protein provided on this diet limits end products of protein metabolism—an important consideration in kidney disease.
    1 Steak and milk provide more protein than is desirable for this patient.
    2 Hamburger and milk provide protein not desirable in this case.
    3 Liver, cottage cheese, eggs and cream provide a high-protein diet.

79. Knowledge, planning, physiological integrity (a).
    1 Parenteral nutrition allows the intestines to rest without stimulating pancreatic secretions.
    2, 3, 4 Oral feedings stimulate pancreatic secretions.

80. Knowledge, application, physiological integrity (b).
    3 Although spicy foods can aggravate peptic ulcer disease, the causative agent is the bacterium *H. pylori*.
    1 Although smoking and alcohol use contribute to ulcer development, they are not the primary cause.
    2 Although these aggravate the disease, they are not the causes.
    4 Adequate rest and relaxation enhance the body's natural healing process, but stress does not cause ulcers.

81. Knowledge, implementation, physiological integrity (b).
    1 Soft diets are easier to digest, thereby reducing the workload of the heart.
    2 Decreasing irritation to the digestive tract is not important in the diet therapy for cardiovascular disease.
    3 Unless the patient is overweight, no specific reason exists to reduce calories.
    4 This is not the primary reason for the soft diet in this situation.

82. Application, planning, physiological integrity (b).
    4 A high-fiber diet provides the bulk that stimulates peristalsis, thereby decreasing constipation.
    1 These provide very little residue.
    2 All foods in this meal provide very little residue.
    3 Once again, little fiber or residue is in these foods.

83. Knowledge, planning, health promotion and maintenance (b).
    2 This is the recommended limit of sodium in the diet for all adults.
    1 This is the typical sodium intake of people with heavy use of salt.
    3 This is inadequate sodium intake and is unlikely to be achieved with normal food intake.
    4 This is typical of persons with a light taste for salt, but it is greater than the recommended daily allowance.

84. Knowledge, assessment, physiological integrity (b).
    2 Aspirin may cause low-level blood loss from erosions in the stomach.
    1 Vitamin C is not likely to cause iron deficiency.
    3 Antacids are not likely to cause iron deficiency
    4 Anticonvulsants are not likely to cause iron deficiency.
85. Comprehension, planning, physiological integrity (b).
    1 Fat is the principal cause of contraction of the diseased gallbladder.
    2 The patient will still need to consume adequate intake for energy and metabolism.
    3 Dairy products tend to be high in fat and may aggravate the pain of gallbladder disease.
    4 Carbohydrates should be the primary source of energy, especially during the acute phase of gallbladder disease.
86. Application, planning, physiological integrity (b).
    1 Including high-fiber foods in menu planning facilitates lowered blood glucose and blood cholesterol.
    2 Fiber slows intestinal transit time.
    3 Fiber helps clear LDL cholesterol in the colon.
    4 Fiber delays gastric emptying time.
87. Knowledge, planning, physiological integrity (b).
    3 Because of anorexia, many patients with chronic renal disease do not have adequate intake of calories or protein.
    1 Patients with chronic renal disease need to maintain normal serum potassium and sodium blood levels.
    2 Patients with chronic renal disease need to maintain acceptable levels of phosphate and calcium.
    4 Fluid balance is needed to prevent dehydration or fluid overload.
88. Application, implementation, physiological integrity (b).
    4 This option provides soothing texture and temperature along with essential nutrients.
    1 Fatty sauces such as gravy are easier to swallow and add taste appeal to food items.
    2 These foods might irritate his mouth and make him less likely to want to eat.
    3 Snacks and frequent small meals are a good way to provide nutrition with less energy expenditure on the part of the patient.
89. Knowledge, assessment, physiological integrity (b).
    1 Purging after eating can cause irreversible damage to the enamel of teeth caused by increased acid content of the mouth.
    2, 3 These are not commonly associated with bulimia.
    4 The person with bulimia is more likely to experience hypoglycemia because of inadequate intake or retention of food.
90. Knowledge, evaluation, physiological integrity (b).
    4 Normally, the caloric needs of individuals with hay fever do not increase.
    1 Severe burns require the greatest increase in calories to maintain body weight.
    2 Healing fractures requires increased calories, in addition to calcium, phosphorus, and vitamin D.
    3 Any surgery places stress on the body, increasing the body's need for calories.
91. Knowledge, assessment, physiological integrity (a).
    2 Raw eggs can be contaminated with Salmonella, and vulnerable groups such as older adults, persons who are ill, babies, and pregnant women should avoid them.
    1 *E. coli* infections are associated with undercooked beef or raw milk.
    3 Botulism is associated with inadequately processed or preserved foods.
    4 Staphylococcus infections are associated with skin contaminants.
92. Knowledge, implementation, physiological integrity (b).
    3 AquaMEPHYTON is the pharmacologic term for vitamin K and is given shortly after birth.
    1 The pharmaceutical term for vitamin A is retinoic acid.
    2 The pharmaceutical name for vitamin D is ergocalciferol.
    4 The pharmaceutical term for vitamin C is ascorbic acid.
93. Comprehension, planning, health promotion and maintenance (b).
    2 Increasing dairy products will increase the woman's calcium intake, which can prevent the development of osteoporosis.
    1 This does not have a significance in preventing osteoporosis.
    3 This will not affect the development of osteoporosis.
    4 Protein will not prevent osteoporosis, but increasing calcium-rich protein foods will.
94. Application, planning, physiological integrity (b).
    2 Postoperative nutrition depends on the patient's condition and the type of surgery involved.
    1 Not all patients need TPN after surgery, although it is used commonly after large GI surgeries.
    3 The patient will need increased calories, vitamins, and proteins to facilitate healing after the surgical experience.
    4 Not all surgeries require IV fluids and a high-protein diet.
95. Application, planning, physiological integrity (b).
    2 Based on kilocalories and carbohydrates, green and leafy vegetables contain more potassium compared with bananas and orange juice.
    1, 2, 3 These foods are not good food sources of potassium.
96. Knowledge, assessment, physiological integrity (b).
    2 This accurately describes the role of trace elements in the body.
    1 Trace elements are essential to health.
    3 This is not accurate.
    4 Most of the minerals can be detected in the body's fluids.
97. Comprehension, evaluation, physiological integrity (b).
    4 The average life span of a hemoglobin molecule is 3 months, and this test provides average glucose readings over that time interval.
    1 Fasting blood glucose tests should be done on a daily basis for the patient who is insulin dependent.
    2 Postprandial blood glucose levels determine the level of blood sugar after eating and are affected by additional intake of food or beverage.
    3 The glucose tolerance test is a measurement of the body's ability to appropriately handle the excess sugar presented after drinking a high glucose drink.
98. Knowledge, planning, physiological integrity (b).
    3 These vitamins reduce the levels of homocysteine, but the low-protein, low-potassium diet for patients with end-stage renal disease reduces the food sources of these.
    1, 2, 4 These would not help reduce the levels of homocysteine.

99. Comprehension, assessment, physiological integrity (b).
    1 When bone resorption exceeds bone formation in later life, patients with greater bone density are at less risk for development of osteoporosis.
    2 This is a metabolic bone disease characterized by inadequate amounts of calcium or phosphorus, or both, for mineralization.
    3 This is inflammation of the bone marrow and adjacent bone.
    4 This is a malignancy of the bone tissue.

100. Comprehension, planning, health promotion and maintenance (b).
    4 These beliefs will shape the choices teens make in selecting foods to eat.
    1, 2 Studies show that these do not influence adolescents' eating habits.
    3 This may not influence adolescents' eating habits.

101. Knowledge, planning, physiological integrity (b).
    1 The risk factors most directly associated with CHD are elevated serum TC and LDL and reduced HDL.
    2, 3, 4 These are not the risk factors most directly associated with CHD.

102. Comprehension, planning, health promotion and maintenance (b).
    3 A diet high in fat and energy and low in fruits, vegetables, and dietary fiber strongly predisposes humans and animals to the development of colon cancer.
    1, 2 These diets are likely to help prevent colon cancer.
    4 This diet is not likely to help prevent or promote colon cancer.

103. Knowledge, assessment, physiological integrity (b).
    2 As lean body mass declines after age 30, a gradual, but accelerating, decrease occurs in the BMR.
    1, 3, 4 These do not necessarily decrease with age.

104. Knowledge, assessment, physiological integrity (b).
    2 This disorder is characterized by recurrent episodes of bingeing, purging, fasting, and excessive exercise.
    1 This disorder does not feature episodes of overeating.
    3, 4 These disorders are characterized by overeating without the compensatory purging behaviors.

105. Knowledge, assessment, physiological integrity (b).
    3 A 30% excess of body weight is associated with a 25% to 40% increase in mortality and mortality increases as weight increases.
    1, 2 These are lower than the risk rate published by the National Heart, Lung, and Blood Institute.
    4 This is higher than the risk rate published by the National Heart, Lung, and Blood Institute.

106. Knowledge, implementation, physiological integrity (b).
    1 This is the result not only because of the weaknesses of hair analysis procedures, but also the questionable integrity of some companies who offer the service.
    2 No standard laboratory values exist for the mineral content of hair.
    3 The relationship between hair levels and blood levels is not known for many nutrients.
    4 Keratin is so rich in sulfur that it may mask the presence of some minerals and attract others in levels that exceed those found in other body tissues.

107. Knowledge, planning, physiological integrity (b).
    3 This brings the total to approximately 2500 to 2700 calories per day.
    1 Additional energy is needed for both production of milk and assuring adequate calorie content of the fluid.
    2 Ample fluid intake, in the range of 8 to 10 glasses daily, is needed before and during lactation.
    4 This does not contribute to the health of the mother or the baby.

108. Knowledge, application, physiological integrity (b).
    2 Tea causes diuresis and will increase the body's need for water.
    1 Tea is not a good substitute, and adding sugar to the diet is not a healthy choice.
    3 Tea can reduce the amount of iron that the body absorbs.
    4 Tea contains nearly as much caffeine as coffee and is considered a stimulant.

109. Knowledge, planning, health promotion and maintenance (b).
    2 Carbohydrates and fat are the primary fuels the body uses to maintain energy reserves.
    1, 3 Protein has only a small role as a fuel substrate in energy production; it may be used only when fuel supply from carbohydrates and fats is insufficient.
    4 See rationale for 1 and 3; vitamins are not macronutrients.

110. Comprehension, implementation, safe, effective care environment (b).
    4 The source of contamination for most *S. aureus* food poisonings is from an infection on the hand of a worker preparing food.
    1 Clostridium infections are usually caused by inadequately prepared or preserved foods.
    2 Salmonella poisonings usually result from eating contaminated raw eggs.
    3 *E. coli* infections are usually the result of improperly cooked contaminated beef.

111. Comprehension, planning, health promotion and maintenance (b).
    1 Infants have not yet developed the ability to resist the small amount of botulism spores in honey.
    2 Adolescents are able to resist the small amount of botulism spores in honey.
    3 Middle-aged adults are able to resist the small amount of botulism spores in honey.
    4 Elderly adults are able to resist the small amount of botulism spores in honey.

112. Comprehension, assessment, physiological integrity (b).
    2 Although eating balanced meals at regular times is a prudent approach, nutrition has no known effect on premenstrual syndrome.
    1, 3, 4 Nutrition has no known effect on premenstrual syndrome.

113. Comprehension, assessment, health promotion and maintenance (b).
    3 Other reasons include blood loss caused by parasites among young children who do not practice good hand washing.
    1 Trace minerals are not needed for iron absorption.
    2 This is not a true statement.
    4 Growing children absorb iron at a very high rate and can often be induced to take supplemental iron in the form of multiple vitamin and mineral tablets.

114. Comprehension, assessment, physiological integrity (b).
    These are warning signals of severe dehydration.

115. Knowledge, planning, physiological integrity (b).
    1 Five to ten bread exchanges are allowed per day on an 1800-calorie diet.
    2, 3, 4 These exceed the allowance of the exchange diet for bread and grains.

116. Comprehension, assessment, safe, effective care environment (b).
    3 This can be unsafe because of the possibility of infection or fermentation of retained substances, as well as the fact that the patient is deprived of the benefit of the nutrition or therapeutic effect of medication. It is common in children, psychiatric patients, or confused patients.
    1 This process is known as diverticulosis.
    2 This is associated with increased morbidity and mortality related to obesity.
    4 Although this is a prudent practice, it is not known as "pouching."

117. Knowledge, implementation, health promotion and maintenance (b).
    1, 2 The WIC Program is designed to provide nutrition education and vouchers for prescribed supplemental foods and is aimed at promoting the growth of the young child.

118. Knowledge, planning, physiological integrity (b).
    4 Substances on the list meet strict guidelines for inclusion.
    1 Food additives come from many different sources.
    2 Substances on the list are determined to be generally safe for consumption.
    3 Some of the food additives designed to retain freshness may not be on the GRAS list.

119. Application, planning, physiological integrity (b).
    2 These agents emulsify tiny particles of one liquid in another to improve texture and consistency.
    1 Typical additives in this category are vitamins, minerals, milk, and iodized salt.
    3 Typical additives in this category are spices, citrus oils, and amyl acetate.
    4 Typical additives in this category are butylated hydroxytoluene, benzoates, and propionic acid.

120. Application, assessment, health promotion and maintenance (b).
    3 Food choices are often poor, and absorption of nutrients such as vitamin B_{12} is compromised.
    1 Alcohol decreases the secretion of pancreatic enzymes.
    2 Alcohol causes a decrease in the liver stores of vitamins.
    4 Alcohol causes a decrease in the secretion of pancreatic enzymes.

121. Application, assessment, physiological integrity (b).
    3 In addition, most antipsychotic drugs will also have this effect caused, in part, by increased appetite.

    1 This is a false statement and would frighten the patient.
    2 This does not address the issue of the side effect of the medication.
    4 This is not a prudent comment for the nurse to make under the circumstances; and it does not address the issue of the side effect of the medication.

122. Application, planning, physiological integrity (b).
    1 In many instances, desserts such as trifle will have a liqueur poured over them, or tiramisu may have a coffee liqueur incorporated into it. Patients must be educated to avoid all sources of alcohol, not just alcoholic beverages.
    2 This statement is not addressing either the patient's concerns or the real risk of ingesting alcohol that is not obvious.
    3, 4 These statements address neither the patient's concerns nor the real risk of ingesting alcohol that is not obvious.

123. Application, implementation, physiological integrity (b).
    1 The patient need not continue the prescribed diet until otherwise instructed. Although modifications may be made, it is unlikely that he will be able to maintain reduced LDL cholesterol levels on his previous diet.
    2, 3, 4 These are not prudent comments for the nurse to make. Dietary modifications will most likely be a permanent part of this patient's diet from now on.

124. Application, implementation, physiological integrity (b).
    2 Stopping diabetes medication, whether oral hypoglycemic agents or insulin, is best done only with a physician's supervision.
    1, 3 These can lead to a hyperglycemic reaction if the patient has soft or liquid foods without medication.
    4 This is not a prudent comment for the nurse to make. Stopping diabetes medication, whether oral hypoglycemic agents or insulin, is best done only with a physician's supervision.

125. Comprehension, planning, physiological integrity (b).
    4 Saturated fatty acids raise blood cholesterol, which raises the risk of coronary heart disease and stroke.
    1 TFAs, or hydrogenated fats, tend to raise total blood cholesterol levels and LDL ("bad") cholesterol and lower HDL ("good") cholesterol.
    2 Monounsaturated fatty acids seem to lower blood cholesterol when substituted for saturated fats.
    3 These foods do not contribute to raising the serum cholesterol.

CHAPTER 5　Medical-Surgical Nursing

This chapter presents the nursing assessment of medical-surgical patients and is grouped according to the body system affected. Following the nursing process, frequent patient problems and recommended nursing care are identified and discussed. A selected group of major diagnoses, medical management, and nursing care plans is included. Although assessment of each system's functioning and problems is isolated, the student must remember that total patient assessment is necessary each time a patient is given care. The chapter begins with a brief overview of anatomy and physiology before moving on to the anatomy and physiology of the individual body systems, which precede the respective medical diagnoses. Nursing assessment, care, and responsibility for the patient before and after surgery, diagnostic testing, and nursing care procedures are discussed. Medications, the specific nursing responsibilities they entail, and their adverse effects are addressed in Chapter 3.

ANATOMY AND PHYSIOLOGY: AN OVERVIEW

A. Anatomy: the study of the structure of the body, its many parts, and their relationship to one another
B. Physiology: the study of how the body and its many parts function
C. Homeostasis: a state of constancy or dynamic equilibrium within the body
D. Anatomical terminology
　1. Anatomical position: the body is erect, with arms at sides and palms turned forward
　2. Anterior: toward the front of the body
　3. Posterior: toward the back of the body
　4. Cranial: near the head
　5. Superior: toward the head
　6. Inferior: toward the lower aspect
　7. Medial: toward the midline
　8. Lateral: toward the side
　9. Proximal: nearest the origin of a structure (elbows are proximal to the fingers, shoulder is proximal to the elbow)
　10. Distal: farthest from the origin of a structure
E. Body cavities
　1. Dorsal: pertaining to the back; has two subdivisions that are continuous with each other
　　a. Cranial: the space inside the skull; contains the brain
　　b. Spinal: extends from the cranial cavity nearly to the end of the vertebral column; contains the spinal cord
　2. Ventral: pertaining to the front; contains structures of the chest and abdomen; has two subdivisions
　　a. Thoracic: chest cavity; contains the heart, lungs, and large blood vessels; separated from the lower cavity by the diaphragm

　　b. Abdominopelvic: one large cavity, with no separation
　　　(1) Abdominal: upper portion; contains stomach, liver, gallbladder, pancreas, spleen, kidneys, and most of the intestines
　　　(2) Pelvic: lower portion; contains urinary bladder, lower part of intestines, and internal reproductive organs

Structural Units
Cell

A. Definition: the basic unit of structure and function of all living things; made of protoplasm (meaning "original substance"), which is composed of oxygen, hydrogen, nitrogen, carbon, sulfur, and phosphorus; vary in size and shape
B. Structure and function
　1. Structural parts
　　a. Cytoplasmic membrane: keeps cell whole and intact; allows certain substances to pass through and prevents others from entering (semipermeable membrane)
　　b. Cytoplasm: area in which most cellular activity occurs; the working and storage area
　　c. Nucleus: the control center; directs cell activity and is necessary for reproduction; the site of the genetic material, deoxyribonucleic acid (DNA)
　2. Characteristics of cells
　　a. Irritability: responds to stimuli
　　b. Growth and reproduction: gets larger in size and is able to increase in number
　　c. Metabolism: chemical reaction consisting of:
　　　(1) Anabolism: forming new substances to build new cell material; constructive
　　　(2) Catabolism: breaking down of substances into simpler substances and disposing of waste; destructive
　　d. Contractility: the ability to shorten and thicken in response to a stimulus
　　e. Conductivity: ability to transfer an electrical charge or impulse
　3. Functions
　　a. Movement of substances through cell membranes
　　　(1) Diffusion: movement of dissolved particles through a semipermeable membrane from an area of high concentration of particles to an area of low concentration of particles. Diffusion continues until the particles are evenly distributed.
　　　(2) Osmosis: movement of water through a semipermeable membrane from an area in which a large amount of water (dilute solution) exists to an area of a low concentration of water (a concentrated solution). Osmosis occurs until the water is evenly distributed.

(3) Filtration: movement of water and particles through a membrane because of a greater pushing force on one side of the membrane

b. Reproduction mitosis: process of cell division; distributes identical chromosomes (DNA molecules) to each cell formed; enables cells to reproduce their own kind

Tissues

A. Definition: groups of similar cells having like functions
B. Classifications and functions
1. Epithelial: cells are packed close together; contain no blood vessels; three main types
   a. Simple squamous: single layer of cells through which substances can pass; function is absorption; lines air sacs of lungs, lines blood vessels, and covers membranes that line body cavity
   b. Stratified squamous: several layers of closely packed cells; protect the body against invasion of microorganisms; outer layer of skin, epidermis
   c. Simple columnar: single layer of cells; lines the stomach, intestines, and respiratory tract; specializes in secreting mucus and in absorption
2. Connective: cells are separated by intercellular material; located in all parts of the body; various types include areolar, adipose, bone, and cartilage; functions to support and protect
3. Muscle: three types of muscle tissue
   a. Skeletal or striated (voluntary): cells have striations; attach to bones; contractions are controlled voluntarily; cause movement
   b. Cardiac or striated (involuntary): cells have cross-striations; cardiac muscle cells have the inherent power of rhythmic contraction.
   c. Visceral or nonstriated (smooth involuntary): cells appear smooth; help form walls of blood vessels and intestines; contractions cannot be controlled; cause movement
4. Nerve: composed of cells called neurons; all neurons receive and conduct electrochemical impulses; important in control of the entire body

Membranes

A. Definition: thin, soft sheets of tissue that cover, line, lubricate, and anchor body parts
B. Classification and functions
1. Epithelial: lubricate and protect the body against infection; two types
   a. Mucous: line body cavities that open to the exterior (mouth, nose, intestinal tract, and urinary tract); secrete mucus, which protects against bacterial invasion
   b. Serous: line cavities that do not open to the exterior; cover the lungs, stomach, and heart; secrete thin fluid that prevents friction
2. Connective: cover bone or hold body parts in place
   a. Skeletal: cover bones and cartilage; support the bony structure
   b. Synovial: line joint cavities and secrete synovial fluid, which lubricates
   c. Fascial or fibrous: hold organs in place; superficial—connects the skin to underlying structures; deep—supports the internal organs (the viscera)

Organs

Organs are structures composed of several tissues grouped together. They perform a more complex function than does a single tissue. The composition and structure depend on their function.

Systems

A. Definition: groups of organs that contribute to the function of the whole; they perform a more complex function than does a single organ; no system can function independently of another system.
B. Body systems and functions
1. Integumentary (skin): covers and protects the body
2. Musculoskeletal: supports and allows movement; body's framework
3. Circulatory: transports food, water, oxygen, and waste
4. Digestive: processes food and eliminates waste
5. Respiratory: supplies oxygen and eliminates carbon dioxide
6. Urinary: excretes waste
7. Nervous: controls and coordinates body activities
8. Endocrine: regulates body activities
9. Reproductive: increases the number of the species

MUSCULOSKELETAL SYSTEM

Anatomy and Physiology of the Skeletal System
(Figure 5-1)

A. Functions
1. Support: forms framework for body structures and provides shape
2. Protection: protects the internal organs
3. Movement: serves as levers that are activated by the contraction of an attached muscle
4. Mineral storage: stores calcium and minerals used by the body when needed
5. Produces blood cells: forms erythrocytes and thrombocytes and red marrow of bone
B. Bone composition
1. Composed of 33% organic material and 67% inorganic mineral salts
2. Collagen: organic part derived from a protein; fibrous material with a jellylike substance between the fibers; gives bone flexibility
3. Inorganic substance consists of large amount of mineral salts, calcium phosphate, calcium carbonate, calcium fluoride, magnesium phosphate, sodium oxide, and sodium chloride; these minerals give bone its hardness and durability.
C. Classification of bones
1. Long bone: consists of diaphysis, epiphysis, and medullary cavity (e.g., femur)
2. Short bone: contains more spongy bone than compact; generally cube shaped (e.g., wrist bone)
3. Flat bone: thin and flat; has two thin layers of compact bone with a spongy bone between them; red blood cells (RBCs) are manufactured here (e.g., sternum)
4. Irregular: do not fall into preceding categories; are not symmetrical (e.g., vertebrae)

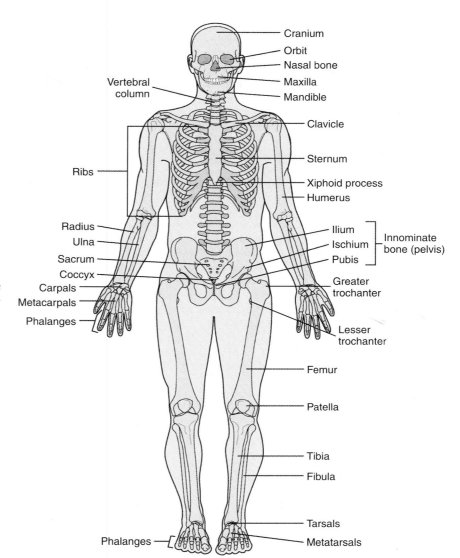

FIGURE 5-1. Bones of the body. *(From Sorrentino SA:* Mosby's textbook for nursing assistants, *ed 6, St Louis, 2004, Mosby.)*

Labels on figure: Cranium, Orbit, Nasal bone, Maxilla, Mandible, Clavicle, Sternum, Xiphoid process, Humerus, Ilium, Ischium, Innominate bone (pelvis), Pubis, Greater trochanter, Lesser trochanter, Femur, Patella, Tibia, Fibula, Tarsals, Metatarsals, Vertebral column, Ribs, Radius, Ulna, Sacrum, Coccyx, Carpals, Metacarpals, Phalanges, Phalanges

D. Structure of long bones
1. Similar to other bones in the body as to structure, development, and function
2. Longer than wide; have a shaft with heads at both ends; bones of extremities are long bones
3. Diaphysis or shaft: hollow cylinder of hard compact bone; contains medullary canal, which is filled with yellow bone marrow; in the adult, it is primarily a storage area for adipose fat.
4. Epiphysis: the ends of the diaphysis composed of spongy bone covered by a thin layer of compact bone; contains red marrow where some RBCs are manufactured during childhood and adolescence; erythropoietic activity in the adult occurs mainly in flat bones and vertebrae.
5. Periosteum: strong fibrous membrane that covers the bone; contains blood vessels, lymph vessels, nerves, and bone cells necessary for growth, repair, and nutrition
6. Epiphyseal disk (flat plate of hyaline cartilage): allows for lengthwise growth of long bones; at puberty when growth stops, it calcifies and becomes the epiphyseal line.

7. Haversian canals: run lengthwise through bone matrix, carrying blood vessels and nerves to all areas of the bone; nourish the osteocytes or bone cell
E. Processes: bony prominences that serve as landmarks
1. Acromion: highest point of the shoulder
2. Olecranon: the upper end of the ulna; forms the point of the elbow
3. Iliac crest: curved rim along the upper border of the ilium
4. Ischial spine: lies at the back of the pelvic outlet
5. Acetabulum: the deep socket in the hipbone
6. Greater trochanter: the large protuberance located at the top of the shaft of the femur
F. Factors that affect bone growth and maintenance
1. Heredity: each person has a genetic potential for height with genes inherited from both parents
2. Nutrition: nutrients such as calcium, phosphorus, and proteins are raw materials of which bones are made; without nutrients, bones cannot grow properly.
3. Hormones: produced by endocrine glands; help regulate cell division, protein synthesis, calcium metabolism, and energy production

4. Exercise: bearing weight, such as walking; without exercise, bones become thin and fragile.

G. Joints: point at which bones meet; classification is determined by the extent of movement.
   1. Synarthroses: fibrous connective tissue holds joining bones close together; no movement (e.g., sutures in skull)
   2. Amphiarthroses: slight movement (e.g., joints between the vertebrae)
   3. Diarthroses: free movement; all have a joint capsule, a joint cavity, and a layer of cartilage.
      a. Ball-and-socket joint: ball-shaped head of one bone fits into a concave socket of another bone (e.g., hip joint)
      b. Hinge joint: allows movement in only two directions, flexion and extension (e.g., knee)
      c. Pivot joint: small projection of one bone pivots in an arch of another bone (e.g., vertebrae of the neck)
      d. Saddle joint: exists only between the metacarpal bone and a carpal bone of the wrist (e.g., thumb and wrist)
      e. Gliding joint: bone surfaces slide over one another (e.g., wrist, ankle)

H. Ligaments: connective tissue bands that hold bones together

I. Tendons: connective tissue bands that attach bones to muscles

J. Bursa: a sac or cavity filled with fluid that reduces friction

Anatomy and Physiology of the Muscular System
(Figure 5-2)

A. Functions
   1. Produces movement by contraction (Table 5-1)
   2. Maintains posture
   3. Produces heat and energy
B. Structure and types
   1. Striated: skeletal, voluntary muscle; attached to bones and accounts for body movement; controlled consciously
   2. Smooth: visceral, nonstriated, involuntary muscle; found in the walls of internal organs and blood vessels; works automatically
   3. Cardiac: found only in the heart; striated, branched, and involuntary
C. Characteristics
   1. Excitability: capacity to respond to stimulus
   2. Contractility: ability to shorten and thicken in response to a stimulus
   3. Extensibility: ability to stretch
   4. Elasticity: ability to regain original size and shape
   5. Tonicity: ability to maintain steady contraction
D. Contraction and movement
   1. Muscles move bones by pulling on them; as muscle contracts, it pulls insertion bone toward its original bone.
      a. Origin: attached to fixed structure of bone
      b. Insertion: attached to movable part
   2. Several muscles contract at the same time to produce movement.
      a. Agonist: prime mover; responsible mainly for producing movement
      b. Antagonists: responsible for relaxing when the prime mover is contracting
      c. Synergists: aid the prime mover in producing movement

3. To contract, muscle must first be stimulated by nerve impulses
   a. Subminimal stimulus: does not cause contraction
   b. Minimal stimulus: does cause contraction
   c. Maximal stimulus: causes all muscle fibers in muscle to contract
   d. Supramaximal stimulus: strength of stimulus is above maximal; no effect on strength of contraction
4. Types of contraction
   a. Isometric: increases the tension without causing movement
   b. Isotonic: produces movement
   c. Tonic: does not produce movement but increases firmness of muscles that maintain posture
   d. Twitch: a quick, jerky contraction
   e. Tetanic (tetanus): sustained contraction
5. Types of movement
   a. Flexion: makes angle at joint smaller
   b. Extension: makes angle at joint larger
   c. Abduction: moves part away from midline
   d. Adduction: moves part toward midline

MUSCULOSKELETAL CONDITIONS AND DISORDERS

Musculoskeletal disorders may be acute or chronic. Acute problems are usually related to simple injuries. Chronic disorders may be more distressing to the patient because of loss of mobility and changes in self-image. The nurse needs to possess good skills in observation, positioning the patient safely, and use and care of equipment. The nurse is probably the most important health care provider in preventive care associated with complications of immobility.

Nursing Assessment

A. Nursing observation (objective data)
   1. General appearance
      a. Age
      b. Weight loss or weight gain
      c. Height changes: loss
      d. Abnormal gait
      e. Absence of extremity
      f. Deformity
      g. Malalignment
      h. Use of assistive devices
      i. Spinal curvature
   2. Respirations
      a. Rate
      b. Depth
      c. Character: any difficulty
   3. Pulse
      a. Presence of pulse above and below injured or casted part
      b. Rate, quality, character
   4. Neurovascular status
      a. Assessment of skin color and temperature
      b. Pulses, presence of
      c. Intact sensation (noting numbness)
      d. Motor function
      e. Sensation and capillary refill
   5. Motor function
      a. Compare affected and unaffected sides

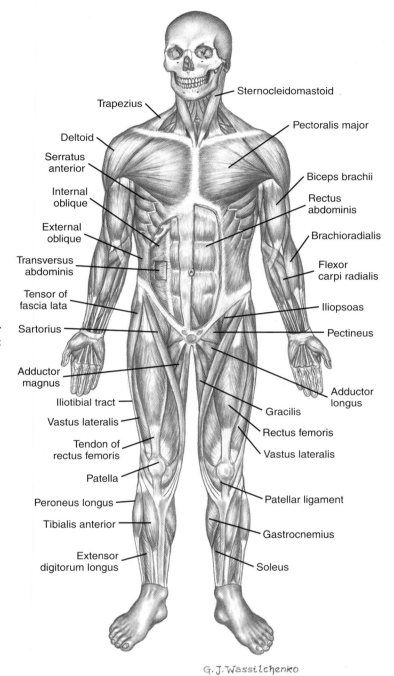

FIGURE 5-2. Skeletal muscles of the body, anterior view. *(Phipps, Monahan, Sands, et al.* Medical-Surgical Nursing health and illness perspectives, *ed. 7, St. Louis, 2003, Mosby.)*

Trapezius
Sternocleidomastoid
Deltoid
Pectoralis major
Serratus anterior
Biceps brachii
Internal oblique
Rectus abdominis
External oblique
Brachioradialis
Transversus abdominis
Flexor carpi radialis
Tensor of fascia lata
Iliopsoas
Sartorius
Pectineus
Adductor magnus
Adductor longus
Iliotibial tract
Gracilis
Vastus lateralis
Rectus femoris
Tendon of rectus femoris
Vastus lateralis
Patella
Peroneus longus
Patellar ligament
Tibialis anterior
Gastrocnemius
Extensor digitorum longus
Soleus

G. J. Wassilchenko

b. Limited ability or loss of ability to move body part
c. Diminished muscle strength to passive resistance
d. Limited range of motion (ROM)
e. Degree of ability to perform activities of daily living (ADL)
6. Pain and swelling
   a. Location, character, frequency, duration, alleviating or aggravating factors
   b. Bony enlargements or soft tissue swelling
B. Patient description (subjective data)
1. Pain
   a. Patient's account of location, character, frequency, duration, onset

b. May use the PQRST method of assessment
   P: provoking incident; What initially caused the pain?
   Q: quality of pain; Is the pain throbbing, stabbing, or burning?
   R: region; Where is the pain? Does the pain radiate? What measures relieve the pain?
   S: Severity of the pain. Is the pain mild, moderate, or severe?
   T: timing of pain; When is the pain worse?
2. Stamina
   a. Weakness, fatigue
   b. Changes in ability to perform ADL

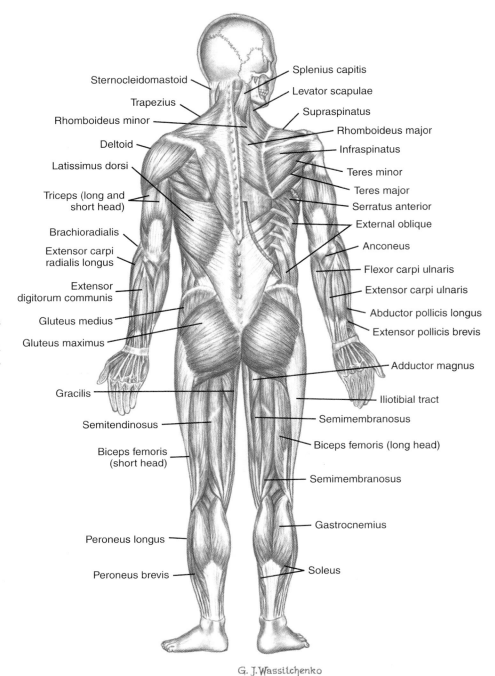

Sternocleidomastoid
Trapezius
Rhomboideus minor
Deltoid
Latissimus dorsi
Triceps (long and short head)
Brachioradialis
Extensor carpi radialis longus
Extensor digitorum communis
Gluteus medius
Gluteus maximus
Gracilis
Semitendinosus
Biceps femoris (short head)
Peroneus longus
Peroneus brevis

Splenius capitis
Levator scapulae
Supraspinatus
Rhomboideus major
Infraspinatus
Teres minor
Teres major
Serratus anterior
External oblique
Anconeus
Flexor carpi ulnaris
Extensor carpi ulnaris
Abductor pollicis longus
Extensor pollicis brevis
Adductor magnus
Iliotibial tract
Semimembranosus
Biceps femoris (long head)
Semimembranosus
Gastrocnemius
Soleus

G. J. Wassilchenko

FIGURE 5-2. cont'd   **Skeletal muscles of the body, posterior view.** *(Phipps, Monahan, Sands, et al.* Medical-Surgical Nursing health and illness perspectives, *ed. 7, St. Louis, 2003, Mosby.)*

3. Report of recent injury
   a. Description
   b. Evaluation and treatment
4. Motor function
   a. Pain with movement
   b. Limited movement; difficult gait
5. General
   a. Maintenance of weight
   b. Changes in appetite
   c. Tolerance of ADL

Diagnostic Tests and Methods

A. Serum laboratory studies
   1. Complete blood count (CBC): an aid in determining anemia or the presence of infection
   2. Erythrocyte sedimentation rate (ESR): elevation is evidence of an inflammatory process.
   3. Rheumatoid factor: a protein found in the blood of most persons afflicted with rheumatoid arthritis
   4. Uric acid: high concentration is found in persons who have gout

TABLE 5-1   The Skeletal Muscles

Muscle	Location	Function
Sternocleidomastoid	Neck	Flexion and rotation of head
Trapezius	Upper Back	Helps hold head erect; also assists in moving the head sideways
Latissimus dorsi	Lower back	Extension and adduction of upper arm
Pectoralis major	Chest	Flexion and abduction of upper arm
Deltoid	Shoulder	Adduction of upper arm
Biceps brachii	Anterior upper arm	Flexion of arm and forearm
Triceps brachii	Posterior upper arm	Extension of arm and forearm
Gluteus maximus	Fleshy part of hips and buttocks	Extension of thigh
Gluteus medius	Lateral part of hips and buttocks	Abduction of thigh when limb is extended
Hamstring group	Posterior thigh	Flexion of lower leg and extension of thigh
Quadriceps femoris	Anterior thigh	Flexion of thigh and extension of lower leg
Gastrocnemius	Calf of leg	Helps in extension of foot and flexion of leg

5. Lupus erythematosus (LE) cell
   a. A cell identified in persons with lupus
   b. Normally, no LE cells are in the blood.
B. Procedures
   1. Roentgenogram (x-ray): a film to determine the presence of a deformity, fracture, or tumor of the skeletal system
   2. Aspiration: withdrawal of fluid from a joint to obtain a specimen for diagnostic purposes
   3. Bone biopsy: removal and examination of bone tissue
   4. Myelogram: x-ray examination of the spinal cord after injection with radiopaque dye
   5. Bone scan: isotope imaging of the skeleton
   6. Computed tomography (CT): use of roentgen rays to provide accurate images of thin cross-sections of the body
   7. Magnetic resonance imaging (MRI): aids in diagnosing musculoskeletal conditions through the clear differentiation of various types of tissue, such as bones, fat, and muscle
   8. Arthroscopy: endoscopic examination that allows for direct visualization of a joint
   9. Electromyography (EMG): used to evaluate nerve conduction in skeletal muscle
   10. Positron emission tomography (PET): using an isotope, scans the brain for evaluation of structure function
C. Nursing intervention for myelogram
   1. After procedure, have patient remain flat in bed for 12 to 24 hours before allowing him or her to resume usual activities.
   2. Encourage fluids to 2000 to 3000 ml every 24 hours.
   3. Observe for alterations in normal motor and sensory states.
   4. Observe for nausea and vomiting.

Frequent Patient Problems and Nursing Care

A. Disturbed body image related to immobility
   1. Provide atmosphere of acceptance.
   2. Express empathy, warmth, and friendliness.
   3. Encourage acceptance of self-limitations.
   4. Encourage self-performance.
B. Impaired skin integrity: potential breakdown related to immobility and assistive devices
   1. Change the patient's position frequently.
   2. Keep the skin clean, dry, and lubricated.
   3. Massage bony prominences.
   4. Provide sheepskin or polyurethane foam padding.

C. Risk for injury: joint contracture related to incorrect body alignment
   1. Place hands, feet, and knees in the natural position of function.
   2. Provide devices to protect against poor alignment of body part.
   3. Assist in performing active and passive ROM exercises.
   4. Provide trapeze over the patient's bed.
   5. Avoid knee gatch position or pillow under knee.
D. Ineffective airway clearance related to increased secretions
   1. Change the patient's position frequently.
   2. Encourage coughing and deep breathing.
   3. Observe for coughing, fever, and green-yellow sputum.
E. Impaired tissue perfusion: potential for thrombi and emboli related to impaired physical mobility or edema
   1. Encourage patient to move lower extremities.
   2. Encourage adequate hydration.
   3. Avoid use of knee gatch or pillow under knee.
   4. To avoid release of emboli, never rub legs.
   5. Encourage use of elastic stockings.
   6. Take daily calf measurements.
F. Acute pain related to bone fracture or disease
   1. Inspect and palpate the painful site looking for inflammation, edema, bruising, tenderness, and skin warmth.
   2. Support the affected body part.
   3. Apply warm, moist compress to affected body part where prescribed.
   4. Give prescribed analgesic.
   5. Evaluate effectiveness of pain relief measures.
G. Impaired physical mobility related to cast or traction confinement, joint pain, stiffness, or inflammation
   1. Explain the reason for and intended effect of ROM exercises.
   2. Have the patient maintain body alignment.
   3. Provide total exercising of muscles and joints, except if severe pain or inflammation is present; movement is contraindicated if recent surgery was performed on or near the joint.
H. Acute pain related to cast
   1. Massage the area around the cast, except for leg casts.
   2. Pad rough edges.
   3. Elevate extremity to reduce swelling.
   4. Inspect the skin for irritation.

5. Observe for cyanosis and assess capillary refill times of the casted extremity.
6. Observe for complaints of numbness and tingling of casted extremity.
7. Observe cast for indentations.

I. Self-care deficits (feeding, bathing, and hygiene) related to impaired physical mobility
1. Assist with ADL.
2. Provide self-care aids or devices.
3. Teach self-care activities.

Major Medical Diagnoses
Rheumatoid Arthritis

A. Definition: a chronic, systemic disease in which inflammatory changes occur throughout the body's connective tissue destroying joints internally; joints most involved are hands, wrists, elbows, knees, and ankles.
B. Pathology: cause is unknown; related theories include autoimmune, microorganisms, viruses, and genetic predisposition.
C. Signs and symptoms
1. Subjective
a. Sore, stiff, swollen joint or joints
b. Fatigue
c. Weakness
d. Malaise
e. Loss of appetite
2. Objective
a. Low-grade fever
b. Weakened grip
c. Anemia
d. Weight loss
e. Subcutaneous nodes
f. Enlarged lymph nodes
g. Joint deformity
h. Muscle atrophy
i. Limited ROM
j. Edema and tenderness of joint
k. Extraarticular symptoms: lung, heart, blood vessels, muscle, eye, and skin
D. Diagnostic tests and methods
1. Elevated ESR
2. Slightly elevated white blood cell (WBC) count
3. Presence of serum rheumatoid factors
4. Synovial fluid aspiration
5. X-ray film to reveal joint deformity
6. Low hemoglobin (Hgb) and hematocrit (Hct)
E. Treatment
1. Antiinflammatory agents, analgesics, corticosteroids, gold salts, and immunosuppressive drugs
2. Heat applications such as paraffin dip, hot packs, and warm tub baths or showers for analgesia or muscle relaxation
3. Surgical intervention to prevent deformities or remove damaged joints
4. Physical therapy to maintain optimal function
F. Nursing intervention
1. Provide undisturbed periods of rest.
2. Use firm mattress, footboards, splints, and sandbags to maintain proper body alignment.
3. Encourage self-performance activities such as combing hair, feeding self, and brushing teeth.
4. Assist with ROM exercises within limits of pain tolerance.

Osteoarthritis

A. Definition: a local joint disorder affecting weight-bearing joints; results in disintegration of the cartilage covering the ends of bones
B. Pathology: cause is unknown; predisposing factors include aging, joint trauma, and obesity.
C. Signs and symptoms
1. Subjective
a. Pain after exercise; relieved by rest
b. Morning stiffness
c. Muscle spasms
d. Reduced strength
2. Objective
a. Limited ROM
b. Crepitant joint
c. Prominent bony enlargement
D. Diagnostic tests: x-ray studies reveal joint abnormalities.
E. Treatment
1. Weight reduction to relieve strain
2. Heat and massage for aching and stiffness
3. Physical therapy to maintain optimum level of functioning
4. Drugs to relieve symptoms
a. Analgesics
b. Antiinflammatory agents
c. Steroids
5. Surgical intervention to prevent deformity, relieve inflammation, delay progression, or replace affected joint
F. Nursing intervention
1. Encourage the patient to express feelings concerning disorder.
2. Provide moist heat, massage, and prescribed exercise, if ordered, to relax muscle and relieve stiffness or discomfort.

Gouty Arthritis (Gout)

A. Definition: a disorder in which excessive amounts of uric acid are retained in the blood
B. Pathology
1. Cause is related to a disorder of purine metabolism.
2. Uric acid crystals are deposited in the joints and cartilage and form lumps (tophi).
3. Deposits cause local irritation and an inflammatory response.
4. Men older than 30 years of age are most commonly affected.
C. Signs and symptoms
1. Subjective
a. Acute pain, swelling, and inflammation of great toe (most affected joint)
b. Headache
c. Malaise
d. Anorexia
e. Pruritus (local)
2. Objective
a. Skin over joint is swollen, warm, and red
b. Limited ROM
c. Tophi located in cartilage of ears, hands, and feet
D. Diagnostic tests and methods
1. Elevated serum uric acid level
2. Elevated ESR and WBC count
E. Treatment
1. Dietary restriction of foods high in purine
2. Uricosuric drugs to increase uric acid excretion; Allopurinol to inhibit uric acid formation

3. Weight loss and periodic blood glucose screening because a relationship may exist between gouty arthritis and insulin resistance
4. Colchicine to reduce pain and relieve swelling
5. Alkaline ash diet to increase urinary pH

F. Nursing intervention
1. Instruct the patient to avoid foods high in purine content.
2. Encourage physical activity to promote optimal muscular and skeletal function.
3. Use bed cradle (or tent sheets over side rails) to prevent pressure of linen on feet and legs.
4. Encourage fluid intake of 2000 to 3000 ml daily to avoid renal calculi, unless contraindicated.
5. Instruct patient to limit alcohol intake, which may precipitate an acute attack.
6. Instruct patient to avoid salicylates because of antagonistic actions of uricosuric drugs.

Systemic Lupus Erythematosus (SLE)

A. Definition: a chronic multisystem inflammatory disorder involving the connective tissues, such as the muscles, kidneys, heart, and serous membranes; may affect the skin, lungs, and nervous system
B. Pathology
1. Cause is unknown; believed to be an autoimmune disorder
2. Inflammation produces fibroid deposits and structural changes in connective tissue of organs and blood vessels.
3. Results in problems with mobility, oxygenation, and elimination
C. Signs and symptoms
1. Subjective
a. Abdominal, joint, and muscle pain
b. Weakness; fatigue
c. Depression
2. Objective
a. Low-grade fever
b. Weight loss
c. Butterfly skin rash over bridge of nose and cheeks, which increases with exposure to the sun
d. Anemia
e. Alopecia
D. Diagnostic tests
1. Positive LE test
2. Elevated ESR
3. Increased gamma globulin levels
4. Positive antinuclear antibody titer
5. High anti-DNA test
E. Treatment
1. Corticosteroids, analgesics, and medications for anemia
2. The drug hydroxychloroquine is indicated in some individuals.
3. Avoidance of exposure to sunlight
F. Nursing intervention
1. Provide emotional support to patient and family in coping with poor prognosis.
2. Encourage alternative activity and planned rest periods.
3. Instruct to avoid persons with infections, undue exposure to sunlight, and emotional stress, which can cause exacerbations.

4. Encourage intake of foods high in iron content: liver, shellfish, leafy vegetables, and enriched breads and cereals.

Scleroderma (Progressive Systemic Sclerosis)

A. Definition: fiberlike changes in the connective tissue throughout the body caused by collagen deposits and subsequent fibrosis
B. Pathology
1. An insidious, chronic, progressive disorder, usually beginning in the skin
2. Skin becomes thick and hard; fingers and toes become fixed in a position.
3. Other disorders that occur are difficulty in swallowing, impaired gastrointestinal (GI) mobility, cardiac and renal problems, and osteoporosis.
C. Signs and symptoms
1. Subjective
a. Sweating of hands and feet
b. Stiffness of hands
c. Muscle weakness
d. Joint pain
e. Dysphagia
2. Objective
a. Increased pigmentation or dyspigmentation
b. Dilated capillaries of lips, fingers, face, and tongue
D. Diagnostic tests and methods
1. Positive LE cell test
2. False-positive syphilis test
E. Treatment
1. Skin care to prevent formation of decubiti
2. Physical therapy
3. Analgesics for joint pain
4. Corticosteroids
F. Nursing intervention
1. Provide emotional support to patient and family in addressing physical and psychological needs.
2. Encourage moderate exercise to promote muscular and joint function.
3. Force fluids; encourage fluid intake of at least 1500 to 2500 ml/day, unless contraindicated by patient's condition.
4. Advise to avoid cold temperatures; use gloves to remove items from freezer.
5. Plan rest periods.
6. Provide assistive devices to help with ADL (eating, grooming)

Osteomyelitis

A. Definition: bone inflammation caused by direct or indirect invasion of an organism
B. Pathology: bacteria enter bloodstream through an open fracture, open wound, or by secondary invasion from blood-borne infection from a distant site such as bone or infected tonsils.
C. Signs and symptoms
1. Subjective
a. Tenderness over the bones
b. Painful movement; limited mobility
c. Malaise
2. Objective
a. Fever
b. Chills

c. Heat, swelling, and redness of the skin over the bone
d. Signs of sepsis
e. Wound drainage

D. Diagnostic tests and methods
1. Positive blood cultures
2. Elevated ESR
3. Elevated WBC count
4. X-ray film may not reveal abnormalities for 5 to 10 days from onset.

E. Treatment
1. Long-term antibiotic therapy
2. Drainage from abscess with continuous irrigation of wound
3. Surgical removal of necrotic bone

F. Nursing intervention
1. Use strict aseptic technique when changing dressings.
2. Keep affected limb in proper alignment with pillows and sandbags.
3. Maintain drainage and secretion precautions for disposal of dressings.
4. Provide a high-calorie, high-protein diet and adequate hydration.
5. Provide undisturbed rest periods.
6. Move affected body part gently, because of severe pain.

Osteoporosis

A. Definition: metabolic bone disorder in which bone mass is decreased. Bones become weak and brittle. Prevention is crucial; adequate calcium intake must be maintained throughout life.

B. Pathology
1. Common in postmenopausal women
2. May be result of deficit of estrogen and androgens, prolonged immobilization, insufficient calcium intake or absorption, or endocrine disorder
3. Sites usually affected are vertebrae, pelvis, hip, wrist, and femur.

C. Signs and symptoms
1. Subjective: backache that worsens with sitting, standing, coughing, and sneezing
2. Objective
a. Kyphosis
b. Loss of height
c. Pathological fractures

D. Diagnostic test: x-ray film reveals bone demineralization and compression of vertebrae.

E. Treatment
1. Physical activity and exercise to prevent atrophy
2. Estrogen replacement to provide calcium balance
3. Diet high in protein and calcium
4. Vitamin-D supplements
5. Support of spine with brace or corset
6. The medication Fosamax is used to help alleviate bone loss.

F. Nursing intervention
1. Encourage the patient to use a walker or cane to stabilize balance when ambulating.
2. Encourage fluid intake of 2000 to 3000 ml daily, unless contraindicated, to avoid formation of renal calculi.
3. Give instruction on foods that are high in protein and calcium content.

4. Emphasize need to follow prescribed daily activity and exercise.
5. If confined to bed, give passive and assist with active ROM exercises.
6. Teach safety measures to protect from fractures.

Osteogenic Sarcoma

A. Definition: a tumor located in the bone composed of cells derived from connective tissue

B. Pathology
1. Highly malignant tumor that may metastasize to the lungs
2. Affects children, adolescents, and young adults
3. Usually occurs in shaft of long bones, especially affecting the femur

C. Signs and symptoms
1. Subjective: pain
2. Objective
a. Restricted ROM
b. Swelling
c. Weight loss
d. Anemia

D. Diagnostic tests and methods
1. X-ray examination to reveal lesion in the extremity and chest; CT scan
2. Biopsy examination to evaluate cells
3. Frozen section for rapid diagnosis of possible malignant lesion

E. Treatment
1. Chemotherapeutic agents to reduce and retard growth
2. Radiation therapy to destroy malignant tissue
3. Amputation of affected limb or resection of tumor
4. Use of cadaver limb to preserve function after bone removal

F. Nursing intervention
1. Provide emotional support to patient and family to reduce fear and anxiety.
2. Provide diet high in protein and caloric content.
3. If patient undergoes amputation procedure, follow special nursing actions. (Refer to amputations.)
4. If patient is receiving radiotherapy:
a. Provide noninfectious environment.
b. Avoid ointments, lotions, powders, and washing of port (treated) areas.
c. Do not remove markings on skin.
d. Observe site for redness, swelling, itching, and drying.

Osteomalacia

A. Definition: a disorder in which widespread softening and demineralization of bones occur

B. Pathology
1. Possible causes
a. Vitamin D-deficiency resulting from poor dietary intake of vitamin D
b. Body's inability to absorb or use vitamin D
c. Lack of ultraviolet rays
2. The effect of parathyroid hormone on bone resorption and calcium absorption is decreased.
3. Most affected bones are spine, pelvis, and lower extremities.

C. Signs and symptoms
   1. Subjective
      a. Rheumatic-type pain
      b. Weakness
   2. Objective
      a. Waddling gait
      b. Spontaneous fractures
      c. Bone deformities
D. Diagnostic tests and methods
   1. Reduced calcium and phosphorus serum levels
   2. X-ray examination to reveal fracturelike lines of affected bones
E. Treatment
   1. Therapeutic doses of vitamin D
   2. High dietary intake of calcium and phosphorus
F. Nursing intervention
   1. Change patient's position gradually.
   2. Teach good body mechanics.
   3. Encourage intake of foods high in calcium: meat, shellfish, and dark-green leafy vegetables.
   4. Emphasize need to maintain weight in normal range.
   5. Instruct on avoidance of heavy lifting.
   6. Safety measures to prevent fractures.

Osteitis Deformans (Paget's Disease of Bone)

A. Definition: an inflammatory condition in which certain bones become soft, thick, and deformed
B. Pathology
   1. Unknown cause; occurs mainly in men of middle age or older
   2. Disease disturbs new bone tissue with bones becoming enlarged and coarse in texture.
C. Signs and symptoms
   1. Subjective
      a. Bone pain; worsens at night
      b. Tenderness on pressure of the bones
      c. Back pain
      d. Headache from enlarged skull
      e. Deafness or blindness caused by pressure from overgrowth of bone
   2. Objective
      a. Pathological fractures
      b. Decrease in height
      c. Bowing of femur and tibia
      d. Enlarged skull
D. Diagnostic tests and methods
   1. Skeletal x-ray film to reveal bone enlargement and denseness
   2. Elevated serum alkaline phosphate value
   3. Urinary excretion of hydroxyproline is increased.
E. Treatment
   1. Androgen therapy for men; estrogen therapy for women to reverse hypercalciuria, if present
   2. Salicylates for pain
F. Nursing intervention
   1. Observe for stress fractures.
   2. Emphasize need for maintenance of normal weight.
   3. If fracture occurs and patient becomes immobilized:
      a. Limit calcium intake to avoid renal calculi.
      b. Provide high fluid intake to avoid hypercalcemia.
   4. Explain safety measures to prevent fractures.

Herniated Nucleus Pulposus (Slipped Disk or Rupture of Intervertebral Disk)

A. Definition: protrusion of the nucleus pulposus, which compresses the nerve roots of the spinal cord
B. Pathology
   1. Site usually affected is between L4 and L5, L5 and sacrum, C5 and C6, or C6 and C7.
   2. Causes may be straining of the spine in an unnatural position, degenerative changes, heavy lifting when bending from the waist, and accidents.
C. Signs and symptoms
   1. Subjective
      a. Cervical disk
         (1) Stiff neck
         (2) Shoulder pain descending down the arm into the hand
         (3) Numbness of arm and hand
      b. Lumbosacral disk: low-back pain radiating down the posterior thigh
   2. Objective
      a. Cervical disk
         (1) Sensory disturbances of the hand
         (2) Atrophy of biceps and triceps
      b. Lumbosacral disk
         (1) Difficulty in ambulating
         (2) Lasègue sign: pain in back and leg while raising heel with knee straight; numbness of leg and foot
         (3) Foot drop
D. Diagnostic tests and methods
   1. X-ray examination to reveal narrowing disk space
   2. Myelogram to localize site
   3. EMG
   4. CT scan of the spine
   5. MRI of spine
E. Treatment
   1. Cervical traction (cervical disk); traction to lower extremities (lumbosacral disk)
   2. Bed rest, heat application, and analgesics
   3. Surgical intervention
      a. Laminectomy: removal of a portion of the vertebra and excision of the ruptured portion of the nucleus pulposus
      b. Spinal fusion: permanent binding of the vertebrae
      c. Chemonucleolysis: dissolving of the affected disk through the injection of chymopapain
F. Nursing intervention
   1. Encourage patient to verbalize feelings related to immobility, fears, and future impairment.
   2. Observations for traction:
      a. Check that it is hanging free and has not fallen or become caught in bed grooves.
      b. Observe for frayed cords and loosened knots.
   3. Give back care to promote circulation and relax muscles.
   4. Have the patient maintain proper body alignment.
   5. Provide diet high in fiber, with adequate hydration to avoid constipation and straining.
   6. Instruct patient on principles of body mechanics.
   7. If patient has myelogram procedure:
      a. Position flat for period prescribed by physician.
      b. Encourage adequate hydration.

8. If patient undergoes surgical intervention, follow general postoperative nursing actions.
   a. Observe for leakage of cerebrospinal fluid on surgical dressing; reinforce dressing until inspected by physician.
   b. Change position by log rolling to prevent motion of spinal column.
   c. Provide straight-backed chair for patient to sit in; feet must be on floor.
   d. Discharge instructions
      (1) Avoid heavy lifting and climbing stairs.
      (2) Avoid riding in car.
      (3) Avoid forward flexion of head (cervical laminectomy).

Fractures

A. Definition: a break in the continuity of bone that may be accompanied by injury of surrounding soft tissue, producing swelling and discoloration
B. Pathology
   1. Most fractures are a result of trauma; pathological fractures result from disorders such as osteoporosis, malnutrition, bone tumors, and Cushing's syndrome.
   2. Types of fractures
      a. Closed (simple): skin is intact over the site.
      b. Open (compound): break in skin is present over the fracture site; the ends of the bone may or may not be visible.
      c. Complete: fracture line extends completely through the bone.
      d. Incomplete (partial): fracture line extends partially through the bone; one side breaks while the opposite side bends.
      e. Comminuted: more than one fracture, with bone fragments either crushed or splintered into several pieces
      f. Greenstick: splintering of one side of a bone (most often seen in children because of soft bone structure)
      g. Impacted: one bone fragment that is driven into another bone fragment
C. Signs and symptoms
   1. Subjective
      a. Pain on movement of body part
      b. Tenderness
      c. Loss of function
      d. Muscle spasms
   2. Objective
      a. Deformity
      b. Edema
      c. Bruising
      d. Crepitus
D. Diagnostic test: x-ray examination to confirm location and direction of fracture line
E. Treatment
   1. Reduction of the fracture consists of pulling the broken bone ends to correct alignment and regain continuity; a cast is usually applied, or the part may be placed in a traction device.
      a. Closed reduction: manual manipulation to bring ends into contact
      b. Open reduction: surgical intervention to cleanse the area and attach devices to hold the bones in position

2. Cast application to immobilize, support, and protect the part during the healing process
3. Traction to apply a pulling force in two directions to realign the bones
   a. Skin traction is temporarily applied: light weights that are attached to the skin with strips of adhesive tape
      (1) Buck's extension: exerts a straight pull on the limb; used for fractures of upper and lower leg, hip dislocation, and pelvic injuries
      (2) Bryant's traction: vertical extension of lower extremities, hip flexed 90 degrees, knees extended, and buttocks clear of the bed (see Figure 8-16) for reduction of femur or hip dislocation in very young children
      (3) Russell traction: a sling is placed behind the knee to create an upward pull of the knee; and at the same time, a horizontal force is exerted on the tibia and fibula; used for fractures of femurs
   b. Skeletal traction provides continuous reduction by the attachment of a device to the bone.
      (1) Kirschner wires or Steinmann pins are surgically inserted through the skin and bone; a traction bow or stirrup is attached to the wire or pin to exert a longitudinal pull and control rotation.
      (2) Crutchfield tongs are inserted into parietal areas of the skull to obtain hyperextension; used for spinal fractures
      (3) Halo traction-halo loop for alignment of cervical area; loop is attached to a halo vest or cast.
F. Nursing intervention
   1. Provide emergency nursing care of fractures (see Chapter 10).
   2. Provide nursing care for the patient with a cast.
      a. Observe for neurovascular impairment of limb (Box 5-1).
      b. Elevate (use palms of hands) extremity in cast on pillow to reduce edema.
      c. Promote drying of cast by exposing it to air.
      d. Inspect for skin irritation under edges of cast: apply lotion, pad edges, and apply tape to edge of cast.
      e. If drainage is present on the cast, measure and note.
      f. Observe for possible infection: increased temperature, foul odor from cast, edema, and "hot spots" over the cast.
      g. May apply ice for first 24 hours to reduce edema.
      h. Observe for complications.
         (1) Pulmonary emboli: if emboli lodges in the lungs, patient may experience dyspnea, anxiety, restlessness, chest pain, cough, hemoptysis, and increase in temperature.

BOX 5-1   Signs of Neurovascular Impairment

Compare casted extremity to other extremities when assessing the following:
   Cyanosis
   Slow capillary refill times (greater than 3 seconds)
   Poor pulse
   Lack of sensation
   Complaints of numbness and tingling

(2) Fat emboli: similar to pulmonary emboli, except the emboli are a fat globule, probably arising from central area of the fractured bone

(3) Compartment syndrome occurs when circulation to the muscles is compromised; look for changes in neurocirculatory status.

   i. Educate the patient on home cast care.

3. Provide nursing care for the patient in traction.

   a. Inspect and maintain ropes, knots, and pulleys; taut rope rides easily over pulleys; knots should not slip and should be unobstructed.

   b. Inspect and maintain weights: hang freely, off the floor and free of bedding.

   c. Observe for skin traction.

    (1) Inspect skin condition at distal ends of bandages (wrist and heel) for possible skin breakdown.

    (2) Ensure that tapes do not encircle a limb, are applied smoothly, and are applied on skin that is free of irritation.

    (3) Assess neurovascular status: color, pulses, warmth, and sensation.

   d. Observe for skeletal traction.

    (1) Inspect insertion points daily for signs and symptoms of infection.

    (2) Provide dressing change or wound care aseptically to prevent infection.

    (3) Inspect pins, wires, and skeletal apparatus for sharp ends that may catch on bed linen.

    (4) Assess neurovascular status.

   e. Examine and give skin care to all pressure points on which the patient rests.

   f. Provide foot support to prevent foot drop, especially for patients with Russell traction or Buck's extension.

   g. Observe for thrombophlebitis, especially for the patient with Russell traction because of pressure to the popliteal space.

   h. Encourage diet high in protein and vitamins to promote healing.

   i. Encourage 2000 to 3000 ml fluid intake daily to prevent complications such as constipation, renal calculi, and urinary tract infections.

   j. Encourage patient to perform ROM and isometric exercises.

   k. Have the patient maintain proper position and good alignment.

Fractured Hip

A. Definition: fracture of the hip joint

B. Pathology

   1. Site of fracture

    a. Inside the joint (intracapsular or neck of the femur)

    b. Outside the joint (extracapsular or base of the neck of the femur)

   2. Elderly women experience high incidence because of osteoporosis.

C. Signs and symptoms

   1. Subjective: pain

   2. Objective

    a. Leg appears shorter than unaffected extremity.

    b. Foot points upward and outward on affected side (external rotation).

    c. Edema

    d. Discoloration

D. Diagnostic test: x-ray study to confirm discontinuity of the bone

E. Treatment

   1. Russell traction or Buck's extension: before open reduction to prevent muscle spasms if surgery is not contraindicated

   2. Closed reduction with application of hip spica cast if the fracture occurred in the intertrochanteric site

   3. Open reduction and implantation of a prosthesis to replace head and neck of femur or fixation device to secure fragments of the fracture

    a. Austin Moore prosthesis

    b. Thompson prosthesis

    c. Neufeld nail and screws

    d. Smith-Petersen nail

    e. Ziekel nail

F. Nursing intervention

   1. Provide nursing care of the patient in traction as outlined previously in the section on fractures.

   2. Be aware of coexisting problems such as diabetes or cardiac, vascular, or neurological disorders.

   3. Considerations for the older adult patient

    a. Complications of immobility

    b. Reduced tolerance to drugs

    c. Delayed healing because of nutritional problems related to the aging process

   4. Keep side rail up, and provide trapeze to facilitate movement.

   5. Encourage patient to participate in ADL: eating, bathing, and combing hair.

   6. Provide postoperative care.

    a. Inspect dressings and linen for drainage and bleeding.

    b. Provide trochanter roll to prevent external rotation of legs.

    c. Provide and maintain proper alignment. Use an abductor pillow to prevent adduction; adduction, external rotation, or acute flexion of the hip can dislocate hip before it is healed.

    d. Encourage quadriceps-setting exercises.

    e. Assist the patient in learning to use walker and ambulating with a non–weight-bearing technique.

    f. Instruct on the use of an elevated toilet seat to prevent hip flexion.

Arthroplasty

A. Definition: replacement of a joint, which may be necessary to restore function, relieve pain, and correct deformity

B. Pathology: arthritic changes damage the joint, resulting in impaired mobility, pain, and deformity; hip, knee, fingers, elbow, and shoulder are commonly affected.

C. Signs and symptoms

   1. Subjective

    a. Pain

    b. Limited ROM

    c. Limited weight-bearing ability

   2. Objective

    a. Limited ROM

    b. Edema and skin character changes around affected joint

D. Diagnostic tests and methods
1. X-ray studies to confirm joint changes and damage
2. Arthroscopy to provide direct visualization and inspection of joint changes
E. Treatment: a prosthetic device used to replace the articulating joint surfaces (hip, knee, shoulder, elbow, and fingers)
F. Nursing intervention
1. Maintain proper positioning postoperatively (e.g., if hip is replaced, maintain affected leg in abduction).
2. Wound care: monitor drains, note blood loss, and monitor dressing status.
3. Monitor continuous passive ROM machine, if used for knee replacement.
4. Assist with prescribed activity, and encourage prescribed exercise.
5. Monitor pain; provide pain control.
6. Assess neuromuscular function.
7. Monitor skin integrity.

Amputation

A. Definition: surgical removal of part or all of an extremity
B. Pathology
1. Majority of amputations result from blood vessel disorders, causing inadequate oxygen supply to the tissue.
2. Other indications for amputation are gas gangrene, malignant tumors, septic wounds, severe trauma, and burns.
3. A skin flap is usually constructed for prosthetic equipment.
C. Signs and symptoms
1. Subjective
a. Gas gangrene and septic wounds: pain
b. Peripheral vascular diseases
(1) Pain
(2) Tingling
2. Objective
a. Gas gangrene and septic wounds
(1) Fever
(2) Edema
(3) Foul odor
(4) Bronze or blackened wound due to necrosis
b. Peripheral vascular diseases
(1) Edema
(2) Pallor
(3) Shiny, hairless skin
(4) Hyperpigmentation
(5) Ulcer formation
c. Arterial diseases
(1) Pallor
(2) Cyanosis
(3) Diminished pulses
(4) Pain on pressure
D. Diagnostic tests and methods
1. Oscillometry
2. Arteriography
3. Skin temperature studies
4. X-ray examination
5. Doppler flow studies
E. Treatment
1. Psychological preparation
2. Rehabilitation preparation

3. Nutritional status buildup
4. Prosthetic device
F. Nursing intervention
1. Provide preoperative care.
a. Encourage expression of feelings by providing honesty concerning loss of limb.
b. Explain to the patient the possibility of experiencing pain in the amputated limb (called phantom limb pain).
c. Explain to the patient that he or she will undergo a program of exercises that includes strengthening of upper extremities, transferring from bed to chair, and ambulating with a walker or crutches.
2. Provide postoperative care.
a. Provide routine postoperative care.
b. Monitor for hemorrhage; if it occurs, apply manual pressure and notify physician.
c. Apply elastic (Ace) bandages in a crisscross or figure-8 pattern only.
d. Elevate the residual limb 8 to 12 hours on a pillow; remove after 12 hours to prevent hip contracture; place in prone position 1 hour out of every 4 hours to prevent hip contracture.
e. Prevent outward rotation by placing trochanter roll along the outer side of the residual limb.
f. Instruct the patient not to hang the residual limb over the edge of the bed, wheelchair, chair, or handrail of his or her crutches to avoid residual limb contracture.
g. When conditioning of the residual limb is ordered, begin by having the patient push the residual limb against a pillow and progress to pushing against a firmer surface.
h. Teach the patient to massage the residual limb to soften the scar and improve vascularity.
i. Use transcutaneous electrical nerve stimulator (TENS) for relief of phantom limb pain.
j. Encourage progressive ambulation and physical therapy.

RESPIRATORY SYSTEM

Anatomy and Physiology

A. Respiration: the taking in of oxygen, its use in the tissues, and the giving off of carbon dioxide; has two stages
1. External: exchange of oxygen and carbon dioxide between body and outside environment; consists of inhalation and exhalation; also known as ventilation
2. Internal: exchange of carbon dioxide and oxygen between the cells and the interstitial fluid surrounding the cells
B. Organs (Figures 5-3 through 5-6)
1. Nose
a. Divides into two cavities separated by nasal septum
b. Ciliated mucosa lines the cavities and traps inhaled foreign particles.
c. Filters, warms, and moistens air
d. Serves as organ of smell
(1) Receptors located in olfactory epithelium of upper part of nasal cavity
(2) Stimulates appetite and flow of digestive juices
(3) Senses of smell and taste work together to give flavor to food.

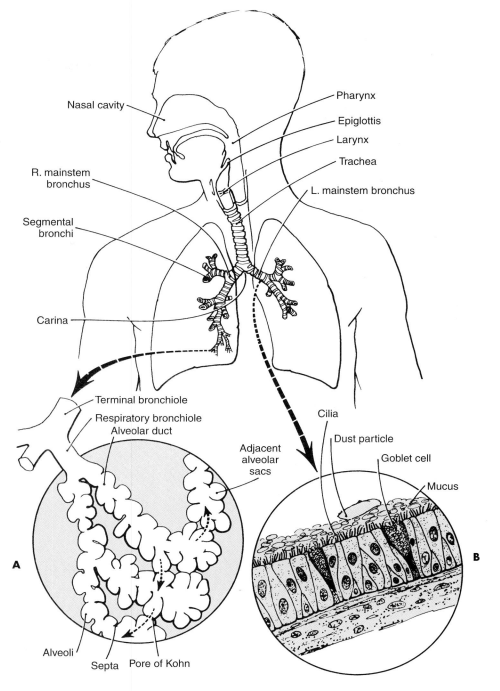

FIGURE 5-3. Structures of the respiratory tract. A, Pulmonary functional unit. **B,** Ciliated mucous membrane. *(From Phipps, Monahan, Sands, et al. Medical-Surgical Nursing health and illness perspectives, ed. 7, St. Louis, 2003, Mosby.)*

e. Paranasal sinuses: lighten skull, act as resonance chamber in speech

2. Pharynx: passageway for food and air; divided into three parts
   a. Nasopharynx (behind nose): contains adenoids; eustachian tube, which drains the middle ear, opens into the nasopharynx
   b. Oropharynx (mouth): contains tonsils, which are lymphatic tissue
   c. Laryngopharynx: opens into larynx toward front and into esophagus toward back

3. Larynx (voice box)
   a. Formed by nine cartilages in boxlike formation

b. Thyroid cartilage that forms the Adam's apple
   c. Epiglottis: flap of elastic cartilage that closes off the larynx when swallowing food
   d. Produces sound; vocal cords vibrate with expelled air
   e. Passageway for air to the trachea

4. Trachea (windpipe): tube reinforced by C-shaped rings; open ends of rings face posteriorly toward the esophagus and allow esophagus to expand when swallowing food; solid portion keeps the trachea open for the passage of air.

5. Bronchi
   a. Formed by the division of the trachea into two branches; distribute air to the lungs' interior; called bronchial tree

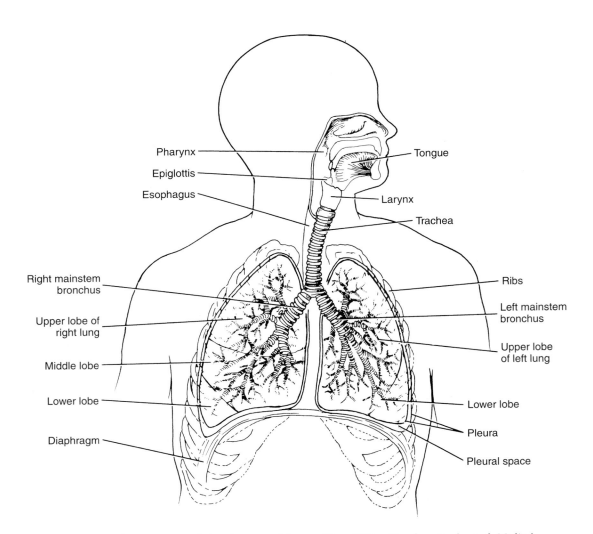

FIGURE 5-4. **Anatomy of the thorax and lungs.** *(From Phipps, Monahan, Sands, et al. Medical-Surgical Nursing health and illness perspectives, ed. 7, St. Louis, 2003, Mosby.)*

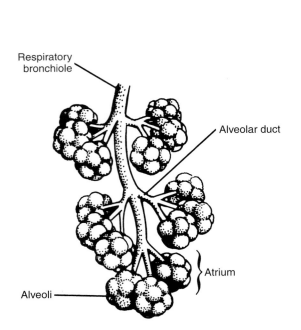

FIGURE 5-5. **Respiratory unit.** *(From Phipps, Monahan, Sands, et al. Medical-Surgical Nursing health and illness perspectives, ed. 7, St. Louis, 2003, Mosby.)*

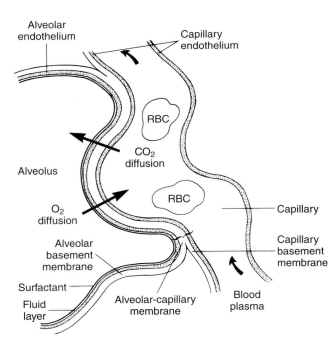

FIGURE 5-6. **Alveolar-capillary membrane.** *(From Long BC, Phipps WJ, Cassmeyer VL: Medical-surgical nursing: a nursing process approach, ed 3, St Louis, 1993, Mosby.)*

b. Right main bronchus is larger and more vertical; aspiration is more common by this route.

c. Bronchi divide into smaller branches called bronchioles.

d. Bronchioles divide into smaller tubes and terminate in the alveoli.

e. Alveoli: microscopic air sacs that resemble bunches of grapes; composed of a single, thin layer of squamous epithelium; external surface surrounded with spider webbed pulmonary capillaries; here, gas exchanges occur, oxygen passes from the alveoli into the capillary blood, and carbon dioxide leaves the blood to enter the alveoli.

6. Lungs

a. Cone shaped; upper part is the apex; broad lower part is the base; base is concave and rests on diaphragm.

b. Tissue is porous and spongy.

c. Pleura: thin, moist, slippery membrane covering lungs; prevents friction during breathing movement

C. Physiology

1. Two phases of breathing: inspiration and expiration

2. Respiration is controlled by respiratory center in medulla oblongata.

3. Carbon dioxide stimulates respiration.

4. Muscles of respiration

a. Diaphragm: dome shaped; separates thoracic and abdominal cavities; contracts and relaxes

b. Intercostals: between the ribs; elevate the ribs and enlarge the thorax during inspiration

5. Mechanism of inspiration

a. Contraction of diaphragm causes the thorax to expand.

b. The lungs cling to the thoracic wall as a result of the attachment of the pleural membranes.

c. Intrathoracic pressure decreases.

d. The volume within the lungs (intrapulmonary) increases, and gases in the lungs spread out to fill the space.

e. Result is a decrease in gas pressure, and a partial vacuum sucks air into the lungs; air continues to move into the lungs until intrapulmonic pressure equals atmospheric pressure.

6. Mechanism of expiration

a. Respiratory muscles relax, and thorax decreases in size.

b. Intrathoracic and intrapulmonary volumes decrease.

c. As volume decreases, gases are forced closer together, and intrapulmonary pressure rises higher than atmospheric pressure.

d. Gases flow out of lungs and equalize pressure inside and outside the lung.

7. Volumes of air exchanges

a. Total lung capacity (TLC): total volume of air present in the lungs after maximum inspiration

b. Vital capacity (VC): volume of air that can be expelled after maximum inspiration

c. Tidal volume (TV): volume of air exhaled after normal inspiration

d. Residual volume (RV): amount of air remaining in lung after maximum expiration

RESPIRATORY CONDITIONS AND DISORDERS

All cells of the body depend on adequate oxygenation and removal of carbon dioxide for health. The respiratory system is dependent on central nervous system regulation and on the cardiovascular system for blood supply. Respiratory distress or dysfunction may be secondary to disease in another system. Many pulmonary diseases are chronic. Therefore the nurse must make a complete respiratory assessment of all patients and include this in nursing care planning, even when the primary diagnosis is unrelated to the respiratory system.

The following are terms used to describe respirations:

Bradypnea: slow respirations

Cheyne-Stokes: periods of apnea alternating with rapid respirations

Dyspnea: difficulty breathing; may be subjective or objective

Dyspnea on exertion (DOE)

Kussmaul breathing: fast, deep, and labored respirations

Orthopnea: difficulty breathing in a supine position; relieved by sitting up

Paroxysmal nocturnal dyspnea: transient episodes of acute dyspnea that occur a few hours after falling asleep

Short of breath (SOB)

Tachypnea: rapid respirations

Wheeze: sound as air moves out through bronchi and bronchioles that have been narrowed by spasm, swelling, and secretions

Nursing Assessment

A. Nursing observations (objective data)

1. Respirations

a. Rate

b. Depth

c. Characteristics (wheezing); any difficulty breathing; DOE

2. Oxygen deprivation (note any)

a. Restlessness

b. Yawning

c. Anxiety

d. Drowsiness

e. Confusion

f. Disorientation

g. Flaring nostrils

h. Retractions

3. Cough

a. Frequency

b. Relationship to activity and precipitating factors

c. Production of sputum

d. Describe completely (e.g., dry, productive, nonproductive, hoarse, barking, moist, or hacking)

4. Lung sounds (adventitious)

a. Crackles

b. Wheezes

c. Friction rub

d. Stridor

e. Rhonchi

5. Sputum (note the following):

a. Consistency (e.g., thick, tenacious, watery, frothy)

b. Amount (e.g., scant, moderate, copious)

     c. Color (e.g., white, yellow, pink, rust, blood tinged, green)

     d. Odor

  6. Skin color

     a. Pallor, ashen, or ruddy

     b. Cyanosis (bluish discoloration): observe lips, nail beds, and mucous membranes

  7. Skin

     a. Temperature

     b. Diaphoresis

  8. Vital signs

     a. Pulse: note rate, quality, and characteristics

     b. Blood pressure

     c. Temperature (rectal; tympanic)

     d. Pulse oximetry

  9. Nasal discharge

  10. Voice: huskiness

B. Patient description (subjective data)

  1. Cough

  2. Pain

  3. Difficulty breathing

  4. Fatigue or weakness, dizziness or fainting

  5. Sputum

C. Patient history

  1. History of orthopnea—use of extra pillows needed to sleep

  2. Respiratory illness or difficulty

  3. Injuries

  4. Use of medications or respiratory aids

  5. Smoking

  6. Seasonal exacerbations

  7. Exposure to environmental irritants

  8. Known allergies

  9. Coexisting, chronic illness (i.e., human immuno-deficiency virus [HIV], diabetes, immunocompromised conditions, therapies)

Diagnostic Tests and Methods

A. Chest x-ray examination: a picture of lung tissue from different angles; based on a knowledge of normal anatomy and usual changes in disease, diagnosis of many conditions can be made (e.g., tumors, pneumonia); no preparation and no special care or observations are required after x-ray examination.

B. Bronchoscopy

  1. Direct inspection of the trachea and bronchi through a scope passed via the nose or mouth; with this procedure, specimens are obtained for biopsy and culture; foreign bodies can be removed (e.g., fish bones).

  2. Nursing responsibilities: provide general preparation as that for a surgical procedure (see Chapter 2); after the procedure, monitor vital signs, provide oral hygiene, and observe for cough and blood-streaked sputum; do not allow patient to eat or drink until gag reflex returns.

C. Bronchogram

  1. Visualization of bronchial tree through x-ray examination after introducing radiopaque dye; patient is given sedative and antispasmodic.

  2. Nursing responsibilities: provide postural drainage to aid in removal of dye; encourage deep breathing and coughing; do not allow patient to eat or drink until gag reflex returns.

D. CT scan: produces clear, anatomic images of the chest cavity

E. Ultrasound: image of area is created by high-frequency sound; used for specific data relative to lung capacities

F. MRI: image created by magnetic resonance, a noninvasive procedure

G. Thoracentesis

  1. Needle aspiration of fluid from pleural cavity (space); local anesthesia is used.

  2. Nursing responsibilities: maintain proper positioning; support and reassure patient during the procedure; monitor vital signs during and after the procedure.

H. CBC: WBC count changes from normal values may indicate infection.

I. Arterial blood gas analysis

  1. Measurement of the partial pressure of oxygen and carbon dioxide in the blood; arterial puncture is performed.

  2. Nursing care: once the blood sample is obtained, apply constant pressure to the site for 5 minutes; apply pressure dressing; inspect site frequently for hematoma and pain; distally for skin temperature, and color.

J. Culture and sensitivity

  1. Throat or nasopharynx

  2. Sputum

     a. Identifies organisms and specific medication to which patient will respond

     b. Nursing responsibilities: obtain before starting antibiotics; first sputum in the morning usually has the most organisms.

K. Sputum analysis

  1. Acid-fast bacillus (AFB): determines presence of *Mycobacterium tuberculosis*

  2. Cytology: assists in the diagnosis of lung carcinoma

L. Pulmonary function test: determines extent of respiratory difficulty and evaluates function of respiratory system; no special preparation or nursing care is required after testing; a spirometer is used to diagram air movement, lung volumes, and airflow; the computer determines the actual value, predicted value, and percentage of the predicted value; examples of these tests are:

  1. Volumes: Tidal volume (TV), expiratory reserve volume, residual volume (RV), and inspiratory reserve volume

  2. Capacities: Total lung capacity (TLC), functional residual capacity, vital capacity (VC), inspiratory capacity

M. Lung scan, Positron emission tomography (PET): radioisotopes are inhaled or administered intravenously; a scanning device records the pattern of radioactivity; used in diagnosing vascular diseases (e.g., pulmonary embolism); no special preparation or nursing care is required.

N. Biopsy examination

  1. Removal of a small amount of tissue to identify disease; biopsy may be of a lymph node to determine if the disease has spread into the lymphatic system.

  2. Nursing care: provide general preoperative and postoperative care (see Chapter 2)

Frequent Patient Problems and Nursing Care

A. Activity intolerance related to fatigue related to body cells' demand for oxygen is not met; the patient tires easily and becomes short of breath.

1. Protect from exertion; provide care; space activities appropriately.
2. Plan care to include rest periods.
3. Leave call bell and all personal belongings within easy reach.
4. Provide oxygen with humidity as ordered.
5. Limit conversation.
B. Risk for injury related to dizziness, caused by diminished oxygen to the brain cells
   1. Provide all care as in preceding list.
   2. Maintain safety; use side rails.
   3. Perform neurological assessment every 4 hours (q4h).
   4. Assist when patient is out of bed.
C. Impaired oral mucous membrane related to mouth breathing
   1. Encourage fluids if allowed.
   2. Provide oral hygiene every 2 hours (q2h).
   3. Lubricate lips with non–petroleum-base product.
D. Ineffective breathing pattern related to orthopnea
   1. Place a pillow longitudinally under back.
   2. Provide table with pillow for headrest in extreme difficulty.
   3. Use footboard to prevent slipping down in bed.
   4. Semi- to high-Fowler's position.
E. Impaired tissue perfusion (cardiopulmonary); impaired gas exchange related to dyspnea and coughing
   1. Oxygen therapy: maintain safety of equipment and proper care and observations.
   2. Organize care and work efficiently to conserve patient's energy.
   3. Plan rest periods.
   4. Position in semi- to high-Fowler's position; use two pillows.
   5. Provide soft diet and small, frequent feedings.
   6. Avoid gas-forming foods.
   7. Prevent constipation and straining.
   8. Use rectal thermometer; take tympanic temperature.
   9. Make accurate observations about cough and sputum.
   10. Obtain specimens as needed.
   11. Provide tissues and bag for disposal within easy reach for infection control.
   12. Provide sputum cup if specimen needed.
   13. Change position every 2 hours (q2hrs)
   14. Encourage deep breathing.
   15. Encourage fluids every 2 hours (q2hrs).
   16. Provide oral hygiene every 2 hours (q2hrs).
   17. Provide postural drainage if ordered (see Chapter 2).
   18. Give expectorants as ordered (see Chapters 2 and 3).
   19. Suction as necessary (prn).
F. Anxiety related to dyspnea, fatigue, and weakness
   1. Maintain quiet environment.
   2. Help the patient remain calm.
   3. Explain everything slowly and carefully.
   4. Provide physical and mental rest.
   5. Answer call lights promptly.
   6. Provide frequent contacts.
   7. Offer realistic encouragement.
   8. Provide restful diversion (e.g., music).
   9. Encourage the patient to express feelings and concerns.
G. Impaired nutrition, less than body requirements, related to dry mouth from mouth breathing, foul taste and odor from sputum, and fatigue; may affect desire for food
   1. Make mealtime pleasant.
   2. Provide oral hygiene before each meal.
   3. Remove used tissues and sputum cups.
   4. Request food preferences.
   5. Give small, frequent, attractively served meals.

Major Medical Diagnoses
Sinusitis

A. Definition: inflammation of one or more of the sinuses of the frontal, ethmoid, sphenoid, or maxillary bones; secretions become infected; is acute but becomes chronic if not treated or leads to complications: septicemia, meningitis, brain abscess
B. Cause: results from the spread of organisms from the nose or trapped secretions interfering with drainage (e.g., nasal polyps, edema from allergy)
C. Signs and symptoms
   1. Subjective: pain and headache
   2. Objective
      a. Nasal secretions, possibly purulent and blood tinged
      b. Elevation of temperature; mild leukopenia
D. Diagnostic tests and methods
   1. Patient history and physical assessment
   2. X-ray examination, transillumination
E. Treatment
   1. Irrigation and inhalation of steam
   2. Antibiotics and decongestants (see Chapter 3)
   3. Surgery (e.g., Caldwell-Luc [infected maxillary sinus is removed through an incision under the upper lip] or ethmoidectomy)
F. Nursing intervention
   1. Administer nonnarcotic analgesics or nasal constrictors (see Chapter 3).
   2. Provide moist steam; a hot, dry environment will increase congestion; a vaporizer may thin secretions and soothe passages.
   3. Provide hot wet pack; may relieve pain and congestion of over-involved sinus.
   4. Give general preoperative and postoperative care (see Chapter 2); note specific orders for care or observations.

Epistaxis (Nosebleed)

A. Definition: bleeding from the nose
B. Cause: may be spontaneous, related to direct trauma, or a result of systemic diseases (e.g., hypertension, blood dyscrasias); may be caused by local irritation from chronic infections or low-humidity environment
C. Sign: bleeding; shock if profuse
D. Diagnostic tests and methods: patient history and physical examination; platelet, Hct, and Hgb if profuse
E. Treatment (only if bleeding cannot be stopped)
   1. Nasal packing
   2. Cauterization of site with 10% silver nitrate stick
   3. Epinephrine spray
   4. Treatment of systemic disease
   5. Hemostatic agents
F. Nursing intervention
   1. Maintain patent airway (direct patient to breathe through mouth); have suction available.
   2. Control bleeding: pinch nose firmly with fingers on soft part of nose; position in high-Fowler's with head forward.

3. Instruct patient to expectorate blood (swallowing will cause vomiting).
4. Apply ice or cold compresses to nasal area to constrict blood vessels.
5. Monitor vital signs.
6. Avoid hot liquids.
7. Provide oral hygiene.
8. Reassure patient and family.

Deviated Septum

A. Definition: airway obstruction caused by deflection of bone and cartilage in the nasal septum
B. Causes
   1. Trauma
   2. Congenital
C. Diagnostic tests and methods
   1. Patient history
   2. Physical assessment
   3. X-ray examination
D. Treatment: surgery-submucous resection (SMR), performed through the mucous membrane within the nares; bone and cartilage are removed.
E. Nursing intervention
   1. Provide general preoperative and postoperative care (see Chapter 2).
   2. Before surgery, inform patient that nasal packing will be in place 24 to 48 hours; nasal breathing will not be possible; a temporary loss of smell will occur; sneezing must be avoided; and pain, discoloration, and swelling around the eyes will be present.
   3. Maintain airway; place patient on side or in semi-Fowler's position; monitor respirations.
   4. Provide oral hygiene every 1 to 2 hours.
   5. Provide ice compresses; note bleeding on dressing; inspect back of throat for trickle of blood.
   6. Use rectal or tympanic thermometer.
   7. Provide liquid diet when tolerated; encourage fluids; prevent constipation.
   8. Discourage forceful coughing.

Polyps

A. Definition: grapelike swellings of tissue; nasal polyps obstruct breathing and block sinus drainage (see sinusitis).
B. Treatment: surgical removal
C. Nursing intervention
   1. Surgical preparation
   2. Close check on postoperative bleeding

Laryngitis

A. Definition: an inflammation and swelling of the mucous membrane lining of the larynx
B. Cause: local irritation (e.g., smoking, spread of infection from elsewhere in the upper respiratory tract, abuse of vocal cords)
C. Signs and symptoms
   1. Subjective: pain
   2. Objective
      a. Hoarseness
      b. Loss of voice
      c. Cough
D. Diagnostic tests and methods
   1. Physical assessment
   2. Patient history
   3. Indirect laryngoscopy
E. Treatment and nursing intervention
   1. Rest voice; provide alternate means of communication.
   2. Removal of cause
   3. Provide steam inhalations.
   4. Administer astringent or antiseptic spray (see Chapter 3).

Carcinoma of the Larynx

A. Description: squamous cell carcinoma grows, spreads, and metastasizes; the rate of growth is determined by location of the lesion in the larynx.
B. Causes: related to heavy smoking, chronic laryngitis and vocal abuse, and alcohol consumption
C. Signs and symptoms
   1. Subjective: anxiety (i.e., concerning surgery, confirmation of diagnosis, disfigurement)
   2. Objective
      a. Hoarseness
      b. Signs of metastasis: pain, lump in throat, difficulty swallowing, dyspnea, and enlarged, painful lymph nodes
D. Diagnostic tests and methods
   1. Patient history
   2. Visual examination (laryngoscopy)
   3. Biopsy examination
   4. Laryngeal tomography
E. Treatment: surgery
   1. Removal of larynx (laryngectomy) (partial or complete)
   2. Radical neck dissection: wide excision, including lymph nodes, epiglottis, thyroid cartilage, and muscle tissue; a permanent tracheostomy is performed
   3. Radiotherapy with surgery
F. Nursing intervention
   1. Provide general preoperative and postoperative care (see Chapter 2).
   2. Provide immediate postoperative care.
      a. Maintain patent airway; patient may have a permanent tracheostomy (see Chapter 2); there will be a shorter tube (laryngectomy tube); place patient in semi-Fowler's position; provide frequent mouth care.
      b. Observe dressing every hour; connect wound drains to suction as ordered; prevent movement of head.
   3. Provide continued postoperative care.
      a. Provide method of communication (e.g., magic slate), leave call bell close to hand, and answer promptly in person.
      b. Assist and be supportive as alternate methods of speech are learned (e.g., esophageal speech, use of mechanical voice box).
      c. Provide high-calorie, high-protein diet (tube feedings may be required at first).
      d. Arrange for a visit from someone who has had a similar operation and satisfactory rehabilitation.
      e. Investigate lifestyle changes (i.e., smoking, alcohol consumption) to decrease further risk of complications.

Pneumonia

A. Definition: an inflammation of the lungs or part of the lung (e.g.; left lower lobe [LLL] pneumonia); secretions fill the alveolar sacs, which is a good medium for bacterial growth;

the inflammation spreads to adjacent sacs; spaces of the lung consolidate with thick exudate; irritation may cause bleeding, and sputum has the characteristic rusty color; exchange of air is difficult and, in advanced conditions, not possible.
B. Causes: bacterial infections and viruses are spread by respiratory secretions (droplets); chemical irritation; fungi and other organisms; aspirations; patients with poor health and low natural resistance to infection are more susceptible (e.g., older adults, persons with chronic illness, and immunocompromised individuals should consider receiving Pneumovax vaccine as a preventative measure for the most common type of bacterial pneumonia).
C. Signs and symptoms
   1. Subjective
      a. Dyspnea, shortness of breath
      b. Pain on inspiration
      c. Shallow breathing, signs of air hunger, orthopnea, and oxygen deprivation
   2. Objective
      a. Marked elevation in temperature
      b. Cough: painful and dry at first, then productive with copious amounts of thick sputum (color according to organism)
      c. X-ray results
D. Diagnostic tests and methods
   1. Patient history
   2. Physical assessment with auscultation of chest
   3. Chest X-ray examination
   4. Sputum culture and sensitivity
   5. CBC
E. Treatment
   1. Specific and broad-spectrum antibiotics (see Chapter 3)
   2. Antipyretics, analgesics (codeine), expectorants, and bronchodilators (see Chapter 3)
   3. Intravenous (IV) fluids; encourage oral fluids.
   4. Oxygen with humidity; incentive spirometer
F. Nursing intervention
   1. Provide optimum rest: provide care; help patient conserve energy; schedule rest periods; limit conversation; keep personal items and call bell within easy reach; alleviate anxiety.
   2. Maintain oxygen with humidity.
   3. Isolate as indicated, especially patients with oral and nasal secretions; provide for proper disposal (see Chapter 2).
   4. Liquefy secretions: encourage fluids (3000 ml daily or more); observe and document production of sputum; suction as necessary.
   5. Provide oral hygiene every 2 hours.
   6. Monitor vital signs every 4 hours; use rectal thermometer; monitor lung sounds.
   7. Assist with loosening of secretions: have patient turn, cough, and deep breathe every 2 hours (splint chest if painful); observe and document cough; may need aerosol treatment.
   8. Maintain adequate nutrition: provide liquid-to-soft diet high in protein and calories.
   9. Maintain IV fluids and medication schedule to ensure continued blood levels.
   10. Position for comfort (high-Fowler's or lying on affected side).

Pleurisy

A. Definition: inflammation of the pleural membranes (local or diffuse); may or may not have fluid exudate; when fluid is present, the condition is pleural effusion; when purulent, the condition is empyema.
B. Cause: infections (e.g., pneumonia, lung abscess, trauma, fungus, tuberculosis, lung cancer, CHF, ascites)
C. Signs and symptoms
   1. Subjective
      a. Sharp pain on inspiration (referred to shoulder, abdomen, or affected side)
      b. Dyspnea
      c. Anxiety
   2. Objective
      a. Cough
      b. Elevation of temperature
      c. Decreased breath sounds
      d. Pleural rub
D. Diagnostic tests and methods
   1. Chest x-ray examination
   2. Patient history
   3. Physical assessment, including auscultation of chest
   4. Examination of pleural fluid obtained via thoracentesis and laboratory analysis
E. Treatment (according to cause)
   1. Analgesics and antibiotics
   2. Drainage of fluid: thoracentesis, then chest tubes to underwater-seal drainage with suction
   3. Oxygen if dyspnea is severe; alleviate pain by turning patient to affected side.
F. Nursing intervention: see plan for patient with chest tubes (Box 5-2); provide diet high in protein, calories, minerals, and vitamins; alleviate anxiety.

Pneumothorax, Hemothorax

A. Definition
   1. Pneumothorax: air in pleural space allowing for partial or complete collapse of the lung
   2. Hemothorax: blood in pleural space
B. Causes
   1. May be spontaneous
   2. Trauma (e.g., knife wound, fractured rib that punctures lung)
   3. Postoperative (e.g., where the thoracic cavity has been entered)
   4. Diagnostic (e.g., central venous pressure [CVP] line, thoracentesis, pleural biopsy)
C. Signs and symptoms
   1. Subjective
      a. Sudden, sharp chest pain (when spontaneous)
      b. Vertigo
   2. Objective
      a. Diaphoresis, rapid pulse, and rapid respirations
      b. Decreased blood pressure
      c. Decreased breath sounds
      d. Dyspnea
D. Diagnostic tests and methods
   1. Patient history and physical assessment
   2. Chest x-ray examination
   3. Auscultation
   4. Observation

BOX 5-2　Patient With Chest Tubes

Description
Drainage tubes are inserted between the ribs into the pleural cavity to allow for drainage of secretions, blood, or air; the tube(s) is attached to an underwater seal system to allow for expansion of the lung and to prevent air from entering the pleural cavity; the drainage system may or may not be attached to suction

Indications
- Chest surgery
- Stab wounds to the chest
- Pleural effusion
- Spontaneous pneumothorax

Nursing Intervention
- Do complete assessment of the respiratory system q2h; place patient in semi-Fowler's position; provide oxygen with humidity
- Prevent complications of immobility; have patient turn, deep breathe, and cough q2h; encourage patient to ambulate as ordered and as condition allows; splint chest to cough
- Encourage fluids to liquefy secretions; provide tissues and bag for proper disposal; provide sputum cup
- Provide oral hygiene q2h
- Anticipate pain; medicate as needed; observe respirations 30 minutes after administration of sedative or analgesic
- Observe underwater seal system qh:
  Drainage color and amount
  Rise and fall of water in bottle (or suction) going to patient
  Bubbling (if connected to suction)
- Alleviate anxiety
- Pace activities to allow for periods of rest
- Monitor chest tube drainage

E. Treatment
　1. Closure of wound with airtight dressing
　2. Aspiration of fluids and air; water-seal drainage
　3. Analgesics
　4. Thoracentesis
F. Nursing intervention
　1. Provide nursing care and observations as necessary for primary diagnosis.
　2. Place patient in high-Fowler's position.
　3. Monitor vital signs.
　4. Administer oxygen.
　5. Provide nursing care for a patient with chest tubes as described in Box 5-2.
　6. Provide instructions on tube or dressing care if discharged with chest tube in place.

Influenza

A. Definition: acute disease that may occur as an epidemic; recovery is usually complete; no permanent immunity results; complications and death may occur in patients with chronic or debilitating conditions, especially cardiac or pulmonary conditions.
B. Cause: virus
C. Signs and symptoms
　1. Subjective
　　a. Headache, chest pain, muscle ache
　　b. Dry throat
　2. Objective
　　a. Nuchal rigidity
　　b. Elevated temperature
　　c. Coughing, sneezing, nasal discharge, and herpetic lesions
　3. GI symptoms; nausea, vomiting, and anorexia
　4. Weakness
D. Diagnostic tests and methods: patient history and physical assessment
E. Treatment
　1. Prevention with vaccines; influenza vaccine recommended on a yearly basis
　2. Relief of symptoms
　3. Antiviral therapy: amantadine hydrochloride for the prophylaxis and treatment of influenza A virus
F. Nursing intervention
　1. Provide rest, assist with care; provide quiet environment and dim lighting.
　2. Encourage fluids.
　3. Relieve symptoms: provide antipyretics, analgesics.

Pulmonary Tuberculosis

A. Definition: a chronic, progressive infection; alveoli are inflamed, and small nodules are produced called primary tubercles; the tubercle bacillus is at the center of the nodule (these become fibrosed); the area becomes calcified and can be identified on x-ray film; the person who has been infected harbors the bacillus for life; it is dormant unless it becomes active during physical or emotional stress.
B. Cause: *Mycobacterium tuberculosis,* Koch bacillus, an AFB spread by droplets from an infected person
C. Signs and symptoms
　1. Subjective
　　a. Malaise; patient is easily fatigued.
　　b. Chest pain
　　c. Anorexia and weight loss
　　d. Anxiety (i.e., fear of chronic disease, fear of public rejection)
　2. Objective
　　a. Cough and hemoptysis (coughing up blood from the respiratory tract)
　　b. Elevation of temperature and night sweats
D. Diagnostic tests and methods
　1. Patient history and physical assessment, coexisting chronic illness
　2. Chest x-ray examination
　3. Sputum specimen for AFB; aspiration of gastric fluid for AFB if unable to obtain specimen
　4. Tuberculin skin testing (e.g., Mantoux test)
E. Treatment
　1. Antituberculin drugs for 18 to 24 months (see Chapter 3)
　2. Rest (physical and emotional)
　3. Diet high in carbohydrates, proteins, and vitamins (especially vitamin B_6)
　4. Surgical resection of affected lung tissue or involved lobe (only when necessary)
F. Nursing intervention
　1. Provide rest; assist with or provide care; plan rest periods; limit conversation; leave personal items in easy reach.

2. Prevent transmission: ensure proper isolation (AFB, tuberculosis); provide tissues and bag for disposal; encourage proper use of tissues; insist on patient covering mouth and nose when coughing or sneezing; provide mask for patient if necessary; room must be equipped with special means of ventilation.

3. Provide frequent, small meals and nutritious snacks; provide mouth care after meals.

4. Help the patient avoid chills; keep patient's skin dry and clean; protect from drafts, especially at night.

5. Allay fears of patient and family about transmission: encourage proper adherence to drug maintenance; explain how organism is carried, transmitted, and destroyed (nurse must be aware that a tuberculin test is recommended for all contacts with a person with tuberculosis); a positive test result does not mean the disease has developed but indicates that the organism has entered the body and that the body has produced antibodies at some point; explain need for multiple, long-term drug therapy.

Chronic Obstructive Pulmonary Disease

Chronic obstructive pulmonary disease (COPD) includes chronic and frequently progressive pulmonary disorders that affect expiratory air flow; asthma, chronic bronchitis, and pulmonary emphysema may occur independently or together.

Asthma

A. Definition: spasms of the bronchial muscle; edema and swelling of the mucosa produce thick secretions; air flow is obstructed; air enters and is trapped; a characteristic wheeze accompanies attempts to exhale through narrowed bronchi; breathing is labored; coughing is attempted, but patient fails to expectorate satisfactory amounts; patient experiences great anxiety; the attacks last 30 to 60 minutes, often with normal breathing between attacks; an attack that is difficult to control and is resistant to all forms of treatment is called status asthmaticus.

B. Causes
  1. Recurrent respiratory infection
  2. Allergic reaction
  3. Physical or emotional stress may provoke attack in a person with asthma

C. Signs and symptoms
  1. Subjective: anxiety or feeling of suffocation, dyspnea
  2. Objective
    a. Shortness of breath, expiratory wheeze, labored respirations, diaphoresis, use of accessory muscles, and flaring nostrils
    b. Thick, tenacious sputum (after acute attack)

D. Diagnostic tests and methods: patient history and physical examination, arterial blood gas analysis, allergy testing, pulmonary function; peak flow meter

E. Treatment
  1. Removal of cause (source of allergy) or desensitization
  2. Low-flow, humidified oxygen
  3. Bronchodilators, mast cell inhibitors, corticosteroids, or sedatives (see Chapter 3); metered-dose inhalers

F. Nursing intervention
  1. Reduce anxiety: provide time to listen; do not leave patient alone during attack.

2. Remove cause: keep environment free from dust and other allergens.
3. Provide continuous humidity as ordered.
4. Encourage fluids; maintain IV as ordered.
5. Position for maximal comfort and breathing: have patient sit in high-Fowler's position with arms supported by an over-bed table.
6. Prevent secondary infections: avoid staff and visitors with upper respiratory infections.
7. Teach abdominal breathing.
8. Do not allow smoking; refer patient for help in quitting.
9. Avoid exposure to cold, wet weather.
10. Instruct on preventive treatment for exertional asthma.
11. Instruct on medications, use of inhalers.

Chronic Bronchitis

A. Definition: chronic, progressive infection accompanied by hypersecretion of mucus by the bronchioles; without treatment and prevention of acute attacks, the alveolar sacs and capillaries will extend and destruct.

B. Causes
  1. Asthma
  2. Acute respiratory tract infections (e.g., pneumonia, influenza, smoking, and air pollution contribute to incidence)
  3. Familial tendency

C. Signs and symptoms
  1. Subjective
    a. Worsening dyspnea
    b. Exertional dyspnea
  2. Objective
    a. Results of diagnostic tests
    b. Cough, productive with thick, white sputum; sputum is blood tinged as disease progresses (cough is greatest on arising).
    c. May progress to wheezing, prolonged expiratory time, use of accessory muscles

D. Diagnostic tests and methods
  1. Patient history
  2. Pulmonary testing to rule out other disease (e.g., tuberculosis, malignancy)
  3. Chest x-ray analysis

E. Treatment
  1. Preventing irritation of bronchial mucosa: encouraging patient to discontinue smoking and to change aggravating conditions in occupation or home environment
  2. Preventing upper respiratory tract infection: maintaining optimum health, adequate rest, and high-protein, high-vitamin diet
  3. Providing bronchodilators, antibiotics, corticosteroids, and influenza vaccine during epidemics (see Chapter 3)

F. Nursing intervention
  1. Provide care to relieve patient problems. (See discussion on frequent patient problems and nursing care outlined earlier in this chapter.)
  2. Loosen, liquefy, and remove secretions: provide postural drainage and chest percussion as ordered; encourage fluids.
  3. Involve patient and family in care and care planning.
  4. Do not allow smoking; refer patient for help in quitting.

Emphysema

A. Definition: a chronic, progressive condition in which the alveolar sacs distend, rupture, and destroy the capillary beds; the alveoli lose elasticity, inspired air is trapped; inspiration is difficult and expiration is prolonged; the lung tissue becomes fibrotic; exchange of gases is not possible; anxiety increases; signs of oxygen deprivation are evident.

B. Cause (see bronchitis)

C. Signs and symptoms
   1. Subjective
      a. DOE (later, dyspnea on slightest exertion and orthopnea)
      b. Anorexia and weakness
   2. Objective
      a. Results of diagnostic tests
      b. Wheezing, prolonged expiratory time
      c. Chronic cough; productive, purulent sputum in copious amounts
      d. Speaks in short, jerky sentences
      e. Cerebral anoxia: is drowsy and confused; may become unconscious and go into coma
      f. Barrel chest
      g. Weight loss

D. Diagnostic tests and methods
   1. Patient history and physical examination
   2. Chest x-ray examination
   3. Pulmonary function tests
   4. Arterial blood gas analysis, CBC
   5. Sputum analysis

E. Treatment (see bronchitis)

F. Nursing intervention
   1. Loosen, liquefy, and remove secretions: provide postural drainage and chest percussion as ordered; encourage fluids; administer expectorants as needed.
   2. Promote respiratory function: breathing exercises and coughing.
   3. Administer oxygen; oxygen is administered in low concentrations only (1 to 2 L); oxygen can be dangerous when the carbon dioxide level of the blood is high; the respiratory center of the brain becomes accustomed to the low blood oxygen level; if oxygen increases, respiratory rate will slow significantly.
   4. Prevent and control infections: administer antibiotics; avoid contact with people with upper respiratory tract infections; avoid smoking.
   5. Provide rest: limit exertion of any type; provide care; minimize conversation; assist with all movements (e.g., turning, getting into chair).
   6. Include family in care and care plan; be understanding that this condition is chronic.
   7. Teach pursed-lip breathing and abdominal breathing.
   8. Encourage small, frequent meals.

Cancer of the Lung

A. Definition: primary or secondary (from metastasis [e.g., from prostate]) malignant tumor; bronchogenic carcinoma is the most common primary tumor; usually without symptoms until late stages when metastasis has occurred to brain, spinal cord, or esophagus; treatment is difficult in late stages, and treatment is based on symptoms; prognosis is poor unless detected and treated early.

B. Cause: strongly related to smoking, air pollution, and chemical irritants

C. Signs and symptoms (occur in late stages)
   1. Subjective
      a. Dyspnea and chest pain
      b. Fatigue, anorexia
   2. Objective
      a. Results of diagnostic tests
      b. Productive cough with blood-streaked sputum
      c. Weight loss

D. Diagnostic tests and methods
   1. CT scan, MRI
   2. Examination of sputum for cells (cytology)
   3. Bronchial biopsy examination

E. Treatment
   1. Surgery: procedure depends on size and location of tumor (lobectomy, pneumonectomy, or laparoscopic thoracotomy)
   2. Radiation
   3. Chemotherapy
   4. Photodynamic therapy with laser

F. Nursing intervention
   1. Provide nursing care for symptoms. (See discussion on frequent patient problems and nursing care earlier in chapter.)
   2. Provide preoperative and postoperative nursing care (see Chapter 2).
      a. Maintain patent airway; administer oxygen; have patient turn, cough, and deep breathe every 2 hours; a patient with a pneumonectomy must not cough; do not turn on operative side until physician orders (prevent mediastinal shift).
      b. Provide special care for a patient with chest tubes (rarely used but still a possibility).

CARDIOVASCULAR, PERIPHERAL, AND HEMATOLOGIC SYSTEMS

Anatomy and Physiology of the Circulatory System

A. Functions
   1. Major function: transports oxygen, carbon dioxide, cell wastes, nutrients, enzymes, and antibodies throughout the body
   2. Secondary function: contributes to the body's metabolic functions and maintenance of homeostasis

B. Heart (Figure 5-7)
   1. Hollow, cone-shaped muscular organ the size of a man's fist; functions as a pump
   2. Positioned in thoracic cavity between the sternum and thoracic vertebrae
   3. Apex extends slightly to the left and rests on the diaphragm, approximately at the level of the fifth rib; point where apical pulse is assessed
   4. Layers
      a. Pericardium: outer covering; consists of two layers of serous membrane that is lubricated and prevents friction when the heart beats
      b. Myocardium: dense fibrous connective tissue; the wall of the heart

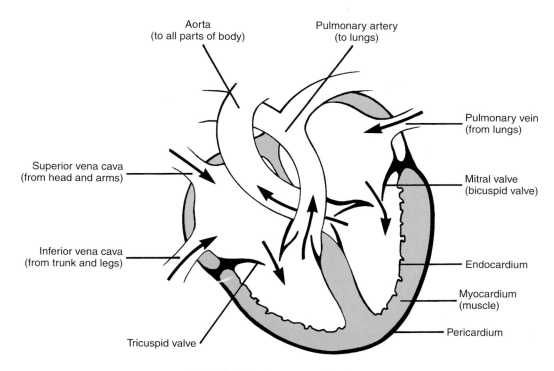

FIGURE 5-7. Structures of the heart.

c. Endocardium: a thin, serous lining that helps the blood flow smoothly through the heart; lines the heart chamber

5. Chambers
   a. Atria: upper chambers—primarily receiving chambers; mostly receiving chambers, they do not exert the major pumping force of the heart.
      (1) Right atrium: receives deoxygenated blood from the coronary sinus and the superior and inferior vena cava
      (2) Left atrium: receives oxygenated blood from the lungs by way of the four pulmonary veins
   b. Ventricles: lower chambers—the pumping chambers; they have the major responsibility of forcing blood out into large arteries.
      (1) Right ventricle: receives blood from right atrium and pumps blood to lungs by way of the pulmonary artery
      (2) Left ventricle: does the major work of the heart; has the thickest muscular wall; pumps blood to all parts of the body by way of the aorta
      (3) Interventricular or interatrial septum: divides the heart longitudinally

6. Valves: permit flow of blood in only one direction
   a. Atrioventricular (AV) valves
      (1) Tricuspid: allows blood to flow from right atrium into right ventricle
      (2) Mitral or bicuspid: allows blood to flow from left atrium to left ventricle
   b. Semilunar valves
      (1) Pulmonary semilunar: allows blood to flow out of right ventricle into pulmonary artery
      (2) Aortic semilunar: allows blood to flow out of left ventricle into aorta

7. Physiology
   a. Cardiac cycle: refers to one complete heartbeat, consisting of contraction or systole and relaxation or diastole of the atria and ventricles
   b. Auscultatory sounds: heard through a stethoscope; the first sound, systolic, is longer and louder because of the closure of the cuspid valves; the second sound, diastole, is shorter and softer because of the closure of the semilunar valves
   c. Conduction system
      (1) Functions: initiates heartbeat; conducts electrical impulses around heart; coordinates heartbeat
      (2) Components
         (a) Sinoatrial (SA) node: the pacemaker of the heart; sets and regulates the beat by sending electrical impulses to the atria and the AV node
         (b) Atrioventricular (AV) node: receives impulses from SA node; transmits electrical impulses by way of bundle of His to the ventricles
         (c) Bundle of His: fibers that begin at AV node and follow the interventricular septum; divides into Purkinje fibers
         (d) Purkinje's fibers: conducting fibers; stimulate the ventricles to contract
   d. Heart rates: controlled by internal and external factors
      (1) Bradycardia: slower than normal rate, less than 60 beats per minute (bpm)
      (2) Tachycardia: faster than normal rate, more than 100 bpm
      (3) Extrasystole: premature beat
      (4) Sinus arrhythmia: a deviation from the normal pattern of the heartbeat resulting from changes in the rate and depth of breathing or other benign causes

C. Blood vessels
  1. Arteries: elastic, muscular-conducting tubes; carry blood away from the heart and to the capillaries; all arteries (except pulmonary) carry oxygenated blood
     a. Aorta: the largest artery, from which all other arteries branch out and become smaller and smaller
     b. Arterioles: extremely small arteries; branch into the capillaries
  2. Veins: thin-walled tubes that have one-way valves to prevent backflow of blood; transport blood back to the heart; all veins (except pulmonary) carry deoxygenated blood.
     a. Venae cavae: largest veins; enter the right atrium
        (1) Superior vena cava: returns blood from the head, arms, and thoracic region
        (2) Inferior vena cava: returns blood from body regions below the diaphragm
     b. Venules: extremely small veins; collect blood from the capillaries
  3. Capillaries: microscopic vessels; carry blood from arterioles to venules; exchange of nutrients and waste products occurs in capillaries
D. Types of circulation
  1. Systemic: blood flows from the left ventricle into the aorta, through the body, and back to the right atrium; provides oxygen-rich, nutrient-laden blood to body organs
  2. Pulmonary: blood flows from the right ventricle into the pulmonary artery, to the lungs, and then back to the left atrium through the pulmonary vein; its function is to carry blood to the lungs for gas exchange and return it to the heart
  3. Portal: detour of venous blood from stomach, pancreas, intestines, and spleen through the liver, where it is processed, and returned by way of the inferior vena cava; excess glucose is removed and stored in the liver as glycogen; poisonous substances are removed and detoxified
E. Blood
  1. Functions
     a. Transports oxygen and carbon dioxide to and from lungs
     b. Transports nutrients, hormones, and waste products
     c. Helps maintain acid-base balance, electrolyte balance, and fluid balance
     d. Carries substances that help fight infection
     e. Acts to maintain homeostasis
  2. Composition
     a. Plasma: liquid, straw-colored portion of blood
        (1) Approximately 90% water
        (2) Contains blood proteins (fibrinogen, prothrombin, albumin, gamma globulin)
        (3) Contains mineral salts (electrolytes), hormones, nutrients, oxygen, carbon dioxide, and waste products (urea, lactic acid, and uric acid)
     b. Formed elements
        (1) Erythrocytes: RBCs
           (a) Contain hemoglobin, which carries oxygen to cells and carbon dioxide from cells
           (b) Originate in red bone marrow
           (c) Life span is 100 to 120 days
           (d) Destroyed by the spleen, liver, and bone marrow
           (e) Normal range: male, 4.5 to 6.2 million per cubic millimeter; female, 4 to 5.5 million per cubic millimeter

        (2) Leukocytes: WBCs
           (a) Principal function is to fight infection
           (b) Able to multiply rapidly
           (c) Classified according to whether they contain visible granules in their cytoplasm
               Granulocytes: include neutrophils, eosinophils, and basophils
               Agranulocytes: include lymphocytes and monocytes
           (d) Formation is in red bone marrow and by lymphatic tissue in lymph nodes, thymus, and spleen
           (e) Normal range: 5000 to 10,000 per cubic millimeter (ml^3)
        (3) Thrombocytes: platelets
           (a) Aid in clotting process
           (b) Originate in bone marrow
           (c) Normal range: 200,000 to 400,000/ml^3
  3. Blood types
     a. Every person belongs to one of the four groups: type A, type B, type AB, or type O; and is classified as either Rh positive or Rh negative
     b. Type A blood: type A antigens in RBCs, anti-B antibodies in plasma
     c. Type B Blood: type B antigens in RBCs, anti-A antibodies in plasma
     d. Type AB blood: type A and type B antigens in RBCs; no anti-A or anti-B antibodies in plasma; a person with type AB is called a universal recipient.
     e. Type O blood; no type A or type B antigens in RBCs; both anti-A and anti-B antibodies in plasma; a person with type O is called a universal donor.
     f. Rh-positive blood: Rh-factor antigen in RBCs
     g. Rh-negative blood: no Rh factor in RBCs; no anti-Rh antibodies in plasma
     h. Harmful effects can result from a blood transfusion if donor's RBCs become agglutinated by antibodies in the recipient's plasma.
F. Lymphatic system: represents an accessory route for return of fluid from interstitial spaces to cardiovascular system; consists of lymphatic vessels, lymph nodes or glands, and spleen
  1. Lymph: transparent fluid in surrounding spaces between tissue cells; made of water and end products of cell metabolism; referred to as intercellular or interstitial fluid
  2. Function of system
     a. Lymphatic vessels: return fluid and proteins to blood
     b. Lymph nodes: filter injurious particles, such as microorganisms and cancer cells
     c. Tonsils: filter and remove bacteria or pathogens entering the throat
     d. Thymus: most active during early life; relates immune reaction through puberty; atrophies at adulthood
  3. Spleen: consists of lymphoid tissue
     a. Forms lymphocytes and monocytes
     b. Destroys old RBCs
     c. Stores blood until needed and then releases it into circulation
G. Immunity: the body's defense system against diseases and substances interpreted as nonself; mediated by T and B lymphocytes of the circulatory system; the functions of lymphocytes in immunity by cell type are:
  1. T lymphocytes: originate from stem cells in thymus; responsible for cellular immunity (a slow response) to an

antigen; act against most bacteria, viruses, tumor cells, and foreign organs or grafts; clone into types of regulatory cells-helper and suppressors
  a. Helper T cells: interact directly with B cells by stimulating activity of B cells on killer T cells
  b. Killer T cells: directly attack virus-infected cells, promote lysis
  c. Suppressor T cells: terminate normal immune response
2. B lymphocytes: originate mainly in fetal liver and lymphoid tissue during first few months of life; responsible for humoral immunity (a rapid response) to an antigen
  a. Clone antibody-producing plasma cells
  b. Protect against toxin
3. Naturally acquired immunity
  a. Active: acquired through contact with disease
  b. Passive: acquired from antibodies obtained through placenta and mother's milk
4. Artificially acquired immunity
  a. Active: immunization with vaccines
  b. Passive: administration of immune serum

CARDIOVASCULAR CONDITIONS AND DISORDERS

Diseases related to the cardiovascular system are the leading cause of death in the United States. Cardiovascular health problems occur along the age continuum. To reduce death and disability, three major objectives include early detection of the disease, appropriate treatment to control the disease progression, and reduction of predisposing factors by promoting screening, education, and patient care of cardiovascular health.

Nursing Assessment

A. Nursing observations
  1. Vital signs
    a. Temperature
    b. Pulse: character, rate, rhythm, and any irregularities
    c. Respiration: character, rate; noting abnormalities
  2. General appearance
    a. Noting skin temperature, character, and color (jaundice, cyanosis, pallor); noting clamminess
    b. Distended neck veins
    c. DOE (dyspnea on exertion)
    d. Limited or reduced ability to perform ADL
    e. Clubbing of fingers
    f. Presence of edema; pedal, pulmonary, ascites, or sacral (if supine)
  3. Heart sounds
    a. Noting bruits (whooshing sounds caused by turbulent blood flow) in carotids
    b. Abnormal heart sounds, dysrhythmias, murmurs
    c. Precordial movements, thrills
B. Patient description (subjective data)
  1. Chest pain
    a. Onset, location, frequency, duration, radiation
    b. Alleviating or aggravating factors
    c. Chest pain may occur during periods of physical and emotional stress (emotions, eating, exercise, environment); pain may radiate to arm or jaw, or may occur at rest.

2. Easily fatigued
  a. Can no longer perform usual activities without frequent rest periods
  b. Intolerance of exercise or exertion
3. Palpitations
4. Dizziness, feelings of fatigue, especially when arising or standing
5. Cough
  a. Frothy or blood tinged (hemoptysis)
  b. Nocturnal cough
6. Family history of heart disease and hypertension
7. DOE (dyspnea on exertion)

Diagnostic Tests and Methods

A. Electrocardiogram (ECG)
  1. Tracing of the electrical activity of the heart
  2. Tool used to identify abnormal cardiac rhythms (dysrhythmias) and coronary atherosclerotic heart disease
  3. Reassure the patient that the ECG is recording the electrical impulses of the heart and is not delivering any electrical impulses to the body
  4. May be done on ambulatory patients through the use of telemetry units; signals from a box that the patient carries with him or her is conveyed to a monitor at a nurses' station.
B. Stress test
  1. A procedure designed to detect cardiac ischemia that develops during exercise or exertion
  2. A heart tracing (ECG) is recorded and monitored while a patient performs an activity such as stair climbing, pedaling a stationary bicycle, or walking on a treadmill.
C. Blood tests
  1. CBC: analyzes components of the blood
    a. Low Hgb and Hct indicate anemia.
    b. Elevated WBC count indicates inflammation, infection.
  2. Erythrocyte sedimentation rate (ESR): may indicate inflammation
  3. Blood urea nitrogen (BUN) and creatinine: to detect the effects of heart disease on the kidneys
  4. Serum enzymes and isoenzymes (serum glutamic oxaloacetic transaminase [SGOT], creatine phosphokinase [CPK], and lactate dehydrogenase [LDH]): Troponin will elevate in a myocardial infarction.
  5. Serum lipids: elevated blood lipids have been associated with coronary disease.
  6. Blood cultures: if bacterial endocarditis is suspected
  7. Coagulation studies: prothrombin time (PT) and partial thromboplastin time (PTT); useful in monitoring anticoagulant therapy
  8. Serum electrolytes: detect imbalances in sodium, potassium, and calcium
  9. Arterial blood gas analysis: monitors oxygenation and acid-base balance
D. Urinalysis: to determine the effects of heart disease on the kidney
E. Holter monitoring
  1. Portable monitor designed and equipped to record the patient's heartbeat during a 24-hour period; a written record of the patient's activity is kept simultaneously; helpful in determining dysrhythmias
  2. Assists the patient in the recording of activity
F. Coronary angiography

1. A roentgenogram of the coronary circulation facilitated by introducing contrast medium into the artery to outline the vessel and determine the extent of the disease process
2. After the study, the patient must be observed for bleeding from the puncture site and have a cardiovascular status check of the involved area (pulses and skin temperature).

G. Chest x-ray examination: a standard chest roentgenogram is used to determine heart size and shape.

H. Echocardiography (ultrasound cardiography)
   1. Echoes from sound waves are used to study the movements and dimensions of cardiac structures; determines abnormalities
   2. Information derived includes size of cardiac structures.

I. Radionuclide studies
   1. Tracing material is injected IV, and the radioactivity concentration over a body part is recorded.
   2. Size, shape, and filling of the heart chambers can be recorded; heart damage, as well as cardiac circulation, can also be evaluated.

J. Cardiac catheterization
   1. A cardiac catheter is introduced through a vein or artery and is advanced through the system; pressures of the heart chambers and pulmonary arteries are recorded, and blood is analyzed; a contrast dye can be injected for visualization of certain structures to detect defects.
   2. Patient may feel a warm flushing sensation on injection of the dye; some patients experience chest pain.
   3. Patient observations after examination: monitor bleeding at the insertion site, check pulses and skin warmth in the involved area, and check heart rate and rhythm.

K. Oscillometry: a noninvasive test that measures the amplitude of pulsations over an artery

Frequent Patient Problems and Nursing Care

A. Acute or chronic pain related to decreased cardiac output; overactivity
   1. Evaluate and record onset, duration, and intensity.
   2. Note any associated symptoms (nausea, vomiting, dyspnea).
   3. Monitor vital signs and record.
   4. Give vasodilators as prescribed; monitor for effectiveness, and observe for side effects.
   5. If pain is unrelieved in 15 minutes by drugs or rest, notify physician.
   6. Reinforce patient teaching regarding diet, drugs, planned exercise, and stress management.
   7. Administer oxygen as prescribed.
   8. Record reactions to treatment and nursing care.

B. Ineffective breathing pattern related to dyspnea
   1. Monitor vital signs and record.
   2. Note character and rate of respirations.
   3. Elevate the head of the bed at least 30 degrees.
   4. Help patient assume an orthopneic position when necessary.
   5. Auscultate chest and note the presence of abnormal lung and heart sounds.
   6. Monitor oxygen therapy.
   7. Monitor intake and output.
   8. Record reactions to treatment and nursing care.
   9. Give diuretics, cardiotonics, and bronchodilators as prescribed, and monitor for side effects.
   10. Note color, character, and amount of sputum.

C. Decreased cardiac output related to dysrhythmias
   1. Monitor vital signs and record.
   2. Note and report any changes in the vital signs.
   3. Auscultate chest, noting any abnormal heart sounds and report abnormalities.
   4. Give antidysrhythmic drugs as prescribed, and monitor for side effects.
   5. Monitor for and report any associated symptoms.

D. Risk for peripheral neurovascular dysfunction related to edema
   1. Note and record location and degree of edema.
   2. Elevate legs.
   3. Change positions when in bed.
   4. Note degree of pitting.
   5. Note "weeping" of skin areas.
   6. Monitor for skin breakdown.
   7. Give prescribed diuretics and cardiotonics.
   8. Note the presence of tenderness in the upper quadrant of the abdomen.
   9. Note the presence of ascites.
   10. Note daily weight.
   11. Record intake and output.
   12. Limit fluid intake as prescribed.
   13. Reinforce teaching for reduction of dependent edema.

E. Activity intolerance related to reduced cardiac reserve
   1. Encourage progressive ambulation.
   2. Encourage progressive resuming of ADL.
   3. Provide for planned activity and rest periods.
   4. Monitor for signs of fatigue.
   5. Stop activity at the first sign of intolerance.
   6. Encourage ROM exercises.
   7. Provide prescribed diet.
   8. Reinforce patient instruction of planned exercise.

F. Impaired tissue perfusion related to decreased cardiac output.
   1. Observe for presence of postural hypotension-orthostatic vital signs. (Note if blood pressure drops when standing.)
   2. Assist patient to dangle legs over the side of the bed before standing to reduce dizziness.
   3. Instruct patient to get up slowly.
   4. Assess patient's pulse when standing.

G. Excess fluid volume related to decreased cardiac output
   1. Daily weight; report weight changes.
   2. Record intake and output.
   3. Monitor serum electrolytes.
   4. Limit fluids as indicated.
   5. Provide salt-restricted diet if ordered.
   6. Give diuretic medication as prescribed.
   7. Reinforce instructions regarding diet, drugs, and weight control.

H. Impaired tissue perfusion related to hypertension
   1. Monitor vital signs and report changes.
   2. Provide sodium-restricted diet as prescribed.
   3. Provide cholesterol-controlled diet if prescribed, and monitor for side effects.
   4. Instruct in the avoidance of risk factors (smoking, stress, and obesity).
   5. Reinforce teaching in the areas of diet, weight control, avoidance of risk factors, and home monitoring of blood pressure.

Major Medical Diagnoses
Arteriosclerosis and Atherosclerosis

A. Definition
1. Arteriosclerosis: a process in which the arterial walls harden, thicken, and lose their elasticity, resulting in restricted blood flow
2. Atherosclerosis: one form of arteriosclerosis; fatty plaques that form on the intima (inner layer) of the arteries

B. Pathology
1. The underlying mechanism is the formation of fatty plaque deposits in the arteries.
2. The plaque increases in size and ultimately obstructs blood flow to vital areas.

C. Arteriosclerosis is associated with the following health problems:
1. Coronary artery disease
2. Angina pectoris
3. Myocardial infarction
4. Hypertension
5. Peripheral vascular disease
6. Cerebrovascular accidents (strokes)

D. Signs and symptoms vary, depending on the arteries affected by the sclerosing process.
1. Extremity involvement
   a. Cramping pain (intermittent claudication)
   b. Numbness and tingling
   c. Reduced circulation, causing ulceration or pain
   d. Outward changes: skin pallor, cool skin, reduced or absent pulses, loss of leg hair, and skin ulceration
2. Coronary involvement
   a. Chest pain
   b. Dyspnea
   c. Palpitations
   d. Fainting (syncope)
   e. Fatigue

E. Diagnostic tests and methods
1. Patient history and physical examination
2. Arteriograms
3. ECG
4. Oscillometry

F. Treatment
1. Dietary restriction of fat and cholesterol
2. Vasodilating drugs
3. Cholesterol-lowering drugs
4. Elimination or reduction of risk factors (Box 5-3)
5. Weight management
6. Planned exercise
7. Prevention of pressure in extremities
8. Use of special devices such as bed cradles

9. Bypass surgery or removal of plaques may be considered

G. Nursing intervention
1. Assess and document signs and symptoms.
2. Protect the extremity from trauma.
3. Monitor protective devices (bed cradles, pads, and so forth).
4. Provide skin care to ulcerated areas or areas affected by reduced circulation.
5. Monitor pulses and skin character of involved extremities.
6. Report changes in the involved extremities.
   a. Absence of pulse
   b. Cyanosis
   c. Increased pain
   d. Temperature change (coldness)
7. Monitor for signs and symptoms of infection in ulcerated areas.
8. Provide slow, progressive physical activity as prescribed.
9. Administer prescribed diet.
10. Administer prescribed drugs.
11. Relieve pain from ischemia.
12. Avoid cold and provide adequate warmth to prevent vasoconstriction.
13. Avoid constrictive clothing.
14. Educate the patient and family regarding avoidance of risk factors, dietary management, medication, and activity.

Angina Pectoris

A. Definition: episodes of acute chest pain resulting from insufficient oxygenation of myocardial tissue, caused by decreased blood flow to the area (ischemia)
1. Episodes occur most frequently during periods of physical or emotional exertion.
   a. Exercise
   b. Eating a heavy meal
   c. Environmental temperature extremes
2. Episodes seldom last more than 15 minutes.

B. Causes
1. The major cause is atherosclerosis.
2. Narrowed coronary arteries obstruct blood flow; thus oxygen carried by the blood cannot sufficiently meet tissue demands, particularly during periods of exertion.

C. Signs and symptoms
1. Substernal chest pain, usually brought on by exertion
2. Radiation of pain to the jaw or an extremity
3. Dyspnea
4. Anxiety or feeling of impending doom
5. Tachycardia
6. Diaphoresis
7. Sensation of heaviness, choking, or suffocation
8. Indigestion

D. Diagnostic tests and methods
1. Patient history and physical examination
2. ECG
3. Holter monitoring
4. Coronary angiography
5. Stress testing
6. Chest x-ray examination
7. Serum lipid and enzyme values

BOX 5-3	Risk Factors in the Development of Atherosclerosis

Obesity
Sedentary lifestyle
Smoking
Stress
High-fat diet

E. Treatment
1. Relieving chest pain through by using vasodilating drugs (e.g., nitrates, beta-blockers, calcium channel blockers), sedatives, and analgesics
2. Dietary restriction of fat and cholesterol
3. Planned exercise
4. Weight management
5. Stress management
6. If conservative measures are unsuccessful, coronary bypass surgery or an angioplasty may be considered.
F. Nursing intervention
1. Assess and document signs and symptoms and reactions to treatment.
2. Administer vasodilating medication and monitor for side effects.
3. Instruct patient to inform the nursing staff at the onset of an anginal attack.
4. Provide emotional support and assurance.
5. Provide prompt relief of pain.
6. Monitor vital signs, particularly during an attack.
7. Educate the patient and family regarding diet, activity, drug therapy, and avoidance of risk factors.

Hypertension (High Blood Pressure)

A. Definition: characterized by persistent elevation of blood pressure. (See Box 5-4 for current classification system.)
1. Primary hypertension (essential): a persistent elevation of blood pressure without an apparent cause
   a. Actual cause is unknown; known as the "silent killer" because the patient frequently does not experience symptoms until organ damage has occurred.
   b. Primarily, small blood vessels are affected; peripheral resistance increases, and blood pressure rises.
   c. Constricted blood vessels eventually cause damage to organs that rely on a blood supply from these vessels.
2. Secondary hypertension: a persistent elevation of blood pressure associated with another disease state
   a. Renal disease
   b. Toxemia
   c. Adrenal dysfunction
   d. Atherosclerosis
   e. Coarctation of the aorta
B. Predisposing factors
1. Smoking
2. Obesity
3. Heavy salt and cholesterol intake
4. Heredity
5. Aggressive, hyperactive personality
6. Age: develops between 30 and 50 years of age

7. Sex: primarily men over 35 years of age and women over 45 years of age
8. Race: blacks have twice the incidence of whites
9. Birth-control pills and estrogens
C. The heart brain, kidney, and eyes can be damaged if the hypertensive state continues without correction.
D. Signs and symptoms may be insidious and vague; a person can have the disorder and not know it.
1. Tinnitus
2. Light-headedness
3. Blurred vision
4. Irritability
5. Fatigue
6. Tachycardia and palpitations
7. Occipital, morning headaches
8. Nosebleeds (epistaxis)
9. DOE (dyspnea on exertion)
E. Diagnostic tests and methods
1. Patient history and physical examination
2. Series of resting blood pressure readings
3. Routine urinalysis, BUN, and serum creatinine to screen for renal involvement
4. Serum electrolytes to screen for adrenal involvement
5. Blood sugar levels to screen for endocrine involvement
6. Lipid profile
7. Chest x-ray examination
8. ECG
9. Holter monitoring
10. Funduscopic eye examination
F. Treatment
1. Lifestyle modifications such as exercise, smoking cessation, heart-healthy diet
2. Lowering blood pressure by using diuretics and antihypertensive drugs
3. Sodium-restricted diet (Box 5-5)
4. Cholesterol-controlled diet
5. Weight management
6. Stress management
7. Reduction or elimination of smoking
8. Planned exercise
G. Nursing intervention
1. Assess and document signs and symptoms and reactions to treatments.
2. Administer prescribed medication.
3. Observe for and report drug-related side effects.
4. Monitor weight every day to evaluate initial diuretic therapy.
5. Monitor intake and output to evaluate initial diuretic therapy.

BOX 5-4   How to Classify Hypertension

Take two or more blood pressure readings and average the results. Use this average as well as averages from other blood pressure readings to classify your patient's risk for hypertension.

Category	Systolic Reading mm/Hg	Diastolic Reading m/Hg
Normal	<120 and	<80
Prehypertension	120-139 or	80-89
Stage I	140-159 or	90-99
Stage II	≥160 or	≥100

Joint National Committee on Prevention, Detection, Evaluation, and Treatment of High Blood Pressure (2003). National Institutes of Health.

BOX 5-5   Foods High in Sodium

Processed meats (luncheon meats)
Processed cheese
Shellfish
Canned vegetables
Milk
Snack foods such as potato chips and french fries
Salted nuts

---

6. Monitor vital signs, particularly blood pressure, under the same conditions every day.
7. Provide planned activity and rest periods.
8. Provide prescribed diet.
   a. Calorie controlled
   b. Sodium restricted
   c. Cholesterol controlled
9. Educate the patient and family.
   a. Drug therapy and side effects
   b. Dietary restrictions; weight management
   c. Elimination of risk factors, such as smoking
   d. Activity
   e. Blood pressure monitoring
   f. Need for participation in and compliance with the prescribed regimen

Myocardial Infarction (Heart Attack)

A. Definition: the obstruction of a coronary artery or one of its branches
   1. The obstruction results in the death of the myocardial tissue supplied by that vessel.
   2. The myocardial tissue dies because of oxygen deprivation (infarction or necrosis).
   3. The heart's ability to regain or maintain its function depends on the location and size of the area of infarction.
B. A myocardial infarction can occur whenever a coronary artery or branch of the artery becomes occluded by a thrombus, emboli, or the atherosclerotic process.
C. Signs and symptoms
   1. "Crushing" chest pain lasting longer than 15 minutes and unrelieved by rest or drugs
   2. Shortness of breath
   3. Nausea and vomiting
   4. Tachycardia
   5. Diaphoresis and pallor
   6. Temperature rise after 48 hours
   7. Elevation of the cardiac enzymes
   8. Dysrhythmias
   9. Anxiety
D. Diagnostic tests and methods
   1. Patient history and physical examination
   2. ECG
   3. Cardiac enzyme studies (Troponin, SGOT, LDH, CPK-MB)
   4. Chest x-ray examination
E. Treatment
   1. Analgesic drugs to relieve pain
   2. Oxygen to relieve respiratory distress
   3. Vasopressor drugs to prevent circulatory collapse (cardiogenic shock)

4. Cardiac monitoring to detect dysrhythmias
5. Hemodynamic monitoring: internal monitoring of the blood pressure and pulmonary artery pressure
6. Bed rest with progressive activity to allow the damaged myocardium to heal
7. IV fluids to provide for IV drug administration
8. Cardiopulmonary resuscitation in the event of cardiac standstill (arrest)
9. Pacemaker insertion
10. Anticoagulant therapy
11. Thrombolytic therapy to dissolve blood clot and restore blood flow
12. Nitrates
F. Nursing intervention
   1. Provide pain relief.
   2. Provide ongoing assessment and documentation of symptoms and reactions to treatment.
   3. Administer and monitor oxygen.
   4. Record vital signs hourly during the acute period.
   5. Record intake and output hourly during the acute period.
   6. Provide bed rest during the acute period and progressive activity as prescribed.
      a. Apply antiembolism stockings.
      b. Allow patient out of bed to use bedside commode (less taxing to the cardiovascular system).
      c. Monitor pulse during periods of activity.
   7. Avoid activities that produce straining (Valsalva maneuver) to avoid stimulation of the vagus nerve, which will induce bradycardia.
      a. Administer stool softeners as prescribed.
      b. Caution patient against straining when attempting a bowel movement.
   8. Provide diet as prescribed.
      a. The patient may start out on liquids and then progress.
      b. Sodium and cholesterol may be restricted.
      c. Caffeine may be restricted.
   9. Give prescribed antidysrhythmics and monitor for side effects.
   10. Give prescribed cardiotonics and diuretics and monitor for side effects.
   11. Monitor for complications.
      a. Cardiogenic shock: circulatory collapse caused by decreased cardiac output; the vital organs are not being perfused.
         (1) Monitor vital signs every 15 minutes.
         (2) Record intake and output hourly.
         (3) Report changes in rate, rhythm, and conductivity.
         (4) Observe and report signs and symptoms of restlessness, diaphoresis, pallor, low blood pressure, and tachycardia.
         (5) Administer and monitor prescribed vasopressors and antidysrhythmics.
         (6) Administer oxygen as prescribed.
         (7) Provide cardiac and hemodynamic monitoring. (Hemodynamic monitoring refers to the internal monitoring of blood pressure and pulmonary artery pressure.)
      b. Pulmonary edema: left ventricle failure (pumping mechanism) caused by strain on a diseased heart; cardiac output (the amount of blood pumped out by

the heart to the body per minute) is reduced, resulting in lung congestion.

(1) Observe and report symptoms of anxiety, dyspnea, orthopnea, frothy, pink-tinged sputum, crackles in the lungs, decreased urine output, and dependent edema.

(2) Record vital signs every 15 minutes.

(3) Record intake and output hourly.

(4) Place bed in high-Fowler's position.

(5) Administer cardiotonics and diuretics as prescribed and monitor for side effects.

(6) Administer and monitor oxygen therapy.

(7) Be prepared to administer analgesics to allay anxiety and reduce respiratory rate.

(8) Provide emotional support to patient and family.

Heart Failure

A. Definition: failure of the pumping mechanism of the heart, resulting in an insufficient blood supply to meet the body's needs

B. Causes
1. The underlying mechanism in heart failure (HF) involves the failure of the pumping mechanism of the heart to respond to the metabolic changes of the body.
2. The result is a heart that cannot supply a sufficient amount of blood in relation to the body's needs and to the amount of blood returning to the heart (venous return); pressure builds up in the vascular beds on the affected side of the heart.

C. HF is described in terms of left-sided or right-sided failure, depending on which ventricle is affected.

D. Signs and symptoms are divided into left-sided failure and right-sided failure, although both sides may be affected.
1. Left-sided failure leads to pulmonary congestion.
   a. Dyspnea
   b. Orthopnea
   c. Nonproductive cough that worsens at night
   d. As severity of failure increases, frothy, blood-tinged sputum is noted (pulmonary edema).
   e. Anxiety and restlessness
   f. Fatigue
2. Right-sided failure may follow left-sided failure and results in systemic venous congestion.
   a. Weight gain caused by fluid accumulation in the tissues
   b. Dependent edema in the form of ankle edema or sacral edema
   c. Ascites caused by the collection of fluid in the abdominal cavity; ascites may also hinder respiration
   d. Fatigue
   e. GI symptoms such as nausea, vomiting, and anorexia
   f. Decreased urine output
   g. Distended neck veins

E. Diagnostic test and methods
1. Patient history and physical examination, including the findings of edema, abnormal heart sounds, and the presence of crackles with dyspnea
2. Chest x-ray examination
3. ECG
4. Arterial blood gas studies
5. Liver function studies
6. Renal function studies

F. Treatment
1. Drug therapy: digitalization, diuretics, and sedatives
2. Recording of weight daily
3. Monitoring intake and output
4. Oxygen therapy
5. Hemodynamic monitoring
6. Restricting fluids
7. Restricting dietary sodium
8. Bed rest with progressive activity
9. Elevating the head of the bed on blocks
10. Monitoring vital signs

G. Nursing intervention
1. Provide ongoing assessment and documentation of signs, symptoms, and reactions to treatment.
2. Monitor oxygen therapy.
3. Record vital signs every 15 minutes to 2 hours during the acute phase.
4. Record intake and output hourly during the acute phase.
5. Weigh patient daily.
6. Administer and monitor prescribed cardiotonics, diuretics, and sedatives; observe for side effects.
7. Determine the amount of activity that produces the least discomfort to the patient.
8. Monitor for dependent edema.
   a. Ankle edema when sitting upright
   b. Sacral edema when in supine position
9. Raise the head of the bed as prescribed.
10. Observe for complications of bed rest.
    a. Have patient turn, cough, and take deep breaths.
    b. Apply antiembolism stockings.
11. Provide emotional support to the patient and family.
12. Provide a diet low in sodium, if prescribed.
13. Educate the patient and family concerning dietary management, drug therapy, and activity.
14. Restrict fluids as ordered.

Valvular Conditions

A. Valvular dysfunction results in either stenosis or insufficiency of the heart valves.
1. Valvular stenosis results from cardiac infections; the valve leaflets (cusps) become fibrotic and thicken and may even fuse together, thus hindering blood flow.
2. Valvular insufficiency occurs in much the same way as does valvular stenosis; after repeated infections, the valve leaflets (cusps) become inflamed and scarred and can no longer close completely; the incomplete closure allows blood to leak from the left ventricle into the left atrium during systole.

B. Blood flow through the heart is altered, resulting in decreased cardiac output, systemic and pulmonary congestion, and dilation of the heart chambers.

C. Causes
1. Rheumatic heart disease is the primary cause of valvular dysfunction.
2. Other causes include syphilis, bacterial endocarditis, and congenital malformations.

D. Signs and symptoms
1. Mitral stenosis
   a. DOE (dyspnea on exertion)
   b. Orthopnea

c. Pink-tinged sputum
d. Fatigue
e. Palpitations
f. Heart murmur
2. Mitral insufficiency
   a. Fatigue
   b. DOE (dyspnea on exertion)
   c. Heart murmur
   d. Orthopnea
   e. Pulmonary congestion
3. Aortic stenosis
   a. Fatigue
   b. Angina
   c. Syncope
   d. Heart murmur
   e. HF (heart failure)
4. Aortic insufficiency
   a. Palpitations
   b. Dyspnea
   c. Fatigue
   d. Orthopnea
   e. Anginal pain occurring even at rest
E. Diagnostic tests and methods
   1. Patient history and physical examination; a murmur is a common finding of the examination.
   2. ECG
   3. Chest x-ray examination to determine heart size
   4. Cardiac catheterization to reveal possible pressure changes
   5. Echocardiogram: provides information concerning structure and function of valves
   6. Laboratory studies
F. Treatment
   1. Mitral stenosis
      a. Antibiotics administered prophylactically to prevent recurrences of causative agents
      b. Drug therapy: diuretics, cardiotonics, and antidysrhythmics
      c. Restricted sodium diet
      d. Planned activity and avoidance of symptom-producing activity
      e. Surgical correction of the defect
         (1) Mitral commissurotomy: the fused valve leaflets are separated, and the mitral opening may be dilated.
         (2) Valve replacement: diseased valve is replaced with a prosthetic valve.
   2. Mitral insufficiency
      a. Planned exercise and avoidance of symptom-producing activity
      b. Sodium-restricted diet
      c. Drug therapy; diuretics, cardiotonics, antidysrhythmics, and vasodilators
      d. Surgical correction
         (1) Valvuloplasty: repair of the existing valve
         (2) Valve replacement
   3. Aortic stenosis
      a. Prevention of infective endocarditis
      b. Treatment of symptoms
      c. Drug therapy: diuretics, nitrates, and cardiotonics
      d. Sodium-restricted diet
      e. Valve replacement

G. Nursing intervention
   1. Assess and document signs and symptoms and reaction to treatments.
   2. Administer prescribed medication, and observe patient for side effects.
   3. Provide a calm, quiet environment.
   4. Allow patient and family to verbalize their anxieties and fears.
   5. Monitor vital signs and report changes.
   6. Weigh the patient daily.
   7. Provide the prescribed diet.
      a. Nutritionally well balanced
      b. Sodium restricted to prevent fluid retention
   8. Encourage progressive activity as prescribed.
      a. Consider the patient's limitations.
      b. Provide rest periods.
   9. Monitor intake and output if diuretics are used.
   10. Educate the patient and family concerning diet, drugs, activity, and need for compliance.
   11. Vocational counseling may be needed if the patient has a demanding job.

Inflammatory Disorders of the Heart

A. Definition: diseases resulting from acute or chronic inflammation of the lining of the heart and valves caused by bacteria or viruses, trauma, or other factors
   1. Pericarditis: an inflammation of the pericardium
      a. The result is a loss of elasticity or fluid accumulation within the pericardial sac.
      b. Heart failure and cardiac tamponade may result.
   2. Myocarditis: an inflammation of the myocardium
      a. The result is impairment of contractility.
      b. Myocardial ischemia and necrosis may result.
   3. Endocarditis: an inflammation of the inner lining of the heart and valves associated with a streptococcal infection
   4. Rheumatic heart disease
      a. Usually associated with rheumatic fever
      b. Rheumatic fever is an inflammatory process that can affect all the layers of the heart.
      c. Cardiac impairment results from swelling and scarring of valve leaflets, leading to valvular changes (mitral insufficiency, aortic insufficiency, and pericarditis).
B. Signs and symptoms
   1. Chest pain
   2. Dyspnea
   3. Chills and intermittent fever
   4. Weakness and fatigue
   5. Diaphoresis
   6. Anorexia
   7. Dysrhythmias
   8. Elevated cardiac enzymes
   9. Friction rubs (auscultatory sound created by the rubbing together of two serous surfaces)
   10. Presence of Aschoff bodies (collection of cells and leukocytes in the interstitial layers of the heart)
   11. New heart murmur or an abnormal heart sound
   12. Existing streptococcal infection
   13. Cardiac enlargement
   14. Joint involvement
C. Diagnostic tests and methods
   1. Patient history and physical examination
      a. History of recent infections

b. History of heart disease
2. ECG
3. Chest x-ray examination
4. Cardiac enzyme studies
5. Blood cultures
6. Echocardiogram to assess valvular disease and vegetation (growth of scar tissue)
7. Laboratory studies: CBC, electrolytes, ESR
8. Radionuclide studies to assess heart structure and heart damage

D. Treatment
1. Identification and elimination of the infecting agent
2. Drug therapy: antibiotics, cardiotonics, antiinflammatory agents, analgesics, and corticosteroids
3. Blood cultures
4. Oxygen
5. Rest and planned activity
6. Well-balanced diet
7. Prevention of exposure to other infectious agents

E. Nursing intervention
1. Assess and document signs and symptoms and reactions to treatment.
2. Maintain a calm, quiet environment.
3. Administer prescribed drugs, and monitor for side effects.
4. Evaluate the patient's understanding of the disease process and the need for compliance.
5. Alleviate pain.
6. Allay patient and family's fears and anxieties.
7. Monitor vital signs and report changes.
8. Observe for signs and symptoms of complications (tachycardia, dyspnea, and orthopnea).
9. Educate the patient concerning the illness, diet, drugs, activity, avoidance of infections, dental care, vocational counseling, and compliance to the regimen.

PERIPHERAL VASCULAR CONDITIONS AND DISORDERS

Peripheral vascular disease refers to vascular disorders exclusive of those affecting the heart. The underlying factor in peripheral vascular disease is the arteriosclerotic process. Blood flow is slowed because of vessels that are narrowed or obstructed. The lack of normal blood flow causes tissue changes (see section on arteriosclerosis). Vascular disease related to the lower extremities is discussed in this section.

Nursing Assessment

A. Nursing observation
1. Skin of the lower extremities
a. Redness (hyperemia) of the leg when in a dependent position
b. Cold or blue feet
c. Varicose veins
d. Sparse hair distribution
e. Lesions or stasis ulcers
f. Edema
g. Dermatitis or brown pigmentation of the skin
2. Delayed capillary filling
3. Diminished or absent pulses
a. Rigidity (hardness) of the vessels

b. Palpable vibration of the vessels (thrill)
4. Assessing major arteries for bruits (an auscultatory sound taking the form of a whooshing, buzzing, or humming sound caused by turbulent blood flow)
5. Differences in leg circumference
6. Thickening of nail beds

B. Patient description (subjective data)
1. Leg cramps
2. Aching calves
3. Leg numbness
4. Leg pain occurring during exercise (claudication)
5. Loss of sensation in one or both legs
6. Past or present history
a. Alcohol excess
b. Diabetes mellitus
c. Hypertension
d. Thrombophlebitis

Diagnostic Tests and Methods

A. Chest x-ray examination for abnormalities
B. Oscillometry: a noninvasive test that measures the amplitude of pulsations over an artery
C. Doppler ultrasonography: a device that emits sound waves that can be used to measure the amount of blood flow through a vessel
D. Arteriography: used to determine the location and extent of the disease process
E. Venography: radiographic study used to determine the location and size of a blood clot, vessel distention, and development of collateral circulation
F. Trendelenburg test
1. Used to determine valvular competency
2. The leg is elevated to 90 degrees, and a tourniquet is placed around the thigh.
3. The patient stands, and the vein-filling pattern is observed.
4. Normally, the veins fill slowly from below in 20 to 30 seconds; the rate of filling should not greatly accelerate when the tourniquet is removed.
G. Lung scan
1. Used to assess the presence of pulmonary embolism and lung damage
2. An intravenous radiographic isotope is injected into the patient.
3. Pulmonary circulation is assessed with a scanning device.
4. The patient also inhales a radioactive gas and is scanned to determine lung distribution of this gas.
H. Arterial blood gas analysis: used to assess the adequacy of ventilation
I. X-ray examination of the abdomen: may show evidence of an aneurysm
J. Blood tests
1. CBC: for routine evaluation
2. ESR to determine the presence of an inflammatory process
3. Coagulation studies (platelet count, bleeding time, PT, and PTT) to determine the existence of blood disorders

Frequent Patient Problems and Nursing Care

A. Pain related to intermittent claudication
1. Evaluate and record onset, duration, and intensity.
2. Provide rest during the episode.

3. Determine the amount of exercise the patient can tolerate before claudication occurs.
4. Assess for and report claudication occurring without activity.
5. Educate the patient on avoiding exposure to cold and maintaining warmth.

B. Excess fluid volume as evidenced by edema of the lower extremities or decreased cardiac output, or both
1. Note and record location and degree.
2. Instruct patient to avoid activity that places the legs in a dependent position for prolonged periods.
3. Instruct patient to avoid wearing constricting clothing around the legs.
4. Monitor for skin breakdown.
5. Elevate legs.

C. Impaired skin integrity related to stasis ulcers
1. Note location and character of ulceration.
2. Maintain bed rest with leg elevation.
3. Perform prescribed wound care.
4. Instruct the patient to avoid trauma to the legs.
5. Instruct the patient in proper skin care measures.
6. Reinforce patient teaching in the area of drugs, diet, activity, and skin care.

Major Medical Diagnoses
Arteriosclerosis Obliterans

A. Definition: a chronic arteriooclusive disease
1. Progression is slow and insidious.
2. The medial and intimal layers of arteries become inflamed and thrombosed.
3. Vessels lose elasticity, and plaques obstruct blood flow.
4. Vessels primarily affected are the femoral and carotid arteries.

B. Causes
1. Associated with atherosclerotic process
2. Predisposing factors include hypertension, smoking, hyperlipidemia, obesity, and a positive family history.

C. Signs and symptoms
1. Intermittent claudication
2. Pain in the legs at rest
3. Impotence
4. Paresthesia
5. Pallor or blanching on elevation of leg
6. Hyperemia (redness) or dusky appearance of the leg or legs when dependent
7. Loss of hair on extremities
8. Absent or diminished pulses

D. Diagnostic tests and methods
1. Patient history and physical examination
2. Oscillometry
3. Doppler ultrasonography
4. Arteriography
5. Laboratory studies

E. Treatments
1. Protection of extremity from injury
2. Prevention and control of infection
3. Drug therapy: vasodilators, analgesics, and antibiotics
4. Weight-reduction diet if patient is obese
5. Bed rest
6. Avoidance of smoking
7. Surgical management: endarterectomy (removing the obstructing plaque) or a bypass graft

F. Nursing intervention
1. Assist the patient in obtaining body warmth and warmth to the extremity.
   a. Warm room
   b. Warm bath
   c. Warm clothes, such as socks
2. Avoid applying direct heat to the affected part.
3. Protect the affected part from trauma and pressure.
   a. Use bed cradle.
   b. Assess skin lesions and monitor for signs of infection.
   c. Caution patient against wearing anything that constricts.
4. Give prescribed drugs and monitor for side effects.
5. Assess the affected part daily.
   a. Assess skin color, temperature, and circulation.
   b. Monitor for pain.
6. Provide emotional support.
7. Educate the patient and family regarding:
   a. Hygiene and avoidance of infection
   b. Rest and planned exercise
   c. Protection from injury
   d. Diet
   e. Drugs
   f. Improvement of circulation

Buerger Disease (Thromboangiitis Obliterans)

A. Definition: an inflammatory process affecting primarily arteries that causes occlusion, thrombosis, and ultimately ischemia
1. Medium-sized distal arteries of the legs are primarily affected.
2. Veins can also be affected.

B. Causes
1. Exact cause is unknown.
2. Associated with smoking
3. Men in the 25- to 40-year age group who smoke are at risk.
4. Familial tendency

C. Signs and symptoms
1. Coldness of the extremities
2. Diminished or absent pulses
3. Numbness and tingling
4. Cramping pain (intermittent claudication)
5. Pain at rest, not associated with activity
6. Skin ulceration
7. Aggravation of symptoms by exposure to cold environment
8. Change in appearance of extremities
9. Muscle atrophy
10. Slow-healing cuts
11. Gangrene
12. Sensitivity to cold

D. Diagnostic tests and methods
1. Patient history and physical examination
2. Oscillometry
3. Doppler ultrasonography
4. Arteriography
5. Laboratory studies
6. ECG
7. Chest x-ray examination

E. Treatment
1. Restricting smoking

2. Drug therapy: vasodilating drugs, analgesics, and anti-coagulants
3. Moderate exercise
4. Avoidance and treatment of infection
5. Protection from trauma
6. Sympathectomy (disruption of nerve impulses to a particular area)
7. Nerve blocks (drug injections to block nerve impulses)
8. Amputation, as a last resort
F. Nursing intervention
1. Support the patient in his effort to stop smoking.
2. Give prescribed vasodilators, analgesics, and anticoagulants; monitor for side effects.
3. Document location and character of pain.
4. Assist the patient in maintaining warmth.
5. Educate the patient and family concerning drug therapy, activity, and avoidance of smoking, exposure to cold, constricting clothing, and trauma.

Raynaud's Disease

A. Definition: a peripheral vascular disease affecting digital arteries
1. Disease occurs primarily in women.
2. Exposure to environmental cold, emotional stress, or tobacco use produces spasms of the arteries.
3. Hands and arms are usually affected.
B. Cause
1. Exact cause is unknown.
2. Associated with collagen diseases in women
C. Contributing factors
1. Pressure to the fingertips such as that encountered by typists and pianists
2. Using hand-held vibrating equipment on a regular basis
D. Signs and symptoms
1. Numbness and tingling
2. Blanching of digits and cyanosis
3. Hyperemia
4. Coldness
5. Dryness and atrophy of the nails
6. Pain
7. Punctate (small hole) lesions of the fingertips
8. Eventual gangrene of the fingertips
E. Diagnostic tests and methods
1. Patient history and physical examination
2. Doppler ultrasonography
3. Arteriography
4. ECG
5. Chest x-ray examination
F. Treatment
1. Drug therapy with vasodilators
2. Sympathectomy: in advanced cases
3. Elimination of smoking
4. Avoidance of stressful situations
5. Avoidance of exposure to cold
G. Nursing intervention
1. Document location and characteristics of pain.
2. Observe affected areas daily.
3. Administer prescribed vasodilators and analgesics; monitor for side effects.
4. Instruct patient to avoid activities that precipitate spasms.
5. Instruct patient to avoid exposing the hands to the cold without proper protection.

6. Support patient's effort to give up smoking.
7. Offer emotional support and allay anxiety.
8. Educate the patient and family concerning drug therapy, avoidance of cold, protection from trauma and infection, and prevention of spasms.

Aneurysms

A. Definition: the enlargement or ballooning of an artery, usually caused by trauma, congenital weakness, arteriosclerosis, or infection; aorta is the most frequently affected artery.
B. Causes
1. Causes are varied, but the prime culprit is arteriosclerosis; plaque formation causes degenerative changes, leading to loss of vessel elasticity, weakness, and dilation.
2. Syphilis
3. Infections
4. Congenital disorder
5. Trauma
6. Risk factors: obesity, smoking, hypertension, stress, high blood cholesterol levels
C. Signs and symptoms
1. Abdominal
   a. Increased blood pressure
   b. Visible or palpable pulsating mass
   c. Pain or tenderness in the abdominal area
2. Thoracic
   a. Dyspnea
   b. Dysphagia
   c. Hoarseness or cough
   d. Severe chest pain
3. Ruptured aneurysm
   a. Anxiety
   b. Restlessness
   c. Pain
   d. Diminished pulses
   e. Hypotension and shock
D. Diagnostic tests and methods
1. Patient history and physical examination
2. Chest x-ray examination
3. Abdominal x-ray examination
4. Ultrasonography
5. Angiography, arteriography
6. Routine ECG
7. Laboratory studies
E. Treatment
1. Conservative measures
   a. Drug therapy: antihypertensives, pain relievers, and negative inotropic agents
   b. Correct hydration and electrolyte imbalances
   c. Decreased activity
2. Surgical repair
   a. Resection and replacement with a prosthesis of Teflon or Dacron
   b. Resection and replacement with a graft
F. Nursing intervention
1. Provide immediate postoperative care.
   a. Assess vital signs and peripheral pulses every 15 minutes; then decrease the frequency as ordered.
   b. Record intake and output hourly.
   c. Compare extremities for warmth and color.
   d. Administer IV fluids at prescribed rate.
   e. Relieve pain with prescribed analgesic.

f. Monitor oxygen therapy.

g. Give prescribed prophylactic antibiotics as ordered.

h. Assess level of consciousness every 1 to 2 hours.

i. Auscultate lung sounds and bowel sounds at least every 4 hours.

j. Monitor for dysrhythmias.

k. Have patient turn, cough, and deep breathe at least every 2 hours.

2. Other postoperative considerations

a. Provide antiembolism stockings.

b. Provide emotional support, and allay anxiety.

c. Encourage early ambulation as prescribed.

d. Instruct patient to observe for changes in the extremities such as color and warmth.

e. Instruct patient on assessments of peripheral pulses.

Phlebitis and Thrombophlebitis

A. Definition: inflammatory disorders of the veins

1. Phlebitis: inflammation of a vein

2. Thrombophlebitis: inflammation of a vein with clot formation

B. Causes

1. The inflammation and clot formation are associated with venous stasis, vessel damage, and enhanced blood coagulability.

2. Situations that produce venous stasis include decreased mobility, prolonged periods of sitting and standing, wearing confining clothing, and increased abdominal pressure.

C. Signs and symptoms

1. Redness and pain along vein path

2. Elevation of temperature

3. Swelling

4. Positive Homans' sign (pain on dorsiflexion of the foot)

5. Area is sensitive to the touch

D. Diagnostic tests and methods

1. Patient history and physical examination

2. Doppler ultrasonography

3. Venography

4. Laboratory studies: CBC, ESR, and coagulation studies

5. Lung scan to rule out pulmonary embolism

E. Treatment

1. Bed rest

2. Anticoagulant therapy

3. Thrombolytic therapy

4. Vasodilators

5. Warm, moist packs to the affected leg (some physicians prefer ice packs to the area)

6. Antiembolism stockings

7. Elevation of affected extremity

8. Surgical intervention is required in only a small percentage of patients

F. Nursing intervention

1. Assess and document signs and symptoms.

2. Administer analgesics as ordered, and monitor for side effects.

3. Elevate leg as ordered; avoid using a knee gatch or pillow under the affected knee; avoid crossing legs.

4. Apply warm, moist heat as ordered.

5. Assess thigh and calf measurements daily.

6. Monitor vital signs every 4 hours.

7. Maintain bed rest as ordered.

8. Apply antiembolism stockings on unaffected leg.

9. Avoid massaging calf of affected leg.

10. Avoid constrictive clothing.

11. Monitor anticoagulant therapy.

12. Monitor for bleeding tendencies.

a. Bleeding gums

b. Epistaxis

c. Bruising easily

d. Melena

e. Petechiae

13. Monitor Hgb and Hct levels.

14. Educate the patient and family concerning drug therapy, avoiding activities that aggravate the existing state, and monitoring for signs and symptoms of complications.

15. Monitor patient for complications such as an embolism.

Embolism

A. Definition: a blood clot circulating in the blood

B. Causes

1. The clot may be a fragment of an arteriosclerotic plaque, or it may have originated in the heart.

2. If large, an embolism may lodge in a vessel bifurcation and obstruct the flow of blood to vital organs or tissues.

3. Most emboli arise from deep-vein thrombi; the embolus travels in the bloodstream until it lodges in a narrowed area, usually the lungs.

C. Signs and symptoms: dependent on the area involved

1. Pain at the site

2. Shock

3. Areas supplied by the involved vessel evidence pallor, coldness, numbness, tingling, and cyanosis.

4. Sudden onset of dyspnea

5. Cough and hemoptysis

6. Chest pain

7. Tachycardia

8. Tachypnea

D. Diagnostic tests and methods

1. Patient history and physical examination

2. Lung scan

3. Chest x-ray examination

4. Arterial blood gas analysis

E. Treatment

1. Oxygen therapy

2. IV fluids

3. IV anticoagulants

4. Analgesics

5. Thrombolytic agents

F. Nursing intervention

1. Assess and document signs and symptoms and reactions to treatments.

2. Monitor vital signs.

3. Monitor arterial blood gas reports.

4. Administer prescribed analgesic and monitor for side effects.

5. Administer anticoagulants as prescribed and monitor for bleeding tendencies.

6. Monitor oxygen therapy.

7. Give ROM exercises.

8. Provide antiembolism stockings.

9. Educate the patient and family concerning drug therapy, monitoring for bleeding tendencies, and restriction of activities.

Varicose Veins

A. Definition: dilated, tortuous leg veins resulting from blood backflow caused by incomplete valve closure leading to congestion and further enlargement
B. Causes
   1. Basic cause of varicosities is unknown
   2. Predisposing factors: heredity, pregnancy, obesity, and aging
C. Signs and symptoms
   1. Leg fatigue and aching
   2. Leg cramping and pain
   3. Heaviness in the legs
   4. Dilated veins
   5. Ankle edema
D. Diagnostic tests and methods
   1. Patient history and physical examination
   2. Venography
   3. Trendelenburg test
E. Treatment
   1. Rest with elevation of legs
   2. Exercise
   3. Support stockings
   4. Avoidance of prolonged standing, sitting, and crossing the legs
   5. Weight management
   6. Surgical vein stripping, ligation; vein sclerosing
   7. Laser
F. Nursing intervention
   1. After surgery, check legs for color, movement, temperature, and sensation.
   2. Provide leg exercises as prescribed.
   3. Reinforce the importance of weight management.
   4. Instruct the patient to avoid prolonged sitting and standing.
   5. Avoid constrictive clothing.

HEMATOLOGIC CONDITIONS AND DISORDERS

Disorders of hemopoiesis refer to problems of the blood-forming tissues such as the blood cells, bone marrow, spleen, and lymph system. This discussion includes descriptions of the anemias, leukemia, and acquired immunodeficiency syndrome (AIDS).

Nursing Assessment

A. Nursing observations
   1. Pulse
     a. Character, rate, rhythm
     b. Noting tachycardia or periods of palpitations
   2. Respirations
     a. Character, rate, rhythm
     b. Tachypnea
     c. DOE (dyspnea on exertion)
     d. SOB (shortness of breath)
   3. Blood pressure: hypotension, perhaps orthostatic
   4. Temperature: unexplained occurrences of elevation, sometimes accompanied by chills and sweating
   5. Skin
     a. Color: pallor, cyanosis
     b. Pruritus

     c. Bruising
     d. Slow to heal cuts
     e. Bleeding from nose or mouth
   6. Oral mucosal changes
     a. Mouth ulcerations
     b. Bleeding gums
     c. Smooth tongue
   7. Motor
     a. Lack of coordination
     b. Loss of usual stamina
     c. Changes in ability to perform activities
     d. Intolerance to exertion (climbing stairs, usual housework, walking)
B. Patient description (subjective)
   1. Changes in ability to perform ADL
   2. Self-reported increase in weakness and fatigue
   3. DOE (dyspnea on exertion)
   4. Changes in appetite
     a. Weight loss
     b. Anorexia
     c. Nausea and vomiting
   5. Skin
     a. Easily bruises
     b. Bleeding from gums, nose
   6. Mood changes: irritable
   7. Progressive symptoms
     a. Onset of headaches
     b. Onset of fatigue
     c. Numbness, tingling, burning feet
     d. Intermittent swollen, tender lymph nodes

Diagnostic Tests and Methods

A. Red blood cell (RBC) count
   1. The blood study is used in routine screenings and provides information about the hematologic system.
   2. Circulating RBC counts rise in conditions such as anemia and hypoxia.
B. Erythrocyte indexes (mean cell volume, mean cell Hgb concentration, and mean cell Hgb)
   1. Aid in describing the anemias
   2. Provide a relationship among the number, size, and Hgb content of the RBCs
C. Hemoglobin and Hematocrit levels
   1. Provide an index to the severity of the anemia
   2. Hematocrit refers to the number of packed RBCs found in 100 ml of blood.
   3. Hemoglobin is the oxygen-carrying component of the RBC and is more reliable in determining the severity of the anemia.
D. Reticulocyte count: number of newly formed RBCs
   1. Provides information concerning the cause of the anemia
   2. Indicates whether the anemia is a result of diminished production or excessive loss or destruction of RBCs
E. Erythrocyte sedimentation rate (ESR)
   1. Not specific to anemias
   2. Elevated ESR suggests the presence of an underlying disease process; therefore further studies may be indicated.
F. Serum iron
   1. Helpful in classifying the anemia
   2. Useful in differentiating an acute from a chronic disorder

G. Total iron-binding capacity (TIBC): helpful in classifying the anemia and differentiating between an acute and a chronic disorder
H. Serum bilirubin
   1. Useful in evaluating the degree of RBC hemolysis
   2. Bilirubin is formed from the hemoglobin of destroyed RBCs.
   3. Elevations may indicate the increased destruction of RBCs caused by a particular disease process.
I. Schilling test
   1. Used in classifying anemias, particularly a vitamin-B$_{12}$ disorder
   2. Helps differentiate between an intrinsic factor deficiency and an intestinal absorption disorder
   3. Patient preparation
      a. The patient may be instructed to take nothing by mouth (NPO) before the test.
      b. Oral radioactive vitamin B$_{12}$ is administered.
      c. Nonradioactive parenteral dose is given 2 hours later.
      d. Urine collection follows.
      e. A third of the vitamin appears in the urine; little or no radioactivity in the urine suggests a GI malabsorption problem.
      f. Procedure may be repeated with the addition of intrinsic factor to the oral vitamin B$_{12}$.
      g. Nonabsorption of vitamin B$_{12}$ without intrinsic factor but absorption with the intrinsic factor is suggestive of pernicious anemia.
   4. Nursing intervention
      a. Explain the basic procedure to the patient.
      b. Maintain NPO.
      c. Collect the urine at the specified time.
J. Vitamin-B$_{12}$ level
   1. Used to help identify pernicious anemia
   2. Provides an index for determining the adequacy of vitamin-B$_{12}$ levels and the need for further evaluation
   3. Vitamin-B$_{12}$ is important for normal hematopoiesis.
K. Serum folate level
   1. Folic acid is another important factor in hematopoiesis.
   2. Useful in folic acid deficiency anemia.
L. Gastric analysis
   1. Nasogastric tube is inserted and then histamine is injected to stimulate gastric secretions.
   2. Gastric contents are aspirated and analyzed.
   3. Achlorhydria (absence of hydrochloric acid) is a feature of pernicious anemia because of a lack of intrinsic factor in the stomach.
M. Sickle cell preparation
   1. The reaction of the blood specimen in hypoxia is observed.
   2. Sickling of cells in hypoxia suggests sickle cell trait or sickle cell anemia.
N. Hemoglobin electrophoresis
   1. An electric field separates the specimen into the various types of Hgb present.
   2. Hemoglobin S and A suggest sickle cell anemia or trait.
   3. Hemoglobin F suggests thalassemia.
O. Bone marrow biopsy
   1. Bone marrow aspiration provides information about blood cell production.
   2. Test may be used in patients suspected of having leukemia, aplastic anemia, and other hematologic disorders.

3. Sample of marrow may be obtained from the sternum, iliac crest, vertebrae, or vertebral body.
4. Procedure
   a. The skin over the designated area is prepared and anesthetized.
   b. The needle is inserted into the center of the bone, and a small amount of marrow is aspirated.
5. Nursing intervention
   a. Allay patient's anxiety before the examination.
   b. Assist with the marrow as instructed.
   c. Place patient in a comfortable position after the procedure.
   d. Monitor pain status (soreness remains for several days).
   e. Monitor puncture site for bleeding.
P. WBC count and differential
   1. Determines the total number of leukocytes
   2. The differential helps analyze each type of WBC and determine if the amount present is in proper proportion.
   3. Aids in the diagnosing of infection and blood disorders such as leukemia
Q. Platelet count
   1. Evaluates adequacy of platelet levels
   2. If platelet levels drop below a certain level, spontaneous hemorrhage is possible.
R. Serum for HIV: determines the presence of the HIV antibodies
S. Lymphangiography: radiologic examination used to detect lymph node involvement

Frequent Patient Problems and Nursing Care

A. Activity intolerance related to weakness and fatigue
   1. Provide planned activity and rest periods.
   2. Monitor for signs of fatigue.
   3. Reinforce patient teaching of planned activity and exercise.
   4. Assist patient with activities of daily living (ADL).
   5. Assess vital signs as ordered.
B. Impaired tissue perfusion related to hypotension
   1. Observe for evidence of postural hypotension.
   2. Assist patient in dangling legs over the side of the bed before standing.
   3. Instruct patient to get up slowly.
   4. Assess patient's pulse when standing.
C. Ineffective breathing pattern related to DOE (dyspnea on exertion)
   1. Note the degree or kind of activity that causes dyspnea.
   2. Note character and rate of respirations during the episodes.
   3. Instruct the patient to stop the activity and relax when dyspnea is experienced.
   4. Assist the patient in planning activities so that dyspnea will not occur.
   5. Reinforce patient teaching regarding planned exercise and rest periods.
D. Impaired oral mucous membranes caused by ulcerations of the mouth and tongue
   1. Assess the ulcerated areas daily.
   2. Provide mouth care with a soft-bristle brush or cotton swab.
   3. Offer soothing mouthwashes every 2 to 4 hours.
   4. Instruct the patient to avoid ingesting food or drink that may aggravate the ulcers.

E. Deficient fluid volume related to hemorrhage
   1. Assess for signs of bleeding.
      a. Tarry stools
      b. Hematuria
      c. Bleeding gums
      d. Bleeding tendency
      e. Petechiae
      f. Epistaxis
   2. Protect from trauma and injury.
   3. Avoid parenteral injections.
   4. Have patient use soft-bristle brush for mouth care.
   5. Monitor vital signs at least every 4 hours.
   6. Monitor Hgb and Hct values.
   7. Encourage intake of fluids and the prescribed diet.
F. Risk for infection related to interference with the immune system
   1. Prevent exposure to others with infection.
   2. Monitor for signs and symptoms of infection.
   3. Give prescribed drugs, and monitor for side effects.
   4. Place in protective isolation (may be known as neutropenic precautions) if ordered.

Major Medical Diagnoses
Anemia Caused by Decreased RBC Production

A. A balance normally exists between RBC production and RBC destruction; however, alterations do occur that significantly affect RBC production.
   1. Iron-deficiency anemia
      a. Results from insufficient dietary intake of iron, which is needed for the formation of hemoglobin and RBCs
      b. Other causes: malabsorption, blood loss, and hemolysis
   2. Pernicious anemia
      a. Caused by a lack of intrinsic factor in the GI tract
      b. Intrinsic factor is needed for the absorption of vitamin-B_{12}.
      c. Anemia usually results from a loss of the mucosal surface of the GI tract, which secretes intrinsic factor.
      d. Patients undergoing total gastrectomies and small-bowel resections are at risk.
   3. Folic acid–deficiency anemia
      a. Folic acid is required in the synthesis of DNA, which, in turn, is necessary for the production of RBCs.
      b. Common causes: poor diet (lacking in green, leafy vegetables, citrus fruits, liver, grains, and dried beans), malabsorption, and drugs that interfere with the absorption of folic acid
   4. Thalassemia
      a. Unlike the other three anemias, thalassemia is a genetic disorder resulting in abnormal hemoglobin synthesis.
      b. The main problem is an inadequate production of normal Hgb; hemolysis is a secondary problem.
      c. People of Mediterranean ancestry are at risk.
      d. Mild forms of this anemia (thalassemia minor) may be asymptomatic.
      e. Patients with a more severe hemolytic form (thalassemia major) may experience hepatomegaly, splenomegaly, jaundice, and bone marrow hypertrophy.
B. Signs and symptoms
   1. Skin changes
      a. Pallor
      b. Jaundice
      c. Pruritus
      d. Dermatitis
   2. Eye and visual disturbances
      a. Blurred vision
      b. Scleral icterus
   3. Mouth
      a. Glossitis
      b. Smooth tongue
      c. Ulcerations of the mucosa
   4. Cardiovascular
      a. Tachycardia
      b. Murmurs
      c. Angina
      d. Congestive heart failure (CHF)
      e. Hypotension
   5. Respiratory
      a. Tachypnea
      b. DOE (dyspnea on exertion)
      c. Orthopnea
   6. Neurological
      a. Dizziness
      b. Headaches
      c. Irritability
      d. Depression
      e. Incoordination
      f. Impaired thought processes
   7. GI
      a. Nausea and vomiting
      b. Anorexia
      c. Hepatomegaly
      d. Splenomegaly
   8. General
      a. Weight loss
      b. Weakness and fatigue
      c. Bone pain
      d. Numbness, tingling, and burning of the feet
C. Diagnostic tests and methods
   1. Patient history and physical examination
   2. Routine chest x-ray examination
   3. Routine ECG
   4. Schilling test
   5. Gastric analysis
   6. CBC and RBC indexes
   7. Bone marrow aspiration or biopsy
   8. Serum iron level
D. Treatment
   1. Iron therapy
   2. Increase dietary iron intake
   3. Vitamin B_{12} replacement (pernicious anemia)
   4. Folic acid replacement
   5. Hematinics
   6. Blood transfusions (thalassemia)
E. Nursing intervention
   1. Assess and document signs and symptoms and reactions to treatments.
   2. Provide planned activity alternated with rest periods.
   3. Assist patient with ADL to avoid fatigue.
   4. Monitor supplemental oxygen therapy in use.
   5. Administer prescribed drugs, and monitor for side effects.
   6. Monitor blood transfusions.
   7. Provide oral hygiene, particularly if mouth ulcers are present.

8. Provide the prescribed diet.
9. Instruct patient to get up from bed or chair slowly to avoid dizziness.
10. Educate the patient on avoiding and preventing exposure to infection.
11. Support patient and allay anxiety.
12. Educate the patient and family concerning drugs, diet therapy, and planned activity.

Anemia Caused by RBC Destruction

A. Definition: a process in which RBCs are destroyed faster than they are produced
B. Known causes of RBC destruction
1. Snake venom
2. Infections
3. Drugs or chemicals
4. Heavy metals or organic compounds
5. Antigen antibody reaction
6. Splenic dysfunction
7. Congenital causes
a. Thalassemia: a group of hereditary hemolytic anemias characterized by a defect or defects in one or more of the Hgb polypeptide chains
b. Sickle cell anemia (see Chapter 8)
c. Spherocytosis: a hemolytic anemia characterized by spherocytes (small, globular erythrocytes without the characteristic central pallor) in the blood; the spleen destroys abnormal cells.
d. Glucose-6-phosphate dehydrogenase (G6PD) deficiency: a hemolytic disorder brought on by stressors such as infection, certain drugs, acidosis, and toxic substances; individuals with this genetic disorder are relatively symptom free until they experience the stressor that initiates the hemolytic process.
C. Signs and symptoms
1. Anemia
2. Jaundice
3. Splenomegaly
4. Hepatomegaly
5. Weakness and fatigue
6. Skin pallor
7. Anorexia
8. Weight loss
9. Dyspnea
10. Tachycardia
11. Tachypnea
12. Hypotension
13. Cholelithiasis (gallstones): caused by excessive bilirubin
D. Diagnostic tests and methods
1. Patient history and physical examination
2. Laboratory studies
3. Routine chest x-ray examination
4. Routine ECG
5. Bone marrow biopsy
6. Renal studies to monitor kidney status
E. Treatment
1. Identifying the causative agent
2. Blood or blood product replacement
3. Supportive care
4. Genetic counseling
5. Splenectomy to halt the destruction of abnormal RBCs by the spleen

6. Maintaining renal function
7. Maintaining fluid and electrolyte balance
F. Nursing intervention
1. Assess and document signs and symptoms and reactions to treatment.
2. Monitor vital signs as ordered, and report abnormalities.
3. Allay fears and anxieties.
4. Provide planned exercise and rest periods.
5. Caution patient to get up slowly from the bed or chair to avoid postural hypotension.
6. Assist patient with ADL.
7. Monitor intake and output.
8. Monitor laboratory studies.
9. Encourage intake of fluids.
10. Provide prescribed diet.
11. Administer prescribed drugs, and monitor for side effects.
12. Educate the patient and family concerning drugs, diet, activity, and compliance to the prescribed regimen.

Aplastic Anemia (Hypoplastic)

A. Definition: a failure of the bone marrow to produce adequate amounts of erythrocytes, leukocytes, and platelets
B. Exact cause is unclear (idiopathic).
1. May be congenital
2. Related to radiation exposure
3. Results from a disorder that suppresses bone marrow (cancer)
4. Exposure to toxic substances may be a contributing factor.
C. Signs and symptoms
1. General symptoms of anemia; refer to the preceding outlines in this section.
2. Susceptibility to infection
3. Fever
4. Bleeding tendencies
D. Diagnostic tests and methods
1. Patient history and physical examination
2. Laboratory studies, particularly WBC count and platelet count; a reduced WBC count predisposes the patient to infection; a low platelet count predisposes the patient to a bleeding disorder.
3. Bone marrow biopsy examination to evaluate blood cell production
4. Routine chest x-ray examination
5. Routine ECG
E. Treatment
1. Identifying the causative agent
2. Supportive care
3. Administration of blood or blood products
4. Hydration with IV fluids
5. Protection from injury and infections
6. Prevention of hemorrhage
7. Splenectomy
8. Bone marrow transplant
F. Nursing intervention
1. Assess and document signs and symptoms and reactions to treatment.
2. Monitor vital signs at least every 4 hours.
3. Monitor for and report signs of bleeding.
4. Give prescribed medication and monitor for side effects.
5. Avoid fatiguing the patient; provide planned exercise and rest periods.

6. Prevent injury and exposure to infection.
7. Neutropenic precautions may be necessary.
8. Monitor supplemental oxygen if ordered.
9. Provide and encourage the prescribed diet.
10. Allay fears and anxiety.
11. Provide oral hygiene, avoiding aggravation of bleeding gums.
12. Provide skin care using protective devices and frequent repositioning.
13. Educate the patient and family concerning drug therapy, diet, planned activity, avoidance of injury and infection, monitoring for bleeding tendencies, and compliance with the regimen.

Leukemia

A. Definition: a disorder of the hematopoietic system characterized by an overproduction of immature WBCs
  1. As the disease progresses, fewer normal WBCs are produced.
  2. The abnormal cells continue to multiply and eventually infiltrate and damage the bone marrow, spleen, lymph nodes, and other organs.
B. Classification of leukemias
  1. Two major categories: acute and chronic
    a. Acute leukemia has a rapid onset; cells in this phase are young, undifferentiated, and immature.
    b. Chronic leukemia has a gradual onset; cells are mature and differentiated.
  2. Further classification: identifying the type of WBC involved
    a. Acute granulocytic leukemia (nonlymphocytic): the myeloblasts proliferate; myeloblasts are the precursors of granulocytes.
    b. Acute lymphoblastic leukemia: immature lymphocytes proliferate in the bone marrow.
    c. Chronic granulocytic leukemia (nonlymphocytic): excessive neoplastic granulocytes are found in the bone marrow.
    d. Chronic lymphocytic leukemia: characterized by inactive, mature-appearing lymphocytes.
C. Leukemia is considered a neoplastic process; cause is unknown.
D. Predisposing factors
  1. Familial tendency
  2. Viral origin
  3. Exposure to chemicals
  4. Exposure to radiation
E. Once leukemia is diagnosed, the aim of therapy is to prolong survival by attaining a state of remission.
  1. Management of acute leukemia is aggressive.
  2. Management of chronic leukemia aims to control the disorder and maintain remission.
  3. All forms of leukemia are fatal if untreated.
F. Signs and symptoms
  1. General symptoms of anemia
  2. Decreased resistance to infection
  3. Fever
  4. Bleeding tendencies
  5. Enlarged lymph nodes
  6. Splenomegaly
  7. Hepatomegaly
  8. Elevated WBC count
  9. Low platelet count and low Hgb and Hct levels
  10. Poor appetite
  11. Mouth ulcers
  12. Diarrhea
G. Diagnostic tests and methods
  1. Patient history and physical examination
  2. Laboratory studies to evaluate peripheral blood
  3. Bone marrow biopsy
  4. Routine chest x-ray examination
  5. Routine ECG
  6. Lymph node biopsy examination
H. Treatment
  1. Drug therapy: chemotherapeutic agents, analgesics, sedatives, and antibiotics
  2. Radiation therapy (prophylactic measure)
  3. Bone marrow transplants are still under investigation.
  4. Hydration with IV fluids
  5. Replacement of blood and blood products
  6. Monitoring renal status
  7. Protection against infection (neutropenic precautions if needed)
  8. Prevention of hemorrhage
I. Nursing intervention
  1. Assess and document signs and symptoms and reactions to treatment.
  2. Prevent patient from being exposed to infection.
    a. Screen visitors.
    b. Monitor WBC counts.
    c. Practice good hand washing.
    d. Neutropenic precautions may be required.
  3. Avoid fatigue.
    a. Provide planned exercises and rest periods.
    b. Assist patient with ADL.
  4. Monitor for bleeding tendencies.
  5. Administer blood or blood components as ordered, and monitor for side effects.
  6. Monitor intake and output.
  7. Encourage intake of fluids.
    a. Keep fluids at the bedside.
    b. Provide patient with favorite fluids.
  8. Administer prescribed medication as ordered, and monitor for side effects.
    a. Analgesics and sedatives
    b. Antiemetics
  9. Monitor IV fluids.
    a. Monitor the IV site for infiltration.
    b. Monitor rate.
  10. Allay anxieties and fears.
  11. Monitor vital signs at least every 4 hours, and report abnormalities. (An elevated temperature may be the only sign of infection in an immunocompromised patient.)
  12. Monitor supplemental oxygen if ordered.
  13. Provide and encourage the prescribed diet.
  14. Provide oral hygiene, which protects against aggravation of bleeding and drying of the mouth; carefully monitor oral status.
  15. Provide skin care to include the use of protective devices and frequent repositioning.
  16. Educate the patient and family concerning drug therapy, diet, activity, monitoring for bleeding tendencies, avoidance of injury and infection, and compliance with the regimen.

Acquired Immunodeficiency Syndrome

A. Definition: a viral disorder that disrupts the balance of T lymphocytes and ultimately destroys them, rendering the body incapable of defending itself against infection; course is progressive and fatal.
B. Cause: infection with HIV (Human immunodeficiency virus)
   1. The virus is spread by sexual contact, sharing of infected needles, and contact with infected blood and blood products.
   2. Infected mothers can pass the virus to the unborn baby during the gestational period, the birth process, or breast-feeding.
   3. The virus may also enter the body when contaminated blood or body fluids come in contact with broken skin surfaces.
C. Signs and symptoms (vary with each patient; may harbor the virus but be asymptomatic for months or years)
   1. Swollen lymph glands
   2. Recurrent fever, night sweats
   3. Weight loss, diminished appetite
   4. Chronic diarrhea
   5. Fatigue
   6. White patches or lesions in the mouth
   7. Presence of opportunistic infections such as *Pneumocystis carinii* (pneumonia) and Kaposi sarcoma (purplish skin lesions)
   8. Dry cough, shortness of breath
   9. Centers for Disease Control and Prevention clinical categories (Table 5-2)
      a. Category A: categories B and C have not occurred; asymptomatic HIV infection; persistent, generalized lymphadenopathy; acute HIV infection
      b. Category B: category C has not occurred; presence of conditions commonly associated with HIV
      c. Category C: once in this category, person remains in this category; all clinical conditions listed as associated with advanced HIV disease or AIDS
   10. Symptoms may occur as early as 2 to 6 weeks after exposure, or individual may be asymptomatic for months or years; seroconversion (when the blood work changes from a *negative* to a *positive* for HIV antibodies) may not occur for 8 to 12 weeks or longer; retesting is advisable 6 months after exposure, then at 1 year; further testing is left up to the health care provider.
D. Diagnostic tests and methods
   1. Patient history and physical examination
   2. Serum for HIV antibodies

TABLE 5-2   1993 Revised Classification System for HIV Infection and Expanded AIDS Surveillance Case Definition for Adolescents and Adults

CD4 Cell Categories	Clinical Categories*		
	(A) Asymptomatic or PGL	(B) Symptomatic, Not (A) or (C) Conditions	(C) AIDS-Indicator Conditions
>500/mm³	A1	B1	C1
200-499/mm³	A2	B2	C2
<200/mm³ AIDS-indicator cell count	A3	B3	C3

Adapted from Harkness G, Dincher JR: *Medical surgical nursing: total patient care*, ed 9, St Louis, 1996, Mosby.
Centers for Disease Control and Prevention: Impact of the expanded AIDS surveillance case definition on AIDS case reporting–US first quarter, 1993, *MMWR* 42(16):308-310, 1993a.
*Description of Clinical Categories
  A: One or more of the conditions listed below with documented HIV infection. Conditions listed in categories B and C must not have occurred.
      —Asymptomatic HIV infection
      —Persistent generalized lymphadenopathy (PGL)
      —Acute (primary) HIV infection with accompanying illness or history of acute infection
  B: Symptomatic conditions that meet at least one of the following criteria: (a) the conditions are attributed to HIV infection and/or are indicative of a defect in cell-mediated immunity; or (b) the conditions are considered by physicians to have a clinical course or management that is complicated by HIV infection. Examples of conditions in clinical category B include, but are not limited to the following:
      —bacterial endocarditis, meningitis, pneumonia, or sepsis
      —candidiasis, vulvovaginal that is persistent (greater than one month duration) or poorly responsive to therapy
      —candidiasis, oropharyngeal (thrush)
      —cervical dysplasia, severe; or carcinoma
      —constitutional symptoms, such as fever (38.4° C) or diarrhea lasting more than one month
      —hairy leukoplakia, oral
      —herpes zoster (shingles), involving at least two distinct episodes or more than one dermatome
      —idiopathic thrombocytopenic purpura
      —listeriosis
      —*Mycobacterium tuberculosis,* pulmonary
      —nocardiosis
      —pelvic inflammatory disease
      —peripheral neuropathy
  C: Any condition listed in the 1993 surveillance case definition for AIDS. The conditions in clinical category C are strongly associated with severe immunodeficiency, occur frequently in HIV-infected individuals, and cause serious morbidity or mortality.

3. Presence of opportunistic infections
   a. *Pneumocystis carinii* pneumonia
   b. Kaposi sarcoma
4. Bronchial biopsy (tests for presence of opportunistic infections)
5. Lumbar puncture (tests for neurological evidence of infections)
6. CT scan
7. Enzyme-linked immunosorbent assay (ELISA); detects antibodies for HIV; false positives may occur.
8. Western blot test to confirm the results of a positive ELISA test; detects HIV antibodies
9. CD-4 cell counts: if less than 200, the risk for opportunistic infections increases (see Table 5-2)

E. Treatment
1. Treatment is instituted according to the symptoms.
2. Protecting the patient from opportunistic infections
3. Zidovudine (azidothymidine [AZT], Retrovir)
4. Didanosine
5. Zalcitabine
6. Nutritional support
7. Treatment of opportunistic infections

F. Nursing care
1. Assess and document signs and symptoms and reactions to treatment.
2. Monitor vital signs.
3. Monitor arterial blood gas, CBC, and platelet count.
4. Administer prescribed medication, and monitor for side effects.
5. Employ blood and body fluid precautions. (Note: this should be followed when caring for all patients.)
   a. Wear protective clothing (gloves, masks, goggles, gowns, and so forth) as needed for the procedure.
   b. Wash hands thoroughly.
   c. Label specimens accordingly.
   d. Dispose of contaminated articles properly.
6. Plan activity followed by rest periods.
7. Encourage physical independence.
8. Monitor oxygen therapy.
9. Monitor pain status, and provide analgesia and comfort measures.
10. Offer support to the patient and allay anxiety.
11. Educate the patient and family concerning mode of spread, protective measures, and home care.

Lymphoma

A. Definition: a group of malignancies originating in the stem cell of the bone marrow
B. Causes: unknown, possibly linked to viruses, genetics, environmental exposures, and possibly autoimmune links
C. Two main types
1. Hodgkin's disease
2. Non-Hodgkin's lymphoma
D. Signs and symptoms
1. Swollen, painless lymph nodes
2. Fever, chills
3. Weight loss
4. Night sweats
5. Fatigue
6. Loss of usual stamina; changes in ability to perform ADL

E. Diagnostic tests and methods
1. History and physical examination
2. CBC and RBC indexes
3. Blood chemistry: alkaline phosphatase, gamma globulin
4. Serum protein electrophoresis
5. Urine electrophoresis
6. Lymph node biopsy
7. Bone marrow biopsy
F. Treatment
1. Staging laparotomy with splenectomy (to improve response to chemotherapy)
2. Chemotherapy
3. Radiation therapy
G. Nursing care
1. Assess and document signs and symptoms and reactions to treatment.
2. Monitor vital signs.
3. Monitor laboratory studies.
4. Assist in preventing infection and recognize early signs.
5. Assist in planning activity; provide rest periods.
6. Monitor oxygen therapy if ordered.
7. Monitor pain status and provide comfort measures.
8. Give support and allay anxiety.
9. Maintain hydration.

GASTROINTESTINAL SYSTEM

Anatomy and Physiology

A. Organs (Figure 5-8)
1. Mouth (buccal cavity)
   a. Receives food; aids in digestion; aids in speaking
   b. Consists of hard and soft palate, teeth, tongue, and salivary glands
      (1) Teeth
         (a) Deciduous: baby teeth
         (b) Permanent: appear at approximately 6 years of age
         (c) Incisors: cut food
         (d) Canines: tear food
         (e) Molar: grind food
      (2) Salivary glands, parotid, submandibular, sublingual manufacture saliva, which contains ptyalin to begin the chemical breakdown of starches
      (3) Tongue: also organ of taste
         (a) Receptors (taste buds, located in tongue): stimulated only if substance is in solution
         (b) Four kinds: sweet (tip of tongue); sour (side of tongue); salty (tip of tongue); bitter (back part of tongue)
         (c) Stimulates appetite and flow of digestive juices
   c. Functions
      (1) Ingestion of food
      (2) Mastication of food
      (3) Lubrication of food
      (4) Digestion of starch with salivary amylase
2. Pharynx: transports food
3. Esophagus: muscular tube; uses peristalsis to conduct food from pharynx to stomach
4. Stomach

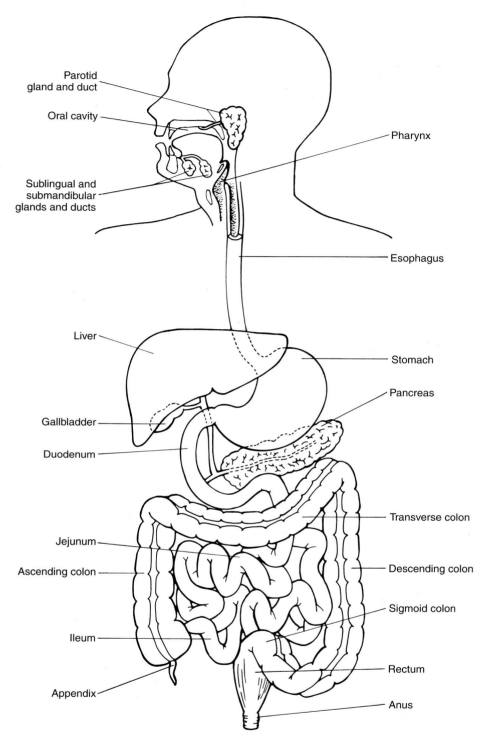

FIGURE 5-8. Digestive system. *(Modified from Phipps, Monahan, Sands, et al.* Medical-Surgical Nursing health and illness perspectives, *ed. 7, St. Louis, 2003, Mosby.)*

a. J-shaped pouch; varies in size, depending on contents; stores food and changes it into chyme
b. Three divisions
  (1) Fundus: upper portion; the cardiac sphincter between the esophagus and fundus; controls the entrance of food
  (2) Body: the largest, central portion

  (3) Pylorus: lower portion above the small intestine; the pyloric sphincter controls the passage of food into the duodenum
c. Special cells in the stomach secrete gastric juices and enzymes (including hydrochloric acid): the chemical breakdown of protein begins in the stomach.
  (1) Pepsin: begins digestion of protein

(2) Lipase: acts on emulsified fat

(3) Renin: acts on casein (a protein) in milk

(4) Gastrin (hormone): related to the control of gastric secretions; not an enzyme

(5) Hydrochloric acid: makes stomach content acid and activates enzymes

d. Chyme: the semiliquid contents of the stomach, consisting of partially digested food and gastric enzymes

e. Functions

(1) Storage of food

(2) Breakdown of food by churning

(3) Liquefying of food with hydrochloric acid

(4) Digestion of protein with enzyme (pepsin)

5. Small intestine: extends from the pyloric sphincter to the ileocecal valve, which prevents backflow of material and regulates forward flow

a. Size: approximately 20 ft (600 cm) long and 1 inch (2.5 cm) in diameter

b. Three major divisions

(1) Duodenum: approximately 10 inches (25 cm) long; curves around head of the pancreas; pancreatic and common bile duct enter below pyloric sphincter.

(2) Jejunum: approximately 8 ft (240 cm) long

(3) Ileum: approximately 12 ft (360 cm) long; terminal part

c. Functions

(1) Digestion of food

(2) Absorption of food

d. Intestinal glands, pancreas, liver, and gallbladder secrete digestive enzymes that complete the chemical breakdown of food.

(1) Bile (formed in the liver and stored in the gallbladder): not an enzyme; emulsifies fat

(2) Trypsin (pancreas): digests proteins into amino acids

(3) Amylase (pancreas): digests starches into sugars

(4) Lipase (pancreas): digests fat into simplest forms (fatty acids and glycerol)

(5) Erepsin (intestine): digests proteins into amino acids

(6) Lactase, maltase, sucrase (secretions of the small intestine): digest sugar into simplest forms (glucose, fructose, galactose)

6. Large intestine

a. Size: approximately 5 to 6 ft (150 to 180 cm) long and 2-1/2 inches (6 cm) in diameter

b. Divisions

(1) Cecum: a blind pouch approximately 3 inches (7.5 cm) long; appendix attaches to distal end; located in right lower quadrant

(2) Colon: ascending, continues up right side; transverse, extends across to the left; descending, descends on left side of pelvis

(3) Sigmoid: S-shaped portion; extends to rectum

(4) Rectum: approximately 8 inches (20 cm) long

(5) Anus: terminal opening, guarded by internal and external sphincters

c. Functions

(1) Reabsorption of fluids

(2) Temporary storage of fecal matter; defecation

B. Accessory organs (see Figure 5-8)

1. Liver: largest organ in body; lies below diaphragm in upper right quadrant of abdominal cavity

a. Metabolizes carbohydrates, fats, and proteins

b. Detoxifies harmful substances

c. Produces and stores heparin and fibrinogen

d. Stores glycogen and vitamins A, B, B_{12}, and K

e. Manufactures bile; hepatic duct drains bile into gallbladder.

2. Gallbladder: small sac embedded in the interior surface of the liver

a. Concentrates and stores bile

b. Releases bile through the common bile duct into the duodenum when fat enters the small intestine

3. Pancreas: long, triangular gland; lies behind the stomach; produces enzymes that break down food particles; secretes enzymes into the duodenum; has two functions

a. Exocrine gland; secretes digestive enzymes that neutralize chyme

b. Endocrine gland: islets of Langerhans; secretes insulin for utilization of glucose; secretes glucagons to regulate blood sugar level

C. Functions

1. Digestion: two processes

a. Mechanical: chewing, swallowing, and peristalsis of food; ends with elimination

b. Chemical: breakdown of food into simpler compounds by the action of enzymes

2. Absorption

a. Occurs in small intestine

b. Most water is absorbed in large intestine.

3. Metabolism: the sum of all body functions to convert simple compounds into living tissue

a. Catabolism: process in which substances are broken down into simpler substances, resulting in the release of heat and energy

b. Anabolism: the building phase in which simpler substances are combined to form more complex substances (conversion of food into living tissues)

c. Basal metabolism: the amount of energy (calories) used by the body when at rest

GASTROINTESTINAL CONDITIONS AND DISORDERS

The GI system provides a means by which food and fluids enter the body and are converted into elements that help maintain the human organism. Important to note is that other systems of the body influence this system. The endocrine system, central nervous system, and autonomic nervous system all serve as regulators to the GI system.

Nursing Assessment

A. Nursing observations (objective data)

1. Vital signs

2. Skin and mucous membrane character and color

a. Gingivitis

b. Stomatitis

c. Jaundice

3. Hematemesis: emesis is as coffee grounds in appearance, signifying digested blood.

4. Stool changes

a. Melena (tarry stool)
b. Clay-colored (lack of bile pigment)
c. Frothy, foamy, foul smelling (seen in pancreatitis)
d. Constipation
e. Diarrhea
f. Changes in size or shape, or both (may indicate colon lesion)
5. Urine color: dark urine (tea colored)
6. Hemorrhoids
7. Abdominal distention
8. Edema
9. Bowel sounds
B. Patient description (subjective data)
1. General
a. History of GI-related problems
b. Family history of GI-related problems
2. Weight
a. Loss or gain
b. Appetite changes: increase or decrease
3. Dietary and eating changes
a. Presence of nausea and vomiting
b. Difficulty chewing
c. Dysphagia
d. Occurrence of indigestion or dyspepsia
e. Intolerance to certain foods
f. Presence of pain: relationship to meals and eating
4. Changes in bowel habit
a. Diarrhea
b. Constipation
c. Alternating diarrhea and constipation
d. Gas formation
5. Easily bruised

Diagnostic Tests and Methods

A. Patient history and physical examination
B. Examination of stool
1. Examination of stool for occult (hidden) blood
2. Fecal analysis: analysis of stool for mucus, pus, blood, parasites, and fat content
3. Stool for ova and parasites must be taken to the laboratory while it is still warm.
4. Nursing intervention
a. Instruct the patient in the proper collection of the specimen.
b. Take the specimen to the laboratory promptly.
C. Radiographic examination
1. Upper GI series
a. Patient ingests contrast medium (barium).
b. Movement of the medium through the esophagus and into the stomach is observed by fluoroscopy; x-ray films are also taken.
(1) Aids in identification of esophageal and stomach pathology
(2) Nursing intervention
(a) Explain procedures to the patient.
(b) Patient is usually NPO before the examination.
(c) Enemas or cathartics may be given before and after the examination.
(d) Allay patient's anxiety.
2. Lower GI series (barium enema)
a. The filling of the colon with barium is observed by fluoroscopy; x-ray films of the colon are also taken.

b. Aids in the detection of abnormalities or defects in the colon, such as lesions, polyps, tumors, and diverticula
c. Nursing intervention
(1) Explain procedures to the patient.
(2) Patient is usually NPO before the examination.
(3) Enemas or cathartics may be given before and after the examination.
(4) Allay patient's anxiety.
3. Gallbladder series (oral cholecystography)
a. Patient is given an oral radiographic dye to ingest the evening before the examination.
b. The gallbladder is visualized to detect gallstones and obstruction of the biliary tract.
c. Nursing intervention
(1) Explain procedures to the patient.
(2) Administer the radiographic dye as prescribed.
(3) Maintain NPO after the dye is given.
(4) Allay patient's anxiety.
4. Ultrasound of the gallbladder
5. Cholangiography
a. Aids in the visualization of the biliary duct system
b. Three methods
(1) Intravenous cholangiography (IVC): a radiographic dye is administered IV, and x-ray films are taken.
(2) Percutaneous transhepatic cholangiography: under fluoroscopy, a cannula is inserted into the liver and bile duct; a radiographic dye is injected into the duct, and filling is observed.
(3) Operative or T-tube cholangiography: contrast medium is instilled into the common bile duct, cystic duct, or gallbladder using a fine needle or catheter during surgery or via an existing T tube postoperatively.
c. Nursing intervention
(1) Explain procedures to the patient.
(2) Maintain NPO as ordered.
(3) Monitor the patient for bleeding or bile leakage if the percutaneous approach was used.
6. Barium swallow: barium contrast study used to detect esophageal abnormalities and reasons for dysphagia
D. Endoscopy
1. Endoscopy of the upper GI tract (esophagoscopy, gastroscopy, gastroduodenoscopy, esophagogastroduodenoscopy)
a. Visualization of the esophagus, stomach, or duodenum with a lighted scope
b. Useful in detecting inflammation, ulceration, tumors, and other lesions
c. Nursing intervention
(1) Explain procedures to the patient.
(2) Obtain signed consent.
(3) Maintain NPO as ordered.
(4) Administer preoperative medication as ordered.
(5) After the examination, maintain NPO until the gag reflex returns.
2. Colonoscopy, sigmoidoscopy
a. Visualization of the internal structures of the colon with a fiberoptic scope
b. Lesions, tumors, and polyps may be visualized, and a biopsy may be performed.
c. Nursing interventions

(1) Explain procedures to the patient.
(2) Prepare patient with enemas and cathartics as ordered.
(3) After the examination, observe for rectal bleeding and signs of perforation (malaise, distention, and tenesmus).
E. Ultrasonography
  1. Noninvasive test that uses echoes from sound waves to visualize deep structures of the body
  2. Requires no special preparation
  3. Useful in detecting masses, fluid accumulation, cysts, tumors, and so forth
F. Scans (liver and pancreas)
  1. Assessment of size, shape, and position of the organ
  2. Radionuclide is injected IV, and a scanning device picks up the radioactive emissions, which are recorded on paper.
  3. Nursing intervention
    a. No preparation is required for liver scanning.
    b. Fasting and dietary preparation may be ordered for pancreatic scanning.
    c. Explain procedures to the patient.
    d. Allay patient's anxiety.
G. CT scan
  1. Noninvasive, radiological imaging technique that takes exposures of the body or body part at different depths
  2. Requires no special preparation
H. Liver biopsy
  1. Invasive procedure in which a needle is inserted into the liver through a small incision in the skin and a sample of liver tissue is obtained
  2. The incision is usually made on the right side, at the sixth, seventh, eighth, or ninth intercostal space.
  3. Nursing interventions
    a. Obtain signed consent.
    b. Explain procedure to the patient.
    c. Take baseline vital signs.
    d. Provide assistance during the procedure.
    e. After the procedure, monitor the vital signs every 15 minutes to 1 hour; carry out prescription for bed rest (position flat or on the right side), assess the site and monitor for complications.
I. Laboratory studies
  1. Serum amylase
    a. Measures the secretion of amylase by the pancreas
    b. Useful in diagnosing pancreatitis
  2. Serum lipase
    a. Measures the secretion of lipase by the pancreas
    b. Useful in diagnosing pancreatitis
  3. Serum bilirubin and spot urine amylase: indicates the liver's ability to conjugate and excrete bilirubin
  4. Coagulation studies (PT and PTT): useful in analyzing hemostatic functions
  5. Liver enzyme studies (SGOT, serum glutamic-pyruvic transaminase [SGPT], and LDH): elevations usually indicate liver damage
  6. Hepatitis-associated antigen (HAA): presence suggests hepatitis
  7. Ammonia levels: elevated in advanced liver disease
  8. Urine amylase: elevated amylase levels indicate pancreatic dysfunction.

J. Gastric analysis
  1. Gastric contents are analyzed primarily for hydrochloric acid content.
  2. Acidity (pH), volume, and cytology may also be determined.
K. D-xylose tolerance test
  1. This study evaluates absorption.
  2. Xylose in water is given orally.
  3. A urine collection of several hours follows; the amount of D-xylose in the urine is measured.
  4. Abnormal amounts of D-xylose in the urine indicate a malabsorption problem.
  5. Nursing interventions
    a. Explain procedure to the patient.
    b. Maintain npo before the examination.
    c. Give patient instructions on collecting the urine.

Frequent Patient Problems and Nursing Care

A. Pain related to impaired oral mucous membranes
  1. Give soft, bland foods.
  2. Encourage intake of fluids that do not aggravate the condition.
  3. Encourage the use of soothing mouth rinses.
  4. Administer topical medication as prescribed.
B. Impaired swallowing related to gingivitis
  1. Give mouth irrigations as prescribed.
  2. Offer soft, bland foods and liquids.
  3. Instruct the patient in the benefit of good oral hygiene and professional dental cleaning.
C. Deficient fluid volume related to nausea and vomiting
  1. Observe character and quantity of emesis.
  2. Observe for associated symptoms.
  3. Observe for precipitating factors.
  4. Administer antiemetics as prescribed.
  5. Offer ice chips.
  6. Maintain cool environment.
  7. Apply a cool compress to the neck and forehead for comfort.
  8. Offer sips of clear liquids, such as 7-Up or ginger ale.
  9. Reduce environmental stimuli such as noise, unpleasant odors, and unpleasant sights.
  10. Encourage rest and deep breathing.
  11. Serve patient's favorite foods.
  12. Limit food servings.
  13. Provide mouth care after episodes of emesis.
D. Risk for aspiration related to dysphagia
  1. Provide patient with favorite foods arranged attractively.
  2. Provide soft, bland foods that can easily be chewed.
  3. Provide small, frequent feedings.
  4. Avoid irritating food and fluid.
  5. Monitor intake.
  6. Administration topical medication as ordered.
  7. Follow aspiration precautions.
E. Impaired nutrition, less than body requirements, related to anorexia
  1. Assess status of the anorexia.
  2. Monitor intake of food and fluid.
  3. Determine patient's food likes and dislikes.
  4. Prepare patient for meals.
    a. Relieve pain.
    b. Provide mouth care.
    c. Assist patient to a comfortable position.

d. Use patient screen for privacy.

e. Remove unpleasant stimuli from patient's view.

5. Prepare food tray.

a. Serve food at the proper temperature.

b. Make the tray attractive.

c. Serve appropriate quantities. (Large quantities may reduce the appetite.)

F. Deficient fluid volume related to diarrhea

1. Document character, consistency, number, and appearance of stools.

2. Assess for associated symptoms.

3. Monitor intake and output.

4. Administer antidiarrheals as prescribed, and monitor for side effects.

5. Avoid milk and milk products.

6. Increase fluid intake to at least 3000 ml daily.

7. Monitor vital signs at least every 4 hours.

8. Identify symptoms of electrolyte imbalance.

9. Monitor laboratory reports for electrolyte values.

G. Constipation related to decreased peristalsis or activity

1. Administer enemas, stool softeners, and cathartics as ordered.

2. Encourage fluids to at least 3000 ml daily.

3. Provide hot drinks to stimulate peristalsis.

4. Encourage a diet high in fiber.

5. Check for an impaction.

6. Encourage exercises.

7. Instruct patient concerning proper diet, increased fluid intake, exercise, and avoidance of laxative abuse.

Major Medical Diagnoses
Esophagitis

A. Definition: an inflammation of the esophagus; more common in middle age

B. Causes

1. Inflammation of the esophagus may be brought on by irritants (food and tobacco), bacteria, or trauma (also see hiatal hernia).

2. Fungal: Candida

3. Gastroesophageal reflux disease (GERD): term for reflux esophagitis; an incompetent lower esophageal sphincter allows a reflux of gastric contents into the esophagus.

4. Malignancy

5. Prolonged nasogastric intubation

6. Repeated vomiting

C. Signs and symptoms

1. Heartburn (epigastric distress)

2. Pain with eructation or regurgitations

3. Dysphagia

4. Pain associated with ingestion of citrus liquids, alcohol, or hot or cold fluid

5. Symptoms aggravated by lying down after meals

6. Bleeding

D. Diagnostic tests and methods

1. Patient history and physical examination

2. Barium swallow

3. Esophagoscopy and biopsy

4. Routine chest x-ray examination

E. Treatments

1. Avoid food and fluids that aggravate the symptoms.

2. Administer antacids, analgesics, and sedatives.

3. Elevate head of bed on shock blocks.

4. Maintain bland diet.

5. Medications are used to decrease the amount of gastric acid produced (Pepcid, Zantac, Axid, among others).

6. Surgery may be necessary if conservative measures fail.

a. Fundoplication: plication (making tucks) in the fundus of the stomach around the lower end of the esophagus

b. Vagotomy and pyloroplasty: interruption of the impulses carried by the vagus nerve to reduce gastric secretions; the pylorus is also surgically manipulated to provide a larger conduit between the stomach and the duodenum.

F. Nursing intervention

1. Assess signs and symptoms and reactions to treatments.

2. Provide small, frequent feedings of bland, low-roughage foods.

3. Discourage intake of food close to bedtime.

4. Administer medication as prescribed and monitor for side effects.

5. Place the patient in semi-Fowler's position.

Esophageal Varices

A. Definition: dilated vessels that occur at the lower end of the esophagus

B. Causes

1. Dilation of these vessels is usually a complication arising from cirrhosis of the liver.

2. Veins in the lower esophagus become distended as a result of increased portal pressure; the varices may rupture, causing hemorrhage and subsequent shock.

C. Signs and symptoms

1. Usually, no signs and symptoms appear until the varices become ulcerated.

2. Hematemesis and coffee-ground emesis.

3. Melena

4. Tachycardia

5. Hypotension

6. Low Hgb and Hct levels

D. Diagnostic tests and methods

1. Patient history and physical examination: history of alcoholism may exist.

2. Fiberoptic endoscopy

3. Laboratory studies: Hgb, Hct, and liver function studies

4. Angiography

5. Barium swallow

6. CT scan

7. Ultrasound

E. Treatment

1. Blood and blood product replacement

2. Control of bleeding through ice water lavages, insertion of Sengstaken-Blakemore tube, and vitamin-K therapy

3. Laboratory studies to monitor bleeding status and effectiveness of treatments

4. Hydration with IV fluids

5. Monitoring intake and output

6. Surgery if needed to control bleeding

7. Injection of the bleeding varices with a sclerosing agent to control the bleeding

F. Nursing intervention

1. Provide ongoing assessment of signs and symptoms and reactions to treatment.

2. Monitor vital signs at least every 4 hours, and monitor vital signs every 30 minutes if bleeding is occurring.
3. Record intake and output hourly if varices are bleeding.
4. Monitor fluids: assess the site and monitor flow rate.
5. Give prescribed medication as ordered, and monitor for side effects.
6. Allay patient's anxieties and fears.
7. Assess all emesis and stool for the presence of blood.
8. Monitor laboratory studies and inform physician of incoming laboratory test values.
9. Keep head of bed elevated.
10. Monitor the Sengstaken-Blakemore tube if in use; keep scissors taped to the head of the bed in case of emergency.
11. Note the character of respirations.

Hiatal Hernia

A. Definition: a protrusion of the proximal area of the stomach through a weakened area of the diaphragm into the thoracic cavity (Figure 5-9)
B. Causes
  1. Congenital weakness
  2. Increased abdominal pressure
  3. Trauma
  4. Relaxation of the musculature
  5. Gastric reflux may flow into the esophagus, causing inflammation and ulceration.
C. Signs and symptoms
  1. Heartburn (pyrosis)
  2. Sternal pain after a heavy meal
  3. Regurgitation
  4. Feeling of fullness
  5. Dysphagia
  6. Dyspnea
D. Diagnosis tests and methods
  1. Patient history and physical examination
  2. Upper GI series (barium swallow)
  3. Esophagoscopy
  4. Routine chest x-ray examination
E. Treatment
  1. Conservative
    a. Elevation of the head of the bed on shock blocks
    b. Bland diet with frequent small feedings
    c. Avoidance of caffeine, alcohol, and chocolate

    d. Drug therapy with anticholinergics, histamine blockers, and antacids
    e. Weight management
    f. Avoidance of activities that increase intraabdominal pressure
  2. When conservative measures fail, surgery is indicated: fundoplication—"wrapping" the upper part of the stomach around the esophageal sphincter to prevent reflux
    a. Nasogastric tube
    b. IV therapy
    c. Drug therapy with analgesics and antiemetics
    d. Monitoring vital signs
    e. Monitoring intake and output
F. Nursing intervention
  1. Assess and document signs and symptoms and reactions to treatments.
  2. Administer prescribed drugs, and monitor for side effects.
  3. Monitor vital signs at least every shift and more often if surgery was performed.
  4. Monitor intake and output if surgery was performed.
  5. Provide the prescribed diet.
  6. Inform the physician if the patient reports gastric reflux after surgery.
  7. Educate the patient and family concerning drug therapy, diet, activities to avoid, and the need for compliance.

Gastritis

A. Definition: an inflammation in the mucosal lining of the stomach; the condition may be acute or chronic.
B. Gastritis may be caused by bacteria, alcohol, drugs, or toxins that cause the lining of the stomach to become inflamed and edematous
C. Signs and symptoms
  1. Nausea and vomiting
  2. Anorexia
  3. Epigastric tenderness
  4. Feeling of fullness
  5. Cramping
  6. Diarrhea
  7. Fever
D. Diagnostic tests and methods
  1. Patient history and physical examination
  2. Identification of a causative agent

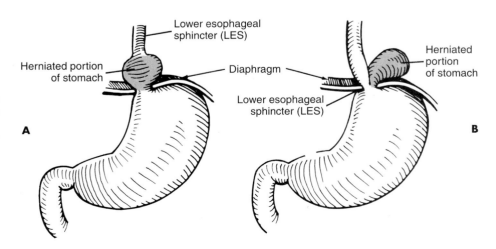

FIGURE 5-9. Hiatal hernia. **A,** Sliding hernia. **B,** Paraesophageal hernia. *(From Phipps, Monahan, Sands, et al. Medical-Surgical Nursing health and illness perspectives, ed. 7, St. Louis, 2003, Mosby.)*

3. Laboratory studies
4. Stool culture
5. Endoscopy with biopsy
6. Gastric analysis

E. Treatment
   1. Supportive care
   2. Bed rest
   3. Continued NPO if nausea or vomiting is severe
   4. Hydration with IV fluids
   5. In severe cases, a nasogastric tube is inserted.
   6. Drug therapy: antiemetics, antacids, and H2-receptor antagonists
   7. Progressive diet when acute symptoms subside
   8. Restriction of smoking

F. Nursing intervention
   1. Assess and document signs and symptoms and reactions to treatments.
   2. Monitor vital signs at least every 4 hours.
   3. Monitor intake and output.
   4. Provide the prescribed diet.
   5. Administer medication as prescribed and monitor for side effects.
   6. Note amount and character of emesis and diarrhea.
   7. Monitor IV fluids.
   8. Educate the patient and family concerning drug therapy, diet, activities, and any restrictions.

Cancer of the Stomach

A. Cancer can develop anywhere in the stomach.
B. Causes
   1. Exact cause is unknown
   2. Familial tendency is suspected.
   3. Predisposing conditions: chronic gastric ulcers and gastritis
C. Signs and symptoms
   1. Loss of appetite, early satiety
   2. Weight loss
   3. Weakness and fatigue
   4. Pain
   5. Melena
   6. Anemia
   7. Hematemesis
   8. Dizziness
   9. Indigestion or dysphagia
   10. Constipation
D. Diagnostic tests and methods
   1. Patient history and physical examination
   2. Laboratory studies
   3. Stool analysis
   4. Gastric analysis
   5. Barium studies
   6. Gastroscopy
E. Treatment
   1. Preoperative therapy
      a. Correct nutritional deficiencies
      b. Treat anemias
      c. Blood replacement
      d. Gastric decompression with a nasogastric tube
   2. Surgery: removal of the cancerous lesion or tumor along with a margin of normal tissue
   3. Radiation therapy and chemotherapy may be used if the patient is not expected to undergo surgery.

a. Combination therapy has a better response rate.
b. Single-agent therapy has proved to be of little value.

F. Nursing intervention
   1. Preoperative care
      a. Offer support to the patient and family.
      b. Assess and document signs and symptoms and reactions to treatments.
      c. Provide and encourage the prescribed diet.
      d. Monitor vital signs at least every 8 hours.
      e. Monitor blood and fluid replacement therapy.
      f. Provide preoperative teaching.
   2. Postoperative care (immediate)
      a. Have patient turn, cough, and breathe deeply.
      b. Monitor nasogastric suctioning and tube patency.
      c. Monitor vital signs as ordered.
      d. Record intake and output.
      e. Administer prescribed medication, and monitor for side effects.
      f. Assess dressing.
      g. Assess for bowel sounds.
      h. Encourage early ambulation and ROM exercises to prevent thrombosis.
      i. Provide antiembolism stockings.
      j. Relieve pain with drugs and supportive measures.
   3. Postoperative period
      a. Provide six to eight small feedings.
      b. Weigh patient daily while in hospital to monitor weight loss.
      c. Reduce fluids taken with meals if not tolerated.
      d. Educate the patient and family concerning drug therapy, dietary restrictions, activity, wound care, and compliance with the regimen.

Peptic Ulcers

A. Definition: ulcerations in the mucosal lining of the distal esophagus, stomach, or small intestine (duodenum or jejunum); duodenal ulcers are more common than gastric ulcers, and men are more prone to ulcers than are women.
B. Cause: exact cause is unknown; recurrent or refractory ulcers linked to *Helicobacter pylori* infections.
C. Predisposing factors
   1. Stress
   2. Smoking
   3. Heavy caffeine ingestion
   4. Ingestion of certain drugs (acetyl salicyclic acid [ASA], steroids, nonsteroidal antiinflammatory drugs [NSAIDs])
   5. Infection of the mucosa by *H. pylori*
D. Signs and symptoms
   1. Loss of appetite
   2. Weight loss or gain
   3. Pain (gnawing, burning)
   4. Melena
   5. Anemia
   6. Hematemesis; coffee-ground emesis
   7. Occasional nausea or vomiting
   8. Dark, tarry stools
E. Diagnostic tests and methods
   1. Patient history and physical examination
   2. Gastroscopy and duodenoscopy
   3. Barium studies
   4. Gastric analysis
   5. Laboratory studies

F. Treatment
1. Conservative
   a. Rest
   b. Drug therapy: antacids, anticholinergics, histamine receptor antagonists, sedatives, and analgesics
   c. Elimination of smoking and caffeine
   d. Reduction of stress
   e. Bland diet with small, frequent feedings
   f. In acute situations, the patient may be NPO and have nasogastric tube inserted.
2. Surgical intervention
   a. Closure if perforation has occurred
   b. Pyloroplasty and vagotomy if the gastric outlet is obstructed
   c. Total or partial resection of the stomach to remove the ulcerated areas
G. Nursing intervention
1. Conduct ongoing assessment of signs and symptoms and reactions to treatments.
2. Monitor vital signs at least every 4 hours.
3. Administer the prescribed medication, and monitor for side effects.
4. Provide the prescribed diet.
5. Provide physical and emotional rest.
6. Monitor for signs and symptoms of complications (perforation, hemorrhage, and obstruction).
7. Instruct patient regarding elimination of smoking, avoidance of certain foods, and reduction of stress.
8. Educate the patient and family concerning drug therapy, diet and dietary restrictions, avoidance of stress, and the need for compliance with the prescribed regimen.

Obstruction

A. Definition: a mechanical or neurological abnormality inhibiting the normal flow of gastric or intestinal contents
B. Obstructions may result from scar tissue formation, cancer, or strangulated hernias; all are mechanical barriers to the normal flow of gastric or intestinal contents.
C. A neurological obstruction, in the form of a paralytic ileus, causes interference with innervation, thus hindering normal peristaltic activity.
D. Signs and symptoms
1. Abnormal pain and distention
2. Projectile vomiting
3. Nausea
4. Possible absence of bowel sounds or increase in bowel sounds
5. Cramping
6. Abdomen may be tense (distended)
7. Obstipation (chronic constipation)
E. Diagnostic tests and methods
1. Patient history and physical examination
2. Flat plate of the abdomen
3. Laboratory studies
F. Treatment
1. Surgery for treating mechanical obstructions
2. Gastric or intestinal decompression to decrease nausea and vomiting
3. Hydration with IV therapy
4. Prophylactic antibiotics
5. Monitoring intake and output
6. Supportive care

G. Nursing intervention
1. Assess and document signs and symptoms and reactions to treatments.
2. Monitor vital signs at least every 4 hours.
3. Record intake and output.
4. Monitor the decompression tube, and assess quantity and character of drainage.
5. Provide mouth care while patient is intubated.
6. Administer prescribed medication, and monitor for side effects.
7. Maintain NPO.
8. Monitor the states of distention and hydration.
9. Provide routine postoperative care if patient undergoes surgery.

Crohn's Disease (Regional Enteritis)

A. Definition: an inflammatory disease affecting primarily the small bowel and also possibly the large bowel; the intestinal lining ulcerates, and scar tissue forms; bowel becomes thick and narrow.
B. Cause is unknown; stricture, obstruction, and perforation can occur as a result of this disorder; malabsorption of fluid and nutrients is also associated with this disorder.
C. Signs and symptoms (aggravated by illness or stress)
1. Abdominal pain and cramping
2. Diarrhea
3. Weight loss
4. Fever
5. Anemia
6. Weakness and fatigue
7. Anorexia
8. Abdominal tenderness
D. Diagnostic tests and methods
1. Patient history and physical examination
2. Laboratory studies: CBC, electrolytes, clotting studies
3. Stool examination
4. Endoscopy
5. Proctosigmoidoscopy and biopsy examination
6. Barium studies
E. Treatment
1. Drug therapy: sedatives, antidiarrheals, antibiotics, steroids, hematinics, anticholinergics, and analgesics
2. Hydration with IV therapy
3. Correcting nutritional deficiencies
4. Providing symptomatic relief
5. In severe cases, the patient may be NPO, have a nasogastric tube, and require blood transfusions.
6. High-calorie, high-protein, low-residue diet
7. Surgery is indicated if fistula formation, bleeding, perforation, or obstruction is present.
F. Nursing intervention
1. Assess and document signs and symptoms and reactions to treatments.
2. Monitor vital signs every 4 hours.
3. Record intake and output.
4. Provide and encourage the prescribed diet.
5. Assist with ADL.
6. Monitor the number, amount, and character of stools.
7. Monitor hydration status.
8. Assess for abdominal distention.
9. Maintain skin integrity, and monitor for anal excoriation.

10. Provide support to the patient.
11. Administer prescribed medication and monitor for side effects.
12. Educate the patient and family concerning drug therapy, dietary restrictions, and compliance; provide information on ostomy care if applicable.

Ulcerative Colitis

A. Definition: an inflammatory disorder of the large bowel; the inflammatory process begins in the distal segments of the colon and ascends.
   1. The mucosa ulcerates, bleeds, and becomes edematous and thickens.
   2. Perforations and abscesses can occur.
   3. The colon eventually loses its elasticity, and its absorptive ability is reduced.
B. Cause is unknown, although it has been associated with stress, autoimmune factors, and food allergies.
C. Signs and symptoms
   1. Abdominal cramping pain with diarrhea
   2. Nausea
   3. Dehydration
   4. Cachexia
   5. Weight loss
   6. Anorexia
   7. Bloody diarrhea
   8. Anemia
D. Diagnostic tests and methods
   1. Patient history and physical examination
   2. Laboratory studies to reveal anemia and electrolyte imbalance: CBC, electrolytes
   3. Stool examination
   4. Proctosigmoidoscopy
   5. Barium studies
E. Treatment
   1. Drug therapy: sedatives, antidiarrheals, antibiotics, steroids, hematinics, anticholinergics, and analgesics
   2. Correction of malnutrition
   3. Hydration with IV therapy
   4. Colectomy with ileostomy if other medical treatment fails
   5. Providing symptomatic relief
   6. Monitoring weight
   7. Monitoring intake and output
   8. Parenteral hyperalimentation if necessary
   9. Psychotherapy
F. Nursing intervention
   1. Assess and document signs and symptoms and reactions to treatments.
   2. Provide emotional and physical rest.
   3. Monitor number, amount, and characteristics of stools.
   4. Provide skin care measures to avoid anal excoriation.
   5. Monitor intake and output.
   6. Monitor vital signs every 4 hours.
   7. Weigh patient daily.
   8. Increase intake of fluids.
   9. Provide the prescribed diet.
   10. Administer prescribed medication, and monitor for side effects.
   11. Assess bowel sounds every 4 hours.
   12. Assist with ADL.
   13. Provide emotional support.

14. Educate the patient and family concerning drug therapy, dietary restrictions, avoidance of stress, and compliance with the prescribed regimen.

Diverticulosis, Diverticulitis

A. Definition: diverticulum—an outpouching of the mucosa of the colon
   1. Diverticulosis: the existence of diverticula in the large intestine
   2. Diverticulitis: an inflammation of the diverticulum
B. Cause of diverticulosis is unknown; theories include a congenital weakness of the colon, colon distention, constipation, and inadequate dietary fiber.
C. Signs and symptoms
   1. Abdominal cramps
   2. Lower-quadrant tenderness
   3. Constipation or constipation alternating with diarrhea
   4. Fever
   5. Occult bleeding
   6. Elevated WBC count
D. Diagnostic tests and methods
   1. Patient history and physical examination
   2. Laboratory studies
   3. Stool examination for occult blood
   4. Sigmoidoscopy
   5. Colonoscopy
   6. Barium studies
E. Treatment
   1. High-residue diet
   2. Drug therapy: bulk laxatives, antibiotics, stool softeners, and anticholinergics
   3. In more severe cases, the patient may be NPO and require IV therapy.
   4. Surgery: colon resection for obstruction and hemorrhage
F. Nursing intervention
   1. Assess and document signs and symptoms and reactions to treatments.
   2. Provide increased fiber in the diet.
   3. Increase intake of fluids.
   4. Administer prescribed medication, and monitor for side effects.
   5. Instruct patient to avoid activity that increases intraabdominal pressure (straining at stool, lifting, bending, and wearing restrictive clothing).
   6. Educate the patient and family concerning drug therapy, dietary restrictions, and avoidance of constipation and activity that increases intraabdominal pressure.

Colon and Rectal Cancer and Polyps

A. Definition: the cancerous process can invade the large intestine; cancer of the colon and rectum may take the form of well-defined tumor or cancerous polyp: a polyp is a pouch-like structure projecting from the wall of the bowel; polyps may be cancerous or benign.
B. Cause of colon cancer is unknown; persons with colon polyps, lesions, diverticula, or ulcerative colitis are monitored closely for malignant changes in the bowel.
C. Signs and symptoms
   1. Changes in bowel pattern
   2. Rectal bleeding
   3. Changes in the shape of stool
   4. Weakness and fatigue

5. Weight loss
6. Rectal pain
7. Abdominal pain
8. Anemia

D. Diagnostic tests and methods
   1. Patient history and physical examination
   2. Laboratory studies
   3. Barium studies
   4. Proctosigmoidoscopic examination

E. Treatment
   1. Surgical resection of the affected area, creation of a colostomy if necessary
   2. Chemotherapy
   3. Radiation therapy
   4. Supportive therapy

F. Nursing intervention (also see nursing care plan for cancer of the stomach)
   1. Assess and document signs and symptoms and reactions to treatments.
   2. Monitor vital signs at least every 4 hours and more often during the postoperative periods.
   3. Record intake and output.
   4. Monitor dressings and wound drainage.
   5. Relieve pain.
   6. Administer prescribed medication, and monitor for side effects.
   7. Provide psychological support.
   8. Monitor colostomy site.
   9. Monitor perineal area if drain or packing has been inserted.
   10. Assist patient with sitz baths if ordered.
   11. Assist patient with ADL as needed.
   12. Monitor hydration status.
   13. Encourage increased fluid intake.
   14. Educate the patient and family concerning drug therapy, diet, activities, colostomy care, and adaptation to everyday activity.

Hemorrhoids

A. Definition: varicosities or dilated vessels in the rectal and anal area

B. Cause: hemorrhoids result from increased abdominal pressure, such as that during pregnancy and from prolonged periods of sitting and standing; constipation and obesity are also predisposing factors.

C. Signs and symptoms vary from no symptoms at all to pain, itching, and bleeding.

D. Diagnostic tests and methods
   1. Patient history and physical examination
   2. Digital examination
   3. Proctoscopy

E. Treatment
   1. Symptomatic relief in mild cases
      a. Topical medication to shrink the mucous membrane
      b. Stool softeners and laxatives to keep stool soft and avoid straining
      c. Sitz baths to relieve pain
      d. High-fiber diet to keep stools soft
   2. Rubber-band ligation of internal hemorrhoids: the constriction impairs circulation; the tissues become necrotic and slough off.
   3. Hemorrhoidectomy: the surgical excision of hemorrhoids

a. Removal may be by clamp, excision, or cautery.
b. Postoperative treatments are similar to those identified previously for symptomatic relief.

F. Nursing intervention
   1. Assess and document signs and symptoms and reactions to treatments.
   2. Alleviate pain with analgesics, positioning, and sitz baths.
   3. Administer prescribed medication, and monitor for side effects.
   4. Monitor vital signs at least every 4 hours.
   5. Monitor dressings for drainage.
   6. Monitor voiding after surgery.
   7. Assist with gradual return to activity.
   8. Encourage increased fluid intake.
   9. Provide patient with rationale for avoiding constipation and prolonged sitting and standing.
   10. Educate the patient and family concerning drug therapy, high-fiber diet, activity, and avoidance of constipation.

Cholelithiasis, Cholecystitis

A. Definition
   1. Cholelithiasis: the presence of gallstones in the gallbladder or biliary tree
   2. Cholecystitis: an inflammation of the gallbladder usually associated with the presence of gallstones

B. Cause
   1. Cholelithiasis is believed to be precipitated by chemical changes in bile.
      a. Bile stasis, infections of the gallbladder, and metabolic changes can precipitate stone formation.
      b. Stones may lodge in the biliary tree, causing obstruction and biliary colic (Figure 5-10)
   2. Cholecystitis: may be brought on by cholelithiasis or the presence of an organism in the gallbladder

C. Signs and symptoms
   1. Indigestion after a meal high in fat
   2. Nausea and vomiting
   3. Flatulence
   4. Belching
   5. Right upper-quadrant pain radiating to the back or shoulder
   6. Fever
   7. Jaundice
   8. Clay-colored stools
   9. Dark-colored urine
   10. Elevated WBC count

D. Diagnostic tests and methods
   1. Patient history and physical examination
   2. Laboratory studies
   3. Oral cholecystography
   4. IV cholangiography
   5. Ultrasound of gallbladder

E. Treatment
   1. Hydration with IV fluids
   2. Drug therapy: analgesics, antibiotics, and antispasmodics
   3. Drug therapy to dissolve stones has been effective in certain patients
   4. Low-fat diet
   5. Lithotripsy (use of shock waves to disintegrate gallstones) has been attempted in patients having few stones

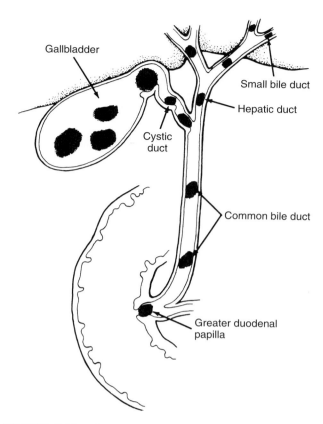

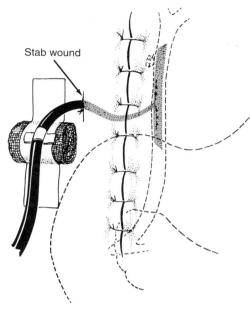

FIGURE 5-11. Section of T-tube emerging from stab wound may be placed over roll of gauze anchored to skin with adhesive tape to prevent its lumen from being occluded by pressure. *(From Phipps, Monahan, Sands, et al.* Medical-Surgical Nursing health and illness perspectives, *ed. 7, St. Louis, 2003, Mosby.)*

FIGURE 5-10. Common sites of gallstones. *(From Phipps, Monahan, Sands, et al.* Medical-Surgical Nursing health and illness perspectives, *ed. 7, St. Louis, 2003, Mosby.)*

    6. Surgical removal of the gallbladder (cholecystectomy) or gallstones (cholecystostomy)

    7. Laparoscopic cholecystectomy (removal through an endoscope inserted through the abdominal wall)

F. Nursing intervention

    1. Assess and document signs and symptoms and reactions to treatments.

    2. Administer prescribed medication, and monitor for side effects.

    3. Alleviate pain and promote comfort.

    4. Monitor IV therapy.

    5. Provide the prescribed diet.

    6. Monitor the state of hydration.

    7. Assess vital signs at least every 4 hours.

    8. Provide postoperative care: monitor dressing, nasogastric tube, and T tube (tube is inserted into the common bile duct during surgery if the common bile duct is explored) (Figure 5-11).

    9. Educate the patient and family concerning drug therapy, dietary restrictions, and wound care if surgery was performed.

Hepatitis

A. Definition: inflammation of the liver

B. Causes

    1. Drugs or chemicals (toxic hepatitis)

    2. Viral origin

    3. Multiple blood transfusions

    4. Hepatitis A

       a. Transmitted by the fecal-oral route

       b. Incubation period is approximately 2 to 7 weeks

       c. May be spread by contaminated food, water, milk, and shellfish

    5. Hepatitis B

       a. Associated with contaminated needles and syringes

       b. Transmitted through blood or blood products and pricking of the skin with contaminated equipment

       c. May also be spread through feces, urine, saliva, and semen

       d. Patients are prone to exacerbations and complications (cirrhosis) from the disease,

       e. Incubation period is approximately 6 to 26 weeks,

       f. Immunization available: given to newborn, then again at 2 and 6 months of age,

    6. Hepatitis C virus (HCV; formerly known as non-HAV and non-HBV) and hepatitis E

       a. Name given to forms of hepatitis caused by a virus genetically different from hepatitis A or B

       b. Associated with blood transfusions, particularly from paid donors; previous IV drug use

       c. No specific antigen is associated with the form

       d. Similar to hepatitis B in characteristics, but the course is insidious in the beginning.

       e. All blood donors are now tested for HCV.

C. Signs and symptoms: (early symptoms of hepatitis A may be more severe)

    1. Fever and chills

    2. Headache

    3. Respiratory symptoms

    4. Anorexia

    5. Nausea and vomiting

6. Liver tenderness
7. Jaundice and itching
8. Elevated liver enzymes
9. Elevated PT values
10. Elevated bilirubin levels
11. Presence of hepatitis virus in feces and serum
12. Presence of the hepatitis surface antigen (HBsAg)
13. Clay-colored stools and dark-colored urine

D. Diagnostic tests and methods
1. Patient history and physical examination
2. Laboratory studies: Hepatitis associated antigen (HAA), liver profile
3. Stool examination
4. Urinary bilirubin and urobilinogen
5. Liver biopsy
6. Serum ammonia levels: protein is restricted if ammonia levels are elevated.

E. Treatment
1. Monitoring liver function studies
2. Bed rest with bathroom privileges
3. High-calorie, high-carbohydrate, high-protein, moderate-fat diet
4. Topical lotions to alleviate dry, itchy skin
5. Hydration with IV therapy
6. Administration of vitamin-K preparations
7. Monitoring for bleeding tendencies and progression of the illness
8. Blood and body fluid precautions
9. Passive immunity

F. Nursing intervention
1. Assess and document signs and symptoms and reactions to treatments.
2. Monitor skin, stool, and urine color.
3. Promote balanced activity and rest periods.
4. Maintain blood and body fluid precautions.
5. Monitor IV therapy.
6. Assess intake and output.
7. Monitor vital signs at least every 4 hours.
8. Provide and encourage the prescribed diet.
9. Offer support to the patient and family.
10. Administer prescribed medication, and monitor for side effects.
11. Monitor for bleeding tendencies.
12. Educate the patient and family concerning drug therapy, the prescribed diet, activity level, and monitoring for complications.

Cirrhosis

A. Definition: cell degeneration occurring in the liver wherever scar tissue replaces normally functioning tissue
B. Cirrhosis is a complication of alcoholism, hepatitis, biliary disease, and certain metabolic disorders.
C. Whatever the cause of the liver destruction, the course of cirrhosis is the same.
1. Liver parenchyma dies and regenerates, and fibrous tissue (scarring) occurs.
2. This alteration in structure progresses in the liver, causing problems in hepatic blood flow and normal liver function; in time, the liver fails.
D. Major complications of cirrhosis
1. Portal hypertension: hypertension resulting from the obstruction of normal blood flow through the portal system; the obstruction is caused by changes in the liver from the cirrhotic process.
2. Esophageal varices (see esophageal varices)
3. Ascites: the accumulation of fluid in the peritoneal or abdominal cavity, which is a later symptom in cirrhosis
4. Hepatic coma (encephalopathy): a condition of advanced liver disease; blood enters the general circulation without being properly detoxified by the liver.

E. Signs and symptoms
1. Headache
2. Nausea and vomiting
3. Weight loss
4. Anorexia
5. Jaundice
6. Abdominal pain
7. Fatigue and weakness
8. Liver enlargement and fibrosis
9. Bleeding disorders caused by disruption in the manufacture of vitamin K–dependent factors
10. Edema
11. Telangiectasis (blood vessels develop a spiderlike appearance)
12. Ascites
13. Esophageal varices
14. Hepatic coma

F. Diagnostic tests and methods
1. Patient history and physical examination
2. Laboratory studies to assess liver function
3. Liver scan
4. Liver biopsy; monitoring for bleeding at site

G. Treatment
1. Rest with activity as tolerated
2. Nutritious diet with protein level determined by liver functioning
3. If ascites is present, restricting fluid and sodium, monitoring weight, and taking abdominal girth measurements daily
4. Monitoring for complications such as ascites, esophageal varices, and hepatic coma
5. Drug therapy to reduce ammonia levels, prevent bleeding, reduce edema, and provide comfort

H. Nursing intervention
1. Assess and document signs and symptoms and reactions to treatments.
2. Administer prescribed medication, and monitor for side effects.
3. Provide and encourage the prescribed diet.
4. Promote comfort.
5. Monitor vital signs at least every 4 hours, and report abnormalities.
6. Monitor status of ascites.
   a. Record weight.
   b. Assess measurements of extremities and abnormal girth.
   c. Monitor intake and output.
7. Provide planned exercise and rest periods.
8. Assist patient with ADL.
9. Monitor skin status and take measures to prevent skin breakdown.
10. Protect against infection.
11. Provide diversional activity.
12. Offer emotional support.

13. Provide ongoing assessment for evidence of hepatic encephalopathy.
    a. Monitor for symptoms of lethargy, confusion, twitching, tremors, sweetish breath odor, fever, and increasing somnolence.
    b. Eliminate dietary protein-decreases serum ammonia levels, which contribute to the encephalopathy.
    c. Administer prescribed drugs and enemas to reduce ammonia levels.
    d. Monitor IV fluids.
    e. Give narcotics and sedatives cautiously.
14. Also see care of patient with esophageal varices at the beginning of this section.
15. Educate the patient and family concerning homebound care.

Pancreatitis

A. Definition: an acute or chronic inflammation of the pancreas
B. Pancreatitis is associated with biliary disease, infections, drug toxicity, nutritional deficiencies, and ingestion of alcohol. Some cases may be idiopathic.
C. The digestive enzymes of the pancreas are released into the pancreatic tissue, causing inflammation.
   1. As the condition progresses, ischemia, duct obstruction, and necrosis may occur.
   2. Bleeding occurs if tissue necrosis affects vessels.
   3. Pancreatic abscesses may occur if bacteria invade the necrotic tissue.
   4. In chronic pancreatitis, the tissue becomes fibrotic and normal function is compromised.
D. Signs and symptoms
   1. Acute pancreatitis
      a. Severe epigastric pain that radiates to the back
      b. Eating tends to aggravate pain.
      c. Patient may assume a side-lying position with knees bent for comfort.
      d. Nausea and vomiting
      e. Low-grade fever
      f. Hypotension
      g. Tachycardia
      h. Jaundice
      i. Elevated WBC count
      j. Shock: if blood vessel or tissue erosion is present
   2. Chronic pancreatitis
      a. Abdominal pain
      b. Weight loss
      c. Steatorrhea (foul-smelling, foamy stool)
      d. Diabetes mellitus if beta cell function is affected
E. Diagnostic tests and methods
   1. Patient history and physical examination
   2. Laboratory tests, particularly electrolytes, amylase, lipase, and liver enzymes
   3. Pancreatic scan and sonography
   4. Visualization of the pancreatic duct (endoscopy)
   5. X-ray studies
F. Treatment
   1. Control of pain
   2. Hydration with IV fluids
   3. Correction of any bleeding
   4. Nasogastric tube and NPO to reduce pancreatic secretions

5. Drug therapy: analgesics, antibiotics, steroids, vitamins, and pancreatic extracts
6. Diet that does not stimulate pancreatic secretions
7. Control of blood glucose levels if beta cells are affected
G. Nursing intervention
   1. Assess and document signs and symptoms and reactions to treatments.
   2. Administer prescribed medication, and monitor for side effects.
   3. Provide the prescribed diet.
   4. Explain dietary restrictions to patient.
   5. Monitor vital signs at least every 4 hours.
   6. Monitor IV therapy.
   7. Promote comfort and relieve pain.
   8. Provide emotional support.
   9. Assess intake and output.
   10. Relieve nausea and vomiting if present.
   11. Note color, character, and amount of urine and stool.
   12. Monitor jaundice if present.
   13. Monitor the nasogastric tube and secretions.
   14. Educate the patient and family concerning drug therapy, diet and dietary restrictions, avoidance of alcohol, monitoring steatorrhea, blood glucose monitoring (glucometer), and compliance with the regimen.

Cancer of the Pancreas

A. Cancer of the pancreas can affect any portion of the pancreas, including the beta cells; metastasis readily occurs to adjacent structures.
B. Cancerous tissue impairs normal pancreatic function, primarily by causing obstruction and hindering the flow of pancreatic secretions.
C. Signs and symptoms
   1. Early symptoms may be vague.
      a. Nausea and vomiting
      b. Anorexia
      c. Weight loss
      d. Weakness and fatigue
   2. Later symptoms
      a. Pain
      b. Jaundice
      c. Diabetes mellitus
D. Diagnostic tests and methods
   1. Patient history and physical examination
   2. Laboratory studies
   3. Pancreatic scan and sonography
   4. X-ray studies
   5. Visualization of the pancreatic duct
E. Treatment
   1. Supportive therapy
   2. Surgical excision: Whipple's procedure may be performed, removing the head of the pancreas, lower portion of the common bile duct, distal portion of the stomach, and the duodenum.
   3. Palliative surgery to restore bile and pancreatic output
   4. Chemotherapy
F. Nursing intervention: see cancer of the stomach

Appendicitis

A. Definition: inflammation of the appendix
B. Signs and symptoms
   1. Right lower-quadrant pain with rebound tenderness

2. Periumbilical pain
3. Nausea and vomiting
4. Anorexia
5. Fever
6. Elevated WBC count
C. Diagnostic tests and methods
   1. Patient history and physical examination
   2. Laboratory tests, particularly a WBC count
D. Treatment
   1. Supportive therapy
   2. Immediate surgical removal (appendectomy)
E. Nursing intervention
   1. Assess and document signs and symptoms and reactions to treatments.
   2. Monitor IV fluids.
   3. Provide comfort measures such as an ice pack to the abdomen and analgesia.
   4. Administer prescribed drugs, and monitor for side effects.
   5. Monitor vital signs as ordered.
   6. Encourage progressive ambulation after surgery.
   7. Monitor the dressing and operative site after surgery.
   8. Educate the patient and family concerning drug therapy, activity restrictions, and care of the operative site.

Peritonitis

A. Definition: infection and subsequent inflammation of the peritoneal membrane by trauma or bacterial invasion
B. The inflammation may be localized or widespread and may affect the organs of the abdominal cavity; adhesions, abscesses, and obstructions may occur.
C. Signs and symptoms
   1. Nausea and vomiting
   2. Abdominal pain
   3. Abdominal rigidity and distention
   4. Fever
   5. Paralytic ileus
   6. Fluid and electrolyte imbalance
   7. Elevated WBC count
   8. Constipation, diarrhea
D. Diagnostic tests and methods
   1. Patient history and physical examination
   2. Laboratory tests including a WBC count, electrolytes, and blood cultures
E. Treatment
   1. Identification of the causative agent
   2. Intestinal decompression
   3. Hydration with IV therapy
   4. Pain control
   5. Drug therapy: analgesics and antibiotics
   6. Monitoring vital signs
   7. Monitoring intake and output
   8. Controlling the spread of infection
F. Nursing intervention
   1. Assess and document signs and symptoms and reactions to treatment.
   2. Assess vital signs every 1 to 2 hours during the acute period.
   3. Monitor intake and output.
   4. Administer prescribed medication, and monitor for side effects.
   5. Provide comfort and relief of pain.

6. Assess bowel sounds.
7. Maintain NPO during the acute period.
8. Maintain nasogastric tube, and monitor output during the acute period.
9. Offer support to patient, and allay anxieties.
10. Place patient in semi-Fowler's position.
11. Have patient turn, cough, and deep breathe at least every 2 hours.

Hernia

A. Definition: a protrusion of an organ or structure through the muscle wall of the containing cavity
B. Hernias may occur around the umbilical area, inguinal area, diaphragm, femoral ring, and at the site of an incision.
C. Hernias are categorized as:
   1. Reducible: can be returned to the normal position
   2. Irreducible: cannot be returned to the normal position
   3. Incarcerated: obstruction of intestinal flow
   4. Strangulated: blood supply is cut off (occluded)— surgical emergency
D. Causes
   1. Congenital weakness in the containing wall
   2. Weakness in containing wall is related to straining and the aging process.
   3. Trauma
   4. Increased intraabdominal pressure (obesity or pregnancy)
E. Signs and symptoms
   1. Protrusion of a structure without symptoms
   2. Appearance of a protrusion when straining or lifting
   3. Pain in certain instances
   4. If the intestine is obstructed, distention, pain, nausea, and vomiting may occur.
F. Diagnostic methods: patient history and physical examination
G. Treatment
   1. Surgery is the treatment of choice.
      a. Herniorrhaphy: surgical repair of the hernia
      b. Hernioplasty: the surgical reinforcement of the weakened area
   2. Use of a truss (a support worn over the hernia to keep it in place)
H. Nursing intervention
   1. Assess and document signs and symptoms and reactions to treatments.
   2. Assess vital signs every shift before surgery.
   3. Report any symptoms of coughing, sneezing, or upper respiratory tract infection noted before surgery because this will weaken the surgical repair.
   4. Apply ice packs as ordered to control pain and swelling.
   5. Monitor voidings following inguinal hernia repair.
   6. Educate the patient and family concerning care of the operative site, activity restrictions, and avoidance of constipation.

NEUROLOGICAL SYSTEM

Anatomy and Physiology

The nervous system acts as a coordinated unit, both structurally and functionally.
A. Functions

1. Regulates system; responsible for coordinating body functions and responding to changes in or stimuli from the internal and external environment
2. Controls communication among body parts
3. Coordinates activities of body system

B. Divisions
   1. Central nervous system (CNS): brain and spinal cord; interprets incoming sensory information and sends out instruction based on past experiences
   2. Peripheral nervous system (PNS): cranial and spinal nerves extending out from brain and spinal cord; carry impulses to and from brain and spinal cord
   3. Autonomic nervous system: functional classification of the PNS; regulates involuntary activities
   4. Somatic nervous system: functional classification of the PNS; allows conscious or voluntary control of skeletal muscles

C. Structure and physiology
   1. Neurons or nerve cells: respond to a stimulus, connect into a nerve impulse (irritability), and transmit the impulse to neurons, muscle, or glands (conductivity); consists of three main parts
      a. Cell body: contains nucleus and one or more fibers or processes extending from cell body
      b. Dendrites: conduct impulses toward cell body; neuron has many dendrites.
      c. Axons: conduct impulses away from cell body; neuron has one axon.
   2. Types of neurons
      a. Motor (efferent) neurons: conduct impulses from CNS to muscle and glands
      b. Sensory (afferent) neurons: conduct impulses toward CNS
      c. Connecting (internuncial) neurons: conduct impulses from sensory to motor neurons

3. Synapse: chemical transmission of impulses from axon to dendrites
4. Myelin sheath: protects and insulates the axon fibers; increases the rate of transmission of nerve impulses
5. Neurilemma: sheath covering the myelin; found in PNS; function is regeneration of nerve fiber.
6. Neuroglia: connective or supporting tissue; important in reaction of nervous system to injury or infection
7. Ganglia: clusters of nerve cells outside the CNS
8. White matter: bundles of myelinated nerve fibers; conducts impulses along fibers
9. Gray matter: clusters of neuron cell bodies; fibers not covered with myelin; distributes impulses across selected synapses

D. Central nervous system (CNS)
   1. Brain (Figure 5-12)
      a. Cerebrum: largest part of brain; outer layer called cerebral cortex; cortex composed of dendrites and cell bodies; controls mental processes; highest level of functioning (Table 5-3)
      b. Cerebellum: controls muscle tone coordination and maintains equilibrium
      c. Diencephalon: consists of two major structures located between cerebrum and midbrain
         (1) Hypothalamus: regulates the autonomic nervous system; controls blood pressure; helps maintain normal body temperature and appetite; controls water balance and sleep
         (2) Thalamus acts as a relay station for incoming and outgoing nerve impulses; produces emotions of pleasantness and unpleasantness associated with sensations
      d. Brain stem: connects the cerebrum with the spinal cord
         (1) Midbrain: relay center for eye and ear reflexes

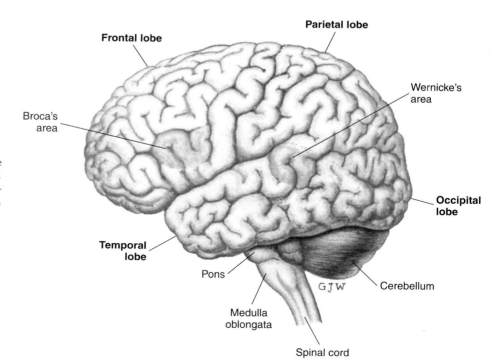

FIGURE 5-12. Lateral view of the brain. *(From Phipps, Monahan, Sands, et al. Medical-Surgical Nursing health and illness perspectives, ed. 7, St. Louis, 2003, Mosby.)*

(2) Pons: connecting link between cerebellum and rest of nervous system

(3) Medulla oblongata: contains center for respiration, heart rate, and vasomotor activity

2. Spinal cord
   a. Inner column composed of gray matter, shaped as an H, made up of dendrites and cell bodies; outer part composed of white matter, made up of bundles of axons called tracts
   b. Function: sensory tract conducts impulses to brain; motor tract conducts impulses from brain; center for all spinal cord reflexes

3. Protection for central nervous system
   a. Bone: vertebrae surround cord; skull surrounds brain
   b. Meninges: three connective tissue membranes that cover brain and spinal cord
      (1) Dura mater: white fibrous tissue; outer layer
      (2) Arachnoid: delicate membrane, middle layer; contains subarachnoid fluid
      (3) Pia mater: inner layer; contains blood vessels
   c. Spaces
      (1) Epidural between dura mater and the vertebrae
      (2) Subdural space: between dura mater and arachnoid
      (3) Subarachnoid space: between arachnoid and pia mater; contains cerebrospinal fluid
   d. Cerebrospinal fluid: acts as a shock absorber; aids in exchange of nutrients and waste materials

E. Peripheral nervous system (PNS)
   1. Carries voluntary and involuntary impulses
   2. Cranial nerves (Table 5-4)
   3. Spinal nerves: 31 pairs; conduct impulses necessary for sensation and voluntary movement; each group is named for the corresponding part of the spinal column.

F. Autonomic nervous system
   1. Part of PNS; controls smooth muscle, cardiac muscle, and glands
   2. Two divisions
      a. Sympathetic: "fight or flight" response; increases heart rate and blood pressure; dilates pupils
      b. Parasympathetic: dominates control under normal conditions; maintains homeostasis

---

TABLE 5-3	Specific Functions of Cerebral Cortexes
Frontal cortex	Conceptualization Abstraction Judgment formation Motor ability Ability to write words Higher level centers for autonomic functions
Parietal cortex	Highest integrative and coordinating center for perception and interpretation of sensory information Ability to recognize body parts Left versus right Motor movement
Temporal cortex	Memory storage Auditory integration Hearing
Occipital cortex	Visual center Understanding of written material

From Phipps WJ, Monahan FD, Sands JK, Marek JF, and Neighbors M: *Medical-surgical nursing: Health and illness perspectives,* ed 7, St. Louis, 2003, Mosby.

TABLE 5-4	Cranial Nerves	
Cranial Nerves	**Conducts Impulses**	**Function**
I Olfactory	From nose to brain	Sense of smell
II Optic	From eye to brain	Vision
III Oculomotor	From brain to eye and eye muscles	Contraction of upper eyelid; maintain position of eyelid; pupillary reflexes
IV Tochlear	From brain to external eye muscles	Eye movements
V Trigeminal	From skin and mucous membranes of head and teeth to chewing muscles	Sensations of head and teeth; muscles of chewing
VI Abducens	From brain to external eye muscles	Eye movements
VII Facial	From taste buds of the tongue and facial muscles to muscles of facial expression	Taste; facial expression
VIII Acoustic	From organ of Corti to brain	Hearing
Vestibular branch	From semicircular canals to brain	Balance
IX Glossopharyngeal	From pharynx and posterior to third of tongue to brain; also from brain to throat muscles and salivary glands	Sensations of tastes, sensations of pharynx; swallowing; secretion of saliva
X Vagus	From throat and organs in thoracic and abdominal cavities to brain; to muscles of throat and abdominal cavities	Important in swallowing, speaking, peristalsis, and production of gastric juices
XI Accessory	From brain to shoulder and neck muscles	Rotation of head and raising shoulders
XII Hypoglossal	From brain to muscles of tongue	Movement of tongue

NEUROLOGICAL CONDITIONS AND DISORDERS

Pathologic conditions of the CNS arises from injuries, new growths, vascular insufficiency, infections, and as complications secondary to other diseases. Patient problems are related to interference with normal functioning of the affected tissue.

The following terms are used in describing the patient with a neurological impairment.

Anesthesia: complete loss of sensation

Aphasia: loss of ability to use language

Auditory or receptive aphasia: loss of ability to understand

Expressive aphasia: loss of ability to use spoken or written word

Ataxia: uncoordinated movements

Coma: state of profound unconsciousness

Convulsion: involuntary contractions and relaxation of muscle

Delirium: mental state characterized by restlessness and disorientation

Diplopia: double vision

Dyskinesia: difficulty in voluntary movement

Flaccid: without tone, limp

Neuralgia: intermittent, intense pain along the course of a nerve

Neuritis: inflammation of a nerve or nerves

Nuchal rigidity: stiff neck

Nystagmus: involuntary, rapid movements of the eyeball

Papilledema: swelling of optic nerve head

Paresthesia: abnormal sensation without obvious cause, with numbness and tingling

Spastic: convulsive muscular contraction

Stupor: state of impaired consciousness with brief response only to vigorous and repeated stimulation

Tic: spasmodic, involuntary twitching of a muscle

Vertigo: dizziness

Nursing Assessment

A. Nursing observations
1. Mental status: drowsiness or lethargy, ability to follow commands
2. Level of consciousness (LOC): ability to be aroused in response to verbal and physical stimuli; ranges from awake and alert to "coma"; Glasgow coma scale (Table 5-5) is the usual guide for assessing and describing the degree of conscious impairment, based on three determinants.
   a. Eye opening
   b. Motor response
   c. Verbal response
3. Orientation
   a. Time: knows month or year
   b. Place: has general knowledge of where patient is (e.g., hospital)
   c. Person: knows own name; is able to name relative or friend
4. Behavior: is it appropriate for the situation?
5. Emotional response: is it appropriate for the situation?
6. Memory: capability for early and recent recall, remote, recent, and new learning ability
7. Speech: presence of aphasia, appropriate speech, words distinct or slurred, quality, rate, loudness, and fluency
8. Vital signs: temperature, pulse, respirations, and blood pressure; note pulse pressure.

TABLE 5-5	Glasgow Coma Scale	
	Stimuli	**Score**
Eyes open	Spontaneously	4
	To speech	3
	To pain	2
	None	1
Best verbal response	Oriented	5
	Confused	4
	Inappropriate words	3
	Incomprehensible	2
	None	1
Best motor response	Obeys commands	5
	Localizes to pain	4
	Flexes to pain	3
	Extends arm to pain	2
	None	1

Adapted from Phipps WJ, Monahan FD, Sands JK, Marek JF, and Neighbors M: *Medical-surgical nursing: Health and illness perspectives,* ed 7, St. Louis, 2003, Mosby.

9. Ability to follow simple directions
10. Eyes
    a. Pupillary reaction to light: the pupils are periodically assessed with a flashlight to evaluate and compare size, configuration, and reaction; differences between both eyes and from previous assessments are compared for similarities and differences.
    b. Movement of lids and pupils
11. Motor function: coordination, gait, balance, posture, strength, functioning, and muscle tone
12. Bladder and bowel control
13. Ears for drainage (may indicate cerebrospinal fluid leak)
14. Facial expression for symmetry
15. Sensation for:
    a. Pain
    b. Light touch, pressure
    c. Smell
16. Rancho Los Amigos scale: a scale of cognitive functioning that was developed to aid in assessment and treatment after traumatic brain injury (TBI)
    a. No response: completely unresponsive to any stimuli
    b. Generalized response: reacts inconsistently and nonpurposefully to stimuli
    c. Localized response: reacts specifically yet inconsistently to stimuli
    d. Confused-agitated: is in agitated state yet has decreased ability to process information
    e. Confused-inappropriate: appears alert; is able to respond to simple commands fairly consistently
    f. Confused-appropriate: has goal-directed behaviors; needs cues
    g. Automatic-appropriate: oriented; does daily routine; has shallow recall of actions
    h. Purpose-appropriate; aware and oriented; is able to recall and integrate past and recent events
17. Grooming, personal hygiene
18. Thoughts, perceptions, attention span

B. Patient description (subjective data)
   1. History of head injury, loss of consciousness, vertigo, weakness, headache, sleep problems, paralysis, seizures, or diplopia
   2. Complaints of pain, numbness, problems with elimination, memory loss, difficulty concentrating, drowsiness, or visual problems
   3. Medications taken
C. History from family
   1. Medical
   2. Activities of daily living (ADL)
   3. Behavior

Diagnostic Tests and Methods

A. Computerized tomography CT (CAT) scan: computer analysis of tissues as x-rays pass through them; has replaced many of the usual tests; no special preparation or care after test
B. Lumbar puncture (spinal tap)
   1. Description: under local anesthesia, a puncture is made at the junction of the third and fourth lumbar vertebrae to obtain a specimen of cerebrospinal fluid; cerebrospinal fluid pressure can be measured; this procedure is also used to inject medications (e.g., spinal anesthesia) and in diagnostic x-ray examination to inject air or dye (e.g., myelogram).
   2. Nursing intervention
      a. Monitor vital signs.
      b. Keep patient supine 4 to 8 hours.
      c. Observe for headache and nuchal rigidity.
      d. Monitor site for leakage.
C. Cerebral angiography
   1. Description: intraarterial injection of radiopaque dye to obtain an x-ray film of cerebrovascular circulation
   2. Nursing intervention after procedure
      a. Related to dye: observe for allergic reaction—urticaria, decreased urinary output, respiratory distress, and difficulty swallowing; have tracheostomy set available.
      b. Related to injection site
         (1) Provide ice pack and bed rest.
         (2) Monitor vital signs.
         (3) Observe for pain, tenderness, bleeding, temperature, and color.
D. Electroencephalography (EEG)
   1. Description: electrodes are placed on unshaven scalp with tiny needles and electrode jelly.
   2. Nursing intervention
      a. Anticipate patient's fears about electrocution; do not give stimulants or depressants before test.
      b. No smoking or caffeinated beverages; patient needs to eat a full meal before the test; fasting may cause hypoglycemia and alter brain waves.
      c. Antiseizure medications or tranquilizers may need to be withheld, if ordered.
      d. Stress need for restful sleep before test; sleep deprivation may cause abnormal brain waves.
      e. Wash hair and scalp after procedure to remove jelly.
      f. Patient may resume all previous activities.
E. Brain scan
   1. Description: after an IV injection of a radioisotope, abnormal brain tissue will absorb more rapidly than will normal tissue; this can be detected with a Geiger counter to diagnose brain tumors.

   2. Nursing intervention
      a. No observations
      b. Patient may resume all previous activities.
F. Magnetic resonance imaging (MRI)
   1. Description: MRI uses a combination of radio waves and a strong magnetic field to view soft tissue (does not use x-rays or dyes); produces a computerized picture that depicts soft tissues in high-contrast color
   2. Nursing intervention
      a. Before the procedure, instruct the patient to remain perfectly still in the narrow cylinder-shaped machine.
      b. Inform the patient that no pain or discomfort will occur, but movement during the MRI must not be made.
      c. No specific care or observations are necessary after the procedure.
G. Myelography (MEG)
   1. Description: injection of a radiopaque dye into the subarachnoid space via a lumbar puncture; performed to locate lesions of the spinal column or ruptured vertebral disk
   2. Types of agents used: metrizamide and Pantopaque; if metrizamide is used, the patient should not take phenothiazines, tricyclic antidepressants, CNS stimulants, or amphetamines for 24 to 48 hours before test; after the procedure is completed, Pantopaque dye is removed; leaving it in would cause meningeal irritation; metrizamide is water soluble and does not need to be removed.
   3. After procedure with Pantopaque, the patient lies flat in bed for 6 to 8 hours; after procedure with metrizamide, patient's head must be elevated 30 to 50 degrees for 6 to 8 hours; fluids are encouraged; common side effects include nausea, vomiting, and possibly seizures; check with physician when medications withheld before test may be given; with both types of agents observe site for leakage of cerebrospinal fluid; strength and sensation in lower extremities should be assessed; encourage fluids; maintain bed rest; monitor vital signs; observe for headache, pain, and dizziness.
H. Positron emission tomography (PET) scan
   1. The patient inhales or is injected with a radioactive substance.
   2. The computer can diagnose and determine level of functioning of an organ.
   3. Exposure to radiation is minimal, and no special care is indicated.
I. Skull x-ray examination: no preparation; no nursing care or observations are indicated afterward.

Frequent Patient Problems and Nursing Care

A. Impaired physical mobility related to progression of primary disease
   1. Give specific care and perform assessment as required (see Chapter 2).
   2. Perform neurological assessment every 2 to 4 hours.
   3. Initiate nursing care measures to prevent complications of immobility.
   4. Use assistive devices.
B. Risk for injury or infection related to "fixed eyes" (no blinking)
   1. Protect with eye shields.
   2. If needed, remove dried exudate with warm saline solution and mineral oil.

3. Have patient close eyes.

4. Inspect for inflammation.

C. Ineffective breathing pattern related to neuromuscular impairment

1. Maintain patent airway, suction as needed, and elevate head 20 to 30 degrees.

2. Have tracheostomy set available.

3. Provide oxygen with humidity.

4. Monitor vital signs every 2 hours.

5. Provide oral hygiene every 2 hours.

6. Lubricate the patient's lips.

D. Risk for hyperthermia, hypothermia related to neuromuscular impairment

1. Assess rectal temperature every 2 hours.

2. Use external heating and cooling, (e.g., hypohyperthermia machine)

E. Risk for aspiration related to neuromuscular impairment

1. Maintain NPO.

2. Position patient on side; turn every 2 hours.

3. Provide nasogastric tube feedings.

4. Monitor IV fluids.

F. Risk for injury related to restlessness, involuntary motions, or seizures

1. Maintain safety (e.g., padded side rails, bed in low position).

2. Follow precautions, care, and observations for a patient with seizures (see convulsive disorders, pp. 248-249).

G. Risk for impaired urinary elimination related to neuromuscular impairment

1. Urinary retention

a. Provide indwelling catheter care.

b. Monitor intake and output hourly.

2. Incontinence

a. Wash, dry, and inspect skin as needed.

b. Implement measures to prevent skin breakdown.

c. Implement bladder training.

H. Bowel incontinence, constipation related to neuromuscular impairment

1. Incontinence

a. Wash, dry, and inspect skin as needed.

b. Implement measures to prevent skin breakdown.

c. Implement bowel training.

2. Constipation

a. Record bowel movements.

b. Provide stool softeners, laxatives, and enemas as ordered.

c. Check for impaction; disimpact as needed.

d. Encourage fluids as tolerated.

e. Encourage activity as tolerated.

f. Increase fiber in the diet.

I. Fear and anxiety related to pain; complications; surgery; possible disfigurement, disability, or dependency; fatal prognosis

1. Explain nursing actions thoroughly.

2. Encourage patient to express feelings.

3. Report to health team.

4. Involve family or significant others in care.

J. Other possible patient problems include:

1. Self-care deficit: perform own ADLs related to sensory-motor impairments.

2. Imbalanced nutrition; less than body requirements related to dysphagia and fatigue

3. Grieving related to actual or perceived loss or uncertain future or both

4. Impaired swallowing related to chewing difficulties, muscle paralysis

5. Activity intolerance related to fatigue and difficulty in performing ADLs

6. Fatigue related to weakness, spasticity, fear of injury, and stressors

7. Risk for social isolation related to spasticity, change in body image

8. Risk for injury related to visual field, motor, or perception deficits

9. Interrupted family processes related to physiological deficits, role disturbances, uncertain future

10. Disturbed sensory perception specifically related to hypoxia secondary to trauma, progression of disease process

11. Impaired communication related to dysarthria or aphasia secondary to physiological changes

12. Risk for deficient fluid volume related to vomiting secondary to increased intracranial pressure (IICP)

Special Situations

A. The patient in coma

1. Unconscious state in which the patient is unresponsive to verbal or painful stimuli; this occurs with many primary diseases; the patient depends on the nurse for maintenance of all basic human needs, nourishment, bathing, elimination, respiration, prevention of complications, and assessment and provision of care for problems (see the preceding section).

2. Nursing intervention

a. Include family in nursing care and care planning as much as possible.

b. Note level of consciousness (LOC) (see nursing assessment of the neurological patient) every 15 minutes if LOC decreases; assess every 1, 2, or 4 hours as LOC improves.

c. Demonstrate respect in patient's presence.

d. Provide a quiet, restful environment.

e. Speak to patient; use proper name; introduce self, and explain all care before starting.

f. Provide privacy.

B. The patient with paralysis

1. Paraplegia: paralysis of the lower extremities from sudden injury (e.g., automobile accident) or progressive degenerative disease (e.g., multiple sclerosis) to the spinal cord; no motion or sensory function or reflexes may be evident; uncontrollable muscle spasms may occur; perspiration ceases and then becomes profuse; a loss of bladder and bowel control occurs; sexual dysfunction, anxiety, fear, depression, anger, and embarrassment are major patient problems; patient may be totally dependent.

2. Quadriplegia (tetraplegia): paralysis of all four extremities from sudden injury (e.g., diving accident) or progressive degenerative disease (e.g., amyotrophic lateral sclerosis [ALS]); symptoms and patient problems include those encountered with paraplegia, as well as autonomic dysreflexia.

3. Nursing intervention

a. Take measures to prevent complications of immobility.

b. Provide bowel and bladder training.

c. Prevent deformity: maintain joint mobility, and correct alignment.

d. Encourage fluid intake.

e. Provide high-protein diet.

f. Encourage independence according to ability.

g. Communicate and work closely with the physiatrist, physical therapist, occupational therapist, and other members of the rehabilitation team.

h. Include family in nursing care and planning.

Major Medical Diagnoses
Increased Intracranial Pressure (IICP)

A. Description: fluid accumulation or a lesion takes up space in the cranial cavity producing IICP; the brain is gradually compressed, or life-sustaining functions cease; onset may be sudden or progress slowly.

B. Causes: tumors, hematoma, edema from trauma or stroke, and abscesses from infections

C. Signs and symptoms: related to primary diagnosis
1. Headache, restlessness, and anxiety
2. Vomiting: recurrent, projectile, and not related to nausea or meals
3. Change in pupil response to light
4. Seizures
5. Respiratory difficulty: irregular, Cheyne-Stokes, or Kussmaul breathing
6. Elevated blood pressure, with wide pulse pressure
7. Increases in pulse at first then slowing to 40 to 60 beats per minute (bpm), regular and strong
8. Altered LOC: becomes lethargic, speech slows, becomes confused, and shows decreased level of response
9. Visual disturbances: diplopia and blurred vision
10. Progressive weakness or paralysis
11. Loss of consciousness, coma, and death

D. Diagnostic tests and methods: neurological assessment by physician and nurse

E. Treatment: depends on cause
1. Surgical intervention (craniotomy)
2. Steroids, anticonvulsants, mannitol, dexamethasone (Decadron), or urea to decrease edema

F. Nursing intervention
1. Elevate head to semi-Fowler's position; never place in Trendelenburg's position.
2. Monitor vital signs every 15 minutes.
3. Prevent aspiration; place patient on side.
4. Maintain airway; provide oxygen therapy as necessary.
5. Observe pupillary response (usually unequal and may not react to light).
6. Report any change in LOC immediately.
7. Provide special care and observation when a patient has a seizure.
8. Provide care and safety for an unconscious patient.
9. Monitor IV fluids closely to prevent overhydration.

Convulsive Disorders

A. Description: frequently, a convulsion or seizure is not a disease but a symptom of a neurological disorder; epilepsy is a disease characterized by a disposition for seizures; the following are types of seizures:
1. Tonic-clonic (formally grand mal): a premonition or sign (aura) may occur; the individual cries out, loses consciousness, and enters a tonic phase (the body is rigid, and the jaw is clenched); then a clonic phase occurs, with jerking movements of muscles, cessation of respirations, and fecal and urinary incontinence; seizure lasts 1 to 2 minutes, followed by a short period of unresponsiveness.
2. Absence (formally petit mal): loss of consciousness that lasts 5 to 30 seconds, during which time normal activities may or may not cease; amnesia concerning this time may occur.

B. International Classification of Epileptic Seizures (Box 5-6)

C. Causes
1. May be secondary to another condition: cerebrovascular accident (CVA), head injury, brain tumor, markedly elevated temperature, toxins, or electrolyte imbalance
2. Epilepsy may have no known cause; onset is usually in childhood, before 30 years of age.

D. Patient problems
1. Related to primary disease
2. Fear of injury
3. Anxiety related to a chronic disease
4. Embarrassment
5. Fear of public rejection
6. Side effects of drug therapy

E. Diagnostic tests and methods
1. Specific tests to identify lesions
2. EEG, CT scan, MRI, and brain mapping
3. Serum chemistries

F. Treatment
1. Treatment and removal of cause, if known
2. Anticonvulsant drugs (see Chapter 3)
3. Surgery: stereotactic (electrical stimulation to locate and resect [destroy] epileptogenic focus)

G. Nursing intervention
1. Provide accurate observation and documentation, including the following: aura, time of onset, whether seizure is generalized or focal, specific parts of body involved, progression of seizure; duration of seizure, eye movement, loss of consciousness, loss of bowel and bladder control, condition after seizure, memory loss, weakness, and any injury caused by seizure.
2. Encourage patient to wear medical identification tag.
3. Have suction available.
4. Secure airway for easy accessibility.
5. During generalized (grand mal) seizure:
   a. Insert airway between teeth before seizure (do not force).

BOX 5-6   International Classification of Epileptic Seizures

Partial (focal) seizures (consciousness may not be impaired): with motor symptoms, with special sensory symptoms, with autonomic symptoms, with psychic symptoms. May become complex partial seizures. May evolve to generalized seizures.

Generalized seizures (involve the entire brain; consciousness is lost): may last from several seconds to minutes. Types: absence seizures, tonic-clonic seizures, atonic seizures

Unclassified seizures: unable to classify because of incomplete or inadequate data

b. Maintain airway.

c. Prevent head injury.

d. Place patient on side if possible.

e. Protect extremities from injury by guiding movements.

f. Do not restrain.

g. Loosen clothing.

h. Remove pillows.

i. Maintain safety until fully conscious.

Transient Ischemic Attacks (TIAs)

A. Definition: altered cerebral tissue perfusion related to a temporary neurological disturbance

1. Exhibited by sudden loss of motor or sensory function

2. Lasts for a few minutes to a few hours

3. Caused by a temporarily diminished blood supply to an area of the brain

4. Patient is at high risk for developing a stroke.

B. Medical management is indicated (control of hypertension, low-sodium diet, possible anticoagulant therapy, smoking cessation).

C. Nursing care would include close observation and assessment; specific care is based on treatment.

Cerebrovascular Accident (Stroke, Brain Attack) and Cerebrovascular Disruptions

A. Description: decreased blood supply to a part of the brain caused by rupture, occlusion, or stenosis of the blood vessels; onset may be sudden or gradual; symptoms and patient problems depend on location and size of area of brain with reduced or absent blood supply (left CVA results in right-sided involvement often associated with speech problems; right CVA results in left-sided involvement often associated with safety and judgment problems).

B. Causes: increased incidence with aging

1. Atherosclerosis

2. Embolism

3. Thrombosis

4. Hemorrhage from a ruptured cerebral aneurysm

5. Hypertension

C. Signs and symptoms

1. Subjective

a. Change in mental status: decreased attention span, decreased ability to think and reason, difficulty following simple directions

b. Headaches

2. Objective

a. Altered level of consciousness

b. Communication: motor or sensory aphasia, difficulty reading, writing, speaking, or understanding

c. Bowel or bladder dysfunction: retention, impaction, or incontinence

d. Seizures

e. Limited motor function: paralysis, dysphagia, weakness, hemiplegia, loss of function, or contractures

f. Loss of sensation or perception

g. Loss of temperature regulation and elevated temperature, pulse, and blood pressure

h. Absent gag reflex (aspiration)

i. Unusual emotional responses: depression, anxiety, anger, verbal outbursts, and crying; emotional lability

j. Problems related to immobility (see Chapter 2)

D. Diagnostic tests and methods

1. Physical assessment and patient or family history

2. EEG, CT scan, lumbar puncture, cerebral angiography, or carotid ultrasonography, Doppler flow studies

E. Treatment

1. Removing cause, preventing complications, and maintaining function; rehabilitation to restore function

2. Providing antihypertensives, anticoagulants, antiplatelet aggregation, antifibrinolytics, and stool softeners (see Chapter 3)

3. Surgical removal of clot, repair of aneurysm, carotid endarterectomy, balloon angioplasty, stents

F. Nursing intervention

1. Maintain bed rest; provide complete care; use turning sheet, foot board, firm mattress, pillows; use trochanter rolls to maintain proper body alignment; anticipate needs, and leave things within reach (e.g., call bell).

2. Reposition patient every 2 hours; provide passive and active ROM exercises; place patient in chair as soon as allowed; use flotation mattress or sheepskin.

3. Provide bath, inspect skin, and provide nursing measures to prevent decubitus ulcers.

4. Provide oxygen with humidity; have patient cough and take deep breaths every 2 hours if possible; maintain airway; suction as needed; prevent aspiration; keep head turned to side; place in semi-Fowler's position.

5. Ensure adequate nutrition and fluid and electrolyte balance; provide nasogastric or gastrostomy tube feeding; maintain IV fluids; provide soft diet when tolerated; use total parenteral nutrition (TPN); follow aspiration precautions.

6. Establish means of communication: call bell, pad and pencil, and nonverbal gestures; use simple commands; speak slowly, explain all care; provide speech therapy.

7. Be nonjudgmental about personality changes; encourage family participation; provide diversional activities; praise accomplishments realistically.

8. Assess LOC; maintain safety in environment; use side rails; restrain only as necessary.

9. Observe for IICP.

10. Monitor vital signs every 4 hours.

11. Ensure elimination; check bowel sounds; monitor bowel movements; monitor intake and output; provide indwelling catheter care; then, conduct bowel and bladder training.

12. Provide care, safety, and precautions for a patient with seizures.

13. Provide support for family.

14. Schedule physical and occupational therapy as soon as possible.

15. Provide nursing measures to prevent complications of immobility (see Chapter 2).

16. Encourage self-care.

Brain Tumor

A. Definition: a benign or malignant growth that grows and exerts pressure on vital centers of the brain, depressing function and causing increased pressure

B. Cause: unknown

C. Signs and symptoms: individual, depending on location and size

1. Personality changes, fear, and anxiety

2. Headaches, dizziness, and visual disturbance (e.g., double vision)
3. Seizures
4. Pituitary dysfunction
5. Signs of IICP
6. Local paresthesia or anesthesia
7. Aphasia
8. Problems with coordination, gait

D. Diagnostic tests and methods
   1. Patient history and physical examination
   2. Neurological assessment including EEG, CT scan, angiography, MRI, PET scan

E. Treatment: surgical removal if possible (craniotomy), frequently combined with radiotherapy and chemotherapy

F. Nursing intervention
   1. Perform timely neurological assessment and documentation.
   2. Provide safety and assist with care as needed.
   3. Be nonjudgmental about personality changes; encourage the patient to express feelings.
   4. Provide postoperative care
      a. Anticipate and provide care as needed to maintain airway
      b. Provide safety and observation during a seizure
      c. Regulate body temperature
      d. Position on unoperated side
      e. Elevate head only under medical order
      f. Inspect dressing every 30 minutes for hemorrhage or drainage (leakage of cerebrospinal fluid)
      g. Make neurological assessment hourly until patient is stable and then every 4 hours; observe for IICP
      h. Provide care for the patient in coma as indicated earlier in this section

Head Injuries

A. Definition: trauma to scalp, skull, or brain; a fracture to the skull may result, either a simple break in the bone or bone fragmentation that penetrates the brain tissue; hemorrhage, concussion, or contusion can also result.
   1. Cerebral concussion: injury to the head; patient may be dazed or unconscious for a few minutes; some functions (e.g., memory) may be impaired for as long as several weeks.
   2. Cerebral contusion: head injury causing bruising of brain tissue; person experiences stupor, confusion, or loss of consciousness; if severe, the person may go into coma.
   3. Cerebral laceration: a break in continuity of brain tissue

B. Cause: blow to the head (e.g., from a fall or automobile accident)

C. Signs and symptoms: individual, according to location and extent of blow
   1. Nausea and vomiting, dizziness, vertigo
   2. Lethargy: increasing loss of consciousness to impending coma
   3. Disorientation
   4. Drainage of cerebrospinal fluid from ear or nose (Battle's sign)
   5. Convulsions
   6. Problems related to IICP

D. Diagnostic tests and methods
   1. Patient history and physical and neurological assessment
   2. X-ray examination

3. Angiography, Doppler studies
4. CT scan, MRI
5. PET scan

E. Treatment
   1. Anticonvulsants, corticosteroids, mannitol (if cerebral edema)
   2. Maintenance of fluid balance
   3. Surgery

F. Nursing intervention
   1. Provide care as discussed for a patient with IICP (see p. 248).
   2. Take neurological assessment hourly.
   3. Maintain airway.
   4. Give care as required for the unconscious patient if necessary.
   5. Take precautions for a patient with seizures.
   6. Observe for serous or bloody discharge from ears or nose.

Multiple Sclerosis

A. Description: a chronic, progressive disease of the brain and spinal cord; lesions cause degeneration of the myelin sheath and interfere with conduction of motor nerve impulses; periods of remissions and exacerbations occur; onset occurs in young adults; progression is unpredictable.

B. Cause: unknown; exacerbates with stress

C. Signs and symptoms vary with individual.
   1. Ataxia
   2. Paresthesia, numbness, tingling
   3. Weakness and loss of muscle tone, fatigue
   4. Loss of sense of position
   5. Vertigo
   6. Blurred vision, diplopia, nystagmus, patchy blindness that may progress to total blindness
   7. Inappropriate emotions: euphoria, apathy, depression
   8. Dysphagia
   9. Slurred speech
   10. Bladder and bowel dysfunction: incontinence or retention
   11. Sexual dysfunction: impotence, diminished sensation
   12. Spasticity as disease progresses

D. Diagnostic tests and methods
   1. Patient history and physical and neurological assessment
   2. CT scan
   3. MRI
   4. Examination of cerebrospinal fluid
   5. PET scan
   6. Evoked responses

E. Treatment: symptomatic; corticosteroids during acute exacerbations

F. Nursing intervention
   1. Provide care to prevent complications of immobility (see Chapter 2).
   2. Encourage patient to maintain independence.
   3. Encourage patient to participate in care plan.
   4. Encourage high-caloric, high-vitamin, high-protein diet; provide nutrition that can be swallowed easily.
   5. Provide bowel and bladder training (may have indwelling catheter).
   6. Provide diversional activities.
   7. Provide safety measures.
   8. Allow time for patients to express concerns about disabilities and dependencies: be supportive.

9. Avoid precipitating factors that cause exacerbations (fatigue, cold, heat, infections, stress).

10. Provide patient and family education.

Parkinson's Disease

A. Definition: a progressive, degenerative disease causing destruction of nerve cells in the basal ganglia of the brain caused by a deficiency of dopamine; limbs become rigid, fingers have characteristic pill-rolling movement, and head has to-and-fro movement; the patient has a bent position and walks in short, shuffling steps; facial expression becomes blank, with wide eyes and infrequent blinking (Parkinson's mask); intelligence is not affected.

B. Cause: unknown

C. Signs and symptoms
1. Tremor
2. Voluntary movement is slow and difficult; coordination is poor (ataxia).
3. Impaired chewing and eating; excessive salivation and drooling occurs.
4. Speech is slow and patient is soft spoken; written communication is difficult.
5. Excessive sweating
6. Emotional changes: depression, paranoia, and eventually confusion
7. Dependency
8. Results of diagnostic tests
9. Side effects of drugs
10. Autonomic manifestations, such as urinary incontinence, constipation, hypotension

D. Diagnostic tests and methods
1. Patient history and physical assessment
2. Neurological assessment, CSF, CT scan

E. Treatment: many patients respond to drug therapy, and the disease is controlled with medication for the remainder of their lives; others have no response, and the disease progresses to a state of invalidism and immobility (usually treated with a combination of drugs) (see Chapter 3) ; surgeries (stereotaxic, fetal dopamine transplant, adrenal medullary transplant)

F. Nursing intervention
1. Encourage patient to maintain independence as much as possible in hygiene and dressing; include patient in planning all aspects of care as much as possible.
2. Encourage participation in previous work and social and diversional activities (avoid social withdrawal).
3. Help patient avoid embarrassment while eating; use straws, wipe drooling saliva, use bib, and keep clothing clean; use utensils with large handles for easy grip.
4. Recommend a soft diet or one of a consistency the patient is able to chew.
5. Provide diversion (activity therapy).
6. Encourage daily exercises as tolerated, especially walking; take safety measures.
7. Encourage patient to avoid fatigue.
8. Help patient to avoid frustration; emphasize capabilities rather than limitations.
9. Reinforce speech, physical, and occupational therapy treatment protocols.
10. Administer stool softeners to avoid constipation.
11. Provide bowel and bladder training.
12. Be patient when patient is slow or clumsy.

13. Establish a means of communication.
14. Enhance cognitive skills (reorient frequently).
15. Prevent pneumonia; force fluids; turn patient when in bed, and encourage patient to be out of bed as much as possible.
16. Provide mouth care every 4 hours.
17. Encourage family participation in all aspects of rehabilitation.

Amyotrophic Lateral Sclerosis (ALS)

A. Definition: also known as Lou Gehrig's disease, ALS is a degenerative disease that affects the upper or lower motor neurons of the brain, the spinal cord, or both.

B. Cause: unknown; a genetic link or a slow-moving viral infection is suspect.

C. Signs and symptoms
1. Fatigue, weight loss
2. Difficulty doing fine motor tasks (buttoning a shirt)
3. Progressive muscle weakness; muscle wasting; atrophy
4. Dysphagia (difficulty swallowing)
5. Dysarthria (difficult speech)
6. Tongue fasciculation (twitching)
7. Jaw clonus (involuntary tightening/relaxing of muscles)
8. Spasticity of flexor muscles
9. Respiratory difficulty
10. Involvement of upper or lower extremities; one side of body affected more than other (late in disease process)
11. No sensory loss; patient remains alert.
12. Death usually occurs 5 to 10 years from onset; caused by respiratory or bulbar paralysis

D. Diagnostic tests and methods: no specific test is available to diagnose ALS; an EMG may be done initially to rule out other neuromuscular diseases.

E. Treatment: symptomatic relief as disease progresses; surgery may be necessary to insert a gastrostomy tube during the latter stages of the disease.

F. Nursing intervention
1. Provide care to prevent complications of immobility.
2. Promote adequate nutrition; implement safety measures.
3. Provide adequate rest periods; instruct to avoid hot baths or traveling in hot weather.
4. Provide alternative means of communication.
5. Prevent bowel and bladder problems with adequate diet; provide medications to prevent urinary tract infections and constipation; bowel and bladder training programs may be necessary.
6. Promote skin integrity.
7. Assist in maintaining activities of daily living.
8. Assist in maintaining a clear airway; encourage use of a tucked chin position when eating or drinking; use of a suction machine; ventilator may be used for respiratory assist during latter stages of disease.
9. Provide patient and family education.
10. Facilitate coping and adjustment; be supportive, and allow patient and family to express their concerns; refer to local support group.

Spinal Cord Impairment

The vertebral column houses the spinal cord. A small cartilage disk acts as a cushion between the vertebrae. All sensory and motor nerves to the neck, trunk, and extremities branch out from the spinal cord. The degree of disability and patient problems is related to the part of the body controlled by the injured or diseased nerves. For herniated intervertebral disk, see musculoskeletal conditions.

Spinal Cord Lesion

A. Definition: a growth compressing the spinal cord; may be benign or malignant; interferes with nerve function
B. Cause: unknown
C. Signs and symptoms: individual, according to area involved
D. Diagnostic tests and methods
    1. Patient history
    2. Myelography (MEG), CT, MRI
    3. Neurological assessment
E. Treatment: surgical removal
F. Nursing intervention: see care of a patient with a laminectomy (p. 200).

Spinal Cord Injuries

A. Description: trauma to spinal cord may cause complete or partial severing of the spinal cord; if severing is complete, permanent paralysis of body parts below site of injury occurs; when partial damage occurs, edema may cause a temporary paralysis.
B. Cause: accident (e.g., automobile, shooting, diving)
C. Signs and symptoms: individual, according to level of spinal cord involved (signs of spinal shock)
    1. Respiratory distress
    2. Paralysis
D. Diagnostic tests and methods: physical examination
E. Treatment
    1. Immobilization: Crutchfield tongs, halo traction, back brace, or body cast
    2. Surgery, corticosteroids, mannitol
F. Nursing intervention
    1. See care of a patient with paralysis, pp. 252-253; observe for complications of spinal shock.
    2. Maintain airway and respiratory function.
    3. See emergency care of a patient with a spinal cord injury, Chapter 10.

ENDOCRINE SYSTEM

Anatomy and Physiology

A. Classification and secretions
    1. Exocrine glands: have ducts (tubes); secretions are carried to an external or internal surface of the body by ducts (e.g., lacrimal gland).
    2. Endocrine glands: ductless; secretions by glands (hormones) are carried to body tissue by blood and lymph.
B. Endocrine glands and hormones (Figure 5-13 and Table 5-6)
    1. Pituitary: located at base of the brain in a saddlelike depression of the sphenoid bone at the base of brain;

called the master gland, approximately the size of a grape; composed of two parts
    a. Anterior lobe: secretes many hormones
    b. Posterior lobe: secretes two hormones
  2. Thyroid: located in the neck inferior to the Adam's apple; easily palpated; the largest of the endocrine glands; consists of two lobes joined by a narrow band (isthmus)

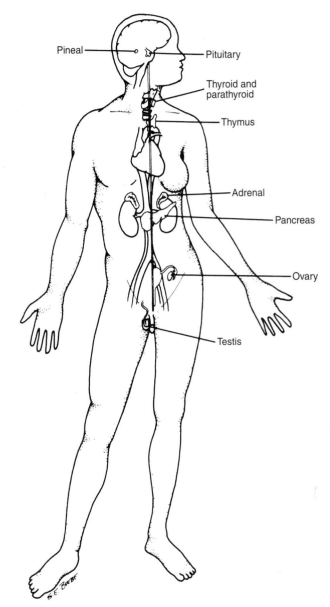

FIGURE 5-13 Endocrine system. (*From Phipps, Monahan, Sands, et al. Medical-Surgical Nursing health and illness perspectives, ed. 7, St. Louis, 2003, Mosby.*)

3. Parathyroid (four glands): located on posterior surface of the thyroid; regulates calcium level in the blood
4. Adrenal
   a. Two small glands; curve over the top of the kidneys
   b. Each gland has two separate parts: inner area (medulla) and outer area (cortex); produces different hormones
   c. Medulla: mimics the action of the sympathetic nervous system
   d. Cortex: outer part of the adrenals: produces three major groups of steroid hormones
5. Gonads (sex glands)
   a. Ovaries in woman: located in pelvic cavity; produce ova and two hormones, estrogen and progesterone; do not function until puberty
   b. Testes in man: suspended in a sac called the scrotum outside the pelvic cavity; produce sperm and sex hormone, testosterone
6. Islets of Langerhans: located within the pancreas; consist of alpha and beta cells
   a. Alpha cells: produce glucagon
   b. Beta cells: secrete hormone insulin
7. Pineal: lies just above midbrain; secretes melatonin, which inhibits gonadotropic hormone (GTH) secretion; exact function in humans is unclear.
C. Functions: regulators of body functions
   1. Growth and development
   2. Reproduction
   3. Metabolism
   4. Fluid and electrolyte balance

ENDOCRINE SYSTEM CONDITIONS AND DISORDERS

The endocrine system is composed of numerous glands and hormones. These hormones are chemical messengers for other target glands or cells. A disturbance in one of the secreting glands may affect the regulation of another gland; therefore the patient may experience multiple problems and have varying needs. Some of the hormonal disturbances may affect patient appearance, personality, and stamina. Part of the nursing intervention is aimed at providing support and education for the patient and the family. Some patients must undergo lifelong hormonal therapy as the result of the endocrine disorder that affects them.

Nursing Assessment

A. Nursing observations
   1. General appearance
   2. Vital signs
   3. Weight
   4. Skin
      a. Color
         (1) Pallor
         (2) Flushed
         (3) Yellow pigmentation
         (4) Bronze pigmentation
         (5) Purple striae over obese areas
      b. Temperature
      c. Dry
      d. Moist
      e. Excess diaphoresis
      f. Poor wound healing
   5. Hair
      a. Dry
      b. Brittle
      c. Thin
   6. Nails
      a. Dry
      b. Thin
      c. Thick
   7. Musculoskeletal
      a. Muscle mass distribution
      b. Fat distribution
      c. Change in height
      d. Changes in body proportions: enlarged ears, nose, jaws, hands, and feet
      e. Diminished muscle strength
   8. Central nervous system (CNS)
      a. Personality changes
      b. Alterations in consciousness
         (1) Listlessness
         (2) Slowed cognitive ability
         (3) Stupor
         (4) Seizures
         (5) Confusion
         (6) Coma
      c. Slowed, hoarse speech
      d. Reflexes
         (1) Trousseau's sign
         (2) Chvostek's sign
   9. Eyes
      a. Periorbital edema
      b. Protruding eyeball (exophthalmos)
      c. Drooping eyelids (ptosis)
   10. GI system
      a. Anorexia
      b. Polyphagia
      c. Polydipsia
      d. Constipation
      e. Diarrhea
      f. Nausea and vomiting
   11. Cardiovascular system
      a. Hypertension
      b. Hypotension
      c. Tachycardia
      d. Bradycardia
   12. Respiratory system
      a. Tachypnea
      b. Acetone breath
      c. Kussmaul's respirations
   13. Renal system
      a. Polyuria
      b. Oliguria
   14. Reproductive system
      a. Menstrual disturbances
      b. Libido disturbances

TABLE 5-6   Endocrine Glands, Hormones, and Actions

Endocrine Glands and Hormones	Actions of Hormones
Anterior Pituitary	
Corticotropin (andrenocorticotropic hormone [ACTH])	Stimulates the adrenal cortex to produce and secrete glucocorticoid hormones
Somatotropic hormone (STH)	Stimulates growth of body cells
Thyroid-stimulating hormone (TSH)	Stimulates the thyroid gland to produce and release thyroid hormone

Gonadotropic hormones (GTH)
   Luteinizing hormone (LH)
   Follicle-stimulating hormone (FSH)
   Lactogenic hormone (prolactin)
	Affect growth, maturity, and function of primary and secondary sex organs

Posterior Pituitary	
Antidiuretic hormone (ADH)	Promotes sodium and water retention in the kidney; increases blood pressure
Oxytocin	Initiates and maintains labor; influences the breasts to release milk
Thyroid	
Thyroxine	Regulates the metabolic rate of all body cells
Pancreas	
Insulin	Promotes glucose use by the cell and decreases blood sugar level
Glucagon	Promotes glucose release from the liver and increases blood sugar level
Adrenal Cortex	
Glucocorticoids (includes cortisol and cortisone)	Assist the body to respond to stress; concerned with carbohydrate, fat, protein metabolism; reduces inflammation
Mineralocorticoids (includes aldosterone)	Promote sodium and water retention in the kidney and potassium excretion
Sex hormones (androgens, estrogen, and progesterone)	Mainly affect development of secondary sex characteristics
Adrenal Medulla	
Epinephrine (adrenaline) and norepinephrine (noradrenaline)	Constrict blood vessels and channel the blood to vital internal organs to prepare the body for emergency situation
Ovaries	
Estrogen	Promotes development of female sex characteristics, growth of female sex organs, and development of the uterine wall for implantation of the fertilized ovum; regulates menstruation
Progesterone	Prepares the uterine wall for implantation of the fertilized ovum; maintains the placenta and pregnancy; regulates menstruation
Testes	
Androgens (includes testosterone)	Stimulates development of the secondary male sex characteristics; essential for normal functioning of male sex organs

c. Galactorrhea (excess mammary gland secretion in women)

d. Gynecomastia (increased breast tissue in men)

B. Patient description (subjective data)

  1. Pain

    a. Headache

    b. Skeletal pain

    c. Back pain

    d. Muscle spasms

  2. Appetite

    a. Anorexia

    b. Polyphagia

  3. Weakness

  4. Numbness

  5. Tingling

  6. Mood swings

  7. Nausea

  8. Intolerance to heat or cold

  9. Polydipsia

  10. Polyuria, nocturia, and dysuria

  11. Decreased libido and impotence

  12. Frequent infections

Diagnostic Tests and Methods

A. Serum laboratory studies

  1. Protein-bound iodine (PBI)

    a. The thyroid hormone, thyroxine, contains iodine that binds itself to blood proteins; therefore the function of the thyroid gland is evaluated by measuring the amount of this iodine.

    b. Factors that may alter test findings

      (1) Ingestion of drugs or administration of dyes containing iodine

      (2) Mercurial diuretics or estrogen

      (3) Pregnancy

  2. Iodine 131 uptake (radioactive iodine thyroid uptake)

    a. Measures the amount of radioactive iodine that has concentrated in the thyroid gland after ingestion of the iodine preparation

    b. Test findings may be altered by recent ingestion of iodides or use of radiographic dyes.

    c. A normal thyroid gland removes 15% to 50% of iodine from the bloodstream.

  3. Basal metabolic rate (BMR): measures the amount of oxygen consumed by the body while the patient is in a state of complete mental and physical rest

  4. Triiodothyronine (T3): measures thyroid function indirectly by evaluating whether radioactive triiodothyronine binds to a serum specimen

  5. Thyroxine (T4): measures the amount of thyroxine in the circulation

  6. Thyroid-stimulating hormone (TSH) radioimmunoassay: indicator of TSH production based on pituitary function; measures TSH levels

  7. Fasting blood sugar (FBS)

    a. Measures the amount of glucose in the bloodstream during a fasting period

    b. No food is permitted for 12 hours before the test.

    c. Normal value: 80 to 120 mg/dl

  8. Postprandial blood sugar

    a. Evaluates the patient's ability to dispose of blood glucose after a meal

    b. Normal value: 80 to 120 mg/dl serum

  9. Glucose tolerance test (GTT)

    a. Determines patient response to a measured dose of glucose

    b. Normal value: blood glucose climbs to a peak of 140 mg/dl serum in the first hour and returns to normal by the second or third hour.

  10. Glycosylated hemoglobin

    a. Determines patient's control of blood glucose over a 3-month period

    b. Normal value for a person without diabetes is 5% to 7 %; patients with diabetes mellitus have ranges from 7% to 9% or more.

  11. Serum potassium

    a. Measures the amount of potassium in the bloodstream

    b. Normal range: 3.5 to 5.5 mEq/L

  12. Serum sodium

    a. Measures the amount of sodium in the bloodstream

    b. Normal range: 135 to 145 mEq/L

  13. Total serum calcium

    a. Measures the amount of calcium in the bloodstream

    b. Normal range: 4.8 to 5.2 mEq/L (9 to 11 mg/dl)

  14. Serum ketones: determines the amount of ketones produced by the metabolism of fat

  15. Blood pH

    a. Measures the acid-base status of the blood

    b. Normal arterial blood findings: pH 7.35 to 7.45

    c. Normal venous blood findings: pH 7.31 to 7.41

  16. Serum phosphorus: measures the amount of serum phosphorus in the bloodstream

  17. Adrenocorticotropic hormone (ACTH) stimulating test (or glucocorticoid-stimulating test)

    a. Evaluates the changes in adrenocortical function produced by the administration of ACTH

    b. ACTH is administered intramuscularly (IM) or IV.

    c. For the IM methods, a blood specimen is obtained 1 hour after administering ACTH.

    d. For the IV method, a 24-hour urine specimen is collected and analyzed.

  18. Cortisone suppression test: used to differentiate between Cushing's syndrome and Cushing's disease

  19. Plasma cortisol

    a. Hormonal study of the adrenal cortex

    b. Low levels are seen in Addison's disease.

    c. Elevated levels indicate Cushing's syndrome.

  20. Plasma cortisol response to ACTH

    a. Hormonal study of the adrenal cortex

    b. Patient's blood specimen is drawn in a fasting state and examined for plasma cortisol levels.

    c. Next, ACTH is administered IM, and a second blood sample is withdrawn.

    d. Rise in the plasma cortisol level in the second specimen is normal.

  21. Urine 17-ketogenic steroids

    a. Measures adrenocortical function

    b. Urine specimen is collected for a 24-hour period and should be kept cold.

B. Urine laboratory studies

  1. 24-hour quantitative sugar specimen

    a. Evaluation of the patient's glucose loss over a 24-hour period

    b. The urine is normally free of sugar.

c. Nursing intervention
  (1) Have the patient void, and discard the specimen at the beginning of the 24-hour period.
  (2) Save all urine voided in a container provided by the laboratory.
  (3) At the end of the 24 hours, have the patient void again, and save the specimen in the container.
2. Urine pH
  a. Measures the acid-base balance of the urine
  b. Normal range: pH 4.8 to 7.5
3. Quantitative urinary calcium: measures the amount of calcium in a 24-hour urine specimen after a period of calcium deprivation
4. Vanillylmandelic acid (VMA) test
  a. Determines the amount of urinary excretion of the end product of catecholamine metabolism
  b. Factors that may alter test findings
    (1) Ingestion of coffee, tea, chocolate, bananas, vanilla-containing food, or aspirin
    (2) Stress
C. Scans
  1. Thyroid scan: radionucleotide study of the thyroid to determine function
  2. CT scan: used to visualize cross sections of tissue

Frequent Patient Problems and Nursing Care

A. Risk for situational low self-esteem related to changes in appearance from fluctuating hormones
  1. Observe the patient for loss of appetite, insomnia, disinterest in self, and unwillingness to discuss alteration in body image.
  2. Encourage patient to express feelings.
  3. Encourage communication with significant other.
B. Imbalanced nutrition, less than body requirements, related to noncompliance with therapeutic diet
  1. Observe the patient for diet intolerance such as refusal to eat, complaints of foods, and eating of foods that are contraindicated.
  2. Explain to the patient and family the reason for and intended effect of therapeutic diet and necessity of maintaining it until discontinued by physician.
  3. Instruct the patient and family on prescribed food selection.
C. Deficient knowledge related to prescribed medication
  1. Explain to the patient and family the dosage and method of administering prescribed drugs.
  2. Provide information about the purpose of the drug and potential side effects.
  3. Describe symptoms that should be reported to the physician.
  4. Explain where therapeutic supplies may be obtained.
  5. Evaluate the patient's response to teaching.
D. High risk for injury related to toxic effects of iodine preparations; discontinue iodides if evidence of the following exists:
  1. Swelling of buccal mucosa
  2. Excessive salivation
  3. Swelling of neck glands
  4. Skin eruptions
E. High risk for injury related to hypoglycemia
  1. Observe for complaints of headache, nervousness, hunger, dizziness, pallor, and sweating (diaphoresis).
  2. Assess vital signs.

3. Give quick-acting carbohydrate.
  a. Orange juice
  b. Cola
  c. Granulated sugar
  d. Crackers
  e. Hard candy
4. If patient is unconscious: give instant glucose (buccally); glucagon (subcutaneously [SC]); IV glucose
5. Have laboratory withdraw serum specimen for glucose assessment.
6. Assess reason for reaction after situation has been controlled.
  a. Length of time since last meal
  b. Correct amount of food eaten or meal omitted
  c. Correct dosage of insulin
  d. Kinds of activities or situation before reaction
F. High risk for injury (seizures) related to hypocalcemia
  1. Observe for complaints of numbness, tingling, cramping, or spastic movements of extremities.
  2. Emergency treatment requires administration of IV calcium.
  3. Prevent airway obstruction.
    a. Keep airway (seizure stick) at bedside.
    b. Provide suction machine at bedside.
    c. Provide tracheostomy set at bedside.
  4. Prevent injury by putting padding along side rails, easing patient to floor, or removing constrictive clothes.
  5. Monitor and record vital signs.
  6. Note frequency, time, level of consciousness, and length of seizure.

Major Medical Diagnoses
Hyperpituitarism

A. Definition: overproduction of growth hormone by the anterior pituitary gland
B. Pathology
  1. Increased activity of the gland usually results from a secreting pituitary tumor.
  2. Two major disorders arise from hypersecretion.
    a. Gigantism: develops in children; hypersecretion before the growth plate closes, results in bone and tissue growth
    b. Acromegaly: a disorder in adults caused by hypersecretion after closure of the epiphyses of the long bones
C. Signs and symptoms
  1. Subjective
    a. Headache
    b. Visual disturbances
    c. Weakness
  2. Objective
    a. Coarse facial features: enlarged ears, nose, lips, tongue, and jaws
    b. Broad hands, fingers, and feet
    c. Palpable, enlarged visceral organs
    d. Disturbances in carbohydrate metabolism, menstruation, and libido
    e. Gynecomastia in men; galactorrhea in women
    f. Symmetrical bone overgrowth (gigantism)
    g. Increased heights; 8 to 9 ft (gigantism)
D. Diagnostic tests and methods
  1. X-ray studies of jaws, sinuses, hands, and feet
  2. Changes in physical appearance

3. CT scan to identify tumor
4. Cerebral arteriography to identify tumor
5. Growth hormone assay
E. Treatment
  1. Surgical intervention: hypophysectomy (excision of the pituitary gland); excision of tumor with laser
  2. Irradiation of the pituitary gland
  3. Medication to treat symptoms related to other hormonal disturbances as a result of hypersecretion
F. Nursing intervention
  1. Assist the patient to accept altered body image emphasizing person's value as an individual.
  2. Explain the basis for altered sexual functioning.
  3. Emphasize need for lifelong medical follow-up.
  4. If the patient has undergone hypophysectomy:
    a. Follow nursing care as for the patient who has undergone intracranial surgery.
    b. Observe for potential postoperative complications.
      (1) Adrenal insufficiency
      (2) Hypothyroidism
      (3) Diabetes insipidus

Hypopituitarism (Simmonds' Disease)

A. Definition: total absence of all pituitary secretions
B. Pathology: occurs after destruction of the pituitary gland by surgery, infection, injury, hemorrhage, or tumor
C. Signs and symptoms
  1. Subjective
    a. Lethargy
    b. Loss of muscle strength
    c. Weakness
    d. Menstrual irregularities
  2. Objective
    a. Emaciation
    b. Pallor
    c. Dry, yellow skin
    d. Diminished axillary and pubic hair
    e. Decreased muscle size
    f. Increased susceptibility to infection
D. Diagnostic tests and methods
  1. T3 and T4
  2. Urine 17-ketogenic steroids
E. Treatment
  1. Replacement hormones
  2. Surgical ablation if tumor is present in pituitary gland
F. Nursing intervention
  1. Emphasize need for lifelong medical follow-up.
  2. Teach the patient self-administration of drug: purpose, proper dosage, and potential side effects.
  3. Follow nursing care as for the patient who has undergone intracranial surgery.

Hyperthyroidism (Graves' Disease and Thyrotoxicosis)

A. Definition: overactivity of the thyroid gland with hypersecretion of T4
B. Pathology
  1. Metabolic rate is increased, resulting in a high amount of energy and oxygen expenditure
  2. May be caused by decreased production of TSH by malfunctioning pituitary gland, which results in high T4 serum concentration

3. May be attributed to enlarged thyroid gland caused by decreased iodine intake
C. Signs and symptoms
  1. Subjective
    a. Polyphagia
    b. Hyperexcitability, personality changes
    c. Heat intolerance
    d. Insomnia
    e. Amenorrhea
    f. Diarrhea, constipation
    g. Increased appetite
    h. Fatigue, weakness
  2. Objective
    a. Weight loss
    b. Exophthalmos
    c. Excessive sweating
    d. Increased pulse rate
    e. Fine hand tremors
    f. Warm, flushed skin
    g. Elevated blood pressure
    h. Bruit over thyroid
D. Diagnostic tests: increased laboratory values of T3, T4, 131I uptake, PBI, and BMR confirm hyperthyroidism; thyroid scan
E. Treatment
  1. Medication to inhibit T4 production
  2. Radioactive iodine to destroy thyroid gland cells to decrease T4 secretion
  3. Drugs to control tachycardia and hyperexcitability
  4. Subtotal or total thyroidectomy
F. Nursing intervention
  1. Teach the patient and family signs and symptoms of hypothyroidism when patient is receiving thyroid-inhibiting drugs.
    a. Increased body weight
    b. Sensitivity to cold
    c. Fatigue
    d. Dry skin, hair, and nails
    e. Slow, hoarse speech
    f. Constipation
  2. Encourage adequate nutrition for increased energy expenditure.
    a. High-calorie, high-vitamin, and high-carbohydrate intake
    b. Between-meal snacks
    c. Increased fluid intake
    d. Avoidance of caffeine
  3. Plan undisturbed rest periods to restore energy; provide cool, quiet, nonstressful environment.
  4. Advise the patient to elevate the head of bed while recumbent to improve eye drainage.
  5. If the patient has undergone surgery:
    a. Place patient on back in a low-Fowler's or semi-Fowler's position to avoid strain on sutures.
    b. Observe dressing for hemorrhage or constriction of the throat; examine back of neck for pooling of blood.
    c. Keep tracheostomy set at bedside in event of respiratory obstruction caused by hemorrhage, edema of glottis, laryngeal nerve damage, or tetany.
    d. Encourage patient to cough and expectorate secretions from throat and bronchi.

e. Observe for signs of thyroid storm (may occur as a result of gland manipulation during surgery): fever, tachycardia, and restlessness.

f. Observe for signs of tetany (may occur if parathyroids are accidentally removed): numbness and tingling around mouth, carpopedal spasms, and convulsions.

Hypothyroidism

A. Definition: absence or decreased production of T4 by the thyroid gland

B. Pathology
  1. The disorder causes a depression of metabolic activity, resulting in physical and mental sluggishness.
  2. Three classifications of hypothyroidism
    a. Cretinism: total absence of T4 from birth
    b. Hypothyroidism without myxedema: mild thyroid failure in older children and adults
    c. Hypothyroidism with myxedema: a severe form of gland failure in adults

C. Signs and symptoms
  1. Subjective
    a. Lethargy
    b. Fatigues easily
    c. Cold intolerance
    d. Constipation
  2. Objective
    a. Increased body weight with loss of appetite
    b. Coarse facial features
    c. Slow, hoarse speech
    d. Dry skin, hair, and nails
    e. Bradycardia
    f. Impaired memory
    g. Slowed thought process
    h. Personality changes

D. Diagnostic tests: decreased laboratory values of T3, T4, 131I uptake, PBI, and BMR confirm hypothyroidism; thyroid scan

E. Treatment: thyroid-replacement drugs

F. Nursing intervention
  1. Educate the patient on self-administration of drug: purpose, proper dosage, and potential side effects.
  2. Emphasize need for lifelong medical follow-up.
  3. Teach the patient and family signs and symptoms of hyperthyroidism when receiving thyroid-replacement drugs: chest pain, tachycardia, nervousness, headache, excessive sweating, heat intolerance, and weight loss.
  4. Encourage decreased caloric intake to avoid weight gain.
  5. Encourage application of emollients to soothe dry skin.

Hyperparathyroidism

A. Definition: oversecretion of parathormone by one or more parathyroid glands

B. Pathology
  1. Results in calcium loss from the bones and an increased secretion of calcium and phosphorus by the kidneys
  2. Usually the result of a parathyroid tumor

C. Signs and symptoms
  1. Subjective
    a. Fatigue
    b. Thirst; poor appetite
    c. Nausea
    d. Back pain
    e. Skeletal pain
    f. Pain on weight bearing
    g. Constipation
    h. Visual disturbances
  2. Objective
    a. Pathological fractures
    b. Vomiting
    c. Kidney stones composed of calcium phosphate

D. Diagnostic tests
  1. Quantitative urinary calcium
  2. Total serum calcium
  3. Serum phosphorus
  4. X-ray film to reveal skeletal changes

E. Treatment: surgical resection of parathyroid gland

F. Nursing intervention
  1. Observe for postoperative conditions (refer to postoperative nursing intervention under diseases of the thyroid gland: hyperthyroidism).
  2. Observe for tetany: tingling of hands and feet, facial muscle spasms, and muscle twitching.
  3. Protect from accidents: position carefully, keep bed low, keep side rails up, and assist to ambulate.
  4. Explain rationale for low-calcium, low-phosphorus diet.
  5. Encourage adequate hydration and dietary fiber to avoid constipation.

Hypoparathyroidism

A. Definition: undersecretion of parathormone by the parathyroid glands

B. Pathology
  1. Insufficiency of parathormone causes a decrease of the serum calcium level and slows bone resorption
  2. Increased serum phosphorus value
  3. Increased neuromuscular irritability that results in tetany

C. Signs and symptoms
  1. Subjective
    a. Lethargy
    b. Painful muscle spasms
    c. Tingling of hands and feet
    d. Visual disturbances
  2. Objective
    a. Dry skin, hair, and nails
    b. Respiratory distress caused by laryngeal spasms
    c. Convulsions

D. Diagnostic tests and methods
  1. Quantitative urinary calcium
  2. Total serum calcium
  3. Positive Trousseau's sign (spasms of fingers and hands after application of blood pressure cuff to arm)
  4. Presence of Chvostek's sign (hyperactivity of facial muscle in response to tapping near the angle of the jaw)
  5. X-ray studies reveal increased bone density

E. Treatment
  1. Calcium replacement in chronic cases
  2. Calcium gluconate IV for emergency treatment
  3. Diet high in calcium and low in phosphorus
  4. Vitamin-D preparation

F. Nursing intervention
  1. Keep endotracheal tube and tracheostomy set at bedside at all times when caring for patients with acute tetany.

2. Promote rest with a quiet, calm, and low-lit environment.

3. Explain need for diet high in calcium but low in phosphorus: encourage avoidance of milk, cheese, and egg yolks.

4. Emphasize importance of lifelong medical follow-up; serum calcium level should be assessed at least three times a year.

Diabetes Mellitus

A. Definition: insufficiency or absence of insulin production by pancreatic islets, creating a disturbance in carbohydrate metabolism, as well as a deficiency in protein and fat conversion

B. Pathology

  1. Develops when a persistent deficiency of insulin occurs

  2. May be caused by trauma, infection, or tumor of the pancreas or increased insulin requirements attributable to obesity, pregnancy, infection, or stress

  3. Persons at risk: women over 40 years of age and individuals who are obese or who have a familial tendency to diabetes

  4. Two classifications

    a. Type 1: insulin-dependent diabetes mellitus (IDDM) (formerly juvenile diabetes): rapid onset, with no production of insulin; affects children and adolescents; is controlled with insulin

    b. Type 2: non–insulin-dependent diabetes mellitus (NIDDM) (formerly adult onset): gradual onset; may be controlled by diet, oral hypoglycemic drugs, or insulin injection

  5. Lack of insulin disrupts transportation of glucose into cells, and cells become energy exhausted; cells must use proteins and fats as a compensatory mechanism.

  6. Blood sugar level becomes elevated because of lack of insulin in the cells.

  7. Cellular dehydration occurs because blood sugar pulls water from the cells into the bloodstream.

  8. Glucose builds up in urine, creating osmotic pull; kidneys cannot reabsorb water.

C. Signs and symptoms

  1. Subjective

    a. Polyuria and nocturia

    b. Polydipsia

    c. Polyphasia

    d. Weakness

    e. Blurred vision

  2. Objective

    a. Hyperglycemia

    b. Glycosuria

    c. Polyuria

    d. Ketosis

    e. Weight loss

    f. Retarded wound healing

D. Diagnostic tests and methods

  1. Presence of polyuria, polydipsia, and polyphagia

  2. Family and medical history

  3. Laboratory studies: FBS, postprandial blood sugar, GTT, and glycosylated hemoglobin

  4. 24-hour urine quantitative sugar specimen

E. Treatment

  1. Drug therapy for hyperglycemia; refer to Chapter 3 for indicated nursing actions.

  2. Therapeutic diet with controlled calories to correct and avoid obesity

    a. American Diabetes Association (ADA) food exchange list; widely prescribed by physicians

    b. Identifies calorie intake of protein (15% to 20%), carbohydrates (50% to 60%), fats (no more than 30%)

F. Nursing intervention

  1. Assist patient in adjusting to condition: allow verbalization of feelings, offer reassurance, and give support at patient's own pace.

  2. Emphasize need to comply with diet and eat meals at prescribed times.

  3. Instruct the patient and family on signs of impending hypoglycemia: diaphoresis, pale, cold, and clammy skin, nervousness, hunger, mental confusion; give orange juice, sugar, or hard candy.

  4. Encourage prompt treatment of minor injuries or irritation to skin.

  5. Emphasize importance of continued medical follow-up, regular vision examinations, and foot care.

  6. Patient teaching should include:

    a. Self–blood-glucose-level monitoring

    b. Self-injection of insulin: selection of equipment, sites of injection, rationale for rotation, accurate withdrawal of insulin, injection technique, and peak action time of insulin

    c. How to use food substitution

    d. Instructions on foot care: hygiene, proper trimming of toenails, proper fit of shoes and stockings, and treatment of minor abrasions

    e. Relationship between exercise and blood glucose

  7. Instruct the patient and family on signs and symptoms of impending ketoacidosis: hot, dry, flushed skin, polydipsia, fruity odor of breath, nausea, and abdominal pain.

  8. Administer insulin by way of pump.

    a. Method of needle insertion and filling of syringe

    b. Instruction on site rotation and needle change every 4 to 8 hours

    c. Removal of pump and covering needle and tubing for bathing

Diabetic Coma (Ketoacidosis)

A. Definition: excess glucose and acid (ketones) in the bloodstream

B. Pathology

  1. A response to insufficient insulin levels primarily seen in type 1 diabetes mellitus

  2. Fats are mobilized for energy; fatty acids are rejected by muscles, resulting in buildup of acids in the bloodstream.

  3. Body's buffer system becomes exhausted.

C. Signs and symptoms

  1. Subjective

    a. Weakness

    b. Polydipsia

    c. Abdominal pain

    d. Nausea

    e. Headache

    f. Polyphagia

  2. Objective

    a. Hot, dry, flushed skin

    b. Listlessness and drowsiness

c. Kussmaul's respirations
d. Sweet or acetone breath
e. Hypotension
f. Confusion
g. Polyuria
h. Nausea and vomiting
i. Coma

D. Diagnostic tests
1. Elevated serum glucose level
2. Elevated serum and urinary ketones
3. Lowered blood pH

E. Treatment
1. Insulin replacement
2. Correcting electrolyte and pH imbalance
3. Fluid replacement

F. Nursing intervention
1. Give insulin as ordered; have another person check to prevent error.
2. Monitor and record vital signs and intake and output.
3. Test for glucose and acetone levels; record on diabetic flow sheet.
4. Position patient with head of bed elevated 30 degrees.
5. Maintain patent airway.
6. Give oral care every 4 hours and prn; keep lips and mouth moist.
7. Assess LOC.
8. Observe patient for signs of hypoglycemia: pale, cool, clammy skin, lethargy, and hypotension.
9. Instruct the patient and family on factors and signs of impending ketoacidosis.
10. Explain the importance of balance among diet, exercise, and insulin.
11. Before discharge, provide diabetic alert band or chain.

Hyperglycemic Hyperosmolar Nonketotic Coma (HHNC)

A. Definition: similar to ketoacidosis but occurs primarily in type 2 diabetes mellitus (NIDDM); ketosis does not develop.
B. Pathology: high serum glucose levels increase osmotic pressure, leading to polyuria; dehydration occurs at the cellular level.
C. Signs and symptoms
1. Subjective
a. Polyuria
b. Polydipsia
c. Drowsiness
d. Confusion
2. Objective
a. Dry, hot skin
b. Flushed skin
c. Hyperglycemia
d. Glycosuria
e. Hypotension
D. Diagnostic tests (see ketoacidosis)
E. Treatment (see ketoacidosis)
F. Nursing intervention (see ketoacidosis)

Hypoglycemia (Insulin Shock)

A. Definition: abnormally low level of glucose in the bloodstream
B. Pathology

1. Accelerated glucose is removed from the serum.
2. May be caused by overproduction or overdosage of insulin
3. Omission of a meal or too little food eaten by a patient receiving insulin
4. Too much exercise without extra food; rapid onset

C. Signs and symptoms
1. Subjective
a. Hunger
b. Weakness
c. Visual disturbances
d. Tingling lips and tongue
e. Nervousness
2. Objective
a. Pale, moist skin
b. Tremors
c. Tachycardia
d. Hypotension
e. Muscle weakness
f. Disorientation
g. Coma

D. Diagnostic test: lowered serum glucose level

E. Treatment
1. Sweetened fluids or sugar given orally; oral glucose preparations
2. Glucagon SC or IM
3. Glucose IV

F. Nursing intervention
1. Give medications as ordered.
2. Monitor and record vital signs and intake and output.
3. Patient teaching should include the following:
a. Always carry and ingest quick-acting carbohydrate when initial signs appear; fruit juices, sweetened sodas, granulated sugar, or hard candy.
b. Prevent medication error by having another person check dosage.
c. Record each administration of medication to avoid duplication.
d. Always wear medical identification tag.
e. Remember to eat a regular meal after raising glucose level to prevent a rebound effect.

Diabetes Insipidus

A. Definition: water metabolism disorder related to hyposecretion of antidiuretic hormone (ADH) by the posterior pituitary lobe
B. Pathology
1. Renal tubules are unable to reabsorb water, resulting in elimination of large amounts of water.
2. Hyposecretion may occur in conjunction with lung cancer, head injuries, pituitary tumor, myxedema, or encephalitis.
3. Other causes may result from malfunctioning, surgical removal, or atrophy of the pituitary gland.
C. Signs and symptoms
1. Subjective
a. Polydipsia
b. Polyuria
2. Objective
a. Signs of dehydration (loss of skin turgor, dry skin and mucous membranes, and cracked lips)
b. Low specific gravity (sp gr) (1.001 to 1.006)

c. Increased fluid intake (5 to 40 L/24 hr)

d. Increased urine output (5 to 25 L/24 hr)

e. Electrolyte imbalance

D. Diagnostic method: restriction of fluid intake to observe changes in urine volume and concentration

E. Treatment: vasopressin replacement

F. Nursing intervention

1. Monitor and record intake and output.

2. Monitor specific gravity

3. Weigh patient daily

Primary Hyperaldosteronism (Conn's Syndrome)

A. Definition: hypersecretion of aldosterone by the adrenal cortex

B. Pathology

1. Usually caused by a tumor or tumors, which results in renal retention of sodium and excretion of potassium

2. Leads to inability of kidneys to concentrate urine (acidify)

C. Signs and symptoms

1. Subjective

a. Headache

b. Polyuria and polydipsia

c. Paresthesia

2. Objective

a. Hypertension with postural hypotension

b. Signs of kidney damage: flank pain, chills, fever, and increased frequency of voiding

c. Low specific gravity

D. Diagnostic tests

1. Low serum potassium level

2. Elevated serum sodium value

3. Elevated urinary aldosterone level

4. Increased urine pH

5. X-ray study reveals cardiac hypertrophy caused by chronic hypertension.

E. Treatment: surgical removal of adrenal tumor

F. Nursing intervention

1. Monitor and record blood pressure, specific gravity, and intake and output.

2. Identify and explain diet high in potassium and low in sodium.

3. Provide fluids to meet excessive thirst.

4. If the patient has undergone adrenalectomy:

a. Protect the patient from exposure to infections.

b. Follow general postoperative nursing actions.

5. Once patient is convalescent, teach the patient self-administration of drugs: purpose, proper dosage, and potential side effects.

6. Before discharge, obtain medical identification tag.

Cushing's Syndrome

A. Definition: hyperactivity of the adrenal cortex

B. Pathology

1. Excessive cortisol is secreted.

2. Disorder results from abnormal growth of cortices or tumor to one of the glands.

3. May occur because of pituitary gland dysfunction, causing excessive production of ACTH

C. Signs and symptoms

1. Subjective

a. Weakness

b. Bruises easily

c. Amenorrhea

d. Decreased libido

e. Changes in secondary sex characteristics

2. Objective

a. Fat deposits to face, back of neck, and abdomen

b. Decreased muscle mass on limbs

c. Unusual growth of body hair

d. Purple striae over obese areas

e. Impaired wound healing

f. Hypertension

g. Mood lability

D. Diagnostic tests

1. Increased plasma cortisol levels

2. ACTH stimulating test

3. Cortisone suppression test

E. Treatment

1. Drugs to inhibit cortisol production

2. Bilateral adrenalectomy

3. Resection of pituitary gland

4. Potassium supplements

5. Diet with sodium restriction

F. Nursing intervention

1. Assist patient in adjusting to altered body image.

2. Place in noninfectious environment.

3. Maintain diet low in calories, carbohydrates, and sodium and high in potassium.

4. Weigh patient daily.

5. Monitor glucose and acetone levels.

6. Follow general postoperative nursing actions if patient undergoes adrenalectomy.

7. Once the patient is convalescent, instruct on self-administration of replacement hormones and drugs: proper dosage, purpose, and potential side effects.

Addison's Disease

A. Definition: hypofunction of adrenal cortex

B. Pathology

1. As a result of dysfunction, adrenal cortex shrinks and atrophies.

2. Disorder usually originates within itself or may result from destruction of the adrenal cortex.

3. Results in disturbances of sodium and potassium

C. Signs and symptoms

1. Subjective

a. Weakness and fatigue

b. Anorexia and nausea

c. Depression

d. Diarrhea

e. Abdominal pain

2. Objective

a. Weight loss

b. Hypotension

c. Hypoglycemia

d. Bronze or tan skin pigmentation

e. Susceptibility to infection

f. Dysrhythmias

D. Diagnostic tests

1. 8-hour IV ACTH test

2. Plasma cortisol response to ACTH

3. Low serum sodium level

4. High serum potassium level

E. Treatment
1. Replacement of adrenal cortex hormones
2. Restoring sodium and potassium balance
3. Diet high in sodium and low in potassium, with adequate fluids
F. Nursing intervention
1. Monitor and record vital signs and intake and output.
2. Weigh patient daily.
3. Observe for sodium imbalance: increased body weight, pitting edema, puffy eyelids, coughing, and diaphoresis.
4. Observe for potassium imbalance: lethargy, flaccid muscles, anorexia, hypotension, and dysrhythmias.
5. Provide small, frequent feedings.
6. Observe for hypoglycemia: weakness, clammy skin, tremors, and mental confusion.
7. Before discharge, obtain medical identification tag.
8. Emphasize need for compliance to diet and medication regimen.
9. Observe for addisonian crisis (causes: stress, surgery, trauma, infection, withdrawal of medication): hypotension, asthenia, abdominal pain, confusion, shock, and vascular collapse.
10. Teach patient to avoid infections and stressful situations.

Pheochromocytoma

A. Definition: hyperactivity of the adrenal medulla
B. Pathology: caused by tumor in adrenal medulla, resulting in increased secretion of epinephrine and norepinephrine
C. Signs and symptoms
1. Subjective
a. Headache
b. Visual disturbances
c. Nervousness
d. Heat intolerance
2. Objective
a. Hypertension (blood pressure may be as high as 220/140 mm Hg)
b. Orthostatic hypotension
c. Tachycardia
d. Hyperglycemia
e. Blanching of skin
f. Weight loss
g. Dysrhythmias
h. Diaphoresis
D. Diagnostic tests
1. Chemical and pharmacological drug tests to differentiate from hypertension or hyperthyroidism
2. X-ray studies to reveal adrenal medullary tumor
3. 24-hour urine collection for VMA and metanephrines
4. Arteriography
5. CT scan
6. Intravenous pyelogram (IVP)
E. Treatment
1. Surgical excision of tumor
2. Drugs to control hypertension and dysrhythmias
F. Nursing intervention
1. Monitor blood pressure every 4 hours and record.
2. Plan undisturbed rest periods: cool, quiet, nonstressful environment.
3. Encourage adequate hydration; record intake and output.
4. If patient undergoes adrenalectomy, follow general postoperative nursing actions: observe for adrenal

crisis—falling blood pressure, tachycardia, elevated temperature, restlessness, convulsions, and coma.
5. Patient teaching should include:
a. Self-administration of medications: purpose, proper dosage, and potential side effects
b. Signs of impending adrenal crisis
c. Avoidance of exposure to infection; report symptoms of infections to physician.
d. Avoidance of stressful situations
e. Emphasis on the need for adequate rest and good nutrition
6. Provide medical identification tag.

RENAL (URINARY) SYSTEM

Anatomy and Physiology

A. Organs (Figures 5-14 and 5-15)
1. Kidneys: bean shaped and reddish brown; lie against posterior abdominal wall; right kidney is slightly lower than the left.
a. External structure
(1) Hilus: concave notch; blood vessels, nerves, lymphatic vessels, and ureters enter the kidneys at this point.
(2) Renal capsule; protective fibrous tissue surrounding kidneys
b. Internal structure
(1) Cortex: outer portion; the greater portion of the nephron is located here.
(2) Medulla: inner portion; consists of 12 cone-shaped structures (pyramids); tip of pyramid points toward renal pelvis and drains waste and excess water into pelvis.
(3) Pelvis: funnel shaped; forms upper end of ureter and receives waste and water
c. Nephron: basic unit of function; microscopic structure composed of capillaries; approximately 1 million per kidney; control the processes of filtration, reabsorption, and secretion (Figure 5-16)
(1) Glomerulus: filtering unit; process of urine formation begins here.
(2) Renal tubules: reabsorption occurs in the proximal convoluted tubules, through Henle's loops, and the distal convoluted tubules; the collecting tubules then pass the final urine product into the pelvis.
2. Ureters: two long, narrow tubes; transport urine from kidney to bladder by peristalsis
3. Bladder: elastic, muscular organ, capable of expansion; stores urine; assists in voiding (micturition: the release of urine or voiding)
4. Urethra: narrow, short tube from bladder to exterior; exterior opening called the meatus
a. In women: approximately 1 1/4 to 2 inches (3 to 5 cm) long; transports urine
b. In men: approximately 8 inches (20 cm) long; transports urine and is a passageway for semen
B. Functions
1. Excretion: nitrogen-containing waste (urea, uric acid, and creatinine) is excreted; normal daily output is 1200 to 1500 ml; primary function is to regulate the volume and composition of extracellular fluid.

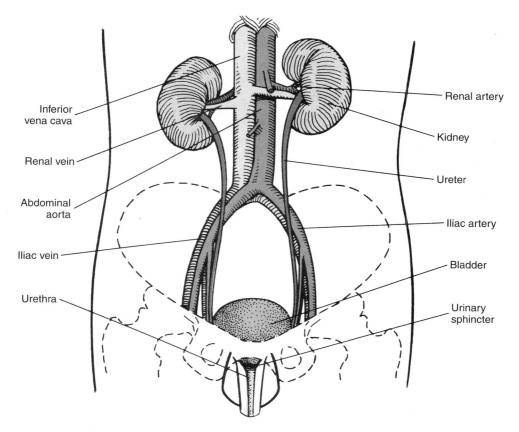

FIGURE 5-14. Organs and other structures of the urinary system. *(From Phipps, Monahan, Sands, et al.* Medical-Surgical Nursing health and illness perspectives, *ed. 7, St. Louis, 2003, Mosby.)*

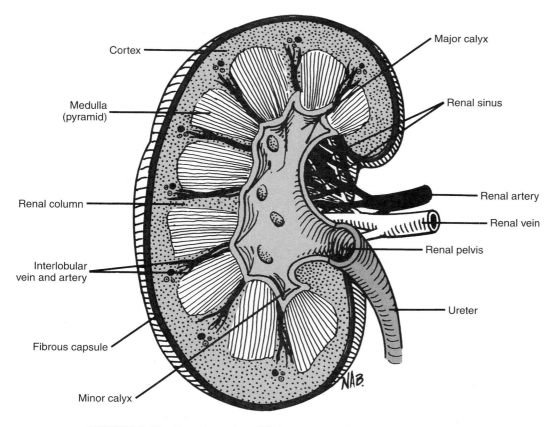

FIGURE 5-15. Frontal section of kidney. *(From Phipps, Monahan, Sands, et al.* Medical-Surgical Nursing health and illness perspectives, *ed. 7, St. Louis, 2003, Mosby.)*

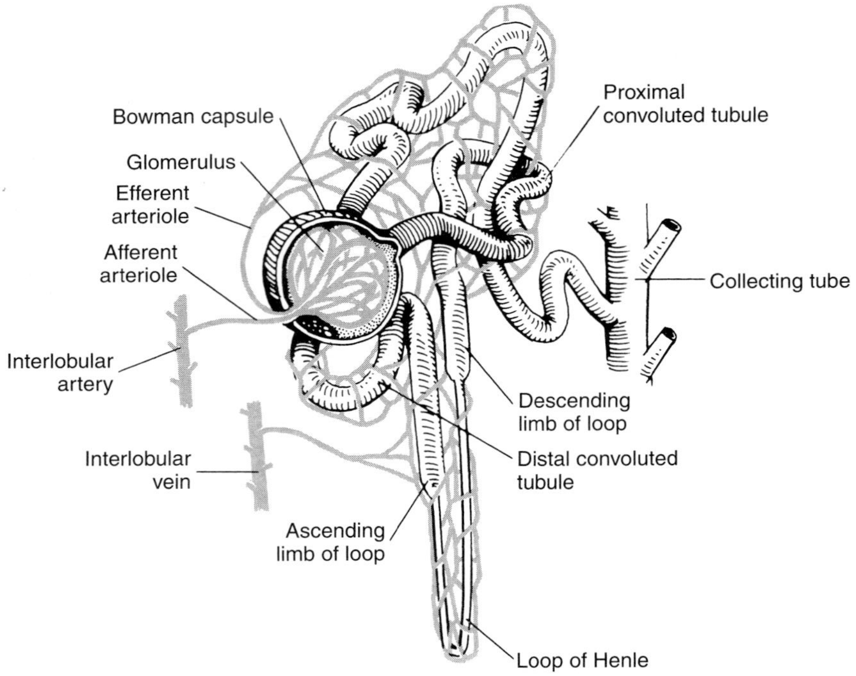

FIGURE 5-16. Nephron. *(From Phipps, Monahan, Sands, et al.* Medical-Surgical Nursing health and illness perspectives, *ed. 7, St. Louis, 2003, Mosby.)*

2. Maintenance of water balance: absorbs more or less water depending on intake; normally, intake is approximately equal to output.
3. Other major functions include renin secretion and blood pressure control, erythropoietin production, vitamin-D activation, and acid-base balance.
C. Urine composition
   1. Clear, yellowish, slightly aromatic, and slightly acid
   2. Contains 95% water and 5% solids, which includes urea, uric acid, creatinine, ammonia, sodium, and potassium; specific gravity indicates amount of the dissolved solids; normal range: 1.003 to 1.035.
   3. Abnormal substances: glucose, blood protein, RBCs, bile, and bacteria

RENAL (URINARY) SYSTEM CONDITIONS AND DISORDERS

The urinary system regulates the composition and volume of the blood. It excretes metabolic wastes and fluids and maintains fluid and electrolyte balance and acid-base balance. Malfunction of this system has generalized effects on the body's normal physiology. Frequently, patients are older and have chronic medical problems (e.g., cardiac conditions); these problems must be considered when nursing care is planned (e.g., many diagnoses and procedures require additional fluids as a natural irrigation; increased fluids might be contraindicated in the patient with a cardiac condition). Problems of the male reproductive system are discussed in this section.

The following terms are used to describe urine output:

Anuria: absence of urine output

Bacteriuria: bacteria in the urine

Costovertebral angle tenderness: examiner strikes one or more light blows to the area where the lower ribs meet the vertebrae (flank); tenderness in this area may indicate renal disorders.

Dribbling: voiding without stream, in small amounts, frequently or constantly

Dysuria: painful or difficult urination

Enuresis: involuntary voiding while asleep

Frequency: voiding often and in small amounts

Hematuria: blood in the urine

Hesitancy: the inability to immediately empty the full bladder when the desire is present

Hydronephrosis: dilation of the pelvis and calices of one or both kidneys, resulting from obstruction to the flow of urine

Incontinence: partial or complete inability to control urine output

Micturition: voiding, urination

Nocturia: awakening to void

Overflow incontinence: leakage of urine in small amounts while bladder remains full and distended

Polyuria: excessive production and excretion of urine

Residual urine: urine remaining in the bladder after voiding

Retention: inability to excrete urine from bladder

Urgency: an intense stimulus to void (may cause incontinence)

Voiding: micturition, elimination of urine

Nursing Assessment

A. Nursing observations
   1. Observe bladder for distention: lower abdominal area will be rigid, tense, swollen, and sensitive to the touch.
   2. Assess urine: amount, color, odor, opacity (clear or cloudy), and presence of sediment, mucus, or clots.
   3. Check catheter (if indwelling) for drainage and meatus for irritation or secretions.
   4. Check genitals (scrotum, labia, and anal area) for irritation, rashes, and lesions.
   5. Monitor fluid and electrolyte balance.
   6. Check eyes, extremities, presacral area, and scrotum for edema.

7. Monitor vital signs: note elevation of temperature and blood pressure.
8. Note problems related to aging (i.e., urgency, stress incontinence).

B. Patient description (subjective data)
1. Change in voiding habits
2. Problems with elimination or changes in patterns of urination
   a. Frequency
   b. Nocturia
   c. Hesitancy of stream
   d. Urgency
   e. Retention
   f. Incontinence
   g. Enuresis
   h. Dribbling
3. Urethral discharge
4. Burning on voiding
5. Pain: suprapubic or flank

C. Obtain patient history regarding:
1. Normal urinary and bowel elimination habits
2. Medical problems with the urinary system (e.g., stones, sexually transmitted diseases [STDs])
3. Medical problems with other body systems (e.g., cardiac conditions), trauma
4. Medications
5. Diet
6. Food or medication allergies
7. Decreased urinary stream
8. Pain or spasms: what precipitated this and what relieved it?
9. Discharge
10. Edema

Diagnostic Tests and Methods

A. Blood studies
1. BUN: normal level is 10 to 20 mg/dl; urea is an end product of protein metabolism and is excreted by the kidneys in urine; an increase indicates impaired renal function.
2. Creatinine: normal level is 0.5 to 1.3 mg/dl; elevation indicates decreased renal function.
3. Acid and alkaline phosphatase: normal value varies with laboratory; increase may indicate metastasis to bone or liver from the kidney; nurse must assess for bone fracture or pathologic conditions of the liver.
4. Albumin: globulin ratio is usually 2:1; a change indicates damage to nephron and loss of albumin in the urine; patient retains fluid and has edema.

B. Urine studies
1. Routine urine: a single voided specimen to observe and compare to known normal specimens; results give information about renal function and systemic health.
2. Specific gravity: normal value 1.003 to 1.035; change indicates dehydration or inadequate kidney function; a single voided specimen is required.
3. Urine culture and sensitivity (see Chapter 2)
4. Creatine: 24-hour urine collection to measure creatinine excreted; oral fluids are encouraged (see Chapter 2).

C. X-ray procedures, radiographic studies
1. Kidneys, ureter, bladder (KUB): an abdominal x-ray study that gives baseline information about size, shape, and placement of organs; flatus and stones are visualized; no preparation or care after procedure is required.
2. Intravenous pyelogram (IVP): an IV injection of a radiopaque dye that is rapidly excreted by the kidney; this tests renal function, and the x-ray films outline renal pelvis, ureters, bladder, and urethra; nursing responsibilities: maintain NPO status before procedure; after procedure, observe for allergic reaction to dye; note voiding.
3. Retrograde pyelogram: visualization of upper genitourinary (GU) tract by injecting radiopaque dye through ureteral catheters to locate obstruction (e.g., stone, tumor); nursing responsibilities: preparation is the same as for preoperative preparation (see Chapter 2); after procedure, monitor vital signs, anticipate pain, and administer analgesics; note voiding, and observe urine.
4. Cystoscopy: a direct visualization of the bladder and urethral orifices; a cystoscope is inserted through the urethra into the bladder; the bladder is distended with sterile solution; stones, tumors, and polyps can be diagnosed; urine can be observed entering the bladder from each ureter to evaluate renal function; instruments may be passed through the cystoscope to crush stones, take biopsy specimens, or pass catheters into ureters; nursing responsibilities: provide general preoperative and postoperative care (see Chapter 2); after procedure, determine what was done during procedure; assess urinary function, observe urine; provide care and observation of a patient with indwelling catheter (see Chapter 2).
5. Renogram: also called renal angiogram; for before and after procedure; see pyelogram.
6. CT scan

D. Other procedures
1. MRI
2. Urodynamic studies

Frequent Patient Problems and Nursing Care

A. Incontinence (types: urge, total, stress, reflex, and functional) related to catheter use, infection, tissue damage, immobility
1. Minimize embarrassment; provide privacy.
2. Wash, dry, and inspect skin, and take measures to prevent decubitus ulcers (pressure sores).
3. Provide bladder training.

B. Impaired skin integrity related to retention of metabolic wastes and resulting toxicity (uremia)
1. Urea is excreted through the skin, causing odor and pruritus: provide frequent and thorough skin care; wash and pat dry.
2. Confusion and disorientation; may progress to state of unconsciousness and coma; provide all care; maintain safety (see comas).
3. Nausea and vomiting: provide mouth care every 2 hours.
4. Renal failure: see nursing care for patient with chronic renal failure, pp. 269-270.

C. Pain related to bladder spasms: bladder spasms caused by catheter irritation are intermittent in the suprapubic area, radiating to the urethra.
1. Assess type, location, and severity of pain.
2. Check catheter for obstruction; irrigate as ordered.
3. Administer medication as ordered (see Antispasmodics, Chapter 3).
4. Reassure patient that spasms are not abnormal.

D. Deficient fluid volume related to dehydration
   1. Use hydration methods (encourage fluids).
   2. Monitor intake and output.
E. Risk for infection or injury (hematuria) related to surgery or pathogens
   1. Monitor signs and symptoms, vital signs.
   2. Administer medication as ordered.
   3. Note characteristics of urine at each voiding.
   4. Encourage fluids if not contraindicated.
   5. Report and document clots noted in urine.
   6. Maintain patency and gravity drainage of catheters.
   7. Assess for signs of anemia (weakness and fatigue).
   8. Provide nursing care and safety as indicated.
   9. Reassure the patient that blood-tinged urine is not unusual after instrumentation or surgery.
F. Urinary retention related to surgery
   1. Take nursing measures to assist the patient with voiding (see Chapter 2).
   2. Monitor intake and output.
   3. Encourage fluids if not contraindicated.
G. Anxiety related to sexual dysfunction, impending surgery, or possible change in body image or function
   1. Provide time to listen to patient express feelings.
   2. Explain all care and procedures; reassure often.
   3. Be honest; provide privacy; avoid embarrassing situations.
   4. Praise patient's progress toward discharge goals.
H. Risk for excess fluid volume related to inability to filter urine
   1. Assess deep skin (e.g., sacral, feet).
   2. Monitor lung sounds.

Major Medical Diagnoses
Cystitis

A. Definition: inflammation of the bladder mucosa; difficult to cure; recurs and may be chronic
B. Pathology: usually from a bacterial infection
   1. May be secondary to infection elsewhere in urinary system (e.g., urethritis)
   2. Contamination during catheterization or instrumentation
   3. An obstruction causing urinary stasis in the bladder (e.g., enlarged prostate, urethral stricture)
C. Signs and symptoms
   1. Subjective
      a. Burning, dysuria, urgency, frequency, nocturia, hematuria, and pyuria
      b. Low-back pain and bladder spasms
   2. Objective: elevation of temperature
D. Diagnostic tests and methods
   1. Patient history and assessment
   2. Urine culture, IVP, voiding cystoureterogram
E. Treatment: systemic medications, urinary antiseptics, antibiotics, sulfonamides, and antispasmodics (see Chapter 3)
F. Nursing intervention
   1. Encourage fluids: 3000 ml daily over that of dietary intake unless contraindicated.
   2. Provide and supervise proper perineal care.
   3. Provide diet that acidifies urine (e.g., cranberry juice).
   4. Monitor temperature, and administer antipyretics as ordered.
   5. Provide sitz baths.

6. Teach preventive measures.
   a. Taking full course of antibiotic therapy as prescribed
   b. Emptying bladder completely
   c. Maintaining a consistent fluid intake of 2 L per day
   d. Voiding after sexual intercourse

Urethritis

A. Definition: inflammation of the urethra; may develop scar tissue and stricture, causing obstruction, cystitis, and nephritis
B. Pathology
   1. Prostatitis; injury during instrumentation or catheterization
   2. Gonococcus infection; chlamydial infection
C. Signs and symptoms
   1. Subjective
      a. Urgency
      b. Frequency
      c. Dysuria
      d. Burning on urination
   2. Objective
      a. Purulent discharge
      b. Results of urine culture
D. Diagnostic tests and methods
   1. Patient history and physical examination
   2. Culture of discharge
E. Treatment
   1. Antibiotics
   2. Dilatation for stricture
F. Nursing intervention
   1. Provide sitz baths.
   2. Demonstrate and supervise thorough hand washing.
   3. Monitor and care of Foley catheter.
   4. Avoid unnecessary catheterization and instrumentation.

Pyelonephritis

A. Definition: infection of the kidney; may be acute or become chronic; kidney becomes edematous, mucosa is inflamed, and multiple abscesses may form; the kidney will become fibrotic, and uremia may develop.
B. Pathology
   1. Ascending infection from an infection lower in the GU tract
   2. Staphylococcal or streptococcal infection carried in the blood
C. Signs and symptoms
   1. Subjective
      a. Nausea
      b. Chills
      c. Dysuria, burning, frequency
      d. Costovertebral angle (CVA) tenderness
   2. Objective
      a. Markedly elevated temperature (102° to 105° F)
      b. Vomiting
      c. Pyuria, hematuria
      d. Increased WBC count
      e. Results of urine cultures and IVP
D. Diagnostic tests and methods
   1. Urine culture and sensitivity
   2. Patient history and physical examination
   3. IVP

E. Treatment: urinary antiseptics and specific antibiotics (see Chapter 3); follow-up care for at least 1 year

F. Nursing intervention
1. Prevent dehydration: encourage fluids and maintain IV therapy.
2. Provide rest and conserve energy.
3. Prevent chill; keep skin dry and clean.
4. Provide mouth care every 2 hours.
5. Provide soft diet.
6. Provide and assist with pericare; demonstrate proper technique and hand washing.
7. Anticipate pain: administer analgesics and local heat.
8. Administer antiemetic as needed.
9. Control temperature: administer antipyretics.

Calculi (Lithiasis)

A. Definition: formation of stones in the urinary tract caused by deposits of crystalline substance that normally remain in solution and are excreted in the urine; may be found in the kidney, ureters, or bladder; vary in size from renal calculi that can be as large as an orange or as small as grains of sand; can obstruct urine flow, causing chronic infection, backflow, hydronephrosis, and gradual destruction of kidney; many small stones pass spontaneously.

B. Cause
1. Infection
2. Urinary stasis
3. Dehydration and concentration of urine
4. Metabolic diseases (e.g., gout, hyperparathyroidism)
5. Immobility (see Dangers of Immobility, Chapter 2)
6. Familial tendency
7. Elevated uric acid
8. Excessive calcium intake

C. Signs and symptoms
1. Subjective
   a. Pain (can be extreme) radiating down flank to pubic area
   b. Frequency and urgency
2. Objective
   a. Hematuria and pyuria
   b. Diaphoresis, nausea, vomiting, pallor (related to pain)
   c. Results of diagnostic tests

D. Diagnostic tests and methods: x-ray studies (KUB, IVP), urine studies (ultrasonography, cystoscopy, serial blood calcium and phosphorus levels)

E. Treatment: depends on location—removal of stones, restoring normal urine production and elimination, preventing recurrence
1. Cystoscopy and crushing of stones (lithotripsy)
2. Dislodging ureteral stone by passing ureteral catheter; laser lithotripsy
3. Surgery to remove ureteral or kidney stone
   a. Pyelolithotomy: removal of stones from renal pelvis
   b. Nephrolithotomy: incision through kidney and removal of stone
   c. Ureterolithotomy: removal of ureteral calculus
   d. Transcutaneous shock wave lithotripsy: ultrasonic waves used to disintegrate renal calculi
   e. Percutaneous stone dissolution: chemical agents injected into a nephrostomy tube to dissolve the stone

F. Nursing intervention
1. Provide general preoperative and postoperative nursing care (see Chapter 2).
2. Supervise and explain diet restrictions as ordered according to type of stone.
3. Provide analgesics as ordered.
4. Observe, describe, and strain all urine.
5. Maintain gravity drainage; never clamp ureteral or nephrostomy catheters.
6. Observe patency of catheters; in most cases, never irrigate renal or ureteral catheters.
7. Record output from each catheter separately; immediately report scanty output from one tube.
8. Encourage fluids (but keep NPO if nausea, vomiting, or abdominal distention occur).

Hydronephrosis

A. Definition: an accumulation of fluid in the renal pelvis; distention of the renal tubules, calyces, and pelvis is present; renal tissues are destroyed from pressure; leads to uremia (azotemia)

B. Pathology
1. Congenital defective drainage; blockage from stones or scar tissues
2. Reflux (backup) from obstructed bladder neck in benign prostatic hypertrophy

C. Signs and symptoms
1. Subjective
   a. Related to cause; in some patients, no symptoms, or mild pain
   b. Severe colicky renal pain
   c. Flank pain radiating to groin
   d. Dysuria
   e. Oliguria to anuria
   f. Nausea
   g. Abdominal fullness
   h. Dribbling, hesitancy
2. Objective
   a. Hematuria, pyuria
   b. Results of diagnostic tests

D. Diagnostic tests and methods
1. Patient history and physical examination
2. Blood serum tests (urea, creatinine)
3. IVP, ultrasonography

E. Treatment
1. Removing the cause
2. Providing for adequate urinary drainage (e.g., bladder catheter, nephrostomy tube)
3. Antibiotics

F. Nursing intervention
1. Provide rest.
2. Provide medication, and care as needed for symptoms (e.g., elevation of temperature, pain).
3. Assess for and provide care as indicated for patient with uremia.

Bladder Tumors

A. Definition: benign or malignant lesions that ulcerate into the mucous membrane; bladder capacity is decreased; benign tumors tend to recur and become malignant.

B. Pathology
1. Related to cigarette smoking and exposure to dyes (environmental: nitrates, benzene, rubber, petroleum)

2. Chronic bladder irritation (e.g., stones, infection)
3. Related to aging

C. Signs and symptoms
  1. Subjective: signs of bladder infection: dysuria, frequency, urgency, chills
  2. Objective
    a. Painless, gross hematuria
    b. Anemia

D. Diagnostic tests and methods
  1. Patient history and physical examination
  2. X-ray studies: IVP, KUB, and retrograde pyelogram
  3. Cystoscopy and biopsy examination
  4. Renoscan, ultrasonography, CT, MRI

E. Treatment
  1. Removing the tumor through cystoscopy if benign
  2. Administering antineoplastic agents into bladder through urinary catheter
  3. Surgery
    a. Partial cystectomy
    b. Cystectomy: total removal of the bladder and provision for urinary diversion
    c. Radiation, intravesicular, external
    d. Chemotherapy, intravesicular
    e. Fulguration (coagulation)
    f. Experimental therapy (photodynamic therapy: use of photosensitivity agent and laser destruction of tumor cells)
    g. Interferon (Roferon-A)

F. Nursing intervention: give according to method of treatment (see specific sections).
  1. Be supportive of patient concerns expressed.
  2. Provide general pre- and postoperative care (see Chapter 2).

Urinary Diversion

A. Definition: surgical intervention to allow for urinary elimination; the bladder is removed; the procedure is permanent.
  1. Ileal conduit (ileal passageway): a small segment of ilium is separated from the intestine, and the distal end is brought out of the abdomen to form a stoma; the ureters are implanted into this ileal pouch; urine flows continuously from the renal pelvis through the ureters into the ileal pouch and into a collecting bag.
  2. Ureterointestinal implant: the ureters are anastomosed into the sigmoid colon or rectum; urine is mixed with feces, and evacuation is controlled from the anal sphincter.
  3. Cutaneous ureterostomies: the ureters are implanted on the abdomen, forming one or two stomas that drain urine continuously into drainage bags.
  4. Continent ileal urinary reservoir (Koch pouch): the ureters are anastomosed to an isolated segment of ileum, which has a one-way valve; urine is drained by periodic insertion of a catheter.
  5. Nephrostomy (may be long term): tubes are inserted in the pelvis of each kidney, brought through the skin, and connected to a closed drainage system.

B. Indication: cancer of the bladder

C. Patient problems (depends on procedure)
  1. Susceptibility to infection
  2. Anxiety or depression about diagnosis and change in body image

3. Inability to control elimination
4. Embarrassment
5. Odor if urine leaks onto skin; risk for impaired skin integrity
6. Impaired skin integrity resulting from the incision and ostomy
7. Pain from surgical incision or urinary obstruction or both

D. Nursing intervention (varies with procedures)
  1. Provide general preoperative and postoperative care (see Chapter 2).
  2. Provide time to listen to patient fears and anxieties.
  3. Assess for fluid and electrolyte imbalance.
  4. Maintain integrity of the skin: clean, inspect, and change drainage bag as needed.
  5. Monitor temperature.
  6. Monitor urine output from each catheter or tube; maintain separate output records for each; if nephrostomy tubes are used, contact physician if tube fails to drain urine, if urine is grossly bloody, or if patient complains of sudden severe flank pain.
  7. Provide stoma care (see ileostomy, colostomy); stoma may need to be dilated in postoperative period.
  8. Monitor fluid and electrolyte balance.
  9. Prevent infection: maintain asepsis; encourage fluids; patient must know when to seek medical attention for pain or elevation of temperature.
  10. Do not give patient laxatives or enemas.
  11. Arrange a visit from a person who has undergone a similar procedure (with permission of physician and patient).
  12. Provide elimination of odor in drainage bags; use weak solution of vinegar or a liquid appliance deodorant.
  13. Empty or change pouch when one-third to one-half full.
  14. Instruct the patient to avoid odor-producing foods such as onions, fish, eggs, cheese; drink cranberry juice.

Kidney Tumor

A. Definition: most tumors of the kidney are malignant; no early symptoms are presented.

B. Cause: unknown

C. Signs and symptoms (only in late stages)
  1. Hematuria with no pain
  2. Low-grade temperature
  3. Weight loss
  4. Anemia
  5. Symptoms related to metastasis (e.g., bone pain)

D. Diagnostic tests and methods
  1. Renal arteriogram: IVP, KUB
  2. Renal biopsy examination

E. Treatment
  1. Surgery: radical nephrectomy
  2. Radiation
  3. Chemotherapy
  4. Biological response modifiers (interferon)

F. Nursing intervention
  1. Provide nursing care for individual symptoms.
  2. Provide general nursing care: before and after surgery, during radiation (see Chapter 2), and for a patient receiving chemotherapy (see Chapter 3).

Acute Renal Failure

A. Definition: sudden damage to the kidneys, causing cessation of function and retention of toxins, fluids, and end products of metabolism; patient may recover, or disease may become chronic or be fatal; may be prerenal, intrarenal, or postrenal

B. Causes: blood transfusion reaction, shock, toxins, burns, renal ischemia, nephrotoxins, trauma, reaction to chemotherapy

C. Signs and symptoms
1. Subjective
   a. Nausea, weakness
   b. Metallic taste in mouth
2. Subjective
   a. Lethargy, headache, drowsiness; convulsion; may go into coma
   b. Vomiting and diarrhea
   c. Sudden oliguria or anuria
   d. Increased bleeding time
   e. Electrolyte imbalance
   f. Abnormal BUN and creatinine levels
   g. Paresthesia
   h. Hypotension

D. Diagnostic tests and methods
1. Patient history and physical examination
2. Blood serum tests, especially potassium
3. Renal scan, renal biopsy, KUB
4. Nephrotomography
5. Retrograde pyelogram
6. Ultrasonography, CT, MRI
7. Urinalysis, CBC

E. Treatment
1. Removal of cause
2. Peritoneal dialysis
3. Hemodialysis

F. Nursing intervention
1. Provide nursing observations and care as indicated for primary problem.
2. Provide care and observations as indicated for patient with chronic renal failure (see chronic renal failure).
3. Provide nursing care as indicated for patient receiving peritoneal dialysis (see peritoneal dialysis).
4. Provide nursing care as indicated for patient receiving hemodialysis (see hemodialysis).
5. Offer emotional support.

Chronic Renal Failure (End-Stage Renal Disease)

A. Definition: progressive kidney damage; the nephron deteriorates; the kidneys stop functioning; this is the final stage of many chronic diseases (e.g., hypertension).

B. Causes
1. Glomerulonephritis, pyelonephritis, polycystic kidney, or urinary tract obstruction, diabetes
2. Essential hypertension
3. Lupus erythematosus
4. Toxic agents
5. Vascular disorders

C. Signs and symptoms (Figure 5-17)
1. Subjective
   a. Malaise
   b. Nausea
   c. Headaches and visual disturbances

2. Objective
   a. Anemia
   b. Oliguria
   c. Hyperkalemia
   d. Twitching (from low serum calcium and increased phosphorus levels); pathological fracture
   e. Hypertension (from fluid retention)
   f. Very susceptible to infection: delayed wound healing and ulcers in the mouth
   g. Bleeding tendency
   h. Uremic frost: urea is excreted in perspiration onto the skin, and small crystals can be seen; this causes severe pruritus.
   i. Vomiting
   j. Decreased erythropoietin
   k. Disorientation, convulsions, coma
   l. Results of diagnostic tests

D. Diagnostic tests and methods
1. Patient history and physical examination
2. Serum blood tests
3. Kidney function tests. BUN, creatinine level
4. X-ray studies
5. Renal arteriograms, renal ultrasound
6. Nephrotomograms
7. Kidney biopsy

E. Treatment
1. Removing (treating) cause
2. Hemodialysis
3. Peritoneal dialysis
4. Kidney transplant

F. Nursing intervention
1. Monitor fluid balance: weigh patient daily; record intake and output.
2. Maintain asepsis: provide catheter care, prevent infections, and encourage frequent hand washing; do not expose patient to staff or visitors with upper respiratory tract infections.
3. Instruct the patient to conserve energy: provide care; maintain rest periods.
4. Provide safety (see care of patient in coma).
5. Relieve pruritus: wash patient frequently with tepid water; do not use soap; handle skin gently; use skin lotion; cut nails; apply calamine lotion.
6. Assist with administration of transfusion; biologic response modifiers; epoetin alfa (erythropoietin).
7. Provide oral hygiene every 1 to 2 hours; use cotton swabs and soft toothbrush; hard candy and mouthwash minimize bad taste in mouth and alleviate thirst.
8. Provide soft, high-carbohydrate, low-potassium, low-sodium, low-protein diet in small feedings.
9. Restrict fluids as ordered.
10. Anticipate cardiac arrest: monitor vital signs.
11. Assess LOC: orient as necessary.
12. Provide nursing care and precautions as indicated for a patient with seizures (see convulsive disorders).
13. Provide nursing measures to prevent dangers of immobility (see Chapter 2).
14. Anticipate and prevent bleeding.
    a. Observe stool, urine, sputum, and vomitus.
    b. Monitor vital signs, laboratory values.
    c. Use soft swab for mouth care.
    d. Avoid injections, if possible.

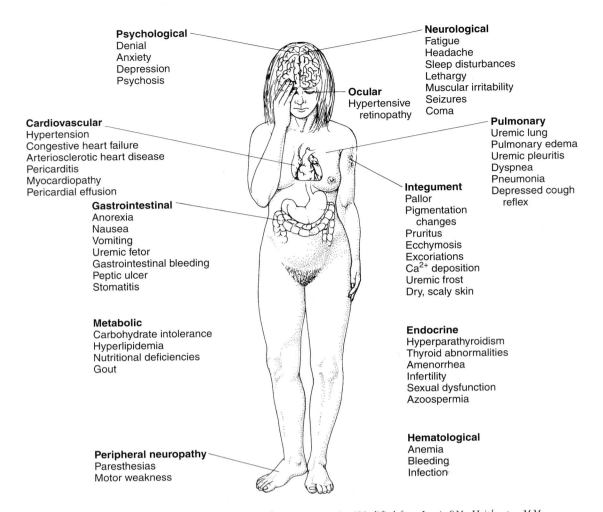

Psychological
Denial
Anxiety
Depression
Psychosis

Neurological
Fatigue
Headache
Sleep disturbances
Lethargy
Muscular irritability
Seizures
Coma

Ocular
Hypertensive
retinopathy

Cardiovascular
Hypertension
Congestive heart failure
Arteriosclerotic heart disease
Pericarditis
Myocardiopathy
Pericardial effusion

Pulmonary
Uremic lung
Pulmonary edema
Uremic pleuritis
Dyspnea
Pneumonia
Depressed cough
reflex

Gastrointestinal
Anorexia
Nausea
Vomiting
Uremic fetor
Gastrointestinal bleeding
Peptic ulcer
Stomatitis

Integument
Pallor
Pigmentation
changes
Pruritus
Ecchymosis
Excoriations
Ca^{2+} deposition
Uremic frost
Dry, scaly skin

Metabolic
Carbohydrate intolerance
Hyperlipidemia
Nutritional deficiencies
Gout

Endocrine
Hyperparathyroidism
Thyroid abnormalities
Amenorrhea
Infertility
Sexual dysfunction
Azoospermia

Hematological
Anemia
Bleeding
Infection

Peripheral neuropathy
Paresthesias
Motor weakness

FIGURE 5-17. Clinical manifestations of chronic uremia. *(Modified from Lewis SM, Heitkemper MM, Dirksen SR: Medical-surgical nursing: assessment and management of clinical problems, ed 5, St Louis, 2000, Mosby.)*

15. Reinforce instructions for kind of drug therapy (i.e., erythropoietin, iron, minerals, antihypertensives, phosphate binders, ion-exchange resins).

Peritoneal Dialysis (Figure 5-18)

A. Description: toxins, end products of metabolism, and fluids are removed from the blood through the peritoneal membrane; a catheter is passed into the peritoneal cavity; dialyzing fluid, which is similar to plasma, is instilled by gravity into the abdominal cavity, and the catheter is clamped; toxins and electrolytes, which are in greater concentration in the blood vessels of the peritoneal membrane, pass into the dialyzing fluid; after a specified dwell time, the catheter is unclamped, and the fluid drains out by gravity.

B. Types
1. Intermittent peritoneal dialysis (IPD)
2. Continuous ambulatory peritoneal dialysis (CAPD)
3. Continuous cycling peritoneal dialysis (CCPD)
4. Access devices may be temporary or permanent.

C. Patient problems
1. Risk for infection related to dialysis procedure
2. Self-care deficit related to discomfort and immobility
3. Fluid volume excess or deficit
4. Body image disturbance

D. Nursing intervention
1. Record baseline vital signs; complete assessment; carefully measure fluid instilled or drained.
2. Maintain surgical asepsis; prevent peritonitis.
3. Assist patient with self-care activities.
4. Observe for complications (hypotension, pain, respiratory distress, hypovolemia, peritonitis, atelectasis).

Hemodialysis

A. Description: blood leaves the patient through an arterial cannula and travels through coils placed in a solution; dialysis takes place, and the detoxified blood returns to the patient's venous circulation; a surgically created arteriovenous fistula (connection) is necessary for repeated dialysis.

B. Patient problems
1. Self-esteem disturbance related to threatened self-image
2. Powerlessness related to dependency on machine
3. Risk for infection related to the hemodialysis procedure
4. Anxiety related to lifelong, life-threatening disease

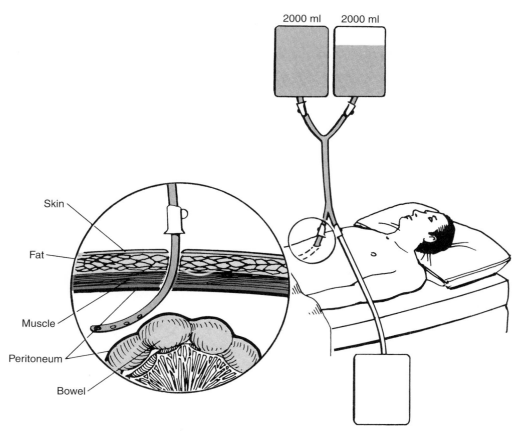

Skin

Fat

Muscle

Peritoneum

Bowel

2000 ml   2000 ml

FIGURE 5-18. **Patient receiving peritoneal dialysis.** Dialysis fluid is being infused into the peritoneal cavity. *(From Phipps WJ, Sands JK, Lehman MK, Cassmeyer VL:* Medical-surgical nursing: concepts and clinical practice, *ed 5, St Louis, 1995, Mosby.)*

5. Fluid volume excess related to fluid accumulation, inadequate dialysis
6. Fluid volume deficit related to rapid removal of body fluid during treatment
C. Nursing intervention
 1. Maintain surgical asepsis.
 2. Assess AV fistula, graft, or shunt for patency; normally, a thrill can be felt by palpating the area of anastomosis and a bruit can be heard with a stethoscope; the bruit and thrill is created by arterial blood rushing into the vein.
 3. Provide emotional support; alleviate anxiety.
 4. Provide patient teaching.

Kidney Transplant

A. Removal of the diseased kidney and transplantation of a normal kidney is sometimes performed for patients with advanced renal failure; restores normal function; less expensive than dialysis after first year
B. Patient problems
 1. Risk for infection related to altered immune system secondary to medications
 2. Anxiety related to possibility of organ rejection
 3. Fear of pain, rejection
 4. Body image disturbance
 5. Knowledge deficit (surgery, drug therapies, nutrition, activities, follow-up care)

MALE REPRODUCTIVE SYSTEM

Anatomy and Physiology (Figure 5-19)

A. External genitals
 1. Scrotum: skin-covered pouch; lies outside of pelvic cavity; contains testes, epididymis, and lower part of vas deferens; lower body temperature here is necessary for reproduction.
 2. Penis: erectile tissue; organ of coitus (sexual intercourse); serves as passageway for urine and semen
B. Testes: small oval glands in scrotum; produce spermatozoa; secrete testosterone
C. Ducts
 1. Seminiferous tubules: formation of sperm
 2. Epididymis: narrow, tightly coiled tubes; provides temporary storage space for immature sperm
 3. Vas deferens: continuation of the epididymis; lies near surface of scrotum; called the spermatic cord
 4. Ejaculatory: pass through prostate; ejaculate semen into urethra
D. Accessory glands
 1. Seminal vesicles: located on each side of the prostate; empty secretion into the prostatic ampulla
 2. Prostate: encircles the upper area of the urethra; secretes alkaline fluid; increases sperm motility
 3. Cowper's gland: located below prostate; produces an alkaline secretion that is primarily a lubricant during sexual intercourse

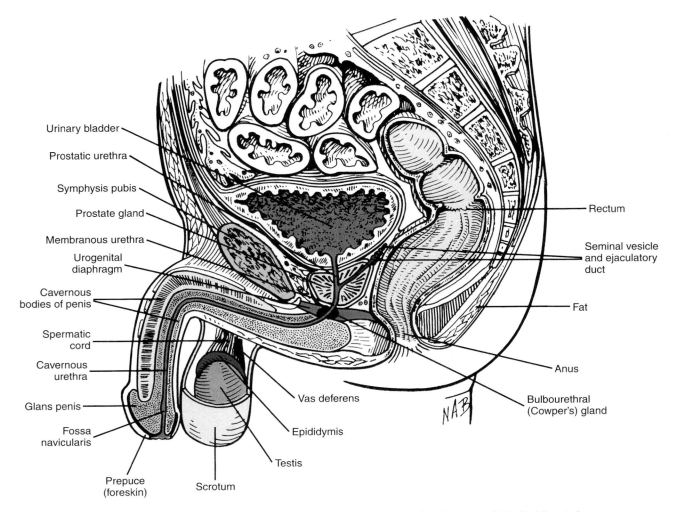

FIGURE 5-19. Male organs of reproduction. (*From Phipps, Monahan, Sands, et al.* Medical-Surgical Nursing health and illness perspectives, *ed. 7, St. Louis, 2003, Mosby.*)

E. Semen: alkaline fluid (pH 7.5); the major bulk (60%) is secreted by the seminal vesicles; the remaining 40% is secreted by other accessory organs.

F. Function
  1. Reproduction
  2. Production of testosterone

MALE GENITOURINARY SYSTEM CONDITIONS AND DISORDERS

The male reproductive and urinary systems are so closely related that disorders that occur in one system greatly influence the other. Aging changes in the male reproductive system predispose them to many disorders. Collecting information about these body systems is often difficult because of embarrassment of the patient in discussing such matters. The nurse should project an open, nonjudgmental attitude during data collection.

Nursing Assessment

A. Nursing observations (objective data)
  1. General appearance
  2. Vital signs
  3. Weight
  4. External genitalia: penis
    a. Lesions
    b. Drainage
    c. Tenderness
  5. Scrotum
    a. Enlargement
    b. Presence of testes in scrotum
  6. Urine
    a. Color, clarity, amount
    b. Incontinence
B. Patient description—subjective data
  1. Pain
  2. Change in urinary stream, urgency
  3. Impotence
  4. Swelling

Frequent Patient Problems and Nursing Care

A. Anxiety related to modesty
  1. Keep the patient's body covered at all times.
  2. Provide privacy.
  3. Speak with the patient during the examination or procedure.

B. Deficient knowledge related to diagnostic examinations
1. Provide factual information related to the examination process.
   a. Teach testicular self-examination.
      (1) Should be done on a monthly basis
      (2) More comfortable if done in shower
      (3) Check each scrotal sac for any abnormalities in size and shape.
2. Risk for sexual dysfunction
   a. Allow patient to express emotions, fears.
   b. Provide literature on aids or medications to assist in achieving satisfactory sexual experiences.

Benign Prostatic Hypertrophy, Hyperphasia (BPH)

A. Description: the prostate gland slowly enlarges (hypertrophies) and extends upward into the bladder; outflow of urine is obstructed; the urinary stream is smaller, and voiding is difficult; a pouch is formed in the bladder as the gland continues to enlarge; stasis of urine occurs; obstruction causes gradual dilation of ureters and kidneys; may cause hydronephrosis; when obstruction is complete, acute urinary retention occurs.
B. Cause: unknown; increased incidence with age, usually over 50 years of age; related to smoking
C. Signs and symptoms
1. Subjective
   a. Dysuria, frequency, nocturia, urgency, retention, hesitancy
   b. Burning on urination, decreased force of stream, end-stream dribbling
2. Objective
   a. Urinary tract infection
   b. Acute urinary retention
   c. Hematuria
   d. Enlarged prostate gland
   e. Results of diagnostic tests
D. Diagnostic tests and methods
1. Patient history and assessment; palpation through rectal examination
2. IVP, cystoscopy, retrograde pyelography
3. Urine culture
4. BUN, CBC
5. Serum creatinine
6. Transrectal ultrasonography
E. Treatment
1. Immediate
   a. Bladder drainage with indwelling catheter
   b. Decompression
   c. Antibiotics as indicated
   d. Suprapubic cystotomy and insertion of catheter for long-term drainage
2. Surgery: type depends on patient's age and size of enlargement (open approaches).
   a. Transurethral resection of the prostate (TURP): an instrument is passed through the urethra to the prostate; under direct visualization, small pieces of the obstructing gland are removed with electric wire; the bleeding points are cauterized; no incision is required; bleeding is a common postoperative problem.
   b. Suprapubic (transvesical) prostatectomy: a low incision is made over the bladder; the bladder is opened, and the prostatic tissue is removed through an incision into the urethral mucosa; two drainage tubes are inserted (a cystotomy tube and a Foley catheter); these tubes are connected to a continuous bladder irrigation setup.
   c. Retropubic prostatectomy: a low abdominal incision is made; the bladder is not entered.
   d. Perineal prostatectomy: the gland is removed through an incision in the perineum; the entire gland and capsule are removed.
   e. Bilateral vasectomy may be performed with a prostatectomy to reduce risk of epididymitis.
3. Other treatment methods
   a. Finasteride (Proscar), an androgen hormone inhibitor, can be used to decrease symptoms; may arrest prostate enlargement
   b. Transcystoscopic urethroplasty: balloon dilatation of prostatic urethra
   c. Transurethral incision (TUIP) at bladder neck
   d. Short-term effects treatment involving microwaves
   e. Implantation of intraurethral prostatic stent
F. Nursing intervention
1. On admission, complete assessment related to:
   a. Aging
   b. Possible infection
   c. Anxiety
   d. Medical problems associated with aging: diabetes, cardiovascular, hearing, sight, GI problems
2. Encourage fluids if not contraindicated; monitor intake and output.
3. Maintain gravity drainage of indwelling catheter.
4. Provide general preoperative and postoperative care (see Chapter 2).
5. Provide specific postoperative care; depends on the procedure performed
   a. Continue to maintain gravity drainage of indwelling catheter.
   b. Keep irrigation flowing (note clots); maintain a closed, continuous irrigation; ensure that drainage not obstructed.
   c. Maintain asepsis; change dressing when it becomes wet (may need physician's order); fecal incontinence may be present if a perineal prostatectomy were performed.
   d. Monitor vital signs; hematuria is expected; report frank bleeding or clots.
   e. Use an oral thermometer (no rectal treatments).
   f. Encourage patient to avoid straining; encourage fluids; provide stool softeners.
   g. Observe for bladder spasms; note if catheter is draining freely; irrigate by syringe as ordered; administer antispasmodics.
   h. Administer analgesic as needed for postoperative pain.
   i. Monitor intake and output; record all drainage tubes separately.
   j. Provide sitz bath for pain and inflammation if perineal prostatectomy were performed.
   k. Provide care instructions if patient is discharged with indwelling catheter.

Cancer of the Prostate

A. Definition: a malignant tumor; no symptoms occur until it has become large or metastasized.

B. Cause: unknown; increased incidence with age (all men older than 40 years should have rectal examinations yearly)
C. Signs and symptoms
   1. Early tumor has no symptoms.
   2. Subjective
      a. Back pain
      b. Frequency, nocturia, dysuria, urinary retention
   3. Objective: symptoms from metastasis
D. Diagnostic tests and methods
   1. Rectal examination
   2. Biopsy examination
   3. Acid phosphatase
   4. Transrectal ultrasonography
   5. Prostate-specific antigen (PSA) level
   6. Serum alkaline phosphatase level (elevated in bone metastasis)
   7. Bone scan to assess metastasis
   8. MRI, CT
E. Treatment surgery
   1. Radical perineal prostatectomy (removal of prostate, capsule, and seminal vesicles)
   2. Bilateral orchiectomy (removal of both testicles)
   3. TURP
   4. Estrogen therapy
   5. Agonists of luteinizing hormone–releasing hormone
   6. Radiation (external, interstitial, spot)
F. Nursing intervention
   1. See nursing intervention for a patient with BPH.
   2. Be supportive as concerns are expressed about a malignancy and feminization from estrogens; answer questions; refer problems to physician.
   3. Control pain for terminally ill patient; hospice care may be considered.

Hydrocele

A. Definition: a cystic mass filled with fluid that forms around the testicle
B. Causes
   1. Infection
   2. Trauma
C. Signs and symptoms
   1. Swelling of testicle
   2. Discomfort in sitting and walking
D. Diagnostic tests and methods: assessment by physical examination
E. Treatment
   1. Aspiration (usually only in children)
   2. Injection of a sclerosing solution
   3. Surgical removal of the sac (hydrocelectomy)
F. Nursing intervention
   1. Provide usual preoperative and postoperative care (see Chapter 2).
   2. Scrotal support (elevation) may be necessary during postoperative period.
   3. Be supportive to concerns expressed by patient.

Cancer of the Testes

A. Definition: an uncommon malignancy; usually, no systemic symptoms are present until metastasis occurs; can be diagnosed early only by examination and finding a hard, non-tender mass (testicular self-examination should be done monthly); age of incidence is usually in early 30s.

B. Treatment
   1. Surgery: orchiectomy
   2. Radiotherapy
   3. Chemotherapy
   4. Possibly radical: lymph node dissection
C. Nursing intervention: related to treatment selected
D. Teach monthly preventative testicular self-examination.

FEMALE REPRODUCTIVE SYSTEM

Anatomy and Physiology

A. External genitals
   1. Vulva
      a. Labia majora: two long folds of skin on each side of the vaginal orifice outside of the labia minora
      b. Labia minora: two flat, thin, delicate folds of skin that are highly sensitive to manipulation and trauma; enclose the region called the vestibule, which contains the clitoris, the urethral orifice, and the vaginal orifice
      c. Clitoris: very sensitive erectile tissue; becomes swollen with blood during sexual excitement
      d. Vaginal orifice: opening into vagina; hymen, fold of mucosa, partially closes orifice and is generally ruptured during first sexual intercourse.
      e. Bartholin's glands: located on each side of vaginal orifice; secrete lubrication fluid
   2. Perineum: between vaginal orifice and anus; forms pelvic floor
B. Internal organs (Figure 5-20)
   1. Ovaries: main sex glands
      a. Located on either side in pelvic cavity
      b. Produce ova, which form in the Graafian follicles
      c. Graafian follicle produces estrogen.
      d. Rupture of a follicle releases an ovum (ovulation).
      e. Ruptured follicles become glandular mass called corpus luteum.
      f. Corpus luteum secretes estrogen, but mainly progesterone.
   2. Fallopian tubes
      a. Extend from point near ovaries to uterus; no direct connection between ovaries and tubes
      b. Fimbriae: fingerlike extensions on tubes; pick up ova and transport into fallopian tubes
      c. Fertilization occurs in outer one third of the fallopian tubes.
   3. Uterus
      a. Upper portion rests on upper surface of bladder; the lower portion is embedded in pelvic floor between the bladder and the rectum.
      b. Pear-shaped, hollow organ that expands tremendously to accommodate a fetus
      c. Divisions
         (1) Body: upper main part
         (2) Fundus: bulging upper surface of the body
         (3) Cervix: neck of the uterus
      d. Endometrium: uterine lining; sloughs off during menstruation
      e. Functions
         (1) Menstruation
         (2) Pregnancy
         (3) Labor

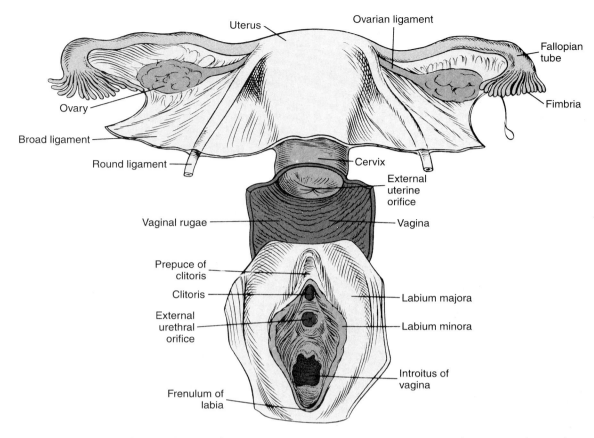

FIGURE 5-20. Female internal organs of reproduction. Major ligaments are shown. *(From Phipps WJ, Sands JK, Lehman MK, Cassmeyer VL: Medical-surgical nursing: concepts and clinical practice, ed 5, St Louis, 1995, Mosby.)*

4. Vagina
   a. Located between rectum and urethra
   b. Structure: wrinkled mucous membrane (rugae); capable of great distention
   c. Functions
      (1) Lower part of birth canal
      (2) Receives semen from male
      (3) Passageway for menstrual flow
C. Breasts (mammary glands)
   1. Located over pectoral muscles
   2. Size depends on adipose tissue rather than glandular tissue.
   3. Consists of lobes, lobules, and milk-secreting cells (acini)
   4. Ducts lead to the opening called the nipple.
   5. Areola: pigmented area surrounding the nipple
D. Function
   1. Reproduction
   2. Production of estrogen and progesterone
E. Menstrual cycle (Figure 5-21)
   1. Phases: regulated primarily by the hormonal control of pituitary gland, ovaries, and uterus
      a. One ovum discharged each month from an ovary; ripens in the Graafian follicle; follicle-stimulating hormone (FSH) from anterior lobe of pituitary stimulates the formation of the follicle.
      b. Estrogen produced by the follicle builds up the endometrium in expectation of a fertilized ovum.

   c. Ovum is discharged into the fallopian tube by luteinizing hormone (LH) from the anterior lobe pituitary; follicle is converted into the corpus luteum.
   d. Postovulation: corpus luteum secretes progesterone and estrogen for final preparation of the endometrium.
   e. Premenstrual: the gradual drop in progesterone and estrogen leads to menses.
   2. Length of cycle: usually 28 days; highly variable; ovulation occurs midway.
   3. Menopause (climacteric) the gradual cessation of menstrual cycle; the ability to bear children ends; occurs at approximately 45 years of age
      a. Ovaries lose their ability to respond to hormones.
      b. Decrease in levels of estrogen and progesterone
         (1) Failure to ovulate
         (2) Monthly flow is less, is irregular, and gradually ceases.
         (3) Reproductive organs atrophy.

FEMALE REPRODUCTIVE SYSTEM CONDITIONS AND DISORDERS

Childbearing is the major physiological function of the female reproductive system. Disorders of this system are distressing to the patient because of interference with sexuality, conception,

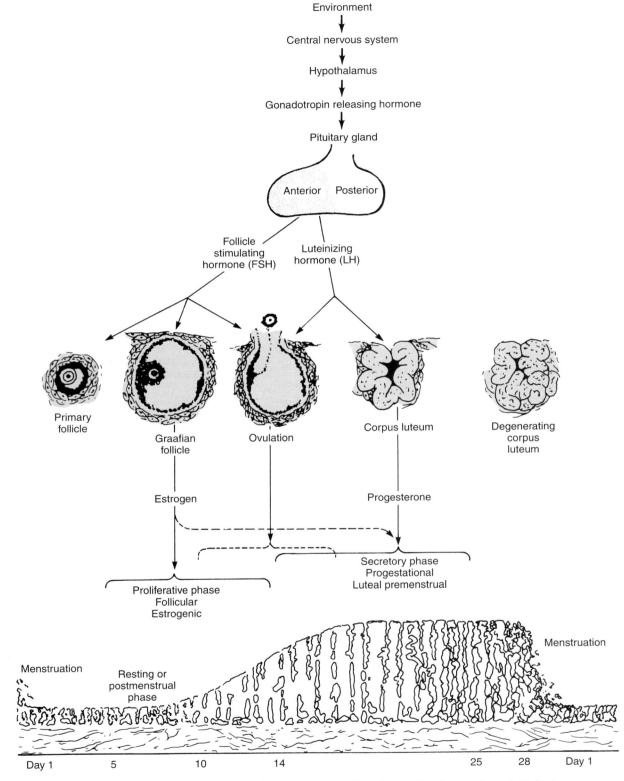

FIGURE 5-21. Hormonal control of menstrual cycle. *(From Phipps, Monahan, Sands, et al.* Medical-Surgical Nursing health and illness perspectives, *ed. 7, St. Louis, 2003, Mosby.)*

and self-image. The nurse plays an important role by clearly providing information to the concerned patient.

Nursing Assessment

A. Nursing observations (objective data)
1. General appearance
2. Vital signs
3. Weight
4. Breasts
   a. Contour
   b. Skin dimpling
   c. Nodules
      (1) Size
      (2) Consistency
      (3) Mobile or fixed
   d. Nipples
      (1) Asymmetry
      (2) Retraction
      (3) Rash
      (4) Ulceration
      (5) Discharge
5. External genitalia
   a. Irritation
   b. Redness
   c. Excoriation
   d. Bulge
6. Introitus
   a. Irritation
   b. Redness
   c. Excoriation
   d. Nodules
7. Discharge
   a. Color
   b. Malodorous
   c. Consistency
B. Patient description (subjective data)
1. Lower abdominal pain and cramping
2. Backache
3. Stress incontinence
4. Urinary frequency and urgency
5. Urine or fecal material draining from vaginal tract
6. Breasts
   a. Tenderness
   b. Burning
   c. Swelling
   d. Pain
   e. Nipples: tenderness, burning
7. External genitalia
   a. Itching
   b. Burning
8. Introitus
   a. Burning
   b. Itching
   c. Tenderness
   d. Dyspareunia (painful intercourse)
9. Menstrual cycle
   a. Duration of cycles
   b. Number of days between cycles
   c. Associated symptoms
      (1) Pain
      (2) Headache
      (3) Irritability
      (4) Depression
      (5) Insomnia

Diagnostic Tests and Methods

A. Serum laboratory studies
1. Luteinizing hormone (LH)
   a. Stimulates progesterone secretion
   b. Diminished levels may relate to prolonged, heavy menses.
   c. Elevated levels may result in short, scanty menses.
2. Follicle-stimulating hormone (FSH)
   a. Stimulates estrogen secretion
   b. Diminished levels may relate to bleeding between cycles.
   c. Elevated levels may result in excessive uterine bleeding.
3. Thyroid function tests
   a. Used to rule out menstrual abnormality secondary to thyroid dysfunction
   b. Diminished thyroid hormone secretion may result in bleeding between cycles, irregular menses, or absence of menstrual flow.
4. Adrenal function tests
   a. Used to rule out menstrual abnormality secondary to adrenal dysfunction
   b. Elevated or decreased production of adrenal cortex hormone secretion may result in amenorrhea.
B. Procedures
1. Pelvic examination: to inspect and assess the external genitalia, perineal and anal areas, introitus, vaginal tract, and cervix
   a. Have patient empty bladder.
   b. Place patient in the lithotomy position.
   c. Flex and abduct patient's thighs.
   d. Place patient's feet in stirrups.
   e. Extend patient's buttocks slightly beyond the edge of the examining table.
2. Laparoscopy: visualization of the pelvic structures with a lighted laparoscope inserted through the abdominal wall
3. Culdoscopy: visualization of the ovaries, fallopian tubes, and uterus with a lighted instrument inserted through the vaginal tract
   a. After procedure, position patient on abdomen to expel air.
   b. Monitor for vaginal bleeding.
   c. Instruct patient to abstain from intercourse, douching, and using tampons until advised by physician.
4. Colposcopy: visualization of the cervix with an instrument that magnifies tissue
5. Papanicolaou smear test (Pap smear): a sample of cervical scrapings is obtained for study under a microscope for evidence of malignant cell changes
   a. Follow nursing actions as those in a pelvic examination.
   b. Write patient's name on the frost side of the slide, handling edges only.
   c. Smear the specimen on a glass slide.
   d. Place a drop of a fixative, dry, and send to laboratory.
   e. Reinforce importance of Pap smears as recommended by the American Cancer Society.
6. Cervical biopsy examination: removal of tissue to examine for presence of malignancy

a. After procedure, advise patient to rest and avoid strenuous activity for 24 hours.

b. Leave packing in place until physician permits removal (usually 12 to 24 hours).

c. Monitor for vaginal bleeding.

d. Instruct patient to abstain from intercourse, douching, and use of tampons until advised by physician.

e. Explain that a malodorous discharge that may last 3 weeks will occur; daily bath should help control this discharge.

7. Conization

a. Removal of cone-shaped tissue of the cervix for analysis of cancerous cells

b. Indicated for removal of diseased cervical tissue

c. Nursing interventions

(1) Maintain packing 12 to 24 hours.

(2) Monitor for bleeding.

(3) Instruct patient to abstain from intercourse, douching, and using tampons until advised by physician.

8. Schiller's test

a. Application of a dye to the cervix to aid in detecting cancerous cells

b. Normal vaginal cells will stain a deep brown.

c. Abnormal cells with not absorb the dye.

d. Nursing intervention: recommend to patient that a perineal pad be used to protect clothes from stain.

9. Ultrasonography

a. A sound frequency that reflects an image of the pelvic structures

b. An aid in confirming ovarian and uterine tumors

10. Culture and sensitivity

a. The culture of a specimen of exudate suspected of infection

b. The sensitivity of an antibiotic to the micro-organism

11. Dilatation and curettage (D & C)

a. A diagnostic and therapeutic procedure

b. The cervix is dilated to scrape the lining of the uterine cavity with a curet.

c. Nursing intervention

(1) After procedure, provide sterile perineal pads and record amount of drainage.

(2) Encourage voiding to prevent urinary retention.

(3) Instruct patient to abstain from intercourse, douching, and using tampons until advised by physician.

12. Mammography: an x-ray examination of the breasts to detect tumors; screening test is done yearly for women over 40 years of age.

13. Thermography: infrared photography used to detect breast tumors

14. Xerography: an x-ray examination of the breasts and skin that provides good definition of the tissue

15. CT, MRI

Frequent Patient Problems and Nursing Care

A. Anxiety related to modesty

1. Keep the patient's body covered at all times.

2. Provide privacy.

3. Speak with the patient during the examination or procedure.

B. Deficient knowledge related to understanding of menstruation

1. Provide factual information related to the process of menstruation.

2. Describe abnormalities associated with menstruation.

3. Describe emotional changes associated with menstruation.

4. Teach menstrual hygiene.

a. Change perineal pad or tampon every 3 to 4 hours.

b. Remove napkin front to back.

c. Alternate sanitary napkins and tampons daily to prevent toxic shock syndrome or backflow of menstruation.

C. Deficient knowledge related to menstrual abnormalities: explain which menstrual symptoms are considered abnormal.

1. Flow occurring more frequently than every 21 days

2. Flow occurring less frequently than every 35 days

3. Duration of less than 3 days

4. Duration of more than 7 days

5. Use of 12 or more perineal pads per 24 hours

D. Acute pain related to menstruation

1. Assess location, duration, onset, and quality of pain.

2. Apply heating pad to the abdomen.

3. Provide warm liquids of patient's choice.

4. Provide massage to lumbar area.

5. Provide pain relief medication as ordered by physician.

E. Deficient knowledge related to breast self-examination (BSE)

1. Recommend that breasts be examined 7 days after onset of menstruation every month (Figure 5-22).

2. Instruct patient on technique of BSE.

a. Inspect breasts in front of mirror with arms at sides.

b. Observe breasts with arms raised above the head.

c. With hands on hips, lean forward and contract chest muscles.

3. Lying supine, palpate each breast with flat part of fingers, and continue in a circular movement to nipple.

4. Observations of the breasts

a. Size

b. Symmetry

c. Skin texture

d. Color

e. Nipple position

f. Nipple discharge

F. Deficient knowledge related to menopause

1. Describe accompanying symptoms associated with menopause.

a. Irregular menses

b. Hot flashes

c. Night sweats

d. Insomnia

e. Depression

f. Anxiety

2. Onset is usually after age 40 years.

3. Explain that menopause does not interfere with sexuality.

4. Recommend use of lubricant before intercourse.

5. Recommend use of contraception for 6 months after the last menstrual period.

How to do BSE
1. Lie down and put a pillow under your right shoulder. Place your right arm behind your head.
2. Use the finger pads of the three middle fingers on your left hand to feel for lumps or thickening. Your finger pads are the top third of each finger.

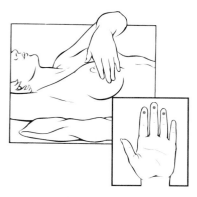

3. Press hard enough to know how your breast feels. If you're not sure how hard to press, ask your health care provider. Or try to copy the way your health care provider uses the finger pads during a breast exam. Learn what your breast feels like most of the time. A firm ridge in the lower curve of each breast is normal.

4. Move around the breast in a set way. You can choose either the circle (A), the up and down line (B), or the wedge (C). Do it the same way every time. It will help you to make sure that you've gone over the entire breast area and to remember how your breast feels each month.

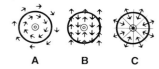

5. Now examine your left breast using right hand finger pads.
You might want to check your breasts while standing in front of a mirror right after you do your BSE each month. You might also want to do an extra BSE while you're in the shower. Your soapy hands will glide over the wet skin making it easy to check how your breasts feel.

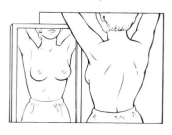

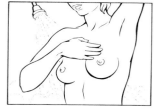

FIGURE 5-22. Breast self-examination. (*Courtesy American Cancer Society.*)

Major Medical Diagnoses
Menstrual Abnormalities
Dysmenorrhea
A. Definition: intense pain at the time of menses
B. Cause: uterine spasms cause cramping of the lower abdomen.
C. Signs and symptoms
  1. Subjective
    a. Headache, backache
    b. Abdominal pain
    c. Chills
    d. Nausea
  2. Objective
    a. Fever
    b. Vomiting
D. Diagnostic method: pelvic examination to rule out other physical disorders
E. Treatment
  1. Analgesics, such as nonsteroidal antiinflammatory agents
  2. Local application of heat
  3. Pelvic exercises
  4. D & C

F. Nursing intervention
  1. Instruct patient on avoidance of fatigue and overexertion during menstrual period.
  2. Instruct patient on ingestion of warm beverages before onset of pain to prevent attack.

Premenstrual tension syndrome (PMS)
A. Definition: a large number of symptoms occurring a few days before menstruation
B. Cause: cause is unclear; may be related to fluid retention combined with emotional tension; usually disappears with onset of menstruation
C. Signs and symptoms
  1. Subjective
    a. Breast tenderness
    b. Headache
    c. Nausea
    d. Depression
    e. Insomnia
    f. Irritability
    g. Fatigue
  2. Objective: weight gain 2 to 10 days before onset of menstruation

D. Diagnostic method: assessment of specific symptoms and psychological health
E. Treatment
1. Diuretics
2. Mild sodium restriction
3. Mild tranquilizers
4. Well-balanced diet
5. Exercise
F. Nursing intervention
1. Assist patient in following a diet with decreased sodium content.
2. Instruct patient to decrease consumption of coffee, alcohol, and nicotine during latter half of menstrual cycle.

Amenorrhea

A. Definition: absence of menstrual periods
B. Causes
1. Diabetes
2. Debilitating illness
3. Malnutrition
4. Obesity
5. Extreme anxiety
6. Anemia
7. Oral contraceptives
8. Chronic nephritis
9. Tumors of the endocrine glands
C. Signs and symptoms
1. Subjective: anxiety
2. Objective
a. Absence of menses by age 17 years (primary amenorrhea)
b. Failure of a menstrual period (secondary amenorrhea)
D. Diagnostic tests and methods
1. Pelvic examination
2. LH level
3. FSH level
4. Thyroid function test
5. Adrenal function test
E. Treatment: according to cause
F. Nursing intervention
1. Encourage the patient to follow prescribed orders to ensure success of therapeutic plan.
2. Provide clear explanations related to cause of disorder to decrease anxiety.

Menorrhagia (Hypermenorrhea)

A. Definition: excessive menstrual flow (amount or duration)
B. Causes
1. Uterine tumors
2. Pelvic inflammatory disease
3. Endocrine disturbances
C. Signs and symptoms
1. Subjective
a. Feeling of pelvic heaviness
b. Fatigue
2. Objective
a. Profuse menstrual bleeding with clots
b. Pale, tired appearance
D. Diagnostic tests and methods
1. Pelvic examination
2. LH level
3. FSH level

4. Thyroid function test
5. Adrenal function test
6. RBC count
E. Treatment
1. According to cause
2. D & C
F. Nursing intervention
1. Encourage intake of foods high in iron content.
2. Encourage planned rest periods.
3. Instruct the patient to count number of pads used during an abnormal period.
4. Weigh each pad before and after use to estimate blood loss.

Metrorrhagia

A. Definition: bleeding between menstrual intervals
B. Pathology
1. Causes are similar to those of menorrhagia.
2. Breakthrough bleeding may occur with use of contraceptive pills.
3. May be early symptom of cervical cancer
C. Signs and symptoms
1. Subjective
a. Feeling of pelvic heaviness
b. Fatigue
2. Objective
a. Spotting or bleeding between menstrual periods
b. Tired appearance
D. Diagnostic tests and methods
1. Pelvic examination
2. LH level
3. FSH level
4. Thyroid function test
5. Adrenal function test
6. RBC count
7. Pap smear
E. Treatment: according to cause
F. Nursing intervention
1. Instruct the patient on how to keep accurate records of bleeding episodes.
2. Encourage continued medical follow-up because of possible cervical changes associated with cancer.

Vaginitis

A. Definition: inflammation of the vaginal mucosa
B. Pathology
1. Invasion of virulent organisms permitted by changes in normal flora; pH becomes alkaline.
2. Causes
a. Trichomoniasis: parasitic organism
b. *Candida albicans* (moniliasis): fungal organism
c. Atrophic (senile): occurs in postmenopausal women because of atrophy of vaginal mucosa
d. Bacterial: invasion by staphylococci, streptococci, *Escherichia coli,* Chlamydia, or *Gardnerella vaginalis*
e. Foreign body
f. Allergens or irritants
C. Signs and symptoms
1. Trichomoniasis: thick, white or yellow, frothy, malodorous discharge causing itching, burning, and excoriation of vulva
2. Monilial: thick or watery, white or yellow, curdlike discharge; mucosa becomes reddened.

3. Atrophic: blood-flecked discharge with burning and itching of the vagina and dyspareunia

4. Bacterial: profuse, yellow mucoid discharge with irritation to vulva and urethra; fishy or foul odor

5. Foreign body: blood-tinged serosanguineous or purulent discharge; foul odor; may be thin or thick

6. Allergens, irritants: increase in usual secretions, itching, burning, rash

D. Diagnostic tests and methods: culture and sensitivity, pelvic examination

E. Treatment

1. Trichomoniasis: metronidazole (Flagyl), Floraquin tablets administered vaginally, and carbarsone suppositories administered rectally; sitz baths to relieve itching

2. Candidiasis: nystatin (Mycostatin) or miconazole (Monistat) creme daily for 14 days; sitz baths to relieve itching

3. Atrophic: antibiotics and estrogen therapy

4. Bacterial: antibiotics and sulfonamide creams

5. Foreign body: removal of object; use of antibiotics

6. Allergens or irritants: removal of cause; use of topical steroid ointment if necessary

F. Nursing intervention

1. Reassure the patient during vaginal examination to decrease anxiety.

2. Instruct patient on perineal hygiene: cleansing front to back.

3. In the event of trichomoniasis, instruct patient to abstain from intercourse, or have partner wear a condom, because this infection can be transmitted.

4. Advise patient to use perineal pads because of increased discharge.

5. Teach patient importance of compliance with treatment.

Uterine Cancer (Endometrium)

A. Definition: new growth of abnormal cells in the uterine lining

B. Pathology

1. Spreads to cervix, fallopian tubes, ovaries, bladder, and rectum

2. Associated factors are women over 50 years of age, obesity, diabetes, and hypertension

3. Prognosis is good if identified in early stages.

C. Signs and symptoms

1. Subjective

a. Postmenopausal bleeding

b. Bleeding between cycles

c. Bleeding after intercourse

d. Watery vaginal discharge

2. Objective

a. Uterine enlargement

b. Suspicious Pap test results

D. Diagnostic tests and methods

1. D & C

2. Tissue biopsy examination

E. Treatment

1. Surgical intervention

a. Panhysterectomy (removal of uterus and cervix)

b. Oophorectomy (removal of ovaries)

c. Salpingectomy (removal of fallopian tubes)

2. Chemotherapy

3. Radiation

F. Nursing intervention: see cancer of the cervix.

Uterine Fibroid Tumors

A. Definition: a benign tumor located in the uterus

B. Pathology

1. Develops slowly; symptoms occur only in relation to size, location, and number of tumors present.

2. Occurs in 25% of women over 35 years of age

C. Signs and symptoms

1. Subjective

a. Menstrual disturbances

b. Backache

c. Frequent urination

d. Constipation

2. Objective; uterine enlargement

D. Diagnostic tests and methods

1. Pelvic examination

2. Laparoscopy

E. Treatment

1. Excision of the myoma is indicated for small tumors

2. Hysterectomy (removal of uterus) with preservation of ovaries is indicated for large tumors

F. Nursing intervention

1. Explain to the patient that tumors may decrease in size after menopause.

2. Encourage the patient to verbalize concerns.

3. If patient undergoes myomectomy, follow general postoperative nursing measures related to abdominal surgery.

4. If the patient undergoes a hysterectomy, follow nursing interventions, cancer of the cervix.

Endometriosis

A. Definition: tissue resembling the endometrial membrane grows in another location in the pelvic cavity

B. Pathology

1. During menstrual period, endometrial cells are stimulated by ovarian hormone.

2. Bleeding into surrounding tissue occurs, causing inflammation.

3. Condition may result in adhesions, fusion of pelvic organs, bladder dysfunction, stricture of bowel, or sterility.

C. Signs and symptoms: symptoms usually appear in women over 30 years of age.

1. Subjective

a. Discomfort of pelvic area before menses, becoming worse during menstrual flow, and diminishing as flow ceases

b. Dyspareunia

c. Fatigue

2. Objective: infertility

D. Diagnostic tests and methods

1. Laparoscopy

2. Culdoscopy

E. Treatment

1. Hormonal therapy to suppress ovulation

2. Surgical intervention: hysterectomy, oophorectomy, or salpingectomy

F. Nursing intervention

1. Provide emotional support.

2. If patient is young, advise not to delay having a family because of risk of sterility.`

3. Explain that hormonal drug may cause pseudopregnancy and irregular bleeding.

4. If patient is middle aged, advise her that menopause may stop progression of condition.
5. Follow general postoperative nursing actions if the patient undergoes surgical procedure.
   a. Observe for vaginal hemorrhage, malodorous vaginal discharge, or vaginal discharge other than serosanguineous discharge.
   b. Observe for urine retention, burning, frequency, or urgency to void.
   c. Listen for renewed bowel sounds.
6. Provide patient teaching on discharge.
   a. Heavy lifting, prolonged standing, walking, and sitting are contraindicated.
   b. Sexual intercourse should be avoided until approved by physician.

Pelvic Inflammatory Disease (PID)

A. Definition: inflammation of the pelvic cavity
B. Pathology
   1. Pathogenic organisms are introduced into the cervix.
   2. PID may be confined to one or more structures: fallopian tubes, ovaries, pelvic peritoneum, pelvic veins, or pelvic tissue.
   3. May result in adhesions, strictures, or sterility
   4. Most common causative organism: gonococcus
   5. Also caused by staphylococci or streptococci
C. Signs and symptoms
   1. Subjective
      a. Abdominal pain
      b. Pelvic pain
      c. Low-back pain
      d. Nausea
   2. Objective
      a. Malodorous, purulent discharge
      b. Fever
      c. Vomiting
D. Diagnostic tests and method: culture and sensitivity test, CBC, pelvic examination, laparoscopy
E. Treatment
   1. Antibiotic therapy
   2. Analgesics
F. Nursing intervention
   1. Provide nonjudgmental, accepting attitude.
   2. Place patient in semi-Fowler's position to provide dependent pelvic drainage.
   3. Apply heat to abdominal area if ordered to improve circulation and provide comfort.
   4. Patient teaching should include the following:
      a. Take shower instead of tub bath.
      b. Perform perineal hygiene: wipe from front to back.
      c. Learn how to recognize if sexual partner is infected with gonococcus: discharge from penis of whitish fluid with painful urination (not all males are symptomatic).
      d. Learn the importance of routine physical examinations because gonococcal infection is asymptomatic in women.
      e. Reinforce "safe sex" guidelines.

Vaginal Fistula

A. Definition: tubelike opening between two internal organs
B. Pathology
   1. Causes include radiation therapy, gynecological surgery, or traumatic childbirth.
   2. Results in impaired blood supply and sloughing of tissue, leading to abnormal opening
   3. Four types affect female reproductive organs
      a. Ureterovaginal: between ureter and vagina; urine leaks into vagina.
      b. Vesicovaginal: between bladder and vagina; urine leaks into vagina.
      c. Urethrovaginal: between urethra and vagina; urine leaks into vagina.
      d. Rectovaginal: between rectum and vagina; flatus and fecal matter leak into vagina.
C. Signs and symptoms
   1. Subjective
      a. Leakage of urine, flatus, and fecal matter
      b. Pain in affected area
   2. Objective
      a. Excoriation
      b. Malodor
D. Diagnostic methods
   1. Symptoms and physical examination
   2. Patient history of radiation therapy
   3. Intravenous pyelogram (IVP)
   4. Cystoscopy
E. Treatment
   1. Small fistula may heal spontaneously.
   2. Surgical excision
   3. Temporary colostomy for rectovaginal fistula
F. Nursing intervention
   1. Provide psychological support: offer reassurance and acceptance.
   2. Encourage patient to verbalize feelings; express empathy.
   3. Observe vaginal discharge and record.
   4. Change perineal pad every 4 hours and prn.
   5. Instruct on perineal hygiene.
   6. Provide sitz bath and irrigation solutions for hygiene if ordered.
   7. Follow general postoperative nursing actions if patient undergoes surgery.
      a. Observe Foley catheter for drainage at all times.
      b. Caution patient not to strain when having a bowel movement.

Prolapsed Uterus

A. Definition: downward displacement of the uterus through the vaginal orifice
B. Pathology
   1. A result of weakened supporting muscles and ligaments of the pelvis
   2. Causes include childbirth injuries, repeated pregnancies with short intervals between, menopausal atrophy, and congenital weakness
C. Signs and symptoms
   1. Subjective
      a. Pain in lower abdomen
      b. Feeling of pressure within pelvis
      c. Stress incontinence
      d. Dyspareunia
      e. Backache
   2. Objective
      a. Urinary stasis

b. Elongated cervix
D. Diagnostic methods
1. Signs and symptoms
2. Pelvic examination
E. Treatment
1. Placement of a pessary in the vagina to support uterus
2. Surgical suspension of the uterus
3. Hysterectomy if condition is postmenopausal
F. Nursing intervention
1. Approach unhurriedly, demonstrate calmness, and encourage expression of feelings to decrease anxiety.
2. Explain all procedures.
3. Follow general postoperative nursing actions.
   a. Chart number of perineal pads used during 8-hour period.
   b. Observe for hemorrhage.
   c. Observe for vaginal discharge other than serosanguineous fluid.
   d. Listen for renewed bowel sounds.
   e. Observe for urinary retention and pelvic congestion.

Cystocele and Rectocele

A. Definition
1. Cystocele: abnormal protrusion of the bladder against the vaginal wall
2. Rectocele: abnormal protrusion of part of the rectum against the vaginal wall
B. Pathology
1. Result of weakened supporting muscles and ligaments of the pelvis
2. Causes include childbirth injuries, repeated pregnancies with short intervals between, menopausal atrophy, and congenital weakness.
C. Signs and symptoms
1. Subjective
   a. Pelvic pressure, backache
   b. Stress incontinence, dysuria (cystocele)
   c. Constipation or incontinence of feces and flatus (rectocele)
2. Objective
   a. Residual urine after voiding (cystocele)
   b. Hemorrhoids (rectocele)
D. Diagnostic methods
1. Signs and symptoms
2. Pelvic examination
E. Treatment
1. Anterior colporrhaphy to adjust cystocele
2. Posterior colporrhaphy to adjust rectocele
F. Nursing intervention
1. Administer catheter care twice a day (bid) and prn.
2. Splint abdomen when coughing.
3. Place in low-Fowler's position or flat in bed to avoid pressure on suture line.
4. Explain to the patient that she should respond to bowel stimuli to avoid suture strain.
5. After each bowel movement, clean perineum with warm water and soap; pat dry anterior to posterior.
6. Apply heat lamp, anesthetic spray, or ice packs if ordered to relieve discomfort.
7. Provide patient teaching.
   a. Heavy lifting and prolonged standing, walking, and sitting are contraindicated.

b. Sexual intercourse should be avoided until approved by physician.
c. Perform pelvic exercises.

Ovarian Tumors

A. Definition: a mass of tissue growing on the ovary; usually asymptomatic until large enough to cause pressure
B. Pathology: two classifications
1. Ovarian cyst: a benign condition but may transform to a malignancy; may be small, containing clear fluid, or may be filled with a thick, yellow fluid; size varies
2. Malignant tumors: a cancerous growth found on the ovary; can be the primary site of the cancer or secondary site caused by metastasis from the GI tract, breast, pancreas, or kidneys
C. Signs and symptoms
1. Subjective
   a. Pelvic pain
   b. Menstrual disturbances
   c. Abdominal distention
   d. Constipation
   e. Dyspareunia
2. Objective: palpable mass
D. Diagnostic tests and methods
1. Culdoscopy
2. Ultrasonography
3. Biopsy examination
E. Treatment
1. Cyst may be observed for regression in size.
2. Oophorectomy (removal of ovaries)
3. Removal of all reproductive organs
4. Estrogen replacement therapy
5. X-ray therapy and chemotherapy
6. Radiation therapy
F. Nursing intervention
1. If patient undergoes oophorectomy, follow general postoperative nursing care related to abdominal surgery.
2. If the patient undergoes surgery for removal of all abdominal reproductive organs, follow nursing intervention covered later under cancer of the cervix.
3. Assist the patient in dealing with changes of body image.

Cancer of the Cervix

A. Definition: new growth of abnormal cells in the neck of the uterus
B. Pathology
1. Early stage is confined to epithelial cervical layer
2. Will continue to invade surrounding area such as bladder and rectum
3. Metastasizes to lungs, bones, and liver
4. Relationship exists between cervical cancer and infection with the human papilloma virus (HPV)
C. Signs and symptoms
1. Subjective
   a. Asymptomatic in early stage
   b. Menstrual disturbances
   c. Postmenopausal bleeding
   d. Bleeding after intercourse
   e. Watery discharge
2. Objective: suspicious Pap test result
D. Diagnostic tests and methods
1. Pap smear

2. Cervical biopsy examination
3. Colposcopy
4. Schiller's test
5. Conization

E. Treatment
1. Panhysterectomy (excision of uterus and cervix)
2. Radiation in advanced case
3. Chemotherapy

F. Nursing intervention
1. Reassure the patient and family that adjustment to illness can be slow.
2. Acknowledge that the patient must adapt to illness according to her age, developmental stage, and past life experiences.
3. If patient is to receive internal radium implant:
   a. Provide isolation.
   b. Instruct the patient to maintain supine or side-lying position.
   c. Explain to the patient and visitors that the amount of time spent with patient will be limited to avoid overexposure to radiation.
   d. Provide high-protein, low-residue diet to avoid straining of bowels, which may dislodge implant.
   e. Maintain high fluid intake: 2000 to 3000 ml daily.
   f. Insert Foley catheter to prevent bladder distention.
   g. Administer antiemetics as ordered.
4. If the patient undergoes surgery, follow general postoperative nursing actions.
   a. Observe for vaginal hemorrhage, malodorous vaginal discharge, or any vaginal discharge other than serosanguineous discharge.
   b. Observe for urinary retention.
   c. Change perineal pads every 3 to 4 hours and prn.
   d. Listen for renewed bowel sounds.

Bartholin Cysts

A. Definition: a tumorlike capsule formed from retained secretions
B. Pathology
1. May develop as a consequence of an earlier bacterial infection of these structures
2. Formation of these cysts results from obstruction in the outlet of these glands.
C. Signs and symptoms
1. Subjective
   a. Pain on walking
   b. Dyspareunia
2. Objective: mobile nodule
D. Diagnostic methods
1. Pelvic examination
2. Palpable nodule
E. Treatment
1. Incision and drainage
2. Antiseptic wound packing
F. Nursing intervention
1. Reassure the patient that normal function of the gland will be regained after the procedure.
2. After surgery, provide a sterile perineal pad every 4 hours and prn.
3. Provide sterile wound care as ordered.
4. Instruct on perineal hygiene.
5. Provide sitz baths for increased circulation and comfort.

6. On patient's discharge from the hospital, explain that the surgical wound is susceptible to bacterial infection until healing has taken place.

Fibrocystic Breast Disease

A. Definition: fiberlike tumors of the breast tissue with cyst formation
B. Pathology
1. Cause is unknown; possible hormonal imbalance
2. Condition occurs during reproductive years and disappears with menopause.
3. A benign condition affecting 25% of women over 30 years of age
C. Signs and symptoms
1. Subjective: breast tenderness and pain
2. Objective: small, round, smooth nodules
D. Diagnostic tests and methods
1. Mammography
2. Thermomastography
3. Xerography
E. Treatment: conservative
1. Aspiration
2. Biopsy examination to rule out malignancy
F. Nursing intervention
1. Explain importance of monthly breast self-examination.
2. Encourage patient to seek medical evaluation if nodule forms, because cystic disease may interfere with early diagnosis of breast malignancy.

Cancer of the Breast

A. Definition: small, painless, fixed lump most frequently located in the upper, outer portion of the breast
B. Pathology
1. Risk factors increase with age.
2. Influenced by heredity
3. Sites of metastasis: lymph nodes, lungs, liver, bone, brain
4. Other risk factors
   a. Obesity
   b. Diet high in fat and protein
   c. Nulliparity
   d. Parity after age 35
   e. Menarche before 11 years of age
   f. Menopause after 55 years of age
   g. History of cancer in one breast
C. Signs and symptoms
1. Subjective: nontender nodule
2. Objective:
   a. Enlarged axillary nodes
   b. Nipple retraction or elevation
   c. Skin dimpling
   d. Nipple discharge
D. Diagnostic tests and methods
1. Mammography
2. Thermography
3. Xerography
4. Breast biopsy examination
E. Treatment
1. Lumpectomy: removal of the lump and partial breast tissue; indicated for early detection
2. Mastectomy
   a. Simple mastectomy: removal of breast

b. Modified radical mastectomy: removal of breast, pectoralis minor, and some of adjacent lymph nodes (the pectoralis major is preserved)

c. Radical mastectomy: removal of the breast, pectoral muscles, pectoral fascia, and nodes

3. Oophorectomy, adrenalectomy, or hypophysectomy to remove source of estrogen and the hormones that stimulate the breast tissue

4. Radiation therapy to destroy malignant tissue

5. Chemotherapeutic agents to shrink, retard, and destroy cancer growth

6. Corticosteroids, androgens, and antiestrogens to alter cancer that is dependent on hormonal environment

F. Nursing intervention

1. Provide atmosphere of acceptance, frequent patient contact, and encouragement in illness adjustment.

2. Introduce a person who has successfully undergone the same experience: arrange contact from Reach to Recovery representative.

3. Encourage grooming activities such as hair, nails, teeth, and skin.

4. Arrange attractive environment.

5. If the patient is receiving radiation or chemotherapy, explain and assist her with potential side effects.

a. Nausea and vomiting

b. Anorexia

c. Diarrhea

d. Stomatitis

e. Malaise

f. Itching

g. Hair loss (alopecia)

6. If the patient has undergone surgical intervention, follow postoperative nursing actions.

a. Elevate affected arm above level of right atrium to prevent edema.

b. Drawing blood or administering parenteral fluids or taking blood pressure on affected arm is contraindicated.

c. Monitor dressing for hemorrhage; observe back for pooling of blood.

d. Empty Hemovac and measure drainage every 8 hours.

e. Assess circulatory status of affected limb.

f. Measure upper arm and forearm, twice daily, to monitor edema.

g. Encourage exercises of the affected arm when approved by physician; avoid abduction.

h. Assist with brushing hair.

i. Assist with squeezing ball.

j. Assist with feeding self.

7. Patient teaching on discharge

a. Exercise to tolerance.

b. Sleep with arm elevated.

c. Elevate arm several times daily.

d. Avoid injections, vaccinations, and taking of blood pressure in affected arm.

e. Never allow blood to be drawn from or IV started in affected arm.

Paget's Disease of the Breast

A. Definition: cancer of the nipple

B. Pathology

1. Rare occurrence affecting women over 40 years of age

2. Spreads from nipple to areola to part of the breasts; ulcerates

C. Signs and symptoms

1. Subjective

a. Itching

b. Swelling

2. Objective

a. Blistering

b. Discharge

c. Nipple retraction

D. Diagnostic method: biopsy examination

E. Treatment: mastectomy

F. Nursing intervention: see nursing intervention, cancer of the breast.

Sexually Transmitted Infectious Diseases

Syphilis

A. Description: caused by a spirochete, *Treponema pallidum;* appears in three stages; transmitted through sexual contact or warm blood

1. Primary stage: after an incubation period of 10 to 60 days (usually 3 weeks), during which no symptoms occur, an ulcer or chancre appears at the site of entry; it contains many organisms and is highly infectious; minor local discomfort or mild generalized symptoms may occur (e.g., headache, lymph node enlargement); without treatment, the condition heals in 3 to 5 weeks.

2. Secondary stage: 3 weeks later, it appears as a mild rash on skin (usually palms of hands and soles of feet) and as papules on mucous membranes; all lesions contain organisms and are highly contagious; symptoms may be mild or generalized (e.g., bone pain, sore throat, hair loss in patches, lymph node changes); lasts a few weeks and becomes dormant if not treated; patient is infectious for approximately 1 year.

3. Third or latent stage: 10 to 30 years later, the spirochetes, which have been deposited in tissues and organs, are in lesions (gummas); these destroy the tissue; common sites are the CNS, eyes, and the aorta.

B. Signs and symptoms: relate to organ involved

C. Diagnostic tests and methods

1. Primary stage: microscopic examination of smear

2. Second and third stages: blood serum tests (e.g., Venereal disease research laboratory [VDRL] and Rapid plasma reagin [RPR])

D. Treatment: penicillin or tetracycline (patient and partner)

Gonorrhea

A. Definition: a highly communicable disease; inflammation of the urethra occurs and spreads to other organs of the genital tract; incubation period is 3 to 4 days.

B. Cause: *Neisseria gonorrhoeae;* transmitted by sexual contact

C. Signs and symptoms

1. Female patients may have no early symptoms or purulent vaginal discharge, dysuria, or urgency; untreated, it may spread to other organs in the pelvic cavity (see PID).

2. Male patients have purulent urethral discharge and burning on urination; may develop urethral stricture, epididymitis, prostatitis

D. Diagnostic tests and methods

1. Patient history and physical examination
2. Smear or culture

E. Treatment: penicillin or tetracycline; ceftriaxone (a cephalosporin) for penicillinase-resistant strains

Herpes genitalis

A. Description: fluid-filled vesicles on genitalia form crusts, causing generalized symptoms such as elevated temperature; pain; may have no symptoms; recurrent episodes occur; problems arise in pregnancy; believed to predispose to cervical cancer
B. Cause: herpesvirus hominis type 2 (herpes simplex virus [HSV])
C. Treatment: symptomatic; topical or oral antiviral agents (acyclovir [Zovirax]); no cure
D. Recommend use of barrier forms of contraception

Chlamydia trachomatis

A. Definition: most common STD in the United States; causes symptoms similar to gonorrheal infections.
B. Cause: *Chlamydia trachomatis*
C. Signs and symptoms
   1. In men: urethritis, dysuria, frequency, watery mucoid discharge; complications include epididymitis, prostatitis, and infertility.
   2. In women: often asymptomatic; mucopurulent cervicitis, dysuria, frequency, local soreness; complications include salpingitis, PID, ectopic pregnancy, and infertility.
D. Diagnostic tests and methods: urogenital smear analysis for enzyme or antibody
E. Treatment: antibiotic therapy (doxycycline, tetracycline, erythromycin)

Condylomata acuminata

A. Definition: also referred to as genital or venereal warts; often seen with other STDs such as gonorrhea and trichomoniasis; highly contagious
B. Cause: Human papilloma virus (HPV)
C. Signs and symptoms: initially, single, small papillary growths that grow into large cauliflower-like masses, profuse foul-smelling vaginal discharge, bleeding; may progress to genital and cervical dysplasia, cancer
D. Diagnostic tests and methods: inspection of urinary meatus, vulva, labia, vagina, cervix, penis, scrotum, anus, perineum; culture and biopsy
E. Treatment
   1. Cryotherapy with liquid nitrogen or cryoprobe
   2. Laser therapy
   3. Acid treatments
   4. Surgery
   5. Chemotherapy (5FU)

Trichomoniasis, Candidiasis

A. Definition: very common STD; symptoms frequently seen only in women
B. Cause: *Trichomonas vaginalis* and *Candida albicans,* respectively
C. Signs and symptoms: itching, discharge
D. Diagnostic tests and methods: culture and inspection of affected tissues
E. Treatment: antifungals, antiprotozoal drugs (metronidazole [Flagyl])

INTEGUMENTARY SYSTEM

Anatomy and Physiology

A. Structure of skin: (Figure 5-23) includes epithelial, connective, and nerve tissue; consists of sweat and oil glands; is soft and has elasticity
   1. Epidermis: outermost layer; cells are flat and tough; no blood supply
      a. Cells undergo constant cellular change by mitosis.
      b. Contains pigment (melanin); amount of pigment varies among races and individuals.
   2. Dermis: "true skin," the inner layer, composed of living cells
      a. Connective tissue framework
      b. Contains blood vessels, nerves, hair roots, and oil and sweat glands
      c. The ridges and grooves form the pattern for fingerprints, unique to each individual.
      d. Nerve endings provide sensation (touch)
         (1) Receptors: small, round bodies (tactile corpuscles)
         (2) Located in dermis; numerous in tips of fingers, toes, and tongue
         (3) Allows perception of heat, cold, and pain
   3. Subcutaneous tissue: lies under dermis
      a. Contains fat cells, which give the skin its smooth appearance
      b. Serves as a shock absorber and insulates deeper tissues
   4. Glands
      a. Sebaceous (oil glands)
         (1) Excrete oily substance (sebum)
         (2) Keep skin soft and moist
      b. Sudoriferous (sweat glands)
         (1) Secrete perspiration
         (2) Part of the body's heating and regulating equipment
   5. Appendages
      a. Hair: covers the skin except on the palms of the hands and the soles of the feet; composed of dead keratinized cells
         (1) Shaft: the hair above the skin
         (2) Follicle: a tiny sac from which the hair root grows
      b. Nails: tightly packed cells of scaly epidermis
         (1) Roots are living cells; visible ends are dead cells.
         (2) They protect the tips of the fingers and toes.
         (3) The pink coloring comes from the blood supply in the nail bed.
B. Functions
   1. Protection: protects deeper tissues from pathogenic organisms and harmful chemicals
   2. Excretion: limited to water and urea; only a small amount of waste products are eliminated.
   3. Regulation: helps regulate body temperature and fluid content
   4. Sensory: contains millions of nerve endings that provide sensory reception to pressure, touch, pain, and temperature
   5. Vitamin-D production—effect of sunlight
C. Effects of aging: skin, hair, nails (Table 5-7)

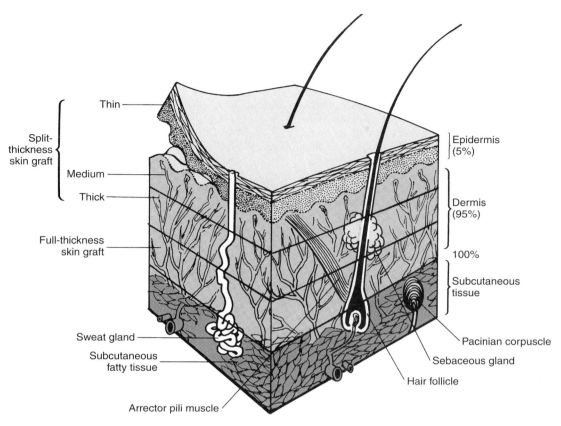

FIGURE 5-23. Structures of the skin and skin layers. *(From Phipps, Monahan, Sands, et al.* Medical-Surgical Nursing health and illness perspectives, *ed. 7, St. Louis, 2003, Mosby.)*

TABLE 5-7	Changes from Aging in Skin, Hair, and Nails	
Parameters	**Observable Changes**	**Cause**
Skin		
Color	Paleness in white skin	Decreased vascularity of dermis; loss of melanocytes
	Brown spots (senile lentigines)	Hyperpigmentation
	Purple patches (senile purpura)	Blood leaking from poorly supported, fragile capillaries
Moisture	Dry skin, decreased perspiration	Decreased sebaceous and sweat gland activity
Elasticity, turgor	Decreased elasticity	Loss of collagen and elastic fibers
	Loose folds and wrinkles	
	Decreased turgor	
Texture	Some rough areas	Environmental effects over time and decreased moisture
	Thinner, more transparent skin	Thinning of epidermis from decreased vascularity of dermis; loss of underlying tissue
Hair		
Color	Grayness	Decreased number of melanocytes in hair
Consistency	Thinner on head and body	Decreased density and rate of hair growth
	Coarser in nose of men	Increased density of nasal hair
Distribution	Loss of hair on head and body	Decreased rate of hair growth; decreased hormones; decreased peripheral circulation
	Increased hair on face of women	Higher androgen-to-estrogen ratio
Nails	More brittle	Slowing of nail growth; decreased peripheral circulation
	Longitudinal ridges	
	Thickening and yellowing of toenails	

From Phipps WJ, Monahan FD, Sands JK, Marek JF, and Neighbors M: *Medical-surgical nursing: Health and illness perspectives*, ed 7, St. Louis, 2003, Mosby.

INTEGUMENTARY SYSTEM CONDITIONS AND DISORDERS

The skin is the body's barrier and protection from the environment. It prevents loss of body fluids and protects tissues and organs from external injury and organisms. Temperature regulation, sensation, and excretion of small amounts of water and sodium chloride are functions of the skin. Maximum health and healing of the skin are maintained by proper nutrition, hydration, electrolyte balance, exercise, and rest. Problems arise from systemic allergies (e.g., food and medication; exposure to external irritants such as chemicals, plants, and cosmetics; exposure to sun, parasites, microorganisms, injury, and new growths).

The following terms are used to describe skin lesions:

Atheroma: fatty patch or thickening on skin

Bleb: blister filled with fluid

Bulla: large blister filled with fluid, as occurs with burns

Comedo: blackhead or acne

Cyst: sac or capsule containing fluid or semisolid material (e.g., sebaceous cyst of scalp)

Erythema: red area (e.g., sunburn)

Excoriation: abrasion of the outer layer of skin (e.g., friction trauma)

Exudate: fluid, usually containing pus, bacteria, and dead cells (e.g., fluid from infected wound)

Fissure: groove, crack, or slit, as occurs with ulceration

Furuncle: painful erythematous raised lesion (e.g., boil)

Hive: solid, raised, and itchy area (wheal), usually the result of allergy

Macule: small, flat discolored area (e.g., freckle)

Maculopapular: multiple lesions consisting of both macules and papules (e.g., early chickenpox)

Mole: flat or raised pigmented growth (e.g., birthmark)

Nevus: congenital raised, pigmented growth (e.g., birthmark or mole)

Nodule: small, solid mass (e.g., swollen lymph node)

Papule: small, red, raised elevation (e.g., measles)

Petechia: red pinpoint hemorrhage; seen in some blood diseases

Pustule: small elevation on the skin containing purulent fluid (e.g., acne)

Ulcer: depression (e.g., open lesion on skin)

Urticaria: hives (e.g., blood transfusion reaction)

Vesicle: small sac containing serous or sanguineous fluid (e.g., pimple)

Wheal: raised lesion, usually accompanied by itching (e.g., mosquito bite)

Nursing Assessment

A. Nursing observations
  1. Skin
    a. Color: any deviation from normal (e.g., pallor, cyanosis, jaundice, blanching), general pigmentation, vascularity, bruising
    b. Turgor: evaluate hydration, elasticity, and mobility.
    c. Lesions and rashes: size, location, color, drainage, crusts, pattern or shape, distribution
    d. Skin temperature for inconsistency: areas cool or warm to the touch
    e. Cleanliness and hygiene
    f. Odor
    g. Pressure areas for existing or potential decubitus ulcers
  2. Hair and scalp
    a. Unusual distribution or absence of scalp and body hair; lesions
    b. Texture: smooth or coarse
    c. Parasites: scalp and pubic
  3. Nails
    a. Cleanliness
    b. Brittleness
    c. Length
    d. Pitting
    e. Shape, contour, clubbing
    f. Color, splinter hemorrhages
B. Patient description (subjective data)
  1. History to include onset, changes, and presence of itching, pain, or burning
  2. Factors that make condition worse or better
  3. Allergies
  4. Recent changes in environment and diet
  5. Medications taken
  6. Concerns about appearance, change in body image, and disfigurement
  7. Changes in activities or lifestyle caused by disease
  8. Environmental or occupational hazards (sun exposure, toxic chemicals, insect bites)
  9. History of systemic disorders

Frequent Patient Problems and Nursing Care

A. Body image disturbance related to disfigurement
  1. Show acceptance by being nonjudgmental.
  2. Plan time to allow patient to express feelings.
B. Pain related to pruritus (itching)
  1. Administer antipruritics and antihistamines (see Chapter 3).
  2. Keep nails short.
  3. Use cotton bedding and clothing; avoid rough fabrics.
  4. Encourage use of cotton gloves when sleeping.
  5. Bathe with tepid water; use minimal soap; pat dry using no friction.
  6. Give oil, medicated, or starch baths.
C. Risk for infection or injury related to open lesions
  1. Use aseptic technique in cleaning; teach hand washing.
  2. Monitor for redness, swelling, elevated temperature.
  3. Use dressings only when necessary, and apply loosely with gauze and nonallergenic tape.
D. Impaired skin integrity related to seborrhea: oily scalp with shedding of greasy scales
  1. Give frequent shampoos.
  2. Use medicated shampoos; rinse thoroughly.

Major Medical Diagnoses
Contact Dermatitis

A. Definition: an inflammatory response of the skin with redness, edema, thickening of the skin, and frequent scaling; vesicles and papules may be present.
B. Cause: an allergic reaction or unusual sensitivity when a substance comes in direct contact with the skin (e.g., poison ivy, soaps, cleaning agents, fabrics)
C. Symptoms: pruritus, erythema
D. Diagnostic test and methods
  1. Allergy testing

2. Patient history and assessment

E. Treatment

1. Systemic medication: antihistamines, antipruritics, corticosteroids (see Chapter 3)
2. Topical medication: corticosteroids (see Chapter 3)
3. Removing cause

F. Nursing intervention

1. Prevent scratching.
2. Give tepid baths.
3. Cut nails.
4. Administer prn medications as soon as possible.

Psoriasis

A. Definition: a chronic condition in which patches of inflammation occur that are red and covered with silvery scales that shed; these usually occur on elbows, knees, lower back, and scalp; they may cover the entire body.

B. Cause: unknown; may be a family tendency; symptoms increase during stress and high anxiety; other related factors are alcoholism, trauma, and infection.

C. Signs and symptoms

1. Subjective
   a. Pruritus, mild to severe
   b. Depression related to appearance
2. Objective
   a. Scratching
   b. Sharply demarcated scaling plaques

D. Diagnostic methods: patient history and physical appearance

E. Treatment (individual)

1. Topical medication: coal tars, corticosteroids (see Chapter 3)
2. Systemic medication: corticosteroids, methotrexate (in severe cases) (see Chapter 3)
3. Exposure to ultraviolet light, photochemotherapy
4. Anxiolytics
5. Antimetabolites

F. Nursing intervention

1. During bath, gently remove scales with cloth or brush.
2. Occlusive dressing may be wrapped in plastic.

Herpes Simplex (Cold Sore, Fever Blister) Type 1 (HSV-1)

A. Definition: a group of blisters on a reddened base, usually on or near mouth or genitalia

B. Cause: a viral infection precipitated by an upper respiratory tract infection or elevation of temperature from systemic infection; frequently related to emotional upset, menstrual cycle, or general immunosuppression

C. Signs and symptoms

1. Pain and local discomfort
2. Distress about appearance

D. Diagnostic methods: physical assessment, viral isolation by tissue culture

E. Treatment: lasts approximately 1 week; antiviral agents (acyclovir) administered topically or systemically

F. Nursing intervention: none indicated

Herpes Zoster (Shingles)

A. Definition: crops of vesicles and erythema following sensory nerves on the face and trunk; higher incidence in older adults

B. Cause: varicella zoster virus (chickenpox)

C. Signs and symptoms

1. Subjective
   a. Severe pain
   b. Malaise
   c. Anorexia
   d. Pruritus
2. Objective
   a. Elevation of temperature
   b. Results of diagnostic tests

D. Diagnostic methods: physical examination; vesicles follow sensory nerve paths.

E. Treatment: no specific treatment (symptomatic only); analgesics may be used for pain; usually subsides in 3 weeks (pain may last for months); antivirals, corticosteroids, capsaicin (Zostrix) for temporary relief of pain

F. Nursing intervention

1. Keep patient in isolation while vesicles are present.
2. Apply topical lotions to lesions for itching.
3. Give baths or compresses for cooling and soothing.
4. Prevent scratching and secondary infection.
5. Anticipate pain; medicate as needed.
6. Provide small, frequent, well-balanced meals.

G. Varicella vaccine (Varivax)

Neoplasms

A. Definition: any new and abnormal growth; may be of varied size and location

B. Cause

1. Benign: unknown
2. Malignant: related to exposure to the sun and chemical and physical irritants, such as pipe smoking

C. Signs and symptoms: anxiety related to diagnosis and change in physical appearance; appearance of lesions

D. Diagnostic test: biopsy examination—high cure rate with early detection

E. Treatment: Table 5-8

F. Nursing intervention

1. Assess all patients for skin lesions.
2. Discuss with patient the importance of reporting any changes in moles.
3. Give preoperative and postoperative instructions (see Chapter 2); surgery is usually outpatient.
4. Provide general care for patient receiving radiotherapy (see Chapter 2).
5. Give general care for patient receiving chemotherapy (see Chapter 3).

G. Classification of common skin tumors (see Table 5-8)

Burns

A. Definition: a wound in which the skin layers and underlying tissue is destroyed

B. Causes

1. Heat: dry or moist (e.g., fire)
2. Chemical (e.g., acids)
3. Electrical (e.g., lighting fixtures, electrical wires)
4. Radiation (e.g., sunlight)
5. Mechanical (e.g., friction from rope)

C. Signs and symptoms: depend on depth (Table 5-9) and area involved

1. Infection: destruction of the body's first line of defense and time postburn (hypovolemic and diuretic stage)

TABLE 5-8   Classification of Common Tumors of the Skin

Classification	Description	Treatment
Benign	Nevus, brown or black mole	Observe for changes: remove only if irritated or changes are observed
Premalignant or potentially malignant	Actinic keratosis: common, sun-induced, premalignant (precancerous) lesions; often on the face and backs of hands; ill-marginated, increased vascularity, and rough-textured surface; becomes reddish and scaly	Cryosurgery; topical medication
	Senile keratosis; brownish scaly spots on face and hands of aging persons	Surgical removal or topical medication or cryosurgery
	Leukoplakia: shiny white patches on mucous membranes of mouth and female genitalia	Removal of irritating teeth; oral hygiene. For genitalia: surgical excision; biopsy
	Moles (nevi) that bleed, grow, or are irritated or crusted Black, smooth moles	May become malignant and are surgically removed
Malignant	Squamous cell carcinoma: begin as a warty growth and grow and become ulcerated; found on exposed surfaces of the body (tongue and lip)	Early surgical removal
	Basal cell carcinoma: a slow-growing tumor; results from exposure to the sun	Chemosurgery, electrosurgery, or surgical removal
	Malignant melanoma: black tumor that metastasized	Widespread excision

TABLE 5-9   Description of Burns

Classification	Depth	Description	Possible cause
Superficial or shallow partial thickness	Epidermis	Red and dry; painful; may have edema; no scarring	Sunburn
Deep partial thickness	Epidermis and some dermis	Mottled, pink to red blisters; painful; leave scar	Hot oil
Full thickness partial	Epidermis, dermis, and subcutaneous tissue	Black or bright red eschar forms leathery covering; leaves scar; may have no pain	Fire
Full thickness deep	All of the above plus subcutaneous fat, fascia, muscle, and bone (nerve endings, hair follicles, and sweat glands are destroyed)	Black; there is no pain	Fire

2. Loss of body tissue (protein)
3. Loss of fluid and electrolytes (edema)
4. Pain
5. Respiratory distress
6. Immobilization
7. Disfigurement
8. Impending shock
D. Diagnostic methods: physical assessment
E. Treatment
  1. Respiratory evaluation, maintenance of airway, and possible tracheostomy; edema of lung tissue from smoke inhalation may cause increased secretions.
  2. Replacement of fluids and electrolytes with IV solutions: plasma, blood, dextran, and electrolytes
  3. Emergency wound care: removal of foreign material; avoidance of contamination
  4. Prevention of infection: tetanus immune globulin and antibiotics
  5. Analgesics for pain (see Chapter 3)

  6. Prevention of shock: plasma expanders; keeping patient warm; monitoring vital signs, urine output
  7. Wound treatment method
    a. Open method exposure; wound heals by epithelialization of eschar; this method requires reverse isolation; eschar must be removed by débridement (cutting away), whirlpool baths, and escharotomy (incision into eschar).
    b. Topical medications (see Chapter 3)
    c. Grafts: to minimize infection and fluid loss; may be temporary because they are frequently rejected; this method allows for growth of new tissue underneath the protection of the graft.
      (1) Autograft: transplantation of skin from patient's own body; care must also be given to donor site; can also grow skin in test tube, then do graft procedure.
      (2) Homograft (allograft): transplantation of tissue from living human
      (3) Heterograft: transplantation from animal (pig or cow xenograft)

(4) Synthetic material used in grafting
d. Cosmetic surgery may be performed during recovery phase

F. Nursing intervention
1. Anticipate and prevent respiratory distress; maintain airway, monitor breathing hourly then every 4 hours (see Chapter 2); keep tracheostomy equipment available.
2. Maintain fluid balance: monitor IV fluids; monitor urine output hourly through indwelling catheter; monitor sp gr hourly; weigh patient daily.
3. Anticipate infection: maintain asepsis and reverse isolation; administer antibiotics; monitor temperature every 2 hours; keep patient warm.
4. Anticipate pain: give frequent sedation as ordered, especially before dressing change (administered IV during early phase of treatment).
5. Prevent dangers of immobilization (see Chapter 2); provide proper alignment to prevent deformities (may be uncomfortable or painful); prevent skin surfaces from touching; use turning frames and cradles.
6. To enhance tissue repair, diet must be high in calories (6000 calories daily) and high in protein; tube feeding or TPN may be necessary.
7. Anticipate shock: assess level of consciousness and mental status; monitor pulse rate and blood pressure.
8. Anticipate Curling's ulcer (stress ulcer): at the end of the first week, assess for GI distress or bleeding.
9. Be aware of anxiety: provide diversional activities; allow time for patient to verbalize feelings; encourage contact with family; involve patient as much as possible with planning and self-care; administer tranquilizers and sedation as necessary.

SENSORY SYSTEMS

Visual System
Anatomy and Physiology (Figures 5-24 and 5-25)

A. Lies in a protective bony orbit in the skull
B. Eyebrows, eyelids, and lashes also protect the eye.
C. Sphere consists of three layers of tissue.
1. Sclera: thick, white fibrous tissue (white of eye); a transparent section over the front of the eyeball, the cornea, permits light rays to enter.
2. Choroid: the middle vascular area; brings oxygen and nutrients to the eye; choroid extends to ciliary body (two smooth muscle structures), which helps control shape of the lens; the front is a pigmented section (iris), which gives the eye color; in the center of the iris lies the pupil, the "window of the eye" (allows light to pass to lens and retina).
3. Retina: inner layer; physiology of vision takes place; contains receptors of optic nerve; neurons are shaped as rods and cones; cones permit perception of color, rods permit perception of light and shade.
D. Chambers
1. Anterior: contains aqueous humor, maintains slight forward curve in cornea
2. Posterior: contains vitreous humor, maintains spherical shape of eyeball
E. Conjunctiva: mucous membrane that covers eyeball and eyelid; keeps eyeball moist

F. Lens: transparent structure behind iris; focuses light rays on retina
G. Lacrimal apparatus: gland located in upper, outer part of eye; produces tears to lubricate and cleanse; nasolacrimal duct is located in nasal corner; tears drain into nose.
H. Normal intraocular pressure: 10 to 21 torr (mm Hg)

Conditions and Disorders of the Eye

Sight is the most important sense to most people. Visual acuity is dependent on general good health, CNS regulation of movement and conduction, and condition of the structures of the eye. Changes in vision are frequently indicative of systemic disease; routine examination of the eye can provide information about diseases in other systems. The nurse must assess the eyes of each patient under his or her care. Although the incidence of blindness and visual impairment increases with age, problems are seen in patients of all ages.

Nursing assessment
A. Nursing observations
1. Glasses, contact lenses, or false eyes
2. Tearing, discharge (clear or purulent), and color of sclera (white, yellow, or pink)
3. Accuracy and range of vision
4. Edema of eyelids; crusting; blinking, rubbing; redness
5. Clouded appearance over pupil; protrusion or bulging of one or both eyes; pupil response to light; Pupils equal, round, react to light, accommodation (PERRLA)
6. Squinting or drooping (ptosis) of eyelid
7. Symmetry
B. Patient description (subjective data)
1. Double vision (diplopia), decreased or absent vision in one or both eyes, blurred or clouded vision
2. Sensitivity to light (photophobia), spots, halos around lights, flashes of light, problems seeing in the dark
3. Eye fatigue, itching, pain, tearing, burning, headache, dryness
C. Note patient history of:
1. Stumbling
2. Trauma of face or eyes
3. Contact lenses or eye medication
4. Changes in vision and any related circumstances
5. Any systemic medications taken

Diagnostic tests and methods
A. Ophthalmoscope: assessment of the interior of eye
B. Tonometer: measurement of intraocular pressure; increased pressure may indicate early glaucoma; recommended every 3 years for individuals between 35 and 40 years of age and on a yearly basis for individuals over 40
C. Fields of vision: testing to measure sight on one or both sides (peripheral vision); perimetry
D. Refraction: measurement of light refraction and lenses required for visual acuity
E. Slit lamp: examination of intraocular structures with a high-intensity light beam (corneal abrasions, iritis)
F. Snellen chart: assessment of visual acuity (three times left eye [OS], right eye [OD], both, or each eye [OU])
G. Retinal angiography: retinal vessels

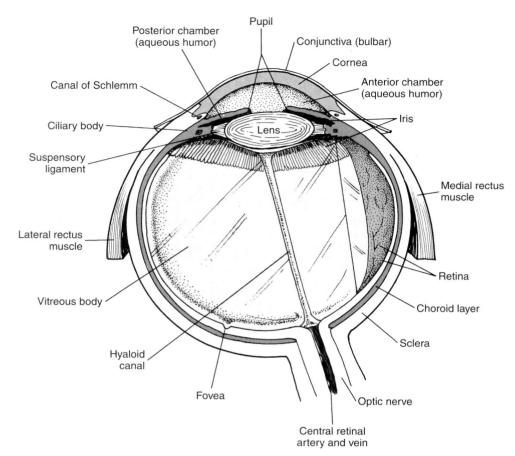

FIGURE 5-24. Horizontal section through left eyeball. *(From Phipps, Monahan, Sands, et al. Medical-Surgical Nursing health and illness perspectives, ed. 7, St. Louis, 2003, Mosby.)*

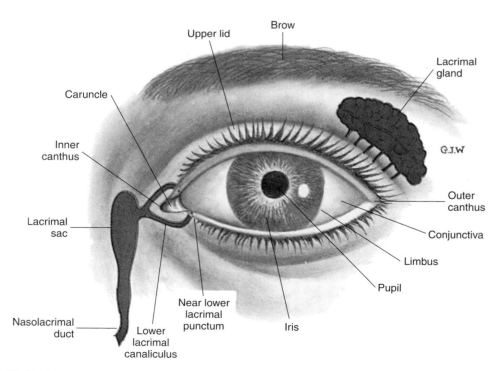

FIGURE 5-25. External eye structures. *(From Thompson JM, McFarland GK, Hirsch JE, Tucker SM: Mosby's clinical nursing, ed 4, St Louis, 1998, Mosby.)*

Eye care professionals

A. Ophthalmologist (also called oculist): a medical doctor who specializes in diagnosis, treatment, and surgery of the eyes, including the prescribing of glasses
B. Optometrist: educated and licensed to test for refractive problems; may prescribe and fit glasses; may, within limits, diagnose disease, prescribe medication, or treat eye diseases (laws vary among states)
C. Optician: fills prescription for corrective lenses as prescribed by physician; fits glasses properly

Frequent patient problems and nursing care

A. Anxiety and fear related to concerns about loss of vision, altered lifestyles, ability to function, employment, plans for the future, and altered body image: allow time for the patient to express feelings.
B. Risk for infection related to drainage, use of eye drops
   1. Clean as necessary with normal saline solution.
   2. Gently apply compresses to loosen if necessary.
   3. Use aseptic technique; wipe from inner canthus to outer canthus.
   4. If drainage is purulent, dispose of properly.
C. Risk for injury related to need for corrective lenses
   1. Glasses must be kept clean and in a protective case.
   2. Contact lenses are kept in a case with R and L to designate which eye the lens fits; obtain directions for soaking from patient.
   3. If patient is dependent on lenses, obtain permission for patient to wear glasses or lenses when going for diagnostic tests.
D. Risk for injury related to photophobia
   1. Keep room dim and evenly lighted.
   2. Keep blinds adjusted to avoid glare.

Major Medical Diagnoses

Low vision

A. Definition: defects that cannot be corrected with lenses
B. Cause: disease of the eye itself, in the visual pathways to the brain, or in the receptors in the brain; macular degeneration
C. Signs and symptoms: vision may be blurred and images distorted; vision may be clear only at close range; shades of color may not be distinguishable.

Total or legal blindness

A. Definition: legal blindness is the ability to see at no more than 20 feet (6 m) what normally should be seen at a distance of 200 feet (60 m) (20/200); this may also refer to severe restrictions in peripheral fields of vision (after corrective lenses are used).
B. Pathology
   1. Macular degeneration, glaucoma, detached retina, diabetic retinopathy
   2. Trauma, laceration
   3. Inflammation, optic neuritis
   4. Vascular or hypertensive retinopathy
   5. Neoplasms of the brain or eye
   6. Cataract
C. Patient problems
   1. Inability to care for self (dependency)
   2. Frustration
   3. Occupational hazards
   4. Boredom

D. Nursing diagnoses
   1. Anxiety related to degree of visual impairment
   2. Risk for injury or trauma related to degree of visual impairment
   3. Body image disturbance
E. Nursing intervention
   1. Allow as much independence as possible; help make use of existing vision; encourage use of any visual aids recommended by physician (e.g., special lenses, large-type books, cane); provide reading material in braille for the patient who has learned this method.
   2. Do not touch patient without talking; always address patient by name; introduce yourself; and tell patient when you are leaving the room.
   3. Explain all care and treatments; encourage patient to participate in planning care.
   4. At mealtime, indicate position of utensils and placement of food on dish by comparing it to numbers on a clock (e.g., "the potato is at 3 o'clock").
   5. Orient patient to room and entire unit; point out hazards and obstacles (doors and windows); explain location of furniture, bathroom, call bell, telephone; keep items in the same place.
   6. Leave bedside table, call bell, and personal items in close reach.
   7. Maintain safety; keep unit uncluttered, floor clean and dry, bed in low position, and side rails up as necessary; tell patient position of bed and side rails.
   8. Guide the ambulatory patient by placing patient's arm on your's while walking slowly.
   9. Provide diversion: radio and books on tapes; be aware of local agencies in your community; many libraries have braille books or tapes available.
   10. Be mindful of patient confidentiality and security.

Refractive disorders

A. Definition: inability of the refractory media to converge light rays and focus on retina
   1. Myopia (nearsightedness): the eyeball is too long; light rays focus at a point before reaching the retina.
   2. Hyperopia (farsightedness): the eyeball is shorter than normal; light rays focus beyond the retina.
   3. Presbyopia: a gradual loss of elasticity of the lens; the ability to focus on near objects is decreased.
   4. Astigmatism: unequal curve in the shape of the cornea or lens; vision is distorted.
B. Cause: unknown; may be inherited
C. Symptoms: diminished or blurred vision
D. Diagnostic tests and methods
   1. Patient history
   2. Refraction
E. Treatment: corrective lenses (glasses or contact lenses); keratorefractive surgery
F. Nursing intervention
   1. Encourage proper care of lenses.
   2. Encourage follow-up checkups as indicated.

Conjunctivitis

A. Definition: infection or inflammation of the conjunctiva

B. Causes: bacteria, usually staphylococci, allergens, chemical reactions, chlamydial or viral infections
C. Patient problems
  1. Very contagious (especially in young children); spread by direct contact with organisms
  2. Purulent drainage and itching
  3. Photophobia
  4. Tearing
D. Diagnostic method: physical assessment, culture and sensitivity of conjunctival scrapings
E. Treatment: ophthalmic antibiotics (see Chapter 3)
F. Nursing intervention
  1. Prevent transmission to others: encourage frequent hand washing.
  2. Provide warm compresses; cleanse eyelids; remove crusts before administering ophthalmic medications.
    a. Discourage rubbing of eyes.
    b. Isolate personal items (towels, washcloths, and pillowcases).

Cataract

A. Definition: the crystalline lens becomes clouded and opaque (not transparent).
B. Causes
  1. Trauma
  2. Congenital
  3. Related to diabetes
  4. High incidence in the elderly (senile cataracts)
  5. Heredity
  6. Infections
  7. Excessive exposure to the sun or ultraviolet rays
C. Signs and symptoms
  1. Loss of vision
  2. Progressive blurring
  3. Haziness with eventual complete loss of sight
D. Diagnostic tests and methods
  1. Examination with ophthalmoscope
  2. Patient history
  3. Ultrasonography
E. Treatment: surgical removal of opaque lens, usually on an outpatient basis; after surgery, corrective lenses are necessary (glasses, contact lenses, or surgical implantation of an artificial lens [IOL])
F. Nursing intervention
  1. Give general preoperative care (see Chapter 2).
  2. Provide nursing care as that for the patient with low vision.
  3. Postoperative management depends on surgical procedure; be careful to adhere to physician's order; general principles are to have patient avoid coughing, bending, or rapid head movements; provide bed rest for a specified time (usually 2 hours); keep patient flat or in low-Fowler's position; have patient deep breathe (avoid coughing); be sure patient avoids straining (give stool softener); help patient avoid vomiting (an antiemetic will be ordered; administer as needed); observe dressing; report pain or bleeding; position patient with unoperated side down.

Glaucoma

A. Definition: intraocular pressure increases because of a disturbance in the circulation of aqueous humor; imbalance between production and drainage as the angle of drainage closes
  1. Acute (closed-angle) glaucoma: dramatic onset of symptoms; immediate treatment is required, usually surgery.
  2. Chronic (open-angle) glaucoma: symptoms progress slowly and are frequently ignored; if disease is not detected early, it may lead to permanent loss of vision.
B. Pathology
  1. Familial tendency
  2. Related to age; incidence increases over 40 years of age
  3. Secondary to injuries and infections
C. Signs and symptoms
  1. Subjective
    a. Loss of peripheral vision (tunnel vision), halos around lights, permanent loss of vision (a leading cause of blindness)
    b. Pain, malaise, nausea
    c. Reduced visual acuity at night
  2. Objective
    a. Pupils fixed and dilated
    b. Vomiting
    c. Results of diagnostic tests
D. Diagnostic tests and methods
  1. History of symptoms
  2. Measurement of visual fields
  3. Measurement of intraocular pressure
  4. Gonioscopy: measures angle of the anterior chamber
  5. Tonometry
E. Treatment
  1. Miotics to decrease intraocular pressure (see Chapter 3)
  2. Surgery: iridectomy (an incision through the cornea to remove part of the iris to allow for drainage), laser trabeculoplasty (relieves excess intraocular pressure), trabeculectomy (new opening made to bypass obstruction and facilitate flow of aqueous humor), laser iridotomy
  3. Continued medical supervision
F. Nursing intervention
  1. Encourage patient to wear medical identification tag.
  2. Administer eye medications on schedule.
  3. Inform the patient to avoid drugs with atropine; discourage straining and lifting.
  4. Give preoperative and postoperative care according to that for a patient with a cataract; pay careful attention to specifics in physician's orders.

Detached retina

A. Definition: the sensory layer of the retina pulls away from the pigmented layer; vitreous humor may leak into the space occupying the position the retina normally assumes.
B. Cause: usually unknown and spontaneous; may be related to sudden blow to the head or follow eye surgery (e.g., removal of cataract)
C. Signs and symptoms
  1. Subjective
    a. Loss of vision in affected area (may be complete loss)
    b. Painless
    c. Visual disturbance (blurring)
    d. Spots and flashes of light
  2. Objective: results of diagnostic tests
D. Diagnostic tests and methods
  1. Patient history and physical assessment

2. Retinal examination with ophthalmoscope
3. Ultrasonography
4. Slit lamp
E. Treatment: depends on area of detachment
   1. Bed rest
   2. Prevention of extension of detachment by restricting eye movements
   3. Mydriatics
   4. Surgical intervention: laser photocoagulation, cryopexy, diathermy, scleral buckling, pneumatic retinopexy, vitrectomy
F. Nursing intervention
   1. Provide individual care according to location of detachment; physician's orders will be specific.
   2. Maintain absolute rest; restrict activity; patch eye to limit eye movement; may use eye shield; patient position is based on location of retinal detachment.
   3. Prepare patient for postoperative care: inform the patient that both eyes may be patched and that he or she may be unable to see.
   4. Postoperative care: position patient exactly as ordered; maintain eye patch or patches; have patient deep breathe and avoid coughing; administer medication for pain; provide care as needed for a person with limited sight.
G. Patient problems, nursing diagnoses
   1. Anxiety related to possibility of permanent vision loss
   2. Self-care deficit related to imposed activity restrictions
   3. Pain related to surgical correction and unusual positioning

Auditory System
Anatomy and Physiology (Figures 5-26 and 5-27)

A. External ear (pinna or auricle): outer, visible portion, shaped as a funnel; gathers sound and sends it into the auditory canal, which is lined with tiny hairs and secretes cerumen, a waxy substance; canal extends to the eardrum, also called the tympanic membrane.
B. Middle ear: small, flattened space; contains three small bones called ossicles: malleus (hammer), incus (anvil), and stapes (stirrup); bones are mobile and vibrate; conduct sound waves; the eustachian tube extends into nasopharynx and equalizes the pressure in the middle ear to that of atmospheric pressure.
C. Internal ear (labyrinth): vestibule; cochlea, snail-shaped bony tube, contains organ of Corti (organ of hearing); semicircular canals are the receptors for equilibrium and head movements.
D. Function
   1. Transmission of sound waves; result is hearing.
   2. Maintenance of equilibrium

Conditions and Disorders of the Ear

Hearing problems are not as obvious initially during assessment as are many other problems. Hearing loss may be misinterpreted. Many people associate hearing aids with dependency or disfigurement or signs of aging and refuse to wear them. However, the sense of hearing contributes to well being and safety. This assessment (hearing) must be made for each patient.

Nursing Assessment

A. Nursing observations
   1. Difficulty hearing or understanding verbal communication
   2. Not responding to loud or sudden noises
   3. Use of hearing aid, lip reading, or sign language
   4. Drainage, dried secretion, or deformities of the ear
B. Patient description (subjective data)
   1. Earache or headache
   2. Difficulty hearing (or lack of hearing) in one or both ears
   3. Itching, drainage, pressure or full feeling
   4. Ringing, buzzing, popping, echoes
   5. Vertigo
   6. Medications taken
C. Note history of:
   1. Ear infections
   2. Ear surgery
   3. Head injury
   4. Medication taken

Diagnostic Tests and Methods

A. Audiometry: a hearing test to determine ability to discriminate sounds, voices, degrees of loudness and pitch
B. Otoscopy: visual examination of the ear canal and tympanic membrane
C. Weber's test: a tuning fork is struck and placed midline on the patient's forehead; the patient is asked where the sound is heard; in this test of conduction, sounds should be heard equally well in each ear.
D. Rinne test: the tuning fork is struck and placed on the mastoid process of the skull behind the ear; the fork is removed, and the patient indicates when the sound can no longer be heard; the still vibrating fork is then placed near the external ear canal; normally, the sound will be heard longer through air conduction than through bone conduction.
E. Caloric stimulation test (CST): tests vestibular reflexes of the inner ear that control balance
F. Electronystagmography: monitors eye movements; done with CST

Patient with Impaired Hearing

A. Definition
   1. Conductive hearing loss occurs when injury or disease interferes with the conduction of sound waves to the inner ear (e.g., cerumen in canal).
   2. Sensory hearing loss occurs when malfunction occurs of the inner ear, auditory nerve, or auditory center in the brain (e.g., toxic effect to eighth cranial nerve from drugs [aspirin]).
B. Patient problems
   1. Inability to communicate
   2. Inability to hear hazards in the environment (e.g., automobiles)
   3. Frustration, anxiety, anger, insecurity
   4. Misinterpretation of communication
C. Treatment: according to cause (cochlear implants, stapedectomy); frequently none
D. Nursing intervention
   1. Find out if a hearing aid can be fitted.
     a. Encourage patient to wear it.
     b. Test batteries for function.
     c. Make sure hearing aid is turned on.
     d. Protect hearing aid from breakage; ask patient or family about usual care and storage.
   2. Attract patient's attention before speaking

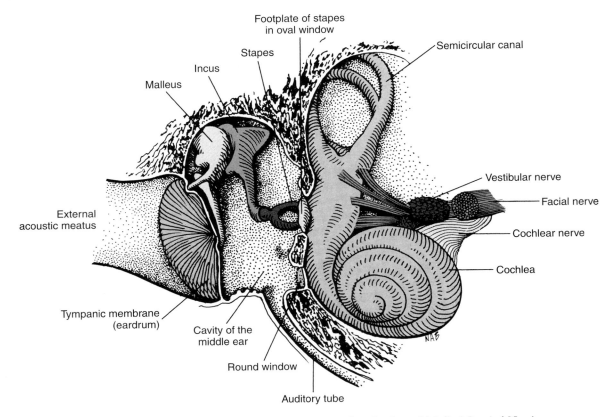

FIGURE 5-26. Structures of the ear. *(From Phipps, Monahan, Sands, et al.* Medical-Surgical Nursing health and illness perspectives, *ed. 7, St. Louis, 2003, Mosby.)*

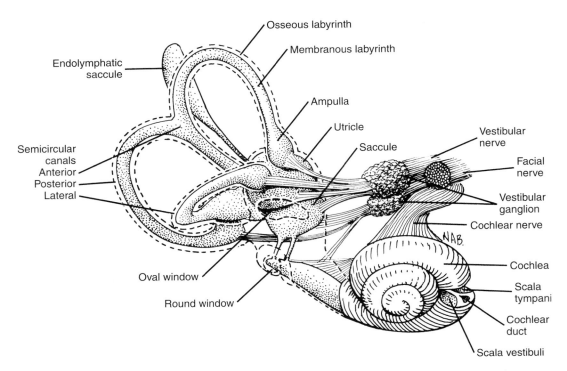

FIGURE 5-27. Structures of the inner ear. *(From Phipps, Monahan, Sands, et al.* Medical-Surgical Nursing health and illness perspectives, *ed. 7, St. Louis, 2003, Mosby.)*

3. Do not touch patient until he or she is aware that you are in the room.
4. Speak face to face; articulate clearly but not too slowly; move close to patient; avoid covering mouth with hand.
5. Provide alternate methods of communication.
    a. Find out if patient lip-reads or uses sign language.
    b. Provide magic slate or pad and pencil.
6. Nursing intervention after surgery
    a. Give general preoperative and postoperative care (see Chapter 2).
    b. Report drainage immediately.
    c. Observe for facial nerve injury: inability to close eyes or pucker lips.
    d. Anticipate vertigo; provide safety.
    e. Be sure patient avoids blowing nose.
    f. Note specific instructions from physician for positioning, activity, and diet.

Major Medical Diagnoses

Ménière's syndrome

A. Definition: a chronic disease with sudden attacks of vertigo and tinnitus (ringing in the ear) with progressive hearing loss; attacks last a few minutes to a few weeks; usually occurs in women over 50 years of age
B. Cause: unknown; related to fluid in cochlea, either increased production or decreased absorption
C. Signs and symptoms
    1. Vertigo
    2. Nausea and vomiting
    3. Ringing in the ears, hearing loss
    4. Disequilibrium
D. Diagnostic tests and methods: patient history, physical examination, neurological assessment, CST, radiography, electronystagmography, audiogram
E. Treatment
    1. Diuretics, low-sodium diet, vasodilators, antihistamines, antiemetics, vestibular depressants, adrenergic agents
    2. Surgery: endolymphatic shunt (reduces pressure and controls vertigo), destruction of the labyrinth as a last resort
F. Nursing intervention
    1. Provide bed rest; position of comfort.
    2. Maintain quiet and safety.
    3. Provide low-sodium diet.
    4. Provide specific nursing care as that for patient with impaired hearing.
    5. Provide general preoperative and postoperative care (see Chapter 2).
    6. Provide nursing care for patient after ear surgery.

Mastoiditis

A. Definition: infection of the mastoid process; may be acute or chronic; not common because of antibiotics
B. Cause: extension of middle ear infection that was inadequately treated
C. Signs and symptoms
    1. Subjective: headache, ear pain, tenderness over mastoid process
    2. Objective
        a. Elevation of temperature
        b. Drainage from ear
D. Treatment
    1. Antibiotics
    2. Surgery
        a. Simple mastoidectomy: removal of infected cells
        b. Radical mastoidectomy: more extensive excision resulting in some degree of hearing loss
E. Nursing intervention
    1. See care of patient with impaired hearing.
    2. Provide general preoperative and postoperative care (see Chapter 2).
    3. Provide nursing care for patient after ear surgery (see section on patient with impaired hearing).

Otosclerosis

A. Definition: a progressive formation of new bone tissue around the stapes preventing transmission of vibrations to the inner ear
B. Cause: unknown
C. Signs and symptoms
    1. Loss of hearing
    2. Ringing or buzzing (tinnitus)
D. Treatment
    1. Hearing aid
    2. Surgery; stapedectomy (removal of diseased bone and replacement with prosthetic implant)
E. Nursing intervention
    1. Provide general care for patient who is hearing impaired.
    2. Give general preoperative and postoperative care (see Chapter 2).
    3. Follow specific orders from physician.
    4. Provide general nursing care for patient after ear surgery (see section on patient with impaired hearing).

SUGGESTED READINGS

Ackley BJ, Ladwig GB: *Nursing diagnosis handbook: a guide to planning care,* ed 5, St Louis, 2002, Mosby.

Dirksen SR, Lewis SL, Heitkemper MM: *Clinical companion to medical surgical nursing,* ed 2, St Louis, 2000, Mosby.

Elkin MK, Perry AG, Potter PA: *Nursing interventions and clinical skills,* ed 3, St Louis, 2004, Mosby.

Harkness GA, Dincher JR: *Medical-surgical nursing: total patient care,* ed 10, St Louis, 1999, Mosby.

Mosby's medical, nursing and allied health dictionary, ed 6, St Louis, 2002, Mosby.

Phipps WJ et al: *Medical-surgical nursing: health and illness perspectives,* ed 7, St Louis, 2003, Mosby.

Physicians' desk reference, Montvale, NJ, Medical Economics (published annually).

Thibodeau GA, Patton KP: *The human body in health and disease,* ed 3, St Louis, 2002, Mosby.

Thompson JM et al: *Mosby's clinical nursing,* ed 5, St Louis, 2002, Mosby.

Tucker SM et al: *Patient care standards: collaborative planning and nursing interventions,* ed 7, St Louis, 2002, Mosby.

REVIEW QUESTIONS

1. A patient who is to undergo a cardiac catheterization communicates to the nurse that he forgot to inform the physician that he is allergic to shrimp. What should the nurse do next?
   1. Inform the physician of the patient's allergy.
   2. Prepare the patient for the catheterization.
   3. Ask the patient what happens when he eats shrimp.
   4. Place an allergy band around the patient's wrist.

2. What are the assessment components for the Glasgow coma scale (GCS)?
   1. Posturing, reflexes, eye opening
   2. Eye opening, verbal and motor response
   3. Voice commands, posturing, reflexes
   4. Seizure activity, motor and verbal response

3. The ability of a cell to reproduce is called:
   1. Lysis
   2. Mitosis
   3. Osmosis
   4. Crenation

4. The immunity that occurs when a person is given a substance containing antibodies or antitoxins is called:
   1. Active
   2. Passive
   3. Permanent
   4. Autoimmune

5. A patient is admitted to the hospital with a possible diagnosis of otosclerosis. Which of the following symptoms did the patient likely exhibit on arrival?
   1. Diplopia
   2. Tinnitus
   3. Nystagmus
   4. Hearing loss

6. A patient has fallen off a horse and is brought to the emergency department for evaluation for a closed head injury. Which of the following assessment findings should the nurse report immediately to the physician?
   1. Vomiting
   2. Headache
   3. Tremors
   4. Pruritus

7. The ovaries produce the hormones:
   1. Estrogen and testosterone
   2. Estrogen and progesterone
   3. Progesterone and prolactin
   4. Progesterone and testosterone

8. A greater amount of body heat is lost when surface blood vessels:
   1. Dilate
   2. Contract
   3. Help the skeletal muscles relax
   4. Increase the production of sweat

9. The pigmented area surrounding the nipple is the:
   1. Areola
   2. Urochrome
   3. Cowper's gland
   4. Bartholin's gland

10. The hormone produced by the testes is:
    1. Estrogen
    2. Progesterone
    3. Testosterone
    4. Aldosterone

11. Connective tissue that attaches muscles to bones is called:
    1. Osseous
    2. Tendons
    3. Cartilage
    4. Ligaments

12. The nurse is caring for a patient with the new diagnosis of Parkinson's disease. Which of the following assessment data would best describe the symptoms of an individual with Parkinson's disease?
    1. Diplopia, tremors
    2. Headache, ataxia
    3. Shuffling gait, dysphagia
    4. Tinnitus, ataxia

13. A patient with diverticulitis makes the following statements. Which statement would indicate to the nurse that further teaching is indicated?
    1. "I can eat popcorn for a snack; the fiber is good for me."
    2. "I should try to avoid constipation as much as possible."
    3. "I should increase my fluids."
    4. "I should take a stool softener every day."

14. Bile is important in the digestive process because it:
    1. Digests simple fats and sugars
    2. Changes complex sugars to glucose
    3. Dissolves meat fibers and makes them easier to digest
    4. Breaks down fat globules so that they can be more easily digested

15. Which of the following tissues forms a protective covering for the body and lines the intestinal and respiratory tract?
    1. Epithelial
    2. Periosteum
    3. Pericardium
    4. Connective

16. Which of the following prevents food from flowing back into the esophagus?
    1. Rugae
    2. Chyme
    3. Cardiac sphincter
    4. Pyloric sphincter

17. Which of the following structures absorbs most of the nutrients that the body uses?
    1. Liver
    2. Stomach
    3. Small intestine
    4. Large intestine

18. Which of the following nursing measures would best alleviate the pruritus and burning that a patient has because of external hemorrhoids?
    1. Sitz bath
    2. Pillows
    3. Acetaminophen
    4. Tapwater enema

19. Tears drain into the nose through the:
    1. Ciliary body
    2. Lacrimal gland
    3. Eustachian tube
    4. Nasolacrimal duct

20. The first eight deciduous teeth to appear through the gums of a baby are the:
    1. Molars
    2. Incisors

3 Canines

4 Eye teeth

21. A patient who has had a cholecystectomy asks the nurse where his T tube is "hooked to." What is the correct response by the nurse?

1 "It is inserted into the area where the gallbladder was to drain blood."

2 "The T tube drains the juices from your liver."

3 "It is inserted into the common bile duct to drain bile while your incision heals."

4 "It drains stomach acid so it does not inflame your incisional area."

22. Which of the following nursing diagnosis is of priority concern for a patient undergoing peritoneal dialysis?

1 Risk for infection

2 Fluid deficit

3 Body image disturbance

4 Self-care deficit

23. The movement that propels food down the digestive tract is called:

1 Rugae

2 Peristalsis

3 Mastication

4 Pylorospasm

24. The end product of protein metabolism is:

1 Ptyalin

2 Glucose

3 Amino acids

4 Hydrochloric acid

25. A patient is scheduled to have his right labyrinth destroyed because of Ménière's disease. Which of the following statements is true regarding this procedure?

1 The patient may still have symptoms from the disease.

2 The patient will be unable to hear on that side after the procedure.

3 The symptoms will likely come back after the procedure.

4 Symptoms will gradually decline after the procedure.

26. Which of the following is a function of the liver?

1 Emulsify fats

2 Absorb nutrients

3 Manufacture trypsin

4 Produce fibrinogen

27. Which of the following minerals would the nurse encourage a patient with hypothyroidism to increase through consumption?

1 Iron

2 Iodine

3 Calcium

4 Phosphorus

28. Which of the following nutrients may increase the discomfort felt by women who are suffering from premenstrual tension syndrome (PMS)?

1 Protein

2 Calcium

3 Sulfur

4 Sodium

29. The chamber of the heart that receives venous blood from body tissues is:

1 Left atrium

2 Right atrium

3 Left ventricle

4 Right ventricle

30. The hormone released by the adrenal medulla during a body emergency is called:

1 Insulin

2 Aldosterone

3 Epinephrine

4 Testosterone

31. The reabsorption of water from the kidney tubules is promoted by:

1 Oxytocin

2 Prolactin

3 Calcitonin

4 Antidiuretic hormone (ADH)

32. A patient has been diagnosed with breast cancer in the early stage. Which of the following surgical procedures would preserve the most breast tissue for this patient?

1 Lumpectomy

2 Mastectomy

3 Needle biopsy

4 Oophorectomy

33. The pacemaker of the heart is the:

1 AV node

2 SA node

3 Bundle of His

4 Purkinje fibers

34. Which of the following arteries carries deoxygenated blood?

1 Aorta

2 Carotid

3 Coronary

4 Pulmonary

35. Which of the following glands secrete oil?

1 Sudoriferous

2 Ceruminous

3 Sebaceous

4 Bartholin's

36. Which of the following describes the rounded portion at the upper and lateral portion of the femur that is most often involved in fractures?

1 Acromion

2 Acetabulum

3 Greater trochanter

4 Olecranon process

37. Which of the following is the major function of the periosteum?

1 Produces RBCs

2 Produces storage for adipose fat

3 Provides for yellow bone marrow

4 Provides a structure for blood, lymph, and nerves

38. A patient is diagnosed with a detached retina. Which of the following symptoms did the patient most likely report?

1 Diplopia

2 Painless loss of vision

3 Tunnel vision

4 Headache on affected side.

39. Which of the following assessment data would be included in an integumentary assessment?

1 Blood sugar levels

2 Blood pressure, pulse

3 Rashes, bruises, decubitus

4 Rashes, bruises, blood sugar levels

40. Which of the following symptoms is associated with the diagnosis of glaucoma?
    1 Painless loss of vision
    2 Diplopia
    (3) Tunnel vision
    4 Strabismus

41. A patient asks the nurse what the purpose is of a miotic. Which of the following is the correct information to include in the answer?
    1 They make pupils small and decrease intraocular pressure.
    (2) They increase the diameter of your pupil to allow more free flow of fluid in the eye.
    3 They are used as a diuretic for the eye.
    4 They are used to treat detached retina.

42. Grooves and ridges that make up fingerprints are located in the:
    1 Elastic skin tissue
    2 Subcutaneous layer of tissue
    (3) Upper surface of the dermis
    4 Upper surface of the epidermis

43. The hormone that regulates blood composition and blood volume by acting on the kidney is:
    1 Oxytocin
    2 Antidiuretic
    (3) Aldosterone
    4 Parathormone

44. Which of the following provide energy for skeletal muscle contraction?
    1 Oxygen and glycogen
    2 Oxygen and acetylcholine
    (3) Glycogen and acetylcholine
    4 Carbohydrates and lactic acid

45. A nurse is caring for a patient who has an injury to the left motor area of the cerebrum. Where would the nurse expect to see paralysis?
    1 Both arms and legs
    2 The left side of the body
    (3) The right side of the body
    4 No paralysis should be observed.

46. A patient is receiving external radiation to treat bone cancer. Which of the following should be stressed during a patient teaching session?
    1 Use cocoa butter oil to lubricate the skin each day.
    (2) Do not allow anyone to wash the markings off of your skin.
    3 Try ice or heat packs if the area becomes sore.
    4 Go to the emergency department right away if the area becomes red.

47. Which of the following is the part of the nervous system that directs the digestion of food and the circulation of blood?
    1 Sensory
    2 Sympathetic
    3 Interneurons
    (4) Parasympathetic

48. Mannitol is used in the treatment of:
    1 Cerebral edema
    2 Pulmonary edema
    3 Ascites
    4 Left-sided heart failure

49. Which of the following is considered the organ of hearing?
    1 Malleus
    2 Organ of Corti
    (3) Tympanic membrane
    4 Semicircular canal

50. Which of the following assessment data would indicate compromised neurovascular function?
    1 Bounding pulse
    (2) Capillary refill time of 6 seconds
    3 Cool extremity
    4 Complaints of pain

51. Which of the following structures is chiefly responsible for fluid and electrolyte balance?
    1 Gonads
    (2) Kidney
    3 Bladder
    4 Islets of Langerhans

52. A patient is diagnosed with a herniated nucleus pulposus. Which of the following facts in the patient's history is significant with regard to the diagnosis?
    1 Smokes one pack a day for 4 years
    2 Plants a garden each year
    3 Eats only two meals per day
    (4) Works as a warehouse manager for a grocery store

53. A patient who is HIV positive asks the nurse what the T cells have to do with immunity. Which of the following statements would best answer the patient's question?
    1 T cells clone into helpers and suppressors.
    2 T cells are responsible for humoral immunity.
    3 T cells clone antibody-producing plasma cells.
    (4) T cells act against bacteria, viruses, tumor cells, and foreign organs.

54. The primary function of the fluid within the eyeball is to:
    1 Produce tears
    2 Dilate the pupil
    (3) Regulate the thickness of the lens
    4 Give and maintain shape of the eyeball

55. A patient should be observed for leakage of CSF _____ after a laminectomy.

56. A patient with continuous bladder irrigation has the following intake and output record. What is the patient's true urine output? _____
    Intake:
       4 ounces of juice
       300 ml of water
       1 cup of milk
       A 24-ounce bottle of cola
       3 ounces of Jello
       3000 ml of irrigant
    Output
       100 ml of emesis
       4000 ml of urine
       200 ml of liquid bowel movement

57. A patient with diabetes is being managed on a split dose of 70/30 isophane insulin suspension (NPH insulin) at 7:30 AM and 4:30 PM. At 2:30 PM one afternoon, the patient calls the nurses' station stating that she is not feeling well. On assessment, the nurse notes that her skin is cool and clammy, her hands are shaking, and she appears very apprehensive. The glucometer blood sugar is 45 mg/dl. The most appropriate nursing intervention for the patient's current symptoms is

to provide:
1 A cube of sugar
2 A large candy bar
3 4 ounces of fruit juice
4 12 ounces of diet drink

58. A patient diagnosed with IDDM is receiving regular insulin (Humulin R) by sliding scale. Glucometer readings show a blood sugar of 250 mg/dl. Based on this finding, the patient will receive 6 units of Humulin R at 3:00 PM. When should the nurse be particularly alert to a possible hypoglycemic episode?
1 5:00 PM
2 7:00 PM
3 8:00 PM
4 10:00 PM

59. Which of the following assessment data may indicate that a patient with an external fixation device has developed osteomyelitis?
1 Chest pain, dyspnea
2 Edema, pain, drainage
3 Numbness, delayed capillary refill
4 Paresthesia, bluish skin around the knee

60. A patient has undergone a craniotomy for removal of a meningioma. Which of the following questions would be the most appropriate in assessing a possible complication of this patient's surgery?
1 "Have you noticed any salty or sweet-tasting drainage coming from your incision?"
2 "Do you have any headache when you turn to your left side?"
3 "Are you hungry or thirsty yet?"
4 "Do you feel that you need to sleep more?"

61. The nurse is preparing to suction the tracheostomy of a patient with AIDS. Which of the following personal protective equipment should the nurse wear?
1 Mask and gown
2 Mask and gloves
3 Gloves and gown
4 Mask with eye shield and gloves

62. The nurse is caring for a patient with a WBC count of 0.2 mm/ml^3. The primary concern of the nurse caring for this patient would be to:
1 Protect the patient from infection.
2 Instruct the patient to wear a facemask.
3 Implement contact isolation precautions.
4 Encourage participation in group activities to build the immune system.

63. A patient with suspected muscular dystrophy has been assigned to your unit. Which of the following observations would be characteristic of this disease?
1 Pillrolling
2 Waddling gait
3 Shuffling gait
4 Tardive dyskinesia

64. When planning care for a patient with ALS, a priority nursing intervention would include:
1 Increased periods of exercise
2 Alternative means of communication
3 Clear airway maintenance
4 Means of adjusting to diagnosis

65. The nurse observes that an elderly patient uses her diaphragm during inspiration and plans to teach her to pursed-lip breathe, based on the understanding that older persons:
1 Need to consciously think about taking deep breaths
2 Are more likely to develop COPD
3 Experience a loss of elastic recoil of the lungs
4 Lose the use of their intercostal muscles

66. The nurse is discussing home care for a patient who is being discharged after an episode of severe angina. Which of the following statements made by the patient requires further teaching?
1 "I should take a nitroglycerin before doing anything strenuous."
2 "I can forget about having sex ever again."
3 "I need to balance exercise with rest."
4 "I am likely to have a heart attack if I don't watch it."

67. A nurse caring for a patient with Amyotrophic lateral sclerosis (ALS) must continually assess for signs and symptoms of disease progression. Which of the following signs and symptoms would indicate disease progression?
1 Aphasia, flexor muscle spasticity, jaw clonus
2 Flexor muscles flaccid, dysarthria, respiratory difficulty
3 Dysphagia, dysarthria, spasticity of flexor muscles
4 Sensory loss, jaw clonus, dysarthria

68. Which of the following types of traction require pin care?
1 Bryant's
2 Kirschner
3 Buck's
4 Russell

69. A nurse is caring for a patient with a suspected diagnosis of osteoarthritis. Which of the following are common characteristics of osteoarthritis?
1 Tenderness and crepitus
2 Bilateral inflammation and immobility
3 Pain resulting from destruction of supportive structures
4 Fluid within the joint along with inflammatory tissue changes

70. The nurse is planning to admit a 90-year old patient for a short-stay cataract removal. An important piece of information for the nurse to obtain in planning his care while in the short procedure unit is:
1 Hobbies and interests
2 Food likes and dislikes
3 Use of alcohol and tobacco
4 Use of a cane, walker, or crutches

71. A nurse is caring for a patient with IDDM. The nurse finds the patient unconscious 2 hours after administering 12 units of regular insulin. A blood glucose reading shows 30 mg/dl. What is the nurse's next course of action?
1 Administer IV insulin.
2 Sit the patient up and place small amount of orange juice in her mouth.
3 Place crushed crackers in the patient's mouth and help her swallow.
4 Place concentrated glucose between the cheek and the gum and allow it to absorb.

72. A patient has been diagnosed with Cushing's syndrome. The nurse is aware that this condition is caused by an overproduction of:
1 Prolactin
2 Cortisol
3 Growth hormone
4 Thyroid hormone

73. The nursing assistant asks the nurse about the turning schedule for a patient who has a right-sided chest tube. The nurse explains that the patient should be turned every hour from:
    1 Back to left side to right side
    2 Back to left side to back
    3 Left side to right side to left side
    4 Back to right side to back

74. A nurse is administering pulse oximetry to a patient receiving oxygen therapy. The patient inquires about the purpose of the test. Which of the following is the nurse's best response?
    1 "This measures how much energy your body uses."
    2 "This determines how fast or slow your heart is beating."
    3 "This test lets us know how much fluid is in your lungs."
    4 "This determines how much oxygen your tissues are receiving."

75. A patient is admitted to the hospital with the diagnosis of cirrhosis of the liver related to alcohol abuse and malnutrition. A nursing assistant asks the nurse what causes the patient's ascites. Which of the following is the most correct statement by the nurse?
    1 The fluid is caused by cardiovascular hypertension.
    2 Low levels of albumin cause fluid to collect in the abdomen.
    3 The fluid is accumulating because of a large obstruction of the patient's common bile duct.
    4 The patient is producing large amounts of ammonia, which cause the fluid collection.

76. A patient pulls out his chest tube. The nurse immediately places petroleum gauze over the puncture site. A dietary aide asks the nurse why she used that dressing. The nurse's most appropriate response is:
    1 "A dressing is used to prevent the patient from infecting the puncture site."
    2 "The petroleum will allow the site to get air circulation."
    3 "The occlusive dressing is done so that air does not enter the lung."
    4 "The dressing is used in case there is any leakage."

77. A patient had a right lower lobectomy at 10:00 AM. It is now 2:00 PM. The nurse knows that the best turning schedule for the patient is:
    1 Right side to back to left side to right side
    2 Left side to back to left side to back
    3 Back to left semiprone to back
    4 Back to right semiprone to back

78. A patient with cholelithiasis is experiencing right upper quadrant pain after eating a meal that was high in fat and asks the nurse for an explanation of how his diet can precipitate pain. The most appropriate response by the nurse would be:
    1 "Foods high in fat are harder to digest."
    2 "The ducts from the liver and pancreas become obstructed."
    3 "Obstructed bile flow limits the amount of bile available to emulsify fat."
    4 "There is an inadequate absorption of both fat and water-soluble vitamins."

79. The nurse is caring for a patient who has had a subtotal thyroidectomy. The nurse is aware that accidental removal of the parathyroid glands can occur and will closely monitor the patient for:
    1 Low calcium levels
    2 Excess cortisol secretion
    3 High urine output
    4 Decreased gag reflex

80. The patient with a hiatal hernia and reflux syndrome reports having pain when he lies down to go to bed at night. An appropriate suggestion by the nurse would be:
    1 Removing high-acid food from the diet
    2 Drinking a hot cup of cocoa before retiring for the night
    3 Abstaining from food or drink before going to bed.
    4 Recommending a sleeping pill one hour before retiring for the night

81. A patient is to have a gynecologic examination in a hospital bed. Which position will the nurse assist the patient in achieving?
    1 Sims'
    2 Prone
    3 Supine
    4 Dorsal recumbent

82. A patient has all of the following in his health history. Which of the following would contribute most to the development of oral cancer?
    1 Alcohol abuse
    2 Poor dental hygiene
    3 Frequent bouts of tonsillitis
    4 Chewing smokeless tobacco

83. The nurse is teaching a patient newly diagnosed with diabetes mellitus about reducing the risk of hypoglycemia. Which of the following will be included in the health teaching?
    1 "Exercise by running each day."
    2 "Space your meals 5 to 6 hours apart."
    3 "Take your diabetes medicine in early afternoon."
    4 "Carry a form of rapid-acting sugar with you at all times."

84. A female patient on antibiotic therapy calls the clinic to speak with the nurse about new onset symptoms. Which of the following patient complaints would lead the nurse to suspect a secondary candidiasis infection?
    1 High fever and swollen lymph nodes
    2 Itching and white discharge from the vagina
    3 Chancres that develop on the outside of the vagina
    4 Excessive bleeding occurring in the absence of a period

85. In planning the nursing care of a patient with dysmenorrhea, the nurse suggests that the patient:
    1 Engage in strenuous exercise to relieve pain.
    2 Eat protein packed foods to delay painful cramps.
    3 Drink warm beverages and use heat to relieve symptoms.
    4 Apply ice packs to the abdomen twice per day.

86. A patient with Addison's disease is being regulated with medication. The nurse knows that the primary goal of medication therapy is:
    1 Restoring electrolyte balance
    2 Reducing the white blood cell count
    3 Increasing bone marrow functioning
    4 Maintaining the red blood cell count level

87. A client with heart failure awakens in the night and calls the nurse complaining of shortness of breath. The nurse can provide relief to the patient by first:
    1 Remaining calm
    2 Elevating the head of the bed

3 Suctioning her

4 Medicating for pain

88. A patient who recently returned to the unit after a bronchoscopy starts to wheeze and appears frightened. What is the nurse's next course of action?

1 Suction the patient.

2 Give the patient pain medication.

3 Call the physician.

4 Call for a respiratory treatment.

89. A neighbor comes to your house after falling on an icy sidewalk. You note that the right lower arm is angulated, but the skin is intact. First-aid measures would include:

1 Calling 911

2 Splinting the affected area

3 Wrapping the area in a warm compress

4 Keeping the affected area below the level of the heart

90. Which of the following hormones stimulates progesterone secretion in the female?

1 FSH

2 LH

3 TSH

4 ACTH

91. A patient's sputum has suddenly become pink and frothy. The nurse has gathered the following data during her assessment. Which of the data is significant and needs to be reported and documented?

1 Decreased appetite

2 Complaints of dull headache

3 Lung sounds with bibasilar crackles

4 Blood pressure of 140/88 mm Hg.

would be HF (L)

92. A nurse is caring for a patient with hypertension and states that he fails to see why he should go on medication when he feels fine. Which of the following is the nurse's best response to the patient's statement?

1 "Your symptoms will get worse, and you should take your pills."

2 "You would be wise to take care of this problem now."

3 "Your hypertension may cause organ damage without creating symptoms."

4 "You should talk to your doctor if you have doubts about the medication."

93. A patient is scheduled for a pulmonary angiogram and wants to know what will happen. The nurse explains that:

1 She will receive a local anesthetic and a tube will be inserted through her nose.

2 She will be placed in a big hollow tube and must remain completely still.

3 She will wear a clip on her nose and breathe into a machine.

4 A dye will be injected through an IV, and an x-ray will be taken.

94. Which of the following subjective symptoms from a patient would lead a nurse to suspect that he may have benign prostatic hypertrophy?

1 Inability to perform intercourse

2 Dizziness

3 Decreased force of urine stream

4 Testicular pain when voiding

95. Which of the following should be included in the plan of care for a patient undergoing a CT scan with contrast?

1 Restricting fluids to 1000 ml 4 hours before the test

2 Placing the patient on npo status for at least 4 hours before the test

3 Allowing the patient to have her usual meal

4 Telling the patient that she will be on bed rest for 4 hours after the test

96. A patient experienced an acute episode of sharp chest pain, breathing difficulty, and change in breath sounds. Which of the following diagnostic procedures would the nurse expect the physician to order for the patient?

1 Ventilation-perfusion scan

2 Angiography

3 Pulmonary function tests

4 Arthroscopy

97. A patient is scheduled for a thoracentesis. The nurse's primary responsibility during this procedure is:

1 Handing the physician collection bottles

2 Keeping the patient still and in proper position

3 Arranging for follow-up x-rays

4 Setting up the three-bottle drainage system

98. The physician has ordered oxygen at 6 L per nasal cannula for his patient. The nurse prepares the humidifier bottle and tubing. The patient asks why the water bottle is necessary. The nurse's best response would be:

1 "The water helps you derive more benefit from the oxygen."

2 "The humidification keeps your nose from becoming dry."

3 "Most patients feel more comfortable when the oxygen is humidified."

4 "Humidity decreases the fire hazard of using oxygen."

99. A nurse is caring for a patient with cirrhosis. Which of the following snacks would help to prevent the development of hepatic coma?

1 Banana and mayonnaise sandwich

2 Cheese and crackers

3 Peanut butter and jelly sandwich

4 Milk and cookies

100. The nurse tells the patient that he needs "coverage" for his blood sugar. The patient asks what kind of insulin he will be getting. The nurse correctly responds that he will receive:

1 Lantus

2 NPH

3 Regular

4 Lente

101. A patient has had a hydrocelectomy because of a severe bacterial infection. Which of the following nursing measures may be necessary postoperatively?

1 Scrotal elevation *to prevent edema*

2 Urinary retention catheter

3 Estrogen therapy

4 Wet-dry saline dressings

102. A nurse is cautioning a patient with diabetes mellitus about the dangers of developing diabetic ketoacidosis (DKA). Which of the following situations should the nurse alert the patient as a possible cause of DKA?

1 Stress

2 Infection

3 Excess insulin

4 Insufficient calories in the diet

103. Many patients with fibromyalgia have difficulty with the diagnosis because:
    1 It is an untreatable disorder.
    2 It is not a "true" disease.
    3 The disorder has few objective symptoms .
    4 They must endure many painful treatments.

104. The nurse is monitoring a patient on bed rest for symptoms of fluid retention. Where would the nurse best assess for edema in this patient?
    1 Feet
    2 Hands
    3 Knees
    4 Sacrum

105. The nurse is teaching a patient about laryngitis. The patient asks if he will still be able to sing in the choir. The nurse's best response is:
    1 "You should really rest your voice for a while."
    2 "If you gargle with saltwater, you should be ok to sing."
    3 "You should practice singing as much as possible before your performance."
    4 "You should probably give up singing in the choir because of the laryngitis."

106. A patient is on a 1500-ml/day fluid restriction. What will the nurse need to take into consideration before dividing up the fluids for the patient for the day?

    _____

    _____

    _____

    _____

107. Which of the following statements made by a patient with sinusitis would indicate to the nurse that further teaching is required?
    1 "I use a warm mist humidifier at night."
    2 "I take my decongestants when the doctor ordered."
    3 "I will call the physician if my fever comes back."
    4 "I will put ice packs on my nose three times a day."

108. Which of the following statements made by a patient who has had a subtotal thyroidectomy may indicate that the patient is experiencing hypocalcemia?
    1 "I have a massive headache."
    2 "My face feels numb."
    3 "I feel nauseous."
    4 "I got dizzy when I went to the bathroom."

109. Which of the following would be a priority nursing diagnosis for a patient who has AIDS?
    1 Risk for infection
    2 Risk for loneliness
    3 Adult failure to thrive
    4 Ineffective sexuality patterns.

110. A patient complained of dizziness immediately after receiving eardrops. This may indicate that:
    1 The eardrops were administered too quickly.
    2 The auditory canal is occluded.
    3 The eardrops were very warm.
    4 He is having an allergic reaction.

111. A patient has been diagnosed with hypertension. Which of the following symptoms did the patient likely experience?
    1 Nausea, vomiting, nosebleeds
    2 Increased urination, fatigue, blurred vision
    3 Chest pain, shortness of breath, nervousness
    4 Blurred vision, irritability, occipital headaches

112. A patient with a head injury has been ordered mannitol IV. The patient is most likely receiving the mannitol because:
    1 The chance for infection is increased.
    2 He has Increased intracranial pressure.
    3 It will help the patient rest more comfortably.
    4 Of the patient's potential for seizures

113. The nurse is reviewing orders for a telemetry patient who has glaucoma. Which of the following orders would the nurse question?
    1 Morphine sulfate, 1 mg IV for complaint of chest pain
    2 Milk of magnesia, 30 ml po for constipation
    3 Ferrous sulfate, 300 mg twice daily
    4 Atropine sulfate, 1 mg IV for symptomatic bradycardia

114. A patient diagnosed with chronic renal failure is becoming more confused. Because all previous laboratory test results were within normal range, which of the following would be of concern to the nurse and should be reported at once?
    1 Potassium of 5.2 mEq/L
    2 Glucose of 90 mg/100 ml
    3 Platelet count of 100,000/mm³
    4 Leukocyte count of 5500/mm³

115. Which of the following nursing interventions would discourage the development of edema in the arm of an individual who has had a mastectomy?
    1 Administer diuretics as ordered.
    2 Elevate the arm above the level of the heart.
    3 Bind the affected arm to the patient's side.
    4 Assess circulatory status frequently.

116. In the acute phase of treatment for a myocardial infarction, the nurse administers supplemental oxygen to the patient. The main goal of oxygen therapy is to:
    1 Prevent ventricular fibrillation.
    2 Decrease anxiety and restlessness.
    3 Prevent the complications of shock.
    4 Increase oxygen supply to myocardial tissue.

117. A patient is to have an autograft to a burn site on his left femur. The nurse knows that the transplanted graft will contain tissue from:
    1 A cadaver
    2 His own body
    3 A living relative
    4 An animal

118. A patient was recently admitted because of a motor vehicle accident. Which of the following observations would cause the nurse to monitor intake and output closely?
    1 Capillary refill less than 3 seconds
    2 Elastic skin turgor
    3 Crackles in lower lobes
    4 Amber aromatic urine

119. A patient is admitted to a medical surgical unit with a diagnosis of acute exacerbation of asthma. Which of the following sounds might the nurse expect to hear when auscultating the lungs?
    1 Rhonchi
    2 Crackles
    3 Rales
    4 Wheezes

120. A nurse is caring for a patient who has undergone arthroplasty of the left knee. Which of the following data, observed in the immediate postoperative period, must be reported immediately?
    1 Nausea and vomiting

2 Slow capillary refill to left foot
3 Infiltration of intravenous fluids
4 Inability to cough productively

121. The nurse is preparing to receive a patient who has been diagnosed with blistered shingles. Which of the following rooms would the nurse choose for the patient?
1 A room with a roommate who has had an arthroscopy
2 A room with a pediatric patient
3 An isolation room
4 It does not matter what room the patient is assigned.

122. The nurse is caring for the stomal area of a patient who had a urinary diversion 2 weeks ago. Which of the following actions is most appropriate?
1 Massaging the area two to three times per day
2 Applying baby oil to the area and stoma
3 Moistening the stoma and area with aloe lotion
4 Cleansing the area with soap and water and patting dry

123. A thoracentesis is done to remove fluid from the:
1 Pleural space
2 Alveolar space
3 Interstitial space
4 Bronchiolar space

124. To best prepare the patient for a cystoscopy during which no x-ray images will be taken, the nurse:
1 Administers enemas until clear
2 Shaves the pubic area
3 Inserts an indwelling catheter
4 Encourages fluid intake

125. A patient has continuous bladder irrigation. When calculating the urine output for the patient, what information will the nurse need to complete the documentation accurately?

_____
_____
_____
_____

126. The nurse assists an elderly patient who has had a hip replacement onto an elevated toilet seat. The patient asks the nurse why she must use this device. Which of the following is the nurse's best response?
1 "The elevation will help the fracture heal properly."
2 "The elevation will keep you from flexing your hip."
3 "The other toilet causes too much pressure on your suture line."
4 "We can keep your hip in better alignment using this seat."

127. A patient diagnosed with varicose veins is reluctant to have surgery to repair them. She asks the nurse what she can do to reduce the pain of the varicosities. The nurse suggests that the patient:
1 Engage in 30 minutes of aerobic exercise every day.
2 Wear knee-high trouser socks.
3 Avoid sitting or standing for long periods.
4 Ride a stationary bike each day.

128. In a patient with myasthenia gravis, which one of the following drugs would the nurse question if they were ordered?
1 Neostigmine (Prostigmin)
2 Neomycin (Mycifradin)
3 Prednisone (Deltasone)
4 Pyridostigmine (Mestinon)

129. Which of the following types of traction contribute most to the development of venous thrombosis?
1 Buck's
2 Russell
3 Halo frame
4 Crutchfield tongs

130. A patient has been prescribed a nonsteroidal antiinflammatory drug (NSAID) for the treatment of osteoarthritis. The patient complains that the drug is causing him gastric distress. What strategies might the nurse suggest to decrease this patient's discomfort?

take c meals
_____
_____
_____

131. When assessing a patient's range of motion, the nurse notices that the patient has trouble extending his right arm out from his side. Moving a body part away from the midline is called:
1 Flexion
2 Abduction
3 Adduction
4 Pronation

132. A nurse is preparing to administer an injection to a non-ambulatory patient. Which IM injection site is appropriate for this client, who has muscle atrophy of both upper and lower extremities?
1 Deltoid
2 Abdomen
3 Ventrogluteal
4 Gluteus maximus

133. The nurse is caring for a patient with a possible diagnosis of Addison's disease. When evaluating the laboratory reports on the patient, which report would indicate this diagnosis?
1 Low cortisol levels
2 Elevation of growth hormone
3 Large amounts of TSH, T3, and T4
4 Serum elevation of the hormone epinephrine

134. A nurse is caring for a patient who is 2 days postoperative appendectomy. The patient complains of incisional pain on ambulation. The nurse suggests splinting the wound with a pillow based on the understanding that:
1 Splinting allows for deeper respirations and coughing.
2 Persons with abdominal incisions are hesitant to ambulate.
3 An abdominal binder would restrict the patient's movements.
4 Sustained stress disrupts wound layers and may impede tissue repair.

135. A patient with hypertension is upset that he has to undergo treatment and states, "I don't feel bad. Why is the doctor making such a fuss?" The best reply by the nurse is:
1 "I will ask the doctor to see you in the morning."
2 "Why do you question our care? We are only trying to help you."
3 "What could I do to help you understand the seriousness of your disease?"
4 "What questions do you have regarding your care? Maybe I can answer them."

136. The nurse is assessing a patient for evidence of a hypoglycemic reaction. Which assessments indicate this reaction?
    1 Polyuria, dysuria, fever
    2 Glycosuria, hematuria, tachypnea
    3 Pale, clammy skin, confusion
    4 Ketonuria, fruity odor to the breath, hot and dry skin

137. An individual who is donating blood is found to be of the type that is considered the "universal donor." The patient's blood type is:
    1 A
    2 B
    3 O
    4 AB

138. Which of the following types of cells may be used in the future to treat Parkinson's disease, spinal cord injury, or rejection of transplanted organs?
    1 Stem cells
    2 Leukocytes
    3 Platelets
    4 Thrombocytes

139. A father is reluctant to allow his child to receive a polio immunization. Which of the following statements made by the nurse is true regarding this procedure?
    1 "This injection will prevent your child from ever contracting polio."
    2 "This injection is mandatory for all children."
    3 "Your child's resistance to polio will be increased from this shot."
    4 "We do not need your consent to treat your child."

140. A nurse is preparing a care plan for a patient who is undergoing chemotherapy for breast cancer. The nurse is aware that many of the drugs used for chemotherapy:
    1 Are given orally
    2 Cause few side effects
    3 Destroy all cells that divide rapidly
    4 Are specific for only cells within the tumor

141. An elderly patient, who is 3 days postpneumonectomy, develops an infection of the surgical site. When securing supplies for the wet-to-dry dressing changes, the nurse orders Montgomery straps, based on the understanding that these:
    1 Are more cost effective
    2 Are less likely to cause additional infection
    3 Will cause less trauma to the skin
    4 Will decrease the need for frequent dressing changes

142. Which of the following devices will assist the patient with a knee replacement to maintain the flexibility of the knee?
    1 A trochanter roll
    2 An abductor pillow
    3 A continuous passive ROM machine
    4 A Hemovac drainage device

143. A nurse is conducting a neurovascular assessment on a client with a leg cast. The nurse charts that the patient's big toe "blanches" well. What was the nurse describing?
    1 The patient's toe has a capillary refill time less than 3 seconds.
    2 The color of the toe
    3 The temperature of the toe
    4 The patient has full mobility.

144. When assessing a patient who is in kidney failure, the nurse suspects the patient is overhydrated. Which of the following assessment data would support the suspicion?
    1 Edema, crackles, low serum osmolarity
    2 Complaints of thirst, weight gain, and high serum sodium levels
    3 Dry cough, weight loss and low serum sodium levels
    4 Dry lips, loss of weight, dark amber urine

145. A patient with arteriosclerosis obliterans asks the nurse how he can best control the pain in his extremity. Which of the following suggestions should the nurse make?
    1 Wear support hose.
    2 Apply hot packs to area.
    3 Wear warm clothing over extremity.
    4 Apply ice to area.

146. The patient with Buerger's disease has the following lifestyle habits. Which health habit probably contributes the most to his diagnosis?
    1 Exercises 10 minutes each day
    2 Smokes two packs a day
    3 Eats a high-fat diet
    4 Drinks one beer each night

147. Which of the following is true when comparing Raynaud's disease and Buerger's disease?
    1 Raynaud's disease affects primarily men.
    2 Buerger's disease is not as serious as Raynaud's.
    3 Raynaud's is triggered by environmental cold.
    4 Buerger's disease affects arteries only.

148. Nursing observations of a patient with severe liver dysfunction with accompanying jaundice would include which of the following?
    1 Dark stools, yellow sclera, dark urine
    2 Clay-colored stools, pruritus, dark urine
    3 Dark stools, pruritus, straw-colored urine
    4 Clay-colored stools, yellow sclera, blood-tinged urine

149. A patient who is very weak secondary to her lung cancer requires frequent suctioning of her nasopharynx. When will the nurse suction the patient?
    1 When the patient requests suctioning
    2 At least every hour
    3 Any time the patient has gurgling in her airway
    4 As prescribed by the physician who wrote the suctioning order

150. A patient has a thoracotomy tube in his left anterior upper thorax. The patient asks the nurse why no blood is draining from the tube? What is the nurse's best response?
    1 "You should probably ask your doctor."
    2 "The blood should begin draining any time now."
    3 "The tube was most likely placed to drain air, not blood."
    4 "Not all chest tubes drain blood."

151. The water-seal chamber of the patient's chest drainage set-up has stopped fluctuating. The chest tube has been in place for 4 days, and the patient is resting comfortably. What is the most probable cause for this development?
    1 The patient's lung has reexpanded.
    2 The tube is dislodged.
    3 The suction has been turned too high.
    4 A kink has occurred in the tubing.

152. A patient has had a coronary artery bypass graft (CABG). The patient's spouse wants to know why her husband has

a tube coming from his chest. What is the nurse's best response to her question?
1 "It drains blood from his lung."
2 "It is a method for delivering oxygen."
③ "It prevents a buildup of blood from around his heart"
4 "It allows us to administer medications, if needed."

153. During a care conference, the head nurse asks if the nursing diagnosis of ineffective airway clearance related to bronchial secretions is still appropriate for the patient. The nurse caring for this patient can best evaluate this by:
1 Taking the patient's temperature
2 Checking the rate and strength of the patient's pulse
3 Counting the patient's respirations for 1 full minute
④ Ascertaining the effectiveness of the patient's cough

154. A patient with a chest tube should be placed in which position?
1 Trendelenburg
② Semi-Fowler's
3 Left lateral
4 Semiprone

155. A patient calls a primary care clinic and asks what he can do to help him get rid of nasal stuffiness and nosebleeds that he has experienced this winter because his furnace has been running. What suggestion would be appropriate for the nurse to make at this time?
1 "You need to make an appointment right away."
2 "Don't let anyone who is sick come into your house."
③ "Run a humidifier in your bedroom while you sleep."
4 "You should buy a carbon monoxide detector for your home."

156. The patient's left thoracotomy tube is connected to water-seal drainage and suction. The patient is to be transported to the x-ray department. How will the nurse transport the patient?
① Disconnect the suction; maintain the water-seal drainage.
2 Disconnect the chest tube from the water-seal drainage system.
3 Ask if the x-ray department can possibly do its procedure in the patient's room.
4 Get a portable suction machine from central supply to transport the patient.

157. Which of the following are symptoms of a true latex allergy?
1 Rash on palms of hands
② Facial swelling and urticaria
3 Sore throat and sneezing
4 Painful blisters on arms and hands

158. A patient with a bee sting allergy is traveling to an out-of-state national park. What should the patient carry with him at all times?

epinephrine pen
_____
_____
_____

159. When planning care for a patient with chronic pain, the nurse remembers that pain medication should be given to a patient:
1 Before bedtime
② Before pain intensity reaches its maximum
3 At least every 4 hours
4 As soon as the client asks for it

160. Damage to the laryngeal nerve may occur following a thyroidectomy. Which of the following assessment data may indicate that the nerve has been damaged?
① Hoarseness
2 Frothy sputum
3 Choking sensation
4 Positive Chvostek's sign

161. Which of the following data collected would support the diagnosis of lower urinary tract infection?
1 Hypertension and somnolence
② Cloudy urine and frequency
3 Unrelenting headache and blurred vision
4 Painful muscle spasms of the abdomen and perineum

162. A nurse is caring for a patient diagnosed with meningitis. The patient is extremely sensitive to light, and her mother sits at her bedside crying. Which of the following should the nurse include in this patient's plan of care?
① Maintaining a calm, relaxed environment
2 Encouraging visitors to help stimulate patient interactions
3 Providing for frequent interactions between the patient and her mother
4 Placing her in a semiprivate room or ward to foster interaction and release tension

163. If 1000 ml of D5W is to infuse over 8 hours, and the drop factor for the tubing is 10 gtts/ml. How many gtt/min should the IV infuse?

_____
_____
_____
_____

164. A patient with hypertension has complaints of headache and weakness. The nurse notices that the patient's face is flaccid on the left side. The nurse should continue to monitor the patient for:
1 Angina
2 Hypertension
3 Myocardial infarction
④ Cerebrovascular accident

165. Which of the following might a patient undergoing a gastrectomy develop postoperatively?
1 Diabetes mellitus
2 Esophageal reflux
3 Pernicious anemia
④ *Helicobacter pylori* infection

166. The nurse is preparing to educate a group of students regarding measures in preventing the spread of hepatitis B. Which of the following does the nurse include in lecture?
① Testing blood donors
2 Avoiding blood donations
3 Adding bleach to the water
4 Avoiding consumption of all shellfish

167. A young patient with a diagnosis of Crohn's disease has had a recent ileostomy. The patient asks the nurse what sports he should avoid when returning to school. In which of the following would the nurse caution the patient against participating?
1 Track
② Football
3 Shot put
4 Swimming

168. A patient is suspected of having a diagnosis of acute appendicitis. Which of the following laboratory tests would most support this diagnosis?
    1 High RBC count
    2 Low platelet count
    3 High serum albumin
    4 High WBC count

169. A nurse is preparing to educate a group of individuals newly diagnosed with diabetes mellitus about the signs and symptoms of hypoglycemia. Which symptoms will the nurse include in her education?
    1 Clammy skin, tremors, confusion
    2 Polyuria, polydipsia, polyphagia
    3 Headache, high blood pressure, nosebleeds
    4 Lethargy, slowed mental processes, hypotension

170. A patient presents to the emergency room with bleeding esophageal varices. For which of the following treatments should the nurse prepare the patient?
    1 Administration of platelets and refrigerated blood
    2 Gastric lavage with room-temperature saline solution
    3 Administration of vasodilators, antibiotics, and antacids
    4 Use of Sengstaken-Blakemore tube and iced saline lavages

171. A patient has a stage-2 decubitus ulcer on the coccyx. Which nursing measure would best prevent the ulcer from progressing to deeper layers of tissue?
    1 Bathing with lanolin based soap
    2 Repositioning patient at least every 2 hours
    3 Administer antiinflammatory drugs as ordered
    4 Placing vitamin A and D ointment on the ulcer

172. A patient with leukemia tells the nurse that he is going to receive a stem cell transplant. The nurse understands that the stem cells may:
    1 Act as an antibiotic within the patient's bloodstream.
    2 Cause the cancer cells to destroy themselves.
    3 Grow new cells that are not cancerous.
    4 Take the place of the destroyed cancer cells.

173. A patient with mastoiditis would have symptoms of:
    1 Pain in and around the ear
    2 Sore throat and tooth pain
    3 Rash and pruritus
    4 Occipital headache

174. The nurse is to administer an antibiotic eye ointment to a patient with a bacterial infection of his right eye. The nurse would:
    1 Place an eye pad on the eye after administering the ointment.
    2 Wear gloves to administer the ointment.
    3 Place the ointment on the eyeball.
    4 Use the unit's stock supply of ointment.

175. The patient returning home after a right cataract extraction with an intraocular lens implant needs to be instructed to avoid:
    1 Excessive fluid intake
    2 Straining at stool
    3 Bathing
    4 Standing near a microwave

176. A patient who has had a tonsillectomy and adenoidectomy complains of having to frequently swallow and asks if she can have some more water to drink. The nurse is concerned because the patient:
    4 May be hemorrhaging

2 Should not be drinking that much water
3 Might damage her incision site by swallowing
4 Should not have discomfort after this surgery

177. A patient, who has noticed that she tends to bump into objects, is being tested for glaucoma. The nurse explains to her that with glaucoma:
    1 Circulation to the brain is decreased.
    2 Blindness is an eventual result.
    3 Her sense of balance is disturbed.
    4 A decrease in peripheral vision is a first symptom.

178. A patient is scheduled for an eye examination and receives mydriatic drops beforehand. After the examination, the nurse advises the patient to:
    1 Wear a patch over her eye.
    2 Wear a pair of sunglasses for the next few hours.
    3 Not lift anything heavier than 5 pounds.
    4 Not sleep on that side of her head for 2 days.

179. A patient with a low WBC count should be protected against:
    1 Hemorrhage
    2 Hyperpyrexia
    3 Jaundice
    4 Infection

180. A 5-year-old patient has an upper respiratory infection. When teaching him how to blow his nose, the nurse tells him to:
    1 Blow with both nostrils open.
    2 Blow one side of his nose at a time.
    3 Keep his mouth open when blowing one side at a time.
    4 Shut his eyes while blowing hard.

181. A patient with the diagnosis of heart failure is being treated with furosemide (Lasix). The patient has complained to the nurse about frequent urination. Which of the following nursing diagnosis is correct for this situation?
    1 Altered tissue perfusion
    2 Fluid excess
    3 Knowledge deficit
    4 Fluid volume deficit

182. A patient has had a hemorrhoidectomy. Which of the following physician orders would be appropriate for this individual?
    1 Encouraging warm showers
    2 Changing occlusive rectal dressings
    3 Using fecal tube to reduce gas pain
    4 Administering laxatives and stool softeners

183. The nurse is assessing a nursing home resident admitted to the emergency department with the tentative diagnosis of "probable right femoral neck fracture." Which assessment finding would support the diagnosis?
    1 The leg is pronated and internally rotated.
    2 The leg is supinated and internally rotated.
    3 The right leg is longer than the left and is laterally rotated.
    4 The right leg is shorter than the left and is externally rotated.

184. A patient is on diuretic therapy for treatment of hypertension. For which electrolyte imbalance is the patient most at risk?
    1 Hypokalemia
    2 Hypocalcemia
    3 Hyperglycemia
    4 Hypoinsulinemia

185. Which of the following assessment findings is an early sign of lymphoma?
    1 High fever
    2 Decreased urine output
    3 Dependent edema
    4 Painless swelling of lymph nodes

186. The nurse is caring for a patient with lymphedema. How can the nurse help relieve the pain associated with this condition?
    1 Encourage long walks.
    2 Elevate the affected extremity.
    3 Encourage liberal fluid intake.
    4 Use an aircast on the affected extremity.

187. Which of the following diets would be best for a patient with hyperthyroidism?
    1 Low-purine, high-fat, 1000-calorie diet
    2 Clear liquids in the form of six small feedings
    3 2-gram low-sodium diet with an evening snack
    4 High-protein, high-calorie, high-carbohydrate diet with snacks

188. A patient who has had a radical thyroidectomy begins to experience extreme nervousness and tachycardia. Which of the following may be occurring?
    1 Thyroid storm
    2 Cushing's syndrome
    3 Hypoglycemia
    4 Hypocalcemia

189. A patient with hypertension is being managed by medication, including a diuretic. Regarding the diet, the nurse would educate the patient to:
    1 Maintain a high-potassium diet.
    2 Drink at least a quart of liquids a day.
    3 Avoid spicy and high-fat, high-cholesterol foods.
    4 Refrain from caffeine and caffeine-containing products.

190. A patient has been diagnosed with primary hypertension. Which one of the following medications is designed to lower blood pressure?
    1 Digoxin (Lanoxin)
    2 Ibuprofen (Motrin)
    3 Cimetidine (Tagamet)
    4 Hydrochlorothiazide (HydroDiuril)

191. The nurse needs to obtain a sterile urine specimen for culture and sensitivity from a patient with an indwelling urinary catheter. Choose all of the following that would apply to this situation.
    1 Disconnect the catheter from the drainage tubing, and let the urine drip into the sterile bottle.
    2 Use a needle and syringe to withdraw urine from the tubing port.
    3 Inject the specimen from the syringe into the sterile bottle.
    4 Place a towel under the bag, and open the drainage valve at the bottom of the drainage bag.
    5 Remove the old Foley, using a straight catheter, and recatheterize.

192. The patient's wife is concerned because her husband, who suffered a CVA 3 days ago, laughs and cries inappropriately. The nurse's best reply is:
    1 "This is a normal healing sign for someone who has had a CVA."
    2 "I ignore him when he starts acting like that."

    3 "He has what is called 'emotional lability.' This may occur after a stroke."
    4 "Men your husband's age like to tease us by acting this way."

193. A patient's spouse calls the day clinic and tells the nurse that his spouse, who has hypothyroidism, is always complaining of being cold. Which statements made by the nurse are correct and would best help the couple? Choose all that apply.
    1 "This is normal for a person who has hypothyroidism."
    2 "Your wife's medication may need to be adjusted."
    3 "Please contact your physician immediately."
    4 "Bring your wife to the emergency department."
    5 "Would you like to make an appointment for your wife?"

194. A patient who had a CVA 2 weeks ago has dysphagia. Based on these data, the nurse tells the aide to:
    1 Keep the patient in bed.
    2 Speak loudly when talking.
    3 Allow extra time for him to answer her.
    4 Make sure he swallows his food.

195. The patient requires nasopharyngeal suctioning. The nurse places the suction catheter into sterile solution. The underlying principle for this action is to:
    1 Maintain sterile technique.
    2 Prevent tissue trauma.
    3 Check patency of the tube.
    4 Check the suction's pressure.

196. A nurse is discharging a patient who has hyperparathyroidism. The nurse advises the patient to contact the physician if she develops flank pain because:
    1 Flank pain can signal a worsening of her condition.
    2 Low calcium levels might be causing the pain.
    3 Kidney stones are a frequent complication of her disorder.
    4 Pain will require immediate surgical intervention.

197. The nurse observes that her patient, age 60, has stress incontinence each time she coughs or gets out of bed. The nurse understands that:
    1 Hormonal changes place older women at risk for stress incontinence.
    2 Her patient is not emptying her bladder completely.
    3 The nerves controlling the bladder are affected.
    4 Her patient's bladder is displaced in her pelvic cavity.

198. A patient who is taking steroids for rheumatoid arthritis complains to the nurse that his stomach has been upset and he has been unable to eat. Which of the following symptoms, if found, would be of most concern to the nurse at this time.
    1 High blood pressure
    2 Cloudy urine
    3 Tarry stools
    4 Nausea

199. A patient sustained an injury to his spinal cord at the C2 level. Based on a spinal cord injury at this level, the nurse would most likely expect the patient to be treated with:
    1 Diuretics
    2 Oxygen via ventilator
    3 Oxygen via nasal cannula
    4 Vasopressors

200. Initial treatment for epistaxis includes which of the following?
 1 Apply pressure to the soft part of the nose with thumb and forefinger.
 2 Pack the anterior nares with sterile, saline-soaked gauze.
 3 Tilt the head back and close mouth while pinching nose.
 4 Blow nose until all blood is removed from both nares.

201. A patient has had a myocardial infarction and is ordered a soft diet. The nurse knows that the soft diet was most likely ordered because:
 1 Most soft diets are also bland and would not fatigue the patient.
 2 Soft diets are easy to chew and digest, decreasing myocardial oxygen demand.
 3 Most patients that have had an myocardial infarction will vomit any other type of diet.
 4 The patient cannot tolerate anything more formed at this time.

202. A patient complains of "skipping sensations" in her chest while she is working at home. The nurse would anticipate that the physician will order for the patient:
 1 A glucometer
 2 Urine collection
 3 A Holter monitor
 4 A Doppler flow study

203. Which of the following is the priority nursing responsibility for a patient who has a tracheostomy?
 1 Suctioning as ordered
 2 Changing the dressing
 3 Maintaining a patent airway
 4 Allaying any anxiety

204. A client who has had an arthroscopy is being monitored for thrombophlebitis. Which nursing measure would best prevent the development of this complication?
 1 Administration of heparin sodium
 2 Early ambulation or ROM exercises
 3 Increased fluids
 4 Administration of diuretics

205. Where will the nurse assess a pacemaker insertion site?
 1 At the neck
 2 On his back
 3 On his upper chest
 4 Midaxillary region

206. When ambulating a patient with right hemiparesis, the nurse should stand on the patient's:
 1 Right side and hold one arm on the gait belt on the patient's waist
 2 Left side and hold one arm around the patient's waist
 3 Right side and 12 inches behind the patient
 4 Left side and hold the patient's right hand

207. Patients that are diagnosed with thalassemia major may present with (check all that apply):
 1 Jaundice
 2 Erythema
 3 Hepatomegaly
 4 Pruritus
 5 Blurred vision

208. Which of the following concerns is a priority in a client with an open head injury?
 1 Infection
 2 Hemorrhage
 3 Increased intracranial pressure
 4 Consciousness

209. A client has been diagnosed with labyrinthitis. Which of the following was probably his primary complaint?
 1 Sinus pain
 2 Dizziness
 3 Cephalgia
 4 Diplopia

210. A patient has otosclerosis and is scheduled for an upcoming surgery. What procedure will the patient most likely undergo?
 1 Stapedectomy
 2 Mastoidectomy
 3 Myringotomy
 4 Cerumen removal

211. A patient with bilateral hearing aids complains of ear pressure and is subsequently diagnosed with impacted ear cerumen. Which physician orders will the nurse anticipate? Check all that apply.
 1 Remove hearing aids during the day.
 2 Provide hydrogen peroxide drops to ears twice each day for 7 days.
 3 Irrigate ears with normal saline once daily.
 4 Leaving the right hearing aid out of the patient's ear.
 5 Do not put hearing aids in until further notice.

212. A patient is to receive 1000 ml of 5% dextrose in water plus 40 mEq potassium chloride in 12 hours. In checking the flow rate, how much should the patient receive per hour?
 1 42 ml/hr
 2 83 ml/hr
 3 100 ml/hr
 4 125 ml/hr

213. A patient is at risk for a pulmonary embolism secondary to deep-vein thrombosis. Which one of the following expected outcomes is appropriate for the patient?
 1 Has no pain with respiratory effort
 2 Participates in ADL
 3 Maintains stable weight
 4 Demonstrates effective coughing techniques

214. Which of the following statements apply to the diagnosis of hypoglycemia, secondary to insulin overdose? Check all that apply.
 1 Change in level of consciousness occurs.
 2 Skin is cold and moist.
 3 Skin is warm and hot.
 4 Patient responds rapidly to treatment.
 5 It occurs suddenly.
 6 It develops gradually over time.

215. A patient scored 5 on the Rancho Los Amigos scale, meaning that she is confused-inappropriate. The nurse expects this patient to:
 1 React inconsistently and nonpurposefully to stimuli.
 2 Appear alert and be able to respond to simple commands fairly consistently.
 3 Show goal-directed behavior but depend on external input for direction.
 4 Be in a heightened state of activity with decreased ability to process information.

216. Which of the following symptoms would alert the nurse to a possible adverse effect to thrombolytic therapy?
 1 Vomiting

2 Epistaxis
3 Back pain
4 Blurred vision

217. Diabetic ketoacidosis is treated with:
1 Oral antidiabetic agents
2 Glucose and water
3 Diuretics
4 Insulin

218. Which of the following interventions will the nurse anticipate implementing for a patient with a diagnosis of a myocardial infarction?
1 Adjusting the bed to Trendelenburg position
2 Maintaining prescription of complete bed rest for at least 5 days
3 Providing clear, room-temperature liquids throughout hospitalization
4 Administering a stool softener to prevent straining with bowel movements

219. A nurse is doing blood glucose screenings at a local mall. In addition to testing capillary blood, the nurse inquires to possible symptoms of diabetes mellitus. Which of the following would the nurse include? Check all that apply.
1 Polydipsia
2 Cold skin
3 Dry mouth
4 Excess urination
5 Lack of appetite

220. A client presents to the emergency department a few days after removing a tick from his skin. He complains of influenza-like symptoms and painful joints. The client may be suffering from:
1 Amyotrophic lateral sclerosis
2 Lyme disease
3 Encephalitis
4 Chronic fatigue syndrome

221. A patient with diabetes is being treated for pneumonia. She received 22 units of regular insulin at 6:30 AM and was unable to eat her breakfast. Which of the actions listed should be included in this patient's plan of care? Choose all that apply.
1 Glucometer checks at 15-minute intervals
2 Intake po as soon as possible
3 More regular insulin should be given.
4 Transfer to intensive care unit.
5 IV fluids if the patient is unable to eat

222. The nurse is determining how well a patient with tuberculosis has achieved the goals for the nursing diagnosis: ineffective breathing pattern related to sputum production. Which of the following expected outcomes is appropriate?
1 Stable weight
2 Clear breathing sounds
3 Negative sputum culture
4 Verbalizes need for isoniazid (INH)

223. A patient has Ménière's disease and is taking medication for the vertigo. The nurse is with the patient during a severe attack. Which of the following helps reduce the vertigo?
1 Encourage the patient to move slowly to a chair.
2 Take an additional dose of meclizine (Antivert).
3 Increase fluid intake to 2000 ml/day.
4 Darken the room.

224. A patient suffers from presbycusis. Based on an understanding of this condition, which of the following best states nursing concerns for the patient?
1 At risk for alteration in comfort (physical)
2 At risk for injury: falls
3 At risk for alteration in family roles
4 At risk for increasing alteration in sensory perception, auditory

225. A patient fell in the bathroom, hitting her head on the commode. In monitoring her vital signs, which of the following blood pressures would indicate that the patient is experiencing an increase in intracranial pressure?
1 Systolic decreasing, diastolic decreasing
2 Systolic decreasing, diastolic increasing
3 Systolic increasing, diastolic decreasing
4 Systolic increasing, diastolic increasing

226. A patient has a seizure that is accompanied by incontinence. The patient sleeps for several hours afterwards. What kind of seizure did the patient most likely have?
1 Partial
2 Focal
3 Absence
4 Tonic-clonic

227. A patient asks the nurse why she must lay flat after her lumbar puncture. The nurse correctly answers the patient by saying:
1 "You may get a bad headache if you sit up now."
2 "You may have leakage of spinal fluid if you sit up."
3 "Let me help you sit up; there is no reason why you can't."
4 "Your blood pressure will bottom out if you sit up now."

228. Which of the following is a common symptom in patients with a herniated nucleus pulposus, lumbar region?
1 Headache
2 Low blood pressure
3 Arm pain
4 Buttock and thigh pain

229. A nurse is presenting a class on hearing difficulties of older adults to the aides. Behavioral clues indicating difficulty in hearing and the need for evaluation by an otolaryngologist include:
1 Complaining of ringing in the ears
2 Avoiding face-to-face contact
3 Changing body positions frequently
4 Speaking while others are talking

230. In a patient who has a stage-2 decubitus ulcer and pneumonia, the nurse makes the following observations. Which one is the priority?
1 Temperature of 99.6° F (37.5° C)
2 Facial flushing
3 Tachypnea
4 Productive cough

231. In distinguishing between a sprain and a fracture, the nurse would be more suspicious of a fracture if which of the following signs were present on assessment?
1 Edema
2 Deformity
3 Limited movement
4 Tenderness to palpation of the area

232. An adult patient is placed in Buck's extension traction to the left leg. The nurse is aware that this type of traction can be useful in which of the following injuries?
    1 Neck sprains
    2 Spinal fractures
    3 Shoulder dislocations
    4 Lower extremity and hip fractures
233. Several complications are associated with Russell traction. Which of the following symptoms may indicate a complication?
    1 Drainage at the cast site
    2 Signs of compartment syndrome
    3 Pressure under the popliteal space
    4 Evidence of undue skin pressure from under the boot
234. A client has had a subtotal thyroidectomy. Which of the following should be available in the room of the patient at all times?
    1 A chest tube tray.
    2 Spinal puncture tray
    3 Tracheostomy tray
    4 Transtracheal oxygen delivery
235. After retinal reattachment, the patient should be discouraged from:
    1 Driving
    2 Sleeping supine
    3 Lifting heavy objects
    4 Watching television
236. Hearing aids are most helpful to patients who have:
    1 Conduction deafness
    2 Sensorineural deafness
    3 Impacted cerumen
    4 Senile dementia
237. Urine is transferred from the kidney to the bladder by the:
    1 Meatus
    2 Kidney pelvis
    3 Ureters
    4 Glomerulus
238. A patient is being treated for acute glomerulonephritis. Which of the following facts in the patient's history may have precipitated the event?
    1 Antibiotic therapy
    2 Upper respiratory infection
    3 Frequent urinary tract infections
    4 Low fluid intake
239. Urine moves down the ureters into the bladder by the process of:
    1 Peristalsis
    2 Filtration
    3 Diffusion
    4 Osmosis
240. Which of the following laboratory findings would support the diagnosis of chronic renal failure?
    1 Low serum sodium
    2 High serum creatinine
    3 Low serum osmolality
    4 Low serum albumin
241. A patient is being observed for increased intracranial pressure. Which classification of drugs, besides anticonvulsants and corticosteroids, would the nurse expect the physician to order?
    1 Narcotic analgesics
    2 Antiemetics
    3 Osmotic diuretics
    4 Antibiotics
242. The nurse is distributing health literature on prostate cancer. Which of the following blood tests is recommended by the American Cancer Society as a screening test for this type of cancer?
    1 Carcinogenic embryonic antigen (CEA)
    2 Prostate-specific antigen (PSA)
    3 Digital rectal examination (DRE)
    4 Enzyme-linked immunosorbent assay (ELISA)
243. Which of the following physician orders would the nurse expect for a patient diagnosed with renal calculi?
    1 Whirlpool baths
    2 Limiting fluid intake
    3 Rack all urine
    4 Straining all urine
244. A patient has just returned to his room after undergoing a myelogram (MEG) using Pantopaque (iodine-based) dye. What position is most therapeutic for this patient?
    1 Up ad lib
    2 Supine for at least 6 to 8 hours
    3 Head of bed elevated 15 degrees
    4 Head of bed elevated 60 degrees
245. When teaching a patient who is experiencing migraine headaches, which of these behaviors indicates that the patient teaching has been successful?
    1 The patient states that she needs to exercise daily.
    2 The patient states that she will wear sunglasses when outdoors.
    3 The patient states that she will take an aspirin daily to prevent the headache.
    4 The patient identifies the factors that trigger her headaches.
246. The nurse is teaching a health class to adolescent men about the testicular self-examination and testicular cancer. Which of the following would the nurse stress as a warning sign that needs to be reported to a physician?
    1 A tight prepuce that cannot be retracted
    2 Urinary urgency and frequency
    3 A dull ache in the lower abdomen
    4 Pain upon urination
247. A nurse is caring for a patient with heart failure who has the symptoms of dyspnea, pedal edema, and increased abdominal girth. Which part of the heart is most likely failing?
    1 Mitral valve
    2 Aortic valve
    3 Left ventricle
    4 Right ventricle
248. The nurse is assessing a client who fell at home. If the client has a hip fracture, which of the following symptoms would you expect to find?
    1 Pain and numbness
    2 External rotation of the leg
    3 Large hematoma at the hip
    4 Lengthening of the extremity
249. A nurse notices that a client with a long leg cast has a "hot spot" on the cast. Which of the following might be wrong with the patient?
    1 Swelling under the cast
    2 The cast is too tight

3 Inflammation under the cast
4 A foreign body under the cast

250. A hypertensive patient has been started on a medication that can cause orthostatic hypotension. The nurse can explain to the patient that this side effect can be minimized by:
1 Resting on the edge of the bed
2 Wearing antiembolic stockings
3 Limiting the sodium in the diet
4 Sitting on the edge of the bed momentarily before arising

251. A patient reports that he has chest pain that increases with exertion. The nurse is aware that this may indicate:
1 A myocardial infarction
2 A thrombosed cerebral artery
3 Problems with the mitral valve
4 Insufficient blood supply to the heart muscle

252. A patient is admitted with transient ischemic attack (TIA). Which of the following symptoms are indicative of this disorder? Check all that apply,
1 Gradual loss of sensory function occurs.
2 Temporary loss of motor or sensory function occurs.
3 It results from a sudden lack of blood flow to the brain.
4 Emergency treatment is required.
5 The patient is at high risk for developing a CVA.

253. If a patient has a stroke in the temporal cortex, what deficits will the patient likely experience?
1 Visual
2 Auditory
3 Agnosia
4 Motor

254. A patient has returned from having a myelogram (MEG) using metrizamide (water-based) dye. Which of the following postprocedure actions is most appropriate?
1 Encourage fluids.
2 Secure a bedside commode.
3 Spray the room with a room deodorizer.
4 Administer all drugs withheld before the procedure.

255. A patient is diagnosed with an abdominal aortic aneurysm. The nurse is planning the activity level for the patient. Which would be an appropriate activity for this patient?
1 Bicycling
2 Putting puzzles together
3 Jogging
4 Tennis

256. A patient has been diagnosed with varicose veins. Which of the following facts in the patient's history would predispose the patient to this disorder? Check all that apply.
1 Pregnancy
2 Obesity
3 Many hours spent driving
4 Mother who had varicose veins
5 High blood pressure

257. Patients with sensory dysfunction, such as those with paraplegia, have many teaching needs. Which one of the following is a high-priority teaching need?
1 Importance of doing own weight shifts for 5 minutes every hour
2 Importance of decreasing calcium intake
3 Importance of avoiding cold or very hot foods
4 Importance of adequate fluid intake of 2000 ml/day

258. Which of the following classifications of medications can be used to treat unstable angina pectoris? Check all that apply.
1 Vasoconstrictor agents
2 Beta-blockers
3 Sulfa antibiotics
4 Vasodilating agents
5 Narcotic analgesics

259. The patient has chronic renal failure. The nurse is evaluating his knowledge of the dietary restrictions. Which of the following statements by the patient reflects his understanding of the dietary restrictions?
1 "I never did eat much meat."
2 "I eat a lot of bread and potatoes."
3 "I'd better watch how many onions and cucumbers I eat."
4 "Bananas give me gas, so I avoid them."

260. A patient just underwent a cystoscopy. Immediately following this procedure, which of the following nursing actions is most appropriate?
1 Taking vital signs
2 Administering the PRN narcotic ordered for pain
3 Applying cool towels to the lower abdomen
4 Assisting the patient off the table to the wheelchair

261. A patient has had a cutaneous ureterostomy performed and has catheters (stents) inserted through the ureters to drain the renal pelvis. One of the nurse's main concerns is:
1 Irrigating the stents
2 Maintaining patency of the stents
3 Testing urine for protein, blood, and glucose
4 Preventing contamination of the stents with stool

262. A patient has Parkinson's disease and takes the following medications: amantadine (Symmetrel) and trihexyphenidyl HCl (Artane). In evaluating the effectiveness of these medications, which of the following therapeutic responses would the nurse expect?
1 Decreased salivation, less tremor of head or hands at rest
2 Expressions of depression, thoughts of suicide
3 Normal vital signs, propulsive gait
4 Less visual blurring, mental confusion

263. A patient who is HIV positive should be educated in the prevention of:
1 Urinary tract infections
2 Opportunistic infections
3 Visual changes
4 T-cell count elevation

264. The patient with type 2 diabetes mellitus may use a variety of the following treatments to control his condition. Choose all of the following that apply.
1 Insulin
2 Oral antidiabetics
3 Diet
4 Exercise
5 Glucometer monitoring

265. Which of the following is the most frequent cause of diabetic ketoacidosis (DKA)?
1 Stress
2 Infection
3 Not enough food
4 Too much insulin

266. What type of insulin would the nurse expect to give to a patient in diabetic ketoacidosis (DKA)?
    1 NPH
    2 Lente
    3 Regular
    4 Ultra-Lente

267. A 76-year-old patient with severe arthritis is taking large doses of an antiinflammatory medication that has a side effect of gastric irritation. Patient teaching should include instructions to:
    1 Avoid driving.
    2 Take with food.
    3 Discontinue if CNS effects develop.
    4 Take on an empty stomach to enhance absorption.

268. Which of the following is true concerning rheumatoid arthritis?
    1 Local joint disease
    2 Self-limited illness
    3 Disease of striated muscles
    4 Systemic disease

269. Which of the following is a first-line pharmacological medication used in the treatment of rheumatoid arthritis?
    1 Muscle relaxants
    2 Narcotic analgesics
    3 Antiinflammatory agents
    4 Calcium channel blocking agents

270. A patient has had a bilateral oophorectomy. Which of the following assessment findings would cause the nurse concern?
    1 Serosanguinous drainage from the vagina
    2 Changing the perineal pads every 3 to 4 hours
    3 Foley catheter draining clear yellow urine
    4 Malodorous vaginal discharge

271. In the patient suspected of having benign prostatic hypertrophy, the most frequent signs to assess for are:
    1 Dysuria, nocturia
    2 Hematuria, groin discomfort
    3 Flank pain, chills
    4 Bladder stones, malaise

272. The patient with a cervical spinal injury exhibits spasticity of the extremities. Which of the following types of medications will assist in decreasing the spasticity for the patient?
    1 Muscle relaxants such as baclofen (Lioresal)
    2 Vasodilators such as terazosin HCl (Hydrin)
    3 Narcotic analgesics such as morphine sulfate (Roxanol)
    4 NSAIDs such as tolmetin sodium (Tolectin)

273. A patient receives hemodialysis treatments through an arterio venous (AV) shunt in the left arm. Which of the following are included in the plan of care?
    1 Keep the patient on bed rest.
    2 Irrigate the fistula every 4 hours.
    3 Take the blood pressure on the right arm.
    4 Monitor input and output hourly.

274. A patient has been diagnosed with bursitis, which can be defined as an:
    1 Inflammation of the friction-reducing fluid-filled sac found in joints
    2 Infection of synarthrotic joints
    3 Inflammation of the head of the femur
    4 Infection of the sacs found between the vertebrae

275. During the fifth day in coronary care, a patient with a diagnosis of myocardial infarction develops dyspnea, has blood-tinged, frothy sputum, and becomes very anxious. These symptoms may indicate:
    1 Emphysema
    2 Pulmonary edema
    3 Pulmonary embolism
    4 Chronic obstructive pulmonary disease

276. A nurse is providing care to a patient with a sprained ankle. Which of the following instructions should be given to the patient in regard to decreasing swelling in the ankle?
    1 Instruct the patient to dangle the foot over the edge of the bed.
    2 Tell the patient to elevate the foot and ankle on a pillow.
    3 Tell the patient to request help in performing active ROM exercises to the foot.
    4 Instruct the patient to soak the foot in a warm-water bath.

277. Which of the following nursing care measures are appropriate for a patient diagnosed with gout? Choose all that apply.
    1 Allopurinol twice a day
    2 Increased intake of organ foods
    3 Acid ash diet
    4 Blood glucose monitoring
    5 Alkaline ash diet

278. A patient is 6 hours postoperative for an open-reduction, internal fixation of a fractured femur. Which of the following symptoms would alert the nurse to a possible fat embolism?
    1 Shortness of breath, restlessness
    2 Dysphagia, aspiration pneumonia
    3 Abdominal distension, clay-colored stools
    4 Abdominal pain, absent bowel sounds

279. A nurse is assisting a physician in the application of a plaster cast to a foot and calf. Which of the following is the correct way for the nurse to handle the extremity?
    1 Instruct the patient to elevate the extremity.
    2 Place a pillowcase under the cast to move the extremity.
    3 Pick up the casted extremity, supporting it with the palms of the hands.
    4 Instruct a nursing assistant to elevate the extremity by pulling up on the patient's toes.

280. A nurse is providing dietary instruction to a patient with gouty arthritis. Which of the patient's favorite foods would the nurse recommend he eliminate from his diet?
    1 Chicken and rice
    2 Liver and onions
    3 Beef and potatoes
    4 Veal Parmesan and garlic bread

281. A patient with osteomyelitis of the right knee is admitted to an orthopedic unit. Which of the following statements would indicate to the nurse that further teaching may be necessary?
    1 "I should only be in the hospital overnight."
    2 "I guess this infection could have came from the accident I had a few weeks ago with the staple gun."
    3 "I need to stay in bed for a while."
    4 "I guess I should expect my knee to hurt when I move it around."

282. A nurse is bathing a patient who is 1 day postoperative total hip replacement. Which of the following statements made by the patient would indicate understanding of the positioning required after this surgery?
    1 "I know I shouldn't point my toes."

2 "I need to have lowered chairs."

③ "It will be hard for me not to cross my legs."

4 "I will have trouble not walking for a long time."

283. A nurse is caring for a patient with a diagnosis of possible rheumatoid arthritis. Which of the following elevated laboratory values would support the patient's diagnosis?

1 WBCs and hematocrit

2 Uric acid and hemoglobin

③ ESR and rheumatoid factor

4 LE and rheumatoid factor

284. A nurse is caring for a patient who has been immobilized for 6 days because of the presence of skeletal traction. Which of the following assessment findings might indicate the patient has developed a thrombosis?

1 Shortness of breath

2 Distended neck veins

③ Calf pain and swelling

4 Pain at the skeletal pin sites

285. A nurse is assisting a patient with an above-the-knee amputation (AKA) into a prone position. Which of the following statements made by the patient would indicate that the patient understands the need for this positioning?

1 "Lying prone will alleviate my phantom limb pain."

2 "I have to lay this way to make sure I have good circulation to my stump."

3 "This position will allow me greater comfort than lying on my back."

④ "I have to do this to make sure my hip doesn't get a flexion contracture."

286. A patient who has undergone a hemigastrectomy has been diagnosed with pernicious anemia. The patient asks the nurse what might have caused her problem. Which of the following should be the nurse's best response?

1 "You are no longer able to absorb vitamin B12 because of your surgery."

2 "You are most likely not receiving enough folic acid in your low-fat diet."

③ "Because you have less hydrochloric acid since your surgery, you will have difficulty absorbing vitamin B12."

4 "You can no longer use iron adequately in your body because of your surgery."

287. A patient asks the nurse about the purpose of a serum ESR. The nurse is correct in responding that:

1 "This test will show if you have an infection in your body."

② "Elevation of the ESR signifies an inflammatory process."

3 "This is a test to measure how well the kidneys are working."

4 "Elevation of the ESR usually means you have a blood dyscrasia."

288. A patient with a diagnosis of iron-deficiency anemia has had a series of dyspneic episodes. The patient asks the nurse why this has occurred. Which of the following is the nurse's best response?

1 "Your disease has decreased blood flow to your lungs."

② "You don't have as much oxygen circulating in your bloodstream because of your low red blood cell count."

3 "You may have had some damage to your brain cells because of your chronic low red blood cell count."

4 "The anemia that you have causes you to become short of breath when exercising."

289. A patient presents to the emergency department with a history of epistaxis and black tarry stools. When evaluating the patient's laboratory reports, which of the following conditions might indicate a reason for the patient's symptoms?

1 Leukopenia

2 Leukocytosis

3 Thrombocytosis

④ Thrombocytopenia

290. A patient with chronic heart failure inquires why he does not become short of breath until he exercises or takes a shower. Which of the following statements made by the nurse would best answer his question?

1 "The shortness of breath is caused by your lung constricting."

2 "You need to condition your heart to be able to tolerate exercise."

③ "When you exercise, your heart can no longer meet the oxygen needs of your body."

4 "The blood vessels of your lungs constrict as you exercise, causing the shortness of breath."

291. A nurse is assessing a patient who has just returned to a telemetry unit after a cardiac catheterization. Which of the following nursing interventions would be the most important in the immediate postoperative period?

1 Coughing, deep breathing, leg exercises

2 Urinary output, early ambulation, cardiac monitoring

③ Monitoring for cardiac arrhythmias, bleeding, shortness of breath

4 Assessing vital signs, physical therapy and ambulation, monitoring intake and output

292. A nurse is educating a patient with heart failure regarding a low-sodium diet. Which of the following dietary practices may the patient need to eliminate from his routine?

① Corned beef sandwiches with canned broth each day

2 Shredded wheat and fruit for breakfast each morning

3 Crispy chicken sandwich and cheesy broccoli once per week

4 Hamburgers and French fries for lunch three times per week

293. An elderly patient has had a myocardial infarction of the right side of the heart. Which of the following signs should the nurse anticipate when assessing for heart failure?

1 Nausea

② Heart murmur

3 Crackles in lungs

④ Edema in feet and legs

294. A nurse is obtaining a history from a patient who has been admitted with a diagnosis of probable mitral insufficiency. Which of the following facts in the patient's history would be most significant?

1 Appendectomy 1 year ago

2 One-pack-a-day smoker for 20 years

③ History of rheumatic fever as a child

4 History of a pacemaker insertion 5 years ago

295. A nurse is assessing a patient with complaints of pain and swelling of the left calf. Which of the following recent histories may be significant in this situation?

1 Atrial fibrillation

② Fractured femur

3 Narrow-angle glaucoma

4 New-onset diabetes mellitus

296. The family of a patient who has just returned from an esophagogastroduodenoscopy attempts to feed the patient a milkshake. Which of the following should be the nurse's first course of action?

1 Check the patient's diet order to see if a full liquid diet is ordered.

2 Explain that the patient must wait at least 6 hours before eating.

3 Monitor the procedure to ensure that the patient swallows the liquid.

4 Ask the family to wait until you have checked the patient's gag reflex.

297. A patient is hospitalized with an acute exacerbation of SLE. If the patient has all of the following in their recent history, which one may have contributed to this hospitalization?

1 Ate seafood the night before

2 Went to the beach the day before

3 Has been constipated for the last few days

4 Began taking prednisone a few days ago

298. Which of the following assessment data would indicate that a patient may be suffering from appendicitis?

1 Hematemesis

2 Sharp back pain

3 Severe abdominal distention

4 Rebound abdominal tenderness

299. A patient, recently diagnosed with cholecystitis arrives at an outpatient clinic complaining of severe, right upper quadrant pain. Which of the following data, obtained from the patient history, may have precipitated this problem?

1 Spent 3 hours mowing the lawn

2 Had a hamburger and French fries for lunch

3 Took three acetaminophen for complaints of a headache

4 Had three beers and a bowl of pretzels after mowing the lawn

300. Which of the following nursing diagnosis is most appropriate for a client with osteoporosis?

1 Alteration in bowel elimination

2 Knowledge deficit

3 Body Image disturbance

4 Risk for Injury

301. A patient is admitted to the hospital with a diagnosis of hepatitis A. The patient asks the nurse how he might have possibly caught the virus. Which of the following is the nurse's most appropriate response?

1 "Did you come into contact with a person who has it?"

2 "You may have ingested some contaminated food or water."

3 "Have you had a transfusion of whole blood or platelets lately?"

4 "You might have inhaled some of the virus in your respiratory tract."

302. A nurse is teaching a patient regarding the proper method for administering pancreatic enzymes. Which of the following methods would the nurse advise?

1 "Take the enzymes between meals."

2 "Take the enzymes only if eating a fatty meal."

3 "Take the enzymes at the same time you eat the meal."

4 "Take the enzymes before you retire to bed each night."

303. A patient is scheduled for an elective herniorrhaphy. The nurse notes that the patient has a cold. The nurse reports the cold to the surgeon because:

1 The cold will increase the chance of a postoperative infection.

2 The patient may have an increased chance of peritonitis because of the cold.

3 Coughing and sneezing may compromise the integrity of the surgical incision.

4 The patient may have a prolonged, more expensive hospital stay because of the cold.

304. A nurse notes that a patient's nasogastric tube has not been draining as much as usual. The patient complains of nausea, and abdominal distention is noted. Which of the following is the nurse's next course of action?

1 Remove the nasogastric tube.

2 Call the physician immediately.

3 Assess the patency of the tube.

4 Call for a portable abdominal x-ray unit.

305. A patient is in the emergency department with a suspected tibial fracture. While the patient awaits an x-ray examination, which nursing actions would help reduce the swelling of the leg? Choose all that apply.

1 Application of warm compresses

2 Ice packs

3 Elevation of the extremity

4 Immobilization of the extremity

5 Application of antithromboembolism stockings

306. A nurse is counseling a patient with hypothyroidism concerning drug therapy. Which of the following statements by the patient would indicate that additional teaching may be needed?

1 "I should discontinue the medicine when I feel better."

2 "I should call the doctor if I have a headache or am nervous."

3 "I should try to take the medicine at the same time each day."

4 "I should let the doctor know if I experience weight loss or sweating."

307. A physician tells a patient that he is going to correct a shoulder dislocation by closed reduction. The nurse is correct when she tells the patient that this procedure involves:

1 Surgery

2 General anesthesia

3 Realigning the join by manually pulling on bones

4 Realigning the bones by placement of an external fixation device.

308. Which of the following would be most important in the teaching of a patient that has undergone an adrenalectomy?

1 "Weigh yourself daily."

2 "Avoid stressful situations."

3 "Maintain a diet high in potassium."

4 "Avoid drinking large amounts of water."

309. Which of the following assessment data may indicate that a patient has the disorder of diabetes insipidus?

1 Bounding pulse and low urine output

2 Increased blood pressure and tachycardia

3 Decreased fluid intake and high specific gravity of urine

4 Increased fluid intake and low specific gravity of urine

310. A patient has been admitted to the hospital with the diagnosis of Addisonian crisis. Which of the following medications when stopped abruptly can precipitate an Addisonian crisis?
    1 Insulin
    2 Cardizem
    3 Prednisone
    4 Diltiazem

311. Which of the following measures would assist in ensuring that a patient with diabetes mellitus would receive proper care outside the hospital or clinic?
    1 Wearing a medical alert tag
    2 Carrying a rapid source of glucose with him or her
    3 Carrying a syringe full of insulin with him or her all times
    4 Reporting his or her condition to the local ambulance service

312. A nurse is caring for a patient with hyperpituitarism. Which of the following nursing diagnoses may be appropriate for this patient?
    1 Alteration in comfort
    2 Alteration in body image
    3 Alteration in fluid and electrolyte balance
    4 Altered nutrition, less than body requirements

313. A patient is admitted with a diagnosis of HHNC. The nurse is aware that HHNC differs from DKA in that:
    1 HHNC is more difficult to treat.
    2 DKA includes the complication of metabolic acidosis.
    3 DKA is mostly found in patients who are not insulin dependent.
    4 HHNC includes elevated serum levels of glucose and ketones.

314. A patient has just returned from a thyroidectomy. Which of the following assessment data would be of priority in the immediate postoperative period?
    1 No bowel sounds
    2 Blood pressure of 160/100 mm Hg
    3 Swelling in the neck region
    4 Dime-sized area of blood on the operative dressing

315. A frantic mother calls a health clinic and says that her son, who has diabetes, has a glucometer reading of 36. The child is conscious but nervous. Which of the following should the nurse suggest?
    1 Give the child a can of diet soda.
    2 Bring the child to the hospital immediately.
    3 Give the child some orange juice with sugar in it.
    4 Let the child eat some cheese and crackers.

316. A nurse is caring for a female patient who has had a conization. Which of the following nursing interventions should the nurse expect to carry out for this patient?
    1 Instruct her to replace tampon every 3 hours.
    2 Maintain vaginal packing for the first 12 to 24 hours.
    3 Assist her in using a sitz bath twice per day.
    4 Provide her with instructions on the use of a medicated, vaginal douche.

317. A 47-year-old female patient who works as a nursing assistant comes to an outpatient clinic for a routine physical. The nurse collects the following group of data. Which of the following needs to be addressed by the nurse?
    1 Gynecological examination 6 months ago
    2 Hepatitis B vaccine 4 months ago

3 Last mammogram 8 years ago
    4 Last tuberculosis test 3 months ago after starting a new job

318. The nurse is educating a group of women on the correct technique for breast self-examination. Which of the following methods should the nurse recommend?
    1 "Examine your breasts when your period first starts."
    2 "Palpate your breasts for lumps while sitting at a table."
    3 "Use the palms of your hands to feel for lumps in your breasts."
    4 "Palpate the breasts while lying, sitting, and standing each month."

319. A patient complains of excessive pain during menstruation. Which of the following interventions might the nurse suggest to alleviate discomfort?
    1 Drink cold beverages early in the morning.
    2 Drink warm beverages before the pain begins.
    3 Exercise rigorously to counteract the uterine contractions.
    4 Recommend that the patient ask her doctor for a narcotic prescription.

320. The nurse is caring for a patient who has developed a possible rectovaginal fistula after delivery of her fifth child. Which of the following symptoms would suggest that the patient had developed a rectovaginal fistula?
    1 Leakage of urine from the vagina
    2 Extreme pain following a bowel movement
    3 Passage of stool and flatus from the vagina
    4 White creamy discharge and extreme pruritus

321. A female patient presents to an outpatient clinic because she is concerned that she may have gonorrhea. The patient states her male partner was diagnosed but she has had no symptoms. Which of the following is the best response by the nurse?
    1 "I am sure there is no reason to worry if you have no symptoms."
    2 "I think we should test you because gonorrhea can be asymptomatic in women."
    3 "You can return to the clinic whenever you have burning on urination or get a fever."
    4 "I think we can prescribe you an antibiotic without even doing a culture because your partner is infected."

322. A nurse is assisting a physician in a gynecological examination. Which of the following interventions would increase the comfort of the patient during the procedure?
    1 Allow the patient to keep wearing her undergarments.
    2 Have the patient void before positioning on the exam table.
    3 Ensure that the patient is menstruating when the examination is done.
    4 Leave the room when the examination begins to reduce embarrassment to the patient.

323. A nurse is preparing a patient for an upcoming panhysterectomy. Which of the following should the nurse caution the patient to expect following the surgery?
    1 The patient will have a catheter after surgery.
    2 The patient should expect to be on bed rest at least 4 days.
    3 It is unlikely that the patient will resume a normal diet for a few days.
    4 Physical therapy will be an integral part of her rehabilitation process.

324. A nurse is caring for a patient who has an internal radium implant in her uterus for treatment of cervical cancer. Which of the following statements made by the patient would indicate that further teaching may be necessary?
   1 "I should be taking stool softeners everyday."
   2 "I can lay on either my back or my side when I sleep."
   3 "I should expect to get sick to my stomach with this type of treatment."
   4 "I can have my daughter come in and sit with me if I get bored being hospitalized."

325. A nurse is educating a group of women on premenstrual tension. The nurse has the participants complete a survey of favorite foods. Which of the following favorite foods of the participants can aggravate PMS?
   1 Pizza
   2 Mineral water
   3 Pasta and sauce
   4 Raw fruits and vegetables

326. A patient admitted with COPD also has psoriasis. Which of the following types of skin lesions does the patient have?
   1 Red patches with silver scales
   2 Large, pus-filled macules
   3 A bright red, blistered rash
   4 Large, ulcerated areas

327. A patient in the clinic has been diagnosed with asthma. Laboratory studies have been done and returned. The nurse knows that the primary antibody affected in asthmatic patients is:
   1 International Normalized Ratio (INR)
   2 Immunoglobulin E (IgE)
   3 Hepatitis C virus (HCV) antibody
   4 Carcino embryonic antigen (CEA)

328. Persons with active tuberculosis disease are usually no longer infectious after being on therapy for how long?
   1 1 to 2 days
   2 2 to 3 weeks
   3 3 to 4 months
   4 They will remain infectious for life.

329. A new admission has asthma and uses inhalers. He takes metaproterenol (Alupent), albuterol (Proventil), and beclomethasone (Vanceril). He complains that he does not like the side effects these inhaled medications cause. The nurse will instruct him that he:
   1 Must sit down when using inhalers
   2 Is overdosing himself if he uses all three inhalers within 1 hour
   3 Needs to use the Alupent and Proventil inhalers before the Vanceril
   4 Needs to stop using the inhalers until his next scheduled clinic appointment

330. A patient is to begin medications for tuberculosis. Which of the following statements made by the patient would require further teaching?
   1 "I should cover my mouth and nose when sneezing."
   2 "I won't ever be able to get a PPD again."
   3 "I am glad I will only take these drugs for a few months."
   4 "I can resume normal activity as long as I plan for rest periods."

331. The patient tells the nurse that the reason he came to the clinic is because he has been having difficulty breathing, especially at night. The nurse would be most correct in documenting this information under which section of the admission sheet?
   1 Chief complaint
   2 Psychosocial history
   3 Past medical history
   4 Review of systems

332. A case of active tuberculosis has been confirmed in the nurse's neighborhood and a neighbor asks how she might have been exposed. The nurse's reply states how tuberculosis is transmitted. This includes:
   1 By using the same door handle as the infected person
   2 By an airborne route; the infected person coughing, sneezing, laughing
   3 By touching a tissue that a person infected with tuberculosis used
   4 By riding the bus after the person infected with tuberculosis was on it

333. A patient has a medical diagnosis of respiratory acidosis. His nursing diagnosis is ineffective airway clearance. Which of the following activities is most directly aimed at his nursing diagnosis?
   1 Encouraging fluid intake by offering fluids every 2 hours
   2 Suctioning him every 2 hours and prn
   3 Walking in the halls twice per day
   4 Planning activities to provide rest periods in between

334. A patient has a possible diagnosis of mitral stenosis. Which of the following symptoms correlate with this diagnosis? Choose all that apply.
   1 Heart murmur
   2 heart failure
   3 Palpitations
   4 Orthopnea
   5 Pulmonary edema

335. The nurse in the clinic is gathering data from a new patient. The nurse documents the data gathered. Vital signs are an example of data that should be recorded as:
   1 Subjective data
   2 Routine data
   3 Objective data
   4 Graphic data

336. Which of the following histories of a patient would relate to a diagnosis of bacterial endocarditis?
   1 Previous heart catheterization
   2 Strep throat 4 weeks earlier
   3 Open reduction, internal fixation (ORIF) of the left hip last year
   4 Smokes two packs a day

337. A patient being seen in the clinic has a history of glaucoma. When gathering data related to chronic glaucoma, which of the following complaints would the nurse expect to hear?
   1 Seeing flashes of light and floaters
   2 Having attacks of double vision
   3 Experiencing sudden onset of eye pain with nausea and vomiting
   4 Bumping into objects

338. A patient is admitted to the clinic for a complete physical examination. To prevent injury during the otoscopic examination, which of the following actions should the nurse avoid?
   1 Inserting the otoscope until it touches the eardrum

2 Tipping the patient's head away from the examiner

3 Bracing the examining hand against the patient's head

4 Pulling the ear being examined up and back

339. A patient has been diagnosed with pernicious anemia. Which of the following should be done for this patient on a monthly basis?

1 Administration of vitamin B$_{12}$ PO

2 Vitamin K given IM

3 Therapeutic multivitamin given IV

4 Injectable form of vitamin B$_{12}$

340. In a morning report, the nurse learns that her patient has an upper urinary tract infection. In assessing the patient, the nurse listens for complaints of:

1 Chills, nausea, flank pain

2 Burning on urination, urgency

3 Frequency, suprapubic pain

4 Pain at the end of urination

341. The nurse is making a home visit on her patient who has nephrotic syndrome. The most recent laboratory results show hypoalbuminemia and hyperlipidemia. Which of the following elements is the major pathophysiological factor in this syndrome?

1 Protein

2 Potassium

3 Calcium

4 Sodium

342. The patient has received a prescription for an antimicrobial drug for his upper urinary tract infection. This therapy is usually prescribed for:

1 1 day

2 3 to 5 days

3 5 to 7 days

4 10 to 14 days

343. A male patient is being evaluated for Chlamydia. Which of the following symptoms would cause the physician to suspect a Chlamydia infection?

1 Urethritis

2 A chancre

3 Anal itching

4 Papular warts

344. A patient has been diagnosed with *Pneumocystis carinii* pneumonia. The patient probably has a history of:

1 Pneumonia

2 HIV

3 Leukemia

4 Thalassemia

345. Which of the following is included in patient teaching before a barium enema? Choose all that apply.

1 Nothing to eat for 2 hours before the test

2 Enemas before the examination

3 Laxatives after the examination

4 No meat for 4 days before the examination

346. A patient has stomatitis and the nurse administers topical lidocaine to her mouth before her meal. The intent of the lidocaine is to:

1 Decrease the pain associated with chewing.

2 Keep the sores from becoming infected.

3 Avoids food becoming lodged in the sores.

4 Allow the patient to absorb the food more readily.

347. The nurse is monitoring a patient with a Sengstaken-Blakemore tube for bleeding esophageal varices. Which of the following is most likely in the patient's history?

1 Bronchitis

2 Esophageal cancer

3 Cirrhosis

4 Gastritis

348. The nurse inspects the abdominal incision of a patient who has returned to the skilled nursing facility. Which type of exudate should be reported to the physician?

1 Serosanguineous

2 Serous

3 Clear

4 Purulent

349. A patient with dysphagia has difficulty swallowing liquids. The nurse is advised by the speech therapist to add a thickening agent to his liquids. The nurse knows that the patient will:

1 Have more difficulty swallowing the thickened liquids

2 Have less difficulty swallowing the thickened liquids

3 Benefit more from a blenderized diet

4 Not eat the food because of the consistency

350. Autonomic hyperreflexia may occur after a spinal cord injury. It is critical that the nurse observe for signs of this state. What are the manifestations of increased sympathetic stimulation that are not mediated by the parasympathetic system?

1 Sweating, hypertension, flushed skin

2 Pallor, hypotension, dehydration

3 Tachycardia, pallor, hypotension

4 Thirst, muscle spasticity, goose flesh

351. A patient is unable to respond appropriately and clearly. He is also disoriented to time and demonstrates an inability to follow commands. Which of the following best describes his level of consciousness (LOC)?

1 Oriented, arousable, difficult

2 Confused

3 Having periods of lethargy

4 In a stuporous state

352. Which of the following is the most common cause of autonomic dysreflexia?

1 Visitors

2 Full bladder

3 Taking tympanic temperatures

4 Taking an apical pulse

353. The nurse is assigned to a newly admitted patient who was burned in an apartment fire. The patient quickly develops edema. Which statement best addresses why the nurse is concerned about the edema?

1 Edema means the patient's kidneys have shut down.

2 Edema means frequent skin care is necessary.

3 Edema may lead to hypovolemic shock.

4 Edema indicates that the IV is being infused too rapidly.

354. An aerobic instructor complains to the nurse that she often gets "heartburn" after her aerobic class. Which of the following would the nurse advise for the patient?

1 Drink a large amount of fluids before the class.

2 Limit the amount of bending over in the class.

3 Lie down for 30 minutes before the class.

4 Do not eat a large meal before the class begins.

355. A nurse is administering PPD tests to the residents on the assisted-living wing of a retirement facility. The nurse should assess the injection sites of these residents:
    1 Within 12 to 24 hours
    2 Within 24 to 36 hours
    ③ Within 48 to 72 hours
    4 Within 96 hours to a week

356. Patients who have a gastrectomy are more susceptible to:
    1 Aplastic anemia
    ② Pernicious anemia
    3 Hemolytic anemia
    4 Folic-acid deficiency

357. A patient has been receiving vancomycin hydrochloride (Vancocin) for a methicillin-resistant *Staphylococcus aureus* (MRSA) infection following a craniotomy. With regard to vancomycin hydrochloride, the nurse should report which of the following laboratory results to the physician?
    1 Hemoglobin 12.4 g
    ② Sodium 137 mEq/L
    3 Potassium 4.2 mEq/L
    4 Creatinine 26 mg/dl

358. New medications and combinations of medications are used to treat active tuberculosis disease. The most predominant side effect the nurse needs to look for with the use of tuberculosis drugs such as Isoniazid (INH) is:
    1 Changes in liver enzymes
    ② Sores in the mouth
    3 Increased urination
    4 Decreased saliva

359. Which of the following is an appropriate short-term goal for a patient with the nursing diagnosis: pain related to humeral fracture?
    1 Patient will be able to move arm freely in 1 week.
    2 Patient will report relief from pain before discharge.
    3 The patient will state a reduction in pain during physical therapy sessions.
    ④ Patient will report reduction in painful stimuli 45 minutes after pain medication is given.

360. A 65-year-old patient is to have chest physiotherapy performed by the respiratory therapist. The nurse should plan to:
    1 Administer her albuterol nebulization treatments after the respiratory therapist finishes.
    ② Serve her tray just before this treatment, and offer to take her to the bathroom.
    3 Assess her tolerance to dependent positions required for lower lobe drainage.
    4 Take vital signs 1 hour after the treatment is completed.

361. The nurse is gathering data from a patient who has a history of cataracts. Which of the following complaints would the patient relate to the nurse?
    ① Floaters
    2 Eye pain
    3 Eye dryness
    4 Blurred vision

362. A patient returns to the unit from a suprapubic prostatic resection. He has an IV and three-way Foley catheter connected to continuous bladder irrigation. At the end of the shift, he had an intake of 725 ml fluid IV, 150 ml fluids PO, 3200 ml of irrigation fluid, and 4000 ml output. His intake for the shift was:
    1 150 ml
    2 725 ml
    ③ 875 ml
    4 3200 ml

363. An incontinent patient is being treated for a urinary tract infection. The nursing assistant asks the nurse how the patient became infected. The nurse is correct in stating that the patient probably acquired the infection because:
    ① Of the proximity of urine and feces to the patient's meatus
    2 The patient is in an immunosuppressive state.
    3 The patient is just more susceptible because of the patient's age.
    4 The patient really needs a urinary catheter.

364. Which of the following patient teaching points should be included in the discharge teaching of a patient who is susceptible to urinary tract infections? Choose all that apply.
    1 Avoid sexual intercourse.
    ② Avoid perfumed feminine hygiene products.
    3 Take tub baths daily.
    ④ Increase daily orange juice to eight 8-oz glasses.
    5 Wipe perineum from back to front.

365. Assessing a patient's current and past use of medications, including over-the-counter drugs and herbs, is important. The nurse might expect a change in the ability to control voiding if the patient, during a patient assessment, said he was taking:
    ① Calcium channel blockers
    2 Anticoagulants
    3 NSAIDs
    4 Antiemetics

366. A patient has a history of urinary tract infections. The nurse is doing patient education and should stress the need to:
    ① Empty her bladder when she feels the urge to void.
    2 Make sure she uses protection during sexual activities.
    3 Test her urine with a dipstick after each voiding.
    4 Drink milk before retiring.

367. A patient with peptic ulcer disease says to the nurse "I guess my stress has gotten the better of me." Which of the following is the nurse's most correct response?
    1 "I know what you mean; we all need to decrease stress."
    ② "Not all peptic ulcers are caused by stress; there are other factors."
    3 "You probably have a streptococcal infection."
    4 "Maybe I can get you into a stress-reduction workshop."

368. When providing care to a patient taking sulfa drugs for a urinary tract infection, the nurse should offer fluids frequently during the day to:
    ① Prevent crystals from forming in the urine.
    2 Provide comfort from the burning sensation.
    3 Maintain constant blood levels of the medication.
    4 Maintain sufficient urine output.

369. A patient complains of abdominal discomfort, has an elevated WBC and has rebound tenderness in the right lower quadrant. The patient is exhibiting signs of:
    ① Appendicitis
    2 Pancreatitis

3 Ulcerative colitis

4 Crohn's disease

370. When caring for a patient with a history of metabolic acidosis, the nurse should assess for:

1 Increased urine output

2 Decreased urine output

3 Increasing respirations

4 Decreasing respirations

371. A 35-year-old patient is admitted following an automobile accident with a Glasgow coma scale (GCS) ranging between 13 and 15 since the accident. The nurse knows that these scores indicate:

1 Coma

2 Mild head injury

3 Moderate head trauma

4 Optimum cerebral functioning

372. The nurse is planning her care for a patient who has edema of his legs following extensive burns to both lower extremities. The nurse knows that intracellular swelling after a severe burn is related to:

1 Decreased circulating immunoglobulin

2 Increased cardiac output

3 Increased metabolic demands

4 Disruption in sodium-potassium at the cellular level

373. A patient has an inguinal hernia. The nurse knows that the most dangerous aspect of a hernia is the chance that it may cause:

1 A bowel obstruction

2 Peritonitis

3 A portion of the bowel to become ischemic

4 Strangulation of the stomach lining

374. A comatose patient has an intact airway and is being fed via a nasogastric tube. Which of the following nursing diagnosis is of priority for this patient?

1 Ineffective airway clearance

2 Ineffective breathing patterns

3 Alteration in elimination

4 Risk for aspiration

375. The nurse in the assisted-living facility has been helping a patient who has Grave's disease. The patient refuses to sit down to eat. The nurse can best meet the nutritional needs of this patient by:

1 Allowing her to eat high-calorie, nutritious food as she walks

2 Instituting tube-feeding supplements

3 Restraining her at the table while she eats

4 Give her an all pureed diet she can drink

376. In the postoperative period for cranial surgery, a variety of drugs may be used to control cerebral edema. Which of the following statements best describes how these drugs act in this postoperative phase?

1 Dexamethasone (Decadron) increases kidney output by acting as a thiazide diuretic.

2 Phenytoin (Dilantin) increases the cerebral metabolic rate, decreasing cerebral blood flow and ICP.

3 Furosemide (Lasix) is a diuretic that also reduces the rate of cerebral spinal fluid production.

4 Mannitol (Osmitrol) induces deep sedation, thereby decreasing cerebral metabolic rate.

377. The patient has been admitted with deep partial-thickness (second-degree) burns to both arms. Which of the following best describes a second-degree deep partial-thickness burn?

1 Erythema of intact skin

2 Blister formation that may have ruptured

3 Loss of subcutaneous tissue down to the bone

4 Tissue destruction, possibly involving the entire dermis

378. A patient with asthma tells the nurse that he does not use his albuterol (Ventolin) inhaler because it is the same thing as his ipratropium (Atrovent). The nurse needs to teach him that both inhalers contain:

1 Medications that cause bronchodilation but in different ways; he should wait 5 minutes after using the one inhaler before using the next.

2 Medications that cause bronchoconstriction but in different ways; he should wait 15 minutes after using one inhaler before using the next.

3 Medications that are used for bronchospasm; he can use either one if he feels an attack coming on.

4 The same medication; the names are different because they are made by a different company. He is acting correctly.

379. A patient has COPD. He has signs of both emphysema and chronic bronchitis. Which one of the following assessment findings is usually present in these two categories of COPD?

1 Diminished breath sounds

2 Bronchospasm

3 Cardiac enlargement

4 Increased residual lung volume

380. Which situation best describes the potential of contracting a tuberculosis infection from a person who has active tuberculosis?

1 Lack of frequent hand washing practices in the work setting

2 Close, frequent, or extended contact

3 Sharing a computer at work

4 Sharing the same bathroom in a restaurant

381. The patient has had nasal surgery with the insertion of posterior nasal packing. Which of the following nursing diagnosis is a priority for this patient?

1 Risk for injury

2 Risk for infection

3 Risk for aspiration

4 Altered breathing patterns

382. The laboratory results for a patient who is being treated for asthma have just arrived. Which of the following results indicate the therapeutic blood level for theophylline?

1 10 to 20 μg/ml

2 20 to 30 μg/ml

3 30 to 40 μg/ml

4 40 to 50 μg/ml

383. A patient has gastroesophageal reflux disease (GERD) and emphysema. She is very thin. The nurse questions her about her usual diet at home and she says that she is so short of breath that she has not eaten very much. The diet the nurse should plan to order for her is a:

1 Low-fat diet with six small feedings a day

2 Regular diet with juice between meals and at bedtime

3 High-calorie, high-protein diet

4 High-carbohydrate, bland diet

384. Diabetes insipidus is best treated by the administration of:
    1 Vasopressin
    2 Insulin
    3 Calcium
    4 Glucose

385. A patient with respiratory failure has ineffective breathing patterns as a nursing diagnosis. The patient is most likely suffering from:
    1 Respiratory alkalosis
    2 Hyperventilation
    3 Metabolic acidosis
    4 Respiratory acidosis

386. The nurse is caring for a patient who has nosocomial pneumonia. According to the Centers for Disease Control and Prevention (CDC), the single most effective way to prevent the spread of disease is:
    1 Using antibiotics
    2 Using protective isolation technique
    3 Frequent hand washing
    4 Using standard precautions

387. Which of the following symptoms are indicative of the diagnosis of pheochromocytoma? Choose all that apply.
    1 Blood pressure of 90/50 mm Hg
    2 Diaphoresis
    3 Heart rate of 50 bpm
    4 Blood pressure of 200/120 mm Hg

388. A patient has cataracts. Patient education that is appropriate for this patient is to:
    1 Teach him to avoid bright light or bright sunlight.
    2 Tell him that special glasses will help him see better.
    3 Tell him that over-the-counter medications will help to reduce eye pain.
    4 Tell him to wear sunglasses at night to reduce glare from the headlights.

389. A patient has a lower urinary tract infection. The nurse should advise her to avoid beverages that may irritate the bladder. These beverages are:
    1 Milk and dairy products
    2 Caffeine and carbonated drinks
    3 Bottled water products
    4 Fruit-flavored drinks

390. The nurse is instructing the patient with asthma about the importance of measuring peak flow rates. Which of the following statements about the purpose for measuring peak flow rates is correct?
    1 They help wean him off his bronchodilator.
    2 They measure his response to bronchodilator therapy.
    3 They eliminate the need for blood test monitoring of the drug level.
    4 They determine when he may return to work.

391. With which of the following data should the nurse be most concerned during assessment of a patient with pneumonia?
    1 Capillary refill of greater than 3 seconds and buccal cyanosis
    2 A Hct of 47% and WBCs of 5500/ml
    3 Nonproductive cough and clear lung sounds
    4 Potassium level of 3.7 mEq/L and clear, amber urine

392. Which of the following is the most likely nursing diagnosis for a patient with an ileal conduit?
    1 Body image disturbance
    2 Alteration in sexual patterns

393. Risk for alteration in skin integrity
    4 Altered patterns of mobility

393. Which of the following interventions is appropriate for a patient who has urolithiasis?
    1 Ambulation
    2 Diuretic medications
    3 Restricting fluids to 1000 ml per day
    4 Low-protein diet

394. The nurse has been told in report that her patient has an upper urinary tract infection. In assessing the patient, the nurse knows that the infection is in her:
    1 Bladder
    2 Urethra
    3 Kidney
    4 Bloodstream

395. A patient has a urinary tract infection, and the nurse encourages her to void every 2 to 3 hours to:
    1 Train the bladder
    2 Reduce the possibility of reflex incontinence
    3 Reduce urinary stasis and the risk of infection
    4 Prevent fluid retention with overflow

396. A patient is admitted for obstructive urinary retention. He is newly diagnosed with adult-onset diabetes mellitus. The nurse checked his blood glucose level before dinner; it was 45 mg/dl. The best action is to:
    1 Give 6 oz of orange juice to drink immediately.
    2 Administer regular insulin according to the sliding scale orders.
    3 Call the physician immediately.
    4 Call the dietary department to have them deliver his dinner as soon as possible.

397. A patient was admitted with second- and third-degree burns over 40% of her body after her house was destroyed by fire yesterday. The nurse is monitoring her condition. Which of the following would the nurse want to report immediately?
    1 Urine output of 200 ml in the last 6 hours
    2 Decrease of body temperature to 98.4° F in the last hour
    3 Edema formation in the upper airway
    4 Complaints of pain during dressing changes

398. Which of the following situations would require a nurse to perform a vaginal douche using sterile technique?
    1 After a vaginal hysterectomy
    2 Before an IVP
    3 Before the patient has an abdominal hysterectomy
    4 When a patient has a yeast infection

399. The nurse needs to assess for the signs of hypocalcemia in a patient who:
    1 Has been taking high doses of vitamin C
    2 Is on hydrochlorothiazide (Esidrix) medication
    3 Is diagnosed with hyperparathyroidism
    4 Is being treated for chronic renal failure

400. A 42-year-old patient is recovering from cranial surgery. It is important to plan nursing interventions to prevent an increase in intracranial pressure. Which of the following actions best helps to decrease the possibility of ICP?
    1 Encouraging her to do deep breathing and coughing
    2 Doing endotracheal suctioning every 4 hours or as needed
    3 Maintaining her bed in a high-Fowler's (90-degree) position
    4 Spreading interventions evenly throughout the day

401. A patient is diagnosed with basal cell carcinoma of the scalp. The client has all of the previous histories listed. Which one of the facts probably contributed to his condition?
1 The patient uses Rogaine.
2 The patient has a family history of colon cancer.
3 The patient smokes cigarettes.
4 The patient is bald.

402. A patient is receiving dressing changes to a burned area on the right leg. Which of the following nursing interventions will best help this patient's comfort level before the procedure?
1 Administer an analgesic.
2 Explain the procedure thoroughly.
3 Reposition the patient on her right side.
4 Turn on the television to distract the patient during the procedure.

403. A patient calls in to the clinic and states that he is having painless hematuria. What advice should the nurse give the patient?
1 Drink a large amount of fluids.
2 Try not to drink any reddish colored fluids.
3 Make an appointment with your physician as soon as possible.
4 Go to the emergency room right away.

404. The nursing assistant notices that a patient with chronic renal failure has a strong odor and a white film on her skin that is difficult to clean. The assistant asks the nurse what is causing the problem. The nurse correctly states that these are:
1 Caused by improper care at a nursing home
2 Nothing about which to be concerned
3 The effects of the skin excreting urinary wastes
4 Important changes of which the physician should be aware

405. A nurse is attempting to gather information from a patient who has a sexually transmitted disease. Which of the following is true regarding this situation?
1 Most individuals speak freely about their sexual contacts.
2 It is not necessary to know with whom the patient has had sex.
3 Patients with asymptomatic STDs cannot transmit the disease.
4 Individuals are reluctant to discuss personal sexual information.

406. The nurse is preparing a dose of digoxin for a patient with heart failure. The patient's apical pulse is 48. What should the nurse do next?
1 Call the physician.
2 Hold the drug, and notify the registered nurse.
3 Give the digoxin; it will raise the heart rate.
4 Check the blood pressure before giving the digoxin.

407. A physician has ordered Tylenol 650 mg PO PRN, for a temperature of 100.4° F or greater. The nurse has on hand 325-mg tablets. How many tablets will the nurse give? 2 Tablets

408. Thrombolytic agents are used to treat patients with myocardial infarction. What is the action of the thrombolytic?
1 Dissolves fresh thrombi
2 Prevents further thrombi from developing
3 Thins the blood
4 Keeps platelets from aggregating in the bloodstream

409. A patient returns to the unit after having a bowel resection. One of the physician orders reads "no straws allowed." What is the rationale behind this order?
1 It may injure the patient's airway.
2 It will create a positive pressure in the lung.
3 It will create swallowing of air and put pressure on the suture line.
4 It will cause the development of diverticula in the patient's colon.

410. Which of the following procedures is used in the diagnosis of esophagitis?
1 EGD
2 ERCP
3 Barium enema
4 Barium swallow

411. A patient has been placed on nitroglycerin. This medication treats angina by:
1 Increasing blood flow to the myocardium
2 Lowering the client's blood pressure
3 Dilating cerebral arteries
4 Decreasing the number of ectopic beats

412. A patient calls a clinic and states that her stools have turned tarry black. She believes that she is bleeding internally. Which question should the nurse ask next?
1 "Are you taking vitamin K?"
2 "Do you have hemorrhoids?"
3 "Do you take ferrous sulfate?"
4 "Why don't you come to the clinic?"

413. Which of the following is the most common cause of low vision in individuals over 70 years of age?
1 Glaucoma
2 Macular degeneration
3 Presbyopia
4 Cataracts

414. Some anticancer medications depress the patient's bone marrow and require careful observation for:
1 Increased platelet counts
2 Anemia
3 High levels of WBCs
4 Metastasis

415. A patient is on a vasodilator. He complains that, when he stands, he becomes dizzy. The patient is experiencing:
1 Vertigo
2 Anemia
3 Bradycardia
4 Hypotension

416. The physician orders Stadol 2 mg IM stat. The pharmacy sends a vial that reads Stadol 5 mg/ml. How much will the nurse give? .5 mL

417. A patient takes all of the following medications. Which one is most likely to cause hypokalemia?
1 Digoxin
2 Tegretol
3 Aspirin
4 Lasix

418. Regarding electrolyte imbalance, patients who are immobile are most at risk for developing:
1 Hypokalemia
2 Hypercalcemia
3 Hypocalcemia
4 Hyperkalemia

419. A patient has had a myocardial infarction. He is most at risk for developing:
    1. Cardiogenic shock
    2. Anaphylaxis
    3. Hypertension
    4. Vascular injury

420. What is the rate of infusion if the order reads to give 1000 ml of IV fluid over 24 hours with a drop factor of 60 gtt/min? __42__

421. A patient asks why he cannot receive anything by mouth after his GI surgery. The nurse is most correct in saying that this order has been given because:
    1. The patient is really not hungry after surgery.
    2. He will become extremely nauseated afterwards.
    3. He might aspirate.
    4. The GI tract is not working because of the anesthesia.

422. The nurse medicates a patient with a narcotic analgesic. Which of the following nursing diagnosis is priority at this time?
    1. High risk for falls
    2. Risk for altered breathing patterns
    3. Pain
    4. Risk for infection

423. A physician orders Demerol 50 mg IM for a patient's postoperative pain. The nurse has Demerol 100 mg/ml on hand. How much will the nurse give? __0.5 mL__

424. A nurse is preparing to deliver nasogastric tube feedings. Which of the following assessments should be carried out before delivering the feedings? Choose all that apply.
    1. Assess bowel sounds.
    2. Assess lung sounds.
    3. Measure blood pressure.
    4. Measure heart rate.
    5. Ensure patency of tube.

425. Which of the following laboratory values would indicate to the nurse that a patient should be placed in protective isolation?
    1. RBC count of 5.8
    2. WBC count of 15
    3. Platelet count of 260,000
    4. WBC count of 1.8

426. After a patient undergoes surgery to the upper respiratory tract, the nurse should monitor the patient for:
    1. Infection
    2. Patent airway
    3. Bleeding tendencies
    4. Septicemia

427. A patient who has had surgery on the thyroid is to wear an ice collar around the neck. What is the most likely reason for this order?
    1. To reduce swelling of the neck
    2. To decrease the pain associated with the surgery
    3. To increase production of thyroid hormone
    4. Decrease the chance of hemorrhage

428. The nurse is addressing a group of high school students regarding the use of tobacco. A student says, "I won't get lung cancer because I don't smoke, I chew snuff." Which of the following is the best response by the nurse?
    1. "Well, you shouldn't do that either."
    2. "You're right, you won't get lung cancer."
    3. "You can still get oral cancer from the smokeless tobacco."
    4. "I don't think you understand the purpose of my speech!"

429. What structure or structures return oxygenated blood from the lungs?
    1. Pulmonary artery
    2. Pulmonary veins
    3. Superior vena cava
    4. Inferior vena cava

430. A patient with a myocardial infarction hears the physician tell the nurse that the patient's "cardiac enzymes are elevated." How should the nurse best explain this statement to the patient?
    1. "The physician meant that your heart is injured badly."
    2. "When you have a heart attack, your blood count goes up."
    3. "The liver signals when you have had a heart attack."
    4. "Injured hearts releases enzymes from their cells that we can measure."

431. A nurse is teaching a patient about Buerger-Allen exercises. These exercises will help the patient who has a diagnosis of:
    1. Pulmonary edema
    2. Thromboangiitis obliterans
    3. Thrombophlebitis
    4. Paget's disease

432. Which of the following patient teaching points should be included in the discharge planning of a patient who has heart failure? Choose all that apply.
    1. Weigh yourself every day.
    2. Take your blood pressure before taking your Digoxin.
    3. Increase your carbohydrate intake.
    4. Take your diuretic early in the morning.

433. A nurse is performing blood pressure screenings at the local mall. A mall walker has a blood pressure of 188/100 mm Hg. What advice should the nurse give the walker?
    1. "Go to the doctor immediately."
    2. "Why don't you drink a glass of water, and then I'll take it again."
    3. "Sit down and rest for a while, and I'll take it again."
    4. "Come back tomorrow, and I'll take it again."

434. A patient who is on a sodium-restricted diet is retaining fluid. She states that she has not been eating salt but has been eating out at a lot of restaurants. Which of the following types of restaurants would have food that is most likely to cause the fluid retention?
    1. Vegetarian
    2. Italian
    3. Chinese
    4. French

435. The physician orders Motrin 600 mg po every 4 hours. The nurse has Motrin 300-mg tablets. How many tablets will the nurse give? __2 tablets__

436. Which of the following is true concerning ulcerative colitis?
    1. Major symptoms are constipation and flatus.
    2. It involves the stomach and duodenum.
    3. It is caused by overuse of laxatives.
    4. Symptoms are caused by inflammation of the colon.

437. The primary purpose of the villi found in the small intestine is to:
    1. Absorb nutrients into the bloodstream.

2 Create a more formed stool.

3 Concentrate fecal material.

4 Reabsorb water back into the intestines.

438. A patient newly diagnosed with hypothyroidism asks the nurse how her disease will be treated. The nurse responds by saying:

1 "You will have to have surgery on your thyroid."

2 "You will need to take hormone replacements."

3 "You can be treated with diet and exercise."

4 "Radiation treatments are the primary therapy."

439. Gigantism and acromegaly are caused by a disorder of the:

1 Thyroid gland

2 Adrenal gland

3 Pituitary gland

4 Pancreas

440. A physician orders Versed 3 mg IM preoperatively for a patient scheduled to have a bowel resection. The nurse has Versed 10 mg/2 ml on hand. How much will the nurse give?

_0.6mL_

441. A patient with IDDM asks the nurse what the new "blood test" is that his physician wants him to have. If the patient is referring to the Hgb A1C, the nurse explains that this test:

1 Gauges how well the patient's blood sugar is controlled over a 3-month period

2 Can show if the patient has been cheating on his diet

3 Can measure the amount of insulin the patient uses over time

4 Is routine before a pancreatic stem cell transplant

442. A patient is scheduled to receive an ERCP. This test will provide information on:

1 Ulcerations of the small intestine

2 Bowel obstructions

3 Liver enzyme studies

4 Obstruction of bile ducts

443. The patient has a large accumulation of fluid in his abdominal cavity. The nurse surmises that this patient has a diagnosis of:

1 Peritonitis

2 Cirrhosis

3 Hepatitis

4 Diverticulitis

444. A patient who has had a bowel resection is to resume his diet. Which of the following diets should be instituted first for this patient?

1 High residue

2 Low fiber

3 Clear liquid

4 Mechanical soft

445. The physician's order reads to infuse 2000 ml of IV fluids over 10 hours. The drop factor of the administration set is 10 gtt/ml. How many drops per minute will the nurse infuse the IV? _33_

446. A patient has had a cholecystectomy. During discharge teaching, which foods would the nurse discourage her from consuming?

1 Raw vegetables

2 Fried foods

3 Tomatoes

4 Pasta

447. A patient is to receive three 8-ounce cans of formula feeding via a tube-feeding pump. If the nurse infuses the feeding at 80 ml/hr, how long will it take to infuse the feeding?

3 Hours

448. A patient states to the nurse, "I don't know why I keep getting hemorrhoids." Which of the following problems in the patient's history would contribute to their development?

1 Sexually transmitted diseases

2 Frequent urinary tract infections

3 Ear infections

4 Periods of constipation

449. A patient has a prolapsed uterus. Which of the following is the priority nursing diagnosis for the patient?

1 Hemorrhage

2 Alteration in sexual patterns

3 Alteration in urinary elimination

4 Alteration in bowel elimination

450. A primary problem in a patient with a vesicovaginal fistula is:

1 Elimination

2 Infection

3 Bleeding

4 Respiratory difficulty

ANSWERS AND RATIONALES

1. Analysis, planning, physiological integrity (c).
   3 Many individuals react differently to foods. By finding out what his reaction entails, you can better inform the physician.
   1 Further action is indicated before the procedure.
   2 You should ascertain the nature of the allergy first.
   4 This will eventually be done but is not a priority.

2. Knowledge, assessment, health promotion and maintenance (a).
   2 These are the identified components of the Glasgow Coma Scale (GCS).
   1 Posturing and reflexes are not components of the GCS.
   3 None of these are components of the GCS.
   4 Best motor and verbal response is part of the GCS, but seizure activity is not.

3. Knowledge, assessment, physiological integrity (a).
   2 The DNA molecules in the nucleus of a cell duplicate themselves, and the cell divides, forming two identical cells.
   1 Lysis is the swelling of RBCs placed in a hypotonic salt solution.
   3 Osmosis is the movement of water through a permeable membrane.
   4 Crenation is the shrinking of RBCs placed in a hypertonic solution.

4. Knowledge, implementation, health promotion and maintenance (b).
   2 In acquiring passive immunity, the body of the recipient plays no active part in response to an antigen.
   1 In active immunity, the resistance to a disease results from the development of antibodies within the body.
   3 Newborn babies receive a short-term immunity as a result of the antibodies of their mother, but it is not considered permanent.
   4 Autoimmune immunity occurs by the body's producing antibodies to its own tissues.

5. Comprehension, assessment, physiological integrity (b).
   4 Loss of hearing of the affected ear is the most likely symptom.
   1 This is double vision and is not a symptom of this disorder.
   2 Although they may complain of ringing in the ears, it is not the primary symptom.
   3 This is common with disorders of the inner ear.

6. Comprehension, assessment, physiological integrity (b).
   1 Vomiting is a sign of IICP, which is a complication of head injury.
   2 A person with head trauma is likely to have a headache.
   3 Tremors are not directly related to closed head injury.
   4 Itching of the skin would not be a complication of closed head injury.

7. Knowledge, assessment, physiological integrity (b).
   2 Estrogen and progesterone promote development of the female sex characteristics and sex organs; they also regulate menstruation for the purpose of reproduction.
   1 Testosterone is produced by the testes of men.
   3 Prolactin is produced by the pituitary gland.
   4 Although progesterone is produced by the ovaries, testosterone is produced by the testes.

8. Knowledge, assessment, physiological integrity (a).
   1 Dilation of the blood vessels brings more blood to the surface so that heat can be dissipated.
   2 Contraction of blood vessels will preserve body heat.
   3 An increase in blood supply constricts muscles, rather than relax them.
   4 The production of sweat is increased by dilation of blood vessels but is not the primary cause of lost body heat.

9. Knowledge, assessment, physiological integrity (a).
   1 The area is located slightly below the center of the breast and contains slightly raised areas.
   2 Urochrome gives urine its color.
   3 Cowper's glands are located on either side of the urethra and just below the prostate gland in men.
   4 Bartholin's glands lie on either side of the vagina.

10. Knowledge, assessment, physiological integrity (a).
    3 The testes produce testosterone, which gives men their secondary sex characteristics.
    1 Estrogen is produced by the ovaries.
    2 Progesterone is produced by the ovaries.
    4 Aldosterone is produced by the adrenal cortex.

11. Knowledge, assessment, physiological integrity (a).
    2 The connective tissue is made of dense fibrous tissue in the shape of a cord and has great strength.
    1 Osseous is another term for bone tissue.
    3 Cartilage makes a slick surface for rotation and shock absorption at joints.
    4 Ligaments attach bone to bone.

12. Application, assessment, health promotion and maintenance (c).
    3 Difficulty swallowing or speaking and a shuffling gait are common symptoms.
    1 Individuals with Parkinson's disease do not usually experience diplopia, although they do have tremors.
    2 Headache is not a common symptom, and ataxia (difficulty walking) may be found in the form of a shuffling walk.
    4 Tinnitus is not normally associated with Parkinson's disease.

13. Application, evaluation, physiological integrity (c).
    1 Popcorn has hulls and seeds, which precipitate a diverticular attack. More teaching on diet is needed.
    2, 3, 4 These are all correct teaching points for a patient diagnosed with diverticulitis.

14. Knowledge, assessment, physiological integrity (a).
    4 The primary purpose of bile is to emulsify fats so that they can be more easily digested.
    1 The liver converts glycogen to glucose.
    2 Bile does not act on sugars, only fats.
    3 Trypsin is the enzyme primarily responsible for digesting meats.

15. Comprehension, assessment, physiological integrity (b).
    1 Epithelial tissue has many forms that are arranged in single or several layers to form a protective covering and lining for the internal organs of the body.
    2 Periosteum is a connective tissue covering of bone.
    3 Pericardium is a fibrous sac lined with serous membrane that surrounds the heart.
    4 Connective tissue supports and connects other tissues and parts of the body.

16. Comprehension, assessment, physiological integrity (b).

3 The cardiac sphincter prevents regurgitation of stomach contents back into the esophagus.

1 Rugae are the folds in the stomach lining that allow for its expansion.

2 Chyme is the semiliquid substance in the stomach that is formed from the combination of hydrochloric acid and food.

4 The pyloric sphincter separates the stomach and duodenum. It determines how long food will stay in the stomach.

17. Comprehension, assessment, physiological integrity (a).

3 The small intestine contains villi that absorb most of the nutrients that are derived from the digestion of food.

1 Absorbed nutrients travel by way of the portal vein to the liver.

2 The stomach absorbs very little nutrients because most food has not been digested into small enough particles for absorption.

4 By the time the food reaches the large intestine, most of the nutrients have been absorbed, and all that remains is the indigestible wastes left from the food.

18. Application, planning, physiological integrity (b).

1 Sitz baths will soothe the patient's itching and burning skin.

2 Pillows may provide comfort but will not soothe itching and burning.

3 Tylenol will not diminish comfort.

4 A tap-water enema will further irritate the area.

19. Knowledge, assessment, physiological integrity (a).

4 The nasolacrimal duct is a small opening into the nose at the inner corner of the eye that allows the fluid to drain through.

1 The ciliary body is a smooth muscle structure to which the lens is attached.

2 The lacrimal gland releases tears into the anterior face of the eyeball.

3 The eustachian tube connects the middle ear chamber with the throat.

20. Knowledge, assessment, physiological integrity (b).

2 Incisors are the four top and bottom front teeth.

1 Molars are the last to appear, usually by 2 to 2½ years.

3 Canines are another name for eye teeth and appear after the incisors.

4 Eyeteeth, or canines, appear later in a baby.

21. Comprehension, implementation, physiological integrity (c).

3 T tubes are used to drain away bile from the incision site.

1 Other types of devices are used to drain blood.

2 The T tube is not inserted into the liver.

4 The T tube is not positioned in such a way as to drain stomach acids.

22. Analysis, planning, physiological integrity (c).

1 Of the nursing diagnoses listed, infection is of paramount importance based on Maslow's hierarchy of needs, owing to the insertion of a catheter into the abdomen.

2 Fluid deficit might be a nursing diagnosis; however, more likely, individuals undergoing peritoneal dialysis have fluid overload.

3 Many patients undergoing peritoneal dialysis have a body image disturbance, but this is not the priority nursing diagnosis.

4 Patients who take peritoneal dialysis do so at home and should not have a self-care deficit.

23. Knowledge, assessment, physiological integrity (a).

2 The progressive, wavelike movement that occurs involuntarily forces food in a forward motion.

1 Rugae are the folds in the stomach that allow for expansion.

3 Mastication is the action of chewing.

4 This is a spasm of the pyloric sphincter.

24. Knowledge, assessment, physiological integrity (a).

3 Amino acids are the digestible form of protein.

1 Ptyalin is an enzyme found in saliva that begins the breakdown of starches.

2 Glucose is the end product of carbohydrate digestion.

4 Hydrochloric acid is a solution found in the stomach.

25. Comprehension, planning, physiological integrity (c).

2 When a patient has his labyrinth destroyed, he will be unable to hear from that side.

1 The patient, although unable to hear, should be free from symptoms.

3 The symptoms should not come back after the procedure.

4 The symptoms should stop when the labyrinth is destroyed.

26. Comprehension, assessment, physiological integrity (b).

4 The liver is responsible for the production of fibrinogen, which aids in the clotting process.

1 Bile is responsible for emulsifying fats and is produced by the liver.

2 The small intestine is responsible for absorbing nutrients.

3 The pancreas manufactures and secretes trypsin, which aids in digesting proteins.

27. Application, planning, physiological integrity (c).

2 Iodine is an element that aids in the formation of thyroxine, which is the hormone produced by the thyroid gland; a lack of it causes hypothyroidism.

1 Iron is essential in the manufacture of hemoglobin.

3 Calcium is essential to the clotting process, muscular function, and bone growth and development.

4 Phosphorus is also essential for bone growth and development.

28. Comprehension, planning, physiological integrity (c).

4 By causing further fluid retention, sodium increases the discomfort felt by women suffering from premenstrual tension syndrome (PMS).

1 Protein foods should not affect the comfort level.

2 Calcium, important for bone growth, does not affect comfort level.

3 Phosphorus does not affect comfort level.

29. Knowledge assessment, physiological integrity (c).

2 The right atrium receives deoxygenated blood from all the body tissues via the superior and inferior vena cava.

1 The left atrium receives oxygenated blood from the four pulmonary veins.

3 The left ventricle receives oxygenated blood from the left atrium and pumps blood to all the body's tissues.

4 The right ventricle receives deoxygenated blood from the right atrium and pumps that blood to the lungs to be oxygenated.

30. Knowledge, assessment, physiological integrity (b).

3 Epinephrine is a hormone manufactured in the adrenal medulla and increases blood pressure and heart rate.

1 Insulin is manufactured in the pancreas and decreases blood sugar levels.
2 Aldosterone is produced in the adrenal cortex and aids in regulating electrolytes and water balance.
4 Testosterone is produced by the testes and stimulates growth and development of the sex organs.

31. Comprehension, assessment, physiological integrity (c).
    4 Antidiuretic hormone (ADH) is produced in the posterior pituitary and promotes reabsorption of water in the kidney.
    1 Oxytocin is produced in the posterior pituitary and causes uterine muscle contraction.
    2 Prolactin is produced by the anterior pituitary and promotes milk formation.
    3 Calcitonin is produced in the thyroid and assists in decreasing serum calcium levels.

32. Comprehension, evaluation, physiological integrity (c).
    1 A lumpectomy is a surgical procedure designed to limit the size of breast tissue removed in patients with an early diagnosis.
    2 A mastectomy, removal of the breast, would not preserve the most breast tissue.
    3 A needle biopsy is a diagnostic examination and not a surgical procedure for removal of breast tissue.
    4 An oophorectomy is removal of an ovary.

33. Knowledge, assessment, physiological integrity (b).
    2 The SA node, located in the right atrium, sets and regulates the rate of the heart rate.
    1 The AV node conducts the electrical impulse of the heartbeat down toward the bundle of His.
    3 The bundle of His receives the electrical impulse of the heartbeat from the AV node and conveys it to the Purkinje fibers.
    4 The Purkinje fibers are the terminal branches of the conduction system of the heart.

34. Knowledge, assessment, physiological integrity (b).
    4 The pulmonary artery carries deoxygenated blood from the heart to the lungs.
    1 The aorta carries oxygenated blood from the heart to all body tissues.
    2 The carotid artery carries oxygenated blood to the brain.
    3 The coronary arteries carry oxygenated blood to the heart muscle itself.

35. Comprehension, assessment, physiological integrity (a).
    3 Sebaceous glands secrete oil.
    1 Sudoriferous glands secrete perspiration.
    2 Ceruminous glands secrete earwax.
    4 Bartholin's glands secrete mucus in the reproductive system.

36. Comprehension, assessment, physiological integrity (b).
    3 The greater trochanter closely articulates with the hip joint and is involved in many fractures.
    1 The acromion process is the highest point of the shoulder.
    2 The acetabulum is the hollowed out area of the hip joint.
    4 The olecranon process forms the point of the elbow.

37. Knowledge, assessment, physiological integrity (c).
    4 The periosteum is a tough covering that provides structure for blood, lymph, and nerve channels.
    1 Red bone marrow produces RBCs.
    2 Adipose tissue is stored in the diaphysis or shaft.
    3 Yellow bone marrow provides a site for storing fatty material.

38. Comprehension, assessment, health promotion and maintenance (c).
    2 A painless loss of vision is one of the predominant symptoms in patients with a detached retina.
    1 Double vision is not a common symptom.
    3 Tunnel vision is common in patients with glaucoma.
    4 Headaches are not a common symptom.

39. Comprehension, assessment, health promotion and maintenance (b).
    3 Rashes, bruises, and decubitus are all data that are derived from assessing the skin and its appendages—the integumentary system.
    1 Blood sugar levels would be an assessment of the endocrine system.
    2 Blood pressure and pulse are considered part of the respiratory and cardiovascular system.
    4 Blood sugar levels are not part of the assessment of the integumentary system.

40. Application, assessment, health promotion and maintenance (c).
    3 Because individuals with glaucoma experience loss of peripheral vision, they have the symptom of tunnel vision.
    1 Painless loss of vision is a common finding with detached retina.
    2 Diplopia is not a common finding in patients with glaucoma.
    4 Strabismus is more common in children and is not common in patients with glaucoma.

41. Comprehension, implementation, physiological integrity (c).
    1 Miotics are used to make the pupil smaller and increase the angle of Schlemm to allow fluid to flow from the eye, decreasing intraocular pressure.
    2 Mydriatics increase the diameter of the pupil and are contraindicated in patients with glaucoma.
    3 Although they reduce intraocular pressure, they are not a diuretic.
    4 These medications are not used to treat detached retina.

42. Comprehension, assessment, physiological integrity (b).
    3 The upper surface of the dermis has raised and depressed areas that are unique to each individual and thus provide a means for identification.
    1 Elastic connective tissue is found in the subcutaneous layer, not on the surface of the skin.
    2 The subcutaneous layer is below the level of the dermis.
    4 The upper surface of the epidermis consists of epithelial cells that are constantly being shed.

43. Comprehension, assessment, physiological integrity (c).
    3 Aldosterone is released by the adrenal cortex in response to decreased blood volume, decreased blood sodium ions or increased potassium ions.
    1 Oxytocin stimulates uterine muscles during birth.
    2 ADH prevents excess water loss in the urine.
    4 Parathormone regulates calcium ion homeostasis of the blood.

44. Knowledge, assessment, physiological integrity (a).
    1 Oxygen prevents the formation of lactic acid, and glycogen is the form of energy that the skeletal muscles use.
    2 Acetylcholine is important in transmitting nerve impulses.
    3 Although oxygen prevents lactic acid buildup, acetylcholine is a neurotransmitter.
    4 Lactic acid is a waste product caused by anaerobic metabolism in the muscles.

45. Comprehension, assessment, physiological integrity (b).
    3 The left motor control center in the brain controls the right side of the body because of the crossing of the nerve tracts within the brain.
    1 Only one side of the body is affected if an injury is to only one side of the brain.
    2 The left side of the body is controlled by the right side of the brain.
    4 Normally, some paralysis is observed when damage occurs to the motor control center of the brain.

46. Application, planning, physiological integrity (c).
    2 The physician has placed the marks on the skin to guide the radiation beam to the tumor; removing the markings may cause inaccurate treatments.
    1 The patient should not apply any oils or lubricants over the skin.
    3 Ice and heat will create further discomfort for the patient.
    4 The area that is irradiated will become red; it is an expected result.

47. Comprehension, assessment, physiological integrity (c).
    4 The parasympathetic division of the autonomic nervous system maintains homeostasis by regulating digestion and circulation.
    1 The sensory neurons carry impulses towards the CNS.
    2 The sympathetic nervous system controls the "fight or flight" response.
    3 Interneurons conduct impulses from the sensory neurons to the motor neurons.

48. Comprehension, planning, physiological integrity (c).
    1 Mannitol is a diuretic used to treat individuals with IICP.
    2 Pulmonary edema is treated by furosemide and morphine sulfate.
    3 Ascites is normally treated by an abdominocentesis.
    4 Left-sided heart failure (HF) is normally treated with a loop diuretic, such as furosemide.

49. Knowledge, assessment, physiological integrity (c).
    2 The snaillike cochlea contains the organ of Corti, which contains the hearing receptors.
    1 The malleus is an ossicle in the middle ear.
    3 The tympanic membrane is the eardrum.
    4 The semicircular canal controls equilibrium.

50. Analysis, assessment, physiological integrity (c).
    2 This assessment finding is the only one listed that is a symptom of neurovascular compromise.
    1 A bounding pulse indicates good arterial blood flow.
    3 A cool extremity may be a sign of decreased neurovascular status, but the patient may simply be cold.
    4 Complaints of pain are not usually associated with neurovascular impairment; numbness and tingling are more common.

51. Knowledge, assessment, physiological integrity (a).
    2 When water intake is excessive, the kidneys excrete generous amounts of urine. If water intake is lost, they produce less urine; the process is regulated by hormones.
    1 The gonads are the sex glands and are not directly involved in fluid and electrolyte balance.
    3 The bladder is the storage center for urine but does not affect fluid and electrolyte balance.
    4 The islets of Langerhans are the functional cells of the pancreas that secrete insulin and glucagon.

52. Analysis, evaluation, physiological integrity (c).
    4 Working in a warehouse, the patient would be required to bend and lift heavy objects, which is one of the predisposing factors for herniated disks.
    1 Although this is not a healthy lifestyle practice, it has little to do with a herniated nucleus pulposus.
    2 This practice should not contribute significantly to this disorder.
    3 This should have little bearing on this diagnosis.

53. Comprehension, implementation, physiological integrity (c).
    4 The primary responsibility of T cells is to destroy any foreign-related protein in the body.
    1 Although correct, this statement does not explain the T cells' role in the immune response.
    2 This is incorrect; B cells are responsible for humoral immunity.
    3 B cells are responsible for cloning antibody-producing plasma cells.

54. Knowledge, assessment, physiological integrity (b).
    4 The primary function of the humors, or fluids of the eye, is to maintain the shape of the eyeball.
    1 The production of tears is regulated by the lacrimal gland.
    2 Dilation of the pupil is the responsibility of the intrinsic muscles of the eye.
    3 The ciliary body regulates the thickness of the lens.

55. Application, assessment, physiological integrity (c).
    Cerebrospinal fluid

56. Application, assessment, physiological integrity (c).
    Intake: 4450 ml
    Output: 300 ml emesis and bowel movement, 4000 to 3000 ml of urine = 1000 ml of true urine

57. Application, implementation, physiological integrity (c).
    3 This should raise the blood sugar to the desired level. The patient is alert and is able to consume the juice.
    1 This will not be a sufficient amount to raise the glucose level.
    2 This can cause the blood sugar to rise quickly and then fall quickly again.
    4 Diet drinks do not contain sugar and will not alter the blood sugar level.

58. Comprehension, planning, physiological integrity (c).
    1 The peak action for regular insulin is 2 to 4 hours after administration; the nurse should therefore be particularly alert around 5:00 PM or 6:00 PM for any hypoglycemic episodes.
    2 The peak action will most likely occur before this time.
    3 Regular insulin should have left the patient's bloodstream by this hour.
    4 By this time, the patient will not have any effect from the regular insulin.

59. Application, assessment, physiological integrity (b).
    2 These are the classic symptoms of osteomyelitis.
    1 These symptoms can signal pulmonary emboli.
    3 These symptoms may indicate neurovascular impairment.
    4 These are symptoms of neurological impairment.

60. Application, assessment, physiological integrity (c).
    1 Salty or sweet-tasting drainage from the operative area may indicate that cerebral spinal fluid is leaking.

2 Headache is frequent after craniotomy, usually caused by stretching or irritation of nerves of the scalp during the operation. Position should not affect headache unless the left is the operative side.

3 Neither hunger nor temporary anorexia would indicate a possible complication. The nurse would anticipate thirst postoperatively.

4 The patient has had general anesthesia so sleepiness is expected but level of consciousness changes are critical.

61. Comprehension, planning, safe, effective care environment (b).

4 A mask with an eye shield and gloves are needed to protect the caregiver's hands and eyes from direct contact or spraying of infected secretions.

1 A plain mask will not offer adequate protection against spraying of material.

2 Gloves are mandatory; however, the mask without an eye shield will not be adequate.

3 A mask with eye shield is indicated; gown and gloves are not adequate protection.

62. Application, planning, safe, effective care environment (c).

1 A WBC count of 0.2 is indicative of immunosuppression. The immunocompromised patient is unable to resist foreign agents and is susceptible to overwhelming infection.

2 The nursing staff wears facemasks to prevent spread of microorganisms to the patient.

3 Protective isolation precautions are indicated.

4 Patients with immunosuppression are encouraged not to be around groups of people because this increases the risk of infection.

63. Comprehension, assessment, physiological integrity (b).

2 The pelvis of a patient with muscular dystrophy widens, causing a waddling gait.

1 Pillrolling is a common behavior associated with Parkinson's disease.

3 Patients with Parkinson's disease also have a shuffling gait.

4 Tardive dyskinesia is an irreversible condition of involuntary muscle movements seen in patients taking antipsychotic medications.

64. Application, planning, physiological integrity (c).

3 A patient diagnosed with ALS needs to maintain a patent airway at all times, a priority for patients with ALS.

1, 2 Periods of exercise are necessary, but they would not be increased. Adequate periods of rest are a necessity for this patient, as are alternative forms of communication. However, these are not a priority at this time.

4 Providing counseling and other means to facilitate coping with the diagnosis also is important, although not as critical as #3.

65. Comprehension, planning, physiological integrity (b).

3 It is true that it takes longer to inspire or expire air because of age-related physiological changes.

1 This is not a proven fact for older adults.

2 This is not a proven correlation.

4 Overall respiratory muscle structure and function decrease in older adults.

66. Comprehension, evaluation, health promotion and maintenance (c).

2 The patient does not have to give up sex if proper precautions are taken.

1 This is true and would assist the patient in regaining his sexual interests.

3 This is also true for this patient.

4 This is a true statement, stated in layman's terms, and shows that the patient is aware of the risks of further myocardial infarction.

67. Comprehension, assessment, physiological integrity (b).

3 These are signs noted during later stages of the disease; others include jaw clonus and respiratory difficulty.

1 Aphasia is not a symptom noted in ALS; the patient can speak but has difficulty doing so.

2 Flexor muscles become spastic, not flaccid.

4 No sensory loss is experienced with ALS; the patient remains alert.

68. Comprehension, implementation, health promotion and maintenance (c).

2 Kirschner traction is a type of skeletal traction that uses pins and wires.

1, 3, 4 These are all forms of skin traction, without wires or pins.

69. Comprehension, assessment, physiological integrity (b).

1 Tenderness and crepitus are common characteristics of joints involved in osteoarthritis.

2 Most joints involved in osteoarthritis are on one side of the body. These findings are consistent with rheumatoid arthritis.

3 In osteoarthritis, pain is caused by the loss of articular cartilage.

4 Rheumatoid arthritis commonly presents with these symptoms.

70. Application, assessment, physiological integrity (b).

4 Given that the patient will be staying a short while, this information appears to be the most pertinent because the nurse will need to ascertain how the patient will ambulate before and after surgery.

1 This data would not be particularly relevant at this time.

2 Although this is important to note, the nurse will need to assess how the patient will ambulate because the priority for the short-stay will be on rapid recovery.

3 Although this data is important, it is not the most pertinent at this time.

71. Application, implementation, physiological integrity (c).

4 Concentrated glucose can be absorbed between the buccal mucosa and gum; when patient fully awakens, give a fast-acting carbohydrate by mouth.

1 Insulin would further lower the blood glucose reading, and LPN/LVNs are not permitted to administer IV insulin.

2 This places the patient in danger for aspiration.

3 This action will most likely result in the patient choking and aspirating.

72. Comprehension, assessment, physiological integrity (b).

2 Cortisol is made by the adrenal cortex and will produce Cushing's syndrome if it is overproduced.

3 An increase in growth hormone after the epiphyseal plates close leads to acromegaly.

1 Prolactin is not associated with Addison's disease.

4 An overproduction of thyroid hormone is referred to as hyperthyroidism.

73. Application, implementation, physiological integrity (c).

4 This direction allows the fluid left in the space to consolidate and lessens the possibility of mediastinal shift.

1, 2, 3 These are inappropriate; they increase risk of mediastinal shift when placed on unaffected side.

74. Comprehension, implementation, physiological integrity (b).

4 The pulse oximetry machine measures how much of the capillary blood is saturated with oxygen.

1 Pulse oximetry does not measure metabolic rate.

2 Although most pulse oximetry machines measure the heart rate, it is not the primary purpose of the machine.

3 Only a chest radiograph will be able to show how much fluid is in the lung.

75. Comprehension, implementation, safe, effective care environment (c).

2 Decreased albumin levels alter the hydrostatic pressure in the liver's portal circulation, forcing fluid into the abdominal cavity.

1 Hypertension may contribute to portal hypertension but does not cause ascites.

3 This may cause jaundice but should not cause ascites.

4 Ammonia levels may be elevated but do not cause ascites.

76. Comprehension, implementation, physiological integrity (c).

3 This is standard practice. The petroleum gauze creates an occlusive dressing that does not allow air to flow into the lung.

1 Infection is not a priority at this time.

2 The petroleum has the opposite effect.

4 Although this is true, this is not the primary reason an occlusive gauze is used.

77. Application, implementation, physiological integrity (b).

1 A patient with a lobectomy may be turned to either side.

2, 3, 4 These do not allow for full expansion and drainage of all remaining lobes.

78. Comprehension, implementation, physiological integrity (c).

3 Bile is needed to emulsify fat. When fat requires bile for emulsification, the gallbladder contracts in an effort to release the bile to be used in this process. A diseased gallbladder that must contract causes a sensation of pain.

1 Foods high in fat require bile released by the gallbladder to aid in the emulsification process.

2 The duct leading from the liver to the gallbladder may possibly become blocked, but it is less likely to involve the pancreas in most acute presentations.

3 Although a portion of this statement is true, this does not explain the mechanism by which pain is produced.

79. Comprehension, assessment, health promotion and maintenance (c).

1 Accidental removal of the parathyroid glands can lead to hypocalcemia.

2 Cortisol is secreted by the adrenal gland and is not associated with a thyroidectomy.

3 This is not associated with parathyroid removal.

4 Although respiratory compromise is a potential problem with a thyroidectomy, loss of the gag reflex is not associated with parathyroid removal.

80. Application, implementation, health promotion and maintenance (b).

3 Abstaining from food or drink decreases the chance of esophageal reflux when she lies down.

1 This suggestion will not reduce bedtime discomfort.

2 This will worsen the symptoms; chocolate is one of the aggravating factors for hiatal hernia.

4 This will cause a worsening of symptoms.

81. Application, implementation, physiological integrity (b).

4 This is the preferred position for an examination that is done in a hospital bed.

1 This is the appropriate position for the patient undergoing a rectal examination.

2 This is not the preferred position for access to the female reproductive system.

3 This will not provide access to the vagina for the procedure.

82. Comprehension, assessment, health promotion and maintenance (b).

4 Smokeless tobacco or snuff is a precipitating factor for oral cancer.

1 Alcohol abuse is not a factor in oral cancer; however, it is for other conditions.

2 Poor dental hygiene is not a predisposing cause for oral cancer.

3 Frequent bouts of tonsillitis are not a precipitating cause for oral cancer.

83. Application, implementation, health promotion and maintenance (b).

4 Hypoglycemia can be countered with the ingestion of a rapid-acting sugar.

1 Running is too strenuous an activity for an individual with diabetes mellitus.

2 Meals should be spaced no further than 4 hours apart.

3 Medication should be taken first thing in the morning.

84. Application, implementation, health promotion and maintenance (b).

2 These are the common symptoms of candidiasis.

1 This is not common in candidiasis, but it is common of some systemic infections.

3 This is common in genital warts.

4 Although a cause for concern, these are not symptoms associated with candidiasis.

85. Application, implementation, physiological integrity (b).

3 The application of heat will alleviate discomfort, and drinking warm beverages will decrease the incidence of abdominal cramps.

1 This will increase discomfort.

2 This will have no bearing on abdominal cramps.

4 Applying ice will not alleviate discomfort.

86. Application, planning, physiological integrity (c).

1 Addison's disease is a failure to produce the needed hormones by the adrenal cortex that help regulate electrolyte balance.

2 Addison's disease does not affect the WBC count, and this goal would cause the patient to be unable to fight off infectious diseases.

3 Because Addison's disease does not affect the bone marrow, this would not be a goal of therapy.

4 The RBC count is not affected in Addison's disease, and this would not be a goal of therapy.

87. Application, implementation, physiological integrity (b).

2 Raising the head of the bed may relieve the dyspnea if it is paroxysmal nocturnal dyspnea.

1 This is helpful but does not physically relieve the underlying cause.

3 This is not necessary based on information given. Additionally, suctioning may cause trauma to mucous membranes.

4 This intervention would not be appropriate. In addition, some pain medication may depress respirations.

88. Application, implementation, physiological integrity (c).

3 Wheezing is not normal after a bronchoscopy; the physician should be alerted.

1 Wheezing is caused by narrowed airways, not by secretions.

2 Pain medication will not correct the wheezing problem.

4 A respiratory treatment may be indicated, but it requires a physician order.

89. Application, implementation, physiological integrity (b).

2 Splinting protects the fracture, immobilizes the arm and may prevent worsening of the situation.

1 Use 911 only in true emergencies.

3 Warmth may actually cause an increase in edema and does not immobilize the fracture.

4 The extremity should be elevated to prevent edema formation.

90. Knowledge, assessment, physiological integrity (b).

1 FSH stimulates the follicle to develop, which will secrete progesterone once ovulation has occurred.

2 LH does not stimulate progesterone secretion.

3 TSH stimulates the thyroid to release thyroxine.

4 ACTH stimulates the adrenal glands.

91. Application, implementation, health promotion and maintenance (c).

3 Crackles may be associated with left-sided heart failure.

1 Decreased appetite is common in a lot of disorders.

2 Although the nurse will alert the physician about the headache, it is not of paramount importance.

4 This blood pressure is not at a danger level.

92. Application, implementation, physiological integrity (b).

3 This is the only true statement and validates the patient's knowledge deficit while providing information.

1 The patient did not refuse anything; the patient requires more information.

2 This may not be true, and it is never a good idea to tell patients what they should do. Provide information so that patients can make an informed choice.

4 This response is trite and does not address the problem. The nurse is being judgmental.

93. Knowledge, implementation, physiological integrity (c).

4 This is the correct definition.

1 This is the definition of a bronchoscopy.

2 This is the definition of an MRI.

3 This is the definition of spirometry.

94. Comprehension, implementation, health promotion and maintenance (c).

3 Men with BPH complain of urgency, frequency, and diminished urine stream.

1 This is not a common problem with BPH.

2 Dizziness is a common symptom for many disorders but not BPH.

4 This is not a common finding.

95. Application, implementation, physiological integrity (c).

2 This is correct based on the use of the contrast medium (dye).

1, 3 These are not proper procedures; patient should be NPO.

4 This is not necessary; patient's activity has nothing to do with standard protocol for this test under normal circumstances.

96. Comprehension, assessment, physiological integrity (c).

1 This is used to determine areas of lung being ventilated, because of an obstruction or clot in the pulmonary circulation. It is a common procedure for this diagnosis.

2, 3 These are inappropriate tests for this medical diagnosis.

4 This is done for joint pain.

97. Application, implementation, physiological integrity (c).

2 The primary responsibility is for the nurse to reduce the risk for an accidental injury by keeping the patient still.

1 This may be a secondary objective for the nurse; however, physicians usually handles this on their own.

3 This can be done before the procedure.

4 If this is indicated, the nurse will have the setup complete before the procedure begins.

98. Application, implementation, physiological integrity (b).

2 Oxygen is very drying, when flow rate is more than 4 L/min; humidification is necessary.

1 This is not really responsive to patient's concern.

3 Although true, this response is incomplete in rationale.

4 Humidity does not increase safety factors when oxygen is in use; additionally, such a statement may be cause for patient concern.

99. Comprehension, planning, physiological integrity (c).

1 Protein is converted to ammonia, and a buildup of ammonia affects brain tissue. Protein should be restricted if ammonia levels rise. This snack is lowest in protein

2, 3, 4 These snack s are high in protein.

100. Application, planning, physiological integrity (c).

3 Regular insulin is fast acting and is used when prompt action is desired.

1 Lente is an intermediate acting insulin that does not provide prompt action and is not used for coverage.

2 NPH is an intermediate acting insulin that does not provide prompt action and is not used for coverage.

4 This is an oral agent that does not provide prompt action and is not used for coverage.

101. Application, planning, physiological integrity (c).

1 After a hydrocelectomy, the scrotum will be elevated to prevent edema.

2 The patient may have a catheter, although this is not always true.

3 Estrogen therapy may be indicated for prostate cancer.

4 A wet-dry saline dressing is not normally indicated.

102. Application, evaluation, health promotion and maintenance (c).

2 Infection can cause fluctuations to occur in blood sugar, usually in the form of elevations.

1 Although stressful situations may precipitate DKA, an infection is more likely to cause it.

3 Excess insulin would cause hypoglycemia.

4 Insufficient calories in the diet would also cause hypoglycemia.

103. Application, assessment, health promotion and maintenance (c).

3 Patients with fibromyalgia have few objective findings.

1 Fibromyalgia can be treated.

2 Fibromyalgia is a true, newly discovered disorder.

4 Patients with fibromyalgia are normally treated with medications and exercise.

104. Application, assessment, health promotion and maintenance (b).

4 In a patient on bed rest, dependent edema will pool in the sacrum, the lowest point of the patient when lying in bed.

1 Because the feet are mostly elevated, edema will not occur in the feet.

2 Edema is normally found in the hands of ambulatory patients.

3 Edema is not normally assessed in the knee region.

105. Comprehension, planning, physiological integrity (b).

1 Patients with laryngitis should rest their voice.

2 Resting the voice is a more effective treatment modality than is gargling with saltwater.

3 Treatment is aimed at resting the voice.

4 This would be very traumatic to tell a patient, and it may not be true.

106. Application, planning, physiological integrity (b).

The nurse will need to consider patient preference and normal drinking patterns, the amount of fluid on their dietary tray, the time and amount of medications that are given to the patient.

107. Application, planning, physiological integrity (c).

4 Application of ice packs is not standard treatment for sinusitis; and this statement needs clarification for the patient.

1 This is standard treatment for sinusitis.

2 Decongestants are a standard treatment.

3 These are standard discharge instructions for a patient with sinusitis.

108. Application, assessment, physiological integrity (c).

2 Facial numbness is the first sign of hypocalcemia; tetany and seizures may follow.

1 A headache is not one of the warning signs of hypocalcemia.

3 Nausea is not a predominant symptom of hypocalcemia.

4 This can be caused by several factors and not merely hypocalcemia.

109. Application, planning, physiological integrity (c).

1 Because of the destruction of T cells, opportunistic is the priority problem for these individuals.

2, 3, 4 Although these all may very well be a problem for patients with AIDS, it is not the priority based on Maslow's hierarchy of needs.

110. Comprehension, implementation, physiological integrity (b).

3 Eardrops should be warmed to body temperature (no more than 100° F [38° C]). Vertigo may result from high or low temperatures.

1 Although eardrops should be slowly instilled and allowed to flow into the canal, the rate most likely did not cause the vertigo.

2 Occluded canal may cause vertigo. However, his vertigo occurred immediately following administration of the eardrops.

4 This is most unlikely although possible if being given for the first time (not the best response).

111. Application, assessment, health promotion and maintenance (b).

4 These are common manifestations of hypertension in patients.

1 Nausea and vomiting are not common symptoms of hypertension.

2 Increased urination is not a common finding in patients with hypertension.

3 These are not common assessment findings for a patient with hypertension.

112. Comprehension, implementation, physiological integrity (c).

2 Mannitol is an osmotic diuretic used to decrease intracranial pressure in patients with head injury.

1 Mannitol is not an antibiotic.

3 Sedatives or pain medications would offer this action.

4 Although mannitol may indirectly reduce the chance for seizures by decreasing intracranial pressure, this is not the primary reason for giving this medication.

113. Analysis, evaluation, physiological integrity (c).

4 Atropine, used for symptomatic bradycardia, causes mydriasis (dilated pupil), which would worsen the patient's glaucoma.

1 Morphine sulfate would not have a negative effect on the patient's glaucoma.

2 Milk of magnesia should not create a problem for a patient with glaucoma.

3 Ferrous sulfate, or iron, should not have a negative impact on the patient's glaucoma.

114. Analysis, implementation, physiological integrity (b).

3 This is considered a low platelet count, which can predispose the patient for bleeding episodes.

1, 2, 4 These are laboratory values within normal range.

115. Comprehension assessment, health promotion and maintenance (b).

2 This would promote venous return and decrease the swelling in the extremity.

1 A diuretic is not normally used for swelling caused by injury or surgery.

3 This technique would not reduce swelling and would limit Range of motion (ROM).

4 Although this is done on a routine basis, it will not decrease edema formation.

116. Comprehension, implementation, physiological integrity (c).

4 The goal of oxygen therapy is to supply the myocardium with additional oxygen, thereby reducing the myocardial oxygen demand and enabling the heart to supply oxygen to the tissues of the body.

1 Oxygen, in and of itself, will not prevent ventricular fibrillation.

2 Hypoxia will increase the patient's anxiety and restlessness.

3 Oxygen will not prevent cardiogenic shock.

117. Application, implementation, physiological integrity (a).

2 An autograph is tissue taken from the patient's own body.

1, 3, 4 These are all derived from substances other than the patient's own skin.

118. Application, assessment, health promotion and maintenance (c).

3 This may indicate overhydration.

1 This is normal capillary refill time.

2 This is normal skin turgor.

4 This is the normal color and odor of urine.

119. Application, assessment, physiological integrity (b).

4 Caused by narrowed airways, wheezes are common in patients with asthma.

1, 2, 3 These are all adventitious breath sounds caused by other disorders.

120. Application, assessment, physiological integrity (b).

2 Changes in the circulatory status of the involved extremity indicate a complication.

1 This is not serious and may be a reaction to the anesthetic.

3 This can be handled by the nurse, in most cases, and is not a serious complication of arthroplasty.

4 This may not be of any concern; the patient may not have any sputum to produce, and as long as the patient does incentive spirometry, and deep-breathing exercises, pulmonary status should be maintained.

121. Application, planning, safe, effective care environment (c).

3 This is the best choice given that the patient's blisters are weeping and still infectious.

1 The chance of infection in the roommate makes this situation a bad choice.

2 Pediatric patients are more susceptible to infection, and adults are not normally placed with a pediatric roommate.

4 Choosing the room for the patient is important because of the chance of contamination.

122. Application, implementation, physiological integrity (b).

4 This maintains cleanliness. Preventive skin care is important in maintaining the integrity of the skin and stoma.

1 Massaging may injure the delicate stoma and is unnecessary unless ordered by the physician.

2 Oils may be irritating to the skin and stoma; it promotes fungal infection.

3 The lotion will provide a medium for fungal growth and may irritate the stoma.

123. Knowledge, planning, physiological integrity (c).

1 A thoracentesis is withdrawal of fluid from the pleural space.

2, 3, 4 No type of puncture is recommended into any of these potential spaces.

124. Application, implementation, physiological integrity (c).

4 This ensures a continuous flow of urine in case specimens are needed. It removes bacteria that may be introduced during the procedure.

1 Bowel preparation is required if x-ray images are taken. Enemas until clear may be unsafe, depending on the number or amount administered.

2 This is unnecessary for this procedure.

3 This is inappropriate; see #1 for correct response.

125. Comprehension, implementation, physiological integrity (b).

The nurse will need to know the amount of irrigant that was used during the continuous bladder irrigation and then subtract that amount from the total urine to get the true urine output.

126. Comprehension, planning, physiological integrity (b).

2 The elevated toilet seat will not allow the patient to flex her hip past 90 degrees, an activity that may dislocate the hip.

1, 3, 4 All of these responses sound logical; however, none of them are based on scientific fact.

127. Comprehension, implementation, physiological integrity (b).

3 Standing and sitting for long periods cause varicose veins to develop and increases pain for the patient. Additionally, blood stasis predisposes the patient to blood clots.

1 This activity would increase pain for the patient.

2 These would not provide support for the patient, as would antiembolism or support stockings.

4 This activity would not decrease the pain of varicose veins and may prompt further development.

128. Application, implementation, physiological integrity (c).

2 This drug potentiates muscle weakness because of effect on myoneural junction.

1 This drug blocks the action of cholinesterase at the myoneural junction and allows acetylcholine to act. It is therapeutic.

3 Corticosteroids are sometimes used as an adjunct therapy. It is therapeutic.

4 Mestinon blocks the action of cholinesterase at the myoneural junction and allows acetylcholine to act. It is therapeutic.

129. Application, assessment, health promotion and maintenance (c).

2 Russell traction is a sling that attaches to the patient's skin under the knee, placing pressure on the popliteal space, increasing the possibility of venous thrombosis.

1 Buck's traction is a type of skin traction that does not predispose patients to thrombosis.

3 A Halo frame is attached in the head region and has little effect on the lower extremities.

4 Crutchfield tongs are a type of skeletal traction that is attached to the skull.

130. Application, planning, physiological integrity (b).

The nurse might suggest that the patient take his medication with milk or juice or with a meal. Taking the medication in the evening may also help the individual's gastric distress. If problems continue to persist, the physician may prescribe medications designed to protect the gastric mucosa from the effects of the medications on the stomach.

131. Application, assessment, physiological integrity (b).

2 Abduction moves a body part away from the midline.

1 Flexion decreases an angle at a joint.

3 Adduction is moving a body part toward the midline.

4 Pronation rotates a part to face downward.

132. Application, planning, physiological integrity (c).

3 The ventrogluteal is a deep muscle located in the upper, outer quadrant of the hip. It has few superficial

blood vessels and makes a good injection site for someone who has muscle atrophy.

1 The deltoid is not a good choice because of the patient's muscle atrophy.

2 Intramuscular injections are not given in the abdomen.

4 The gluteus maximus is not a good choice because of the muscle atrophy.

133. Application, assessment, physiological integrity (c).

1 An underproduction of cortisol from the adrenal medulla is associated with Addison's disease.

2 Overproduction of this hormone leads to acromegaly or gigantism.

3 Elevation of these levels indicates hyperthyroidism.

4 Elevation in epinephrine levels does not indicate Addison's disease.

134. Application, implementation, physiological integrity (c).

4 Additional stress placed on the tissues by movement may disrupt the healing tissue. Splinting lessens the chance for this to occur.

1 This is true, but the question is specific to ambulation.

2 This is too sweeping of a statement. Although more pain is involved from movement with an abdominal incision, not all patients are hesitant to do so.

3 The binder would be a good choice for the patient if it were applied correctly.

135. Application, implementation, psychosocial integrity (c).

4 This is an open-ended question that seeks to explore the patient's feelings. It is always best to allow the patient to express his or her views.

1 This does not address the patient's fears.

2 This is defensive and will not help the patient cope.

3 This statement appears to be patronizing. It is best to ascertain what the patient's questions are first.

136. Comprehension, assessment, physiological integrity (b).

3 These are low blood sugar (hypoglycemic) symptoms.

1, 2 These are not associated with hypoglycemia.

4 These are symptoms of ketoacidosis.

137. Knowledge, assessment, physiological integrity (c).

3 This blood type has no A or B antigens and can be given to individuals who are type A, B, or O, provided the Rh factor is also compatible.

1 Patients with blood type A can receive blood from individuals with A or O blood, if the Rh factors are compatible.

2 Patients with type B blood can receive blood from donors who are type O or B, if the Rh factor is compatible.

4 Patients with type AB blood must receive blood that is type AB or O.

138. Application, planning, health promotion and maintenance (c).

1 Stem cells are cells that can grow and develop into cells and tissues that might correct deficiencies in patient's organs, nerves, muscles, or brain.

2, 3, 4 All of these cells are fully developed, mature cells that are not able to be used in this manner.

139. Application, implementation, health promotion and maintenance (b).

3 This statement is accurate description of how immunizations work and does not give false assurance.

1 This is not a true statement; the chance always exists that a person can contract polio after the injection.

2 Immunizations are mandatory for children in the United States who attend school; however, parents can decline for religious or ethical reasons.

4 Parental consent is required for all but the most emergent of care; this statement is also antagonistic and does not meet the father or the child's learning needs.

140. Comprehension, planning, physiological integrity (a).

3 Chemotherapy agents attack all rapidly dividing cells in the body and normally cause nausea, vomiting, alopecia, and anemia because of this fact. The nurse will need to plan care to alleviate the side effects as much as possible.

1 Not all drugs are given orally, although some are.

2 As previously mentioned, these drugs have many side effects.

4 No medications are available, to date, that target only the cells in the tumor.

141. Application, implementation, physiological integrity (b).

3 Skin of older adults is fragile and may not tolerate adhesive tape. Frequent tape applications should be avoided.

1 Although this is true, #3 explains the physiological rationale for using Montgomery straps, which is given priority over cost.

2 This is an inappropriate response; the method used to secure the dressing would cause and increase in infection.

4 The frequency of dressing changes is based on physician orders or the amount of drainage, or both. The straps secure the dressing in place.

142. Application, implementation, health promotion and maintenance (b).

3 A continuous passive ROM machine allows the patient to regain flexibility to the knee very early after surgery.

1 A trochanter roll would keep the patient's leg from externally rotating.

2 An abductor pillow keeps the patient from adducting the legs after a hip replacement.

4 A Hemovac drainage device will not promote flexibility of the knee.

143. Application, assessment, physiological integrity (b).

1 This common term means that the patient's toe turns white when pushed on. However, the color returns very quickly to the toe; quick capillary refill is defined as less than 3 seconds for color to return.

2, 3, 4 These are all assessments important in a neurovascular assessment.

144. Application, assessment, physiological integrity (b).

1. These are all signs of fluid overload.

2, 3, 4 All of these responses have mixed symptoms for dehydration and fluid overload.

145. Application, implementation, physiological integrity (b).

3 Treatment for this condition revolves around keeping the extremities warm with socks, mittens, and other warm layers.

1 Support hose will not keep this patient from experiencing exacerbations.

2, 4 Patients with this disorder will worsen their condition by application of hot or cold to the areas affected.

146. Comprehension, evaluation, health promotion and maintenance (c).

2 Many patients with Buerger's disease have a history of cigarette smoking. The nicotine in the cigarettes contributes to spasms of the blood vessels.

1, 3, 4 None of these are predisposing factors to Buerger's disease.

147. Application, planning, health promotion and maintenance (b).

3 Raynaud's phenomenon is triggered by contact with cold.

1 This is not true; Raynaud's disease affects primarily women.

2 Both of these diseases cause considerable pain for patients.

4 Buerger's disease affects both types of blood vessels.

148. Application, assessment, physiological integrity (c).

2 Damaged parenchymal cells are unable to metabolize bilirubin, which give the stool its normal color; bilirubin in the circulation causes jaundice, pruritus, and dark urine.

1 Stools are clay colored because of the liver's inability to metabolize bilirubin.

3 Clay-colored stools are common in advanced liver disease; urine is dark in color.

4 Urine is not blood-tinged but dark in color with liver dysfunction.

149. Application, implementation, physiological integrity (b).

3 Patients should not be routinely suctioned unless they are unable to control their secretions. Gurgling in the airway signifies a need for suctioning.

1 If the patient requests suctioning, encouraging her to expectorate her secretions might be appropriate.

2 Suctioning on a routine basis is unnecessary, unless otherwise indicated.

4 Most orders for suctioning are written as prn, and the times are at the discretion of the nurse.

150. Analysis, implementation, physiological integrity (c).

3 Tubes that are placed high in the anterior chest are placed primarily to reestablish normal pressure in the lung by creating an outlet for air.

1 This is a trite response. The nurse should answer the question with the correct answer.

2 This statement is not true.

4 Although this statement is true, it does not meet the learning needs of the patient.

151. Application, evaluation, physiological integrity (c).

1 Given this situation, this scenario is the most likely reason for the fluctuations to have ceased. The nurse will need to perform a complete assessment on the patient to ascertain this.

2 Tube dislodgment is an unlikely scenario and would be immediately apparent to the nurse.

3 Turning the suction up too high would merely create extra bubbling in the suction chamber and should not affect the tidaling in the water-seal chamber.

4 Although this may be a likely reason for this problem, given the patient situation, the reexpansion of the lung is a more likely scenario.

152. Comprehension, planning, psychosocial integrity (c).

3 This is the correct response, presented in terms the wife can understand.

1 This is not a correct response; thoracotomy tubes drain blood from the lung.

2, 4 These are not correct responses.

153. Application, evaluation, physiological integrity (b).

4 The nurse needs to establish if the patient can clear his own airway.

1 This would indicate an infection or dehydration, or both.

2 This is inappropriate for this nursing diagnosis.

3 This would give the opportunity to assess the effort of breathing.

154. Knowledge, implementation, physiological integrity (b).

2 This position promotes full chest expansion and comfort for the patient.

1 This position is not indicated except in emergency situations. It would create respiratory distress in this patient.

3 This is the position for promoting GI comfort and giving enemas and suppositories.

4 Semiprone would not promote good chest expansion.

155. Comprehension, evaluation, physiological integrity (b).

3 The patient's dry nasal passages are probably caused by the dry heat in his home. Running a humidifier would moisturize the air and may stop his discomfort.

1 This is not an emergency situation.

2 No basis exists for this suggestion, and it would alarm the patient.

4 This is true, but it does not relate to the question.

156. Application, planning, physiological integrity (b).

1 This is the only choice that maintains the water-seal drainage. The patient can be off suction for short periods.

2 This would break the closed system and might create a pneumothorax.

3 Although this is possible, and it would depend on the patient's condition, no harm exists in transporting the patient to the x-ray department.

4 This would take much time, and no harm exists in transporting the patient.

157. Comprehension, assessment, physiological integrity (c).

2 Patients who have a true latex allergy react to the resin from the rubber plant. The typical reaction creates angioedema and urticaria.

1, 3 These are reactions to substances that cause superficial histamine release.

4 This is not an allergic reaction.

158. Application, planning, physiological integrity (b).

The patient should carry a dose of self-injectable epinephrine. The patient should also have a medic alert tag on his possession.

159. Knowledge, planning, physiological integrity (b).

2 Most narcotic analgesics work best when given before pain intensity reaches its maximum.

1 Analgesics should not be given at bedtime, if no pain is present, just for the purpose of promoting sleep.

3 Pain medication can be given only when ordered by the physician and should not be given routinely except in cases of terminally ill patients with chronic pain.

4 The nurse must use discretion and assess the patient, also checking to determine when the last dose was given and how often it is ordered.

160. Comprehension, assessment, physiological integrity (b).
  1 Because of damage to the nerve, the nurse would expect hoarseness of the voice.
  2 This may indicate pulmonary edema.
  3 This may indicate hemorrhage.
  4 This indicates tetany and hypocalcemia.

161. Application, planning, physiological integrity (a).
  2 Symptoms of a urinary tract infection include urinary frequency, dysuria, and cloudy urine.
  1 These are symptoms of some systemic disorder, such as renal failure.
  3 These are possible symptoms for IICP.
  4 These are not indicative of a lower urinary tract infection.

162. Application, planning, psychosocial integrity (c).
  1 A calm environment is important; these patients are usually in a hyperactive state.
  2 The number of visitors may need to be limited to avoid overtaxing the patient's energies.
  3 A supportive environment is necessary but does not overstimulate the patient.
  4 A private room ensures better control over the environment.

163. Application, implementation, physiological integrity (c).
  1000 ml divided by 8 hours + 125 ml/hr. 125 ml/hr × 10 gtts/min divided by 60 min/hr = 21 gtts/min.

164. Application, assessment, health promotion and maintenance (b).
  4 Muscle weakness and personality changes herald the possibility of neurological problems.
  1 Chest pain on exertion is a symptom of angina; this patient does not exhibit this.
  2 The patient may have no symptoms at all or symptoms of fatigue and headache.
  3 The presenting symptoms indicate a potential neurological complication, not a cardiac one.

165. Comprehension, assessment, health promotion and maintenance (b).
  3 Following this procedure, a loss of sufficient intrinsic factor may occur.
  1 Diabetes mellitus is a pancreatic problem resulting from insufficient amounts of insulin.
  2 Reflux refers to the backward flow of gastric contents through an incompetent sphincter, allowing juices to flow into the esophagus. This is not a complication of a gastrectomy.
  4 *H. pylori* may be found in the gastric mucosa and may cause peptic ulcers. The incidence of *H. pylori* does not increase after a gastrectomy.

166. Comprehension, planning, health promotion and maintenance (b).
  1 Protection of the blood supply is a sound measure to prevent the transmission of hepatitis B and C and HIV.
  2 Blood donors cannot get a blood-borne disease by donating blood.
  3 This may reduce the risk of ingestion of some pathogens but not the hepatitis B virus.
  4 Shellfish are associated with contraction of hepatitis A.

167. Application, planning, physiological integrity (b).
  2 Contact sports that can result in blunt blows to the abdomen should be discouraged.
  1 This noncontact sport poses a reduced risk of injury.
  3 Although strenuous, this sport poses little risk of injury to the patient's stoma.
  4 If the patient feels comfortable swimming with an ileostomy, it should not be discouraged.

168. Application, assessment, health promotion and maintenance (b).
  4 This is a common laboratory finding in appendicitis.
  1 This is found in polycythemia vera.
  2 A low platelet count is not consistent with appendicitis.
  3 This is not common in appendicitis, but it is in chronic renal failure.

169. Application, planning, health promotion and maintenance (b).
  1 These are symptoms of hypoglycemia.
  2 These are classic symptoms of hyperglycemia.
  3 These are not the cardinal symptoms of diabetes mellitus but are indicative of hypertension.
  4 These symptoms are not indicative of diabetes mellitus.

170. Application, planning, physiological integrity (b).
  4 The tube is a triple-lumen tube with an esophageal balloon to control bleeding of varices. One lumen is for lavage, and another is used for suction.
  1 Platelets do not need to be replaced. Refrigerated blood lacks prothrombin and coagulation factors needed for clotting.
  2 Iced saline solution is used. Gastric lavage would wash out the stomach, not control bleeding in the esophagus.
  3 Vasodilators will not control bleeding. Antibiotics and antacids may be used after the acute phase.

171. Application, planning, physiological integrity (a).
  2 Repositioning will decrease the chance of the ulcer becoming deeper.
  1 Soap is not indicated for patients with this type of ulcer.
  3 This is usually not an effective treatment for this type of ulcer.
  4 Ointments and medications are not going to be effective on skin that is not intact.

172. Application, planning, health promotion and maintenance (b).
  3 Stem cells may begin to produce new cells that will be cancer free.
  1, 2, 4 Stem cells do not exert their effectiveness in this manner.

173. Application, assessment, physiological integrity (a).
  1 Pain in and around the ear, over the mastoid process, is a classic symptom.
  2, 3, 4 These are not common symptoms of mastoiditis.

174. Comprehension, planning, safe, effective care environment (a).
  2 Gloves should be worn.
  1 Eye pads are contraindicated in general eye infections because they enhance bacterial growth.
  3 Ointment should be placed in the conjunctiva.
  4 All patients should have their own tubes of ointment to prevent cross-infection.

175. Comprehension, planning, physiological integrity (a).
  2 Straining at stool increases intraocular pressure and can damage the eye.
  1 Restricting fluids is unnecessary.

3 Bathing is allowed, although showers may be prohibited.

4 This has no bearing on the patient's surgery.

176. Analysis, assessment, physiological integrity (c).

   1 Frequent swallowing is a sign that the patient may be swallowing blood from a hemorrhage.

   2 No restriction in water intake has been ordered.

   3 This is not normally a problem from swallowing, although swallowing after this surgery is difficult.

   4 This surgery is very uncomfortable for both children and adults.

177. Comprehension, implementation, health promotion and maintenance (b).

   4 This is the only true statement.

   1 This is not directly related to glaucoma.

   2 Blindness is not always a result if glaucoma is diagnosed and treated.

   3 This is not directly related to glaucoma.

178. Application implementation, physiological integrity (b).

   2 Mydriatics cause an enlarged pupil that would let too much light into the eye. The effects should last only a few hours and sunglasses should help them.

   1 No need exists for a patch over her eye.

   3 This restriction is imposed on individuals who have had eye surgery.

   4 This is an unnecessary restriction

179. Analysis, planning, safe, effective care environment (b).

   4 Patients with a low WBC count need to be placed in protective isolation (neutropenic precautions) because of their compromised immune function.

   1 Hemorrhage is a priority when a patient has a low platelet count.

   2 Fever may be an indicator of infection, but the protection is against infection.

   3 Jaundice is a sign of liver disease.

180. Application, implementation, physiological integrity (b).

   1 This prevents excessive pressure.

   2 Excessive pressure from nose blowing can force infected secretions up the eustachian tube into the middle ear.

   3 Keeping mouth open is not necessary. The patient should blow with the nostrils open.

   4 Excessive pressure from nose blowing can force infected secretions up the eustachian tube into the middle ear.

181. Application, assessment, physiological integrity (b).

   3 This patient has a knowledge deficit about the desired action of diuretics.

   1 Altered tissue perfusion is not a concern for this patient.

   2 The patient may have a fluid excess, that information was not provided; the paramount concern in this situation is the knowledge deficit.

   4 The patient shows no indication of fluid volume deficit.

182. Application, planning, physiological integrity (b).

   4 This is a measure that will assist the patient with elimination and make the first bowel movement less painful.

   1 Sitz baths are more soothing to the rectum.

   2 Occlusive dressings are not normally used; rectal packing and loose dressings to collect drainage may be used.

3 Gas formation is not a common problem with this procedure.

183. Application, assessment, health promotion and maintenance (c).

   4 The involved leg may be shorter because of the pull of the muscles nearest the fracture site, and the leg rotates outward.

   1 Pronation is a term associated with the upper extremities; the leg will be externally rotated.

   2 Supination is a term associated with the upper extremities; the leg will be externally rotated.

   3 The affected leg is normally shorter than the other and is externally rotated.

184. Comprehension, planning, physiological integrity (b).

   1 Hypokalemia may occur as a result of the diuretic therapy.

   2 Low blood calcium is not a consequence of diuretic therapy.

   3 Hyperglycemia is a concern when a patient is on steroid therapy.

   4 An underproduction of insulin is associated with pancreatic dysfunction.

185. Comprehension, assessment, health promotion and maintenance (b).

   4 The painless swelling of lymph nodes is one of the hallmarks of Hodgkin's disease, and non-Hodgkin's lymphoma.

   1 This is not an early sign of the disorder.

   2 This is a common finding in renal disorders.

   3 This is frequently a problem in many disorders but not lymphoma.

186. Comprehension, implementation, physiological integrity (c).

   2 Elevation of the extremity above the level of the heart will decrease the venous swelling.

   1 This will aggravate the condition.

   3 This will not affect the localized swelling.

   4 This will promote venous return but will continue to trap the fluid within the extremity.

187. Comprehension, planning, physiological integrity (b).

   4 Diet should supply calories, protein, and carbohydrates to compensate for the increased metabolic demands imposed by the disease.

   1 Restriction of purine is not necessary, and calories in this diet are insufficient.

   2 This would provide insufficient calories; it will not meet the metabolic demands of the body.

   3 Restricting sodium is not necessary.

188. Application, assessment, health promotion and maintenance (c).

   1 These are the classic symptoms of thyroid storm.

   2 These symptoms are not typical of Cushing's syndrome.

   3 These symptoms are not typical of hypoglycemia.

   4 These symptoms are not those of hypocalcemia.

189. Application, planning, physiological integrity (b).

   1 Many diuretics cause excretion of both sodium and potassium; maintaining adequate potassium levels is important for proper heart function.

   2 This may potentiate a fluid-retention problem.

   3 These foods would not be restricted because the patient is on a diuretic.

4 Caffeine is a natural diuretic and is not normally restricted in patients taking diuretics.

190. Comprehension, planning, physiological integrity (b).

4 This medication is a diuretic intended to promote fluid loss in an effort to decrease blood pressure in some patients.

1 This is a cardiotonic and is normally given to individuals who have heart failure, arrhythmias, or atrial fibrillation.

2 This is an antiinflammatory.

3 This is a histamine blocker that suppresses gastric acid secretion.

191. Application, implementation, safe, effective care environment (c).

2 This maintains an intact drainage system. It is less likely that urine specimen will become contaminated.

3 This maintains the sterility of the specimen.

1, 4, 5 These are inappropriate to the situation. 1 and 4 will not provide a sterile specimen and there is no need to have the patient endure a repeat and unnecessary catheterization.

192. Comprehension, implementation, psychosocial integrity (a).

3 This is an emotional change that is common after a CVA. Emotional lability may or may not be appropriate to the situation.

1 This is common but normal.

2 This is inappropriate and encourages negative behavior modification technique. The patient has emotional lability.

4 This is inappropriate. The patient is not acting this way on purpose.

193. Application, implementation, health promotion and maintenance (b).

1 This is a true statement.

2 This is also true, but a blood test will be needed to ascertain this situation.

5 This is the correct follow up statement.

3, 4 Situation at hand is not an emergency which makes these statements inappropriate.

194. Comprehension, assessment, physiological integrity (b).

4 Dysphagia means difficulty swallowing. He may need to double swallow between bites.

1 This is an inappropriate, unnecessary restriction.

2 This is not necessary. No indication exists that patient is hearing impaired.

3 This is a good practice for any person who has had a CVA. However, it is not specific to this question.

195. Comprehension, implementation, physiological integrity (b).

2 Lubrication would allow easier insertion.

1 This is a sterile technique but not the underlying principle.

3 This is a result. It is not the underlying principle.

4 This may be a result, but it is not the underlying principle.

196. Comprehension, implementation, health promotion and maintenance (c).

3 Flank pain would signal the presence of kidney stones.

1 This is a trite reason to give; the patient needs more information.

2 Usually high calcium levels are a problem in this disorder.

4 Many times, kidney stones can be treated conservatively.

197. Knowledge, planning, physiological integrity (a).

1 This is true. Weakened pelvic muscles may also be a cause.

2 This is an inappropriate assumption; this is called "residual" and is not usually a factor in stress inconvenience.

3 This is an inappropriate assumption; muscles and nerves are usually involved, not nerves alone.

4 This is an inappropriate assumption; this may be true, but other symptoms would be evident, such as back pain.

198. Analysis, assessment, physiological integrity (c).

3 Tarry stools may indicate bleeding, a complication of peptic ulcer disease, which may signal more serious gastric distress.

1, 2, 4 These would not signal a worsening of the patient's original complaint.

199. Comprehension, planning, physiological integrity (c).

2 Injuries above C3 cause respiratory paralysis and require ventilatory support.

1 Diuretics may be ordered, but patent airway is a more pressing concern.

3 This would not maintain a patent airway for this patient.

4 These may also be indicated, but the patent airway is the immediate concern.

200. Comprehension, implementation, physiological integrity (a).

1 This is the proper procedure for stopping the nosebleed.

2, 3, 4 These measures are ineffective and will worsen the problem. Packing is only done as a last resort.

201. Comprehension, planning, physiological integrity (b).

2 Easily digestible foods are given to patients to lessen the myocardial oxygen demand.

1 This is not the primary purpose for giving a soft diet to this person.

3 This is not true.

4 Although this may be true, the rationale behind giving the soft diet is not given.

202. Analysis, evaluation, physiological integrity (b).

3 The Holter monitor will record a tracing of the heart during various activities and is compared with activities that the patient is documenting as well.

1 A glucometer evaluates capillary blood sugar levels.

2 Urines are used to evaluate various conditions but not heart activity during exertion.

4 This study evaluates blood flow through a carotid artery or extremity.

203. Comprehension, planning, physiological integrity (c).

3 Maintaining a patent airway is the primary concern based on the patient's medical diagnosis and Maslow's hierarchy of human needs.

1 Suctioning will clear the airway, maintaining patency; it is a means of maintaining a patent airway.

2 Changing the dressing around the tracheostomy would be a nursing skill to prevent infection. Airway is the primary concern.

4 Although this is important, airway is still the more immediate concern

204. Application, assessment, health promotion and maintenance (b).

    2 Early exercise will help prevent stasis of blood flow in the legs, which will help prevent blood clots from forming.

    1 This may be a physician order but not a nursing measure.

    3 Increasing fluids will prevent the individual from becoming dehydrated but will not prevent the formation of blood clots.

    4 Diuretics will create a dehydrated condition in an individual who does not have fluid retention.

205. Comprehension, assessment, physiological integrity (a).

    3 Pacemaker generator insertion sites are frequently found near the clavicle in the upper chest.

    1 Transvenous pacemaker insertion sites are frequently found in the upper chest region.

    2 This is not accurate. Only external pacemakers have a lead on the back; it is not an insertion site.

    4 This is not a true response.

206. Application, implementation, physiological integrity (b).

    1 The nurse should stand on the affected side and support with gait belt. The gait belt provides stability and greater control in assisting the patient without putting undue pressure on patient or the nurse's body.

    2 This is inappropriate and does not provide the patient with a base of support.

    3 This is not a safe practice; the patient may hesitate or tip backward.

    4 This is inappropriate. A patient with right-sided weakness requires the nurse to stand on the right side. Reaching over to hold the patient's right hand may change patient's center of gravity and tip her forward. In addition, these body mechanics are awkward for the nurse.

207. Comprehension, assessment, physiological integrity (b).

    1, 3 Jaundice and hepatomegaly are the primary symptoms of thalassemia major.

    2, 4, 5 Erythema, pruritus, and blurred vision are not common in patients with this disorder.

208. Analysis, assessment, safe, effective care environment (c).

    1 Infection is the primary concern based on Maslow's hierarchy of needs. The patient's first line of defense is gone.

    2 Hemorrhage is a problem but is a lesser problem compared with the infection process.

    3 Increased ICP is more of a problem with a closed head injury.

    4 Consciousness would not be the primary concern, although it is a secondary concern.

209. Comprehension, assessment, physiological integrity (c).

    2 Because of pathological changes in the inner ear, patients with labyrinthitis frequently complain of dizziness.

    1 Sinus pain is not associated with labyrinthitis.

    3 Cephalgia may be a complaint, but it is generally not the principal complaint.

    4 Double vision is not a frequent complaint.

210. Comprehension, evaluation, physiological integrity (b).

    1 The surgery most likely to be performed in this situation is removal of the stapes, one of the small bones of the middle ear.

    2 A mastoidectomy is performed to remove an infected mastoid process.

    3 A myringotomy is performed for otitis media.

    4 Cerumen removal is not a surgical procedure and is done for removal of wax because of impacted cerumen.

211. Application, planning, physiological integrity (b).

    2, 3 These are standard treatments for patients with impacted cerumen.

    1, 4, 5 No need exists to remove the hearing aids unless the patient is uncomfortable.

212. Comprehension, planning, physiological integrity (a).

    2 The patient should receive 1000 ml/12 hr, or 83.333 ml/hr.

    1, 3, 4 These are incorrect math calculations.

213. Comprehension, evaluation, physiological integrity (b).

    1 Persons with a pulmonary embolism experience pain related to ischemia caused by obstruction of small pulmonary arterial branches, process in lung, described as pleuritic chest pain.

    2 This relates to activity intolerance or interest in doing own self-care. It may be an indication of lessened anxiety.

    3 Appetite, weight, nutritional status are not usual problems for patients with a pulmonary embolism.

    4 This is related to an ineffective airway clearance problem.

214. Comprehension, evaluation, physiological integrity (c).

    1, 2, 4, 5 These are symptoms of hypoglycemia.

    3 This is a symptom of hyperglycemia.

    6 It occurs suddenly, not gradually.

215. Comprehension, assessment, physiological integrity (b).

    2 This is the correct description.

    1 This describes level II = generalized response.

    3 This describes level VI = confused-appropriate.

    4 This describes level IV = confused-agitated.

216. Application, assessment, physiological integrity (b).

    2 Bleeding is a serious side effect of anticoagulant therapy. Nursing measures focus on monitoring for signs of active bleeding.

    1 This is a common side effect of any medication. Hematemesis would be of serious concern.

    3 This is not a common side effect of this class of medications and is not suggestive of bleeding.

    4 This is a common side effect of many medications.

217. Comprehension, implementation, physiological integrity (b).

    4 Insulin must be given to patients with DKA to correct the hyperglycemia and ketosis.

    1 Oral antidiabetic agents will not correct DKA, although they are helpful in type 2 diabetes mellitus.

    2 Glucose and water would create further problems for the patient with DKA.

    3 Diuretics are used to treat hypertension or HF but not DKA.

218. Application, planning, physiological integrity (b).

    4 This reduces risk of constipation and straining, which may put a strain on damaged myocardium.

    1 This is not a standard of care for a patient having an myocardial infarction.

    2 Prolonged bed rest is no longer advocated for patients with myocardial infarction.

    3 This is no longer a standard of care.

219. Comprehension, assessment, health promotion and maintenance (c).

1, 3, 4 These are the classic signs of diabetes mellitus.

2, 5 These are not seen in patients with diabetes mellitus.

220. Comprehension, evaluation, safe, effective care environment (a).

2 These are the signs and symptoms of Lyme disease.

1 The signs and symptoms and history do not point to a diagnosis of ALS.

3 Patients with encephalitis complain of photophobia and headache.

4 Patients with chronic fatigue syndrome complain of extreme tiredness.

221. Analysis, planning, physiological integrity (b).

1, 2, 5 The nurse should expect to make glucose checks frequently and get the patient something to eat as soon possible. If the patient is unable to eat, then glucose IV fluids would need to be given, and a bolus dose of dextrose 50% may need to be delivered IV.

3, 4 More regular insulin would compound the problem, and the patient is not yet critical enough (and might not be) to be moved to the intensive care unit.

222. Analysis, evaluation, physiological integrity (b).

2 This indicates that sputum has been expectorated from the lungs.

1 This relates to decreased appetite and altered nutrition.

3 This demonstrates effectiveness of therapy.

4 This relates to a knowledge deficit nursing diagnosis.

223. Analysis, implementation, safe, effective care environment (b).

1 To prevent falling and to decrease vertigo sensation, the person has to be still and avoid all head movements that aggravate the spinning sensation.

2 This would be appropriate only if PRN had been ordered.

3 Normal hydration is 2000 ml/day. At times, a diuretic may be prescribed to help decrease fluid volume of endolymph.

4 This may increase sensation of vertigo however, bright, glaring lights should be avoided.

224. Comprehension, planning, physiological integrity (a).

4 Presbycusis is the term used to describe hearing loss associated with aging.

1 This is inappropriate; hearing loss does not usually affect physical comfort.

2 This is possible if the person is unaware of environmental sounds. However, it is not a common cause.

3 This is inappropriate; hearing loss does not usually affect family roles.

225. Comprehension, evaluation, physiological integrity (b).

3 Widening pulse pressure is a sign of IICP.

1, 2, 4 These are not signs of widening pulse pressure.

226. Knowledge, evaluation, safe, effective care environment (b).

4 Tonic-clonic seizures are total body seizures that have the above signs and symptoms.

1, 2, 3 These types of seizure do not usually cause the patient to become incontinent or become sleepy afterwards.

227. Comprehension, implementation, physiological integrity (a).

1 Some patients experience a spinal headache after removal of cerebral spinal fluid.

2 Leakage of spinal fluid can occur even if laying flat.

3 This is an inappropriate response for the nurse to make; the nurse must know why the patient must lay flat.

4 This is inappropriate. Blood pressure is affected by many factors and should not be directly affected by this procedure.

228. Comprehension, assessment, physiological integrity (a).

4 A herniated disk in the lumbar region would create compression of the sciatic nerve, creating buttock and thigh pain.

1, 2, 3 These are not associated with this disorder.

229. Application, assessment, health promotion and maintenance (a).

1 This may indicate a problem in the middle ear.

2 It is important to frequently watch others' faces to lip-read.

3 This may be true if position changes were to lean forward to hear better.

4 This behavior may result from a variety of factors that are not hearing related.

230. Analysis, implementation, physiological integrity (a).

3 Airway, breathing, and circulation are the first priority. Rapid respirations that are shallow and irregular need immediate action.

1 The nurse needs to know patient's previous temperature.

2 This may indicate many things. The nurse needs further data. It is not a priority.

4 This may indicate therapy is effective. The nurse needs further data. It is not a priority.

231. Application, assessment, physiological integrity (b).

2 Angulation, deformities, and shortening of a limb are suggestive of a break in bone continuity.

1 Edema is present with both sprains and fractures.

3 Contused soft-tissue structures are tender, thus limiting mobility as well.

4 Both types of injuries may evidence tenderness.

232. Application, planning, physiological integrity (b).

4 Traction is commonly used to reduce femoral fractures.

1 Buck's traction is not used to treat neck sprains.

2 Patients with spinal fractures are normally placed on Stryker frames.

3 Shoulder dislocations are treated with immobilization devices.

233. Application, assessment, physiological integrity (b).

3 Russell traction uses a sling that may slide up under the knee and cause pressure, compromising circulation.

1 This type of traction does not involve a cast.

2 Compartment syndrome normally develops in cast situations, when an encircling, or constricting device, is used.

4 A boot device is not common in this type of traction.

234. Application, planning, physiological integrity (b).

3 One of the complications of a thyroidectomy is swelling around the trachea, compromising the airway. A tracheostomy set must be in the room for quick intervention if this happens.

1 A chest tube tray would not be necessary. No fear exists of collection of fluid in the pleural space.

2 A spinal tray should not be necessary.

4 Transtracheal oxygen delivery would not be beneficial because the patient's upper trachea would be occluded.

235. Application, planning, physiological integrity (c).

3 Lifting heavy objects would increase the patient's intraocular pressure, which can damage the reattachment.

1, 2, 4 These activities would not elevate intraocular pressure.

236. Comprehension, planning, physiological integrity (b).

1 Hearing aids help assist patients with conduction deafness caused by otosclerosis.

2 Hearing aids will not help individuals with deafness associated with impaired nerves.

3 The impacted cerumen will cause conduction deafness but will need to be removed before a hearing aid can help.

4 Senile dementia does not normally cause hearing loss, although old age might.

237. Comprehension, assessment, physiological integrity (a).

3 The ureters are the structures that transport urine to the bladder.

1, 2, 4 These structures of the renal system have different functions.

238. Comprehension, evaluation, physiological integrity (b).

2 Many times, glomerulonephritis is precipitated by an upper respiratory infection caused by the Streptococcus bacteria. The antigen-antibody complex formed from the infection impairs kidney function.

1 Antibiotic therapy is not a precipitating factor for this disorder.

3 Upper respiratory infections are implicated in this disorder, not urinary tract infections.

4 A low fluid intake, although important to many other kidney disorders, does not predispose a person to this disorder.

239. Knowledge, assessment, physiological integrity (b).

1 Peristalsis, rhythmic, wavelike contractions of visceral muscle propels urine through the ureters.

2, 3, 4 These are methods for moving solutions through a semipermeable membrane.

240. Analysis, evaluation, physiological integrity (c).

2 Creatinine, a component of protein metabolism, is elevated in patients with renal failure because the kidney is unable to excrete this waste, which builds up in the patient's bloodstream.

1, 3, 4 These abnormal laboratory values are indicative of other disorders.

241. Comprehension, planning, physiological integrity (c).

3 These are also known as hyperosmolar drugs. Mannitol (Osmitrol) is an example. These agents draw water from the edematous brain.

1 These should be used carefully; they may mask LOC or cause respiratory depression.

2 These may be ordered if nausea is present.

4 These may be ordered if an open wound is caused by trauma.

242. Application, assessment, health promotion and maintenance (a).

2 This is recommended as an annual test for all men age 50 and older.

1 This is a blood test used as a monitoring tool to evaluate the response to treatment of a patient with cancer or for recurrence of the disease.

3 This is a screening test for BPH or prostate cancer; it is not a blood test. It is an examination recommended for all men over the age of 40.

4 This is one of the diagnostic tests for HIV.

243. Analysis, planning, physiological integrity (c).

4 A common order for anyone admitted with nephrolithiasis would be straining urine to try to collect a stone specimen, which would then be sent to the laboratory for analysis.

1 Whirlpool baths would not be beneficial to this patient and are not usually ordered. When patients have extracorporeal shockwave lithotripsy, they are immersed in a bath for this procedure.

2 The opposite order would be given unless contraindicated. The patient needs to increase fluid intake.

3 Racking urine is a physician order that was common for suspected hematuria. It entails placing urine in test tubes and allowing it to sit for hours until blood would settle out.

244. Comprehension, implementation, physiological integrity (a).

2 Pantopaque is a heavy dye, and the physician strives to remove all the dye to prevent irritation of the meninges. Lying flat may help to lessen chance of headache.

1 This position is unsafe. Besides headache, strength and sensation of lower extremities must first be assessed.

3, 4 These positions are inappropriate. Any remaining dye may rise.

245. Comprehension, evaluation, psychosocial integrity (a).

4 Discovery of triggering factors demonstrates understanding of disease process and preventative health habits.

1 This is not directly related. However, it may relieve stress, which is frequently a trigger of headaches.

2 No proof exists that sunlight triggers these types of headaches.

3 Acetylsalicylic acid (aspirin) is seldom effective for classic migraine. Taking it as a preventive may not be a healthful habit.

246. Application, assessment, health promotion and maintenance (a).

3 The ache may be in the groin. Other signs are a lump or enlargement of a testicle, heaviness or sudden collection of fluid in the scrotum, enlargement or tenderness of the breasts, or any combination of these.

1 This describes phimosis.

2, 4 These are not warning signs of testicular cancer.

247. Comprehension, assessment, physiological integrity (c).

4 Right ventricle problems cause a pooling and backup of blood entering the heart from the systemic circulation. The dyspnea is caused by pressure from the ascites on the lungs. Failure of one of the ventricles normally results in failure of the opposite ventricle.

1 Patients who have mitral valve disease normally have murmurs. Only in advanced disease do ventricular problems develop.

2 Patients who have aortic valve problems have murmurs. Only in advanced cases do ventricular problems develop.

3 Left ventricular failure would exhibit itself as pulmonary edema, dyspnea, and crackles in the lungs.

248. Application, assessment, physiological integrity (b).

2 Patients with a hip fracture generally have shortening and external rotation of the affected extremity.

1 Pain and numbness may be present with sprains, contusions, and other problems.

3 A large hematoma at the hip certainly may be present at the site of a hip fracture; however, the symptoms of #2 are more indicative of this event.

4 Lengthening of the extremity is not seen in a hip fracture.

249. Application, assessment, physiological integrity (c).

3 A hot spot is usually a sign of inflammation under the cast.

1 Swelling causes tightness of the cast and affects the neurocirculatory status.

2 Tightness of a cast would manifest itself in changes in the neurocirculatory status of the extremity.

4 An object or foreign body beneath the cast, if large enough, may initially be evidenced by changes in neurocirculatory status.

250. Application, planning, physiological integrity (b).

4 This gives the body a chance to adjust the circulation to the effects of gravity.

1 This will not prevent hypotension.

2 Antiembolic stockings will not prevent hypotension.

3 Limiting dietary sodium is used in the treatment of hypertension but will not prevent hypotension.

251. Comprehension, assessment, health promotion and maintenance (b).

4 Anginal pain is caused by myocardial ischemia, which is insufficient blood and oxygen to the heart muscle. The pain may be precipitated or exacerbated by exertion.

1 Not enough information is provided to assume that the patient had a myocardial infarction.

2 Angina is a cardiac problem, not a cerebral problem.

3 An incompetent valve does not normally cause this kind of chest pain.

252. Application, evaluation, physiological integrity (a).

2, 3, 4, 5 These are signs and symptoms or statements consistent with a TIA.

1 A TIA has a sudden onset.

253. Application, implementation, physiological integrity (b).

2 The auditory center is in the temporal lobe, as is the olfactory center.

1 The visual center is in the occipital lobe.

3 Agnosia is a symptom of a CVA.

4 The frontal lobe houses the motor cortex.

254. Comprehension, implementation, physiological integrity (c).

1 This aids in absorption of dye. Metrizamide dye is water soluble and does not need to be removed.

2 This is not usually necessary.

3 Common side effects of this dye include nausea, vomiting, and seizures, with the peak time of risk at 4 to 8 hours after the procedure.

4 Phenothiazines, tricyclic antidepressants, CNS stimulants, or amphetamines should not be taken from 24 to 48 hours or immediately after the procedure. These drugs lower seizure threshold.

255. Analysis, planning, health promotion and maintenance (b).

2 Putting puzzles together is a noncontact activity that would be the safest for the individual.

1, 3, 4 These activities can result in contact or would result in jarring of the abdomen, which may cause the aneurysm to rupture.

256. Application, evaluation, health promotion and maintenance (c).

1, 2, 4 These are predisposing factors to the development of varicose veins because they cause pooling of blood in the extremities, which leads to incompetent valve development.

3 This is a risk factor for deep-vein thromboses.

257. Application, planning, physiological integrity (a).

1 The patient is at high risk for decubitus ulcers. Sensory loss prevents perception of pain and pressure, the warning signs of tissue injury. If the patient is able, encourage patient involvement.

2 This is inappropriate; adequate calcium intake is essential for all individuals.

3 This is inappropriate and is not relative to the situation.

4 This is not individualized to persons with sensory or motor loss.

258. Application, planning, physiological integrity (c).

2, 4, 5 These drugs increase the flow of oxygen-rich blood to the myocardium, thereby decreasing chest pain, which is caused by ischemia.

1 These would slow blood flow to the myocardium, increasing chest pain.

3 These drugs are used to treat infections, primarily those that are caused by gram-negative rods.

259. Application, evaluation, physiological integrity (a).

1 The diet is high in carbohydrates and restricted in sodium, potassium, phosphorus, and protein.

2, 3, 4 These do not indicate a change in dietary habits.

260. Application, implementation, physiological integrity (b).

4 Blood that drained from the legs while the person is in the lithotomy position will flow back into vessels of the feet and legs as the person stands. Dizziness and fainting can occur from the sudden change in distribution.

1 Although bleeding, perforation of bladder and sepsis are complications of this procedure; the effect on vital signs would not be immediately evident.

2 This is not usually necessary.

3 This is inappropriate and is not relevant to the situation.

261. Application, planning, physiological integrity (c).

2 Hydronephrosis can occur rapidly if obstruction occurs.

1 Stents are not irrigated.

3 This may be ordered but is not directly related to this situation.

4 The stents are not near the rectum.

262. Analysis, evaluation, physiological integrity (b).

1 If the client had therapeutic effects, they would be exhibited in a decrease of parasympathetic activity.

2 These are not normally present in clients with Parkinson's

3 Vital signs are not affected by Parkinson's disease; propulsive shuffling gait is a sign of muscular rigidity and loss of postural reflexes.

4 These are not symptoms of Parkinson's disease.

263. Application, planning, physiological integrity (b).

2 The patient may have a weakened immune system and should avoid the risk of infection.

1 HIV-positive patients can develop urinary tract infections, however, no fail-safe way exists to prevent them, which is why patient education is critical.

3 The virus can, and often does, affect other body organs and the eyes are no exception, only this usually occurs in the later stages of the disease.

4 T-cell count decreases as disease progresses.

264. Comprehension, planning, physiological integrity (c).

1, 2, 3, 4, 5 These may be part of the treatment plan for persons with type 2 diabetes mellitus.

1 Patients who use insulin are classified as having type I diabetes mellitus, or IDDM.

265. Application, assessment, health promotion and maintenance (b).

2 Infection increases metabolism and increases the demand for insulin.

1 This may affect glucose levels but is not a primary cause.

3 This would cause hypoglycemia.

4 This would also cause hypoglycemia

266. Application, planning, physiological integrity (b).

3 Regular insulin is rapid acting and is given during the acute phase of DKA.

1 This is an intermediate-acting insulin and may be given after the acute phase of DKA is over.

2 This is also an intermediate acting insulin.

4 This is an extended, long-acting insulin and is too difficult to control in treating DKA.

267. Application, implementation, physiological integrity (b).

2 This would reduce gastric irritation.

1 Nothing in antiinflammatory drugs would prevent anyone from driving.

3 Normally, CNS effects are not common when taking an antiinflammatory drug.

4 This would cause a large amount of gastric irritation.

268. Application, assessment, health promotion and maintenance (b).

4 Disorder tends to progress, and involvement of other systems is common with advancement of the disorder.

1 This is characteristic of osteoarthritis.

2 The disease tends to be chronic in nature.

3 This does not describe rheumatoid arthritis.

269. Knowledge, planning, physiological integrity (b).

3 These drugs reduce the inflammatory process.

1 These are not normally used as a first-line drug in treating rheumatoid arthritis.

2 These are not used as first-line drugs in treating rheumatoid arthritis.

4 These are not the drugs of choice for treating rheumatoid arthritis.

270. Application, assessment, physiological integrity (a).

4 Malodorous discharge would signal a possible infectious process. It should be reported and investigated immediately.

1, 2, 3 These are all normal, expected findings.

271. Application, assessment, physiological integrity (a).

1 Awakening at night to void is most common. Pain on urination is a sign of cystitis that most men find disturbing.

2 Hematuria may result from blood vessels that have been overstretched. Groin pain is not present in most men.

3 These may result if urinary tract infection develops because of stasis of urine.

4 These may develop; however, they are not common signs.

272. Comprehension, implementation, physiological integrity (a).

1 These decrease tone and involuntary movements and help relieve anxiety and tension.

2 These are inappropriate; vasodilators will not decrease spasticity.

3 These are inappropriate; narcotic analgesics are not given for spasticity.

4 These are inappropriate; NSAIDs will not decrease tone.

273. Application, implementation, physiological integrity (a).

3 Taking the blood pressure in left arm may cause compression or occlude the fistula, or both. Any compression, tight clothing, or carrying objects with arm bent should be avoided.

1 This is unnecessary; patients are discharged with this in place.

2 This is inappropriate and is not proper procedure.

4 Fluids may be restricted. Some patients may have urine output. Hourly monitoring is usually not appropriate.

274. Comprehension, assessment, physiological integrity (b).

1 Inflammation of the bursa is the term for bursitis.

2 This would be osteomyelitis.

3 Once again, this would be termed osteomyelitis.

4 This is not the correct selection.

275. Application, assessment, physiological integrity (b).

2 These symptoms are indicative of pulmonary edema, a complication of myocardial infarction caused by heart failure.

1 These symptoms do not support a diagnosis of emphysema.

3 These symptoms do not support a diagnosis of pulmonary embolism.

4 COPD does not have these symptoms.

276. Application, implementation, physiological integrity (b).

2 Elevating the foot will reduce the swelling of the sprained ankle.

1 The foot will have increased swelling because of the effects of gravity.

3 Exercise will increase swelling by increasing blood flow to the area.

4 A warm bath will promote vasodilation, increasing the swelling in the area.

277. Application, planning, physiological integrity (c).

1, 4, 5 These may be ordered and should be followed by the patient who has gout. Allopurinol is a medication used to control symptoms. Patients who have gout may also be prone to diabetes, and an alkaline ash diet helps decrease uric acid tophi formation.

2, 3 Organ foods are high in purine, which contributes to uric acid formation. An acid ash diet also contributes to uric acid formation.

278. Comprehension, assessment, physiological integrity (b).

1 The signs and symptoms of fat embolism include shortness of breath and restlessness as a result of hypoxia caused by occlusion of pulmonary blood vessels.

2 Difficulty swallowing and aspiration pneumonia are not symptoms of fat embolism.

3 These are symptoms of cholecystitis.

4 These symptoms may indicate paralytic ileus.

279. Comprehension, implementation, physiological integrity (a).

3 By using the palms of the hands, the nurse is less likely to place indentations in the cast, which can compromise circulatory status when the plaster dries.

1 The patient will not be able to hold the extremity for a prolonged period.

2 The pillowcase will stick to the cast, causing excess pressure that will mold the cast.

4 Not only is this uncomfortable for the patient, it also restricts adequate support of the extremity.

280. Application, planning, physiological integrity (c).

2 Liver is high in purines, which increase uric acid levels and would exacerbate the patient's condition.

1 These foods have no purines.

3 These foods would not exacerbate the patient's arthritis.

4 Veal and garlic bread do not have a high purine content.

281. Comprehension, assessment, physiological integrity (b).

1 Osteomyelitis most often requires extensive long-term antibiotic therapy.

2 This activity can have introduced pathogenic bacteria near the bone.

3 In the acute phase, mobility should be minimized to decrease the spread of the infection.

4 Pain on movement is common in patients with osteomyelitis.

282. Analysis, evaluation, physiological integrity (c).

3 Crossing of the legs may result in displacement of the new femoral head.

1 No restriction on plantar flexion exists; this should be done to increase circulation to the legs.

2 Low chairs would cause a greater than 90-degree hip flexion; elevated toilet seat and chairs are needed.

4 Physical therapy, with limited weight bearing and ambulation, begins soon after surgery.

283. Knowledge, assessment, physiological integrity (a).

3 The presence of an elevated ESR and rheumatoid factor would indicate rheumatoid arthritis.

1 Although the WBCs are slightly elevated, the patient should not have an elevated Hct count.

2 Uric acid is elevated in patients with gout.

4 Although the rheumatoid factor is present, the LE cells are present in patients with SLE.

284. Comprehension, assessment, physiological integrity (b).

3 A patient who has developed a thrombosis will exhibit calf pain and swelling of the affected extremity.

1 This finding is common in a patient with pulmonary emboli.

2 This is an assessment finding in heart failure or hypervolemia.

4 This may indicate loss of skin integrity or a pin tract infection.

285. Application, evaluation, physiological integrity (b).

4 This is the correct rationale behind positioning.

1 The prone position will not alleviate phantom limb pain.

2 Although important, this is not the primary reason for the positioning.

3 Most patients do not feel that the prone position is the most comfortable. This is not the reason for the positioning.

286. Application, implementation, physiological integrity (c).

1 Because of the patient's surgery, hydrochloric acid secretion and intrinsic factor are lacking; the patient will not be able to absorb vitamin B12, which causes pernicious anemia.

2 A lack of folic acid does not cause pernicious anemia.

3 Although technically correct, this question does not adequately explain the rationale to the patient.

4 This is untrue; a lack of iron does not cause pernicious anemia.

287. Application, implementation, physiological integrity (c).

2 This is the correct statement by the nurse.

1, 3, 4 These statements are incorrect, and because of the technical language used in these statements, they would have to be further explained by the nurse.

288. Comprehension, implementation, physiological integrity (b).

2 This statement provides the best explanation for the patient's symptom.

1 This is not a true statement.

3 This is most likely not true, and it does not answer the patient's question.

4 This is a true statement but does not answer the patient's question. It assumes that the patient was exercising.

289. Comprehension, evaluation, physiological integrity (b).

4 A low platelet count, thrombocytopenia, would cause bleeding tendencies.

1 A low WBC count might cause inability to fight infection.

2 A high WBC count would indicate an infectious process.

3 An elevated platelet count would cause a high clot situation.

290. Analysis, implementation, physiological integrity (c).

3 Exercise increases the oxygen demands of the body, which the failing heart is not able to accommodate.

1 Bronchi dilate with exercise.

2 This may be true, exercise must be started gradually, but this statement does not answer the patient's questions.

4 The blood vessels of the heart and lungs dilate, increasing blood flow, which does not cause shortness of breath.

291. Application, assessment, physiological integrity (b).

3 Monitoring for arrhythmias, SOB (which can indicate a pulmonary embolism), and bleeding at the insertion or access site is the most important assessment at this time.

1 Leg exercise is discouraged for the first 6 to 8 hours after the procedure.

2 Early ambulation is discouraged for the first 6 to 8 hours after the procedure.

4 The extremity that is accessed should not be exercised in the immediate period following a cardiac catheterization.

292. Application, evaluation, physiological integrity (b).

1 Corned beef and canned broth have high levels of sodium; eating them each day would not be beneficial.

2 Both shredded wheat and fruit are low in sodium, and consuming them each day should not have an undesirable effect.

3 Broccoli and chicken are relatively low in salt, and having this lunch once a week should not compromise the patient.

4 Although French fries do contain a small amount of salt, consuming this meal three times a week should not adversely effect the patient.

293. Comprehension, assessment, physiological integrity (c).

4 With right-sided heart failure, blood backs up in the systemic circulation, causing swelling of the lower extremities.

1 Nausea is not normally associated with heart failure.

2 An extra heart sound may be heard (S3), but it is not the sound of a murmur.

3 These are symptoms of left-sided heart failure.

294. Application, assessment, safe, effective care environment (c).

3 Rheumatic fever and subsequent heart disease is the prominent cause of valvular insufficiency.

1 An appendectomy should not have any bearing on the patient's present diagnosis.

2 Although significant for heart disease in general, the history of rheumatic fever is more significant.

4 Although significant because of the possible introduction of bacteria into the heart, the history of rheumatic fever is more significant.

295. Analysis, evaluation, physiological integrity (b).

2 A fracture would temporarily restrict mobility in the leg, increasing venous stasis and the chance of a blood clot.

1 Atrial fibrillation may cause clots to form inside the heart.

3 Narrow-angle glaucoma should not have any effect on the development of blood clots.

4 Although small clots eventually effect blood vessels, the fracture is more likely to be significant.

296. Application, implementation, physiological integrity (c).

4 The nurse should first check to see that the patient's gag reflex has returned.

1 The patient will most likely return to his or her pretest diet, but a gag reflex must be intact first.

2 No time restrictions exist on this test; a gag reflex must be intact.

3 This would be done after checking for an intact gag reflex.

297. Application, evaluation, health promotion and maintenance (b).

2 Sunlight is one of the triggers for SLE. Going to the beach may have exposed the patient to too much sunlight.

1, 3, 4 None of these are triggers for SLE.

298. Comprehension, assessment, physiological integrity (b).

4 Patients with appendicitis frequently complain of rebound tenderness of the abdomen on palpation.

1 Hematemesis is a symptom of perforated ulcers.

2 Sharp back pain may be a symptom of aortic dissection or pancreatitis.

3 Abdominal distention is common with intestinal obstruction or ileus.

299. Application, assessment, physiological integrity (b).

2 This high-fat meal may precipitate a gallbladder attack.

1 Physical activity does not normally cause or precipitate gallbladder pain.

3 Taking acetaminophen does not normally precipitate pain in this area.

4 Although alcohol may cause gastritis, it does not normally cause pain in the gallbladder region.

300. Application, planning, safe, effective care environment (b).

4 A client with osteoporosis is at high risk for injury from falling, pathological fractures, or fractures from daily wear and tear.

1 Alteration in bowel elimination is not associated with the diagnosis of osteoporosis, although many elderly clients have problems with bowel elimination.

2, 3 Using Maslow's hierarchy of needs, these diagnoses may be pertinent to patients with osteoporosis; however, safety is the more important consideration here.

301. Comprehension, implementation, psychosocial integrity (a).

2 Hepatitis A is transmitted by ingestion of contaminated food or liquids.

1 Hepatitis A is not transmitted by direct contact.

3 Hepatitis A is not transmitted by blood or blood products.

4 Hepatitis A is not transmitted in this manner.

302. Application, planning, physiological integrity (b).

3 Pancreatic enzymes are taken with meals.

1 The enzymes will not be able to aid digestion if taken between meals.

2 The enzymes need to be taken when eating any carbohydrates, proteins, or fats.

4 This would not allow proper digestion to take place.

303. Comprehension, assessment, physiological integrity (c).

3 Any increased abdominal pressure will place stress on the surgical incision.

1 This may be true but would not be the primary reason for notifying the surgeon.

2 The patient should not have an increased chance for peritonitis because of a respiratory problem.

4 Again, this may be true, but it is not the primary reason for notifying the surgeon.

304. Analysis, evaluation, physiological integrity (b).

3 Assess the patency of the tube by checking with an air bolus.

1 This may be contraindicated and is premature; assess patency first.

2 Assess patency of tube before notifying the physician.

4 This requires a physician order; ascertain whether the tube is patent first.

305. Comprehension, implementation, physiological integrity (b).

2, 3, 4 These are first-aid measures aimed at reducing the swelling of the extremity.

1 This will cause vasodilation and will promote swelling in the limb.

5 This will cause great pain and will not reduce swelling in the limb.

306. Application, evaluation, physiological integrity (b).

1 The need for lifelong thyroid replacement therapy would be necessary, with medical follow-up.

2 This is true and may indicate an overdose of thyroid replacement drugs.

3 This establishes an adequate level of the drug in the bloodstream.

4 This may indicate hyperthyroidism, which can be caused by the thyroid replacement therapy.

307. Application, planning, physiological integrity (b).

3 The definition of a closed reduction is manually pulling on bones to realign the extremity. In some instances, this is done in the emergency room, with some pain medication given before the procedure.

1 This would be an open reduction, internal fixation.

2 This procedure does not involve general anesthesia.

4 This would require a surgical procedure.

308. Application, implementation, physiological integrity (b).

2 Patients who had adrenalectomies must stay stress free because they no longer have the ability to respond readily to these situations.

1 Adrenalectomies do not normally necessitate an accurate intake and output record.

3 This is indicated in a person who has Conn's syndrome.

4 This is advised for patients who have diabetes insipidus.

309. Comprehension, assessment, physiological integrity (b).

4 Individuals with diabetes insipidus have an increased intake of fluids coupled with dilute urine.

1 A bounding pulse and low urine output are signs of a hypervolemic state.

2 Individuals who are hypovolemic have low blood pressure; tachycardia is a significant finding for dehydration.

3 Individuals with diabetes insipidus have an increased urine output and a low urine sp gr.

310. Comprehension, evaluation, physiological integrity (b).

3 The abrupt withdrawal of steroids can cause an addisonian crisis, an inability to respond to stressful situations.

1 The withdrawal of insulin in a patient with diabetes mellitus can cause hyperglycemia.

2 Cardizem is an antiarrhythmic and antianginal and will not cause an addisonian crisis when withdrawn.

4 Diltiazem is a cardiotonic; abrupt withdrawal may precipitate heart failure.

311. Comprehension, planning, physiological integrity (b).

1 Wearing a medic alert tag will ensure that others who are outside the hospital setting will respond appropriately.

2 Although this is advisable, without the medic alert tag, no one would know what to do with the glucose.

3 This practice is not advisable and will not assist personnel without a medic alert tag.

4 Although this is a good idea, it will not ensure proper care in all locations.

312. Comprehension, assessment, psychosocial integrity (a).

2 Patients with hyperpituitarism have structural alterations to their body, which can cause problems with self-esteem and body image.

1 The problems that stem from excess pituitary hormone do not normally cause an alteration in comfort.

3 Alteration in fluid and electrolytes is more common with Addison's disease.

4 This diagnosis more common in hyperthyroidism.

313. Comprehension, assessment, physiological integrity (b).

2 Ketones cause metabolic acidosis in DKA.

1 Both conditions are treated with insulin administration.

3 HHNC is found primarily in patients who are non–insulin dependent.

4 Serum ketones and glucose are elevated in DKA.

314. Application, assessment, physiological integrity (b).

3 Swelling in the neck region is of priority because it can compromise the respiratory status.

1 This is to be expected in the immediate postoperative period.

2 Although a concern, respiratory compromise is of top priority.

4 A small amount of bleeding is to be expected and should not be of great concern; further monitoring is indicated.

315. Comprehension, implementation, physiological integrity (b).

3 The child should be given orange juice with sugar, which will increase his blood sugar level quickly.

1 This will not increase the child's blood glucose because it contains no sugar.

2 It will take too long for the child to go to the hospital, and this is a treatable condition at home. Patient teaching in the prevention of hypoglycemic episodes should follow this occurrence.

4 Cheese and crackers should be given after the orange juice; however, it will not elevate the glucose level quickly enough in this instance.

316. Comprehension, planning, physiological integrity (b).

2 Patients who have had a conization normally have vaginal packing that needs to be maintained. The nurse should also anticipate monitoring for bleeding.

1 The patient should not used tampons until instructed to do so by her physician.

3 This may disrupt the site and can encourage bleeding.

4 Patients should not douche until instructed to do so by their physician.

317. Comprehension, assessment, health promotion and maintenance (b).

3 Mammograms are recommended yearly for individuals over the age of 40.

1 Gynecological examinations should be done on a yearly basis.

2 Hepatitis B vaccine is indicated for this individual because she works in a high-risk occupation.

4 Tuberculosis tests should be done on a yearly basis.

318. Comprehension, implementation, health promotion and maintenance (b).

4 Breasts should be palpated in a variety of positions to ensure that all areas are assessed.

1 Breast self-examinations (BSEs) should be conducted 7 days after onset of menstruation.

2 This can be done, but breasts also need to be palpated while lying and standing.

3 The pads of the fingers should be used to feel for lumps.

319. Comprehension, planning, physiological integrity (b).

2 Drinking warm beverages will help relax the uterine muscles and decrease the pain involved with uterine spasm.

1 This will cause additional cramping and pain.

3 It is recommended that women do not exert themselves during their period.

4 Antiinflammatory medication is more effective, with less side effects, compared with narcotic analgesics.

320. Comprehension, assessment, physiological integrity (b).

3 Patients with rectovaginal fistulas will have leakage of fecal matter and flatus from the vagina. This condition causes extreme anxiety in the patient.

1 This occurs in a ureterovaginal, vesicovaginal, or urethrovaginal fistula.

2 This is common with hemorrhoids.

4 These are common findings in a patient that has *Candida albicans* infection.

321. Comprehension, assessment, health promotion and maintenance (b).

2 Women rarely have any early symptoms of gonorrhea. The patient should be tested because her partner is infected.

1 This is not true; gonorrhea does not always cause symptoms in women.

3 The patient should be tested immediately.

4 The patient should be tested before giving antibiotics; she may not be infected.

322. Comprehension, implementation, physiological integrity (b).

2 Voiding will increase the patient's comfort during the procedure and will keep the patient from voiding during the examination.

1 This will impede the examination.

3 Patients cannot be menstruating during the time of the examination; visualization and culture is difficult.

4 The patient may need support during the examination and may feel abandoned.

323. Comprehension, implementation, physiological integrity (c).

1 Because of the nature of the surgery and the proximity to the urethra, an indwelling catheter is placed during the surgery and will remain for a few days.

2 Because of the complications of immobility, patients are ambulated early after surgery, even the surgeries involving internal organs.

3 The patient will most likely resume a normal diet after the bowel sounds have returned.

4 Unless the patient has a preexisting condition, physical therapy would not necessarily be a part of her postsurgical care.

324. Application, assessment, physiological integrity (b).

4 The general recommendation is that family and visitors spend as little time in the direct proximity to the patient as possible. The amount of time visitors can stay is also limited.

1 This is a true statement; it prevents straining of stool, which can dislodge the implant.

2 These are the preferred positions because the risk of the implant dislodging is less.

3 Nausea and vomiting generally accompany radiation therapy.

325. Comprehension, implementation, physiological integrity (b).

1 Pizza is high in sodium and would aggravate the symptoms of PMS.

2 Mineral water should not aggravate the condition. Beverages with caffeine would worsen the symptoms.

3 Pasta and sauce should not aggravate the condition, unless the sauce contains excessive amounts of salt.

4 Raw fruits and vegetables are a healthy snack and should not aggravate PMS.

326. Comprehension, assessment, physiological integrity (b).

1 Patients with psoriasis experience reddened patches with silvery scales that sometimes slough off; they are very self-conscious concerning this problem.

2 Large pus-filled macules are not normally found in patients with psoriasis.

3 This may be a sign of impetigo or another infectious disease.

4 These are not normally present in psoriasis.

327. Application, assessment, physiological integrity (b).

2 Immunoglobulin E is the antibody most often associated. Many persons with asthma have an allergic component to their disease.

1 INR is a calculated measure as part of a coagulation profile (blood clotting).

3 HCV test is performed to detect the hepatitis C virus and to determine the antibody level.

4 CEA is a measure that may be increased with various cancers such as cancer of the colon, liver, and pancreas. CEA levels may also be increased in persons who are chronic cigarette smokers and in persons who have inflammatory bowel disorders.

328. Comprehension, planning, physiological integrity (b).

2 Persons are usually no longer infectious after 2 to 3 weeks of therapy.

1, 3 These are incorrect timeframes. Cell-mediated immunity to the mycobacteria, which develops 3 to 6 weeks later, usually contains the infection and arrests the disease.

4 If this were true, all persons with tuberculosis disease would need to remain isolated.

329. Application, planning, physiological integrity (b).

3 This is proper technique. Corticosteroid inhalers should be used last because they require gargling after use to prevent oral candidiasis.

1 This may help; it depends on the side effects he is experiencing. Sitting may calm the patient, reduce a sense of panic, and may maximize chest expansion.

2 He should be using as prescribed. A few to 5 minutes are generally recommended between medications.

4 If he is concerned, he needs to call the clinic and make an appointment. He should not stop taking these medications on his own.

330. Application, implementation, physiological integrity (b).
   3 Usually, the patient with tuberculosis will need to be on these medications for as long as needed, generally 6 to 18 months or longer.
   1, 2, 4 These are correct statements made by the patient that signify understanding of the infectious process and the disorder.

331. Comprehension, implementation, safe, effective care environment (a).
   1 The reason for coming as perceived by the patient is defined as the chief complaint. The physician first looks to this part of the admission sheet on which to base the priorities of treatment and care.
   2 This section refers to environmental, spiritual, cultural aspects, and family dynamics.
   3 The past medical history may be important. The reason for seeking treatment today warrants attention. Frequently, the information in this section is not always accurate, depending on how reliable the memory is of the person supplying the information.
   4 The review of systems is a thorough body-system approach of assessment and data gathering. The physician or nurse practitioner fills out this section.

332. Comprehension, implementation, physiological integrity (a).
   2 This bacillus is transmitted in the droplet nuclei formed when the person with active tuberculosis coughs, sings, talks, laughs, or sneezes.
   1, 3, 4 Inspiring the droplet in these situations is highly unlikely. Prolonged contact is necessary.

333. Comprehension, implementation, physiological integrity (b).
   2 These actions will ensure that the patient has a patent airway.
   1, 3, 4 These are more appropriate if the nursing diagnosis stated a respiratory problem.

334. Application, assessment, physiological integrity (b).
   1, 3, 4, 5 These symptoms are caused by the stricture of the mitral valve.
   2 Heart failure may be a complication of this malady; however, it is not a symptom of it.

335. Comprehension, implementation, safe, effective care environment (b).
   3 Vital signs are objective data.
   1 Data stated by the patient is subjective, such as the purpose for the clinic visit.
   2, 4 These are incorrect and nonexistent.

336. Application, evaluation, physiological integrity (b).
   2 Bacterial endocarditis is generally associated with an upper respiratory infection caused by the Streptococcus bacteria.
   1, 3, 4 These are not generally associated with bacterial endocarditis, although a heart catheterization may predispose the patient to other infections.

337. Application, evaluation, health promotion and maintenance (c).
   4 Painless loss of peripheral vision is associated with this type of glaucoma
   1 This is associated with retinal detachments.
   2 Double vision indicates difficulty with both eyes focusing together on an object.
   3 Nausea, vomiting, headache, and eye pain or redness are associated with acute closed-angle glaucoma.

338. Application, implementation, physiological integrity (a).
   1 This is unsafe and can cause damage to the eardrum. This would also cause discomfort. It is best if the otoscope is held in a superior position.
   2, 3, 4 These are safe and appropriate techniques for an otoscopic examination.

339. Application, planning, physiological integrity (b).
   4 Because the patient cannot absorb vitamin B12, they must be injected with it.
   1 Vitamin B12 cannot be given by mouth; it is broken down by gastric juice.
   2, 3 These may be orders, but they are not associated with pernicious anemia.

340. Application, assessment, physiological integrity (c).
   1 Fever, chills, nausea, vomiting, flank pain, bloody urine, are signs of an upper urinary tract infection.
   2, 3, 4 These complaints are prevalent in lower urinary tract infection.

341. Application, assessment, physiological integrity (c).
   1 Nephrotic syndrome is a group of symptoms associated with increased glomerular permeability. The primary symptoms are proteinuria, hypoalbuminuria, and edema. Loss of protein leads to the third tissue spacing of fluids as well as vitamin-D deficiency. Remember, albumin is protein.
   2, 3, 4 These are not identified as major factors in the pathophysiology of this syndrome.

342. Comprehension, planning, physiological integrity (b).
   4 The course of therapy is usually longer for upper urinary tract infection; expect a 10- to 14-day course.
   1, 2, 3 These are possible courses of antimicrobial therapy, especially with lower urinary tract infections.

343. Application, assessment, health promotion and maintenance (b).
   1 In men with Chlamydia, urethritis, conjunctivitis, arthritis, and mucocutaneous lesions (Reiter's syndrome) are the common symptoms.
   2 This is present in syphilis.
   3 This is usually not present in STDs.
   4 This is a manifestation of genital warts.

344. Application, assessment, physiological integrity (b).
   2 A patient with HIV is prone to the development of this pneumonia, which is an opportunistic infection.
   1 Although this may be true, because of the opportunistic causative organism, HIV would be the causative factor.
   3, 4 Leukemia thalassemia do not predispose the patient to this type of pneumonia, although they may be more prone to other infections.

345. Application, assessment, physiological integrity (b).
   1, 2, 3 These are included. The patient should be npo before the examination; the patient will also need laxatives before the examination for the bowel to be cleansed; after the examination, laxatives are given to remove any residual barium that would be left behind.
   4 Eating or not eating meats does not affect examination results. Preparation begins, at most, the day or evening prior to the examination, not 4 days in advance.

346. Application, planning, physiological integrity (b).
  1 The lidocaine will numb the mouth, making it easier for the patient to chew and swallow.
  2, 3, 4 Topical lidocaine will not act as an antibiotic or a barrier, nor will it aid in absorption of the food because that takes place in the small intestine.

347. Comprehension, assessment, health promotion and maintenance (b).
  3 Patients with cirrhosis generally have portal hypertension, which predisposes the patient to esophageal varices.
  1, 2, 4 These do not predispose the client to esophageal varices.

348. Comprehension, implementation, safe, effective care environment (a).
  4 Purulent drainage indicates that an infection of the wound may be present. This needs to be communicated to the physician if this is a new development.
  1, 2, 3 These are expected types of drainage based on the age of the incision. In general, drainage is expected to change from sanguineous (red to serosanguineous [pink]) to serous (straw colored) to clear during a period of hours to days.

349. Application, implementation, physiological integrity (b).
  2 The thickening agent will add texture to the food, making it easier to swallow.
  1 Patients have more difficulty swallowing liquids because they are not able to feel the liquid, and it easily travels into the trachea.
  3 The patient must be started on thickened liquids to ascertain if he can tolerate these foods.
  4 The nurse has no way of knowing this unless she tries.

350. Comprehension, assessment, physiological integrity (c).
  1 The manifestations of this increased stimulation state are hypertension, blurred vision, headache, sweating, flushed skin, and bradycardia.
  2, 3, 4 These are mainly opposite of the increased stimulation manifestations.

351. Application, implementation, physiological integrity (a).
  2 Level of consciousness is defined by both the content of consciousness and the arousal level. Confusion is defined as having the described behaviors, as well as agitation and irritability. Disorientation to time occurs first, followed by place and person.
  1 "Difficult" is a value judgment.
  3 Lethargy is reflective of a patient who is unable to be aroused spontaneously but requires some external stimuli such as touch, voice, and so forth. Confusion may also be present.
  4 Stupor indicates a patient in a deep sleep or unresponsive. Arousal occurs only with vigorous and continuous stimulation.

352. Comprehension, assessment, physiological integrity (b).
  2 Although any stimulation can cause this phenomenon to occur, the most common are a full bladder, full bowel, wrinkled sheets, and so forth.
  1, 3, 4 Skin stimulation may be a stimulus and needs to be done gently, such as when taking vital signs.

Visitors may unknowingly cause a draft, which may stimulate this reaction.

353. Comprehension, planning, physiological integrity (b).
  3 Hypovolemic shock may occur as a result of intravascular volume depletion as fluid moves into the intracellular spaces. Observing and planning for shock is critical. This is a priority. The greatest initial threat to a patient with a major burn is hypovolemic shock.
  1 Monitoring urine output would better indicate kidney status.
  2 Skin care and comfort are important.
  4 A too-rapid IV would increase intravascular volume.

354. Application, planning, physiological integrity (b).
  4 If the patient eats a large meal before the class, she is more likely to have symptoms because of the increased abdominal pressure she experiences while exercising.
  1 This will increase the problem for the patient.
  2 This would be rather difficult to do in an aerobics class! It is unrealistic.
  3 This is likely to contribute to increased heartburn symptoms.

355. Application, implementation, physiological integrity (a).
  3 Most policies recommend assessing the site within 48 to 72 hours (2 to 3 days).
  1, 2, 4 These are not the recommended times. Inaccurate assessments may result.

356. Comprehension, assessment, physiological integrity (b).
  2 Patients who have had all or part of their stomach removed will have decreased amounts of intrinsic factor, which is needed to absorb vitamin B12. Lack of vitamin B12 causes pernicious anemia.
  1, 3, 4 These types of anemias are not caused by hemigastrectomy.

357. Application, implementation, physiological integrity (c).
  4 This value may indicate nephrotoxicity. Many antibiotics, such as vancomycin, are nephrotoxic. Normal finding is 0.5 to 1.5 mg/dl. Increased creatinine indicates impaired kidney function.
  1, 2, 3 These are within normal laboratory findings.

358. Application, assessment, physiological integrity (b).
  1 Hepatitis, with the risk increasing with the age of the patient, needs to be assessed for. Hepatic enzymes are measured before and during therapy.
  2, 3, 4 These symptoms have not been noted with active tuberculosis or vancomycin therapy.

359. Application, planning, physiological integrity (b).
  4 A short-term goal for pain should have a very short time frame, given the severity of the pain. The only one of these distractors that is associated with pain and is of short duration is #4.
  1 This is a goal associated with impaired mobility.
  2 This is a long-term pain goal.
  3 This is not a realistic goal for any nursing diagnosis because most patients will have increased pain during and after physical therapy.

360. Application, planning, physiological integrity (b).
  3 Postural drainage of the lower and middle lobes requires lying in a head-down position that patients in respiratory distress or those who are dyspneic may not be able to tolerate.

1 This should be done immediately preceding the Chest physical therapy (CPT).

2 The procedures of CPT should be performed at least 1 hour before and 3 hours after meals.

4 Waiting a full hour after CPT to take vital signs is unnecessary.

361. Application, assessment, physiological integrity (a).

4 Cataracts lead to progressive blurring of vision.

1 Floaters are characteristics of a retinal detachment.

2, 3 Eye pain or eye dryness is not characteristic of cataracts.

362. Application, implementation, physiological integrity (b).

3 The IV and po intake equals 875 ml.

1, 2, 4 The intake equals the IV and po amounts. A separate area is used to record the amount of bladder irrigating fluid.

363. Application, evaluation, physiological integrity (b).

1 Patients who are incontinent generally get urinary tract infections because of the close proximity of feces to the urinary meatus.

2 No indication exists that the patient is immunosuppressed.

3 This may be true but does not adequately explain the rationale.

4 No indication exists that this is the case; the nurse is second-guessing physician orders.

364. Application, planning, physiological integrity (a).

2 This is the only correct choice. Using scented feminine hygiene products may contribute to urinary tract infections.

1 Avoiding sex is unnecessary. Voiding before and after sex is recommended.

3 Tub baths actually contribute to urinary tract infections.

4 Orange juice has too much sugar to recommend this amount per day, and it will not decrease the incidence of urinary tract infections.

5 The perineum should be wiped from front to back.

365. Application, assessment, physiological integrity (b).

1 Calcium channel blockers may affect the ability of the bladder or sphincter to contract or relax normally.

2 Anticoagulants may cause hematuria.

3 NSAIDs usually do not affect bladder control.

4 Antiemetics have not been shown to affect bladder or sphincter control.

366. Application, implementation, physiological integrity (b).

1 It has been found that resisting the urge to void for longer than 1 hour can result in a urinary tract infection. The distended bladder shortens the urethra.

2 Voiding after sexual intercourse is recommended.

3, 4 These actions are not recommended.

367. Comprehension, evaluation, psychosocial integrity (c).

2 This statement is both knowledgeable and truthful.

1 This statement signifies that no further teaching is needed.

3 *Streptococci* has not been implicated in peptic ulcer disease; *H pylori* has been.

4 This may be very helpful to the individual, but further teaching is required.

368. Application, implementation, physiological integrity (a).

1 Fluid intake is especially important, at least eight 8-ounce glasses a day. Encouraging fluid decreases the potential of the adverse effect of crystal formation.

2, 4 These are indirect effects.

3 This is important and best achieved by giving the drug as scheduled.

369. Application, assessment, physiological integrity (b).

1 These are the classic signs of appendicitis.

2, 3, 4 These signs and symptoms are not indicative of these disorders.

370. Comprehension, assessment, physiological integrity (b).

3 The body attempts to compensate by increasing respirations and blowing off carbon dioxide.

1, 2, 4 Decreasing respirations may cause retention of CO_2. The kidneys act later than does the respiratory system.

371. Comprehension, assessment, physiological integrity (b).

4 The higher the number rating on this scale is, which ranges from 0 to 15, the better will be the prognosis and the likelihood of optimal cerebral functioning.

1, 2, 3 These states would be most likely have rating lower than 13.

372. Comprehension, planning, physiological integrity (b).

4 A disruption of the transmembrane potential at the cellular level causes a sodium potassium–pump impairment, resulting in intracellular swelling.

1 If the immunoglobulins were decreased, this would affect the immune status and not third-tissue spacing.

2 The cardiac output would be decreased.

3 The hypermetabolic state increases the oxygen consumption.

373. Analysis, assessment, physiological integrity (c).

3 If the hernia strangulates, a portion of the bowel may become ischemic, necessitating surgical intervention.

1 The strangulation is not an actual bowel obstruction.

2 Peritonitis would be a result of a perforated bowel.

4 The inguinal hernia does not have any effect on the stomach lining.

374. Comprehension, assessment, physiological integrity (c).

4 Risk for aspiration is the most pressing concern for this patient, given the nasogastric tube feedings.

1, 2 These may be of concern if the patient had a problem with a patent airway or if pneumonia or CHF were present.

3 The tube feedings may cause diarrhea, but it is not the most pressing concern at this time.

375. Application, planning, physiological integrity (b).

1 By allowing the wandering patient to eat high-calorie, nutritious foods as she paces, the nurse will be meeting both needs of the patient.

2 Although this may be indicated at some time, for now, the po route is the preferred method.

3 This is a counterproductive measure and may not cause her to have a higher intake.

4 This diet may not be adequate for the patient, and she is able to chew food.

376. Application, evaluation, physiological integrity (c).
3 This accurately describes the therapeutic actions for using this thiazide diuretic.
1 This agent is thought to stabilize cell membrane and improve autoregulation and blood flow, which is why this agent is ordered.
2 Phenytoin (Dilantin) is believed to prevent the formation of cerebral edema and control ICP.
4 Mannitol (Osmitrol) withdraws fluid from normal tissue but may increase edema if the blood barrier is damaged.

377. Comprehension, assessment, physiological integrity (a).
4 This type of deep partial-thickness burn may involve all layers of the dermis.
1 This best describes a superficial partial-thickness (first-degree) burn.
2 Intact blister formation is indicative of superficial partial-thickness burn.
3 This indicates a full-thickness burn.

378. Application, implementation, physiological integrity (b).
1 The reason stated is correct. In addition, remind him to shake the inhalers before using and to hold his breath for 10 seconds after inhaling the medications.
2, 3, 4 These statements give incorrect rationale and information. Ventolin is a beta-adrenergic agonist that stimulates beta-adrenergic receptors, producing bronchodilation. Atrovent is an anticholinergic that acts by blocking acetylcholine, resulting in bronchodilation.

379. Application, implementation, physiological integrity (a).
4 This finding is present in both of these forms of COPD.
1 This is a finding with emphysema.
2, 3 These usually are present with chronic bronchitis.

380. Comprehension, implementation, physiological integrity (a).
2 This describes the person who is at greatest risk.
1, 3, 4 The spread is by the airborne route. It is highly unlikely that the bacillus lives long outside the host or that a casual contact is a high-risk situation.

381. Application, implementation, physiological integrity (b).
4 Packing in the posterior pharynx may obstruct the patient's airway. Use a flashlight when assessing the back of the throat.
1, 2, 3 These might be pertinent if the client aspirates or obstructs his airway.

382. Comprehension, implementation, physiological integrity (b).
1 Individuals metabolize xanthines at different rates. Dosage is determined by monitoring response, tolerance, pulmonary function, and serum theophylline levels. Serum theophylline concentrations should range from 10 to 20 μg/ml; toxicity has been reported with levels above 20 μg/ml.
2, 3, 4 These levels may be considered toxic. The patient needs to be assessed for theophylline toxicity.

383. Application, planning, physiological integrity (c).
3 A patient with COPD requires additional calories because of the increased work of breathing.
1 The meals should be small and offered six times a day; nonetheless, the patient needs calories to meet body requirements.
2 Fluids should be taken between meals to prevent excess stomach distention; however, plain water would be better than juice because of the GERD.
4 A diet that is high in carbohydrates should be avoided in patients retaining CO_2.

384. Comprehension, planning, physiological integrity (b).
1 Vasopressin is synthetic ADH, which is deficient in individuals who have diabetes insipidus.
2 Insulin is used in treating diabetes mellitus.
3 Calcium is used in treating osteoporosis.
4 Glucose is used to treat hypoglycemia.

385. Analysis, assessment, physiological integrity (c).
4 CO_2 is trapped in the alveoli, the basic problem in emphysema. Respiratory acidosis occurs when the lungs cannot exhale CO_2 adequately. As a result, the partial pressure of carbon dioxide in the arterial blood ($PaCO_2$) and carbonic acid increase, and pH decreases.
2 Hyperventilation causes the rapid blowing off of CO_2.
1, 3 These are potential effects of emphysema, not the basic cause of acidosis.

386. Comprehension, implementation, safe, effective care environment (b).
3 Hand washing for at least 20 seconds is still considered to be the best means of preventing disease transmission.
1, 2 These should be used only when medically indicated.
4 Hand washing is part of standard precautions. Potential for exposure to blood and body fluids determine the need for protective equipment.

387. Application, assessment, physiological integrity (b).
4 High blood pressure, caused by excessive catecholamine secretion, will result from this disorder.
1, 2, 3 These are not symptoms of this tumor formation.

388. Application, planning, physiological integrity (b).
1 Persons with cataracts need to be encouraged to avoid sunlight and wear sunglasses to decrease glare and the scattering of light.
2 Surgical procedures are also available if the patient chooses. The "cataract" glasses are not commonly used today.
3 Eye pain is not associated with cataracts.
4 Persons with cataracts usually have poor night vision. Driving at night is not encouraged.

389. Comprehension, planning, physiological integrity (a).
2 Beverages that irritate the bladder are citrus, alcohol, coffee, tea, colas, and carbonated drinks.
1, 3, 4 These have not been identified as irritating to the bladder.

390. Comprehension, planning, physiological integrity (b).
2 Serial measurements of peak flow rate provide objective data of the therapeutics of drug response.
1, 4 This may be an indirect result.
3 Blood test monitoring should be done while the person is on bronchodilator therapy.

391. Application, assessment, physiological integrity (b).
1 These are indicative of decreased tissue oxygenation.
2, 3, 4 These are all normal assessment data.

392. Application, planning, physiological integrity (b).

3 Ileal conduits may allow leakage of urine onto the skin, altering skin integrity.

1, 2 These may be a result of the ileal conduit; however, alteration in the integrity of the skin is the primary concern.

4 No alteration in mobility should occur from the conduit.

393. Application, planning, physiological integrity (b).

1 Ambulation helps promote passing of the stone, as does encouraging fluids.

2, 3 These measures are contraindicated in the patient with urinary tract stones.

4 Protein restriction is unnecessary.

394. Knowledge, assessment, physiological integrity (a).

3 Upper urinary tract infections affect the ureters and kidneys.

1, 2, 4 These are all lower urinary tract infections.

395. Application, planning, physiological integrity (b).

3 Voiding this often, in addition to having adequate fluid intake, has been shown to reduce the possibility of urinary stasis and reinfection.

1 This is true for patients who need bladder training, such as those with incontinence.

2 Reflex incontinence is seen in neurogenic disorders; it is the loss of urine caused by detrusor hyperreflexia or involuntary urethral relaxation, or both, in the absence of the desire to void.

4 This is dribbling of urine by reason of the inability of the bladder to empty itself. The cause for this problem should be determined. This problem may lead to urinary tract infections.

396. Application, implementation, physiological integrity (c).

1 The orange juice is a simple source of carbohydrate, which would increase his glucose level quickly. Remember that the normal glucose level needs to be between 75 and 110 mg/dl.

2 This is unsafe. This action would increase his potential for insulin shock.

3 The immediate notification of the physician is unnecessary; however, the physician should be made aware of action taken and the patient's response.

4 This action may be appropriate, but it is not the first action.

397. Application, implementation, physiological integrity (b).

3 This is the most life threatening.

1 This is a normal urine output.

2 Hypothermia may result because of fluid evaporation from open wounds.

4 Patient comfort is important. Pain medication may be necessary before dressing changes.

398. Analysis, planning, physiological integrity (b).

1 The only time vaginal douching is a sterile procedure is after perineal surgery.

2, 3, 4 These situations do not require sterile procedure.

399. Application, assessment, physiological integrity (b).

4 Hypocalcemia may occur in patients with chronic renal failure because the kidneys become unable to excrete phosphorus. Serum phosphorus levels increase, and the calcium level decreases.

1 No direct relationship exists between vitamin-C intake and calcium.

2 Potassium is the electrolyte most directly affected by diuretic medications.

3 Hyperparathyroidism results in hypercalcemia and bone demineralization.

400. Application, implementation, physiological integrity (b).

4 Intracranial pressure (ICP) is the pressure produced by the brain tissue, cerebral spinal fluid, and blood volume within the skull. Allowing the patient to rest between nursing activities helps to keep the ICP within 5 and 15 mm Hg. Too many activities may increase metabolic demands that would alter the balance of the three components, which determine ICP and the brain's inherent compensatory capability.

1, 2 Coughing, suctioning, laying flat, bearing down, or the Valsalva maneuver may cause ICP to rise.

3 Neck and hip flexion should be avoided. Maintaining the patient's neck, hips, and knees in alignment promotes venous flow. A high-Fowler's position causes flexion. A semi-Fowler's position improves cerebral perfusion and allows for gravity to drain fluid from the brain.

401. Analysis, evaluation, physiological integrity (c).

4 This is the only answer that includes a possible link to skin cancer. The bald patient has more potential for a sunburned scalp, which increases the risk for this cancer.

1, 2, 3 None of these distractors have been shown to increase the risk of skin cancer.

402. Analysis, planning, physiological integrity (c).

1 Dressing changes that are very painful should be done only after the patient has been medicated with an analgesic, which would increase the comfort of the individual.

2 This will decrease the patient's anxiety but will not contribute to comfort.

3 This may increase the patient's comfort but not to the extent of the analgesic.

4 Although this may distract the client, the analgesic is a better choice for comfort.

403. Analysis, planning, physiological integrity (b).

3 Because the hematuria may be a sign of bladder cancer, the patient should be directed to visit his physician as soon as possible.

1 This is good advice if the patient were having symptoms of a urinary tract infection.

2 This would not affect the color of the patient's urine.

4 This would be good advice if it is not given as an urgent nature. This matter is urgent, but the patient might be frightened with this advice.

404. Analysis, assessment, safe, effective care environment (c).

3 This is the only answer that is truthful and relates the correct information to the assistant.

1 This is not the reason a patient gets uremic frost.

2 The frost should be removed from the patient's skin to control odor.

4 This is something of which the physician can be made aware at his or her next visit; it is not an urgent development.

405. Comprehension, assessment, psychosocial integrity (b).

4 Sexual contact information is extremely personal, and many patients will not be willing to disclose this information.

1 This is generally not the case.

2 Knowing who the contacts are is required so that proper screening and treatment can begin.

3 This is not true; patients who do not have symptoms can still transmit the disease.

406. Analysis, planning, physiological integrity (c).

2 The correct procedure in this situation is to hold the dose and notify the registered nurse; standard practice generally dictates that the dose not be given if the patient has a heart rate of 60 bpm or less.

1 It is not necessary (and may be inappropriate) for the LPN to call the physician, and standards of practice are already in place for this situation.

3 This is not correct; digoxin slows the heart rate.

4 Although this is something the nurse may wish to do, it does not apply to giving the digoxin dose.

407. Comprehension, implementation, physiological integrity (b).

Dose ÷ On Hand × Quantity. 650 ÷ 325 = 2 tablets.

408. Comprehension, evaluation, physiological integrity (a).

1 The action of a thrombolytic agent is to dissolve fresh thrombi that have formed.

2 This is an action of heparin or Coumadin.

3 This drug does not thin the blood; platelet inhibitors keep platelets from adhering to the walls of the blood vessels.

4 This action of a thrombolytic is to dissolve fresh thrombi. Plavix inhibits platelets.

409. Analysis, evaluation, physiological integrity (b).

3 Using straws causes individuals to swallow more air than just drinking from a cup. The extra air may bloat the stomach and cause gas formation that would put pressure on the suture line.

1 This is not a concern with straw use in an adult.

2 This is not a true statement.

4 Constipation contributes to the formation of diverticula.

410. Comprehension, planning, physiological integrity (c).

4 A barium swallow will outline the entire esophagus and pick up any inflammatory conditions.

1 An EGD will detect problems in the lower stomach and duodenum.

2 An ERCP detects abnormalities in the stomach, duodenum, and bowel ducts.

3 A barium enema is useful in detecting lower bowel problems.

411. Comprehension, planning, physiological integrity (c).

1 This is the correct action of this medication.

2 Although this drug does lower the blood pressure, this will not alleviate angina.

3 Although this medication may do this action, it is only a side effect of the medication.

4 This is the action of antiarrhythmics.

412. Comprehension, evaluation, physiological integrity (c).

3 This medication would contribute to tarry stool color.

1 Vitamin K does not contribute to the formation of tarry stools.

2 Bleeding from hemorrhoids is generally bright red in color, not tarry.

4 This may be the nurse's next advice; however, the nurse wants to determine if a reason exists for the stool color before making the patient an appointment.

413. Comprehension, evaluation, physiological integrity (b).

4 Cataracts cause most sight loss in this age group.

1, 2, 3 Although all these conditions can cause sight loss, they are not the primary reason.

414. Analysis, evaluation, physiological integrity (c).

2 Anemia is a common problem in patients who take antineoplastics. Suppression of the Red blood cell-forming bone marrow is the primary reason.

1, 3, 4 Suppression of bone marrow does not create an increase in WBCs or platelets, nor does it contribute to the process of metastasis.

415. Analysis, evaluation, physiological integrity (b).

4 Patients on vasodilators often experience a drop in blood pressure when quickly rising from a seated position.

1 The dizziness experienced by the patient is secondary to the decrease in blood pressure.

2, 3 There is no indication that the patient is anemic or has a slow pulse rate.

416. Application, implementation, physiological integrity (c).

Dosage ÷ On Hand × Quantity. 2 mg ÷ 5 mg × 1 = 0.4 ml

417. Analysis, planning, physiological integrity (c).

4 Lasix creates diuresis through the loop of Henle in the kidney. As water is lost, so are the electrolytes potassium and sodium.

1, 2, 3 These drugs are not diuretics and do not contribute to hypokalemia.

418. Analysis, assessment, physiological integrity (c).

2 Hypercalcemia results from calcium moving out of bones and into the bloodstream. The more immobile the individual is, the better the chance is for developing hypercalcemia.

1 Hypokalemia is not associated with immobility, but it is with diuretic use.

3 Hypocalcemia is not associated with immobility.

4 Hyperkalemia is associated with renal disorders.

419. Analysis, assessment, physiological integrity (b).

1 Cardiogenic shock may develop in patients who have had an myocardial infarction who have a large portion of their left ventricle affected by the infarction.

2 Anaphylaxis stems from an antibody-antigen reaction.

3 Hypertension may contribute to having an myocardial infarction but is not usually caused by one.

4 Vascular injury is not associated with having had an myocardial infarction.

420. Application, implementation, physiological integrity (c).

Calculation: amount of infusion divided by time to deliver = ml/hr; then, ml ÷ hr × gtt factor ÷ 60 minutes. 1000 ml ÷ 24 hours = 42 ml/hr; 42 ml/hr × 60 gtt/min ÷ 60 minutes = 42 gtt/min.

421. Comprehension, implementation, physiological integrity (c).

4 This is the only correct information of which the nurse can be aware. The anesthesia slows peristalsis, and eating after surgery would likely result in an emesis.

1 This may be true; however, it is not the correct response for everyone. Although a patient may be hungry after surgery, food is prohibited until return of peristalsis.

2 This is very true, but the most valid response as to the reason why food is not given is response #4.

3 The risk of aspiration is high when a person has an emesis but is not the primary reason why food is prohibited after surgery.

422. Application, assessment, health promotion and maintenance (c).

2 Narcotics suppress the CNS, slowing respirations, which predisposes the patient to altered breathing patterns.

1 Although this is a valid response, based on Maslow's hierarchy of needs, it is of lesser importance than is respiration.

3 Pain is the diagnosis for which the narcotic is given. If the analgesic is effective, the pain diagnosis should cease to be a problem for the time being.

4 No data in the situation supports this diagnosis.

423. Application, implementation, physiological integrity (b).

Dose ÷ On Hand × Quantity. 50 mg/ml ÷ 100 mg/ml × 1 = 0.5 ml

424. Analysis, implementation, safe, effective care environment (c).

1, 2, 5 Assessments made on the bowel sounds would confirm peristalsis. Lung sounds would alert the nurse of any adventitious sounds (possible aspiration). Ensuring the patency of the tube is imperative before each feeding, as is confirming proper placement of the tube.

3, 4 Measuring heart rate and blood pressure are not necessary assessments prior to a nasogastric tube feeding. 1, 2, and 5 ensure the safety of the procedure.

425. Analysis, evaluation, safe, effective care environment (c).

4 A WBC of 1.8 indicates neutropenia, which increases the patient's chance for infection.

1 This is a normal RBC count.

2 A WBC count of 15 is indicative of infection.

3 This is a low-normal value for platelet counts.

426. Analysis, assessment, physiological integrity (b).

2 Airway is always the primary assessment to be made after surgery.

1, 3, 4 These are assessments that should be made; however, airway remains the most important.

427. Analysis, evaluation, physiological integrity (b).

1 The cold pack will reduce swelling around the neck region. Swelling can compromise the airway.

2 Although the cold may anesthetize the site, it is placed primarily to reduce swelling.

3 Cold will not have any effect on production of hormone.

4 Although cold causes vasoconstriction, it is not the primary purpose for placement of the ice.

428. Application, implementation, health promotion and maintenance (b).

3 This is the only true teaching response that is non-judgmental and meets the needs of the adolescent.

1 This is demeaning and not helpful to the teen.

2 This is true but needs to be expanded with further information.

4 This is argumentative and is not helpful to the learning needs of the adolescent.

429. Knowledge, assessment, physiological integrity (c).

2 The four pulmonary veins return blood from the lungs to the left atrium of the heart.

1 The pulmonary artery carries deoxygenated blood to the lung.

3 The superior vena cava transports deoxygenated blood from above the diaphragm into the right atrium of the heart.

4 The inferior vena cava transports deoxygenated blood from below the diaphragm into the right atrium of the heart.

430. Analysis, implementation, safe, effective care environment (c).

4 This is the most correct response that does not alarm the patient.

1 The physician gave no indication how high the cardiac enzymes were; therefore this response may be incorrect and is certainly alarming to the patient.

2 This is not correct information.

3 Liver enzymes elevate when the patient has cirrhosis.

431. Knowledge, planning, physiological integrity (b).

2 Thromboangiitis obliterans is Buerger's disease. These exercises are designed to assist the individual in promoting arterial circulation to his extremities.

1 The exercises are designed to increase circulation to the extremities.

3 These exercises would be contraindicated in someone with thrombophlebitis.

4 Paget's disease is a condition of the bone, and these exercises would not help this disorder.

432. Application, planning, physiological integrity (c).

1, 4 The patient can assess any fluid retention by weighing himself daily. The patient should also take his diuretic in the morning to decrease the chance that he will have nocturia.

2 The patient should be instructed to take his pulse before taking his digoxin.

3 Increasing carbohydrates will not affect the patient's heart failure and may contribute to weight gain.

433. Analysis, planning, health promotion and maintenance (b).

3 Exercise may elevate the patient's blood pressure. The patient should sit and allow his heart rate and blood pressure to return to normal and have the nurse check it again to get a true reading.

1 This would alarm the patient and is not necessary.

2 This would not necessarily lower the patient's blood pressure.

4 With a blood pressure that high, the nurse will want to check the blood pressure sooner than the next day.

434. Analysis, planning, health promotion and maintenance (c).

3 Chinese food contains monosodium glutamate (MSG), which should be avoided on a salt-restricted diet.

1 Vegetarian diets contain little meat and dairy products, which are high in sodium.

2 Italian foods are not especially high in salt or MSG.

4 French cooking is not especially high in salt or MSG.

435. Application, planning, physiological integrity (a).

Dosage ÷ On Hand × Quantity. 600 mg ÷ 300 mg × 1 = 2 tablets.

436. Comprehension, assessment, physiological integrity (c).

4 This is the only true statement concerning ulcerative colitis.

1 The patient's major symptoms are likely to be cramps and diarrhea.
2 The colitis involves the large intestine.
3 This syndrome is not caused by an overuse of laxatives; it may be an autoimmune disorder.

437. Comprehension, assessment, physiological integrity (b).
1 The villi absorb digested nutrients into the bloodstream to be taken to the liver via the portal vein.
2 This is the action of the large intestine.
3 This also occurs in the large intestine.
4 Water is reabsorbed into the intestines in the small intestine.

438. Application, planning, physiological integrity (b).
2 The patient will need to take hormones for the rest of her life.
1 Surgery is not usually indicated for someone with hypothyroidism.
3 This is not true; hormone replacement is needed.
4 This may be indicated for hyperthyroidism, not hypothyroidism.

439. Knowledge, assessment, physiological integrity (b).
3 The pituitary gland secretes growth hormone, which is the hormone malfunction in these two disorders.
1, 2, 4 These hormones do not secrete growth hormone and are therefore incorrect responses.

440. Application, implementation, physiological integrity (b).
Dosage ÷ On Hand x Quantity. 3 mg ÷ 10 mg x 2 ml = 0.6 ml

441. Comprehension, implementation, physiological integrity (c).
1 The HgbA1C is a marker that measures how well individuals have controlled their blood sugar over a 3-month period. It is much more accurate than fasting blood glucose level.
2 Although this may be true, it is not an adequate explanation.
3 This test cannot measure the amount of insulin a patient has been using.
4 This really has nothing to do with the question; it is not necessarily indicated before this treatment, and whether the patient is being prepared for one is unknown.

442. Knowledge, planning, physiological integrity (b).
4 An ERCP is useful in discovering obstructions in the common bile duct, cystic duct, or hepatic duct.
1 A barium enema or colonoscopy would be more beneficial to detect inflammation.
2 X-ray studies or barium swallows are more useful in determining bowel blockages.
3 Liver enzyme studies are useful in determining liver damage caused by cirrhosis or hepatitis.

443. Analysis, assessment, physiological integrity (c).
2 Cirrhosis creates changes in oncotic pressure within the portal system; this creates ascites, an accumulation of fluid within the abdomen.

1 Peritonitis is an infection of the peritoneum and results in abdominal distention and slowed peristalsis.
3 Hepatitis may cause this problem, but it is much more likely that it will occur with cirrhosis.
4 Diverticulitis contributes to cramping, constipation, and pain but does not result in ascites.

444. Comprehension, planning, physiological integrity (b).
3 Clear liquids are generally the first diet to be resumed for patients who have had abdominal surgery.
1 A high-residue or high-fiber diet would be too difficult to digest for this patient.
2 A low-fiber diet is still too difficult for this patient to digest.
4 A mechanical soft diet is too much consistency for the patient to begin to digest, although the patient may advance to this after tolerating a clear and full liquid diet.

445. Application, implementation, physiological integrity (c).
Calculation: amount of infusion ÷ time to deliver = ml/hr; then, ml/hr × gtt factor ÷ 60 minutes. 2000 ml ÷ 10 hours = 200 ml/hr, 200 ml/hr × 10 gtt/min ÷ 60 minutes = 33 gtt/min.

446. Application, planning, physiological integrity (b).
2 Fried foods would stimulate the gallbladder to contract so as to release its bile. Eating a large, fatty meal after a cholecystectomy may cause the patient to have painful diarrhea.
1 Raw vegetables should not create a problem for the patient.
3 Vegetables are acidic; they do not cause excess bile to be released.
4 Pasta is a carbohydrate but has little fat; therefore it should not create a problem.

447. Application, implementation, physiological integrity (c).
8 oz = 240 ml. 240 ml × 3 cans = 720 ml. 720 ml ÷ 80 m/hr = 9 hours to infuse.

448. Analysis, evaluation, health promotion and maintenance (c).
4 Constipation is a primary factor in the development of hemorrhoids.
1, 2, 3 These are not implicated in the development of hemorrhoids.

449. Analysis, planning, physiological integrity (c).
1 Hemorrhage is the primary risk in the patient who has a prolapsed uterus.
2 Although this may be a concern, it is not the primary problem.
3 Although this may be a problem, it is not a primary problem.
4 This should not be a problem for this patient.

450. Analysis, planning, physiological integrity (c).
2 The patient will have the potential for multiple urinary tract infections because of the fistula.
1, 3, 4 These problems should not develop in this patient.

CHAPTER 6 Mental Health Nursing

The licensed practical/vocational nurse (LP/VN) must understand basic mental health nursing principles to practice nursing safely. Basic mental health concepts are useful in understanding responses to disease and dysfunction, both physically and socially. Each person responds to disease and disorder according to his or her own basic personality, past experiences, intelligence, and coping skills. These concepts are explored and studied in mental health nursing.

HOLISM

A. Definition: this concept of health holds that illness results from a complex interaction among the mind and body and the environment, a concept that views an individual as more than the sum of his or her parts.
B. Approaches to treatment: multifaceted approaches are used to treat disturbances rather than simply relying on treatment aimed at specific symptoms; we are no longer content to treat the illness; we are learning to treat the whole person. Approaches include the following dimensions:
   1. Physical
   2. Emotional
   3. Intellectual
   4. Sociocultural
   5. Spiritual

MENTAL HEALTH CONTINUUM

A. Mental health and mental illness are seen as opposite poles on a continuum.
B. The precise point at which an individual is deemed mentally ill is determined by the specific behavior exhibited and by the context in which the behavior is seen.
C. Some behaviors that are considered inappropriate in one setting may be considered normal in another setting.
D. Variations are based on the culture, the time or era, personality, and other variables.
E. Behaviors of the mentally ill are often exaggerations of normal human behaviors.

MENTAL HEALTH

A. Definition: an individual's ability to cope with life's problems and to draw satisfaction from living throughout various life stages
B. Persons may experience times of greater or lesser satisfaction with life and, at times of lesser satisfaction, may seek the assistance of a therapist or counselor.

C. No clear set of characteristics specific to mental health can be identified.
   1. All behavior is considered meaningful and may be interpreted as the individual's effort to adapt or cope with the environment.
   2. At times, some adaptations fail; others are continued long after the need for them has passed; still others may be directed to an undesired end.

MENTAL ILLNESS

A. Definition: a pattern of behavior that is disturbing to the individual or the community in which the individual resides; behaviors may interfere with daily activities, impair judgment, or alter reality; a mental illness is a disturbance of a person's ability to cope effectively, which results in maladaptive behaviors and impaired functioning.
   1. The person who is mentally ill acts in ways that seem unrelated to current reality.
   2. Relationships with family and friends are disturbed.
   3. The person's ability to work and to contribute to his or her own welfare may be impaired.
   4. The person often experiences subjective discomfort.
   5. The person may exhibit symptoms such as delusions, hallucinations, paranoia, passive-aggressive behavior, or compulsions.
B. Historical perspective of mental illness
   1. Early history
      a. Mentally ill persons were thought to be possessed by supernatural forces, evil spirits, or demons.
      b. Mentally ill persons were removed from society or mistreated in other ways.
      c. These beliefs and practices have lasted many years; some are still practiced today.
   2. Classical era (Greco-Roman)
      a. Certain attitudes about mental illness started to change.
      b. Early scientific interest led to various classification systems.
      c. The idea of divine possession was rejected in favor of the "humoral theory of disease."
      d. Humors were thought to be basic internal fluids capable of controlling behavior.
      e. The terms melancholia and hysteria are derived from these ancient beliefs.
   3. The Middle Ages, the Renaissance, and Protestant Reformation eras saw some reform; however, in general:
      a. Society returned to the idea of divine possession or spiritual explanations for mental illness.

Eighteenth Century

Phillipe Pinel (1745-1826, France): freed mentally ill persons from chains

Benjamin Rush (1745-1813, United States): founded Pennsylvania Hospital; the father of American psychiatry

Nineteenth Century

Florence Nightingale (1860, England): founder of modern nursing

Dorothea Dix (1802-1887, United States): promoted legislation to establish mental hospitals

Linda Richards (1873, United States): first psychiatric nurse

Daniel Tuke (1827-1895, England): founded York Retreat based on Quaker principles

Twentieth Century

Clifford Beers (1876-1943, United States): wrote the book, *The Mind That Found Itself,* generating public concern for the treatment of mentally ill persons

Adolf Meyer (1866-1950, United States): director of the Johns Hopkins Clinic; founder of the mental hygiene movement

Emil Kraepelin (1856-1926, Germany): classified mental disorders

Eugene Bleuler (1857-1939, Switzerland): coined the word *schizophrenia* and classified it into types

Sigmund Freud (1856-1939, Austria): developed psycho-analytic theory; revolutionized psychiatry

Carl Jung (1875-1961, Switzerland): developed a personality theory that included the concepts of introversion and extroversion

Karen Horney (1885-1952, United States): theorized that culture had a great influence on mental illness

b. The mentally ill person was often mistreated by incarceration.

4. The Modern era: numerous reforms are instituted (Box 6-1).

5. Modern developments include:
   a. Discovery of phenothiazines (the major tranquilizers)
   b. Community mental health: 1960s; still in use today; the aim is to provide care of mentally ill persons in their own communities rather than in large institutions; a primary goal of the community mental health concept is to return patients to their home as quickly as possible and to foster the development of support systems in the community.
   c. Patients released from large hospitals: in the late 1970s, a large number of mentally ill persons were released into communities where they often did not receive treatment either because they did not seek it or because adequate types of services were not available; this process is called deinstitutionalization; some people believe that an increase of *street people* or homeless has occurred as a result of the process.
   d. Community mental health centers were established.
   e. Mental health costs decreased in the United States because of the development and use of psychotropic medications.

NURSING ROLE

A. The nursing process
   1. Assessment: the LPN gathers subjective and objective data through observation, interview, and examination; data are obtained through:
      a. Health history
      b. Mental status examination
         (1) General appearance
         (2) Affect and mood
         (3) Intellect and sensorium
         (4) Thought processes
         (5) Insight
      c. Psychological testing
         (1) Intelligence testing
         (2) Personality testing
      d. Self-assessment (e.g., stress scale, decision-making trees)
      e. Physical examination
   2. Diagnosis: nurses diagnose and treat human responses to illness; the nursing diagnosis is formulated by the registered professional nurse; the LPN contributes to this phase of the nursing process by collecting objective and subjective data; potential nursing diagnoses identify the problem and the etiologic factors of the problem; actual nursing diagnoses identify the problem, origin, and signs and symptoms; the North American Nursing Diagnosis Association (NANDA) listing is used; examples of actual and potential nursing diagnoses used in mental health nursing include the following (these are examples, not a complete listing):
      a. Anxiety (panic) related to family rejection; exhibited by chest discomfort, palpitations, dizziness, diaphoresis, and trembling
      b. Impaired social interaction related to negative role modeling; exhibited by verbalized and observed discomfort in social situations
      c. Risk for violence: self-directed activity related to history of suicide attempts
      d. Risk for trauma related to muscular incoordination

The psychiatric–mental health areas of concern for formulating nursing diagnoses appear in Box 6-2.

   3. Planning: the plan of care is based on the nursing diagnosis; specific nursing interventions are devised to attain specifically stated goals; when possible, goals should be developed jointly with the patient and cooperation enlisted; goals may be short term or long term; all goals should be prioritized, emphasizing reduction or elimination of the identified problem; goals usually include the anticipated length of time for accomplishment and the standard for judging whether the goal has been met.
   4. Implementation: the planned nursing actions that assist the patient in achieving the identified goal (e.g., health teaching, activities of daily living [ADL], other prescribed treatments, and medications); this phase is ongoing, and reactions to treatment are observed and documented so that the care plan may be modified periodically as goals are met.
   5. Evaluation: outcome achievement is identified, as well as the factors that affected the goal being met, partially met, or not met; this process is followed by the decision to continue, modify, or terminate the plan; following

BOX 6-2	Psychiatric—Mental Health Nursing's Phenomena of Concern

Actual or potential mental health problems of clients pertaining to the following:
- The maintenance of optimal health and well being and the prevention of psychobiological illness
- Self-care limitations or impaired functioning related to mental and emotional distress
- Deficits in the functioning of significant biological, emotional, and cognitive systems
- Emotional stress or crisis components of illness, pain, and disability
- Self-concept changes, developmental issues, and life process changes
- Problems related to emotions such as anxiety, anger, sadness, loneliness, and grief
- Physical symptoms that occur along with altered psychological functioning
- Alterations in thinking, perceiving, symbolizing, communicating, and decision making
- Difficulties in relating to others
- Behaviors and mental states indicating that the patient is a danger to self or others or has a severe disability
- Interpersonal, systemic, sociocultural, spiritual, or environmental circumstances or events that affect the mental and emotional well being of the individual, family, or community
- Symptom management, side effects or toxicities associated with psychopharmacological intervention and other aspects of the treatment regimen

From American Nurses' Association: *A statement on psychiatric mental health clinical nursing practice and standards of psychiatric mental health clinical nursing practice,* Washington, DC, 1994, the Association.

evaluation of goal achievement, the entire nursing process and care plan are reviewed, modified, or updated to reflect new nursing diagnoses.

B. Principles of mental health nursing; the nurse must:
1. Understand own inner needs, thoughts, and feelings and be aware of how these affect patients.
2. Be aware of own resources and limitations so as to function effectively in mental health nursing.
3. Respect the patient as a person; take time to listen to what is said.
4. Be aware of the patient's dignity; show patience and understanding.
5. Be nonjudgmental and nonthreatening; patients must be accepted; a trusting relationship must be established.
6. Be honest.
7. Reassure patients by being available and allaying fears.
8. Explain routines, rules, and regulations when appropriate.
9. Maintain a calm, hopeful attitude.
10. Encourage reality orientation, and avoid entering into patient's unrealistic thinking.
11. Emphasize strengths that the patient displays by acknowledging healthy behavior; offer warm understanding, but do not encourage overdependency or intimacy.
12. Remember that all staff members are role models and are often viewed as authority figures by patients.
13. Help reduce anxiety by making as few demands as possible on patients.
14. Explain what is happening to the patient in simple, understandable language.
15. Remain objective, but do not display aloofness or distance; maintain your awareness of the patient's humanity and dignity.
16. Maintain a nurse-patient relationship that is always realistic and professional.
17. Remember that a reason exists for all behavior.
18. Note that behavior is changed through emotional experience rather than through rational means.
19. Allow patients to exercise all of their basic human rights.
20. Use the least-restrictive method or methods of controlling behavior, such as communication.
21. Respect the confidentiality of the patient.

C. Communications in mental health nursing
1. Communication: a complex activity consisting of a series of events, each interdependent on the other, which results in a negotiated understanding between two or more people in a given situation.
   a. Communication is not merely the exchange of information.
   b. Each message (input) generates an extremely complex reaction that eventually leads to a selective response (output), which, in turn, becomes a new input for the communicators.
2. Modes of communication
   a. The most apparent form is verbal (written or spoken language) communication; spoken communication is the more important in mental health nursing.
   b. Spoken communication is always accompanied by at least one of the following additional communication forms:
      (1) Paralanguage: voice quality, tones, grunts, and other nonword vocalizations
      (2) Kinesis: facial expression, gestures, and eye and body movements
      (3) Proxemics: the spatial relationship between persons
      (4) Touch and messages to other sensory organs: aromas and cultural artifacts (jewelry, clothing, hairstyle)
   c. Effective communications are:
      (1) Efficient: messages are simple, clear, and timed correctly.
      (2) Appropriate: messages are relevant to the situation.
      (3) Flexible: communication is open to alteration based on perceived response.
      (4) Receptive: feedback is allowed (checking and correcting by either or both parties).
3. Therapeutic communication (Box 6-3)
4. Blocks to communication (Table 6-1)

Text continued on p.363

BOX 6-3　Therapeutic Communication Techniques

Listening

Definition: an active process of receiving information and examining reaction to the messages received

Example: maintaining eye contact and receptive nonverbal communication

Therapeutic value: nonverbally communicates to the patient the nurse's interest and acceptance

Broad Openings

Definition: encouraging the patient to select topics for discussion

Example: "What are you thinking about?"

Therapeutic value: indicates acceptance by the nurse and the value of the patient's initiative

Restating

Definition: repeating the main thought the patient expressed

Example: "You say that your mother left you when you were 5 years old."

Therapeutic value: indicates that the nurse is listening and validates, reinforces, or calls attention to something important that has been said

Clarification

Definition: attempting to put into words vague ideas or unclear thoughts of the patient to enhance the nurse's understanding or asking the patient to explain what he or she means

Example: "I'm not sure what you mean. Could you tell me about that again?"

Therapeutic value: helps clarify feelings, ideas, and perceptions of the patient and provides an explicit correlation between them and the patient's actions

Reflection

Definition: directing back the patient's ideas, feelings, questions, and content

Example: "You're feeling tense and anxious, and it's related to a conversation you had with your husband last night?"

Therapeutic value: validates the nurse's understanding of what the patient is saying and signifies empathy, interest, and respect for the patient

Humor

Definition: the discharge of energy through the comic enjoyment of the imperfect

Example: "That gives a whole new meaning to the word *nervous*"; said with shared kidding between the nurse and patient

Therapeutic value: can promote insight by making conscious repressed material, resolving paradoxes, tempering aggression, and revealing new options, and is a socially acceptable form of sublimation

Informing

Definition: the skill of information giving

Example: "I think you need to know more about how your medication works."

Therapeutic value: helpful in health teaching or patient education about relevant aspects of patient's well being and self-care

Focusing

Definition: questions or statements that help the patient expand on a topic of importance

Example: "I think that we should talk more about your relationship with your father."

Therapeutic value: allows the patient to discuss central issues and keeps the communication process goal directed

Sharing Perceptions

Definition: asking the patient to verify the nurse's understanding of what the patient is thinking or feeling

Example: "You're smiling, but I sense that you are really very angry with me."

Therapeutic value: conveys the nurse's understanding to the patient and has the potential for clearing up confusing communication

Theme Identification

Definition: underlying issues or problems experienced by the patient that emerge repeatedly during the course of the nurse-patient relationship

Example: "I've noticed that in all of the relationships that you have described, you've been hurt or rejected by the man. Do you think this is an underlying issue?"

Therapeutic value: allows the nurse to best promote the patient's exploration and understanding of important problems

Silence

Definition: lack of verbal communication for a therapeutic reason

Example: sitting with a patient and nonverbally communicating interest and involvement

Therapeutic value: allows the patient time to think and gain insights, slows the pace of the interaction, and encourages the patient to initiate conversation while conveying the nurse's support, understanding, and acceptance

Suggesting

Definition: presentation of alternative ideas for the patient's consideration relative to problem solving

Example: "Have you thought about responding to your boss in a different way when he raises that issue with you? For example, you could ask him if a specific problem has occurred."

Therapeutic value: increases the patient's perceived options or choices

Modified from Stuart GW, Laraia MT: *Principles and practice of psychiatric nursing,* ed 7, St Louis, 2001, Mosby.

TABLE 6-1	Ineffective Responses That Hinder Therapeutic Communication		
Response	**Discussion**	**Nontherapeutic Response**	**Therapeutic Response**
Offering false reassurance	The nurse, in an effort to be supportive and to make the patient's pain disappear, offers reassuring clichés. This response is not based on fact. It brushes aside the patient's feelings and closes off communication. It is often the result of the nurse's inability to listen to the patient's negative emotions. No one can predict the outcome of a situation.	"Don't worry; everything will be okay." "Things will be better soon; you'll see."	"I know you have a lot going on right now. Let's make a list and begin to discuss them one at a time. Working toward solutions will assist you to get through this."
Not listening	The nurse is preoccupied with other work that needs to be done, is distracted by noise in the area, is thinking and about personal problems.	"I'm sorry, what did you say?" "Could you start again? I was listening to the other nurse."	"That is interesting. Please elaborate." "I really hear what you are saying; it must be difficult."
Offering approval	How a patient feels about what he or she said or did is most important. The patient must approve of his or her own actions.	"That's good." "I agree; I think you should have told him."	"What do you think about what you said to him?" "How do you feel about it?"
Minimizing problem	The nurse may use this when facing the enormity of a particular problem. This is used in an effort to make the patient feel better. It cuts off communication.	"That's nothing compared to that other client's problem." "Everyone feels that way at times; it's not a big deal."	"That is a very difficult problem for you." "That sounds pretty important for you to deal with."
Offering advice	This response undermines patients' ability to solve their own problems. It serves to render them dependent and helpless. If the solution provided by the nurse does not work, the patient may blame the outcome on the nurse. Patients do not take responsibility for developing outcomes. The nurse maintains control and at the same time devalues the patient.	"I think you should...." "In my opinion, it would be wise to...." "Why don't you do...." "The best solution is...."	"What do *you* think you should do?" "There can be several alternatives; let's talk about some. However, the final decision must be yours." "I will listen to your problem and help you see it clearly." "We can develop a pros and cons list, which may assist you in solving the problem."
Giving literal responses	The nurse feeds into a patient's delusions of hallucinations and denies the patient the opportunity to see reality. This does not provide a healthy response toward growth.	Patient: "That TV is talking to me." Nurse: "What is it saying to you?" Patient: "There is nuclear power coming through the air ducts." Nurse: "I'll turn off the A/C for a while."	"The TV is on for everyone." "There is cool air blowing from the vents. It is the A/C system."
Changing the subject	The nurse changes the topic at a crucial time because the discussion is too uncomfortable. It negates what the patient seems interested in discussing. Communication will remain superficial.	Patient: "My mother always puts me down." Nurse: "That's interesting, but let's talk about...."	"Tell me about that."

From Fortinash KM, Holoday-Worret PA: *Psychiatric-mental health nursing,* ed 3, St Louis, 2004, Mosby.

Continued

TABLE 6-1   Ineffective Responses That Hinder Therapeutic Communication—cont'd

Response	Discussion	Nontherapeutic Response	Therapeutic Response
Belittling	The nurse puts down patient's expressed feelings to avoid having to deal with painful feelings.	Patient: "I don't want to live anymore now that my child is gone." Nurse: "Anyone would be sad; but that's no reason to want to die."	"The death must be very difficult for you. Tell me a little more about how you are feeling."
Disagreeing	The nurse criticizes the patient who is seeking support.	"I definitely do not agree with your view." "I really don't believe that."	"Let's talk about the way you see that." "It seems hard to believe. Please explain further."
Judging	The nurse's responses are filled with his or her own values and judgments. This demonstrates a lack of acceptance of the patient's differences. It will provide a barrier to further disclosures.	"You are not married. Do you think having this baby will solve your problems?" "This is certainly not the Christian thing to do." "You are thinking about divorce when you have three children?"	"What will having this baby provide for you?" "What do you think about what you are attempting to do?" "Let's discuss this option," or "Let's discuss other options."
Excessive probing	This serves to control the nature of the patient's responses. The nurse asks many questions of patients before they are ready to provide the information. This is self-protective to the nurse by avoiding the anxiety of uncomfortable silences. The patient feels overwhelmed and may withdraw.	"Why do you do this?" "What do you think was the real cause?" "Do you always feel this way?" "Why do you think that way?"	"Tell me how this is upsetting you." "Tell me what you believe to be the cause." "Tell me how you feel when that happens." "Explain your thinking on this if you can."
Challenging	This stems from the nurse's belief that if patients are challenged regarding their unrealistic beliefs, they will be coerced into seeing reality. The patient may feel threatened when challenged, holding onto the beliefs more strongly.	"You are not the Queen of England." "If your leg is missing, then how can you walk this hall?"	"You sound like you want to be important." "It seems to you like you are missing a leg. Tell me more about that."
Superficial comments	The nurse gives simple or meaningless responses to patients. It suggests a lack of understanding regarding the patient as an individual. The interactions remain superficial, maintaining distance *between* nurse and patient. Nothing of significance is communicated.	"Great day, huh!" "You should be feeling good; you are being discharged today." "Keep the faith; your doctor should be coming anytime now."	"What kind of day are you having?" "How are you feeling about leaving the hospital today?" "You look worried. Your doctor called and said he would be here within the hour."
Defending	The nurse may believe that he or she must defend him or herself, the staff, or the hospital. The nurse may not take the time to listen to the patient's concerns. Efforts need to be made to explore the patient's thoughts and feelings.	"Your doctor is a good doctor. He would never say that." "We have a very experienced staff here. They would not ever do that."	"What has you so upset about your doctor?" "Tell me what happened on the evening shift."

From Fortinash KM, Holoday-Worret PA: *Psychiatric-mental health nursing,* ed 3, St Louis, 2004, Mosby.

TABLE 6-1	Ineffective Responses That Hinder Therapeutic Communication—cont'd		
Response	Discussion	Nontherapeutic Response	Therapeutic Response
Self-focusing	The nurse focuses attention away from the patient by thinking about sharing his or her own thoughts, feelings, problems. The focus is taken away from the patient who is seeking help. The nurse is more interested in what to say next instead of actively listening to the patient.	"That may have happened to you last year, but it happened to me twice this month, which hurt me a great deal and...." "Excuse me, but could you say that again? I have a response to make, but I want to be sure of what you said."	"Tell me about your incident and how it might relate to your sadness now." "If I heard you accurately, you said...."
Criticism of others	The nurse puts down others.	Patient: "The staff members on the day shift let me smoke two cigarettes." Nurse: "The day shift is always breaking the rules. On this shift, we follow the one-cigarette policy." Patient: "My daughter is hateful to me." Nurse: "She must be just awful to live with."	"The policy is one cigarette, which we must follow." "It sounds like you are having a rough time now with your daughter."
Premature interpretation	The nurse does not wait until the patient fully expresses thoughts and feelings related to a particular problem, which rushes the patient and disregards his or her input. The nurse may miss what the patient wants to explain.	"I think this is what you really mean." "You may think that way consciously, but your unconscious believes...."	"What do you think this means?" "So you think...."

D. Nurse-patient relationship
  1. One-to-one relationship between a nurse and a patient
  2. Patient centered
  3. Goal directed
  4. Not for nurse's satisfaction
  5. The focus is on modification of patient behavior, increasing patient's self-worth, and developing patient's coping strategies.
  6. Therapeutic, not social, relationship
  7. Phases
    a. Preorientation: data collection about the patient; self-analysis of attitudes, biases, and perceptions by the nurse
    b. Orientation: 2 to 10 sessions; the nurse and patient become acquainted; trust and rapport are established; parameters of the relationship are also established; discussions are contracted; patient problems are identified; the plan is built on the patient's strengths.
    c. Working begins when the patient demonstrates responsibility to uphold terms of the contract; establish priorities and goals with patient; help the patient achieve behavior change (e.g., discussion, role-playing); focus on the present; reinforce the contract terms as necessary.
    d. Termination begins during orientation phase; the purpose is to conclude the relationship; focus on

patient growth, and help the patient with expression of feelings about relationship closure.
E. Applications of mental health nursing
  1. Community mental health center
  2. Partial hospitalization setting: day or night hospitals
  3. Mental health clinic
  4. Liaison: use of mental health workers in the general hospital setting
  5. Alcohol and drug abuse facilities and clinics
  6. Inpatient units
  7. Crisis intervention
  8. Health maintenance organizations

PERSONALITY DEVELOPMENT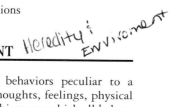

A. Definition: a consistent set of behaviors peculiar to a specific individual; the sum of thoughts, feelings, physical characteristics, and sociocultural biases on which all behavior is built
B. Heredity
  1. Personality is influenced by inherited characteristics, both physical and psychological.
  2. Controversy exists over the extent of genetic influence on specific human behaviors.

C. Environment
1. The environment is a strong determining factor in the individual's development.
2. Environment includes the intrauterine environment, as well as all the external factors that influence the individual after birth.
D. Physical basis: personality develops normally if the necessary physical basis is present.
1. The brain is the major organ of thought and is necessary to the development of personality.
2. Other influential factors include a normally functioning endocrine system, which strongly influences behavior.
E. Major theorists: comparison of Freud and Erickson (Table 6-2)
F. Elements of personality (Freud)
1. Levels of consciousness
a. The unconscious: always outside the awareness of the individual; influences actions in ways the individual may not understand; thought to include dreams
b. The preconscious: usually outside awareness; available to the conscious mind in special circumstances, such as under hypnosis or during therapy
c. The conscious: ordinary awareness
2. Structures: some theorists refer to personality structures.
a. Freud: ego, id, and superego
b. Berne: child, adult, and parent
3. Functions: each structure is thought to perform specific functions (Freud).
a. Id (child): basic, innate psychic energy; emotional
b. Ego (adult): mediates between person's perception and objective reality; always rational
c. Superego (parent): incorporates societal values; judgmental and critical
G. Development levels: various theorists describe levels of development.
1. Freud: oral, anal, phallic, latency, genital
2. Erikson: basic trust versus mistrust; autonomy versus shame and doubt; initiative versus guilt; industry versus inferiority; identity versus role diffusion; intimacy versus isolation; generativity versus stagnation; ego integrity versus despair
H. Development of the self-concept
1. Development through experience with other people (e.g., parents, siblings, relatives, peers, teachers, other adults)
a. Feelings of adequacy or inadequacy
b. Feelings of acceptance or rejection
c. Opportunities for identification
d. Expectations of values, goals, and behaviors
2. Self-concept consists of:
a. Body image: one's perception of one's body
b. Self-ideal: one's idea of what is *good* behavior
c. Self-esteem: personal judgment of one's own worth
d. Role: one's perception of how one fits into the society
e. Identity: the combination of all of these factors into a unified whole

Stress

Hans Selye in 1956 defined stress as *wear and tear on the body*. All people are continuously exposed to varieties of stress: physical, chemical, psychological, and emotional. Almost any situation, pleasant or unpleasant, that requires change leads to some level of stress. Stress produces a clearly identifiable response called the general adaptation syndrome; it is associated with concomitant physical and chemical changes that commonly occur in the body.

EGO DEFENSE MECHANISMS

Ego defense mechanisms are basic psychological tools that individuals use at various times to manage life's crises. These mechanisms may also be referred to as ego defenses, defense mechanisms, or protective mechanisms. As such, they defend the ego or self from untoward anxiety, help resolve conflicts, and return the individual to a point of psychological homeostasis or comfort. These mechanisms are usually outside conscious awareness and are not considered pathological in and of themselves; they should not be removed or challenged until the individual is ready and has adequate strength to tolerate the stressful situation. Common defense mechanisms are listed in Table 6-3, p. 369.

MENTAL DISTURBANCES AND RESOURCES

Anxiety

A. Definition: a state of alertness or apprehension, tension or uneasiness; a major component of all mental disturbances; anxiety is an internal state that the individual experiences when a perceived threat to the physical body or to the psychological integrity of the person exists; it interferes with concentration, focusing attention on the perceived threat; in its mild form, anxiety serves to alert the person to danger and to prepare the body to react to danger; in its severe form, it is debilitating and may immobilize the person and interfere with activities; anxiety is usually described in degrees or levels.
B. Process: coping behaviors
1. Adaptive coping: the problem creating the anxiety is resolved.
2. Palliative coping: the problem creating the anxiety is not resolved but rather temporarily reduced; the problem returns at a later date.
3. Maladaptive coping: energy is channeled toward reducing the anxiety, and no effort is made to solve the problem.
4. Dysfunctional coping: the problem is not solved, and the anxiety not reduced.
C. Levels
1. Mild (1)
2. Moderate (2)
3. Severe (3)
4. Panic (4)
D. Assessment (Table 6-4, p. 370)
E. Interventions
1. Remain with the highly anxious patient; leaving the patient alone increases anxiety.
2. Reduce environmental stimuli, or move the patient to a quiet area; the patient's ability to handle stimuli is compromised. *Text continued on p. 371*

TABLE 6-2   A Comparison of the Development Stages Postulated by Freud, Sullivan, Erikson, and Piaget

Freud	Sullivan	Erikson	Piaget

I. Oral stage (0-18 mo)
A. The mouth is a source of satisfaction
B. Two phases
  1. Passive
   • Only interests are satisfying hunger and *sucking*
   • Completely helpless, *security* the greatest need
   • Narcissistic and egocentric, operates on *pleasure principle*
   • Omnipotent feelings are prevalent
  2. Active
   • Biting is a mode of pleasure
   • Continuous experimentation and associations
   Sensory discriminations
   • Differentiation between mental images and reality
   • Differentiation of others and discovery of self
	I. Infancy (0-18 mo)
	A. The mouth is a source of satisfaction
	B. Mouth—takes in (sucking), cuts off (biting), and pushes out (spitting) objects introduced by others
	C. Crying, babbling, and cooing are modes of communication used by the infant to call attention of adults to self
	D. *Satisfaction response (pleasure principle)*: infant's biological needs are met and a mutual feeling of comfort and fulfillment is experienced by mother and infant (mother gives and infant takes)
	E. *Empathic observation*—capacity to perceive feelings of others as his or her own immediate feelings in the situation
	F. *Autistic invention*—state of symbolic activity in which the infant believes he or she is master of all he or she surveys
	G. Experimentation, exploration, and manipulation are methods used to acquaint self with environment
		I. Oral-sensory stage (0-12 mo)
		A. The mouth is a source of satisfaction and a means of dealing with anxiety-producing situations
		B. Focus is on the development of the basic attitudes of *trust vs. mistrust*
		C. Attitudes are formed through mother's reaction to infant needs
			I. Sensorimotor stage (0-12 mo)
			A. Emphasis is on preverbal intellectual development
			B. Learns relationships with external objects
			C. Focus is on physical development with gradual increase in ability to think and use language

II. Anal stage (1½-3 yr) A. Primary activity is on learning muscular control association with urination and defecation (*toilet-training period*) B. Exhibits more self-control; walks, talks, dresses, and undresses C. *Negativism*—assertion of independence D. Introduction of *reality principle*, ego development E. Superego begins to develop	II. Childhood (1½-6 yr) A. Begins with the capacity for communicating through speech and ends with a beginning need for association with peers B. Uses language as a tool to communicate wishes and needs C. Anus is power tool used to give or withhold a part	II. Anal-muscular stage (1-3 yr) A. Learns the extent to which the *environment* can be influenced by direct manipulation B. Focuses on the development of the basic attitudes of *autonomy vs. shame and doubt* C. Exerts self-control and willpower	II. Preoperational stage (2-7 yr) A. Learns to use symbols and language B. Learns to imitate and play C. Displays egocentricity D. Engages in *animistic thinking*—endowment of objects with power and ability

Modified from Kreigh H, Perko J: *Psychiatric and mental health nursing: commitment to care and concern*, Reston, 1979, Reston Publishing.

Continued

TABLE 6-2 A Comparison of the Development Stages Postulated by Freud, Sullivan, Erikson, and Piaget—cont'd

Freud	Sullivan	Erikson	Piaget

II. Anal stage—cont'd
  F. Engages in parallel play
	...of self to control significant people in his environment
	  D. Emergence and integration of *self-concept* and *reflected appraisal of significant persons*
	  E. Awareness that postponing or delaying gratification of one's wishes may bring satisfaction
	  F. Begins to find limits in experimentation, exploration, and manipulation
	  G. More aggressive
	  H. Uses parallel play and curiosity to explore environment
	  I. Uses exhibitionism and masturbatory activity to become acquainted with self and others
	  J. Demonstrates a beginning ability to think abstractly		

III. Phallic stage (3-6 yr)
  A. *Libidinal energy* focus on the genitals
  B. Learns *sexual identity*
  C. *Superego* becomes internalized
  D. Sibling rivalry and manipulation of parents occurs
  E. Intellectual and motor facilities are refined
  F. Increased socialization and *associative play*
		III. Genital-locomotor stage (3-6 yr)
		  A. Learns the extent to which being *assertive* will influence the environment
		  B. Focus is on the development of the basic attitudes of *initiative vs. guilt*
		  C. Explores the world with senses, thoughts, and imagination
		  D. Activities demonstrate direction and purpose
		  E. Engages in first real social contacts through *cooperative play*
		  F. Develops conscience	

IV. Latency (6-12 yr)
  A. *Quiet stage* in which sexual development lies dormant, emotional tension eases
	III. Juvenile stage (6-9 yr)
	  A. Learns to form satisfactory relationship with peers
		IV. Latency (6-12 yr)
		  A. Learns to use energy to create, develop, and
			III. Concrete operations stage (7-11 yr)
			  A. Deals with visible concrete

B. *Normal homosexual phase*
- For boys, gangs
- For girls, cliques

C. Increased intellectual capacity
D. Starts school
E. Identifies with teachers and peers
F. Weakening of home ties
G. Recognizes authority figures outside home, age of *hero worship*

V. Genital stage (12 yr–early adulthood)
A. Appearance of secondary sex characteristics, reawakening of sex drives
B. Increased concern over physical appearance

B. *Peer norms* prevail over family norms
- For boys, gangs
- For girls, cliques

C. Engages in *competition, experimentation, exploration,* and manipulation
D. Able to cooperate and compromise
E. Demonstrates capacity to love
F. Distinguishes fantasy from reality
G. Exerts internal control over behavior

IV. Preadolescence (9-12 yr)
A. Learns to relate to a friend of the same sex—*chum relationship*
B. Concerned with group success and derives satisfaction from group accomplishment
C. Shows signs of *rebellion*—restlessness, hostility, irritability
D. Assumes less responsibility for own actions
E. Moves from egocentricity to a more full social state
F. Uses experimentation, exploration, manipulation
G. Seeks *consensual validation* from peers

V. Early adolescence (12-14 yr)
A. Experiences physiological changes
B. Uses rebellion to gain independence

---

manipulate

B. *Focus is on the development of basic attitudes of industry vs. inferiority*
C. Able to initiate and complete tasks
D. Understands rules and regulations
E. Displays competence and productivity

V. Puberty and adolescence (12-18 yr)
A. Demonstrates an ability to integrate life experiences

---

objects and relationships

B. Increased intellectual and conceptual development—uses logic and reasoning
C. More socialized and rule conscious

IV. Formal operations stage (11-15 yr)
A. Develops true abstract thought

Continued

Modified from Kreigh H, Perko J: *Psychiatric and mental health nursing: commitment to care and concern,* Reston, 1979, Reston Publishing.

TABLE 6-2 A Comparison of the Development Stages Postulated by Freud, Sullivan, Erikson, and Piaget—cont'd

Freud	Sullivan	Erikson	Piaget
C. Striving toward independence	C. Fantasizes, overidentifies with heroes	B. Focuses on the development of the basic attitudes of *identity vs. role diffusion*	B. Formulates hypotheses and applies logical tests
D. Development of sexual maturity	D. Discovers and begins relationships with opposite sex	C. Seeks partner of the opposite sex	C. Experiences conceptual independence
E. Identity crisis	E. Demonstrates heightened levels of anxiety in most interpersonal relationships	D. Begins to establish identity and place in society	
F. Identification of love object of opposite sex	VI. Late adolescence (14-21 yr)	VI. Young adulthood (18-35 yr)	
G. Intellectual maturity	A. Establishes an enduring intimate relationship with one member of the opposite sex	A. Primarily concerned with developing an intimate relationship with another adult	
H. Plans future	B. Self-concept becomes stabilized	B. Focus is on the development of the basic attitudes of *intimacy and solidarity vs. isolation*	
	C. Attains physical maturity	V. Adulthood (35-65 yr)	
	D. Develops ability to use logic and abstract concepts	A. Primarily concerned with establishing and maintaining a family	
	VII. Adulthood (21 yr and older)	B. Focus is on the development of the basic attitudes of *generativity vs. stagnation*	
	A. Assumes responsibility relevant to station in life	C. Displays a marked degree of creativity	
	B. Maintains balance and involvement among self, family, and community	D. Adjusts to circumstances of middle age	
	C. Further develops creativity	E. Reevaluates life's accomplishments and goals	
	D. Reaffirms values in life	VI. Maturity (older than 65 yr)	
		A. Accepts lifestyle as meaningful and fulfilling	
		B. Focuses on the development of basic attitudes of *ego integrity vs. despair*	
		C. Remains optimistic and continues to grow	
		D. Adjusts to limitations	
		E. Adjusts to retirement	
		F. Adjusts to reorganized family patterns	
		G. Adjusts to losses	
		H. Accepts death with serenity	

Modified from Kreigh H, Perko J: *Psychiatric and mental health nursing; commitment to care and concern*, Reston, 1979, Reston Publishing.

TABLE 6-3	Ego Defense Mechanisms

Defense Mechanism	Example
Compensation: process by which a person makes up for a perceived deficiency by strongly emphasizing a feature that he or she regards as an asset	A businessman perceives his small physical stature negatively. He tries to overcome this by being aggressive, forceful, and controlling in business dealings.
Denial: avoidance of disagreeable realities by ignoring or refusing to recognize them; probably simplest and most primitive of all defense mechanisms	Mrs. P has just been told that her breast biopsy indicates a malignancy. When her husband visits her that evening, she tells him that no one has discussed the laboratory results with her.
Displacement: shift of emotion from a person or object to another usually neutral or less dangerous person or object	A 4-year-old boy is angry because his mother just punished him for drawing on his bedroom walls. He begins to play *war* with his soldier toys and has them battle and fight with each other.
Dissociation: the separation of any group of mental or behavioral processes from the rest of the person's consciousness or identity	A man is brought to the emergency room by the police and is unable to explain who he is and where he lives or works.
Identification: process by which a person tries to become like someone he or she admires by taking on thoughts, mannerisms, or tastes of that individual	Sally, 15 years old, has her hair styled similar to that of her young English teacher whom she admires.
Intellectualization: excessive reasoning or logic used to avoid experiencing disturbing feelings	A woman avoids dealing with her anxiety in shopping malls by explaining that she is saving the frivolous waste of time and money by not going into them.
Introjection: intense type of identification in which a person incorporates qualities or values of another person or group into his or her own ego structure. It is one of the earliest mechanisms of the child and is important in formation of conscience.	Eight-year-old Jimmy tells his 3-year-old sister, "Don't scribble in your book of nursery rhymes. Just look at the pretty pictures," thus expressing his parents' values to his little sister.
Isolation: splitting off of emotional components of a thought, which may be temporary or long term	A second-year medical student dissects a cadaver for her anatomy course without being disturbed by thoughts of death.
Projection: attributing one's thoughts or impulses to another person. Through this process, one can attribute intolerable wishes, emotional feelings, or motivations to another person	A young woman who denies she has sexual feelings about a co-worker accuses him without basis of being a "flirt" and says he is trying to seduce her.
Rationalization: offering a socially acceptable or apparently logical explanation to justify or make acceptable otherwise unacceptable impulses, feelings, behaviors, and motives	John fails an examination and complains that the lectures were not well organized or clearly presented.
Reaction formation: development of conscious attitudes and behavior patterns that are opposite to what one really feels or would like to do	A married woman who feels attracted to one of her husband's friends treats him rudely.
Regression: retreat in face of stress to behavior characteristic of any earlier level of development	Four-year-old Nicole, who has been toilet trained for more than a year, begins to wet her pants again when her new baby brother is brought home from the hospital.
Repression: involuntary exclusion of a painful or conflictual thought, impulse, or memory from awareness. It is the primary ego defense, and other mechanisms tend to reinforce it	Mr. R does not recall hitting his wife when she was pregnant.
Splitting: viewing people and situations as either all good or all bad; failure to integrate the positive and negative qualities of oneself	A friend tells you that you are the most wonderful person in the world one day and how much she hates you the next day.
Sublimation: acceptance of a socially approved substitute goal for a drive whose normal channel of expression is blocked	Ed has an impulsive and physically aggressive nature. He tries out for the football team and becomes a star tackle.
Suppression: a process often listed as a defense mechanism but really a conscious counterpart of repression; it is intentional exclusion of material from consciousness. At times, it may lead to subsequent repression.	A young man at work finds that he is thinking so much about his date that evening that it is interfering with his work. He decides to put it out of his mind until he leaves the office for the day.
Undoing: act or communication that partially negates a previous one; primitive defense mechanism	Larry makes a passionate declaration of love to Sue on a date. On their next meeting, he treats her formally and distantly.

From Stuart GW, Laraia MT: *Principles and practice of psychiatric nursing,* ed 7, St Louis, 2001, Mosby.

TABLE 6-4	Levels of Anxiety		
Severity of Anxiety	**Physical**	**Intellectual**	**Social and Emotional**

Minimal (near 0)	Basal levels of
	   Blood pressure
	   Pulse
	   Respiration rate
	   Oxygen consumption
	   Pupillary constriction
	   Muscles relaxed
		Cognitive activity minimal
		Disregard for external environ-
		   mental stimuli; no attempt
		   to actively process information
		Focus typically on single,
		   nonthreatening mental image
		States of altered consciousness
			No social interaction
			No attempt to deal with
			   environmental stimuli
			Minimal emotional activity
			Feelings of indifference,
			   invulnerability, and
			   contentment prevail

Mild (+1)	Low-level sympathetic arousal
	Moderate to low skeletal
	   muscle tension
	Body relaxed
	Voice calm, well modulated
		Perceptual field open; able to
		   shift focus of attention readily
		Passively aware of external
		   environment
		Self-referent thoughts positive;
		   low concern for unexpected or
		   negative outcomes
			Behavior primarily automatic;
			   habitual patterns and
			   well-learned skills
			Positive feeling of security,
			   confidence, and satisfaction
			   dominate
			Solitary activities

Moderate (+2)	Sympathetic nervous system
	   activation
	   ↑ Blood pressure
	   ↑ Pulse rate
	   ↑ Respiratory rate
	Pupillary dilation
	Sweat glands stimulated
	Peripheral vascular
	   constriction
	Increased muscular tension
	Heightened performance of
	   well-learned skills
	Rate of speech increased,
	   pitch heightened
	Increased alertness
		Narrowing of perception;
		   attentional focus on specific
		   internal or external stimuli
		Conscious effort in processing
		   of information; optimal level
		   for learning
		Self-referent thoughts—mixed;
		   some concern about personal
		   ability or available resources
		   necessary to solve problems;
		   probability of positive outcomes
		   increasingly uncertain
			Increased skill in learning and
			   refining of skills; analyzing
			   problematic situations;
			   integrating cognitive and motor
			   domains
			Feelings of challenge; drive
			   to resolve problems or dilemmas
			Mixed sense of
			   confidence/optimism with fear,
			   lowered self-esteem, and
			   potential inadequacy

Severe (+3)	Fight-or-flight response
	Stimulation of adrenal medulla
	   ↑ Catecholamines, accelerated
	   heart rate, palpitations
	   ↑ Blood glucose
	   ↑ Blood flow to digestive
	   system
	   ↓ Blood flow to skeletal
	   muscles
	Muscles extremely tense
	Hyperventilation
	Physical actions increasingly
	   agitated, pacing, wringing of
	   hands, fidgeting, trembling
	May experience loss of
	   appetite, nausea, "cold sweats"
	Rapid, high-pitched speech
	Facial expression: poor eye
	   contact, fleeting eye
	   movements
		Perceptual capacity restricted;
		   exclusive attention to singular
		   stimuli (internal or external) or
		   multifocal, fragmented
		   processing of stimuli
		Problem solving inefficient,
		   difficult
		Some threatening stimuli
		   disregarded, minimized, denied
		Disorientation in terms of time
		   and place
		Expected likelihood of
		   negative consequences or
		   outcomes high; estimates of
		   personal self-efficacy low
			Flight behavior may be
			   manifested by withdrawal,
			   denial, depression,
			   somatization
			Feelings of increasing
			   threat, need to respond to
			   situation are heightened
			Dissociating tendency;
			   feelings are denied

Panic (+4)	Continued physiological
	   arousal
	Actions disorganized,
	   directionless; unable to
	   execute simple motor tasks;
	   fumbling, gross motor
	   agitation, flailing
	May strike out verbally or
		Perception severely restricted,
		   may be impervious to external
		   stimuli
		Thoughts are random,
		   distorted, disconnected, logical
		   processing impaired
		Unable to solve problems;
		   limited tolerance for processing
			Emotionally drained,
			   overwhelmed
			Reliance on earlier, more
			   primitive coping behaviors:
			   crying, shouting, curling up,
			   rocking, freezing
			Feelings of impotence,
			   helplessness, agony and

From Keltner NL, Schwecke LH, Bostrom CE: *Psychiatric nursing,* ed 4, St. Louis, 2003, Mosby.

TABLE 6-4	Levels of Anxiety—cont'd		
Severity of Anxiety	Physical	Intellectual	Social and Emotional
	physically; may attempt to withdraw from situation Eventual depletion of sympathetic neurotransmitters Blood redistributed throughout body Hypotension May feel dizzy, faint, or exhausted Appears pale, drawn, weary Facial expression: aghast, grimacing, eyes fixed Voice louder, higher pitched	novel stimuli (verbal, auditory, or visual) Preoccupied with thoughts of highly probable negative outcomes; conclusions may be drawn, negative consequences seen as inevitable	desperation dominate; may be experienced as horror, dread, defenselessness; may be converted to anger, rage

3. Remain in control and calm; the patient fears losing control and needs to feel secure.
4. Communicate with clear, simple, short sentences because the patient's ability to deal with complex, abstract statements is compromised.
5. Use of as-necessary (PRN) medications may be needed to decrease patients' anxiety to a manageable level (e.g., lorazepam [Ativan], alprazolam [Xanax]).
6. Encourage use of relaxation techniques.
7. When appropriate, assist the patient with recognizing early signs of anxiety and effective ways to prevent its escalation.
8. Provide opportunities for discussion of the relationship of thoughts and verbalizations to anxiety.
9. Implement seclusion or restraints, or both, if patient is a danger to self or others.

Phobias

A. Definition: irrational, continual fear of an activity, situation, object, or event
B. Types
  1. Agoraphobia (literal meaning, *fear of the marketplace*) without panic attacks; fear of being away from a safe environment or person
  2. Social phobia: irrational fear of exposure to the scrutiny of others
  3. Simple phobia: a disabling fear of some specific object or situation, such as the fear of animals or of being in a high place
C. Assessment data
  1. Panic anxiety
  2. Anticipatory anxiety
  3. Recognition of phobia as irrational
  4. Defense mechanisms of displacement and repression
  5. Avoidance behaviors
  6. Interference with demands of daily activities
D. Interventions
  1. Accept the patient and his or her fears.
  2. Encourage involvement in activities that do not increase anxiety.
  3. Help the patient recognize that his or her behavior is an attempt to cope with anxiety.

4. Use a calm, nonauthoritative approach.
5. Reassure the patient that he or she will not be made to confront the phobia in treatment until ready to do so.
6. Use systematic desensitization.

Obsessive Compulsive Disorder (OCD)

A. Definition: obsessive thoughts (troublesome, persistent thoughts) and compulsions (ritualistic behaviors) that are repetitive
B. Assessment data
  1. Compulsive, ritualistic behavior
  2. Obsessive thoughts
  3. Alterations in normal functioning
  4. Fear of loss of control
  5. Feelings of guilt
  6. Suicidal thoughts or feelings
  7. Rumination (persistent meditation on thoughts)
  8. Insight impairment
  9. Feelings of worthlessness
  10. Decreased self-esteem
C. Interventions
  1. Allow patient time to perform rituals.
  2. Ensure that basic daily needs are met.
  3. Redirect rumination positively.
  4. Do not, initially, call attention to or interfere with the compulsive act.
  5. Demonstrate concern for and interest in the patient.
  6. Encourage verbalization of concerns and feelings.
  7. As anxiety decreases and patient feels comfortable talking with the staff, encourage the patient to talk about his or her behavior and thoughts.
  8. Encourage the patient to try to reduce the frequency of compulsive behavior.
  9. Some people respond to antidepressant medication.

Posttraumatic Stress Disorder (PTSD)

Characteristic symptoms after a psychologically traumatic event include numbness of responses, frequently reliving the event, dreams, depression, and anxiety.

Perception

A. Definition: awareness acquired through the five senses

B. Alterations: thought to be pathological conditions resulting from anxiety
  1. Illusion: misinterpretation of a sensory input
  2. Hallucination: a sensation without an external stimulus; these may be:
    a. Auditory: hearing nonexistent voices or sounds
    b. Olfactory: smelling nonexistent odors or aromas
    c. Visual: seeing nonexistent things, people, or animals
    d. Tactile: feeling somatic sensations
    e. Gustatory: experiencing flavors or tastes
  3. Delusion: a false belief, not based in fact, that cannot be changed by reasoning
    a. Delusions of grandeur: feelings of greatness
    b. Delusions of persecution: feelings of being mistreated
    c. Delusions of sin or guilt: feelings of deserving punishment
    d. Somatic delusions: feelings about the body or part of the body
C. Ideas of reference: feeling that certain events or words have special meaning for self

Thought Disorders

Schizophrenia is considered the psychiatric manifestation of thought disorder; this group of illnesses represents the largest number of mentally ill persons. Schizophrenia affects approximately 1% of the population.
A. Types of schizophrenia
  1. Disorganized: includes frequent incoherence, nonsystematized delusions, and inappropriate affect
  2. Catatonic: includes stupor, negativity, rigidity, excitement, and posturing
  3. Paranoid: includes persecutory delusions, grandiosity, delusional jealousy, and hallucinations
  4. Undifferentiated: does not fit criteria of other categories or combines them
  5. Residual: presence of residual symptoms (e.g., marked social isolation, inappropriate affect, odd beliefs) without delusions, hallucinations, or gross disorganization
B. Assessment data
  1. Delusions of being controlled
  2. Somatic delusions (grandiosity, religious, or nihilistic)
  3. Persecutory delusions accompanied by hallucinations
  4. Auditory hallucinations of a running commentary on behavior or thought
  5. Auditory hallucination on several occasions with content of more than one word
  6. Incoherence, looseness of association, illogical thinking with a deterioration in function
  7. Continuation of symptoms for 6 months or more, occurring before 45 years of age
C. Interventions
  1. Establish trust.
  2. Do not enter into the patient's delusions; maintain your own view of reality without demeaning the patient's view of reality.
  3. Do not argue about hallucinations; the patient views them as real.
  4. Offer reassurance: most patients are experiencing pain from their symptoms.
  5. Touch only with permission; the thought-disordered patient may have a distorted sense of his or her own person.

  6. If you are afraid, be aware that the patient will sense this: be sure you have sufficient backup for your own safety and comfort.
  7. Maintain patient safety.

AFFECTIVE DISORDERS

Disturbances in feeling or affective disorders are classified as either depressive disorders or bipolar disorders.

Depressive disorders

A. Major depression is the predominant mental illness in the United States and Canada, with ranges from 7% to 12% in the male population and 26% to 30% in the female population.
B. Assessment data
  1. Persistent sadness, hopelessness, or tearfulness
  2. Loss of interest in some or all usual activities, fatigue, inability to concentrate
  3. Change in appetite: usually decreased
  4. Changes in weight: usually a loss in weight
  5. Sleep disturbances: usually insomnia but may be increased hours of sleep per day
  6. Withdrawal from family and friends; feeling guilty and unworthy
  7. Hopelessness and helplessness that may become profound and may lead to delusions or fantasies of *ending it all*
  8. If left in this pattern, the patient eventually might justify how nonexistence may solve the problems.
  9. The patient may start to dwell on death and to devise a plan of self-destruction.
  10. Self-destruction becomes the goal; this is suicidal ideation.
C. See suicide prevention and suicide intervention.

Bipolar disorders

A. Category used when one or more manic episodes are noted, whether a depressive episode is or has been experienced
B. Mania characterized by unstable mood, pressured speech, and increased motor activity
C. Intervention
  1. Demonstrate sincere interest.
  2. Accept the patient's feelings; anger may be directed to the nearest safe object, often the nurse.
  3. Allow the patient to express feelings; for example, crying in a dignified environment.
  4. Encourage only the expression of feelings that you believe capable of handling; for example, do not encourage ventilation of feelings and then go to lunch.
  5. If the patient is overactive, limit setting or reduction of stimuli may be necessary.
  6. Avoid power struggles: use force only if necessary to protect the patient or others in the environment.

EATING DISORDERS

A. Obesity and compulsive overeating: consuming greater than the required number of calories, which results in weight gain; not burning as many calories as consumed; the person is usually considered obese when weight is 20% greater than is recommended for his or her height.

B. Anorexia nervosa: an eating disorder characterized by refusal to maintain a minimally normal body weight; it is most often seen in adolescent women (may occur with bulimia or separately).

C. Bulimia: an eating disorder characterized by episodes of binging and then purging; person may not appear overweight or underweight; with nonpurging bulimia, the person uses laxatives, diuretics, fasting, or exercise to control his or her weight; bulimia leads to other symptoms, such as menstrual irregularities, gastric dilation, aspiration pneumonia, dental caries (caused by frequent vomiting), and esophagitis.

PERSONALITY DISORDERS

A. Paranoid personality: characterized by suspicion, rigidity, secretiveness, over sensitivity and alertness, distortions of reality, and the use of projection as a major defense mechanism

B. Borderline personality: at times, moderately neurotic; at other times, overtly psychotic; extremely difficult to treat and often unstable after numerous treatment attempts
  1. Assessment data
    a. Combined anger and depression
    b. Anhedonia (inability to experience pleasure)
    c. Social isolation
    d. Poor impulse control
    e. Dependency
    f. Substance abuse
    g. Sexual promiscuity
  2. Interventions
    a. Be honest with patients.
    b. These patients are often manipulative and attention seeking.
    c. They tend to view people or situations as all good or all bad.
    d. Patients need to begin developing meaningful relationships in which they can begin to trust.
    e. Consistency is important; patients may split the staff to play one staff member against another.

C. Codependency: meeting goals successfully by relying on another person for the answers; characteristics of the codependent person include the following:
  1. Partners are dependent on each other to make a whole relationship.
  2. One of the partners in this relationship assumes a passive role.
  3. One or both may have low self-esteem.
  4. One or both may have poor self-image.
  5. One or both may have an addictive disorder (alcohol, drugs, and so forth).
  6. They tend to be manipulative—a constant conflict exists, either between them or within the family.
  7. They tend to operate in a series of delusions.
  8. Because of delusions, they tend to promote their version of any story as the absolute truth.
  9. They exhibit poor boundaries (limits) in relationships.
  10. They are somewhat to totally insensitive to others' emotions and feelings.
  11. If the codependency exists within family, it is highly likely that a dysfunctional family unit will emerge and the children will become a part of the codependency.
  12. Codependency may be intergenerational and therefore cyclical.
  13. The treatment of codependent persons is designed by identifying the underlying emotions that are fostering the codependency.

D. Substance abuse disorders: a pattern of pathological use of substances that entails factors such as the need for daily use, loss of control, efforts to control use, overdoses, impairment of social functioning, family disruptions, legal problems, and so on; abuse is distinguished from dependency by tolerance of the substance (increasing use requires increasing doses to achieve the same effect) and the presence or absence of a withdrawal syndrome.
  1. Alcoholism
    a. Abuse is distinguished from recreational use by features such as daily drinking, frequent need for the chemical, blackouts, social impairment, and decreased ability to function, such as job loss, driving while intoxicated, arrests, and so forth.
    b. Acute alcohol ingestion may result in a condition formerly known as delirium tremens (DTs), now known as acute alcohol withdrawal syndrome; key features are hallucinations, extreme agitation, and disorientation; treatment includes anxiolytics (benzodiazepines), anticonvulsants, and hydration.
    c. Long-term use may lead to peripheral neuropathy, Wernicke's syndrome (confusion, ataxia, and abnormal eye movements), or Korsakoff's syndrome (alcoholic amnesia syndrome), which is manifested by memory loss and confabulation; these effects are largely caused by deficiency of thiamine and may be partially reversed by providing thiamine; Korsakoff's syndrome is usually irreversible but may be arrested by thiamine replacement therapy and cessation of alcohol abuse.
  2. Barbiturate and sedative abuse (barbiturates or minor tranquilizers such as diazepam, benzodiazepines, and so forth)
    a. Cross-tolerant with alcohol
    b. May be used by street addicts when they are unable to obtain opiates
    c. Second most abused substance after alcohol in the United States
    d. Legally obtained drugs are often used by middle-class women who overuse tranquilizers.
    e. Intoxication is similar to that from alcohol.
    f. A withdrawal syndrome occurs that is similar to that from alcohol withdrawal.
  3. Opiates (heroin, morphine)
    a. Includes street addicts using intravenous (IV) heroin, as well as *medical addicts* who use various prescribed substances such as codeine
    b. IV drug users are at a high risk for acquired immunodeficiency syndrome (AIDS).
    c. Intoxication includes pupil constriction, poor attention span, apathy, slurred speech, euphoria, and psychomotor retardation.
    d. A physical withdrawal syndrome occurs.
  4. Cocaine
    a. Stimulant
    b. Increasing use among the middle class
    c. Considered a social drug, many people believe that it is not addictive.

d. May be snorted or smoked as a *free-base* or as crack.
e. Intoxication includes poor judgment, poor impulse control, feeling of confidence, euphoria, talkative, rapid speech, pacing, elevated heart rate and blood pressure, dilated pupils, nausea, and sweating.
f. May lead to hallucinations with prolonged use; severe depression occurs after the substance use is stopped, leading to strong psychological craving.
g. A true withdrawal syndrome may not occur.

5. Amphetamines
a. Abuse may begin in an effort to control weight or to stay awake for long periods.
b. May be used IV by addicts for a *rush;* may be combined with other drugs such as heroin or barbiturates.
c. Intoxication includes elevated heart rate and blood pressure, dilated pupils, chills, perspiration, nausea, and vomiting.
d. Popular drug of abuse used by truck drivers, used to facilitate driving coast to coast without sleep.

6. Hallucinogens (lysergic acid diethylamide [LSD], mescaline, and so forth)
a. Used much less than in the early 1970s
b. Use leads to altered perceptions and hallucinations; distorted perception of colors; illusions and delusions; unpredictable effects
c. Intoxication includes perceptual changes; dilated pupils; increased pulse, sweating, anxiety, tremors; feelings of paranoia; and poor judgment.

7. Cannabis (marijuana, hashish)
a. Widely used by various groups, usually smoked or eaten
b. Intoxication includes increased pulse rate, bloodshot eyes, increased appetite, dry mouth, distorted perception of time, euphoria, and apathy.
c. May precipitate panic attacks.
d. Used with medical approval in some places—counteracts side effects of some chemotherapy.

8. Substance abuse interventions
a. Severe denial is a common defense mechanism.
b. Keep the patient focused on the purpose of treatment.
c. Manipulation may be used to obtain a substance for abuse.
d. The nurse must remain nonjudgmental.
e. These patients may require repeated attempts at treatment before they can conquer their addiction.
f. Adequate diet, rest, and vitamin supplements are helpful.
g. Long-term success is often achieved through a lifelong affiliation with abstinence programs such as Alcoholics Anonymous (AA) and Narcotics Anonymous (NA).
h. Alcoholism is usually treated in several steps, the first being detoxification; in detoxification, the alcoholic is withdrawn from the chemical through the use of a cross-tolerant substance, usually a benzodiazepine, which is administered for 3 to 5 days in decreasing doses; alcoholics are often referred to AA.
(1) Detoxification should occur in a controlled (monitored) setting because detoxification may become life threatening.
(2) After the acute detoxification period of 3 to 5 days, intense counseling occurs.

(3) The patient may find that continuing in a peer group setting on a regular full- or part-time schedule is beneficial.
(4) In some cases, additional treatment may be suggested in the form of halfway houses, which may offer up to 6 months to 1 year of treatment.
i. Other forms of substance abuse are treated similarly, with combinations of detoxification, if needed, and supportive long-term treatment settings; opiate abusers may also be treated with methadone maintenance in attempts to prevent heroin use and allow the addict to return to more socially acceptable behavior patterns.

PHYSICALLY BASED MENTAL DISORDERS

A. Organic brain syndrome (dementia) may result from vascular disorders of the brain, brain infections, trauma, altered metabolism, poisoning, endocrine disorders, and deficiencies.
1. Global involvement: confusion, delirium, and dementia
2. Selective involvement: may be limited to portions of the personality (e.g., amnesia, hallucinations, psychosomatic disorders)
3. Functional impairment: has the features of psychosis (e.g. paranoia, depression, mania)
4. Special needs of the older adult: special consideration is given to the role of declining physical attributes.
a. Prejudices regarding older adults may be present.
b. Most older adults are not senile.
c. Apparent senile-type behavior may be the result of depression or other forms of illness (e.g., alcoholism).
d. The reaction to drugs of all types may be idiosyncratic (unusual response) among older adults.
e. Special techniques
(1) Life review
(2) Group work aimed at socialization, such as remotivation
(3) Touch: many older adults are deprived of touch in the usual manner because of relational losses.
(4) Medication history review
(5) See Chapter 9 for special needs of the aging adult.

B. Mental retardation: sub-average intelligence; numerous causes have been discovered, including inherited defects in metabolism, genetic defects, birth injuries, and developmental anomalies.
1. Mental retardation: classified as follows, with interventions geared accordingly:
a. Profoundly retarded: needs total nursing care in early stages; the person may later develop rudimentary ability to care for self; always requires some care
b. Severely retarded: may be able to care for self in protected environment; requires monitoring
c. Moderately retarded: usually capable of self-care but requires supervision when under stress
d. Mildly retarded: usually self-supporting; may require support of family or others when under stress
2. Special needs of children and adolescents: many similarities and some differences exist in the therapeutics for children and adolescents.
a. Services in hospitals are usually short and aimed at assessment and evaluation.
b. Most ongoing treatment is on an outpatient basis.

c. Treatment is action oriented, using such modalities as play therapy.

d. Many issues of trust versus mistrust are present.

e. Issues of self-image, limit testing, and developmentally specific concerns exist.

f. Treatment is selected based on the child's mental age, not his or her physical age.

C. Other somatic manifestations of mental disturbance: several conditions, some of which are listed here, have defined or suggested psychological bases.

1. Ulcers
2. Bowel disorders
3. Cardiovascular disorders
4. Asthma
5. Allergies
6. Eating disorders: anorexia, bulimia
7. Headaches
8. Certain endocrine disorders: hyperthyroid, hypothyroid, and so forth

DEATH AND DYING

Nursing intervention is aimed at ensuring the transition of the patient through each of the stages listed in this section. Being aware of your own attitude about death and ensuring that you are meeting the patient's needs and not your own are important. Being nonjudgmental and allowing the expression of emotions by the patient are also essential. Patient defenses are necessary in accepting his or her own death and should not be challenged. Elisabeth Kübler-Ross describes dying as a process that proceeds through the following stages:

A. Shock and denial: the patient cannot actually accept or believe that he or she is going to die; he or she may repress information, seek to escape the truth by seeking other opinions, and be unable to hear the real message.

B. Anger and rage: the patient becomes angry with the terrible truth of impending death; he or she may be hypercritical of others, demanding, and resentful; health care workers often bear the brunt of a patient's rage because they represent cure for others but not for him or her.

C. Bargaining: acceptance has begun, and the patient begins to bargain for more time or for some specific request; during this stage, wills may be finalized and legacies of various kinds bestowed; if possible, requests should be granted because they bring comfort to the dying person.

D. Depression: after acceptance of the inevitable has begun, the person feels sad and alone; he or she may speak little and cry often; quiet acceptance is often the most helpful kind of intervention in this stage.

E. Acceptance: once this occurs, the person is often seen as tranquil and at peace with him or herself; again, the patient may speak little because most of what he or she has to say to others has been said; although still sad, the patient has made his or her peace with death and has accepted the inevitable; this phase may last for months or longer.

GRIEVING

George Engel (1964) defined grieving as a process of sequential steps similar to those in the dying process.

A. Shock and disbelief: the person refuses to accept the loss, may feel stunned or numbed; it is similar to the first stage of dying.

B. Developing awareness: the person may experience varying degrees of physical symptoms such as nausea, vomiting, and loss of appetite; crying is common, and anger may be felt and expressed toward the lost person for the act of desertion; anger may be self-directed and recriminations made.

C. Restitution (resolution): acceptance occurs and is aided by the culturally approved modes of grieving, such as funerals and wearing black.

D. The process of grieving may take more than 1 year; all stages must be experienced for grief to be successfully completed; if grieving is not successful, it may lead to one of the following:

1. Delayed reaction: a later reaction to the loss; delay is caused by repressing reality; it may result in more painful experiences than the normal immediate reaction.

2. Distorted reactions: may include the development of symptoms similar to those of the lost person: medical illnesses, social isolation, agitated depression, and increased use of alcohol or other drugs may occur.

CRISIS INTERVENTION

Generally, all crisis situations have common components. With this knowledge, strategies are developed to assist people through a crisis and minimize its detrimental effects.

A. Crisis is an event that disturbs the equilibrium of the individual or family.

B. The disturbance leads to development of certain symptoms, most notably, anxiety and depression.

C. These feelings continue until a need is felt to reduce or alleviate them.

D. If the person or family has adequate coping mechanisms, the problem will be resolved and the balance restored.

E. Without coping mechanisms, anxiety and depression increase to intolerable levels.

F. Interventions are aimed at providing short-term therapy to increase coping behaviors.

G. Most crises are resolved within 6 to 8 weeks.

H. Intervention entails:

1. A thorough assessment of the situation
2. Planned strategies that do not attempt to rearrange a person's life
3. Strategies that increase intellectual understanding, explore current feelings, offer coping mechanisms, and support existing ties and helpful relationships

CRISIS OF RAPE OR INCEST

Assisting survivors of these violent acts requires substantial time. Intervention begins when the victim calls for help in any form or seeks treatment. This type of violence has two possible phases. One is the acute or immediate phase wherein the victim exhibits fear, confusion, disorganization, and restlessness. The second phase is a long-term process of reorganization and usually begins weeks after the attack.

A. Early relevant feelings include:

1. Physical pain

2. Anger
3. Fear of another attack
4. Outrage at the perpetrator
5. Total violation of (emotional) space
6. Fear of involvement with anyone of the same sex as the perpetrator
7. Emotional drain
8. Helplessness
9. Fear of pregnancy
B. If these immediate feelings are not externalized and dealt with, the result may be permanent psychological damage, including but not limited to the following psychosexual dysfunctions:
1. Sexual arousal disorders
2. Sexual deviations (several varieties)
3. Sexual aversions
4. Delusions of violent sexual behavior, which can be incorporated in the patient's lifestyle
C. Interventions include the following:
1. Assess the victim's safety: "Are you in a safe place?" "Is there help for you?"
2. Listen: accept what is said.
3. Respond as appropriate.
4. Refer patient to appropriate agency.

SUICIDE PREVENTION

Suicide ranks as a leading cause of death in the United States. Specific indicators assist in assessing suicidal risk.
A. Risk factors include:
1. Age and sex: more women attempt suicide; more men are successful.
2. Men over 35 are at higher risk; most suicides occur in men between the ages of 35 and 50 years.
3. Anxiety and depression: many potential suicide victims report increasing anxiety and depression; most significant is a recent change in these feelings.
4. Past coping pattern does not work in the current situation.
5. A past suicide attempt is always considered a high-risk factor.
6. Alcohol or drug abuse: many suicides are committed by alcoholics.
7. Concrete plan: if a plan is in place, considerations include the following:
   a. Is it set in a current time frame?
   b. Is it lethal?
   c. Does the potential victim have the necessary resources to carry out the plan?
8. Significant others: a suicide is often committed to communicate with others.
B. Interventions include the following:
1. Focus on clear and present danger.
2. Reduce present hazards.
3. Give clear directions for patient to follow.
4. Assign to constant monitoring in a hospital.
5. Mobilize significant others when possible.
6. Mobilize past coping mechanisms.
7. Assign concrete specific tasks.
8. Explore positive alternatives to suicide.
9. Teach problem-solving techniques.

SUICIDE INTERVENTION

Intervention becomes critical at the point of suicidal ideation. If intervention does not occur, suicide is highly likely. The patient may be having underlying feelings of hopelessness, helplessness, and impending doom. Frequently, the patient will verbalize the need to *end it all*.
A. Always ask:
1. "Do I understand that you want to hurt yourself?" (This confirms suicide ideation.)
2. "Do you have a plan or how will you hurt yourself? Will you share your plan with me?" (Suicidal gesturing may be evident.)
3. If the specific plan calls for using an enabling device or instrument: May I have the _____ that is included in the plan? (Specify item: knife, razor, and rope for example.)
B. Ordinarily, a loud cry for help can be heard before the suicide occurs if others are perceptive enough to hear it.
NOTE: Severely depressed patients are so physically impaired that they rarely have the energy to commit suicide. As the depression begins to lift, the potential to commit suicide increases, that is, especially if they have communicated the need to *end it all*.

TREATMENT MODALITIES

Psychotherapy

A. Individual psychotherapy: one-to-one relationship between a therapist (physician, psychologist, social worker, nurse clinician) and a patient; sessions of 45 to 50 minutes are usually held weekly or more often; the aim is to improve the functioning of the person; it is most effective with the neuroses and in patients who have good verbal skills and high intelligence.
B. Family group therapy: a family is seen as a group by a therapist, based on the premise that disturbance arises as a function of family interactions and that treatment must be aimed at the family as a whole.
C. Group therapy: treatment provided to a group of persons related by age, symptom, or other commonality; treatment occurs on a weekly or biweekly basis and may include more than one therapist.
D. Behavior modification: techniques are based on conditioning; undesired behaviors are ignored, and desired behaviors are rewarded.

Milieu Therapy

Milieu therapy is the use of a controlled environment to influence the treatment of a patient.
A. Interactions between patient and staff, as well as interpatient relationships, are used as a basis for treatment.
B. Therapeutic communications: behavior modeling and some behavior-modification techniques are often used.

Therapeutic Community

Therapeutic community (Maxwell Jones, 1968) is a method of establishing a milieu for treatment wherein all members, staff and patients, have assigned responsibilities and defined roles in the community. The reasoning is that this type of democratic environment prepares the patient for release into the larger community.

Electroconvulsive Therapy

Use of electroconvulsive therapy (ECT, shock therapy) has recently increased for patients with severe depression who have not responded to other therapies. ECT is the application of an electrical current through the brain, resulting in a grand mal seizure. Some patients suffer a short-term memory loss as a result of the treatment. A physician using general anesthesia gives the treatments; the treatment can be given on an outpatient or inpatient basis. Some patients with severe depression can control further episodes with regular periodic treatments.

Psychopharmacological Therapy

Psychopharmacological agents are used in treating mental health disorders. NOTE: When administering medication to the mental health patient, remember to use a tongue blade to examine the interior of the mouth if you suspect the patient is "cheeking" the medication.
A. Anti-extra pyramidal symptoms (anti-EPS): EPS are unusual muscle movement that involves the fine muscles of the body; these symptoms are acute and tonic or dystonic reactions to the antipsychotic medication.
   1. Frequently, EPS appear in the tongue or in the muscles of the upper chest, neck, and shoulders.
   2. Anti-EPS medications used to reverse the muscular effects of the antipsychotics are diphenhydramine hydrochloride (Benadryl) and benztropine mesylate (Cogentin).
B. See Chapter 3 (Pharmacology) for greater detail regarding drugs that are commonly used to treat mental illness.

Adjunctive Therapies

A. Occupational therapy: the use of vocational tasks to allow patients to express various underlying feelings
B. Recreational therapy: the use of recreational activities to allow patients to express feelings
C. Art therapy: the use of the plastic and graphic arts to express feelings
D. Other therapies may include vocational counseling, bibliotherapy (writing or reading), and dance therapy.

ETHICAL CONSIDERATIONS IN PATIENT CARE

A. In most places, patients may sue institutions under habeas corpus proceedings for their release from treatment.
B. Laws guarantee rights to patients.
C. Nurses and other staff members may be sued for assault and battery for forcing treatments on patients.
D. Wrongful death suits have been brought in circumstances in which a patient has died.

E. A narrow line exists between therapeutic treatment and abuse; you may restrict privileges based on noncompliance with plan of care; but you must be careful that these are not viewed or used as threats.
F. Local laws vary in different parts of the country, and nurses should be aware of local statutes.
G. Confidentiality is essential in mental health nursing.
H. Communications between a patient and a nurse may be considered *privileged*, whereas most medical records are open to subpoena.
I. Documents should contain only factual material not conjecture (opinion).
J. If a patient threatens bodily harm to others, such information is no longer considered privileged and is required to be reported to the authorities.
K. Oppressive mental institutions may infringe on a patient's rights, and nurses should be aware of their responsibilities in such situations.
L. If the patient has information and chooses not to comply, he or she is noncompliant; the nurse has allowed the patient his/her rights if the information was provided and questions answered; the nurse cannot force treatment on the patient.

PATIENT'S RIGHTS MOVEMENT

A. Although patients in psychiatric settings are ill, they retain their civil rights and are often specifically protected under special sections of the law.
B. In most places, *commitment* removes only the patient's right to leave the hospital or terminate treatment.
C. Recent legal decisions indicate that patients may expect treatment and may not simply be detained in hospitals where no active treatment is available.
D. In recent years, patient and former-patient groups have formed and demanded access to records of treatment rationales.

CARE AND TREATMENT OF PATIENTS

Basic needs: the basic needs of patients in psychiatric settings are similar to those of other patients; usually, psychiatric patients do not have the accompanying impairments of the physically ill patient.
A. Most patients are ambulatory.
B. The nurse's role is to guide, encourage, and teach by example.
C. Patients may be socially deteriorated and require assistance in ADL such as how to arrange time to complete their own care.
D. Reward such as praise is helpful in guiding patients in these activities.

SUGGESTED READINGS

American Psychiatric Association: *Diagnostic and statistical manual of mental disorders,* ed 4, Washington, DC, the Association.

Bauer B, Hill S: *Mental health nursing: an introductory text,* Philadelphia, 2000, WB Saunders.

Carson VB, Arnold EN: *Mental health nursing: the nurse-patient journey,* Philadelphia, 1996, WB Saunders.

Fontaine KL, Fletcher JS: *Mental health nursing,* ed 4, Upper Saddle River, NJ, 1999, Prentice Hall Health.

Fortinash KM, Holoday-Worret PA: *Psychiatric mental health nursing,* ed 2, St Louis, 1999, Mosby.

Haber J, Krainovich-Miller B, McMahon AL: *Comprehensive psychiatric nursing,* ed 5, St Louis, 1997, Mosby.

Keltner NI, Schwecke LH, Bostrom CE: *Psychiatric nursing,* ed 3, St Louis, 1999, Mosby.

Morrison M: *Foundations of mental health nursing,* St Louis, 1997, Mosby.

Rawlins RP, Williams SR, Beck CK: *Mental health-psychiatric nursing,* ed 3, St Louis, 1993, Mosby.

Stuart GW, Laraia MT: *Principles and practice of psychiatric nursing,* ed 6, St Louis, 1998, Mosby.

Townsend M: *Psychiatric mental health nursing,* Philadelphia, 1999, FA Davis Co.

Varcarolis EM: *Foundations of psychiatric-mental health nursing,* ed 3, Philadelphia, 1998, WB Saunders.

REVIEW QUESTIONS

1. The nurse is assigned to work with a depressed patient and wants to make sure that her initial contact does what?
   1. Addresses the root of depression
   2. Keeps communication open
   3. Establishes trust
   4. Raises the patient's spirits

2. Which of the following reasons would cause a psychiatric patient to be institutionalized? Select all that apply.
   1. Homelessness
   2. Threat to self
   3. Threat to others
   4. Low income

3. A nurse is caring for a patient with major depression. When planning activities, the nurse knows that the patient needs:
   1. Frequent changes in activities
   2. Constant redirection into numerous activities
   3. Behavior modification that restructures feelings
   4. Well-defined, structured interactions at the beginning of treatment

4. A patient was given both verbal and written instructions before his discharge. He verbalized an understanding of his instructions but has made no attempt to take his medication as ordered or to return for a follow-up visit. He may be labeled as noncompliant.

5. How should the nurse reward a patient who has taken an active role in implementing the treatment plan?
   1. Privileges
   2. Extra snacks
   3. Praise
   4. Money

6. The nurse is admitting a schizophrenic patient that has not eaten in 3 days. The nurse arranges for food to be brought to the patient before she begins the admission paperwork. Based on the five dimensions of holism, this meets what basic need? Physical

7. Personality is the result of:
   1. Heredity and environment
   2. Temperament and heredity
   3. Environment and nurturing
   4. Nurturing and heredity

8. In what step of the nursing process do the patient and nurse develop the goals?
   1. Data gathering
   2. Planning
   3. Implementation
   4. Evaluation

9. A patient approaches the nurse and says, "I am omnipotent. Some day soon I'm going to take over this unit, you'll see." The appropriate nursing intervention should be to:
   1. Call a code.
   2. Tell the patient that no one is omnipotent and to calm down.
   3. Redirect the patient.
   4. Ask the patient why he thinks he is omnipotent.

10. In what phase of the nurse-patient relationship does termination begin?
    1. Presentation
    2. Orientation
    3. Working
    4. Termination

11. Suicide is most likely to occur:
    1. On admission
    2. On discharge
    3. As the depression deepens
    4. As the depression lifts

12. Select all the following interventions that may positively impact a patient with obsessive compulsive disorder (OCD).
    1. The nurse shows concern for the patient.
    2. The nurse assists with activities of daily living (ADL).
    3. The nurse hurries the patient through the ritual.
    4. The nurse makes a point of calling attention to the repetitive act.
    5. The nurse encourages the patient to reduce the frequency of the behavior.

13. A hallucination that the patient labels as a "funny smell" is known to the nurse as:
    1. Tactile
    2. Auditory
    3. Gustatory
    4. Olfactory

14. To help a patient cope with death, the nurse must first know:
    1. How she feels about death
    2. How the patient feels about dying
    3. How the family feels about the patient's illness
    4. The meaning of death

15. In what treatment modality does a group of patients meet on a regular basis for treatment?
    1. Individual psychotherapy
    2. Family therapy
    3. Group therapy
    4. Behavior modification

16. The patient is being admitted to the psychiatric unit and is extremely agitated and pacing the floor. Which of the following nursing interventions would have priority at this time?
    1. Placing the patient in a quiet area away from other patients
    2. Encouraging the patient to participate in a group activity
    3. Setting firm limits on the patient's behavior
    4. Orienting the patient to his room and the nursing unit

17. The nurse was told in report that she is to observe a particular patient for extrapyramidal side effects, which includes:
    1. Dry mouth, anorexia
    2. Gastrointestinal (GI) upset, constipation
    3. Heart palpitations
    4. Muscle rigidity, tremors

18. A nurse working in a hospice overhears one of the patients talking with the physician, begging to be kept alive just 1 more year. The nurse recognizes this as what stage of the grief process?
    1. Denial
    2. Bargaining
    3. Depression
    4. Acceptance

19. The patient yells at the nurse after talking on the phone with their spouse. The nurse recognized this as what type of defense mechanism? Displacement
(Feelings for an object/person are transfered to to a less threatening object/person)

20. The nurse is assisting in the discharge plans for an alcoholic patient. To what outpatient support group should she refer the client? **AA**

21. Which of the following statements by the nurse would gain the most information from a patient who is going through a family crisis?
    1 "Do you hate your spouse?"
    2 "Do you and your family get along?"
    3 "Do you see your family often?"
    (4) "What is it like with you and your family?"

22. Which of the following may be seen in a patient diagnosed with anxiety? Select all that apply.
    (1) Pacing
    (2) Hyperventilation
    (3) Muscle tension
    (4) Loss of appetite
    5 Hypotension
    6 Calmness

23. Which of the following may a nurse see in a patient experiencing a panic attack? Select all that apply.
    (1) Feels faint
    (2) Complains of being "dizzy"
    3 Is able to problem solve
    4 Has increased attention span
    (5) Is agitated

24. A patient is admitted to a psychiatric unit following an unsuccessful suicide attempt. He repeatedly tells the nurse, "I want to die, please help me die." The most appropriate nursing response is:
    1 "Don't worry, you're safe here."
    2 "Relax, nobody's going to kill you."
    3 "Why do you want to die?"
    (4) "You must be feeling very sad right now."

25. The nurse is caring for a patient returning to his room following electroconvulsive therapy (ECT). What behavior should the nurse expect him to exhibit?
    1 The patient complains to the nurse that someone is poisoning his food.
    2 The patient goes to the game room to play pool.
    (3) The patient is unable to recall the date. *Amnesia is*
    4 The patient prepares to go on a field trip. *Common p̄ ECT*

26. How is bipolar disorder exhibited? **Depression alternating c̄ mania**

27. Patients who abuse alcohol may become tremulous and have hallucinations when they stop drinking. This is called:
    1 Tolerance
    2 Abstinence
    (3) Withdrawal
    4 Dementia

28. List two nursing diagnoses for a patient in the manic phase of bipolar disorder. **Risk for Injury / Disturbed thought process**

29. What are two priority nursing interventions to use during the manic phase of bipolar disorder?
    (1) Decrease environmental stimuli.
    (2) Ensure a safe environment.
    3 Pace activities to keep patient busy.
    4 Monitor drug levels daily.

30. Which of the following items indicate major depression? Select all that apply.

(1) Hopelessness
(2) Sadness
3 Motivation
4 Increased self-esteem
(5) Weight loss

31. A patient is admitted to a psychiatric unit. After completing the nursing history and assessment, the nurse determines that a tour of the unit and explanation of the unit rules and regulations is appropriate. The nurse's rationale for this intervention is to:
    (1) Reduce the patient's anxiety.
    2 Demonstrate that interaction with others is required.
    3 Ensure that patient rights are not violated.
    4 Make sure that all the other patients know who the new patient is.

32. When the nurse gathered admission data on a patient, it was determined that the patient is on the health end of the mental health–mental illness continuum. Which of the following statements best supports these findings?
    1 The patient is in an abusive marriage.
    2 The patient describes her life as boring.
    (3) The patient is satisfied with her life.
    4 The patient is being checked for terminal disease.

33. The nurse has noted substantial changes in the behavior of a suicidal patient. Which intervention by the nurse would be most therapeutic?
    1 Document the observations.
    2 Ask co-workers if they have also noticed the changes.
    (3) Ask the patient, "Are you thinking of suicide?"
    4 Restrict the patient's privileges.

34. Which of the following best indicates that the patient is at high risk for suicide?
    (1) Patient has a lethal plan.
    2 Patient is in a shaky relationship.
    3 Patient has made verbal threats.
    4 Patient does not have a strong support system.

35. Repetitive behaviors in response to impulses are **Compulsions**.

36. A nurse is caring for a mentally ill patient who is convinced that his wife is trying to kill him. No evidence exists to support this belief. The nurse recognizes the patient is suffering from:
    (1) Delusions
    2 Hallucinations
    3 Illusions
    4 Compensation

37. A nurse is caring for a patient with bulimia; the patient tells the nurse that she has been bulimic for the last 5 years. In assessing the patient, the nurse hears about the following complaints:
    1 GI upset
    (2) Toothache
    3 Diarrhea
    4 Sore throat

38. A patient tells the nurse that electrodes are in her head that are making her arms and legs burn. Which of the following responses is most therapeutic?
    1 "That's silly; your legs are okay."
    2 "Does the fire travel from one leg to the other?"
    3 "If your legs were burning, I would see it."
    (4) "I understand you feel the fire. How can you stop it?"

39. Paranoid thinking is characterized by feelings of:
    1. Anger and aggression
    2. Suspicion and jealousy
    3. Self-pity and self-centeredness
    4. Simultaneous hero worship and hero hating
40. The nurse is caring for a patient who is undergoing electroconvulsive therapy (ECT). In planning his care, what should the nurse expect?
    1. The patient will be incontinent.
    2. The patient will be at risk for suicide.
    3. The patient will cry and be depressed.
    4. The patient will be confused and experience a temporary loss of recent memories.
41. A nursing diagnosis in psychiatric nursing is:
    1. A behavior or problem related to its probable cause
    2. Not used because nurses do not diagnose
    3. Based on the medical condition of the patient
    4. Useful only in general hospital settings
42. An irrational fear is known as a _Phobia_.
43. A patient, admitted with chronic depression, has not responded to antidepressant medications. The physician has ordered electroconvulsive therapy (ECT) treatments. The patient has signed the permission slip and is asking the nurse what to expect following the treatment. Which of the following responses is most appropriate for the nurse to give the patient?
    1. "ECT changes your chemical messengers."
    2. "ECT will change your subconscious thoughts."
    3. "ECT will cause you to have seizure activity."
    4. "ECT will assist in alleviating your depression.
44. Select all of the following findings that would contribute to a diagnosis of anxiety.
    1. Follows directions easily
    2. Apprehension
    3. Uneasiness
    4. Decreased concentration
    5. Pays attention to details
    6. Waits patiently for a turn
45. A patient approaches the nurse and says, "With all my troubles, I feel worthless. I would like to end all this misery. Everyone would be better off if I were gone." The nurse's most appropriate response to this statement would be:
    1. "Tell me more."
    2. "Are you thinking of killing yourself?"
    3. "I can see that you are very upset."
    4. "I have to take blood pressures right now, then we can talk."
46. A patient exhibiting which of the following signs and symptoms would be diagnosed with a paranoid personality disorder?
    1. Is suspicious of others
    2. Is jealous of his or her spouse
    3. Has strong social support
    4. Is able to control his or her temper
47. A nurse is assigned to a patient scheduled for electroconvulsive therapy (ECT) in the morning. The patient tells the nurse that she is fearful and cannot go through with the treatment as scheduled. The best response from the nurse would be:
    1. "You will be all right."
    2. "Tell me how you feel."

3. "Do you wish to stay depressed?"
4. "ECT is safe for most people."
48. A 42-year-old patient was admitted to the unit for alcohol rehabilitation. The patient tells the nurse that he often cannot remember what he does while he is drinking. The nurse asks him additional questions and determines that he is suffering from:
    1. Psychosis
    2. Blackouts
    3. Denial
    4. Alcoholism
49. A patient tells the nurse that the television is cursing her and that electrodes in her head are making her arms and legs burn. The idea of the television cursing the patient is an example of:
    1. Persecutory delusion
    2. Visual hallucination
    3. Incoherence
    4. Flight of ideas
50. In what eating disorders does the patient exhibit insatiable craving for food but is able to keep weight within a normal range?
    Bulimia
51. Nurses working on the admissions unit of a psychiatric facility frequently care for aggressive patients. The best nursing intervention in most cases when caring for an aggressive patient is to:
    1. Apply restraints until the patient calms down.
    2. Take away privileges if behavior is inappropriate.
    3. Schedule activities with limited stimuli.
    4. Plan a variety of activities to keep the patient occupied.
52. What eating disorder is exhibited by an intense fear of becoming obese?
    Anorexia Nervosa
53. If codependency exists within a family unit, how may the family be labeled?
    1. Abusive
    2. Neurotic
    3. Dysfunctional
    4. Psychotic
54. Poor impulse control, confidence, rapid speech, and hypertension are all signs and symptoms of _____ intoxication.
    1. Cocaine
    2. Alcohol
    3. Opiate
    4. Hallucinogenic
55. A patient rushes up to the nurse and says, "They're after me. They want to torture me and kill me." Which of the following is the most appropriate response?
    1. "Tell me who they are."
    2. "There's no one here except you and me."
    3. "I need to go look for myself."
    4. "You are safe here. Can you tell me more?"
56. The nurse is caring for a patient experiencing extrapyramidal side effects from antipsychotic medications. All of the following medications are ordered. Which one should the nurse administer for the side effects?
    1. Furosemide (Lasix)
    2. Benztropine mesylate (Cogentin)
    3. Prochlorperazine (Compazine)
    4. Acetaminophen (Tylenol)

57. Why is it important that detoxification for substance abuse occurs in a hospital setting?
    1 Adequate rest and nutrition are needed.
    2 Panic attacks may occur.
    ③ It may become life threatening.
    4 Other substances can be substituted for the substance of abuse.

58. A newly admitted adolescent on the unit has taken on the mannerisms and hairstyle of a popular singing star. The nurse recognizes this as an example of:
    ① Identification - Taking on characteristics
    2 Compensation of another
    3 Conversion
    4 Displacement

59. Select the nursing intervention that should take priority in a crisis.
    1 Allow friends to visit.
    ② Provide a safe environment.
    3 Rearrange the patient's schedule.
    4 Make decisions for the patient.

60. A patient complains of trouble with control of his tongue. The neck muscles are also beginning to tighten, and the patient is having difficulty keeping his head in an upright position. The nurse's first response should be:
    ① Check the medication administration record.
    2 Call the physician.
    3 Draw blood per standing order.
    4 Fill out an incident report.

61. A 46-year-old patient is admitted to the hospital's psychiatric unit because of an increasingly depressed mood. After a few weeks of treatment, the nurse observes that the patient has started putting on large amounts of makeup, has become seductive with male patients, and stays up very late pacing the floor. The nurse might conclude that the patient:
    1 Was initially diagnosed incorrectly
    ② May be having a manic episode as part of her illness
    3 Is showing signs of recovery
    4 May be having side effects of the medication

62. The nurse is making rounds and finds the schizophrenic patient sitting in a wet bed and singing nursery rhymes. Which action by the nurse should the nurse take first?
    1 Tell the patient to get cleaned up.
    2 Scold the patient for wetting the bed.
    ③ Help the patient get cleaned up.
    4 Tell the patient firmly that the behavior is inappropriate.

63. The nurse is caring for a patient diagnosed with major depression. The patient refuses to come out of his room. Name a primary nursing intervention for this patient.
    spend time c̄ pt
    _____
    _____

64. Extreme mood swings ranging from deep depression to high activity levels is most often seen in:
    1 Paranoid disorders
    ② Bipolar disorders
    3 Schizophrenia
    4 Eating disorders

65. The nurse is caring for a pediatric patient. The child's parents report that she has withdrawn from the gymnastics classes that she once enjoyed. The most therapeutic thing for the nurse to do would be to:
    1 Tell the child she does not have to go back to class.
    2 Ask the child if she wants to return to the class.
    ③ Ask the child what happened at the gymnastics class.
    4 Tell the child everything will be okay.

66. The nurse is completing discharge instructions for a patient being discharged on Antabuse to help avoid using alcohol. Which of the following statements should the nurse include in the teaching?
    1 "You will need bi-weekly blood work to determine blood levels of the medication."
    2 "The Antabuse can cause you to be sensitive to the sunlight."
    3 "This drug causes sedation; do not operate heavy equipment."
    ④ "The Antabuse can stay in your system as long as 14 days after you stop taking the medication."

67. If a nurse were to select a single identifying characteristic of the patient with obsessive compulsive disorder (OCD), it would be:
    1 Seclusiveness
    2 Aggression
    ③ Orderliness
    4 Instant gratification

68. Which of the following is the most appropriate nursing intervention for a patient?
    ① Have the patient explain what the voices are saying.
    2 Medicate the patient so he does not hear the voices.
    3 Direct the patient's attention away from the voices.
    4 Turn up the television and drown out the voices.

69. A nurse is caring for a patient experiencing manic behavior who is too distracted to eat. The most appropriate nursing intervention should be to:
    1 Plan mealtime as a social event.
    2 Plan for meals that include the patient's favorite foods.
    ③ Offer finger foods that the patient can eat on the go.
    4 Provide a calm mealtime.

70. Which group of people listed below should the nurse expect to be most likely to abuse tranquilizers?
    1 Teenage girls
    2 Middle-age men
    3 Older men
    ④ Middle-age women

71. A patient tells the nurse that he is depressed over the recent death of a parent. Which response is the best communication intervention for this patient?
    1 Say nothing.
    2 "Wouldn't you rather talk about something else?"
    ③ "I have some time. Would you like to tell me more about your feelings?"
    4 "I don't have time for sad people."

72. What illegal drug is often snorted to give confidence and euphoria?
    1 Heroin
    ② Cocaine
    3 Marijuana
    4 LSD

73. The nurse is preparing a patient for discharge. Which statement by the patient diagnosed with anxiety would indicate that he understands his diagnosis?
    1 "Wine with my meals may help me cope better with my anxiety."

2 "I understand that anxiety sometimes will help me perform better."

3 "As long as I take my antianxiety medication I can continue to work 16 to 18 hours a day."

4 "I understand my life will be great from now on."

74. A nurse enters a patient's room and stands just inside the door. The patient is obviously agitated and is escalating to the point that physical harm may occur. What would be the nurse's most appropriate action?

1 Take the patient to the seclusion room.

2 Talk to the patient, and try to identify why he or she is so agitated.

3 Go to the nurses' station and report the patient's behavior.

4 Call the physician.

75. A nurse working on an inpatient psychiatric unit is also responsible for operating a 24-hour emergency telephone line. During a short time, four potential suicide calls have come in. Which of the following callers should the nurse rank at greatest risk for carrying out his or her suicide threat?

1 An adolescent who is thinking of cutting his wrist

2 A young adult who agreed to come to the emergency room

3 A young man who plans to use a gun

4 A young woman who is talking of overdosing on pills

76. What defense mechanism do nurses commonly see used by patients admitted for drug abuse?

1 Substitution

2 Rationalization

3 Identification

4 Denial

77. A ___Crisis___ is an event that disturbs the equilibrium of an individual or family unit.

78. A patient on a psychiatric unit makes all the following comments. Which comment suggests that the patient may be suffering from mania?

1 "I get messages from my dead mother."

2 "Leave me alone while I'm playing solitaire."

3 "I don't need to sleep."

4 "My health is very important to me."

79. In assessing suicidal risk, which of the following is a high-risk factor?

1 Long psychotherapeutic treatment

2 A concrete plan that is relatively lethal

3 Past attempts because these usually mean the person is now able to cope better with stresses

4 Deviance in the person's background

80. If a nurse forces a treatment on a patient against his or her will, the nurse may be sued for:

1 False imprisonment

2 Assault and battery

3 Wrongful death

4 Habeas corpus

81. The nurse understands that the patient who has been committed to the hospital may:

1 Not leave or refuse treatment

2 Lose all of his or her civil rights

3 Not have access to his or her records

4 Not make any decisions regarding his care

82. The physician slams the chart down and leaves in a huff shortly after meeting with a young patient to discuss her terminal diagnosis. This is an example of which defense mechanism?

1 Rationalization

2 Undoing

3 Displacement

4 Compensation

83. The nurse recognizes the communication technique of receiving information and examining responses to the message as:

1 Restating

2 Listening (Active)

3 Reflection

4 Clarification

84. The nurse encourages the patient to expand on a given topic, using:

1 Restating

2 Broad openings

3 Reflection

4 Silence

85. Which of the following statements is most true about the difference between a delusion and a hallucination?

1 Delusions are false beliefs; hallucinations are projections.

2 Delusions are systems; hallucinations are beliefs.

3 Delusions are always true; hallucinations are always false.

4 Delusions are based on fact; hallucinations are based on belief.

86. The nurse states, "Don't worry, everything will be all right." This is an example of what type of communication?

1 Offering false reassurance

2 Offering approval

3 Minimizing the problem

4 Offering advice

87. The nurse realizes that a patient has started to do her hair and dress similar to the new medical student assigned to that unit. This patient is using the defense mechanism of:

1 Displacement

2 Identification

3 Compensation

4 Intellectualization

88. The nurse is caring for female patient in the emergency room. The patient complains of heart palpitations and weakness. No physical cause has been identified for her complaints. What should the nurse do when the patient is having an attack?

1 Acknowledge her discomfort and remain with her.

2 Remind her that all her tests were negative.

3 Encourage the patient to explain the severity of her symptoms to her physician.

4 Explain anxiety and panic attacks.

89. When a patient makes a statement that negates what he said to the nurse earlier in the day, the nurse recognizes that the patient is using the defense mechanism:

1 Rationalization

2 Projection

3 Regression

4 Undoing

90. The nurse caring for a young adult with multiple arrests for driving under the influence is trying to determine if the patient is an alcoholic. Which of the following questions should the nurse ask first?

1 "At what age did you start drinking?"

2 "What type of alcohol do you most often drink?"

3 "Are you able to recall the events that occur while you are drinking?"

4 "Why do you drink?"

91. The chief defense mechanism used by the alcoholic (addict) is:
    1 Denial
    2 Compensation
    3 Reaction formation
    4 Sublimation
92. In a crisis, the aim of intervention is to:
    1 Rearrange life elements of the people involved.
    2 Provide treatment for as long as possible.
    3 Offer support and explore alternatives.
    4 Avoid old ties because these led up to the crisis.
93. The nurse is explaining a diagnostic test to the patient. The patient is very anxious about the test. What should the nurse do to reduce the patient's anxiety?
    1 Explain the details of the procedure to the patient.
    2 Explain the treatment the test provides.
    3 Explain the patient's nothing by mouth (NPO) status.
    4 Assure the patient that the test is very accurate in identifying health problems.
94. Which of the following questions by the nurse would best determine if her patient is a victim of abuse?
    1 Ask if she is being abused   *Be direct!*
    2 Ask if the children are being abused
    3 Ask neighbors or relatives if they have witnessed any abuse.
    4 Ask if you can make a home visit to determine if any abuse is occurring.
95. In a psychiatric setting a nurse would understand that Post-traumatic stress disorder (PTSD) patients commonly report:
    1 Auditory hallucinations
    2 Recurring nightmares
    3 Displaced anger
    4 Depression
96. A patient on suicide precautions reports a recent change in mood. The nurse knows:
    1 This is a high-risk factor.
    2 The crisis has probably passed.
    3 The patient may be manic-depressive.
    4 The patient is responding to the added attention of the precautions.
97. Post-traumatic stress disorder (PTSD) is seen not only in the military, but also in persons:
    1 Raised in foster care
    2 With a genetic weakness
    3 With work related failures
    4 Surviving a catastrophe
98. What complication might the nurse expect in a patient withdrawing from alcohol?
    1 Bleeding
    2 Jaundice
    3 Polyphasia
    4 Seizures
99. The nurse is making morning rounds. After entering the room of a patient who had a mastectomy for breast cancer, the nurse notes that the room is dark, the curtains are closed, and the lights are off. What objective data would the nurse include in the nurse's notes?
    1 "Postoperative depression noted"
    2 "Seems to be depressed"
    3 "Grieving loss of breast"
    4 "Sitting in dark room"

100. A severely depressed patient tells the nurse, "There is no reason for me to continue living." Which of the following responses by the nurse would be the most appropriate?
    1 "Are you thinking about suicide?"
    2 "There are a lot of people worse off than you."
    3 "What would your family do?"
    4 "You have a lot to live for."
101. For the nurse to accept the alcoholic patient's behavior, he or she must first:
    1 Look at the patient's motives.
    2 Look at his or her own feelings about alcoholism.
    3 Compare normal and abnormal behavior.
    4 Take a course in crisis management.
102. Which of the following nursing actions takes priority when administering medications to a depressed patient?
    1 Make sure the patient drinks plenty of water.
    2 Make sure the patient swallows the medication.
    3 Give the medication on an empty stomach.
    4 Give the medication exactly on time.
103. The nurse is caring for a client with dementia and memory loss. Which of the following communication techniques would be most effective?
    1 Talk loudly.
    2 Repeat everything three times.
    3 Use short sentences.
    4 Use written communications.
104. An adolescent on the psychiatric unit has threatened another patient. Which nursing intervention is best for controlling this patient?
    1 Apply leather restraints.
    2 Place the patient in seclusion.
    3 Administer Haldol intramuscularly (IM).
    4 Use the least-restrictive means possible.
105. Which of the following statements made by a recovering alcoholic shows that he has a good understanding of his condition?
    1 "I'll be okay if I stick to wine and beer."
    2 "If my wife will get off my case, I will be fine."
    3 "I know this won't be easy; I am taking one day at a time."
    4 "I am recovered. I haven't had a drink in 10 days."
106. The psychiatric patient has decided to leave against medical advice. What must the nurse assess and document first?
    1 The medication he is taking
    2 His ability to perform ADL   *If he does he cannot leave*
    3 The danger he poses to himself or others
    4 His psychotic behaviors
107. A middle-age man patient is in the waiting room of the physician's office. He has come to get the results of his prostate biopsy. He is overheard laughing loudly and telling inappropriate jokes. The nurse should:
    1 Ask the patient to be quiet.
    2 Ignore the patient's behavior.
    3 Move the patient to an examination room as soon as possible.
    4 Recognize that the patient is expressing his anxiety.
108. The nurse is caring for a patient in the manic phase of bipolar disorder. What diversional activity would be appropriate for the nurse to recommend?
    1 Bridge
    2 Reading

3 Cross stitch

④ Exercise class

109. Patients diagnosed with major depression commonly display signs of:

1 Anxiety

2 Agitation

3 Energy

④ Hopelessness

110. The patient states, "I am depressed." What response by the nurse is the most appropriate?

① "Why do you think you feel this way?"

2 "Everyone feels "down in the dumps" every so often."

3 "Everything will be okay, once you snap out of feeling this way."

4 "Let's play cards and you'll forget about being depressed."

111. The nurse has just been given report on a newly admitted patient who has AIDS. Which of the following actions should the nurse take first?

1 Set up wound and skin isolation.

2 Explain the unit policies to the patient.

③ Examine his or her own feeling about AIDS.

4 Warn the other staff members that the patient has AIDS.

112. The nurse collects objective and subjective data from the newly diagnosed mental health patient. Which of the following is a good example of subjective data?

1 Stares into space blankly

2 Looks sad

3 Appears in no acute distress

④ The patient states, "I have no energy and have to drag myself out of bed."

113. The nurse understands that when a patient grunts and groans during their conversation, he is using what communication technique?

1 Proxematics

② Paralanguage

3 Kinesis

4 Confabulation

114. What type of coping mechanism is used when the anxiety is resolved?

① Adaptive

2 Palliative

3 Maladaptive

4 Dysfunctional

115. What is likely to happen when the nurse leaves the highly anxious patient to check on another patient?

1 The patient understands the nurse has other patients to check.

2 The patient becomes depressed.

③ The patient becomes more anxious.

4 The patient seeks someone else with whom to talk.

116. Which of the following is a priority in dealing with a highly anxious patient?

① The need to feel secure

2 The freedom to pace the room

3 The need for increased environment stimuli

4 The need for strict control

117. A schizophrenic patient that appears in a stupor may be:

1 Paranoid

② Catatonic

3 Incoherent

4 Suspicious

118. The nurse is working with a schizophrenic patient, and the nurse is obviously afraid. What should the nurse do first?

① Make sure adequate backup is available.

2 Explain to the patient that his delusions are not real.

3 Agree with the patient's delusions.

4 Let the patient know that you do not agree with his thoughts.

119. The condition in which the patient consumes excessive calories, eats compulsively, and gains a great deal of weight is known as: Obesity   .

120. The nurse knows that care of a mentally retarded child is based on mental age   and not his chronological age.

121. The nurse is caring for a patient recently diagnosed with a severe rare form of bone cancer. In what stage of the grief process would the nurse expect him to be more demanding and resentful?

1 Bargaining

② Anger

3 Denial

4 Acceptance

122. The nurse understands that patients with what type of mental retardation require monitoring when under stress?

1 Profound

2 Severe

③ Moderate

4 Mild

123. During what stage of the grieving process is crying most common?

1 Shock and disbelief

② Developing awareness

3 Restitution

4 Resolution

124. The nurse is preparing to do the discharge teaching on a patient recently started on antianxiety medication. The physician has left a prescription for the patient. What is the first step in teaching process?

1 Give the patient the prescription.

2 Provide the patient with written drug information.

③ Assess the patient's knowledge about the new medication.

4 Explain common side effects of the medication.

125. Prioritize the four phases of the nurse-patient relationship.

4 1 Working phase

2 2 Orientation phase

1 3 Termination phase

3 4 Preorientation phase

ANSWERS AND RATIONALES

1. Comprehension, planning, psychosocial integrity (b).
   3 Trust is essential when working with a depressed patient.
   1, 4 These are ongoing processes.
   2 This is not the first priority.

2. Knowledge, implementation, psychosocial integrity (a).
   2, 3 These are reasons a person may need to be hospitalized for further evaluation and treatment to decrease the threat.
   1 Although this not grounds for hospitalization, homelessness may be an end product of chronic mental illness.
   4 Low income may contribute to noncompliance with treatment but is not a reason to institutionalize someone.

3. Comprehension, planning, psychosocial integrity (b).
   4 The depressed patient may become overwhelmed if too much is offered too soon; the patient should be engaged in structured, goal-directed activities.
   1 This can lead to withdrawal or seclusive behavior.
   2 This is overwhelming to the patient at the beginning of treatment.
   3 Although feelings cannot be restructured, they can be dealt with if the patient will allow.

4. Knowledge, assessment, psychosocial integrity (a).
   Noncompliant: the situation presented clearly demonstrates an informed decision by the patient not to adhere to treatment.

5. Comprehension, implementation, psychosocial integrity (b).
   3 Praise should please the patient and spur him to do even more.
   1 Privileges need to be earned based on more specific criteria.
   2 This may be nontherapeutic for other reasons.
   4 Nurses should never give the patients money.

6. Application, implementation, psychosocial integrity (b).
   Physical: of the five dimensions on which the concept of holism is based, food meets the first or physical dimensions for the patient.

7. Knowledge, assessment, health promotion and maintenance (a).
   1 The two factors most associated with personality development are heredity and environment.
   2 Heredity is associated, but temperament is not.
   3 Environment is correct, but nurturing is not.
   4 Heredity is correct, but nurturing is not.

8. Comprehension, planning, psychosocial integrity (b).
   2 Patient and nurse work together to set goals in this phase.
   1 Much of this phase may occur before the nurse sees the patient.
   3 In this phase, the interventions are carried out.
   4 In this phase, they are evaluating if the goals worked.

9. Application, implementation, psychosocial integrity (c).
   3 This is the most appropriate option; briefly acknowledge the patient's feelings, then distract him by offering a less-threatening topic or activity.
   1 Measures to reduce anxiety should be started at the first sign of anxiety or discomfort.
   2 Never challenge the patient's delusion system; he will have to defend it.
   4 This reinforces the delusion, and the patient is further from reality.

10. Comprehension, assessment, psychosocial integrity (b).
    2 In this phase, the nurse meets the patient and discusses your involvement.
    1 This occurs before the nurse meets the patient.
    3 Patient upholds terms of contract, which establishes goals and priorities of treatment.
    4 The patient may be angry if the nurse does not let him know in advance when the relationship will end.

11. Comprehension, assessment, psychosocial integrity (b).
    4 Most authorities agree that as depression lifts, the patient is at greatest risk for committing suicide.
    1 He will not likely attempt suicide during the admission process.
    2 A patient who is suicidal will not be discharged.
    3 As depression deepens, he will not have energy to commit suicide.

12. Comprehension, implementation, psychosocial integrity (b).
    1, 5 These are therapeutic.
    2 This has no affect on the ritual.
    3 The nurse should allow time for the ritual.
    4 The nurse should not call attention to the act.

13. Knowledge, assessment, psychosocial integrity (a).
    4 This involves a smell, odor or aroma.
    1 This involves touch sensation.
    2 This involves hearing.
    3 This involves flavor or taste.

14. Knowledge, assessment, psychosocial integrity (a).
    1 Nurses must first be in touch with their feelings.
    2 This is Nursing's second priority.
    3 Nursing should also consider this.
    4 This is not a priority.

15. Comprehension, intervention, psychosocial integrity (b).
    3 People with common complaints meet with one or more therapist(s).
    1 Therapist and patient meet one on one.
    2 Patient and family members meet with the therapist.
    4 Desired behaviors are rewarded.

16. Application, implementation, psychosocial integrity (b).
    1 Remove the patient from added stimuli so he can better cope.
    2 The patient does not need added stimuli at this time.
    3 The patient cannot control his anxiety.
    4 Added stimuli are contraindicated.

17. Knowledge, evaluation, physiological integrity (a).
    4 These are common extrapyrimidal side effects.
    1, 2, 3 These are not extrapyrimidial side effects.

18. Knowledge, assessment, psychosocial integrity (a).
    2 This is common in the bargaining phase.
    1 In this phase, the patient says, "No, not me."
    3 In depression, he quietly sits in the dark.
    4 He will be calm and peaceful.

19. Comprehension, assessment, psychosocial integrity (b).
    Displacement: feelings for an object or person are transferred to a less-threatening object or person.

20. Knowledge, implementation, safe, effective care environment (a).
    AA is the most common of several groups that provide long-term assistance to individuals who have problems with alcohol.

21. Application, implementation, safe, effective care environment (b).
    4 You should encourage the patient to express his feelings.

1, 2, 3 These are not appropriate because they are closed questions that will elicit only a yes or no response.

22. Knowledge, assessment, psychosocial integrity (a).

1–4 These symptoms are usually seen in varying degrees.

5 Hypertension may be seen but not hypotension.

6 The patient is more likely to be aggressive.

23. Knowledge, assessment, psychosocial integrity (a).

1, 2, 5 These are expected in panic attack victims.

3 This is incorrect; the patient will be unable to solve problems.

4 Decreased attention span is seen.

24. Application, implementation, psychosocial integrity (b).

4 Recognizing the patient's feelings and encouraging him to verbalize these feelings is appropriate.

1 Although the patient needs to feel safe, recognizing his feelings and letting him talk is more important.

2 He was not afraid that someone was going to kill him; he was thinking of doing it.

3 This does not acknowledge his feelings nor does it encourage discussion.

25. Application, evaluation, physiological integrity (b).

3 Amnesia is common following electroconvulsive therapy (ECT).

1 Paranoid behavior is not seen with electroconvulsive therapy (ECT).

2 The patient will probably be sedated.

4 The patient is more likely to be sedated.

26. Knowledge, assessment, psychosocial integrity (a).

Sadness alternating with euphoria or depression alternating with mania

27. Knowledge, assessment, physiological integrity (a).

3 Symptoms occur after stopping the drug.

1 Tolerance means increasing doses to achieve effects.

2 To abstain is not to drink.

4 Dementia is unrelated.

28. Application, planning, psychosocial integrity (b).

Disturbed thought process

Risk for injury

Disturbed sleep pattern

Impaired social interaction

29. Application, implementation, psychosocial integrity (b).

1, 2 These are therapeutic.

3 Patients in the manic phase are already extremely active.

4 They are not monitored daily, usually biweekly, initially and every 2 to 3 months after becoming stable.

30. Knowledge, assessment, psychosocial integrity (b).

1, 2, 5 These are classic symptoms.

3 Decreased motivation will be noted.

4 Decreased self-esteem will be noted.

31. Knowledge, implementation, psychosocial integrity (b).

1 The unfamiliar is anxiety provoking; a tour and review of expectations will assist in reducing the patient's anxiety.

2 Patients are free to interact with others but are never required to do so.

3 Patients receive a copy of the Patient Bill of Rights on admission and either a written copy of the unit rules and regulations or a verbal explanation of them; this builds trust and security.

4 This is not the purpose; the patient will be introduced to the group at the first community meeting.

32. Comprehension, assessment, psychosocial integrity (a).

3 This is a healthy response.

1 This is unhealthy.

2, 4 These move toward the illness end of the continuum.

33. Application, implementation, psychosocial integrity (b).

3 Be direct; ask the patient what is necessary to know.

1 This takes no actions related to the nurse's suspicions.

2 This does nothing about the nurse's concerns.

4 This may make the patient feel worse, unworthy.

34. Knowledge, assessment, psychosocial integrity (b).

1 Lethal is high risk.

2 This does not indicate that a breakup would lead to suicide attempt.

3 Although this is a warning sign, it is not as serious compared with a lethal plan.

4 This is not high-risk factor.

35. Knowledge, assessment, psychosocial integrity (a).

Compulsions: these acts are usually contrary to the individual's ordinary actions; behavior can result in increased anxiety if not carried out.

36. Knowledge, assessment, psychosocial integrity (b).

1 A delusion is a false fixed idea.

2 A hallucination is a sensory experience.

3 An illusion is a misrepresentation.

4 Compensation is a defense mechanism.

37. Application, assessment, psychosocial integrity (b).

2 Erosion of tooth enamel is common.

1, 3, 4 These complaints are not as common as toothache.

38. Comprehension, implementation, psychosocial integrity (c).

4 This response accepts reality of her experience and suggests self-control.

1 This response denies reality of her experience.

2 This response enters into the delusion.

3 This response denies reality of her experience.

39. Comprehension, assessment, psychosocial integrity (b).

2 Suspicion and jealousy are the predominant thoughts of the paranoid patient.

1 Paranoid patients are so preoccupied with suspicion and jealousy that these are not substantial possibilities.

3 Self-pity and self-centeredness are more closely associated with the depressed patient who is trying to blame self or relieve feelings of guilt.

4 This is the definition of ambivalence.

40. Application, planning, psychosocial integrity (b).

4 Temporary amnesia is expected following electroconvulsive therapy (ECT).

1 This is not an expected outcome following electroconvulsive therapy (ECT).

2 ECT patients are not usually suicidal.

3 ECT treats depression.

41. Comprehension, planning, psychosocial integrity (b).

1 Nurses diagnose and treat human responses to illness, behaviors, or problems related to their probable causes.

2 Nurses diagnose responses and not disease entities.

3 The medical diagnosis may or may not be related to the nursing diagnosis.

4 Nursing diagnosis is useful in many diverse settings.

42. Knowledge, assessment, psychosocial integrity (a).

Phobia is the correct response.

43. Knowledge, evaluation, psychosocial integrity (b).

4 This is the desired effect of the treatment and can be more effective than medications; for this patient, this is the most appropriate response.

1 This is the primary effect of antidepressant medications, although some people believe that ECT causes changes in monoamine neurotransmitter systems.
2 Although ECT may cause amnesia of the previous few days, it will not last. This effects conscious thinking.
3 This occurs during the treatment.

44. Knowledge, assessment, psychosocial integrity (a).
   2, 3, 4 These are symptoms of anxiety.
   1 This is incorrect; anxious people have difficulty with details.
   5 This is incorrect; the person finds details difficult.
   6 This is incorrect; anxious people are usually impatient.

45. Comprehension, planning, safe, effective care environment (b).
   2 Identify the plan, and then intervene; be direct.
   1 "Tell me more" may not identify the plan.
   3 Although this is true, it does not address the plan.
   4 This response is incorrect; if anyone approaches you with statements such as the ones in this question, find out if they have a plan.

46. Application, assessment, psychosocial integrity (b).
   1, 2 These are seen in paranoia.
   3 This is incorrect; the person may lack social support.
   4 This is incorrect; the person has trouble controlling temper.

47. Comprehension, evaluation, psychosocial integrity (b).
   2 This lets the patient vent her fears.
   1, 4 This response offers false assurance.
   3 This is an inappropriate and nontherapeutic remark.

48. Comprehension, evaluation, psychosocial integrity (b).
   2 A blackout is the inability to remember what was done while under the influence of alcohol.
   1 Psychosis would include short-term and long-term memory loss.
   3 Denial is a part of the grieving process.
   4 He may be alcoholic, but this does not explain the memory loss.

49. Comprehension, assessment, psychosocial integrity (c).
   1 In a persecutory delusion, the television actually does not curse the patient; she feels persecuted by it.
   2 This is not a visual hallucination.
   3 This is not incoherent but structured thought.
   4 This is not flight of ideas.

50. Application, assessment, psychosocial integrity (b).
   Bulimia is the correct response.

51. Comprehension, implementation, psychosocial integrity (b).
   3 Excessive stimuli can agitate the patient.
   1 Restraints would be a last resort.
   2 Behavior modification may not be appropriate on an admissions unit.
   4 This would provide too much stimuli.

52. Application, assessment, psychosocial integrity (b).
   Anorexia nervosa is an eating disorder characterized by an intense fear of becoming fat or obese, resulting in extreme eating restrictions, leading to amenorrhea, emaciation, and disturbance in body image.

53. Knowledge, assessment, psychosocial integrity (a).
   3 The family may be labeled as dysfunctional.
   1, 2, 4 These may not necessarily apply.

54. Knowledge, assessment, psychosocial integrity (a).
   1 These are seen with cocaine use.
   2 These do not indicate alcohol abuse.

3 This is not common of opiates.
4 Not seen in hallucinogenic drug use.

55. Comprehension, assessment, psychosocial integrity (b).
   4 Assurance and willingness to listen are key to therapeutic relations.
   1 Your knowledge may intimidate them; do not buy into their false beliefs.
   2 Be nonjudgmental and nonthreatening.
   3 Avoid buying into a false belief.

56. Comprehension, evaluation, physiological integrity (b).
   2 This is the drug of choice.
   1 This is a diuretic.
   3 This is used as a sedative, for nausea.
   4 Acetaminophen is an analgesic.

57. Comprehension, implementation, psychosocial integrity (b).
   3 Life-threatening events may occur.
   1 You do not have to be hospitalized for adequate rest and food.
   2 Not usually seen with withdrawal and detoxification.
   4 This is not necessary.

58. Application, evaluation, psychosocial integrity (b).
   1 Identification is taking on the characteristics of another.
   2 Compensation is making up for feelings of inferiority.
   3 Conversion is channeling anxiety into bodily signs and symptoms.
   4 Displacement is redirecting energies into another person or object.

59. Application, implementation, psychosocial integrity (b).
   2 Safety is always a priority.
   1 May not be appropriate during the crisis.
   3 This is not a good time to attempt to make change.
   4 Not a priority at this time.

60. Comprehension, assessment, physiological integrity (c).
   1 This is the correct answer; the patient may be experiencing the beginning effects called extrapyramidal side effects/symptoms (EPS). These symptoms are associated with the administration of antipsychotic medications. Incidentally, an anti-EPS medication will probably be ordered to reverse the EPS effects.
   2, 3 These are not appropriate as a *first* response.
   4 This should not be a first response but may be required at some point in the event.

61. Comprehension, assessment, psychosocial integrity (a).
   2 The behavioral changes indicate mania.
   1 This may not be true; diagnosis was accurate for the presenting symptoms.
   3 This is not true; change too rapid and extreme.
   4 This is unrelated.

62. Comprehensive, implementation, psychosocial integrity (b).
   3 This offers reassurance and assistance.
   1 This puts the patient down.
   2 This also puts the patient down.
   4 This implies that the patient did these things on purpose.

63. Application, implementation, psychosocial integrity (b).
   Spend some time with the patient. By doing so, the nurse communicates a sense of worth to the patient. In time, the patient may feel comfortable in discussing his feelings with the nurse.

64. Knowledge, assessment, psychosocial integrity (a).
   2 Mood swings are the characteristics of bipolar disorder; manic (elation) and depression are two phases.

1 Paranoid disorders generally do not involve mood swings at all.

3 Schizophrenia is characterized by disorganized thinking.

4 Persons with eating disorders do not suffer from mood swings.

65. Application, implementation, psychosocial integrity (b).

3 Using a broad opening statement helps gather data.

1 This does not deal with the problem.

2 This is not an open-ended question.

4 This gives false assurance.

66. Comprehension, evaluation, physiological integrity (b).

4 This is a true statement.

1 Toxic blood levels are not a concern.

2 Photosensitivity is not a problem.

3 Sedation is not a side effect.

67. Knowledge, assessment, psychosocial integrity (a).

3 Orderliness is the single feature of the patient with obsessive compulsive disorder (OCD); activities are usually done in a ritual format.

1 The patient with OCD is so busy thinking and doing, a time for seclusion would not exist.

2 Aggression is not an obsessive-compulsive characteristic.

4 Instant gratification is related to poor impulse control; the patient with OCD has an overwhelming need to perform activities that release the underlying feelings.

68. Application, implementation, psychosocial integrity (b).

1 Knowing what the patient hears is important because "the voices" may be directing the patient to harm himself and others.

2 Medicating the patient will interfere with full assessment of the patient's status.

3 Attempts to refocus a patient's attention would prove unsuccessful given that voices are *real* to patient and will not *go away;* action also prevents assessment of the patient.

4 Voices cannot be *drowned out* because they are *real* to the patient and will not *go away;* action also prevents proper assessment of patient.

69. Comprehension, planning, physiological integrity (b).

3 During the manic phase, patients have trouble being still but may eat on the go.

1 This will not make the patient comply.

2 This will not make the patient able to comply.

4 The patient will still be experiencing difficulty in focusing.

70. Knowledge, assessment, psychosocial integrity (a).

4 Middle-age women take tranquilizers legally.

1 This group is more likely to experiment with alcohol, street drugs.

2 This group is not commonly seen abusing tranquilizers.

3 This group is more likely to be alcoholic.

71. Application, implementation, psychosocial integrity (a).

3 Open-ended question, with ample time to listen, is the best therapeutic technique in this situation.

1 You should indicate an interest in what the patient has said; saying nothing is the wrong activity.

2 The pressing issue is death of parents; diversion of discussion is not appropriate.

4 This is inappropriate, and it is insulting.

72. Knowledge, evaluation, psychosocial integrity (a).

2 Cocaine increases confidence and decreases judgment; it causes euphoria.

1 This causes euphoria and slurred speech.

3 This causes euphoria and increased appetite.

4 This alters perception and causes paranoia.

73. Comprehension, evaluation, psychosocial integrity (b).

2 Anxiety is sometimes a healthy response to problems.

1 Alcohol is not effective in managing anxiety.

3 Leisure time is necessary for a healthy lifestyle.

4 The patient will still have good and bad days.

74. Comprehension, assessment, psychosocial integrity (b).

2 Verbal intervention is always the first course of action.

1 This action may be required later, depending on the ability to verbally deescalate the situation.

3 Go for the underlying feeling first.

4 Do not do this until it is necessary.

75. Comprehension, assessment, psychosocial integrity (a).

3 A gun would be a very serious weapon.

1 The patient is thinking of it but has no exact plan or weapon.

2 This individual is seeking help.

4 The patient does not necessarily have pills.

76. Compensation, assessment, psychosocial integrity (a).

4 Drug users frequently deny they have a problem.

1 Not commonly seen used by drug abusers.

2 Not seen as often as denial.

3 Not frequently seen.

77. Knowledge, planning, psychosocial integrity (b).

Crisis is the correct response.

78. Comprehension, assessment, psychosocial integrity (a).

3 This is common among patients with mania.

1 This behavior is not seen in manic patients.

2 The patient probably would not be focused enough to remain still to play cards.

4 This attitude is not associated with mania.

79. Knowledge, assessment, psychosocial integrity (b).

2 A concrete, lethal plan is a very high-risk factor.

1 Treatment duration is usually unrelated.

3 Past attempt is high risk but not for reason stated.

4 This is unrelated.

80. Application, implementation, psychosocial integrity (b).

2 Forcing treatment on a patient may result in assault and battery charges.

1 This refers to the patient being held against his or her will.

3 This applies if the patient dies because of treatment error.

4 Patients use this to petition the court for their release.

81. Comprehension, evaluation, psychosocial integrity (b).

1 If the patient were committed by the court, the court must consent for him to be released.

2 He does not lose his civil rights.

3 Many people request access to records.

4 The patient can make some decisions.

82. Comprehension, evaluation, psychosocial integrity (a).

3 The physician is frustrated over the diagnosis and was not able to express this with the patient.

1 No explanation was given.

2 Nothing was undone.

4 He did not try to make up for a deficiency.

83. Comprehension, assessment, psychosocial integrity (b).

2 Active listening is being defined.

1 This is repeating what was said.

3 This is giving back what was said.

4 This means to explain using other words.

84. Comprehension, implementation, psychosocial integrity (b).
    2 This will help the patient expand on what he or she is saying.
    1 This is repeating what the patient has said.
    3 This is directing what the patient said back to him or her.
    4 This is a lack of communication.
85. Knowledge, assessment, psychosocial integrity (a).
    1 These are exact definitions of the respective terms.
    2 Although both are beliefs, hallucinations are based on misconceptions, and delusions are not based on anything real.
    3 Delusions are always false, as are hallucinations.
    4 Both are real to the patient; hallucinations have triggers.
86. Comprehension, implementation, psychosocial integrity (b).
    1 The is an example of offering false hope, which is never therapeutic.
    2 Offering approval does nothing to make the patient feel better about what was said. An example of this would be, "That's good."
    3 Minimizing a problem cuts off communication and does not help build nurse-patient relationships. An example of this would be, "That's okay. It's not a big deal."
    4 Offering advice is not allowing patients to make their own decisions. An example of this would be, "I think you should…."
87. Comprehension, assessment, psychosocial integrity (b).
    2 Identification is taking on characteristic of someone you admire.
    1 Displacement is shifting of emotions from one person or object to another.
    3 Compensation is building up one feature to make up for a weakness in another area.
    4 Intellectualization is explaining using logic.
88. Application, assessment, physiological integrity (b).
    1 This is the best answer; these symptoms are real to her.
    2 This does not improve her feelings.
    3 This will not decrease her symptoms.
    4 The patient is already anxious and in no state to comprehend these explanations.
89. Application, assessment, psychosocial integrity (b).
    4 Undoing is undoing (negating) previous declarations.
    1 Rationalization is offering a socially acceptable explanation.
    2 Projection puts your thought and actions on others.
    3 Regression is retreating to an earlier level of development.
90. Comprehension, implementation, psychosocial integrity (b).
    3 This gives you important information about the patient's drinking pattern.
    1 This will not determine if he or she is alcoholic.
    2 What the person drinks does not determine if he or she is alcoholic.
    4 This does not determine if he or she is alcoholic.
91. Comprehension, assessment, psychosocial integrity (a).
    1 Denial is the chief defense mechanism in that the addict can always find a reason to drink.
    2 The addiction is the weakness and has an underlying cause that is uncompensated.
    3 Although underlying feelings of guilt and sadness are relieved by the addiction, these feelings return once the drug wears off; the addiction is not the expression of an opposite attitude; it is relief from the underlying feelings.
    4 Sublimation does not fit in the discussion of addiction.

92. Knowledge, implementation, psychosocial integrity (a).
    3 A new observer is often helpful in sorting out complexities and offering useful solutions.
    1 This is not a goal.
    2 Treatment is always time limited.
    4 Old ties are often strengthened.
93. Application, implementation, physiological integrity (b).
    1 The more the patient knows, the less anxious he should be.
    2 The treatment may vary, depending on test results.
    3 This may not be all the patient needs to know before the test.
    4 Do not offer false assurance.
94. Comprehension, assessment, psychosocial integrity (b).
    1 Asking directly is the best approach.
    2 Asking about the children does not answer the question about the patient.
    3 This would be second-hand information, not proof.
    4 You would not want to leave the patient in a potentially dangerous situation until you were able to visit.
95. Comprehension, assessment, psychosocial integrity (b).
    2 Recurring nightmares about the traumatic event are common.
    1 Hallucinations are not common, especially auditory ones.
    3 Displaced anger is not common in PTSD.
    4 Depression is not a common concern in PTSD.
96. Comprehension, assessment, psychosocial integrity (c).
    1 This is high risk: mood change may signal behavior change.
    2 The nurse should not assume that the crisis has passed.
    3 This is a medical diagnosis, and nurses do not make medical diagnoses.
    4 This is not necessarily true.
97. Comprehension, assessment, psychosocial integrity (b).
    4 Any major trauma can lead to post-traumatic stress disorder (PTSD).
    1 This is not a reason for trauma.
    2 Genetics does not play into PTSD.
    3 Work-related failures are not necessarily traumatic.
98. Comprehension, assessment, psychosocial integrity (b).
    4 Seizures are common during alcohol withdrawal.
    1 Bleeding is not commonly seen in alcohol withdrawal.
    2 Jaundice is usually seen in liver failure.
    3 Excessive hunger is not seen; the person usually drinks and does not eat.
99. Comprehension, evaluation, psychosocial integrity (a).
    4 This reports what the nurse observed.
    1 The nurse is diagnosing with this written statement.
    2, 3 The nurse is placing judgment with this written statement.
100. Comprehension, evaluation, psychosocial integrity (b).
    1 This will get the information you need.
    2, 3, 4 These are nontherapeutic.
101. Comprehension, assessment, psychosocial integrity (b).
    2 The nurse should first understand her own feelings.
    1, 3, 4 These do not help the nurse accept the patient's behavior.
102. Comprehension, implementation, physiological integrity (b).
    2 You do not want the patient to hoard the medication.
    1 This is not a priority related to administration of medication.

3 Some medications are to be taken with food.

4 A window of time is allowed; you cannot give each patient's medication exactly on time.

103. Comprehension, implementation, psychosocial integrity (b).

3 Using short sentences may help the patient comprehend.

1 The patient does not have a hearing problem.

2 Hearing the words three times will not help the patient comprehend.

4 He will not comprehend written instructions any better than he would verbal ones.

104. Comprehension, implementation, psychological integrity (b).

4 Always try the least-restrictive means first; you can always do more if this is not successful.

1 This may not be necessary; you may need only to separate the two patients.

2 You may be able to settle this without locking up the patient by himself.

3 This will sedate the patient.

105. Comprehension, assessment, psychosocial integrity (b).

3 The patient understands that recovery is a process.

1 He does not need any alcoholic beverages.

2 He cannot blame the problem on his wife.

4 Recovery is a lifelong process; 10 days is only a start.

106. Comprehension, assessment, psychosocial integrity (b).

3 He cannot leave if he poses a safety threat to himself or others.

1 This will not keep him hospitalized.

2 He can get assistance with activities of daily living (ADL) outside the hospital.

4 His behaviors may not pose a safety threat.

107. Comprehension, assessment, psychosocial integrity (b).

4 His loud behavior is a common sign of anxiety.

1 He is probably not aware that he is so loud and inappropriate; it is the anxiety.

2 He needs attention; he may upset or offend other patients.

3 This gets him away from other patients but is not the best way to address the problem.

108. Comprehension, implementation, psychosocial integrity (b).

4 Exercise is a good way to expend some of the energy.

1 Bridge requires that he sit still and concentrate, which is hard to do if the patient is manic.

2 Reading is also a quiet activity.

3 Cross stitch requires close concentration.

109. Comprehension, assessment, psychosocial integrity (b).

4 Hopelessness is a classic symptom of depression.

1 This is another medical diagnosis and may accompany depression.

2 Agitation is more frequently seen with anxiety.

3 Depressed persons are more likely to be fatigued.

110. Comprehension, assessment, psychosocial integrity (b).

1 This is open-ended and invites more discussion.

2 This puts the patient down and is not open-ended.

3 He cannot snap out of it. This ends the discussion.

4 He cannot turn it off and on. This ends the discussion.

111. Comprehension, implementation, psychosocial integrity (b).

3 The nurse needs to examine her own feelings first so she can best interact with the patient.

1 Universal precautions are needed, not wound and skin isolation.

2 This will be part of the orientation and is not a top priority.

4 This may breech confidentiality.

112. Comprehension, assessment, psychosocial integrity (b).

4 Subjective remarks come from the patient.

1, 2, 3 These are the nurse's observations.

113. Comprehension, assessment, psychosocial integrity (b).

2 Paralanguage is voice quality, tones, and grunts.

1 Proxematics deals with space.

3 Kinesis relates to facial expression.

4 Confabulation fills in gaps of information.

114. Knowledge, assessment, psychosocial integrity (a).

1 If the patient adapts, he deals with the problem and resolves the anxiety.

2 Palliative coping may decrease the anxiety.

3 Maladaptive behavior may make the patient more anxious.

4 The problem will not be solved and the anxiety will not be reduced.

115. Comprehension, assessment, psychosocial integrity (b).

3 Leaving the patient alone will make him more anxious.

1 An anxious patient cannot understand that the nurse must care for others.

2 Nothing in the question supports depression.

4 No data exists to support another person being sought out.

116. Comprehension, implementation, psychosocial integrity (b).

1 Feeling secure can reduce anxiety.

2 Anxious patients may need to be moved to an area with less stimuli.

3 He needs reduced stimuli.

4 Strict control may increase the patient's anxiety.

117. Knowledge, assessment, psychosocial integrity (a).

2 In a catatonic state, the patient appears in a stupor and is rigid.

1 Paranoid patients are jealous and suspicious.

3 Incoherent means not making sense.

4 Suspicion goes with paranoia.

118. Comprehension, implementation, psychosocial integrity (b).

1 The patient may sense your fears; make sure adequate backup is available.

2 The delusions are real to the patient, and you cannot convince him otherwise.

3 You should not agree with delusions that you know are false.

4 Do not confront or argue with the patient.

119. Comprehension, assessment, psychosocial integrity (b).

Obesity: experts have debated for some time over whether obesity is an eating disorder. Although obesity has psychological components, many people believe the disorder to be more of a genetic or metabolic nature.

120. Comprehension, assessment, psychosocial integrity (a).

Mental age, developmental stage

121. Comprehension, assessment, psychosocial integrity (b).

2 In the anger phase, the patient is most likely to be demanding.

1 In this phase, he is requesting more time.

3 In denial, he does not think he has the illness.

4 When the patient reaches acceptance, he is at peace.

122. Knowledge, assessment, psychosocial integrity (a).

    3 Moderately retarded persons may perform self-care but may require support and assistance when under stress.

    1 This type needs total nursing care.

    2 This type requires protected environment and continual monitoring.

    4 This type is self-supporting.

123. Application, assessment, psychosocial integrity (b).

    2 This has physical symptoms; crying is common.

    1 The person is numb and stunned.

    3, 4 These indicate acceptance.

124. Application, assessment, physiological integrity (b).

    3 Assessment is always first.

    1 This does not teach.

    2 This alone does not teach.

    4 You need other information first.

125. Knowledge, assessment, psychosocial integrity (a).

    4 Preorientation

    2 Orientation

    1 Working

    3 Termination

CHAPTER 7   Maternity Nursing

The aim of obstetrics is to offer health services to the child-bearing mother, her baby, and her family that will ensure a normal pregnancy and a safe prenatal and postnatal experience. This chapter reviews components of the nursing process. Each topic presents pertinent information helpful in planning the nursing assessment and in analyzing the nursing need of the family. Nursing management is outlined, giving options for selecting appropriate plans for action. The evaluation of whether outcomes and goals of maternity nursing have been met completes the nursing process. The information presented in this review will assist the nurse in understanding how to:

- Plan, implement, and evaluate the nursing process as it relates to the maternity patient, her baby, and her family.
- Integrate selected theoretic information into the nursing process to meet the basic aims of maternity nursing effectively.

EVOLUTION OF MODERN OBSTETRICS

A. Early influences
   1. Middle Ages and early Christianity: pain of childbirth believed to be a means of expiation for sins
   2. Judaism: contributed to public health through its kosher dietary laws and to hygiene through its ritual of circumcision
   3. Renaissance: Leonardo da Vinci (1452-1519, Italy): contributed to understanding human anatomy through his anatomic drawings
B. Western European influence
   1. Ambroise Paré (1510-1590, France): started trend of doctors replacing midwives
   2. Peter Chamberlen (1560-1631, England and Holland): introduced forceps, paving the way for mechanical devices to assist in difficult deliveries
   3. William Smellie (1697-1763, England): published book on midwifery in 1752 and wrote rules for using forceps during a delivery
   4. William Hunter (1718-1783, England): described placental anatomy
   5. Jean Louis Baudelocque (1746-1810, France): described positions, presentations, and pelvic measurements
   6. Ignaz Philipp Semmelweiss (1818-1865, Austria): a pioneer in obstetric asepsis; found that hand washing before attending mothers greatly reduced the incidence of puerperal (child-bed) fever
   7. Louis Pasteur (1822-1895, France): discovered Streptococcus as the causative organism in puerperal fever (1860)
C. Contributors in the United States
   1. Anne Hutchinson (1634): midwife who delivered many babies of early settlers

   2. William Shippen: established first lying-in hospital and midwifery school in the United States in 1762
   3. Oliver Wendell Holmes (1809-1894): stressed cleanliness and hand washing before caring for new mothers
   4. Margaret Sanger Research Bureau (1923): first organization to address question of contraception and planned parenthood
D. United States legislation affecting mothers and children
   1. 1921: Sheppard Towner Act—promoted health and welfare for mothers and children
   2. 1936: Social Security benefits began; later to include entitlement benefits for mothers and their dependent children
   3. 1943: Emergency Maternal and Infant Care Act to assist families of soldiers during World War II
   4. 1973: Supreme Court legalizes abortion
   5. 1974: Women, Infants, and Children (WIC) Program: federally funded nutritional program providing supplementary food to eligible pregnant, lactating, or postpartum women, their infants, and children under 5 years of age
   6. 1995-1996: several states enacted legislation to lengthen a postpartum stay to 48 hours for a vaginal delivery and 96 hours for a cesarean birth; early discharge would be voluntary.

DEFINITIONS COMMONLY USED IN OBSTETRICS

Statistics

Birth Rates: number of live births per 1000 population
Fetal Death (Stillborn): fetus of 20 weeks or more gestational age who dies in utero before birth
Infant Mortality Rate: number of deaths before the first birthday per 1000 live births
Maternal Mortality Rate: number of mothers dying in or because of childbearing per 100,000 live births
Neonatal Death: death within first 4 weeks of life
Neonatal Death Care: number of deaths within the first 4 weeks of life per 1000 live births
NOTE: Statistics are important to identify problem areas and trends in the health care setting.

Abbreviations (Limited Listing)

ABC: alternative birthing center
ARM: artificial rupture of membranes
BOW: bag of waters; amniotic sac
CPD: cephalopelvic disproportion
CS: cesarean section
DIC: disseminated intravascular coagulation
EDC: estimated date of confinement; due date for birth
EDD: estimated date of delivery
FHR: fetal heart rate

FHT: fetal heart tone

G: gravida; number of pregnancies

GTPAL: gravida, term, premature, abortions, living children; identification of pregnancy status

HCG: human chorionic gonadotropin

HELLP: hemolysis, elevated liver enzymes, low platelet count; extension of pathologic factors related to severe preeclampsia

HIV: human immunodeficiency virus

LDRP: labor, delivery, recovery, postpartum: all phases of maternal and child care occur in the same room with the same staff member.

LGA: large for gestational age

LMP: last menstrual period

P: para; number of viable births

PIH: pregnancy-induced hypertension

PROM: premature rupture of membranes

Q: quadrant; one of four equal parts into which the abdomen is divided to designate position of fetus in uterus

RhoGAM: antibody against Rh factor given early prenatally or within 72 hours postpartum to mother

SGA: small for gestational age

TORCHES: a group of intrauterine infections, including toxoplasmosis, rubella, cytomegalovirus, herpes, and syphilis; commonly associated with high infant mortality

Common Obstetric Terminology

Apgar Score: method of evaluating infant immediately after delivery; usually at 1 minute and at 5 minutes

Advanced Maternal Age (Elderly Primipara): pregnant woman over 35 years of age giving birth to her first child

Braxton-Hicks Contractions: painless uterine contractions felt throughout pregnancy, becoming stronger and more noticeable during second and third trimester

Caput: head; cephalic portion of infant

Cyesis: pregnancy

Dystocia: long, painful labor and delivery

Gestation: developmental time of embryo, fetus, in utero

Grand Multipara: more than five children

High Risk: pregnant woman with preexisting problems that can jeopardize the pregnancy, the fetus, or herself; under 18 years of age or over 35 years of age with no prenatal care (any one or more of these conditions)

Lightening: moving of the fetus and uterus downward into the pelvic cavity during the last 2 weeks before EDC (usually just before labor in multiparas)

Low Birth Weight: weight less than 2500 grams because of the baby being preterm (premature) or because of intrauterine growth retardation

Low Risk: pregnant woman with normal history, between ages 18 and 34, with no medical, psychological, or other preexisting problems, and under good prenatal care

Meconium: first bowel movement of the newborn—thick, tarlike, greenish-black substance

Multigravida: pregnant more than one time

Multipara: given birth to more than one child

Postmature Infant: one born after 42 weeks' gestation

Premature Infant: one born anytime before 37 weeks' gestation

Primigravida: pregnant for the first time

Primipara: giving birth to first child

Pseudocyesis: false pregnancy

Quickening: first movements of the fetus felt by the mother (16 to 18 weeks' gestation)

Secundines: afterbirth of placenta and membranes

Term Infant: one born between 38 and 42 weeks' gestation

Vernix Caseosa: cheesy material covering the fetus and newborn that acts as a protection to the skin

Viable: capable of developing, growing, and sustaining life, such as a normal human fetus at 24 weeks' gestation

Vis a Tergo: external pressure on the fundus to assist in the delivery of the infant

TRENDS

A. Cost containment: rising health care costs are a national concern; increased home care, shortened stays, and increased emphasis on prenatal care are interventions to help control cost and maintain quality; regionalization of services for high-risk childbearing families and managed care are newer methods to attempt to control costs.

B. Prenatal care: emphasis must be placed on improving access to prenatal care, particularly for low-income women; prenatal care can avoid many conditions that can be prevented with adequate monitoring during pregnancy.

C. Early discharge: may be discharged home within 12 to 24 hours (uncomplicated labor and delivery) and 3 to 4 days or less for a CS; these shortened stays are an attempt to control health care costs and are creating an increased need for prenatal education materials and follow-up telephone numbers to reinforce education.

D. Early discharges: these have caused an increased demand for home care and other community services; this home follow-up is especially important for adolescents or other families with psychosocial complications; nurse entrepreneurs have helped to bridge this gap for many families.

E. High-technology care: technological developments, including fetal surgery, have often outpaced society's ability to determine ethical implications of their use.

F. Changing demographics: women are waiting longer in life to have their first babies; nurses need to be familiar with effects of pregnancy on older women.

G. Teen pregnancy: nurses need to identify and implement strategies to decrease incidence of adolescent pregnancy.

H. Changing cultures: nurses need to be sensitive to different cultures' ideas and health practices; examples in which culture plays an important part include pain expression, choice of support person, and preference for a female health care provider.

I. Prepared childbirth experience: mother and father (or alternate) jointly attend childbirth education classes to prepare for the child and for the childbearing and childbirth experience.

J. Alternative birth settings
   1. Birthing centers outside of hospital; ABC
   2. Individual's home
   3. Use of the birthing chair instead of traditional table
   4. Birthing room: labor, delivery, and postpartum hospital stay incorporated into one cheerful, homelike room set up with necessary labor and delivery equipment

K. Variety of positions used to assist labor and delivery (e.g., squat, side position)

L. Showering during first or second stage of labor

M. Inclusion of father or alternate: support person stays in labor and delivery area for both vaginal and CS deliveries

N. Rooming in: allows newborn in room with mother for the day; fathers allowed unlimited visiting time

O. Sibling visits: designated hours that children may visit and see baby

P. Use of midwives: many hospitals and birthing centers throughout the United States now have nurse-midwives as the primary care person conducting prenatal, labor, delivery, and follow-up care.

Q. CS: more frequent now because of sophisticated fetal monitoring; the practice is controversial because of a high number of sections in recent years.

R. Breast-feeding: accepted and encouraged; societies such as La Leche League and popularity of *natural* foods encourage breast-feeding.

S. Genetic counseling: increasingly accurate, safe amniocentesis and advances in genetics encourage counselors to advise couples with genetic problems

T. In vitro method of fertilization to assist pregnancy and fetal development: usually chosen by couples with fertility problems after exploring various methods, including fertility drugs and other insemination practices

U. Students are advised to review the U.S. Department of Health and Human Services: *Healthy People 2010: National Health Promotion and Disease Prevention Objectives,* http://odphp.Osophs.dhhs.gov/pubs/hp2000/

PROCEDURES TO DETERMINE MATERNAL AND FETAL PROBLEMS

A. Alpha-fetoprotein (AFP) test
   1. Screening procedure, not diagnostic
   2. Serum from maternal blood sample is tested; best results if sample is taken at 16 to 18 weeks' gestation; identifies unrecognized high-risk pregnancies
   3. Elevated levels of maternal serum indicate 5% to 10% open neural tube defect (spina bifida) in developing fetus
   4. Recommend two samples of test followed by ultrasound and amniocentesis to confirm findings; genetic counseling availability if confirmed
   5. Other causes of elevated AFP levels: multiple gestation, missed abortions, other abnormalities

B. Hemoglobin electrophoresis
   1. Identifies presence of sickle cell trait in women of African or Mediterranean descent

C. Endovaginal ultrasound
   1. Performed when a high risk of fetal loss is suspected

D. Amniocentesis: invasive procedure during which a needle is inserted through abdomen and uterus to withdraw amniotic fluid; usually done after fourteenth week
   1. Used for determining sex, defects in fetus (e.g., Down syndrome), fetal status (Rh isoimmune problem, fetal maturity, other tests as listed in this section)
   2. Lecithin/sphingomyelin ratio (L/S ratio): used to determine fetal lung maturity by testing surfactant by thirty-fifth week of pregnancy; lecithin level two times greater than sphingomyelin level indicates that lungs are mature
   3. Creatinine level: used to test fetal muscle mass and fetal renal function; 0.2 mg/100 ml amniotic fluid at 36 weeks is normal level; large amount may also indicate large fetus, such as fetus of the mother with diabetes.
   4. Bilirubin level: used for determination of fetal liver maturity; should decrease as term progresses; 450 μm is optimal density.
   5. Cytological testing: determines percentage of lipid globules present in amniotic fluid, indicates fetal age

E. Chorionic villi test
   1. Permits first-trimester testing for biochemical and chromosomal defects; invasive and high-risk procedure during which a plastic catheter is inserted vaginally into the uterus; ultrasound guides catheter to chorionic frondosum.
   2. Can be done 9 to 11 weeks after LMP
   3. Done earlier than amniocentesis; recent evidence shows that test may increase risk of babies born with missing toes and fingers or shortened digits.

F. Fetoscopy: invasive procedure using transabdominal insertion of metal cannula into abdomen; visualization of fetus and placenta for developing abnormalities and to obtain fetal skin or blood samples
   1. High-risk procedure; complications include spontaneous abortion and premature labor.
   2. Limited usage, only if defect cannot be detected otherwise

G. Umbilical cord technique: evaluates condition of fetus
   1. Superior technique because fetal blood can be analyzed as early as eighteenth week of gestation
   2. Can evaluate blood count, liver function, blood gases, acid-base status
   3. Invasive procedure; limited use because of risk of injury to fetus

H. Estriol level study: 24-hour urinalysis of urine from mother; determines estriol level to ascertain fetal well being and placental functioning
   1. Performed at third trimester (32 weeks)
   2. 12 mg in 24 hours is good; below 12 mg indicates that infant is in jeopardy (related to decreased placental functioning)
   3. Decreasing estriol levels can be used in combination with other diagnostic tests to indicate a compromised placenta or fetus.

I. Heterozygote testing (mother's blood): done to detect clinically normal carriers of mutant genes
   1. Tay-Sachs disease: common fatal genetic disease affecting children of Ashkenazi Jews (Eastern Europe)
   2. Sickle cell anemia: common disorder among black Americans of African descent; 1 in 10 African Americans is a carrier.
   3. Cooley's anemia (beta thalassemia): genetic disorder frequent among Mediterranean ethnic groups: Italians, Sicilians, Greeks, Turks, Middle Eastern Arabs, Asian Indians, Pakistanis

J. Contraction stress test: late trimester test to measure placental insufficiency and measure fetal reaction to uterine contractions (potential fetal compromise)
   1. Usually done after EDC has passed
   2. Invasive procedure during which intravenous (IV) oxytocin is administered; baseline recorded on monitor; takes 20 minutes to 1 hour
   3. Breast stimulation techniques are done in some health care settings in place of oxytocin infusion during a contraction stress test
   4. Results: late decelerations during contraction for at least three contractions indicate a positive test; no decelerations

during three successive contractions within 10 minutes indicate a negative test; occasionally, inconsistent decelerations indicate suspicious conditions.

K. Nonstress test (NST): assesses and evaluates FHT response to uterine movement or increased fetal activity

L. Ultrasound procedure: use of high-frequency sound waves to determine fetal size, estimate amniotic fluid volume, neural tube defects, limb abnormalities, evaluation of fetal presentation, and diagnosis of breech presentation.
   1. Usually a second-trimester procedure
   2. Risks are still under investigation.
   3. Acoustic sound waves can be used to help stimulate an inactive fetus during a nonstress test.

M. Biophysical profile: using ultrasound and an NST, this profile evaluates five fetal variables—breathing movements, body movements, muscular tone, qualitative amniotic fluid volume, heart rate

N. Doppler flow studies: using ultrasound techniques to evaluate blood flow studies in deep-lying vessels; these are particularly useful in managing high-risk pregnancies.

O. Fetal movement: noninvasive method of determining fetal well being; patterns that deviate from normal pattern may be an indication for further studies.

ANATOMY AND PHYSIOLOGY OF REPRODUCTION

Obstetric Pelvis

A. Types (Figure 7-1)
   1. Gynecoid: "true" female pelvis
   2. Anthropoid: narrow from side to side
   3. Android: male pelvis
   4. Platypelloid: flat pelvis narrow from front to back
   Types 3 and 4 are not adequate for vaginal delivery.

B. Components
   1. Ilium: flat or lateral, flaring part of pelvis or hip; iliac crest is top part of ilium.
   2. Ischium: inferior dorsal or lower part of hip bone; the ischial spines, sharp projections of the ischium, are

important in obstetrics because they are landmarks to measure progress of presenting part of fetus.
   3. Sacrum: triangular bone between the two hip bones; flat part of the lower back (spine)
   4. Coccyx: two to five rudimentary vertebrate that are fused and attached to lower part of sacrum (tailbone)

C. Measurements
   1. Diagonal conjugate: measured through vagina from lower border of symphysis pubis to promontory of sacrum (12.5 to 13 cm)
   2. Conjugate vera (true conjugate): measured from upper margin of symphysis pubis to promontory of sacrum by x-ray examination or sonogram (11 cm)
   3. Transverse diameter: distance between inner surfaces of the tuberosities of ischium (13 to 13.5 cm)
   4. Obstetric conjugate: measured by x-ray examination or sonogram or by subtracting 1.5 to 2 cm from diagonal conjugate (9.5 to 11.5 cm)

Fertilization and Implantation

A. Definitions
   1. Fertilization: occurs when the sperm and ovum join, usually at the distal third of the fallopian tube within 12 to 48 hours after intercourse
   2. Zygote: product of the union of a sperm and ovum
   3. Implantation: occurs when zygote burrows into the endometrium of the uterus, approximately 7 days after fertilization
   4. Nidation: completion of implantation

B. Processes
   1. Mitosis: rapid cell division
   2. Blastoderm: first division of the zygote
   3. Morula: balllike structure of the blastoderm; sometimes referred to as mulberrylike
   4. Blastocyst: as morula enters uterus
   5. Trophoblast: as blastocyst implants in the uterus, the wall becomes the trophoblast.
   6. Chorionic villi: trophoblasts develop villi that become fetal portion of the placenta.

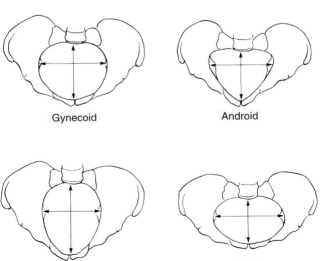

Gynecoid   Android

Anthropoid   Platypelloid

FIGURE 7-1.   Female pelvis: pure types. *(From Burroughs A, Leifer G:* Maternity nursing: an introductory text, *ed 8, Philadelphia, 2001, Saunders.)*

7. Decidua: endometrium undergoes a change when pregnancy occurs.
8. Decidua vera: that portion of the decidua that becomes the lining of the uterus, except for around implantation site
9. Decidua basalis: where implantation occurs and where chorionic villi become frondosum or the beginning of the placental formation
10. Decidua capsularis: covers blastocyst and fuses to form fetal membranes
11. Amnion: inner membrane, which comes from the zygote and blends with the cord
12. Chorion: outer membrane, which comes from the zygote and blends with the fetal portion of the placenta

Development of Human Organism

A. Ovum stage: preembryonic stage from conception until the primary villi appear (first 14 days)
B. Embryo: end of ovum stage to 8 weeks from LMP; period of rapid cellular development; disruption will cause developmental abnormality.
C. Fetus: from end of embryonic stage (8 weeks) to term
D. Placenta: membrane weighing approximately 450 g (1 lb); develops cotyledons that act as areas for nourishing fetus; maternal surface is beefy and red; fetal surface is shiny and gray.
E. Amnionic cavity: fills with fluid (1000 ml) that is replaced every 3 hours; shelters and protects fetus

Sex Determination

A. Normal sperm; carries 22 autosomes and 1 sex chromosome (either an X or a Y chromosome)
B. Normal ovum: carries 22 autosomes and 1 sex chromosome (always an X chromosome)
C. Combined number of chromosomes: 44 autosomes and 2 sex chromosomes (at conception)
D. Genetic component of sperm determines sex of child (Box 7-1)
E. Chromosome carries genes plus deoxyribonucleic acid (DNA) and proteins.
F. Genes: factors in chromosomes carrying hereditary characteristics

PHYSIOLOGY OF FETUS

A. Membranes and amniotic fluid
1. Protect from blows and bumps mother may experience
2. Maintain even heat to fetus
3. Act as an excretory system
4. Supply oral fluid for fetus
5. Allow free movement of fetus
B. Placenta
1. Transport organ: passes nutrients from mother to fetus and relays excretory material from fetus to mother

---

BOX 7-1	Sex Determination

Sperm supplies 22 autosomes and an X sex chromosome
Ovum supplies 22 autosomes and an X sex chromosome
Result: 44 autosomes and an XX = female
Sperm supplies 22 autosomes and a Y sex chromosome
Ovum supplies 22 autosomes and an X sex chromosome
Result: 44 autosomes and an XY = male

---

2. Formation completed by 3 months
3. Functions: kidney, lungs, stomach, and intestines
4. Requirement: adequate oxygen from mother to function well
C. Monthly development
1. Embryonic stage (first to eighth week)
a. Beginning: pulsating heart, spinal canal formation: no eyes or ears; buds for arms and legs
b. By end: little over 1 inch (2.5 cm) long; eyelids fused; distinct divisions of arms, legs; cord formed; tail disappears
2. Fetal stage (ninth week to term)
a. Between 20 and 24 weeks is considered the legal threshold for viability, the age at which the fetus is capable of surviving outside of the uterus
b. The embryo or fetus is most vulnerable to damaging effects of tetragenic agents during the first trimester; tetracycline, caffeine, and many over-the-counter drugs are examples of drugs that are tetragenic.
c. 3 months: 3 inches (7.5 cm) long; weighs 1 oz (28 g); fully formed arms, legs, fingers; distinguishable sex organs
d. 4 months: development of muscles, movement; mother feels quickening; 6 to 7 inches (15 to 17.5 cm) long; weighs 4 oz (112 g); lanugo over body; head large
e. 5 months: 10 to 12 inches (25 to 30 cm) long; weighs ½ to 1 lb (225 to 450 g); internal organs maturing; lungs immature; FHT heard on examination; eyes fused; rarely survives more than several hours
f. 6 months: 11 to 14 inches (27.5 to 35 cm) long; weighs 1 to 1½ lb (450 to 675 g); wrinkled "old man" appearance; vernix caseosa covers body; eyelids separated; eyelashes and fingernails formed
g. 7 months: begins to store fat and minerals; 16 inches (40 cm) long; may survive with excellent care
h. 8 months: beginning of month weighs 2 to 3 lb (900 to 1350 g); by end of month, 4 to 5 lb (1800 to 2250 g); continues to develop; loses wrinkled appearance
i. 9 months: 19 inches (47.5 cm) long; weighs 7 lb (3200 g) (girl) 7½ lb (3400 g) (boy); more fat under skin; vernix caseosa; has stored vitamins, minerals, and antibodies; fully developed
D. Fetal circulation
1. Special structures
a. Ductus venosus: passes through liver; connects umbilical vein to inferior vena cava; closes at birth
b. Ductus arteriosus: shunts blood from pulmonary artery to descending aorta; closes almost immediately after birth
c. Foramen ovale: valve opening that allows blood to flow from right atrium to left atrium; functionally closes at birth; all three fetal structures previously listed allow blood to bypass the fetal lungs and liver.
d. Umbilical arteries (2): transport blood from the hypogastric artery to the placenta; functionally closes at birth
e. Umbilical vein (1): transports oxygenated blood from placenta to ductus venosus and liver, then to the inferior vena cava (IVC); closes at birth
2. Fetal circulation (Figure 7-2)
a. Oxygenated blood from placenta goes through umbilical vein, bypassing portal system of the liver by way of the ductus venosus.

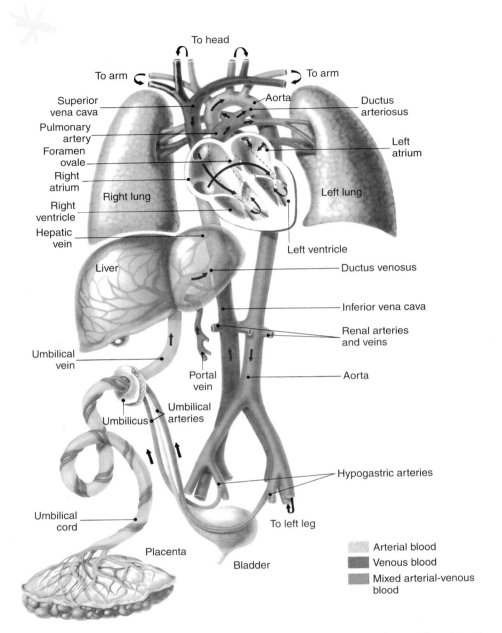

FIGURE 7-2.   Fetal circulation. *Before birth.* Arterialized blood from the placenta flows into the fetus through the umbilical vein and passes rapidly through the liver into the inferior vena cava; it flows through the foramen ovale into the left atrium, soon to appear in the aorta and arteries of the head. A portion bypasses the liver through the ductus venosus. Venous blood from the lower extremities and head passes predominantly into the right atrium, the right ventricle, and then into the descending pulmonary artery and ductus arteriosus. Thus the foramen ovale and the ductus arteriosus act as bypass channels, allowing a large part of the combined cardiac output to return to the placenta without flowing through the lungs. Approximately 55% of the combined ventricular output flows to the placenta; 35% perfuses body tissues; and the remaining 10% flows through the lungs. *After birth.* The foramen ovale closes, the ductus arteriosus closes and becomes a ligament, the ductus venosus closes and becomes a ligament, and the umbilical vein and arteries close and become ligaments. *(Used with permission of Ross Products Division, Abbott Laboratories, Columbus, Ohio.)*

b. From the ductus, venosus blood goes to the ascending vena cava (inferior) to the heart, right auricle.

c. From the right auricle through the foramen ovale

d. To the left auricle, then to the left ventricle

e. Blood leaves the heart through the aorta to the arms and head.

f. The blood then returns to the heart, passing through the descending vena cava (superior).

g. To the right auricle, then to the right ventricle

h. Blood leaves the heart through the pulmonary arteries, bypassing the lungs.

i. Blood goes through the ductus arteriosus to the aorta and down to the trunk and lower extremities.

j. Blood then goes through the hypogastric arteries to the umbilical arteries on to the placenta, carrying carbon dioxide and waste materials.

NORMAL ANTEPARTUM (PRENATAL)

Physiological Changes During Pregnancy

A. Reproductive system
1. External changes
   a. Perineum: increased vasculature; enlarges
   b. Labia majora: change especially in parous woman; separate and stretch
   c. Anal and vulvar varices: caused by increased pelvic congestion
2. Internal changes
   a. Uterus: enlarges to accommodate growing fetus; walls thicken first trimester; Hegar's sign (soft, lower lip of uterus)
   b. Cervix: Goodell's sign (thickens, softens) 6 weeks from LMP because of vascular changes
   c. Vagina: Chadwick's sign (bluish-violet color); mucosal changes approximately 8 weeks from LMP; estrogen activity may cause thick vaginal discharge.

B. Other body system changes
1. Breasts
   a. Increased size, tingling sensations, heavy
   b. Increased pigmentation, darkened areolae
   c. Montgomery's tubercles on areolae
2. Cardiovascular changes
   a. Slight enlargement of heart resulting from increased blood volume
   b. Increased circulation (47%)
   c. Cardiac output increased 30% first and second trimester, then levels off until term; increases during labor and delivery; approximately 13% above normal during postpartum period
3. Hematologic changes
   a. Increased red blood cell (RBC) count; decreased hemoglobin level
   b. Increased tendency for blood to coagulate during pregnancy
   c. Coagulation factors return to normal during postpartum, increasing likelihood of thromboembolism.
4. Respiratory and pulmonary changes: enlarging uterus presses on diaphragm, causing difficulty breathing
5. Skin: increased pigmentation
   a. Linea nigra: darkening line from below breast bone (sternum) down midline of abdomen to symphysis pubis

b. Chloasma gravidarum (mask of pregnancy): dark, frecklelike pigmentation over nose and cheeks; disappears after delivery

c. Stria gravidarum: stretching of skin with silvery to reddish, bluish stretch marks on breasts, abdomen, thighs; never disappears completely; lotion, cocoa butter lubricants may help.

6. Urinary system changes
   a. Traces of sugar in urine resulting from activity of lactiferous ducts
   b. Even though glucosuria is common in pregnancy, all women should be screened for diabetes.
   c. Transitory albumin: may be indication of pending PIH
   d. Cystitis: frequent because ureters lose some compliance or elasticity
7. Endocrine system
   a. Variable production of insulin during pregnancy
   b. Mother's cells become more insulin resistant.
   c. Thyroid gland increases in size, resulting in increased basal metabolic rate (BMR).
8. Digestive system
   a. Morning sickness: nausea and vomiting common during first trimester
   b. Increased appetite after first trimester
   c. Indigestion (heartburn): caused by increasing upward pressure of enlarging uterus or by relaxin hormone, which slows metabolism and keeps food in stomach longer in pregnant women
   d. Constipation: caused by changes in organ positions; pressure of growing uterus on sigmoid colon
9. Musculoskeletal system
   a. Normal lumbar curve becomes more pronounced as weight of pelvic contents tilts the pelvis forward
   b. Extra weight may lead to backache experienced in late pregnancy
10. Weight gain: total weight gain varies from 25 to 30 lb (12 to 13.5 kg) (Table 7-1)

Duration of Pregnancy

A. Length in terms of time
   1. 9 calendar months
   2. 10 lunar months
   3. 280 days (266 days from time of ovulation)
   4. 40 weeks
B. Nagele's rule: to calculate EDC, count back 3 months from the month of the LMP and add 7 days to the first day of LMP

TABLE 7-1	Distribution of Weight Gain During Pregnancy	
Distribution	**Pounds**	**Grams**
Fetus	7½	3400
Placenta	1	450
Amniotic fluid	2	900
Uterus	2½	1125
Increased blood volume	3-4	1350-1800
Breasts	2-3	900-1350
Mother's gain (fat, tissue, etc.)	4-8	1800-3600
Total weight gain	21-28 lb	9.5-12.7 kg

example:

First day of LMP was July 17

Seventh month (July)	17
− 3 months	+7
Fourth month	24 = EDC (April 24)

Signs and Symptoms of Pregnancy

A. Presumptive signs (subjective: mother usually notices)
1. Missed menstrual period
2. Breast changes; nipples tingle, fuller, darker areola in approximately 6 weeks
3. Frequency of urination in approximately 6 weeks
4. Morning sickness: nausea and vomiting in 4 to 6 weeks
5. Skin changes: chloasma, linea nigra, striae (some authors call this a "probable" sign)

B. Probable signs (objective examiner usually notices)
1. Uterus: enlarges; shape changes at 12 to 16 weeks; Hegar's sign: 8 weeks
2. Cervix: Goodell's sign
3. Vagina: Chadwick's sign
4. Implantation site: softens, enlarges (von Fernwald's sign) 6 to 7 weeks
5. Laboratory tests:
   a. Immunological: widely used today; faster, 90% accurate; beta subunit of HCG can be used even before missed period.
   b. Commercially sold pregnancy test: an HAI in-home test, results in 4 minutes; should be confirmed by a physician
6. Braxton-Hicks contractions
7. Ballottement

C. Positive signs (by examiner)
1. Palpate: can feel fetal parts
2. Hearing: FHT
   a. Electronic Doptone scope (audible at 8 to 11 weeks)
   b. Sonogram (can ascertain at 12 weeks)
   c. Auscultation (17 to 24 weeks) with fetoscope (headscope) or Leff stethoscope
3. Ultrasonographic (echographic) evidence of pregnancy visualized on screen
4. Fetal movement palpable after 20 weeks

Prenatal Care

A. Importance
1. Regular assessments and monitoring detect early signs and symptoms disrupting normal, healthy pregnancy.
2. Early evaluation of problem permits development of an appropriate plan of action based on findings.

B. Visits and examinations
1. Initial visits: establish diagnosis of pregnancy
2. Laboratory work drawn during prenatal visits
   a. Alpha-fetoprotein (AFP) measurements in maternal serum are used for early diagnosis of fetal neural tube defects, such as spina bifida and anencephaly.
   b. Estriol levels are assessed as part of a *triple marker test;* in the presence of a fetus with Down syndrome, the AFP levels and estriol levels are low, and the HCG levels are low; these tests in combination with maternal age are used to calculate the risk.
   c. Human placental lactogen (HPL): a placental hormone that may be deficient in certain abnormalities of pregnancy

3. Complete medical history
   a. General personal health, habits, diseases, and medical or surgical problems
   b. History of communicable diseases, especially scarlet fever, measles, rubella, streptococcal infections, kidney conditions that might adversely affect pregnancy, and sexually transmitted diseases, HIV status, tuberculosis
   c. Psychosocial history: assess substance use or abuse (including alcohol, tobacco, illegal prescription or over-the-counter drugs), social support, physical abuse, stress, employment, physical activity, cultural influences, and sibling adjustment; siblings of the baby should be provided with explanations of pregnancy appropriate for the child's age.
   d. Previous pregnancies, miscarriages, abortions, blood transfusions, gynecological problems
   e. Family health status: diabetes, tuberculosis, heart disease, cancer, epilepsy, allergies, mental problems

4. Complete examination to include:
   a. Routine laboratory tests
      (1) Matching blood type and Rh factor
      (2) Antibody screen (rubella, sickle cell) if appropriate
      (3) Complete blood count (CBC), including hemoglobin and hematocrit
      (4) Venereal Disease Research Laboratory (VDRL) test (for syphilis)
      (5) Herpes 1 and 2 tests
      (6) HIV testing for the acquired immunodeficiency syndrome (AIDS) virus
      (7) Hepatitis A and B tests
      (8) Papanicolaou (Pap) smear
      (9) Purified protein derivative (PPD) test used for tuberculosis
      (10) Cervical culture to check for group-B streptococcus
   b. Physical examination to include:
      (1) Pelvic examination and measurements
      (2) Abdominal palpation
      (3) Examination of breasts, nipples
      (4) Vital signs: blood pressure, weight, temperature, respirations
      (5) Urinalysis for sugar and albumin
      (6) Smears (Papanicolaou's [Pap] test) for cytology, gonorrhea, Chlamydia

5. Usual schedule for prenatal visits
   a. Every month for 28 weeks
   b. Every 2 weeks thereafter to thirty-sixth week
   c. Every week from thirty-seventh week to term
   d. Adjusted to individual needs

6. Usual routine for prenatal visits
   a. Perform urinalysis each visit for sugar, acetone, albumin.
   b. Perform capillary blood testing on a glucose oxidase strip for gestational diabetes mellitus (GDM), followed by plasma glucose testing at 12 weeks' gestation on all high-risk pregnancies.
   c. Check vital signs (especially blood pressure).
   d. Check weight gain every visit.
      (1) First trimester: 3 to 4 lb (1.5 to 2 kg) total
      (2) Second trimester: 1 lb (0.5 kg) per week; 12 to 14 lb (6 to 7 kg) total

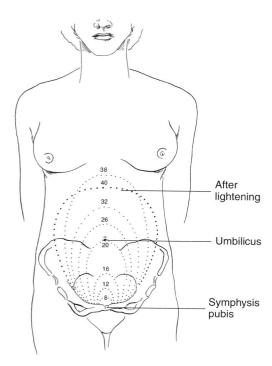

After lightening

Umbilicus

Symphysis pubis

FIGURE 7-3. Height of fundus by weeks of normal gestation with a single fetus. *(From Burroughs A, Leifer G:* Maternity nursing: an introductory text, *ed 8, Philadelphia, 2001, Saunders.)*

(3) Third trimester: 1 lb (0.5 kg) per week; 8 to 10 lb (4 to 5 kg) total
  e. Measure height of fundus to evaluate growth of fetus (Figure 7-3).
  f. Listen to FHT and FHR by Doptone or auscultation.
  g. Ask about fetal activity, attitude of family; answer mother's questions, fears.
  h. Recommend childbirth education classes.
C. Promotion of positive health
  1. Nutritional counseling
    a. Fetus receives all nourishment from mother.
    b. Teenage pregnant mother requires extensive counseling (nutritional pattern poor); focus is on positive effect of good nutrition on adolescent, as well as on fetus.
    c. In the past, sodium restriction was advised to help prevent edema, retention of fluids, and PIH; research has shown that sodium intake in pregnancy helps maintain normal and expanded fluid levels in pregnancy; women may be told to limit foods high in sodium.
    d. Direct relationship exists between maternal nutrition and mental development of the child.
    e. Megavitamins should be avoided during pregnancy; they can be dangerous for the developing fetus.
    f. Long-term users of oral contraceptives may have depleted the body's reserves of vitamin B_6 and folate.
    g. High folic acid intake may disguise vitamin B_{12} deficiency (pernicious anemia), which can lead to neurological damage; folic acid intake should not exceed 400 μg/day.
    h. Energy needs during pregnancy increases little (300 kilocalories/day [kcal/day]) compared with the increased need for nutrients

2. Nutritional needs during pregnancy
  a. See Table 7-2
  b. See Food Pyramid in Chapter 4
3. General health teaching
  a. Daily baths for cleanliness; showers during last 6 weeks for safety's sake
  b. Moderate exercise, especially walking
  c. Douching only on advice of physician
  d. Sexual intercourse is permissible as long as it is not uncomfortable, cervix is closed, and membranes are intact.
  e. Good support bra
  f. Unrestrictive comfortable clothing, hose
  g. Good mental attitude; discuss ambivalent feelings
  h. Smoking: nicotine retards growth of fetus, constricts blood vessels in mother, decreases placental function, and may cause premature labor; growing evidence shows that secondary smoking has damaging effects on the mother, fetus, children, and spouses; research has shown a relationship between mothers who smoke excessively and the incidence of pneumonia and bronchitis in babies at 6 to 9 months of age.
  i. Alcohol: research has yet to determine minimum safe amounts of alcohol (if any) that can be consumed in pregnancy.
  j. Caffeine: caffeine has been shown to cause tetragenic effects in animals; pregnant women should be counseled to avoid foods containing caffeine (found in coffee, tea, chocolate, colas, and some analgesics); newer evidence indicates a higher incidence of sudden infant death syndrome (SIDS) in infants of mothers who consumed significant amounts of caffeine during pregnancy.
  k. Drugs: may pass placental barrier and affect fetus; greatest danger is during first trimester, but effects may not be evident for years after birth; new evidence shows that crack or cocaine may cause significant complications for mother and newborn; pregnant women should be counseled to avoid over-the-counter or prescription medications without the advice of a physician; pregnant women should be counseled about their regular use of vitamins and warned against taking megadoses.
4. Childbirth and parent education classes
  a. Dick-Read method (*Childbirth Without Fear*, 1944): philosophy of relaxation coupled with abdominal and chest breathing and education
  b. Lamaze method, American Society for Prophylaxis in Obstetrics [ASPO]; psychoprophylactic method [PPM], 1960): combines breathing techniques with preparation for childbirth by training mother to anticipate various stages of labor and meet each stage with practiced relaxation and breathing methods; coach to support mother and direct her if necessary.
  c. Bradley method (1965): husband-coached childbirth, emphasizing quiet, darkened atmosphere, no stress
  d. Breathing techniques are more effective if learned before labor; if a woman and her partner are using a technique effectively, do not interfere.
5. Nonpharmacological techniques can be used to augment pain relief; these include breathing, distraction, skin stimulation; practitioners must be trained in these techniques before their implementation with patients.

TABLE 7-2   Nutritional Needs During Pregnancy

Nutrient	Nonpregnant Woman (19-22 yr)	Pregnant Woman	Usage	Food Source

Protein	44 g	74-100 g; needs twice as much	Growth of fetus
			  Placental growth
			  During labor and
			  delivery
			  During lactation
				Milk, cheese, eggs, meat, grains, legumes, nuts

Major Minerals				
Calcium	800 mg	1200 mg; needs one and a half times as much	Fetal skeleton Fetal tooth buds Calcium metabolism in mother	Milk, cheese, whole grains, leafy vegetables, egg yolk
Phosphorus	800 mg	1200 mg; needs one and a half times as much		Milk, cheese, lean meats
Iron	18 mg	30-60 mg supplement; needs almost two to three times as much	Increased maternal blood volume Fetus stores iron in third trimester	Liver, meats, eggs, leafy vegetables, nuts, legumes, whole wheat
Vitamin C (not stored in body so pregnant mother should take at least 1 serving per day)	60 mg	80 mg	Tissue formation Increased iron absorption	Citrus fruits, berries, melon, tomatoes, green peppers, green leafy vegetables, broccoli
Vitamin D	5-10 μg; 200-400 IU	10-15 μg; 400-600 IU; needs almost twice as much	Tooth buds Mineralize bone tissue Aid absorption of calcium and phosphorus	Fortified milk Fortified margarine
Folic acid	180 μg	400 μg	Increase red blood cell formation; prevention of macrocytic and megaloblastic anemia and neural tube defects	Green leafy vegetables, oranges, broccoli, asparagus, liver

μ*g*, Microgram; *IU,* international units.

6. Teaching danger signs (those that must be reported to physician immediately)
   a. Persistent, severe vomiting beyond first trimester
   b. Epigastric or abdominal pain
   c. Edema: face, fingers; especially in the morning
   d. Visual disturbances: blurring, double vision, spots
   e. Frequent or continuous headaches
   f. Bleeding or *leakage of fluid* from vagina
   g. Absence of fetal movements (after quickening)
   h. Chills and fever (signs of infection)
   i. Rapid weight gain (signs of possible preeclampsia)

Normal Discomforts of Pregnancy

See Table 7-3

ABNORMAL ANTEPARTUM

Hypertensive States

A. Definition: a group of conditions that occur during pregnancy, usually after 20 weeks' gestation: symptoms can range from high blood pressure (BP) to headaches, blurred vision, and convulsions with ensuing coma.
   1. Frequent in high-risk mothers
   2. Greater likelihood during first pregnancies
   3. Incidence: 5% to 7% of all pregnancies
B. Types
   1. Pregnancy induced hypertension (PIH): increase of BP to or above 140/90 mm Hg
      a. Increased BP only symptom
      b. Disappears within 10 days following delivery
   2. Preeclampsia: an acute hypertensive condition resulting in elevated BP (increased systolic BP [30 mm Hg] or increased BP [15 mm Hg] over baseline) and proteinuria; edema may also be present.
      a. Mild preeclampsia
         (1) BP 140/90 mm Hg
         (2) Proteinuria 1+
         (3) Rapid weight gain
      b. Moderate-to-severe preeclampsia
         (1) Hospitalize immediately.
         (2) BP 160/110 mm Hg

TABLE 7-3   Normal Discomforts of Pregnancy

Discomfort	Probable Cause	Relief Measures
First Trimester		
Breasts: painful	Hypertrophy of glandular tissue Increased blood flow to area Hormonal effects	Firm, supportive bra, even a nursing bra
Urinary frequency	Pressure on bladder from expanding uterus reduces bladder capacity; increased vascular content	Pads if necessary
Yawning (tired, sleepy)	Whether result of relaxin hormone is questionable; possibly caused by sudden chemical changes in body	Frequent rest periods Balanced diet to prevent anemia
Nausea and vomiting	Hormonal changes Ambivalent feelings regarding pregnancy	Small, frequent meals Limited fluids Dry crackers with tea Avoiding greasy fried foods
Second Trimester		
Heartburn (acid taste in mouth)	Relaxin hormone effect Enlarging uterus displaces stomach upward	Avoiding fatty foods Antacids: Milk of Magnesia, Gelusil, Maalox, Amphojel
Pigmentation	Hormonal	Reassuring the mother that it is temporary and will disappear after delivery
Leg cramps	Calcium-phosphorus imbalance	Position relief Calf stretching Calcium supplements, milk
Constipation	Hormonal: slowing down of peristaltic movements Compression of colon by uterus and baby	Adequate fluids, fruits, foods with roughage Exercises Stool softener but no mineral oil
Third Trimester		
Urinary incontinence	Lightening/dropping of fetus into pelvic cavity pushes presenting part on bladder	Pelvic floor exercise (Kegel): tighten perineal muscles, relax, then repeat
Hemorrhoids	Pressure from fetal presenting part	Increased vascular activity Knee-chest (elevate hips): Kegel exercises Comfort measures: frequent rest periods; sitting in warm tub; supporting legs with pillows
Low back pain	Increased pressure Fatigue Poor weight distribution	Pelvic exercises Pushing, stretching Comfort massaging Good posture
Insomnia	Increased fetal movements Muscular cramping Urinary frequency Dyspnea	Adequate rest periods Warm milk at bedtime Relaxing shower Support with pillows Deep breathing
Varicosities (leg, vulva)	Hereditary disposition Pelvis vasocongestion Pull of gravity Pressure of uterus Forcing stool (constipation)	Support stockings Changing position frequently Abdominal support Keeping legs uncrossed
Edema (legs, feet)	Immobility (staying in one position for a prolonged time)	Periodic resting Moving around Support stockings Elevating legs Plenty of fluids (to serve as a diuretic)
Dyspnea (shortness of breath)	Pressure on diaphragm from expanding uterus	Sitting erect Deep breathing Putting arms above head Keeping weight down

Continued

TABLE 7-3	Normal Discomforts of Pregnancy—cont'd	
Discomfort	**Probable Cause**	**Relief Measures**
Leaking of colostrum	Increased blood supply Prominent nipples	Support bra Pads if necessary (keep clean and dry)
Supine hypotension syndrome (feeling faint)	Pressure on ascending vena cava by uterus	Lying on left side with legs flexed or semi-sitting position
Vaginal discharge	Hormonal	No douching Keeping area clean, dry (perineal care)

    (3) Albumin 2+ to 4+

    (4) Persistent, severe headaches with visual disturbances

    (5) Epigastric pain (late sign)

    (6) Hyperactive deep-tendon reflexes (DTRs) clonus: an abnormal pattern of neuromuscular activity, characterized by rapidly alternating involuntary contraction and relaxation of skeletal muscle

  3. Eclampsia

    a. Definition: most severe form of the hypertensive states, characterized by hypertensive crisis, shock, followed by grand mal seizure and possibly coma

    b. Signs and symptoms

      (1) Alarming weight gain

      (2) Scanty urine (less than 30 ml/hour)

      (3) Proteinuria 4+, RBCs in urine

      (4) BP 200/100 mm Hg or higher

      (5) Edema of retina; can cause blindness

      (6) Severe epigastric pain

      (7) Hyperactive DTRs

      (8) Convulsions: tonic and clonic

NOTE: May start labor prematurely; infant may be severely compromised and die.

    4. HELLP syndrome: a severe form of PIH that involves multiple organ damage; the exact cause is unknown; HELLP syndrome is thought to arise as a result of changes occurring with preeclampsia; arteriolar vasospasm, endothelial damage, and platelet aggregation lead to decreased tissue perfusion and organ damage. The letters stands for Hemoptysis, Elevated Liver function, and Low Platelet level.

C. Treatment and nursing management

  1. According to classification and severity of symptoms; varies from home care precautions to absolute bed rest in a hospital with patient lying on left side

  2. Reduce stimuli

  3. Convulsion precautions

  4. Selective antihypertensive and diuretic therapy may be ordered (e.g., hydralazine [Apresoline] hydrochloride, furosemide [Lasix], magnesium sulfate, mannitol labetalol); nurse should know effects and untoward symptoms.

  5. Monitor edema, BP, FHT, levels of consciousness, DTRs, impending labor signs.

Hyperemesis Gravidarum

A. Definition: pernicious vomiting of pregnancy lasting into second trimester

B. Signs and symptoms

  1. Excessive nausea, vomiting

  2. Considerable weight loss

  3. Severe dehydration

  4. Depletion of essential electrolytes (sodium and potassium)

  5. Vitamin, glucose, protein deficiencies

  6. Ketone bodies in urine: 1 protein

  7. Elevated hemoglobin level, RBC count, hematocrit

C. Treatment and nursing management: untreated will lead to death of mother or fetus, or both

  1. Hospitalize in well-ventilated, private, pleasant environment.

  2. Restrict visitors.

  3. Nothing by mouth (NPO) first 48 hours.

  4. Record intake and output (I & O).

  5. If vomiting occurs, antiemetic medications may be administered.

  6. Provide IV fluids to replace losses in nutrition.

  7. Provide gradual serving of attractive, small portions of food on china dishes, starting with dry toast and tea.

  8. Present nonjudgmental nursing attitudes.

  9. Refer for psychotherapy when appropriate.

Hemorrhagic Conditions

A. Abortion (early pregnancy bleeding)

  1. Definition: the expulsion of uterine contents before viability of the fetus for medical reasons or spontaneously

  2. Types

    a. Induced abortion

      (1) Termination of pregnancy (therapeutic): legal aborting of the fetus for medical or psychological reasons by a licensed physician under controlled, aseptic conditions

      (2) Criminal: an abortion performed under illegal, unsafe conditions

    b. Spontaneous abortion

      (1) Definition: an abortion that occurs naturally (usually in the first trimester)

      (2) Possible causes: hormonal deficiencies, abnormalities of the fetus, incompetent cervix, abnormalities of the reproductive organs, emotional shock, physical injury, acute infections, and growths.

  3. Terminology of abortions

    a. Habitual abortion: three or more consecutive spontaneous abortions for unknown reasons

    b. Threatened abortion: minimal signs and symptoms of abortion, such as bleeding and cramping, but with no loss of uterine contents

    c. Imminent abortion: considerable blood loss, severe contractions; urge to push that without treatment will result in loss of uterine contents.

    d. Inevitable abortion: bleeding, contractions, rupture of membranes, and cervical dilatation in which the uterine contents will be lost; thus treatment will concentrate on the mother.

e. Incomplete abortion: part or parts of uterine contents are retained, necessitating administration of oxytocins to accelerate expulsion of remaining contents, or dilatation and curettage (D & C; a minor surgical intervention) to prevent prolonged bleeding.

f. Complete abortion: entire uterine contents are expelled.

4. Signs and symptoms of abortion
   a. Vaginal bleeding: scant to profuse
   b. Abdominal cramping: slight to severe
   c. Contractions: intermittent, steady, mild, or severe

5. Treatment and nursing management
   a. Prompt and immediate bed rest
   b. Hospitalization when appropriate
   c. Prevention of blood loss and shock
   d. Replacement blood treatment if necessary
   e. Checking vital signs and temperature for 24 hours
   f. Endocrine therapy when appropriate
   g. Surgical intervention when appropriate: Shirodkar operation (purse-string suturing) for known incompetent cervix
   h. Psychotherapy when appropriate
      (1) Prepare for grieving process.
      (2) Provide assistance for burial regulations.
      (3) Let mother vent feelings of love, loss, guilt.
      (4) Provide quiet, supportive, compassionate nursing care.

B. Ectopic pregnancy (early pregnancy bleeding)
   1. Definition: an extrauterine pregnancy in which the products of conception are implanted outside the uterine cavity; 90% occur in the fallopian tube (right tube more frequent); other sites include the abdomen or the ovary.
   2. Signs and symptoms
      a. Abnormal or missed menstrual period
      b. Slight uterine bleeding or spotting
      c. Possible mass on affected side; pain, tenderness, rigid abdomen
      d. If tube ruptures, may be little bleeding externally but massive internal hemorrhaging, with accompanying severe shock
      e. A diagnosis via transvaginal ultrasound is possible before tube rupture; if diagnosed before rupture, a laparoscopy is done to remove portion of the tube; goal is to remove ectopic pregnancy and preserve reproductive function; may also treat with methotrexate
   3. Treatment and nursing management
      a. Immediate hospitalization
      b. Treat shock (warm, quiet, replacement therapy—IV fluids, oxygen).
      c. Cross-match and other blood work: transfusion readiness.
      d. Support mother, who will be extremely frightened.
      e. Prepare for immediate surgery if appropriate.
      f. Arrange for baptism of fetus when appropriate.
      g. Provide postsurgical care with IV fluids, medications, other appropriate treatments (RhoGAM if necessary).
      h. Provide emotional support to mother and family; get assistance of clergy when requested.

C. Gestational trophoblastic neoplasm (formerly known as hydatidiform mole)
   1. Definition: rare degeneration of chorionic villi into a benign neoplasm in which the villi fill with clear viscous fluid and form grapelike clusters; the neoplasm fills the decidua and expands the uterus to larger than normal for gestational age.
   2. Signs and symptoms
      a. Enlarging uterus, greater than for normal gestation
      b. Missed period; spotting to profuse bleeding
      c. Several shiny, tapioca-like "grape clusters" escaping through vaginal tract
      d. Nausea and vomiting
      e. Signs of PIH; usually before 20 weeks' gestation
      f. No FHT
      g. No fetal structures on ultrasound examination
      h. Laboratory findings: HCG titers up to 1 to 2 million (normally 350,000 to 400,000 at 8 weeks)
   3. Treatment and nursing management
      a. Termination as soon as diagnosis confirmed
      b. Blood transfusion if indicated
      c. Assistance in grieving process of mother and family
      d. Follow-up very important
         (1) Contraceptive advice (nothing oral because HCG titers will be distorted)
         (2) HCG titers for at least 6 months

D. Placenta previa (third-trimester bleeding)
   1. Definition: abnormal implantation of a normal placenta for unknown reasons, usually in the lower segment of the uterus; condition usually occurs in multiparas, and incidence appears to increase with age; may also be caused by fibroids
   2. Types (Figure 7-4)
      a. Partial (incomplete): incomplete coverage of the uterine os
      b. Complete (total): entire uterine os completely covered
      c. Marginal (low lying): located in lower uterine segment but away from the os
   3. Signs and symptoms
      a. Painless uterine bleeding: may be intermittent or occur in gushes; scanty to severe; bright red
      b. Third-trimester occurrence
   4. Treatment and nursing management
      a. Diagnosis confirmed by ultrasound or x-ray examination
      b. Avoidance of vaginal examinations
      c. Immediate hospitalization
      d. Quiet environment; fetus uncompromised; station high
      e. Fowler's position (head at 30-degree angle)
      f. Tocolytic therapy with use of magnesium sulfate to manage uterine irritability under certain circumstances
      g. Have double set-up ready so that if vaginal examination is imperative, emergency CS equipment is available and blood is ready for transfusion.
      h. Foley catheter if condition is severe; provide shock care.
      i. Count pads to determine amount, color, duration of bleeding.
      j. Monitor vital signs, especially BP.
      k. Monitor FHT and FHR.
      l. IV fluids; monitor
      m. Support patient and family; keep them informed.

E. Abruptio placentae (third-trimester bleeding)
   1. Definition: premature separation of a normally implanted placenta before the birth of the fetus
   2. Causes
      a. Trauma

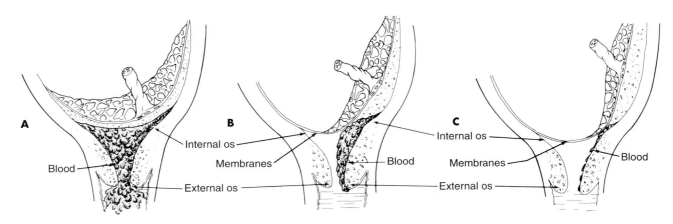

FIGURE 7-4.   Types of placenta previa after onset of labor. A, Complete, or total. **B,** Incomplete, or partial. **C,** Marginal, or low-lying. *(From Lowdermilk DL, Perry SE:* Maternity and women's health care, ed 8, *St Louis, 2004, Mosby.)*

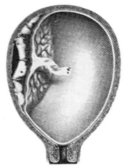

Partial separation
(concealed hemorrhage)

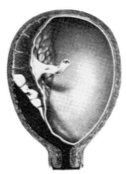

Partial separation
(apparent hemorrhage)

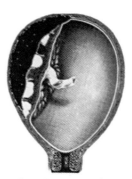

Complete separation
(concealed hemorrhage)

FIGURE 7-5.   Abruptio placentae. Premature separation of normally implanted placenta. *(From Lowdermilk DL, Perry SE:* Maternity and women's health care, ed 8, *St Louis, 2004, Mosby.)*

b. Chronic maternal disease
c. Grand multipara
d. Unknown
3. Types (Figure 7-5)
  a. Complete: separation of the placenta from the uterine wall before birth of the fetus
  b. Partial: separation of a portion of the placenta from the wall of the uterus before the birth of the fetus
4. Signs and symptoms
  a. Severe abdominal pain; sometimes called "exquisite" or unrelenting
  b. Patient is distressed, depressed, and exhibits signs of shock.
  c. Painful bleeding: moderate to severe; internal or external; dark red, not clotted; varying amount
  d. Abdomen tense, boardlike; nurse unable to feel contractions; uterus irritable
  e. Hypovolemic shock possibly resulting in renal failure
  f. Sudden change in heartbeat or bradycardia, or absence of FHT
5. Treatment and nursing management
  a. Depends on stage and intensity of condition; for reasons not clearly understood, partial abruptio placentae may seal off bleeding spontaneously, and labor will proceed normally.

b. Check coagulation profile: fibrinogen and fibrin, platelets.
c. Prevent hypovolemic shock and fetal hypoxia.
d. Cross-match, type, readiness for transfusions.
e. Monitor contractions, FHT, and vital signs.
f. Slight or moderate bleeding may indicate Artificial rupture of membranes (ARM) (or AROM) to hasten delivery or seal off bleeding
g. Severe bleeding (dark red) may indicate immediate CS.
h. Support mother and family.
i. Continued bleeding after delivery may necessitate hysterectomy.
F. Disseminated intravascular coagulation (DIC)
  1. Cause
    a. Unknown
    b. Coincidental with abruptio placentae, postabortal infection, amniotic fluid emboli, placenta previa, and uterine atony
  2. Pathology: not clearly understood; massive clotting, depletion of coagulant factor
  3. Signs and symptoms: excessive bleeding at placental site, incisional site, nose, mouth, gums
  4. Treatment and nursing management
    a. Halt or reverse DIC.
    b. Eliminate cause.

   c. Immediate delivery
   d. Blood replacement
   e. IV fibrinogen, heparin

Medical and Infectious Conditions

A. Chickenpox (varicella)
   1. Causative agent: herpesvirus; *Varicella zoster* virus (VZV)
   2. Effect on mother
      a. May manifest itself as herpes zoster (shingles)
      b. May be fatal if severe
      c. May cause abortion
   3. Effect on fetus
      a. May cause defects of skin, bones, hydrocephalus if contracted during first trimester
      b. Fetal death
B. German measles (rubella or 3-day measles)
   1. Causative agent: virus
   2. Effect on mother
      a. Rash, fever, photophobia
      b. Possible abortion
   3. Effect on fetus if infected during first trimester
      a. Rubella syndrome: heart defects, blindness, deafness, mental retardation
      b. Delayed effect on brain (15 to 20 years of age)
C. Genital herpes
   1. Causative agent: herpes simplex virus 2
   2. Effect on mother
      a. Vaginal discharge
      b. Genital blisters, ulcers
      c. Fever
      d. Painful inguinal lymph nodes
   3. Effect on fetus
      a. Abortion or premature birth
      b. Neonatal infections
      c. Survivors may have central nervous system (CNS) symptoms
D. Group B Streptococcus
   1. Causative agent: Streptococcus bacterium found in the lower genital tract or rectum of 10% to 30% of all healthy pregnant women
   2. Effect on mother
      a. Asymptomatic carriers
      b. Increased risk of abnormal vaginal discharge, urinary tract infection (UTI), endocarditis
   3. Effect on fetus
      a. Pneumonia and sepsis, which can result in death in 12 to 24 hours
      b. Blindness, deafness, mental retardation
   4. Treatment
      a. Prenatal screening: if cultures are positive, the drug of choice is penicillin G.
      b. High-risk women should be offered prophylactic antibiotics in labor.
E. Hepatitis A
   1. Causative agent: virus
   2. Effect on mother
      a. Abortion
      b. Liver failure
   3. Effect on fetus
      a. First-trimester infection: fetal anomalies
      b. Premature birth
      c. Neonatal hepatitis

F. Hepatitis B (serum hepatitis)
   1. Causative agent: hepatitis B virus (HBV); contact with blood and through sexual intercourse
   2. Effect on mother
      a. May be asymptomatic
      b. Low-grade fever, fatigue, joint pain, nausea, vomiting
      c. Liver and spleen enlargement, cirrhosis
      d. Vaccine available for high-risk women and health care workers
   3. Effect on fetus
      a. Avoid exposure of newborn to blood of mother
      b. Preterm at birth
      c. May be asymptomatic at birth
      d. May exhibit signs of acute hepatitis
      e. Possible carrier
      f. Infants born to women who have hepatitis B should receive appropriate vaccinations.
G. Influenza
   1. Causative agent: virus
   2. Effect on mother
      a. Pneumonia
      b. Abortion
      c. Premature labor
   3. Effect on fetus
      a. Abortion or premature birth
      b. Fetal death
   4. Vaccine for pregnant women available; live viral vaccine can infect fetus.
H. Gonorrhea (clap)
   1. Causative agent: *Neisseria gonorrhoeae* bacterium
   2. Effect on mother
      a. Vaginal discharge
      b. Cervical tenderness
      c. Dysuria
      d. Affects ovaries, tubes, causing sterility
   3. Effect on fetus
      a. Ophthalmia neonatorum
      b. Conjunctivitis
      c. Mild-to-severe infections
I. Syphilis (lues)
   1. Causative agent: *Treponema pallidum* bacterium
   2. Effect on mother (if untreated)
      a. Primary chancre
      b. Secondary skin rash
      c. Latent or tertiary CNS problems
   3. Effect on fetus
      a. Rhagades of the corners of mouth and anus
      b. Snuffles
      c. Maceration of palms of hands and soles of feet
      d. Congenital syphilis (symptoms appearing later in life)
      e. Death (stillborn)
J. Cytomegalovirus (CMV)
   1. Causative agent: cytomegalovirus of the herpes group, transmitted by close bodily and sexual contact
   2. May be transmitted by asymptomatic woman to fetus causing fetal damage, retardation, or fetal death
   3. The infant may acquire the virus by exposure to cervical mucus during vaginal birth.
   4. No satisfactory treatment is available for maternal or neonatal CMV.

K. Chlamydia
1. Causative agent: bacterial microorganism *Chlamydia trachomatis* (CT); transmitted by close bodily and sexual contact
2. May initiate pelvic inflammatory disease (PID) leading to ectopic pregnancy and infertility
3. Some evidence suggests relationship between CT and PROM, preterm labor and delivery, low birth weight, increased perinatal mortality, and late onset endometritis.
4. Treatment is extended erythromycin.
5. Transmission from infected birth canal may result in conjunctivitis or pneumonia or both.
L. Cardiac disease
1. Classification
    a. Class I: no limitation of activity
    b. Class II: slight limitation of activity
    c. Class III: considerable limitation of even ordinary activity
    d. Class IV: symptoms of cardiac insufficiency even at rest
2. Treatment and nursing management
    a. Close medical and nursing supervision
    b. Watch for signs and symptoms of fatigue, dyspnea, coughing, palpitations, tachycardia.
    c. Promote rest.
    d. Hospitalize at end of second trimester.
    e. Breast-feeding is contraindicated.
    f. Provide contraceptive education.
    g. Nutrition: offer foods high in iron and protein; avoid raw, deep green vegetables because vitamin K counteracts effects of heparin.
    h. Prevent infections: report first signs of exposure.
    i. Teach comfortable positions: pillows, support, left side.
    j. During labor and delivery: epidural or caudal anesthesia (blocks) block to minimize discomfort on bearing down
    k. Watch for cardiac decompensation (pulse rate over 100 beats per minute [bpm]; respirations over 25)
    l. Vaginal delivery preferred
        (1) Episiotomy, low forceps
        (2) Oxygen to decrease pulmonary edema
        (3) Medication to regulate heart rate
        (4) Diuretic to reduce fluid retention
    m. Postpartal care
        (1) Hospitalization longer than normal to stabilize cardiac output
        (2) Application of abdominal binder (because of rapid change in intraabdominal pressure)
        (3) Bed rest with progressive bathroom privileges dependent on progress
        (4) Prevent overdistention of bladder.

        (5) Encourage bonding; nurse should hold baby at eye level to allow mother to touch and talk to baby.
        (6) Inform mother and family of progress.
M. Diabetes mellitus
1. Definition: inborn error in the transportation and metabolism of carbohydrates
2. Classification: see Table 7-4
3. Effects of diabetes on pregnancy
    a. Difficult to control because of changing patterns of fetal growth and development and maternal demands
    b. Fluctuating insulin requirements
    c. Tendency to develop acidosis (diabetic coma) from lack of insulin
    d. Increased tendency to infection (urinary tract, vaginal tract), preeclampsia, and polyhydramnios
    e. Increased incidence of premature labor
    f. Macrosomia (oversized baby)
    g. Possibility of dystocia
    h. Increased danger of placental deterioration causing hypoxia in fetus
    i. Tendency to abruptio placentae
4. Changing insulin requirements during pregnancy
    a. First trimester: insulin requirement decreased
    b. Second trimester: insulin requirement increased
    c. Third trimester: careful regulation (blood sugar); evaluation of placenta, oxytocin challenge test Contraction stress test (CST)
    d. Intranatal: labor depletes glycogen
    e. Postpartum: insulin reaction resulting from sudden drop in need
    f. Watch for hypoglycemia, shock, infection, bleeding.
    g. No need for insulin 24 to 48 hours after delivery
    h. Hospitalized until insulin balance restored
5. Early recognition of insulin reaction and diabetic coma
6. Treatment and nursing management
    a. Weekly prenatal visits
    b. Regulation of insulin dosage and dietary management
    c. Mother taught to test blood three or four times a day
    d. Testing for placental adequacy: CST (stress test) measures fetal response to uterine contractions; late deceleration indicates problem.
    e. Teach good nutrition.
    f. Help allay fears and anxieties.
N. Addiction and pregnancy
1. Drug addition
    a. Effect on mother
        (1) Abortion
        (2) Premature birth
        (3) Stillbirth

TABLE 7-4	Classifications of Diabetes	
Classification	**Characteristics**	**Treatment During Pregnancy**
Type 1: insulin-dependent diabetes mellitus (IDDM)	Usually juvenile onset; prone to ketosis	Diet control and insulin
Type 2: non–insulin-dependent diabetes mellitus (NIDDM)	Usually adult onset; ketosis resistant; may require insulin for hyperglycemia during stress; requires insulin during pregnancy	Diet control and insulin
Other: gestational diabetes mellitus (GDM)	Develops during pregnancy	Diet control alone or insulin

b. Effect on neonate: see section on Abnormal Newborn, pp. 421-422.
2. Alcohol and pregnancy
   a. Effect on mother
      (1) Poor nutritional habits
      (2) Poor hygiene
      (3) Physical, psychosocial deterioration
   b. Effect on neonate: see section on Abnormal Newborn, pp. 421-422.
3. Treatment and nursing management
   a. Supervised withdrawal
   b. Substitute therapy

Acquired Immunodeficiency Syndrome

Pregnant women whose partners were drug users sharing common needles, high-risk category men (bisexual or homosexual), or men who were infected with the disease have been known to become infected. Transmission of HIV to the unborn fetus has now been confirmed.

A. Confirmed avenues of transmission
   1. Anal or vaginal intercourse
   2. Drug addicts sharing needles of infected users
   3. Contaminated blood transfusions
   4. Transmission to the fetus or neonate can occur transplacentally or by exposure to blood and vaginal secretions at delivery and or by exposure to maternal secretion such as breast milk.
   5. Caesarean section (CS) does not appear to prevent the transmission of the virus totally.
B. Treatment and nursing management
   1. Pregnant HIV-infected women should receive Pneumovax, influenza, and hepatitis vaccines and should be screened for sexually transmitted diseases.
   2. HIV testing is voluntary and must be accompanied by informed consent and counseling; results are confidential.
   3. Immune status needs to be monitored; if immune status falls, physicians may elect to administer azidothymidine (AZT) to delay onset of illness.
   4. HIV-positive women need counseling to practice safe sex to decrease risk of repeatedly exposing fetus.
   5. Infants need to be followed and tested for a minimum of 2 years to determine if they have the disease.
C. The Centers for Disease Control and Prevention (CDC) guidelines for preventing transmission of the AIDS virus
   1. Standard Precautions are required.
   2. Pregnant nurses should be especially careful because an HIV infection can place the fetus at risk.
D. Follow hospital protocol for invasive procedures.

Tuberculosis

Tuberculosis is an increasingly prevalent health problem throughout the world; its resurgence in the United States is attributed to homelessness, drug abuse, poverty, and HIV; rates are particularly high among minorities and recent immigrants to the United States.

A. Confirmed avenues of transmission
   1. Airborne: coughs or sneezes of a person with infectious tuberculosis
   2. Shared air: persons in close air contact for a prolonged period
B. Treatment and nursing management
   1. Preventive therapy, postponed until after delivery

2. A pregnant woman with active disease needs immediate treatment of 2 to 3 antituberculosis drugs.
3. Breast-feeding is permitted; however, infant still needs to undergo prophylactic treatment.

Asthma

A. Definition: chronic lung disease in which airways are overly responsive to stimuli such as allergens, pollutants, exercise, and cold air
   1. Asthma occurs in approximately 1% of all pregnant women.
   2. The incidence of preeclampsia is higher in patients with asthma.
B. Signs and symptoms: cough, wheezing, dyspnea, chest tightness
C. Treatment and nursing management
   1. Pulmonary function tests to monitor lung function
   2. Nonstress tests (NSTs) to monitor fetal well being
   3. Avoiding allergens
   4. Pharmacological therapies
   5. Breast-feeding to provide some neonatal protection against respiratory allergens

Premature Labor

A. Definition: labor occurring before 37 to 38 weeks' gestation
B. Effect on family (focus on psychosocial problems)
   1. Mother not ready for delivery: apprehensive and frightened; feelings of guilt
   2. Family plus professional staff: restrained, quiet, anticipating complications
C. Effect on fetus: see Preterm (Premature) Infant under Abnormal Newborn, pp. 421-422.
D. Treatment and nursing management
   1. PROM usually precedes premature labor; test fluid with nitrazine paper: if alkaline, positive for amniotic fluid
   2. If membranes are intact and cervix is undilated, halt labor if possible; magnesium sulfate and terbutaline are frequently used to halt premature labor.
   3. Immediate bed rest is required.
   4. Monitor maternal pulse and BP.
   5. Know untoward effects of medications.
   6. Prevent infection.
   7. Offer constant emotional support to mother and family: inform, reassure, encourage mother and family.

NORMAL INTRAPARTUM (LABOR AND DELIVERY)

A. Fetal head (passenger)
   1. Two parietal bones: one each side of head
   2. Two temporal bones: one each side of head near temple
   3. Two frontal bones: one each side of forehead
   4. One occipital bone: lower back of head
   5. Sutures: membranous spaces between bones
      a. Sagittal suture: separates parietal bones and extends longitudinally back to front
      b. Frontal suture: between two frontal bones, continuation of the sagittal suture
      c. Coronal suture: as a crown; separates frontal and parietal bones

d. Lambdoidal suture: separates occipital bone from two parietal bones
6. Fontanels: formed by intersection of sutures; allow head bones to override and accommodate to birth passage
   a. Anterior fontanel: membranous, diamond-shaped space (bregma) formed by intersection of sagittal, frontal, and coronal sutures; called "soft spot"; closes within 12 to 18 months
   b. Posterior fontanel: small, membranous triangle-shaped space between occipital bone and two parietal bones; closes within 6 to 8 weeks
7. Principal measurements of the fetal head
B. Presentations, positions, station
   1. Presentation
      a. Definition: refers to that part of the passenger (fetus) that enters the passage (true pelvis, uterine os, vaginal canal) first
      b. Types of presentations
         (1) Cephalic: head, vertex, occiput (93%)
         (2) Breech: buttocks, sacrum, one or both legs, one or both feet (3%)
         (3) Shoulder: scapula (3%)
   2. Lie (Figure 7-6)
      a. Definition: refers to the relationship between the long axis of the passenger and the long axis of the mother
      b. Types
         (1) Longitudinal (99%)
         (2) Transverse (sideways)
   3. Position (Figure 7-7)
      a. Definition: the way in which the presenting part of the fetus lies in relation to the four quadrants of the mother's pelvis and to her back (posterior) and her front (anterior)

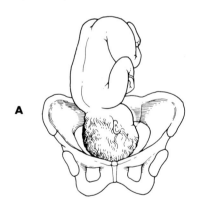
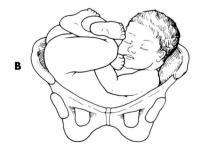

FIGURE 7-6. A, Longitudinal lie. **B,** Transverse lie. *(From Phillips CR: Family-centered maternity and newborn care: a basic text, ed 4, St Louis, 1996, Mosby.)*

b. To determine position, fetal *reference points* are used: these are:
   (1) Occiput (back of fetal head): O
   (2) Chin (mentum): M
   (3) Brow (bregma): B
   (4) Buttocks (sacrum): S
   (5) Shoulder (scapula): Sc
c. Types of position with occiput presentations: LOA, LOT, LOP, ROA, ROT, ROP (see Figure 7-7)
4. Attitude
   a. Definition: relationship of the various fetal parts to one another, or the relationship of the fetal extremities to its body (trunk)
   b. Normal attitude: flexed; fetal head on sternum, arms folded against chest; knees bent, pressing abdomen; legs flexed so toes touch arm
5. Station
   a. Definition: degree to which presenting part is located in the true pelvis; points of reference are the ischial spines, which are designated as 0 (zero)
   b. Levels
      (1) Minus: as in -1, -2, -3 station, means that presenting part is above the ischial spines
      (2) Plus: as in $+1$, $+2$, $+3$ station, means that the presenting part is below the ischial spines
      (3) -5 = floating; $+5$ = presenting part on perineum; or -3 to -5 = floating; $+3$ to $+5$ = presenting part on perineum; check with agency for the numbers used.
C. Mechanisms and stages of labor: labor cannot progress without power.
   1. Definition: the steps or maneuvers the fetus must undertake to accommodate to the passage and be delivered
   2. Process (mechanisms) (Figure 7-8, p. 412)
      a. Engagement: passage of the passenger into the pelvic inlet
      b. Descent: continuous slow progress of the fetus through the pelvis and the birth canal
      c. Flexion: head slowly adapts to birth canal by flexing chin.
      d. Internal rotation: fetal head turns in corkscrew maneuver so the long diameter of the head is parallel to the longest diameter of the pelvic outlet.
      e. Extension: the back of the fetal head goes under the pubic arch; the spine of the fetus extends to adapt itself to the curvature of the birth canal, and the head is delivered.
      f. Restitution: as the head emerges, it rotates back 45 degrees to the position it was before internal rotation, which helps the shoulders accommodate to the outlet.
      g. External rotation: the shoulders drop down and turn to the anteroposterior (AP) position, and the head slowly turns so both head and shoulders are aligned.
      h. Expulsion: the posterior (underneath) shoulder is delivered by lateral flexion (upward motion); then the anterior upper shoulder will slide out (downward motion) from under the pubic arch, and the body is easily expelled.

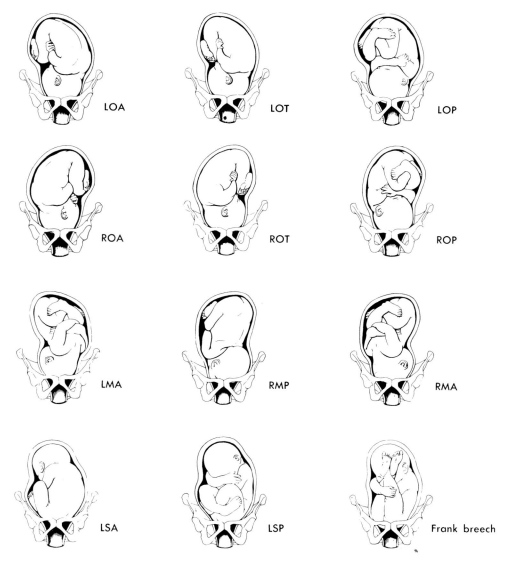

LOA LOT LOP

ROA ROT ROP

LMA RMP RMA

LSA LSP Frank breech

FIGURE 7-7.   Categories of presentations. *(Used with permission of Ross Products Division, Abbott Laboratories, Columbus, Ohio.)*

3. Stages of labor
   a. First stage: begins with the first true labor contraction; ends with complete dilatation and effacement of the cervix
   b. Second stage (expulsion): from complete effacement and dilatation to expulsion of the infant
   c. Third stage (placental): from delivery of the infant to delivery of the placenta and membranes (5 to 20 minutes)
   d. Fourth stage: from delivery of the secundines and repair of the perineum to 1 hour thereafter
D. Fetal evaluation during labor and delivery and immediately after
   1. During labor
      a. Fetal monitoring devices
         (1) Phonotransducer: amplification of fetal heart activity
         (2) Doppler transducer: ultrasonic device
      b. Special stethoscopes for monitoring FHT

   (1) Headscope (fetoscope): stethoscope on a head device; FHT conducted through monitor's frontal bone
   (2) Leff stethoscope: stethoscope with large, heavy conductor
   (3) External fetal monitor (EFM): applied to abdomen; FHT monitored electronically
      c. Direct fetal monitoring: an electrocardiogram (ECG) fetal scalp electrode (FSE) is placed directly to the fetal head.
   2. Evaluation immediately after delivery
      a. Establishment of patent airway
      b. Apgar scoring (Figure 7-9, p. 413): system of evaluating newborn response 1 minute after birth and 5 minutes after birth
      c. Observation for any visible anomalies
E. Nursing assessment
   1. Premonitory (impending) signs and symptoms of labor
      a. Lightening: descent of fetus down pelvic cavity

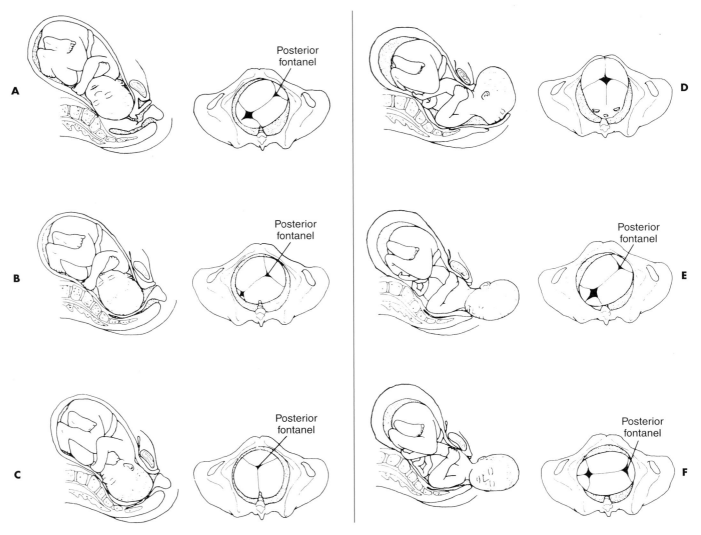

FIGURE 7-8. Mechanism of labor in left occipitoanterior (LOA) presentation. **A,** Engagement and descent. **B,** Flexion. **C,** Internal rotation to OA. **D,** Extension. **E,** Restitution. **F,** External rotation.

b. Braxton-Hicks contractions: painless contractions more frequent, regular
c. Breathing easier; heartburn disappears; hungry
d. Weight loss (decrease in water retention)
e. Frequency (pressure on bladder by presenting part)
f. Bloody show (slight pinkish discharge with or without discharge of mucous plug)
g. Bag of waters (BOW) ruptures spontaneously without prior contractions.

2. Differences between true and false labor
 a. False labor
  (1) Contractions irregular
  (2) No progress in interval or duration of contractions
  (3) Some abdominal discomfort
  (4) No bloody show
  (5) Relief by walking
  (6) No cervical change
  (7) Discomfort mostly in front (lower abdomen)
 b. True labor
  (1) Contractions regular and progressive
  (2) Not relieved by walking

  (3) Cervical changes
  (4) Progressive discomfort starting in back, going around lower abdomen, indentable fundus

3. Spontaneous rupture of membranes
 a. Note time, amount, and color of fluid; note fetal heart tones.
 b. Prevent infection (hand washing, good hygienic practice).
 c. Observe for prolapsed cord (notify physician immediately).
 d. If leakage minimal, spontaneous resealing may occur.
 e. If close to EDC, contractions may begin, usually within 4 to 16 hours.

F. Nursing intervention
 1. Nursing management during first stage of labor
  a. Admit patient to labor room.
  b. Establish rapport; ask pertinent questions regarding labor; observe reaction to labor process.
  c. Offer bedpan frequently (keep bladder empty).
  d. Usually, an IV is started to keep a vein open (KVO). (Prepare equipment, solutions.)

APGAR SCORING CHART

Sign	0	1	2
HEART RATE	Absent	Slow (below 100)	Over 100
RESPIRATORY EFFORT	Absent	Weak cry, hypoventilation	Good strong cry
MUSCLE TONE	Limp	Some flexion of extremities	Well flexed
REFLEX RESPONSE 1. Response to catheter in nostril (tested after oropharynx is clear)	No response	Grimace	Cough or sneeze
2. Tangential foot slap	No response	Grimace	Cry and withdrawal of foot
COLOR	Blue, pale	Body pink, extremities blue	Completely pink

FIGURE 7-9. The Apgar scoring chart. *(From Phillips CR: Family-centered maternity and newborn care: a basic text, ed 4, St Louis, 1996, Mosby.)*

e. Monitor contractions, FHR.
   (1) Hook up to fetal monitoring device.
   (2) Check every 30 to 60 minutes (depending on progress).
   (3) Frequency, duration, and intensity of uterine contractions are assessed to help determine the progress of labor.
   (4) When ominous FHR patterns occur (e.g., late decelerations, lack of variability), the nurse must document interventions and subsequent fetal response.
f. Keep mother, father informed on status and progress.
   (1) Monitor effacement, dilatation, station.
   (2) Encourage father to follow monitor readout.
   (3) Encourage father to use comfort measures for mother.
2. Nursing management during second stage of labor
   a. Uterine muscles bring about effacement and dilatation; abdominal muscles bring fetus down after dilatation and effacement are complete, and levator ani muscles assist in pushing and expelling fetus.
   b. All monitoring equipment is removed from mother.
      (1) Explain procedures.
      (2) Clean perineal area according to hospital policy.
      (3) Computers are frequently used to monitor FHR; EFM or a fetoscope or both are also used; inform physician on rate, strength, position.
      (4) Check BP every 15 minutes as necessary.
      (5) Prepare necessary equipment for delivery readiness and for reception of baby.
      (6) Instruct mother to push with contractions when indicated.
      (7) When infant delivered completely, note time.

(8) Establish patent airway.
(9) Encourage mother and father to see, touch, and speak to infant.
(10) Carefully place prophylactic drops in each eye.
(11) Follow proper identification routine.
(12) Transfer infant into warm crib for further evaluation and care.
3. Nursing management during third stage (placental)
   a. Be sure cord blood specimen is taken.
   b. Placenta delivered within 5 to 20 minutes from expulsion of infant.
   c. Note time and which side of placenta delivered.
      (1) Maternal side, raw and meaty: Duncan delivery
      (2) Fetal side, shiny and neat: Schultze delivery
   d. Administer oxytocin immediately following delivery of placenta to contract uterus and prevent hemorrhage.
   e. Check BP every 15 minutes.
   f. Check fundus for firmness; soft, boggy indicates possible hemorrhaging.
   g. Check and clean perineal area; apply sanitary napkin.
   h. Mother may experience knees shaking, teeth chattering.
      (1) Sudden changes in abdominal pressure plus hormonal changes trigger these symptoms.
      (2) Place several warm blankets over mother.
      (3) Reassure mother and family that it is a normal physiological phenomenon.
   i. Transfer mother to recovery area (if not in birthing room).
4. Nursing management during fourth stage of delivery
   a. Critical hour after delivery; watch for complications, especially hemorrhaging.
   b. Perform fundal check every 5 minutes; massage gently if necessary.
   c. Check BP and vital signs every 10 to 15 minutes until stable.
   d. After approximately 1 hour, when vital signs are stable:
      (1) Offer warm drink, toast, or even meal tray if mother wishes and physician approves.
      (2) Offer bedpan frequently to prevent bladder distention, which will impede involution; if unable to void, catheterization is usually a standing order.
      (3) Give sponge bath to refresh and clean body.
      (4) Teach perineal care with peribottle.
      (5) Transfer to postpartum room.
      (6) Advise mother to request help the first time she wishes to use the bathroom.
5. Commonly used medications during labor and delivery: prepared childbirth has greatly diminished use of analgesics and anesthetics during labor and delivery; patients who experience dystocia may need some medication for relief from exhaustion, fright, or prolonged pain.
   a. Amnesic
   b. Tranquilizer
   c. Analgesic
   d. Regional anesthesia
      (1) Paracervical block: anesthetizes cervical area
      (2) Pudendal block: peripheral nerve block; may also block urge to push for 30 minutes
      (3) Caudal block (spinal): used during first and second stages; continuous or one dose

(4) Saddle block: third, fourth, or fifth lumbar interspace; anesthetizes saddle area (inner groin, perineal area)

(5) Epidural: also administered into lumbar interspace; uses less anesthetic than caudal; blocks urge to push

(6) Spinal block: most commonly used for cesarean birth

e. Nursing management

(1) Encourage urination; encourage fluids.

(2) Observe for postspinal headache; treatment includes bed rest, ibuprofen, IV caffeine; the definitive treatment is a blood patch.

f. General anesthesia: rare

ABNORMAL INTRAPARTUM

Dystocia

A. Definition: prolonged, difficult, painful labor or delivery involving any one or more problems with the three Ps: passage, power, and passenger

B. Problems with passage
1. Inadequate pelvis
2. Soft-tissue deviation: a full bladder is the most common cause.

C. Problems with the power (uterine contractions)
1. Primary uterine inertia: inefficient contractions from the beginning
2. Secondary uterine inertia: well-established labor with good contractions at first; then, progress suddenly or gradually slows and stops altogether.
3. Hypotonic contractions (atonic uterus); most common; no progress in effacement or dilatation
4. Hypertonic uterine contractions
   a. Intense, titanic
   b. No interval between contractions
5. Dystonic contractions
   a. Painful
   b. Ineffective
   c. Asymmetrical (contractions in different segments of the uterus)

D. Problems with passenger (fetus)
1. Excessive size
2. Fetal anomaly
3. Fetal malposition or malpresentation
   a. Occiput posterior (most common)
   b. Breech
   c. Transverse
   d. Face
   e. Soldier (military) presentation
4. CPD (Cephalopelvic disproportion)
   a. Accommodation impossible
   b. May note unusual contour of uterus or abdomen

E. Complications
1. PROM
2. Predisposition to infection
3. Trauma
4. Hemorrhage
5. Prolapse of cord
6. Hypoxia of fetus
7. Severe molding of fetal head: danger of intracranial hemorrhage

8. Extreme backache (posterior positions)
9. Flowering of anus early because of pressure of occiput on lower sacral region, with subsequent residual of hemorrhoids
10. Extreme fatigue

F. Treatment and nursing management
1. Electronic monitoring of fetus and mother
2. Frequent confirmation of cervical progress
3. Sterile techniques during vaginal examination
4. Check status of BOW.
5. Check vital signs.
6. Observe condition of mother.
   a. Need for pain relief
   b. Sometimes after a medicated sleep or rest, dystocia disappears.
7. Support physical and psychological needs.
8. Watch for dehydration.
9. Spontaneous rotation toward end of transition may occur in occiput posteriors.

Supine Hypotensive Syndrome

A. Definition: condition caused by compression of vena cava by heavy uterus for a prolonged period; caused by mother's staying in one position for a long time

B. Signs and symptoms
1. Pallor
2. Light-headedness
3. Dizziness
4. Slight nausea

C. Treatment and nursing management: turn patient on left side to relieve pressure; advise frequent turning and changing of position.

Ruptured Uterus

A. Causes
1. Tetanic, pauseless or continuous contractions
   a. Possible cause: unmonitored pitocin infusion
   b. Unknown
2. Stretching of uterine walls by extensive, rapid growth of hydatidiform mole
3. Attempted vaginal birth after cesarean (VBAC) and uterine scar ruptures during labor
4. Cephalopelvic disproportion (CPD)
5. Forceps delivery

B. Treatment and nursing management
1. Prepare for emergency CS.
2. Monitor for signs of hypovolemic shock and fetal distress.
3. Prepare for all anticipatory nursing responsibilities, surgical or medical.

Prolapsed Cord

A. Definition: displacement of the cord below the presenting part and into the vaginal passage before delivery of fetus

B. Causes
1. Spontaneous rupture of the membranes before engagement
2. Breech presentations
3. Prematurity
4. Polyhydramnios
5. Abnormal presentations

C. Signs and symptoms
1. Cord may be seen, felt, or palpated.

2. Fetal heart pattern is abnormal (baseline bradycardia with decelerations).
D. Treatment and nursing management
1. Do not compress cord; do not try to reposition it.
2. Use sterile saline compress to keep cord moist and protected from infection.
3. Place mother in knee-chest position or in Trendelenburg's position so that presenting part is pushed away from cord by gravity.
4. Prepare for CS, blood cross-match, IV fluids, and so on.
5. Check FHR or use continuous EFM.
6. Support frightened mother and family.
7. If not a standing order, obtain an order for the mother to receive oxygen by mask.

Multiple Pregnancies

A. Definition: simultaneous gestation; twins, triplets, quadruplets, quintuplets, sextuplets, septuplets
B. Signs and symptoms
1. History of multiple gestation (female lineage)
2. Hearing two FHTs, each with own rate
3. Disclosure of multiple limbs, heads, by palpation
4. Larger than normal gestation uterus
5. Weight gain increased more than in normal gestation
6. Striae gravidarum more noticeable early on
7. Confirmation by sonogram
8. X-ray may be done, but only in the third trimester.
C. Types (Figure 7-10)
1. Single-ovum twins (monozygotic, identical)
a. Union of one sperm with one ovum
b. During mitosis, divides into two embryos
c. One placenta, two amniotic sacs
d. Same sex
e. Heredity a factor

2. Fraternal twins (dizygotic, unidentical)
a. Union of two sperm with two separate ova
b. Two amniotic sacs
c. Separate or fused placenta
d. Same or different sex
e. Do not look identical
f. Age of mother a factor; older women tend to release more than one ovum.
3. Formation of triplets and so on is varied.
D. Treatment and nursing management
1. Prenatal care
a. Visits increased
b. Observe for signs and symptoms of preeclampsia.
c. Premature labor common
d. Backaches common: support girdle, longer rest periods.
e. Varicosities common
f. Watch for complications resulting from position, presentation, lie of fetuses.
g. Size of fetuses may cause problems.
h. Be alert for possible CS.
2. Intrapartal care
a. Be prepared for premature labor and premature babies.
b. High-risk second stage
3. Third and fourth stages
a. Possibility of hemorrhage because of oversized uterus
b. Blood loss is greater than that for single births.
c. Oxytocin is not administered to mother until all babies delivered.
d. Risk of infection is greater than that in normal single births.
e. Perinatal mortality is greater than that in single deliveries.

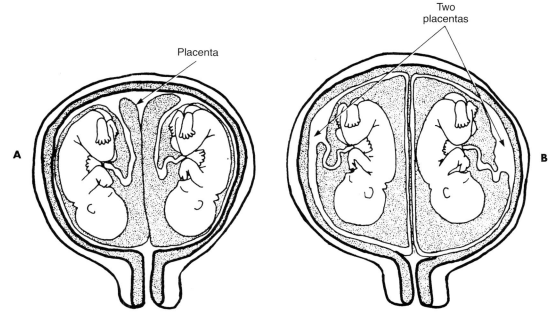

FIGURE 7-10. Multiple pregnancy. A, Identical (monozygotic) twins: two sacs, one placenta. **B,** Fraternal (dizygotic) twins: two sacs, two placentas. *(From Phillips CR: Family-centered maternity and newborn care: a basic text, ed 4, St Louis, 1996, Mosby.)*

Induction of Labor

A. Definition: the use of medication (oxytocin) to stimulate contractions before spontaneous onset
B. Indications
  1. Overdue fetus (over 42 weeks' gestation)
  2. Fetal death
  3. Prolonged rupture of membranes (over 24 hours) if uterine contractions have not begun
  4. PROM
  5. Diabetic mother
  6. Severe preeclampsia (exercise extreme caution)
  7. Steeply rising Rh titer
C. Contraindications
  1. CPD
  2. Fetal distress
  3. Previous CS
  4. Multiple births
  5. Heart conditions
  6. Prematurity
  7. Unengaged presenting part
  8. Placenta previa
  9. Abnormal fetal position (breech or transverse lie)
  10. Active genital herpes
D. Treatment and nursing management
  1. Monitor contractions carefully with external fetal monitor.
  2. If there are no intervals between contractions, stop medication drip and call physician immediately.
  3. Monitor FHR and report any changes immediately.
  4. Check BP: gradual elevation warrants immediate discontinuation of medication and prompt notification of physician.
  5. Keep family and mother informed of progress and procedure.
  6. Monitor vital signs, I&O.
  7. The physician or nurse midwife will assess for cervical dilation as needed and observe for the resting tone of the uterus before increasing the pitocin dose.

Augmentation of Labor

A. Definition: the use of medication to enhance existing contractions
B. Uses
  1. Uterine inertia: primary or secondary
  2. Atonic or hypotonic uterine contractions (may be enhanced by a boost of oxytocin)

Operative Obstetrics

A. Episiotomy
  1. Definition: surgical incision of the perineum during delivery to enlarge the vaginal outlet
  2. Types (Figure 7-11)
  3. Indications
    a. To avoid tearing
    b. To shorten second stage of labor
    c. Fetus or mother in jeopardy
  4. Treatment and nursing management
    a. Provide comfort measures (to promote healing); sitz bath and ice pack first 12 hours.
    b. Encourage Kegel exercises (to lessen pain, promote healing).

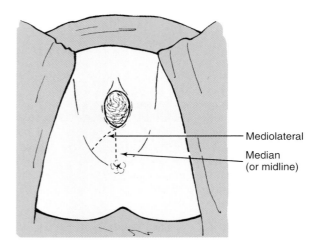

FIGURE 7-11.   Types of episiotomies. *(From Lowdermilk DL, Perry SE:* Maternity and women's health care, ed 8, *St Louis, 2004, Mosby.)*

    c. Apply witch hazel pads to perineal area (to decrease swelling, promote healing).
B. Forceps deliveries
  1. Definition: an operative procedure using various instruments to deliver the presenting part
  2. Indications for use
    a. To shorten second stage
    b. To assist in descent of presenting part when poor progress or fetal distress occurs
    c. Maternal exhaustion
    d. When rotation (of head) is necessary (e.g., left occiput posterior [LOP] to occiput anterior [OA])
    e. To save fetus in jeopardy
  3. Requirements for application
    a. No cephalopelvic disproportion
    b. Presenting part engaged and below ischial spines
    c. Full dilatation and effacement
    d. Ruptured membranes
    e. Empty bladder
    f. FHR checked before and after application
  4. Complications
    a. Lacerations and tears
    b. Hemorrhage
    c. Rupture of uterus
    d. Facial marks or facial paralysis of fetus
    e. Intracranial hemorrhage or brain damage to fetus
C. Vacuum extraction
  1. Definition: a soft, flexible cup placed over the fetal head as a machine exerts suction; allows practitioner to turn or pull the fetal head to assist delivery; an alternative to the use of forceps
  2. Problems for the fetus can be observed at the attachment site, including caput succedaneum or cephalhematoma.
D. Caesarian section (CS)
  1. Definition: an operative procedure to deliver the fetus through a surgical incision made through the abdominal and uterine walls
  2. Indications
    a. Cephalopelvic disproportion
    b. Fetal distress
    c. Prematurity
    d. Dystocia

e. Prolapsed cord
f. Oversized infant (macrosomia)
g. Positions and presentations undeliverable through the vagina
h. Some hypertensive states, placenta previa, abruptio placentae, prolapsed cord abnormalities
i. Maternal exhaustion
3. Types
  a. Elective
    (1) Anticipated difficulties: for example, inadequate pelvis or vaginal deliveries inadvisable because mother has AIDS or herpes
    (2) Previous CSs (selective)
  b. Emergency
    (1) Sudden fetal distress (e.g., rupture of the uterus)
    (2) Accident
    (3) Breech presentation, shoulder presentation (transverse lie)
4. Treatment and nursing management
  a. Routine surgical preoperative and postoperative care plus normal postpartum care
  b. Promote involution.
  c. Provide perineal care.
  d. Monitor lochia; color, amount same as for vaginal delivery.
  e. Support mother and family; allay fears.
  f. Watch for signs and symptoms of infection (chills, fever).
5. VBAC: vaginal delivery after a CS may be encouraged; depends on reason for CS

NORMAL POSTPARTUM

A. Definition: period from end of fourth stage of labor to 6 weeks after day of delivery
B. Immediate care following delivery
1. Continue checking of vital signs.
2. Encourage urination.
  a. Full bladder impedes involution.
  b. Full bladder may cause excessive bleeding.
3. Offer food: if policy permits, offer food and drink to mother after vital signs are stable.
4. Care of fundus
  a. Check for firmness.
  b. Checked lochia for color, amount, and presence of clots.
5. Provide perineal care and care of breasts.
6. Check incision (episiotomy or abdominal).
7. General hygiene: shower may be permissible to clean, refresh mother after vital signs are stable (policies vary).
8. Encourage putting infant to breast for feeding and bonding.
C. Physiological changes during puerperium
1. Reproductive organs
  a. Uterus: involution (return of uterus to normal size and function)
    (1) Walls of uterus return to normal in 3 to 4 weeks.
    (2) Menstruation may return in 3 to 4 weeks.
    (3) Nursing mothers: menstruation may be delayed several months.
    (4) Fundus involutes 1 finger-width every day if umbilicus is used as point of reference (Figure 7-12).

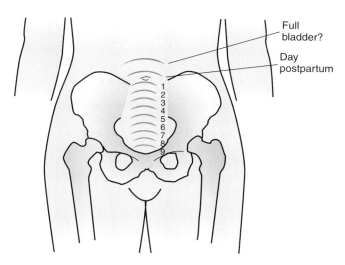

FIGURE 7-12. Involution. Height of fundus as it descends to prepregnant levels postpartum. *(From Lowdermilk DL, Perry SE: Maternity and women's health care, ed 8, St Louis, 2004, Mosby.)*

  b. Vagina
    (1) Returns to normal within 3 to 6 weeks after delivery, depending on type of delivery, length of labor, lacerations, healing process, and so on
    (2) Caesarian sections: vaginal recovery rapid
  c. Perineal area
    (1) Should be intact and clean
    (2) Requires 5 to 7 days for complete healing
2. Return to normal of body system and functions
  a. Hormonal recovery begins immediately.
  b. Lochia: vaginal discharge coming from decidual lining of uterus after delivery
    (1) Lochia rubra: dark red to bright red; occasional clots; flow lasts 2 to 3 days
    (2) Lochia serosa: pale pink to brownish lochia; lighter flow, dependent on ambulation; lasts 2 to 5 days
    (3) Lochia alba: yellowish, creamy discharge consisting of leukocytes and dead cells; lasts 5 to 10 days
    (4) Prolonged or recurring bleeding may indicate a medical problem.
  c. Vascular system
    (1) Average loss of blood at delivery: 250 to 400 ml
    (2) Hemorrhage: blood loss of 500 ml or more
  d. Urinary tract
    (1) Perineal soreness may temporarily reduce voiding reflexes.
    (2) Marked diuresis occurs 8 to 12 hours postpartum.
D. Treatment and nursing management during postpartum
1. Objectives for daily care
  a. Assist in normal process of involution; examples include assessing the fundus and promoting urination.
  b. Assist in preventing infection; examples include proper hand washing and promoting proper breast-feeding technique.
  c. Promote infant bonding with mother and family; examples include sibling visits when appropriate and encouraging partner to participate in care.
2. Nursing techniques for postpartum care

a. Vital signs: watch for symptoms of hypovolemic shock and hemorrhage (fainting); stay with mother who is out of bed (OOB) for the first time since delivery.
b. Check breasts
  (1) Breasts should be soft until milk comes in.
  (2) Encourage daily cleansing in shower.
  (3) Perform daily breast examination to note any complications; nodules may be felt second or third day as milk production begins; teach breast self-examination; report any abnormalities.
c. Engorgement
  (1) Nursing usually prevents this; breast pump; nipple shield
  (2) Nonnursing mother
    (a) Cold compresses or ice bag on breasts
    (b) Supportive bra
    (c) Follow steps a and b only if requested
d. Infections
  (1) Redness, warmth, pain, elevated temperature ≥100.4° F after 24 hr
  (2) May require minor surgical intervention to release drainage
e. Check fundus.
  (1) Height and firmness for proper involution
  (2) Relaxed fundus may indicate problem (hemorrhage or infection)
f. Check lochia: color, amount, odor.
g. Check perineal area: healing and cleanliness.
h. Check legs: pain, tenderness, swelling (thrombi); check for Homans' sign.
i. Check urination: overdistention (subinvolution).
j. Bowels: keep open (encourage fluids with balanced diet); administer stool softener (e.g., docusate sodium sulfosuccinate [Colace]).
k. Afterpains: involution
l. Postpartum blues ("baby blues"): possible hormonal transitory depression; usually noted after discharge
3. Teaching: important component of postpartum nursing management
a. Personal hygiene
b. Weight loss
  (1) Immediately after delivery, 7- to 10-lb weight loss
  (2) Total weight loss of pregnancy may take 6 weeks to 6 months or more to achieve.
c. Phenylketonuria (PKU) tests: requirement by law to test for inborn error of metabolism involving the absence of phenylalanine hydroxylase which acts to convert the amino acid phenylanine to tyrosine, mental retardation would result if left untreated.
d. Discuss with mother and father:
  (1) Importance of bonding
  (2) Readiness for parenthood
e. Postpartum exercises
f. Review methods of holding, bubbling, or burping baby.

ABNORMAL POSTPARTUM

Postpartum Infection

A. Definition: any infection in the reproductive organs during labor, delivery, or up to 1 month postpartum
B. Signs and symptoms

1. Chills, fever, localized back pain (kidney involvement)
2. Malaise
3. Lower abdominal tenderness, lower back pains
4. Foul-smelling lochia (retained placental infection)
5. Fundal height changes abnormal
C. Treatment and nursing management in general
  1. Administration of appropriate antibiotics on time and as directed
  2. Comfort measures appropriate to discomfort
  3. Check of vital signs every 4 hours
D. Specific infections
  1. Urinary tract infection (cystitis, pyelitis)
    a. Cause: trauma (stretching or tearing) or by an organism
    b. Signs and symptoms
      (1) 3 days postpartum
      (2) Low back pain
      (3) Localized pain (pyelitis)
      (4) Chills, high fever, apprehension
      (5) Frequency and burning urination (cystitis)
      (6) Discomfort
    c. Treatment and nursing management
      (1) Bed rest until symptoms subside (1 day)
      (2) Drugs (antibiotics)
      (3) Forced fluids
      (4) Careful hand washing by mother and nursing staff
  2. Mastitis
    a. Definition: inflammation of the glands in one or both breasts; can lead to abscess complications if untreated
    b. Cause
      (1) Staphylococcus infection
      (2) Stasis of milk (usually occurs 2 to 4 weeks postpartum)
      (3) Bruising of breast tissue
      (4) Open cuts in nipple or areola
    c. Signs and symptoms
      (1) High fever (103° F [39.5° C])
      (2) Chills
      (3) Red, tender, painful, hard
    d. Treatment and nursing management
      (1) Support bra
      (2) Antibiotic therapy
      (3) Check incision for drainage
      (4) Heat to area
      (5) Increase fluid intake
      (6) Reassurance of mother
      (7) Continued breast-feeding if permitted by health care provider
  3. Thrombophlebitis
    a. Definition: a clot (thrombus) formed in response to an inflammation of the vessel wall
    b. Signs and symptoms
      (1) Local tenderness: femoral vein
      (2) 1 to 2 weeks postpartum
      (3) Swelling, chills, fever
    c. Treatment and nursing management
      (1) Administration of anticoagulant
      (2) Bed rest
      (3) Antibiotic therapy
      (4) Elevation of legs
      (5) Warm, wet compresses every 15 to 30 minutes
      (6) Massage contraindicated

Postpartum Hemorrhage

A. Definition: any loss of 500 ml or more of blood during first 24 hours following delivery
B. Types
1. Early postpartal hemorrhage resulting from uterine atony (1 to 3 days)
2. Late postpartal hemorrhage resulting from subinvolution (inability of the uterus to involute or return to its prepregnant state) or placental infection
C. Causes
1. Uterine atony
2. Retained placental fragments
3. Overdistention of the uterus
4. Grand multiparity
5. Lacerations
6. Trauma of the uterus caused by forceps delivery
7. Inversion of the uterus (an abnormal condition in which the uterus is turned inside out)
D. Signs and symptoms
1. Visible blood loss
2. Shocklike symptoms: pale, clammy, hypotensive, apprehensive
E. Treatment and nursing management
1. Remaining NPO, warm covers, oxygen as ordered
2. IV fluids (ordered medications; examples include Pitocin and Methergine)
3. Replacement transfusion if ordered
4. Massage boggy uterus until firm.
5. Offer assurance and support to family and mother.
6. Medical management of cause (repair of laceration, possible D&C)

Hematomas

A. Definition: local accumulation of blood caused by injury to a blood vessel from the following:
1. Undue pressure of heavy gravid uterus
2. Bearing down inappropriately
3. Long second stage
4. Primigravida's prolonged pushing
B. Signs and symptoms
1. Severe pain in perineal area
2. Visible vaginal hematoma
3. Vulvular hematoma
4. Large blood-filled sac visible
C. Treatment and nursing management
1. Ice to area for 24 hours (for a small hematoma)
2. Antibiotics if ordered, analgesics if ordered
3. Incision or ligation if necessary, vaginal packing and retention catheter
4. Comfort measures similar to episiotomy care, that is, sitz bath

Subinvolution

A. Definition: inability of the uterus to return to its normal size after delivery; failure to involute; diagnosed 4 to 6 weeks postpartum
B. Causes
1. Retention of placental pieces
2. Infection (endometrium)
C. Signs and symptoms
1. Involution process abnormal
2. Boggy uterus (not firm); foul odor
3. Lochia remains rubra for 2 weeks or longer
D. Treatment and nursing management
1. Surgical intervention (D&C) (for retained placenta)
2. Support and reassurance to mother and family
3. Administration of medications to facilitate involution and cure infection

NORMAL NEWBORN

A. Immediate care following delivery
1. Maintain patent airway.
2. Apply cord clamp, check for bleeding, follow procedure for daily cord care.
3. Maintain warmth.
   a. Wrap in prewarmed receiving blankets or
   b. Place in preheated crib.
4. Preventive care
   a. Instill prophylactic eye drops in each eye as required by law to treat *Chlamydia trachomatis* infection and to prevent ophthalmia neonatorum.
   b. Commonly used prophylactic drugs: erythromycin, penicillin ointments or drops; silver nitrate frequently used in the past is no longer as commonly seen.
   c. Administer intramuscular (IM) injection of vitamin K to reduce likelihood of hemorrhagic disease of the newborn.
   d. Hepatitis B vaccination is recommended for all neonates regardless of hepatitis B surface antigen (HbsAg) status (first dose within 12 hours of birth, second 1 month of age, third 6 months of age)
5. Identification procedures
   a. Complete identification bands as required.
   b. Record footprints of baby and pointer fingerprint of mother.
6. Apgar scoring
7. Initial observation of newborn
   a. Initial observation is the primary responsibility of physician, pediatrician.
   b. Nurse should wear gloves when handling newborn during immediate care and until initial bath; regulations differ for daily routines.
   c. Nurse also makes quick observation, checking for visible anomalies such as cleft lip, cleft palate, extra digits, spinal column, limbs, skin, head.
   d. Reflexes that nurse may check include Moro, sucking, rooting, blinking, grasping.
8. Encourage bonding
   a. After initial delivery room care, wipe off excess blood and debris from baby; wrap securely in clean, warm receiving blanket, and let parents hold baby.
   b. Allow time for mother and father to look at touch and hold infant; allow time to initiate breast-feeding if mother desires.
B. Normal physiology of newborn
1. Vital signs
   a. Temperature
      (1) Axillary: 97.7° to 98.6° F (36.5° to 37° C)
      (2) Rectal: 97.7° to 99° F (36.5° to 37.3° C)
      (3) Rectal temperatures taken only on initial reading, or if temperature elevated, to avoid damage to the large intestine

b. Pulse rate: 120 to 160 bpm
   (1) Apical pulse rate
   (2) Irregular in rate and cadence (normal)
c. Respirations: abdominal and irregular, 30 to 60 per minute
2. Measurements
   a. Weight
      (1) Girls 7 lb (3100 g)
      (2) Boys 7½ lb (3300 g)
      (3) 5.5 to 9 lb (3000 to 4500 g) considered normal
      (4) 5% to 10% weight loss in first 2 to 3 days
      (5) Regains birth weight in 5 to 7 days
   b. Length: 18 to 22 inches (45 to 55 cm) long
   c. Head circumference: 13 to 14 inches (33 to 35 cm)
   d. Chest circumference: 12 to 13 inches (30 to 33 cm)
3. Skin
   a. Milia: small, white sebaceous glands visible about nose, forehead, chin
   b. "Stork bites": telangiectasis or capillary hemangiomas
   c. Red nevi: discoloration, circumscribed, blanch on touch, prominent during crying, disappear in 6 months to a year
   d. Mongolian spots: bluish, bruiselike spots on buttocks, back, shoulders; disappear by toddler or preschool age and found in babies of Hispanic, black, Slavic, or Asian background
   e. Erythema toxicum neonatorum (newborn rash): appears as scratches and pimples; may be nosocomial (hospital-based) infection
   f. Nevi vasculosus (strawberry mark): bright red or dark capillary hemangiomas with raised, rough surfaces; usually disappear by school age
   g. Nevi flammeus (port-wine stain): reddish purple raised capillary hemangiomas; do not blanch on pressure and may not disappear
   h. Lanugo: soft, downy hair on top of skin on ears, forehead, neck, shoulders; disappears in weeks
   i. Vernix caseosa: cheeselike protective material coating fetus, especially under arms, beneath knees, and in folds of thighs and groin
   j. Acrocyanosis: bluish for several hours after delivery (hands and feet)
   k. Physiological jaundice: caused when excessive amounts of hemoglobin needed for intrauterine life decrease to extrauterine levels; the immature liver cannot process the bilirubin fast enough, and jaundice results.
      (1) 50% of normal newborns and 80% of premature newborns have some level of jaundice.
      (2) Treatment includes bilirubin test, increased formula, possible phototherapy.
4. Elimination
   a. Urine: three to four times a day for first few days; usually urinates after every feeding
   b. Bowel movement: five to six times a day for first week
      (1) Meconium: expelled within 2 to 12 hours; black, tarry, thick unformed stool
      (2) Transient stool: blackish or greenish stool expelled after first few feedings
   c. Breast-fed stool: yellow, odorless, slightly runny
   d. Bottle-fed stool: formed, brownish yellow, distinct odor
   e. Each infant establishes own pattern of stool movement

5. Hyperestrogenism and its effect on the newborn
   a. Swelling of the breasts in male or female infant because of hormones from mother; the ensuing discharge is called "witch's milk"
   b. Swelling of the male scrotum: large, with rugae; disappears within days
   c. Pseudomenses with female infant
6. Reproductive organs of the male newborn
   a. Cryptorchidism: testes have not descended into scrotum; often present in premature infants
   b. Occasionally, testes are in inguinal sac at birth but will descend within hours or more; if undescended after 1 month, pediatrician should evaluate.
   c. The foreskin should not be retracted until at least 3 years of age if newborn is circumcised.
7. Circulatory system: pulmonary circulation established within minutes of birth
8. Digestive system: immature at birth but can metabolize nutrients except fats
9. Visual capabilities: immature coordination and muscle control
10. Hearing capabilities: acute hearing within 2 minutes of birth
11. Taste perception: can distinguish sweet and sour in 1 to 3 days
12. Smelling perception: can distinguish smell of mother at 5 days
13. Sleep patterns
    a. Unstable for 6 to 8 hours after birth
    b. Has regular and irregular sleep cycles
14. Newborn reflexes
    a. Sucking, rooting, swallowing, extrusion reflexes
    b. Tonic neck (fencing) should disappear in 3 to 4 months
    c. Grasping (palmar) and plantar lessens in 3 to 4 months
    d. Moro's (startle) disappears in 2 months
    e. Stepping disappears in 3 to 4 weeks
    f. Babinski's (plantar): absence indicates CNS damage.
    g. Blinking, sneezing
15. Immunity in the newborn
    a. Has 3-month supply (passive immunity) from mother if baby is term
    b. Begins own synthesis (active immunity) by 3 months of age
C. Daily observation and nursing care
   1. Newborn nursery care and observation
      a. Constant, careful observation
      b. Place infant in warmer until vital signs are stable.
      c. Check temperature; follow agency policy (e.g., rectal, axilla).
         (1) Infant is placed under warmer to prevent cold stress.
         (2) Heat production becomes normal in 2 to 3 days.
         (3) Newborn loses heat through convection, conduction, radiation, and evaporation.
      d. Check respirations.
      e. Place infant on right side to promote expansion of lungs and drain excess mucus.
      f. Observe for signs and symptoms of respiratory distress syndrome (RDS).
      g. Cord

(1) Cord clamp is removed within 8 to 24 hours.

(2) Antigermicidal agent is applied daily to prevent infections.

h. Check eyes and ears for abnormal drainage.

2. Daily nursery routine

a. Monitoring of daily weight and vital signs, especially temperature

b. Observation and recording condition of skin, cord, eyes, elimination

c. Daily care and changing of crib linen

d. Daily cord care

e. General observation

f. Observation of infant-mother bonding during feeding routine

3. Teaching mothers care of newborn: mothers' classes should incorporate the care, handling, and dressing of the newborn in addition to procedures and demonstrations in sponge baths, tub baths, and cord care.

4. Daily bath routine

a. Purpose

(1) Cleansing

(2) Exercise time

(3) Play, social time with parents (bonding time)

b. Prepare environment: select safe, convenient, warm area.

c. Select and prepare equipment.

(1) Utensils for sponge bath

(2) Necessary articles for procedure

(3) Clean clothing

d. Sponge baths: recommended for babies with cord intact

e. Tub baths: recommended for babies whose cord has fallen off—10 to 14 days after birth

5. Cord care

a. Wipe base of cord with alcohol or designated antiseptic every time diapers are changed and during bath time.

b. After cord falls off:

(1) Wipe with alcohol as instructed after daily bath routine for first day or two.

(2) If drainage persists, cleanse with alcohol and notify pediatrician.

6. Diaper rash

a. Change diapers frequently.

b. Wash area with warm tap water.

c. May apply A & D Ointment as a preventative and protective measure.

d. Expose to air if possible.

(1) Lay infant on abdomen and expose buttocks to air.

(2) Apply Desitin or Balmex if A and D Ointment does not help.

7. Circumcision

a. Definition: the surgical cutting and removal of foreskin; usually done 1 to 3 days after birth

b. Treatment and nursing management

(1) Observe for bleeding, edema.

(2) Treatment may include petroleum jelly (Vaseline) for 3 days depending on the type of instrument used for circumcision.

(3) Check and record first voiding after procedure.

(4) Complications: rare

8. Facts about feeding the newborn

a. Newborn metabolic rate twice that of adult

b. Carbohydrates: needed for brain growth and as source of energy

c. Protein: needed for building tissue; inadequacy results in infection, slow growth, flabby muscles.

d. Fat: difficult to digest and metabolize but needed to maintain integrity of skin

e. Iron: continuous supply needed for growth and development; storage from mother depleted in 4 to 6 months

f. At birth, can take 1 to 2 oz (30 to 60 ml) per feeding

g. By 1 to 2 weeks, can nurse 4 oz (120 ml) per feeding

h. Gradual increase to 6 to 8 oz (180 to 240 ml) per feeding in 1 month

9. Facts about breast milk

a. Less protein than cow's milk; easier to digest

b. More lactose than cow's milk, which facilitates metabolism and is good for bones

c. Lactoferrin decreases dangers to infection

d. Sucking stimulates posterior pituitary of mother to trigger let-down reflex, which allows milk to flow

10. Guidelines for breast-feeding

a. A general rule of thumb is to nurse until breasts are soft once milk is established.

b. To ensure a good supply of breast milk, the mother should:

(1) Obtain adequate rest.

(2) Drink sufficient fluids.

(3) Eat a balanced, nutritious diet.

(4) Maintain psychological equilibrium (maternal-infant bonding).

11. The length of time for breast-feeding varies considerably from infant to infant and is normally 10 to 30 minutes; limiting the time of nursing on each breast is no longer considered effective in preventing sore nipples; it is more important to use correct technique and empty the breasts completely.

12. Contraindications to breast-feeding

a. Mother with AIDS

b. Baby with galactosemia, PKU

ABNORMAL NEWBORN

The Preterm (Premature) Infant

A. Definition: a baby born before 37 weeks' gestation and weighing less than 5½ lb (2500 g)

B. Infants may be Small for gestational age (SGA) because they are preterm or from genetic or intrauterine causes.

C. Statistics

1. Of all live births, 7% are premature.

2. Incidence of prematurity increases to 10% in some minority populations.

3. Prematurity is leading cause of death in infants in the United States.

D. Cause

1. Young, adolescent mothers

2. Elderly primigravidas

3. Multiple births

4. Poor prenatal care

5. Congenital anomalies

6. Diseases or conditions that compromise fetus
   a. Pregnancy induced hypertension (PIH)
   b. Diabetes
   c. Heart disease
   d. Nutritional deficits
   e. Preterm labor
   f. Drug or alcohol addictions
   g. Smoking
   h. Placental insufficiency
E. Characteristics of a premature infant
   1. Central nervous system (CNS)
      a. Poor muscle tone
      b. Poor reflexes
      c. Limp
      d. Assumes froglike position
      e. Weak, feeble cry
      f. Unstable heating mechanism: temperature fluctuates from 94° to 96° F (34° to 36° C)
      g. Poor sucking reflexes
      h. Weak gagging and sucking reflexes
   2. Respiratory system
      a. Insufficient surfactant
      b. Immature lungs, rib cage, muscles
      c. Prone to Respiratory distress syndrome (RDS)
      d. Poor oxygenation
   3. Digestive system: immature gastric system; decreased ability to convert protein and fat to energy, able to digest simple sugars
   4. Integumentary system
      a. Harlequin pattern observed (a temporary flushing of the skin on the lower side of the body with pallor on the upward side); commonly seen in normal infants and disappears as the child matures
      b. Veins and capillaries visible
      c. Lanugo prominent
      d. Vernix prominent
      e. Decreased subcutaneous fat, thinner skin
      f. Skin tight, shiny, taut
   5. Circulatory system
      a. Fragile capillaries
      b. Susceptible to hemorrhages (intracranial)
   6. Renal system
      a. Inability to urinate properly
      b. Easily dehydrated (decreased concentrated urine leading to fluid retention)
      c. Fragile electrolyte balance (metabolic acidosis, sodium bicarbonate decreased and excretion of drugs decreased)
   7. Immune system
      a. Too young to have obtained any immunity from mother
      b. Vulnerable to infection
   8. Endocrine system: a common complication is hypoglycemia
   9. Head
      a. Fontanels large
      b. Suture lines prominent
      c. Old looking
F. Treatment and nursing management
   1. Maintain patent airway.
   2. Frequently monitor blood gases to determine oxygen need.
   3. Maintain body temperature by placing in heater.
   4. Conserve energy: basic care only.
   5. Provide adequate nutrition.
      a. Nasogastric feedings
      b. Special soft nipples
      c. Parenteral fluids
   6. Prevent infection.
      a. Prevent skin breakdown: change positions.
      b. Keep dry and clean.
   7. Length of hospitalization: usually until a weight of 5½ 2 lb (2500 g) is reached
   8. Mothering stimulation taught and practiced
      a. Encouraging parents to stroke, cuddle, talk
      b. Feed, diaper infants
      c. Play soft music
      d. Encourage tapping on isolette and talking
   9. Listen to concerns of mothers and fathers.

Postterm Infant

A. Definition: over 42 weeks' gestation
B. Cause: unknown
C. Characteristics of postmature infant
   1. Old looking
   2. No vernix; no lanugo
   3. Color: yellow-green or meconium stained
   4. Desquamation of hands (palms) and feet (soles)
   5. May have respiratory problems
D. Nursing management
   1. Observe for hypoglycemia.
   2. Observe for RDS.
   3. Look for birth injuries.
   4. Provide symptomatic nursing care.

Neonatal Respiratory Distress Syndrome

A. Definition
   1. A series of symptoms signifying respiratory distress
   2. Synonyms: RDS, hyaline membrane disease (HMD)
B. Statistics
   1. Common in premature babies
   2. Leading cause of death in infants in the United States
C. Causes
   1. Lack or loss of surfactant in lungs
   2. Immaturity
   3. Hypoxia
   4. Hypothermia
D. Signs and symptoms
   1. Appears within minutes to hours after birth
   2. Grunting, rib retraction, nasal flaring (RDS symptoms)
   3. Inadequate oxygen: 60 or more respirations per minute
E. Diagnosis: x-ray examination shows collapsed portions of lungs; arterial blood gases reveal hypoxia.
F. Treatment and nursing management
   1. Transfer to intensive care unit and isolette care.
   2. Initiate oxygen therapy: 60%; hood is best.
      a. Intermittent positive-pressure breathing (IPPB)
      b. Continuous positive airway pressure (CPAP)
      c. Positive end-expiratory pressure (PEEP)
      d. Surfactant replacement
      e. Monitoring blood gases
   3. Endotracheal tube if necessary
   4. IV hydration and nutrition and antibiotic therapy
   5. Elevate head of bed slightly.

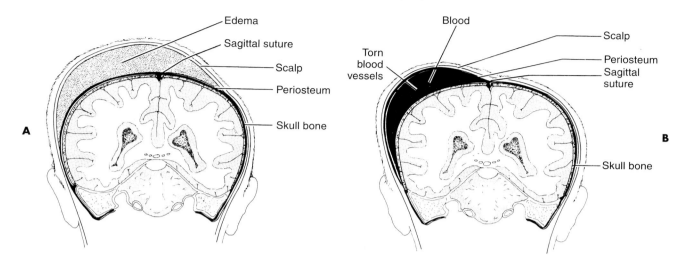

FIGURE 7-13. Differences between caput succedaneum and cephalhematoma. **A,** Caput succedaneum: edema of scalp noted at birth; crosses suture line. **B,** Cephalhematoma: bleeding between periosteum and skull bone appearing within first 2 days; does not cross suture lines.

G. Complication
   1. Retinopathy of prematurity (ROP)
   2. Causes
      a. High arterial oxygen levels
      b. Retinal vascular immaturity

Birth Injuries

A. Normal deviations of the head
   1. Caput succedaneum (Figure 7-13)
      a. Definition: edema (swelling) of soft tissues of scalp
      b. Cause: continuous pressure of the fetal head on cervix
      c. Signs and symptoms
         (1) Crosses suture lines
         (2) Appears at birth
         (3) Disappears in 3 to 4 days
      d. Treatment: none
   2. Cephalhematoma (see Figure 7-13)
      a. Definition: blood between the periosteum and bone
      b. Cause: pressure during delivery (forceps; prolonged labor)
      c. Signs and symptoms
         (1) Never crosses suture lines
         (2) Appears several hours to several days after birth
         (3) Disappears within 3 to 6 weeks
      d. Treatment: none
   3. Molding (Figure 7-14)
      a. Definition: changes in the shape of the head
      b. Cause: accommodation of fetal bones to birth canal during labor and delivery
      c. Signs and symptoms: visual
      d. Treatment: disappears without treatment in 3 days
   4. Soft-tissue injuries (subcutaneous fat necrosis)
      a. Definition: pressure necrosis
      b. Signs and symptoms: purplish, movable mass
      c. Treatment: resolves spontaneously
B. Subconjunctival hemorrhage (scleral or retinal)
   1. Definition: rupture of small capillaries in eye
   2. Cause: increased intracranial pressure of birth

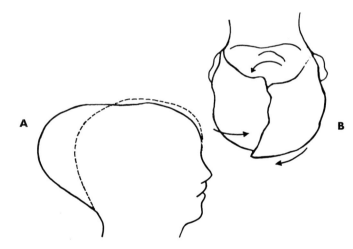

FIGURE 7-14. **A,** Various types of molding. **B,** Bones overlapping during molding. *(From Hamilton PM:* Basic maternity nursing, *ed 6, St Louis, 1988, Mosby.)*

   3. Signs and symptoms: small, red pin dots in white of sclera, or hemorrhaging in retina
   4. Resolves without treatment in 5 days
C. Ecchymosis, petechiae, edema
   1. Definition: blood within tissues; does not blanch with pressure
   2. Cause: forceps, manipulation, pressure
   3. Signs and symptoms: visual in affected areas
   4. Resolves without treatment in 2 days
D. Skeletal injuries
   1. Skull fracture: rare, and unless blood vessels are involved, heals without treatment
   2. Fracture of the clavicle: most common fracture; usually caused by shoulder impaction; dystocia
      a. Treatment: handle infant with care.
      b. Prognosis: good
   3. Fracture of the humerus or femur: rare

a. Cause: dystocia and difficult delivery
b. Treatment
  (1) Immobilize
  (2) Heals rapidly
c. Complications: rare
E. Neurological injuries
  1. Brachial paralysis of upper arm: Erb-Duchenne paralysis (Erb's palsy)
    a. Definition: traumatic injury to the upper brachial plexus, with damage to one or more cervical nerve roots
    b. Cause
      (1) Difficult labor
      (2) Shoulder impaction; dystocia
      (3) Malposition of forceps
    c. Treatment: immobilize with brace or splint.
    d. Nursing management
      (1) Skin care as necessary
      (2) Gentle range-of-motion exercises after healing
  2. Brachial paralysis of lower arm: Klumpke's paralysis (palsy)
    a. Definition: nerves of hand and wrist crushed or severed
    b. Treatment
      (1) Pad wrist and fingers
      (2) Corrective surgery
      (3) Gentle massage after surgery
      (4) Range-of-motion exercises when appropriate
    c. Prognosis: good
  3. Facial paralysis
    a. Definition: crushed or severed nerves of face that cause grimacing and distortion, especially when crying; asymmetric paralysis
    b. Cause: misapplication of forceps
    c. Treatment: condition transitory; reassure parents
F. Central nervous system injuries
  1. Definition: injuries causing intracranial hemorrhaging
  2. Cause
    a. Prematurity
    b. Large full-term babies
    c. Dystocia
    d. Hypoxia
    e. Hypovolemia
  3. Types
    a. In brain itself
    b. Subdural hematoma
  4. Signs and symptoms
    a. Suture line separation
    b. Bulging anterior-fontanel
    c. High-pitched cry
    d. Abnormal respirations
    e. Cyanosis
    f. Irritability or lethargy
    g. Twitching; convulsions
  5. Treatment and nursing management
    a. Head higher than hips
    b. Warmth
    c. Oxygen
    d. IV therapy
    e. Minimal handling
    f. Surgical aspiration (if appropriate)
    g. Measurement of head size weekly
    h. Convulsion precautions

Infections of the Newborn

A. Causes
  1. Dystocia
  2. PROM of 24 hours or more (sepsis neonatorum)
  3. Clinical amnionitis
  4. Maternal infection (toxoplasmosis, syphilis, rubella)
  5. Nosocomial infection (usually staph)
  6. Monilia or yeast infection in mother's vagina
B. Signs and symptoms
  1. Appears within first 48 hours
  2. Vague symptoms
  3. Lethargy, irritability, lack of appetite
  4. Low-grade temperature
  5. Diarrhea
  6. Jaundice
C. Treatment and nursing management
  1. Take cultures of blood, urine, throat.
  2. Administer antibiotic therapy.
  3. Keep warm.
  4. Administer oxygen therapy if necessary.
  5. Isolate if appropriate.
  6. Weigh daily.
  7. Watch for signs of jaundice.
  8. Keep parents informed of progress.

Congenital Malformations

A. Perinatal signs
  1. Polyhydramnios: excessive amniotic fluid; may occur with other congenital anomalies
  2. Oligohydramnios: scant amniotic fluid; indicates urinary tract anomalies and renal disturbances
B. Postnatal congenital malformations
  1. Choanal atresia (gastrointestinal anomaly)
    a. Definition: blockage between the nose and throat; can be unilateral or bilateral
    b. Signs and symptoms
      (1) Cyanotic at rest
      (2) Color improves when crying
      (3) Snorts when feeding
    c. Treatment and nursing management
      (1) Physician may pierce obstruction with a probe if it is only a membrane.
      (2) Minor surgical repair if bone involved; prognosis is excellent.
      (3) Feeding problems; positioning is important.
      (4) Gavage feeding may be necessary.
      (5) Watch closely for aspiration.
  2. Esophageal atresia: refer to Chapter 8.
  3. Congenital laryngeal stridor
    a. Definition: abnormal condition around larynx that causes noisy respiration, especially a crowing sound on inspiration
    b. Cause:
      (1) Flabby epiglottis
      (2) Extraglotteal structures
      (3) Relaxation of laryngeal wall
      (4) Absence of tracheal rings
      (5) Deformity of vocal cords
    c. Signs and symptoms
      (1) Noisy respirations on inspiration
      (2) Most noticeable when crying

(3) Mild-to-severe intercostal or supraclavicular retractions

(4) Cyanosis

(5) Dyspnea

d. Treatment and nursing management

(1) Depends on cause

(2) Mild stridor may subside in 6 to 18 months.

(3) Mother is taught to position baby upright for feeding.

(4) Feed slowly, pausing to let infant catch his or her breath.

(5) Use small nipple.

(6) Watch for aspiration of feedings.

(7) Prevent respiratory complications.

(8) Keep infant warm, dry, away from drafts.

(9) Have oxygen in readiness.

(10) Prepare for tracheotomy.

e. Prognosis: good

4. Cleft lip and cleft palate

a. Definition: bilateral or unilateral fissure or opening on the palate or the upper lips resulting from failure of the bony and soft-tissue structures to unite

b. Cause: developmental failure during the embryonic stage because of heredity, age, or a variety of other factors such as radiation or viral infections

c. Signs and symptoms

(1) Visual on lips

(2) Palate more difficult to notice sometimes

(3) Occurs more frequently in male infants

(4) Difficulty feeding

(5) Choking

(6) Drooling

(7) Milk may drain through nostrils.

d. Treatment

(1) Cleft lips may have butterfly adhesive taping as initial treatment; may be helpful in feeding so milk does not continually drain through fissure

(2) Cleft lip may be surgically repaired at 1 to 2 weeks of age, or at 12 lb (5.5 kg)

(3) Cleft palate; first repair usually by 18 months

e. Nursing management

(1) Feeding precautions

(a) Use soft duck nipple, medicine dropper with rubber tip

(b) Place nipple away from cleft side.

(c) Feed slowly.

(d) Bubble frequently.

(e) Rinse mouth after feedings.

(f) Watch for aspiration, respiratory distress, gastrointestinal disturbances.

(2) Mouth care: prevent cracks, fissures on lips.

(3) Provide postoperative care for cleft lip.

(a) Place infant on side.

(b) Mouth care is important because of Logan bar applied to prevent stretching of sutures.

(c) Prevent crying.

(d) Check swelling (tongue, nose, mouth).

(e) Watch for hemorrhage.

(f) Apply elbow restraints.

(g) Prevent crust formation.

(h) Feed on opposite side of surgery.

(i) Use rubber-tipped dropper (3 weeks).

5. Diaphragmatic hernia

a. Definition: herniation of abdominal viscera into the thoracic cavity as a result of incomplete development during embryonic stage, ranging from minimal to complete herniation

b. Signs and symptoms

(1) Constant respiratory distress

(2) Bowels distended

(3) Bowel sounds heard in chest

(4) Asymmetrical chest contour

c. Treatment and nursing management

(1) Early recognition and prompt surgery

(2) Usual preoperative and postoperative management

d. Prognosis guarded, depending on severity

6. Omphalocele: see Chapter 8.

7. Imperforate anus: see Chapter 8.

C. Congenital anomalies of the Central nervuous system (CNS)

1. Spina bifida occulta

a. Definition: defect in vertebral column without protrusion of spinal cord and meninges; this is one of three types of spina bifida, which is a malformation of the spine, most common in the lumbosacral region, in which the posterior portion of the vertebrae fails to close.

b. Signs and symptoms

(1) Dimple in lower lumbosacral skin

(2) Hair over area (occasionally)

(3) X-ray film confirmation

c. Treatment and nursing management: no treatment is necessary unless neurologic symptoms occur.

2. Meningocele (another form of spina bifida)

a. Definition: defect in spinal cord with protrusion of meninges through an opening in spinal canal; paralysis is present.

b. Surgical correction

3. Myelomeningocele

a. Definition: both spinal cord and meninges protrude through defective bony rings in spinal cord; possible paralysis below sac

b. Signs and symptoms

(1) Look for visual signs.

(2) Observe for change in intracranial pressure.

(3) Check head measurements for hydrocephalus.

(4) Report signs and symptoms of CNS involvement.

c. Preoperative management

(1) Flat on abdomen with sterile gauze, petroleum jelly (Vaseline), Telfa pad, normal saline

(2) No diapers

(3) Keep clean.

(4) Use care to prevent sac from breaking.

(5) Prevent infection: use sterile technique.

(6) Prevent deformity.

(7) Prevent injury.

d. Postoperative management

(1) Vital signs

(2) Symptoms of shock

(3) Oxygen readiness

(4) Head measurements

(5) Cast care if necessary; sometimes casts applied to legs

(6) Importance of good nutrition

(7) Orthopedic and urological habilitation

(8) Encourage normal use of functions.

(9) Minimize disabilities.
(10) Paralysis (if present) may not be alleviated, but further damage can be prevented; aim of surgery is to give infant opportunity for optimal growth and development.
(11) "Crede" bladder to keep it empty and free from infection
4. Hydrocephalus: refer to Chapter 8.
D. Congenital anomalies of the musculoskeletal system (limited)
1. Congenital dislocation of the hip: refer to Chapter 8.
2. Talipes equinovarus (clubfoot): refer to Chapter 8.
3. Phocomelia
a. Definition: developmental congenital anomaly in which only stubs or parts of arms and legs are present; degree of severity varies
b. Cause: interference with embryonic development of long bones; rare and seen as a result of the drug thalidomide taken during early pregnancy to relieve nausea
c. Treatment and nursing management
(1) Psychosocial problems for family and infant
(2) Body surface limited, so heating mechanism overheats rest of body, causing diaphoresis
(3) Personal hygiene; frequent baths
(4) Special education imperative
4. Polydactyly
a. Definition: supernumerary fingers or toes
b. Cause: possibly hereditary
c. Treatment and nursing management
(1) Usually no bone or nerve involvement
(2) Tie digit with silk suture in newborn nursery; it falls off.
(3) Surgical intervention is necessary with bone involvement; x-ray examination is done first to ensure that no bone or ligaments are present.
E. Congenital anomalies of the male genitourinary system
1. Hypospadias: refer to Chapter 8.
2. Epispadias: refer to Chapter 8.

Hemolytic Disease of Newborn

A. Pathological jaundice
1. Cause: Rh factor incompatibility; occurs only when mother is Rh negative and fetus is Rh positive
2. Pathophysiology: the Rh-negative mother is exposed to and develops antibodies against the Rh antigen (sensitization); sensitization to Rh-positive blood can be caused by exposure to the antigen during amniocentesis or when a transplacental bleed occurs during a miscarriage or abortion; the most common time for sensitization to occur is birth.
3. Signs and symptoms
a. Jaundice
b. Anemia
c. Enlarged liver and spleen
d. Generalized edema
e. If untreated, "yellow bodies" will travel to brain, causing brain damage, heart failure, kernicterus, and death.
4. Treatment and nursing management
a. Blood types of mother and father are important for anticipatory guidance.
b. First babies usually do not present a problem.
c. If baby's bilirubin is above 10 or 12 mg/dl, phototherapy may be applied to reduce jaundice; exchange transfusions may be necessary.

d. After birth of Rh-positive baby, an unsensitized Rh-negative mother is given RhoGAM, a specific gamma globulin that will prevent the production of Rh antibodies; this must be given within 72 hours after delivery; the effect is the assurance that subsequent pregnancies will not be harmful to the baby.
e. Rh-antibody titers can be monitored throughout pregnancy (prenatal).
f. Amniocentesis will reveal, by indirect Coombs' test, if mother has antibodies circulating in the maternal plasma or serum.
B. Erythroblastosis fetalis (hydrops)
1. Definition: most severe form of fetal hemolysis
2. Rarely seen since the development of RhoGAM
3. Signs and symptoms include anemia, congestive heart failure, and ascites.
C. ABO incompatibility
1. Definition: an incompatibility of blood groups A and B because of the presence of antigens developed and passed on to the fetus by a type O mother
2. Signs and symptoms
a. Jaundice: mild, occurring during first day or two
b. Slight enlargement of liver and spleen
3. Treatment and nursing management
a. Phototherapy
b. If bilirubin is above 20 mg/dl, an exchange transfusion with group O and appropriate Rh type
c. Observe for progressive lethargy.
d. Monitor level of jaundice (visual and laboratory).
e. Observe color of urine.
f. Observe for edema.
g. Observe for convulsions.
h. Provide symptomatic nursing care.

Down Syndrome (Trisomy 21)

Refer to Chapter 8.

Drug Addiction In Newborns

A. Definition: secondary addiction, caused by drugs being ingested or injected by addicted mother; drugs cross the placental barrier and create a drug-dependent newborn (immature liver unable to excrete drug rapidly during fetal life).
B. Signs and symptoms
1. Low birth weight
2. Premature
3. Immature
4. Withdrawal symptoms within 48 to 72 hours; watch for:
a. Sneezing
b. Respiratory distress
c. Excessive sweating
d. Feeding problems
e. Frantic sucking of fists
f. High-pitched cry
g. Irritable, hyperactive, tremors
h. Fever
i. Diarrhea
C. Treatment and nursing management
1. Prevent infection.
2. Promote good nutrition.
3. Keep quiet (quiet, darkened environment).
4. Offer loving, soothing, cuddling care.
5. Give medications on time.

6. Monitor vital signs.
7. Keep warm.
8. Protect from injury because child is hyperactive.
9. Provide good skin care because of excessive sweating and diarrhea.
10. Provide adequate fluids (prevent dehydration).
11. Encourage mother to assist in care.
  a. Teach holding, diapering, talking, bathing.
  b. Encourage visits.

Infants of Diabetic Mothers

A. Complications
  1. Delivery date may be recommended before EDC or approximately 36 to 37 weeks' gestation to prevent:
    a. Oversized baby (macrosomia)
    b. High-risk infant (babies with diabetes have high rate of infant mortality)
  2. Neonatal hypoglycemia common
  3. RDS complications
  4. Hyperbilirubinemia (severe jaundice)
  5. Intracranial hemorrhage (birth trauma, LGA)
  6. Congestive heart failure
  7. Congenital anomalies in 5% of infants
  8. Hypocalcemia
B. Signs and symptoms
  1. Lethargic
  2. Plump, puffy face
  3. Long and heavy
  4. Respiratory problems
  5. Enlarged heart, liver, and spleen
  6. Symptoms of hypoglycemia
  7. Symptoms of hypocalcemia (tremors)
C. Treatment and nursing management
  1. Medical management is difficult because of rapid, changing growth patterns, nutritional demands, illness.
  2. Parents must be taught techniques for blood glucose monitoring.
  3. Short-acting insulin is best (easier to control).
  4. Treat hypoglycemia and hypocalcemia.
  5. Provide oral feedings when tolerated and blood sugar levels stable.

Cretinism (Congenital Hypothyroidism)

Refer to Chapter 8.

FAMILY PLANNING

A. Trends
  1. Smaller families (except for the poor and disadvantaged)
  2. Delayed parenthood by choice
    a. Career women
    b. Desire for higher education
    c. Alternate living arrangements
  3. Single parents
    a. High divorce rate
    b. Expanding role of father as single parent because custody of children, traditionally awarded to mother, is now being awarded to fathers
    c. Lessening barriers for adoption by single men and women
    d. Cultural and ethnic acceptance of unmarried mothers

e. Opportunities to continue education for pregnant adolescent without pressure of forced marriage
B. Communes: labor and delivery in communal community homes
C. Early sexual encounters (teenage pregnancies)
  1. Need for referrals to family planning centers for guidance and counseling
    a. Teach use of condoms (controversial)
    b. Practice abstinence
  2. Problems originating from early sexual encounters
D. Surrogate mothers
  1. In vitro transplantation of embryo in the uterus of a woman who agrees to have a full-term pregnancy for another woman
  2. Has moral and legal implications

Possible Influential Factors

A. Sex education: incorporation of sex education in public and parochial schools at an early age
B. Freedom of choice
  1. Availability of over-the-counter pregnancy tests
  2. Availability of over-the-counter contraceptives
  3. Abortions mandated as legal by the United States Supreme Court, 1977
C. Postponement of family: using available contraceptive devices
D. Economic factor: high cost of medical care forces young people to consider waiting until affluent enough to *afford* a family.

Common Methods of Birth Control (Contraception)

A. Natural
  1. Rhythm (calendar) method
    a. Based on the principle that ovulation occurs during midcycle of a menstrual period; that is, in a 28-day cycle, ovulation would occur on the fourteenth day.
    b. Accordingly, the most fertile days are considered to be 3 to 4 days before and 3 to 4 days after ovulation.
  2. Basal metabolism method: daily monitoring of early morning temperature for a period of several months and entering it on a graph (Figure 7-15) will establish an ovulation time; *safe* and *fertile* times can be determined, and mother advised on use of this method.
B. Coitus interruptus
  1. Penis withdrawn from vagina just before ejaculation
  2. Least effective of all methods
C. Condom (sheath, snakeskin, rubbers): thin rubber or plastic sheath that fits over penis and acts as barrier, preventing sperm from entering the vagina
D. Diaphragm: mechanical barrier placed at mouth of cervix; used with contraceptive cream or jelly to be effective; may engage in intercourse immediately after placement; should be left in place for 6 hours after intercourse; spermicide must be added each time intercourse occurs.
E. Chemical agents: foam, creams, jelly, vaginal suppositories, and sponges form a chemical barrier in the vagina and render the area unsafe for sperm.
F. Intrauterine devices (IUD)
  1. Devices come in various shapes made of memory plastic inserted in the uterine cavity immediately following the woman's menstrual cycle.

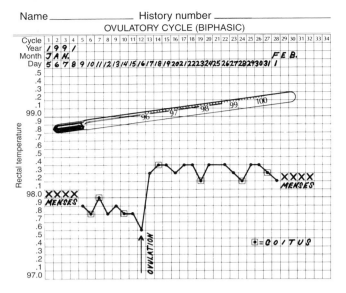

FIGURE 7-15. Basal temperature record shows drop and sharp rise at time of ovulation. *(From Lowdermilk DL, Perry SE: Maternity nursing, ed 6, St Louis, 2003, Mosby.)*

2. Mode of action unclear; thought to interfere with implantation by creating peristaltic waves
3. Disadvantages
   a. Excessive bleeding during menstrual cycle
   b. Extremely controversial; Dalkon Shield was taken off the market because of permanent sterility and multiple gynecological problems.
   c. Possible contamination from IUD string hanging in vaginal orifice
4. Advantage: once IUD is inserted, only periodic checking (usually monthly) to confirm it is still intact.
G. Oral contraceptive (birth control pill)
   1. Most widely used
   2. Considered 90% or more effective
   3. Prevents anterior pituitary from releasing follicle-stimulating hormone (FSH); artificially raises estrogen and progesterone levels and prevents ovulation
   4. Stimulates endometrium, creating hostile environment for sperm
   5. Minor side effects, lasting a few weeks to months: nausea, weight gain, full breasts
   6. Major side effects: thrombophlebitis, hypertension, embolism, cardiovascular disturbances
H. Cervical cap
   1. A small rubber cap fitted over the cervix to prevent sperm from entering the cervical canal
   2. More comfortable than the diaphragm
   3. May be left safely on the cervix for longer periods and remain effective
I. Female condom
   1. A sheath secured by two rings that cover the cervix and vulva; coated with a spermicide preparation
   2. Protects against both pregnancy and disease
   3. May cause a decrease in sensation during intercourse
J. Hormonal injection
   1. Injectable form of progestin
   2. Provides protection for 3 months

K. Hormone Implants
   1. Small capsules placed in upper arm releases progestin
   2. Provides protection for up to 5 years
L. Transdermal patch
   1. Provided effective contraception similar to oral contraceptives
M. Operative sterilization
   1. Vasectomy
      a. Removal of a portion of both vasa deferentia; prevents the transport of sperm into the seminal fluid
      b. Temporary birth control should be used for 2 to 3 months until a semen analysis determines that no viable sperm are present.
      c. Reversal may be possible using microsurgery.
   2. Tubal ligation (bilateral partial salpingectomy)
      a. Fallopian tubes are clipped, cut, or cauterized.
      b. Sexual activity can resume whenever woman is comfortable enough.
      c. Reversal is possible; however, the probability of regaining fertility is seriously decreased.

RESOURCES

Healthy People 2010
Office of Disease Prevention and Health Promotion
200 Independence Avenue SW, Room 738G
Washington, DC 20201
(202) 205-8611
http://www.healthypeople.gov

American Academy of Pediatrics
141 Northwest Point Boulevard
P.O. Box 927
Elk Grove Village, IL 60009-0927
(708) 228-5005
http://www.aap.org

American College of Obstetricians and Gynecologists
409 12th Street SW
PO Box 96920
Washington, DC 20090
http://www.acog.org

Health Resources and Services Administration
Maternal and Child Health Bureau
Parklawn Building, Room 18A-05
5600 Fishers Lane
Rockville, MD 20857
(301) 443-2170
http://mchb.hrsa.gov/

March of Dimes Birth Defects Foundation
1275 Mamaroneck Avenue
White Plains, NY 10605
http://www.modimes.org

National Center for Education and Maternal and Child Health
2115 Wisconsin Avenue NW, Suite 601
Washington, DC 20007
(202) 784-9770
http://www.ncemch.org
National Perinatal Information Center
144 Wayland Avenue, Suite 300
Providence, RI 02906
(401) 274-0650
http://www.npic.org

SUGGESTED READINGS

Burroughs A, Leifer G: *Maternity nursing: an introductory text,* ed. 8, St Louis, 2003. WB Saunders.

Eschleman M: *Introductory nutrition and nutrition therapy,* ed 4, St Louis, 2000, Mosby.

Leifer G: *Introduction to maternity and pediatric nursing,* ed. 4, St. Louis, 2001, WB Saunders.

McKenry LM, Salerno E: *Pharmacology in nursing,* ed 21, St Louis, 2003, Mosby.

Novak JC, Broom BL: *Ingalls and Salerno's Maternal and child health nursing,* ed 9, St Louis, 1999, Mosby.

REVIEW QUESTIONS

1. An additional method of determining the EDD aside from Naegle's rule is:
   1 Rupture of the membranes
   2 Audible fetal heart tones
   3 Lightening
   4 Quickening
2. A couple planning their first pregnancy asks the nurse about the accuracy of home pregnancy tests. The nurse replies that, "Home pregnancy tests are widely used today." However, it is most important that prospective parents:
   1 Wait at least 3 weeks after the first missed period.
   2 Wait at least 9 days after the first missed period.
   3 Make certain that the blood is correctly placed on the stick.
   4 Use a sterile urine specimen to complete the test.
3. A patient who is a mother of a 5-year-old son and is now pregnant again should be classified as:
   1 Gravida I, para I
   2 Gravida II, para II
   3 Gravida II, para I
   4 Gravida II, para 0
4. One of the earliest presumptive signs of pregnancy is:
   1 Hegar's sign
   2 Missed menstrual period
   3 Linea nigra
   4 Braxton-Hicks contractions
5. A couple is thrilled to hear their baby's heart rate with a Doppler transducer. The gestation of the couple's pregnancy at this time is most likely:
   1 4 weeks
   2 10 weeks
   3 18 weeks
   4 24 weeks
6. To confirm a patient's pregnancy, the nurse should give which of the following instructions regarding the required urine specimen?
   1 Give a voided specimen during her first visit.
   2 Instruct her on how to give a sterile specimen in the office.
   3 Tell her to withhold fluid intake during the night and bring in the first voided specimen in the morning.
   4 A catheterized specimen will be required.
7. A prenatal patient asks when she should stop working. The most appropriate response for the nurse is:
   1 "Around the start of the eighth month."
   2 "Everyone is different; it is up to you."
   3 "What do you do for a living?"
   4 "Two weeks before your EDC."
8. Which of the following statements in a prenatal class would indicate to the nurse that a family is beginning to accept the newborn into their world?
   1 A father states, "Everyone is going to have to pitch in and help."
   2 An 8-year-old sibling states, "I can help mommy with the new baby."
   3 A mother states, "I cannot wait to go back to school."
   4 A 3-year-old sibling asks, "Am I going to have to share my toys?"

9. The communicable (childhood) disease most likely to affect pregnancy, with harmful effects to the fetus, is:
   1 Chickenpox
   2 Rubella
   3 Varicella
   4 Rubeola
10. Fetal circulation is different from circulation following birth because:
    1 Blood leaves the heart through the pulmonary arteries, bypassing the lungs.
    2 Blood leaves the heart through the pulmonary veins.
    3 The chambers are not fully developed until after birth.
    4 Blood goes through the ductus arteriosus to the lungs.
11. A student nurse asks, "How is the baby's sex determined?" The nursing instructor responds:
    1 X chromosome from the ovum
    2 A random number of chromosomes
    3 Y or X chromosome from the sperm
    4 Genes that are carried by DNA and protein
12. The basal metabolic rate of a prenatal patient generally increases. An explanation of this would be:
    1 Hormone production is increased.
    2 The thyroid gland increases in size.
    3 Cardiac output and rate increases.
    4 The baby causes a need for excess energy.
13. Which of the following statements by a teenage mom would most indicates to the nurse that the patient is accepting her new role?
    1 "My mom is taking care of the baby so that I can stay in school."
    2 "The baby is going to cause many changes in my schedule."
    3 "She is so cute; I just love her so much."
    4 "My friends have all promised to help."
14. A couple asks why it is so important to the fetus for both of them to stop smoking. The nurse responds:
    1 "Smoking and secondhand smoke causes decreased oxygenation to the fetus."
    2 "Pregnant women who smoke or who are around smoke tend to have larger babies."
    3 "Pregnant women who smoke tend to have babies who are diabetic."
    4 "Pregnant women who smoke tend to have babies with cardiac anomalies."
15. A couple of Eastern European–Jewish heritage is referred for genetic counseling. Which of the following conditions would be of most concern to this couple?
    1 Sickle-cell anemia
    2 Tay-Sachs disease
    3 Thalassemia
    4 Cystic fibrosis
16. A mother in her first trimester confides to the nurse that she is worried she will not be a good mother. She is disappointed that she will not be able to go back to school as she had planned. The nurse should:
    1 Reassure the mother that her feelings of ambivalence are normal in the first trimester.
    2 Tell her that she has to let everyone in the family help her.
    3 Instruct her that she made the baby and she has to take responsibility for it.
    4 Assure her that as the pregnancy progresses, her feelings will become more positive.

17. The patient who is 28 weeks pregnant is having a routine prenatal visit. A trace of albumin is discovered in her urine. The nurse is concerned because this may be an indication of:
    1 PIH
    2 Cystitis
    3 Diabetes
    4 Heart disease

18. A patient in a prenatal class asks about whether Kegel exercises are beneficial in pregnancy. The most appropriate response by the nurse would be:
    1 "Absolutely not! They are dangerous to your heart."
    2 "They help some people, but the benefit is minimal."
    3 "Yes, they can help tighten the pelvic floor muscles."
    4 "Yes, these exercises will help with leg cramps."

19. A couple asks the nurse, "When during the pregnancy do we have to stop having sex?" The nurse responds:
    1 "By the eighth month; it becomes dangerous for the fetus."
    2 "It is safe as long as the patient douches each time."
    3 "Sexual intercourse is okay if the cervix is closed."
    4 "Generally, by the third trimester, it is not advisable."

20. A primigravida in the sixth month of pregnancy is complaining of indigestion. The nurse explains that this is caused by:
    1 A growing uterus pushing on the diaphragm
    2 Eating small frequent meals that increase gastric acid secretion
    3 An increasing basal metabolic rate, leading to increased appetite
    4 Increased nausea and vomiting, common in this trimester

21. A prenatal patient is experiencing leg cramps. A nursing intervention should include:
    1 Advising hot compresses twice daily
    2 Instructing her to elevate her legs at least 15 minutes three times daily
    3 Informing her of the cause (excessive phosphorus) and encouraging her to drink milk
    4 Advising her to chew Tums for calcium

22. A patient is 36 weeks pregnant and in danger of becoming eclamptic. Delivery is induced. She delivers a 5 lb 8 oz (2500 g) boy after just 6 hours of labor. She must continue to be monitored for impending eclampsia for how long?
    1 1 hour
    2 2 hours
    3 24 hours
    4 72 hours

23. Orders for a patient who was recently admitted to the unit include notifying the physician immediately of any changes in status, no vaginal or rectal examinations, fetal monitoring, pad count, oxygen if necessary, and laboratory work (type and cross-match, hemoglobin, hematocrit). These orders would alert the nurse to prepare for which of the following?
    1 Pending abortion
    2 Ectopic pregnancy
    3 Third-trimester bleeding
    4 Missed abortion

24. Estriol testing is a urine test taken at certain intervals to determine:
    1 Fetal age
    2 Lung surfactant of the fetus
    3 Uterine nomenclature
    4 Placental functioning

25. A patient is a chain-smoker. The prenatal nurse has taught her the effect of nicotine and hazards of passive smoke. She does not drink, but the nurse has taught her that fetal alcohol syndrome is a major concern today. In addressing the abuse of tobacco, the nurse would stress that it:
    1 "Is a dirty, nasty habit that yellows your teeth, can cause lung cancer, and can offend nonsmokers."
    2 "Is becoming socially unacceptable and has widespread negative effects on children as well as adults."
    3 "May cause adverse physiological effects on the fetus."
    4 "Retards fetal growth, constricts blood vessels in the mother, decreases placental function, and may cause premature labor"

26. Which of the following statements is correct relative to differences between a stress test and a nonstress test (NST)?
    1 An NST is done by abdominal palpation by the physician.
    2 An NST is done early in pregnancy to determine sex of the infant.
    3 A stress test is usually done late in pregnancy to measure fetal response to uterine contractions.
    4 A stress test is done after the mother has been given orange juice to drink.

27. Mothers are routinely screened during their first prenatal examination for a variety of conditions. One of the most important tests is the alpha-fetoprotein (AFP) test, which:
    1 Determines fetal maturity
    2 Detects a neural tube defect such as spina bifida
    3 Detects Tay-Sachs disease
    4 Detects RDS

28. As a rule, the nurse should schedule the high-risk pregnant mother to be screened for gestational diabetes mellitus (GDM) at:
    1 12 weeks' gestation
    2 20 to 24 weeks' gestation
    3 32 weeks' gestation
    4 40 weeks' gestation

29. Prenatal care is considered the primary means of circumventing complications during pregnancy. Which complication would you consider as most affected by good prenatal care?
    1 Placenta previa
    2 Hyperemesis gravidarum
    3 Pregnancy induced hypertension
    4 Abortion

30. The symptom that is often considered a warning sign of an impending convulsion in the mother with eclampsia is:
    1 Headache
    2 Severe epigastric pain
    3 Scotoma
    4 Puffy face

31. A patient is diagnosed with abruptio placenta. The physician orders fibrinogen levels every 15 minutes. The patient's husband is frightened and asks the nurse why the physician has to withdraw so much blood. The nurse's best response should be:
    1 "You may ask the physician yourself."
    2 "Would you like me to inquire for you?"
    3 "This test determines the status of the clotting factor."
    4 "The physician is determining whether to give her a transfusion or whether to operate."

32. During a nutritional assessment, a nurse is concerned when the patient makes which of the following statements?
    1 "I love vegetables, especially broccoli."
    2 "Some days I am so busy, I eat fast food."
    3 "I take a lot of different vitamins."
    4 "I hate milk, but I guess I need it for the baby."

33. During a class on fetal development, the nurse is asks, "What is the major function of the placenta?" The most appropriate response would be:
    1 "It passes medications from mother to fetus."
    2 "It allows the fetus to develop more rapidly."
    3 "Nutrients are passed from mother to fetus."
    4 "It functions as the kidney and the stomach of the fetus."

34. Which of the following would not be a routine assessment at 10 weeks' gestation?
    1 Goodell's sign felt by the examiner
    2 Complaints of nausea and vomiting
    3 Feelings of quickening by the mother
    4 Increased feelings of tingling in the breast

35. A nurse is teaching a parent's class. She is asked, "When is it appropriate to give my baby a tub bath?" Which of the following statements by the nurse is the most appropriate response?
    1 "A sponge bath or a tub bath is fine at any time, as long as you hold him carefully and support his head."
    2 "A tub bath is fine at any time after the cord falls off, usually in 3 to 5 days."
    3 "A tub bath is fine any time after the cord falls off in 10 to 14 days."
    4 "A tub bath is fine as soon as he can maintain a sitting position."

36. A nurse is caring for a 26-year-old primigravida. She is 24 weeks' gestation. She has been admitted for observation because of premature labor contractions. The patient states, "I feel a rush of fluid between my legs." Which of the following actions should the nurse perform first?
    1 Perform an NST to determine viability of infant.
    2 Perform a nitrazine test for ferning.
    3 Check FHT.
    4 Prepare patient for a vaginal examination.

37. A primigravida who is 30 weeks' gestation is admitted to the maternity unit after having been involved in an automobile accident. She is complaining of dull pain in her lower abdomen. Which of the following assessments would be of the most concern to the nurse?
    1 A FHR of 140 to 160 bpm
    2 Complaints of irregular contractions relieved by walking
    3 Regular contractions occurring at intervals unrelieved by walking
    4 Complaints of shortness of breath

38. A prenatal patient who has had diabetes for 2 years is admitted to a maternity unit for hyperglycemia. She is 9 weeks pregnant and she admits to the nurse that she does not always take her diabetes medications. Which of the following would most likely be ordered for this patient?
    1 Oral hypoglycemics
    2 Regular insulin to cover elevated blood sugars
    3 Oral antibiotics to protect against infection
    4 NPH and regular insulin

39. A newly arrived immigrant woman is being seen by the health care provider for the first time. It is determined that she is pregnant with her first child. The health care provider is concerned, however, because she is also complaining of fever, weight loss, night sweats, and a persistent cough. A diagnosis of active tuberculosis is made. The most appropriate course of action for this patient at this time should be:
    1 Begin a drug treatment regimen according to drug susceptibility and patient's response to treatment.
    2 Do nothing until the pregnancy is over because of the risk of injury to the fetus.
    3 Start with a mild drug and monitor the pregnancy carefully for any signs of complications.
    4 Monitor the pregnancy carefully and begin treatment in the third trimester after the major fetal structures are complete.

40. The patient is 4 weeks pregnant. She is gravida II, para I. Her 3-year-old child was born with spina bifida. In addition to regular vitamin supplements, the health care provider prescribes an additional supplement. The nurse should know that this supplement would most likely be:
    1 Vitamin K
    2 Thiamine
    3 Vitamin E
    4 Folic acid

41. A prenatal patient is diagnosed with group B Streptococcus infection. The treatment should be:
    1 Obtain cultures to identify the organism responsible.
    2 Treat with a course of penicillin.
    3 Wait until labor and then treat with antibiotic.
    4 Educate the patient on how to prevent future infection.

42. A patient in her twentieth week is admitted with hyperemesis gravidarum. The priority nursing intervention should be:
    1 Providing diversion to decrease pain
    2 Monitoring accurate intake and output
    3 Weighing the patient daily
    4 Providing attractive nourishing meals

43. If a patient is truly overdue, her newborn is at risk for:
    1 Polydactyly and jaundice
    2 Desquamated palms of hands and soles of feet
    3 Lanugo and small amounts of ear cartilage
    4 Mongolian spots and milia

44. Which of the following should be of most concern to the nurse caring for a newborn?
    1 A newborn who has not voided in 24 hours
    2 A newborn whose hands and feet are slightly cyanotic
    3 A newborn who passes greenish tarry stool
    4 A newborn who seems to sleep all the time

45. A staff nurse is concerned that the father of the baby is very quiet and does not seem to want to participate in the baby's care. The first priority in this case should be:
    1 Make a special effort to cuddle and care for the baby to set an example for the parents.
    2 Insist that the father sit and hold the baby.
    3 Identify the cultural norms of the couple.
    4 Refer the couple to social services for counseling sessions.

46. During a newborn class the mother asks when the "soft spots" on her baby's head will close. The nurse replies:
    1 "The one on the top will close in 12 to 18 months. The posterior will close in 6 to 8 weeks."
    2 "The posterior will close in 12 to 18 months and the anterior in 6 to 8 weeks."
    3 "The anterior fontanel will close in 4 to 6 weeks and the posterior in 1 year."

4 "You don't have to worry about those spots. They will close."

47. A new mother asks why her baby's breasts are so swollen. The nurse replies:
    1 "You don't have to do anything; the swelling will disappear."
    2 "The doctor is aware and he will speak with you about it."
    3 "It is normal because of exposure to your hormones during pregnancy."
    4 "It is called 'witch's milk,' and some babies produce it."

48. Which of the following statements by a new mom would indicate that she understands the steps necessary for circumcision care?
    1 "I need to check and record every time my baby urinates."
    2 "I need to place petroleum gauze on the penis every time the baby urinates for 3 days."
    3 "A small amount of bleeding is normal."
    4 "I have to keep the penis exposed to air as much as possible."

49. New parents ask why antibiotic ointment is placed in the baby's eyes. The most appropriate response by the nurse is:
    1 "It is administered to prevent gonorrhea from being transmitted."
    2 "It is state law."
    3 "It is administered to prevent infection."
    4 "It prevents blindness caused by infection."

50. The nurse takes an axillary temperature on a 6-hour-old newborn. The most appropriate action for a reading of 96° F should be:
    1 Place the newborn under the warmer until temperature stabilizes at 97.6° to 99° F.
    2 Double wrap the infant and place a hat on his head.
    3 Recheck the temperature in an hour.
    4 Do nothing; this is a normal reading.

51. Which of the following evaluations would be indicative of an infant with RDS? *Resp distress syndrome*
    1 Grunting, rib retraction, nasal flaring
    2 Retrolental fibroplasia
    3 Breathing with abdominal muscles
    4 Breathing irregularly at 38 breaths per minute

52. Signs and symptoms that may indicate a diaphragmatic hernia to the nurse include:
    1 Bowel sounds heard in chest
    2 Difficulty feeding
    3 Dimple in lower lumbosacral skin
    4 Respiratory difficulty

53. Which of the following assessments would indicate a premature infant?
    1 Mongolian spots
    2 Paralysis of lower extremities
    3 "Frog-like" position
    4 Positive Babinski sign

54. Newborn parents are concerned because their baby's eyes seem to be crossed at times. The most appropriate response for the nurse at this time should be:
    1 "This is normal. Newborns eyes often seem uncoordinated for the first few days."
    2 "We have called the eye doctor in on consult."
    3 "This is often caused by the ointment that we put in their eyes at birth."
    4 "New parents worry about everything."

55. Which of the following evaluations would indicate increased intracranial pressure?
    1 Ruptured small capillaries in eye
    2 Bulging anterior fontanel
    3 Edema under the scalp
    4 Difficulty feeding

56. Cocaine is addictive to newborns because of:
    1 The inability of the newborn's immature liver to excrete the drug rapidly
    2 The mother's long-term use of drugs before conception
    3 The mother's ingestion of several different drugs, making it doubly addictive to the newborn
    4 The mother's impaired uterine growth, resulting in the newborn having RDS after birth

57. What Apgar score would be given to a newborn who exhibited the following?
    Heart rate: below 100 bpm
    Respiratory effort: weak cry
    Muscle tone: some flexion
    Reflex response: cough or sneeze
    Color: body pink; extremities blue
    1 4
    2 6
    3 7
    4 8

58. A newborn is diagnosed with pathological jaundice. His sclera is yellow, his bilirubin index is 17, and he is not nursing well. If the newborn's index continues to rise, the nurse should:
    1 Tell the mother that the baby will probably need an exchange transfusion and plan a teaching module of pros and cons.
    2 Prepare unit for possible exchange transfusion procedure; obtain supplies, review procedure, wait for physician's orders.
    3 Place the baby under phototherapy light for longer periods; offer water every 2 hours until jaundice begins to fade.
    4 Suggest that the entire family be tested for proper blood type.

59. After a precipitous delivery in the emergency room, the responsibilities of the emergency room nurse should include:
    1 Performing an admission assessment and giving a bath
    2 Following hospital protocol for nonsterile births
    3 Placing a baby in an isolette for observation
    4 Administering vitamin K to prevent hemorrhage

60. During a vaginal examination, the health care provider states that the fetus is engaged. The nurse explains to the patient that this means:
    1 The fetus is at the ischial spines.
    2 The fetus is floating high in the perineum.
    3 The presenting part is crowning.
    4 The infant has passed into the pelvic inlet.

61. The health care provider is evaluating whether the second stage of labor has begun. The nurse knows that this would be when:
    1 The woman feels the urge to push.
    2 The fetus is at station 1.
    3 The cervix is fully dilated at 10 cm.
    4 The placenta is delivered.

62. A woman is admitted with a history of cardiac disease. Which of these special nursing interventions should be indicated in the course of labor?
    1 Using epidural anesthesia
    2 Checking carefully for signs of cardiac decompensation
    3 Encourage voiding at regular intervals
    4 Monitoring the fetal monitor carefully for any abnormalities

63. After the birth of an infant, the physician examines the umbilical cord carefully. The nurse understands that he is checking for the normal pattern, which is:
    1 Two arteries and one vein
    2 Two veins and one artery
    3 One vein and one artery
    4 Two veins and two arteries

64. A patient in labor is experiencing dystocia. One possible cause for this is:
    1 The cervix is just about to reach full dilation.
    2 The mother is experiencing extreme fatigue.
    3 Excessive size of the fetus
    4 Prolapsed cord

65. The fetal monitoring strip should be evaluated and documented on a regular basis. Which of the following monitor patterns should be considered ominous?
    1 FHR accelerations
    2 Early decelerations
    3 Late decelerations
    4 Isolated variable decelerations

66. The nurse is very careful to evaluate the fundus of the uterus every 15 minutes during the fourth stage of labor. A fundus that indicates a normal finding would be:
    1 Soft to touch but firms up when massaged
    2 Firm and at the umbilicus
    3 Firm and deviated to the right
    4 Soft and deviated to the left

67. To relieve supine hypotensive syndrome in a patient, the nurse should:
    1 Massage her leg.
    2 Instruct her to breathe deeply.
    3 Turn her on left side.
    4 Advise her to walk slowly and carefully.

68. Nursing management during the first stage of labor includes which of the following?
    1 Admit patient to labor room, establish rapport, monitor FHT, keep patient and significant others apprised of progress.
    2 Monitor FHT, monitor BP every 15 minutes, give pushing instructions, maintain patent airway for newborn, follow proper identification routine.
    3 Be sure cord blood specimen is obtained, observe time and delivery of placenta, check perineal area, check fundus, administer oxytocin IV after placenta is delivered, check BP and fundus every 5 minutes.
    4 Watch for hemorrhaging, check fundus every 15 minutes, monitor BP every 15 minutes, offer warm food and fluid, offer bedpan for urination, teach perineal care, transfer patient to postpartum room when condition is stable.

69. After the placenta is delivered and episiotomy suturing is completed, the nurse notices that the patient has begun to shiver. What should the nurse suspect as the probable cause of the shivering?

    1 The sudden emptying of the uterine contents, plus the return of the body chemistry and hormones to the prepregnant state, causes a certain shock to the system.
    2 Loss of blood, length of labor, and a certain tiredness cause the lowering of the body temperature; the warm blankets will help.
    3 Pitocin is given after the delivery of the placenta and may cause the body to respond by shivering.
    4 The shiver is a normal reaction because she has been swallowing ice chips and is covered only with a thin sheet.

70. A couple arrives at the emergency room visibly upset and frightened. She has been in labor for 3 hours and suddenly had a sudden sharp pain that made her gasp for breath. The nurse notices that she is diaphoretic, ashen, cold, and clammy. The nurse also assesses her abdomen to be rigid and boardlike. Judging from the symptoms described, the most likely complication for the nurse to suspect would be:
    1 Low marginal placenta previa
    2 Appendicitis
    3 Premature separation of the placenta
    4 Rupture of the uterus

71. A patient is admitted to the maternity care department. The mother-to-be has been having contractions intermittently at 10- to 20-minute intervals for the last 12 hours. The contractions are relieved by ambulation. Her EDC is 2 weeks away. The physician examines her and finds her to be 0 cm dilated and just slightly effaced. The nurse should know that these contractions are most likely:
    1 True labor and will progress rapidly
    2 True labor and will progress differently for every woman
    3 False labor because they are relieved by activity
    4 False labor that most likely will change to true labor in 24 hours

72. A patient is admitted to the emergency department in active labor. She delivers a baby girl spontaneously after one contraction. The nurse is still alone with the patient. The first responsibility is to:
    1 Ascertain whether the fundus is likely to hemorrhage.
    2 Establish an airway for the baby by milking the trachea and maintaining the head lower than the body.
    3 Quickly tie and cut the umbilical cord.
    4 Look for the uterus to rise, watch the perineum for a trickle of blood, and deliver the placenta.

73. Magnesium sulfate is used for preeclampsia and should not be given if:
    1 BP is elevated.
    2 DTRs are absent.
    3 DTRs are brisk.
    4 Albumin is 3.

74. A patient whose last menstrual period began on May 18 should have an EDC of:
    1 February 9
    2 February 11
    3 February 18
    4 February 25

75. After reviewing prenatal care with a patient, the nurse should instruct the patient to notify the physician immediately if she experiences:
    1 Abdominal pain, bright-red bleeding, chills, fever
    2 Blood-streaked mucus, Braxton-Hicks contractions

3 Constipation, urgency, hemorrhoids

4 Quickening, varicosities, discomfort

76. The patient who is in her third trimester of pregnancy suddenly notices that she is bleeding. At first, the bleeding was scanty but has become heavier. She reports that she has no pain. A nurse should suspect:

1 Abruptio placentae

2 Placenta previa

3 Ruptured uterus

4 Vasa previa

77. In looking over a patient's chart a nurse sees that her hemoglobin is 9.5 g/dl. The patient is 32 weeks' gestation. What does this mean to the nurse?

1 The patient is anemic and needs immediate treatment.

2 This is probably resulting from increased blood volume of pregnancy.

3 This must be her baseline.

4 Z-track iron should be administered to this patient.

78. A patient who is 38 weeks' pregnant is admitted to the maternity ward complaining of headaches and "blind spots" for approximately a week. She complained of upper abdominal pain in the morning. Emergency services brought her to the hospital immediately. Admitting record:

BP: 140/112 mmHg

Albumin: 4

FHT: 140 strong

Cervix: effaced, dilated 3 cm

Presenting part: station 0

Membranes: intact

The admitting nurse, knowing the situation, would place her in:

1 A semi-private room with plenty of sunlight and air

2 A semi-private room, darkened and quiet; restricted visitors

3 A single, darkened room; no visitors; close to nurses' station

4 A single room, plenty of sunlight; no visitors; away from the nurses' station

79. A patient who is 2 months pregnant asks the nurse if it is all right to exercise during pregnancy. The nurse's most appropriate answer should be:

1 "It depends on your previous exercise patterns."

2 "Absolutely. It will help you and your baby feel better."

3 "Do not do any exercise that will jar the baby, such as horseback riding or skydiving."

4 "Make certain that you let your physician know if you experience any pain or discomfort."

80. A patient delivered her first baby, a boy, several hours ago. She has been admitted to her postpartum room in stable condition and is euphoric over her successful implementation of the Lamaze techniques. The nurse finds her uterus firm, slightly above the umbilicus. She has saturated one pad with lochia rubra. Her episiotomy appears clean, but her labia and perineal area are swollen and slightly ecchymotic. The nurse's first priority in nursing care should be to:

1 Apply an ice glove to the perineal area.

2 Massage her uterus so it will go down below the umbilicus.

3 Administer a tranquilizer because she is so euphoric.

4 Watch for hemorrhage because her lochia is so red.

81. A home care nurse is interviewing and assessing a mother who gave birth 10 days ago. Which of the following items should be reported to the physician?

1 A fundus that is not palpable

2 Reports by the mother of problems with constipation

3 Reports by the mother of periods when she just cannot stop crying

4 Reports of the mother of dark red lochia with small clots

82. Which of the following mothers would receive RhoGAM within 72 hours after giving birth?

1 An Rh-negative mother giving birth to an Rh-negative child

2 An Rh-positive mother giving birth to an Rh-positive child

3 An Rh-negative mother who did not receive RhoGAM after a previous miscarriage of a negative fetus

4 An Rh-negative mother giving birth to her first Rh-positive child

83. A patient is a 2-day postoperative cesarean birth. She is of Asian heritage. Because her bowel sounds are positive, she is advanced to a clear liquid diet. She is refusing to drink any clear liquids except for hot water, hot tea, and a special broth that her mother brings her from home. Which of the following interventions is appropriate for the nurse at this time?

1 Insist that the patient consult a dietician for additional clear liquids.

2 Set the patient up and assist as needed with the clear liquids she will drink.

3 Speak with the family about encouraging the patient to drink more of a variety of clear liquids.

4 Explain to the patient that hospital clear liquids are healthier.

84. For the last 3 days, a day-5 postoperative cesarean patient has been experiencing frequent episodes of diarrhea. She is extremely weak and diaphoretic. She is breast-feeding and bonding well with the baby. For infection-control purposes, which of the following interventions would be most appropriate?

1 Have the patient placed on strict respiratory isolation.

2 Discontinue breast-feeding and have the baby remain in the nursery.

3 Have the baby remain in the room with the mother and have one nurse care for both.

4 Contact the physician for blood, sputum, and stool cultures.

85. The nurse evaluates when it is appropriate to let a patient out of bed after epidural anesthesia. The most appropriate time should be:

1 As soon as the catheter is removed from the epidural space

2 When full sensation has returned to the patient's legs

3 When the baby is born and she feels up to it

4 After her first meal

86. Although rare, a spinal headache is often treated conservatively. If conservative treatment is not adequate, which of the following interventions may be attempted?

1 Epidural anesthesia

2 Transcutaneous electrical nerve stimulation

3 A blood patch

4 Antibiotics

87. Which finding in a 10-day postpartum patient would indicate that involution is proceeding at a normal rate?
    1 The uterus is firm, midline, and three fingers below the umbilicus.
    2 The uterus is firm, deviated to the right, and three fingers below the umbilicus.
    3 The uterus is no longer palpable in the abdominal cavity.
    4 The uterus is firm and at the umbilicus.

88. A mother who is 2 weeks postpartum asks, "How can I be certain that my baby is receiving enough nourishment?" The most appropriate reply by the nurse would be:
    1 "When he falls asleep after nursing, he is satisfied."
    2 "If he nurses at least 10 minutes on each side, he is satisfied."
    3 "If he urinates six to eight times a day, he is adequately nourished."
    4 "If he gains weight on a regular basis, he is fine."

89. Which of the following assessments would be of most concern to the nurse? The patient is a 2-day postpartum mother.
    1 A firm fundus two fingers below the umbilicus
    2 Frequency and burning on urination
    3 Breasts that are firm and engorged
    4 Lochia rubra with small clots

90. A patient who is 2 weeks postpartum is admitted to the emergency room. Which of the following evaluations would be indicative of late postpartum hemorrhage?
    1 Boggy uterus, shocklike symptoms
    2 Elevated respirations, back pain
    3 Intermittent abdominal cramping, elevated BP
    4 Foul-smelling vaginal drainage, uterus hard to the touch

91. During evaluation of a midline episiotomy, the nurse suspects that the patient may have a hematoma. Which assessment by the nurse might lead to this conclusion?
    1 The patient had a prolonged second stage.
    2 The patient is complaining of severe perineal pain.
    3 A blood-filled sac is visible in the vaginal area.
    4 The episiotomy is swollen and slightly reddened.

92. A patient is admitted to your medical-surgical unit after delivering a full-term infant who was stillborn. The husband says to the nurse, "I will see my baby and take care of the arrangements. I don't want anyone to say anything to my wife about what happened." The most appropriate action of the nurse should be to:
    1 Reassure the husband that his wishes will be respected.
    2 Explain to the husband that no one will initiate the specific topic with his wife, but they will not stop her from talking about it.
    3 Encourage the husband to talk with his wife so that they can support each other through the grieving process.
    4 Explain politely to the husband that his wife is the patient and it is your responsibility to encourage communication in every way possible.

93. An adolescent who is 1 day postpartum is discussing future birth-control methods with the nurse. She states that she is busy and forgetful and does not want to think about it every day. The most appropriate method for the nurse to recommend would be:
    1 Abstinence
    2 Estrogen patch
    3 Condoms
    4 Depro-Provera injection

94. A nurse is completing her assessments on a postpartum patient. The patient asks the nurse why she had to dorsiflex her foot. The most appropriate response for the nurse would be.
    1 "It is a precautionary assessment to be certain that your circulation is healthy."
    2 "Pain in your inner calf may be an indication of a blood clot."
    3 "Women have extra clotting factors to minimize blood loss during pregnancy."
    4 "Exercise is good for the extremities to help prevent blood clots."

95. A nurse counsels a patient to avoid all medications unless prescribed by a physician because:
    1 Many medications will delay the labor process.
    2 Many medications may trigger an early labor.
    3 Many medications may cause harm to the fetus.
    4 Almost all medications cross the placental barrier.

96. A patient in her third trimester is complaining of shortness of breath when she is trying to rest. The most appropriate intervention for the nurse to suggest would be:
    1 "Rest during the day whenever you have a chance."
    2 "Elevate your legs above the level of your heart."
    3 "Use two pillows when you are trying to sleep."
    4 "Avoid eating too close to your bedtime."

97. Quickening (the first movements of the fetus in utero) is first felt by the:
    1 Tenth to twelfth week
    2 Sixteenth to twentieth week
    3 Eighth to twelfth week
    4 Thirty-second to thirty-sixth week

98. The primary difference between abruptio placenta and placenta previa would be described as:
    1 Presence of pain
    2 Presence of vaginal bleeding
    3 Position of the fetus
    4 Potential for fetal compromise

99. A woman is diagnosed with a possible ectopic pregnancy. Which of the following would not be a possible cause?
    1 Inflammation of the fallopian tubes
    2 A congenital malformation of the fallopian tubes
    3 A history of infection in the fallopian tubes
    4 A chronic vaginal infection

100. An assessment of a primigravida documents the following information: the patient is 2 cm dilated, mild contractions every 15 minutes, lasting 40 seconds, she is alert and talkative. Which phase of labor is she in?
    1 Active
    2 Transition
    3 Latent
    4 Fourth

101. The baby is born in which stage of labor?
    1 First
    2 Second
    3 Third
    4 Fourth

102. A woman diagnosed with gestational trophoblastic neoplasm would most likely have experienced which of the following signs or symptoms in her pregnancy?
    1 Early quickening
    2 Early PIH   BY 20? WK
    3 A missed period
    4 A uterus small for the gestational age

103. Newborns must be protected against infection because:
    1 The immune system of the infant is not fully developed and takes time to do so.
    2 The portals of entry of infection are much more vulnerable than those of an adult.
    3 An infection that is minor to an adult might kill a child.
    4 Babies who are not breast-feeding will not receive protective antibodies from their mother.

104. A pregnant woman is lying on her back during an examination. She begins to complain of lightheadedness and dizziness. The most appropriate nursing intervention at this point would be:
    1 Have the patient change to a sitting position.
    2 Turn patient on her left side.
    3 Elevate the patient's legs.
    4 Elevate her to semi-Fowler's position.

105. A nurse is caring for a high-risk mother who is 8 months pregnant, who states that her membranes ruptured and she is having contractions. The nurse suspects that a prolapsed cord may have occurred. After calling for emergency help, the priority action for the nurse would be:
    1 Place the woman in high-Fowler's position to decrease pressure.
    2 Support the cord to prevent repositioning.
    3 Place the mother in knee-chest position.
    4 Monitor the FHR.

106. A woman is admitted to the maternity unit with a diagnosis of severe PIH. Which of the following medications would the nurse expect to soon order?
    1 Lasix
    2 Aspirin
    3 Magnesium sulfate
    4 Calcium gluconate

107. The normal respiratory rate for a newborn is:
    1 60 to 80 breaths per minute
    2 30 to 90 breaths per minute
    3 12 to 20 breaths per minute
    4 30 to 60 breaths per minute

108. The nurse anticipates that the physician will order which of the following interventions for a 12-hour-old infant with a bilirubin level of 14 mg/dl?
    1 Phototherapy
    2 IV
    3 Radiant warmer
    4 Antibiotics

109. The nurse is concerned because a 12-hour-old infant has a bilirubin of 14 mg/dl. On assessment the infant would show:
    1 Signs of jaundice
    2 Irritability
    3 Signs of infection
    4 A weak cry

110. A new mother is concerned because her baby's eyes appear cross-eyed. The most appropriate response by the nurse would be:
    1 The pediatrician will evaluate this during the baby's first office visit.
    2 This is a genetic characteristic that is more common in boys.
    3 This is the result of poor muscle control and is common in newborns.
    4 Visual stimulation will help correct this problem.

111. All of the following instructions are important following a circumcision, *except:*
    1 Checking carefully for signs of infection
    2 Applying Vaseline jelly and gauze after every voiding
    3 Cleaning the area with alcohol after every voiding
    4 Checking for any oozing or drainage.

112. A new mother asks the nurse about the bruises on her baby's back. The nurse replies:
    1 "These are not bruises; they are called Mongolian spots."
    2 "These are bruises from the birth process, and they will fade."
    3 "These are Mongolian spots and are caused by pigment producing cells."
    4 "I will make certain the pediatrician is informed of these areas."

113. A woman is gravida 3, para 0. The nurse knows that the patient will require:
    1 No special support because she has been pregnant before
    2 A careful assessment to find out the mother's feelings about the pregnancy
    3 Immediate intervention to help her deal with her anxiety
    4 A careful history to determine the outcomes of the previous pregnancies

114. A mother who is breast-feeding asks the nurse how she can be certain that her baby is getting enough to eat. The nurse replies:
    1 "The breast-fed infant should have 3 to 6 stools a day."
    2 "The infant will not lose weight immediately after birth."
    3 "The number of stools will decrease gradually after birth."
    4 "The stools will become more solid."

115. A mother asks the nurse about the "little white pimples" on her baby's cheeks. The most appropriate reply by the nurse is:
    1 "The doctor will order a mild antibiotic cream."
    2 "Washing it very well with soap and water will clear up the rash."
    3 "We will keep an eye on the rash to make sure that it does not spread."
    4 "They are a normal on a newborn and do not require any special intervention."

116. A woman at her second prenatal visit is 8 weeks pregnant. She confides to the nurse that she is worried about her ability to be a mother. The nurse replies:
    1 "Many pregnancies are unplanned."
    2 "It is normal to have concerns about the pregnancy at this point."
    3 "Don't worry; these feelings will pass."
    4 "Your partner will help you work through these anxieties."

117. A patient in the physician's office complains of increased vaginal discharge. The most appropriate nursing intervention would be:
    1 Advise her to decrease sexual intercourse.
    2 Encourage her to wear only cotton underwear.
    3 Ask her if the discharge burns or itches.
    4 Ask her physician to prescribe a douche.

118. A newborn receives an Apgar score of 9 at 1 minute after birth. The reason for this would be:
    1 A heart rate of 110 bpm
    2 Active spontaneous motion
    3 A strong lusty cry
    4 Slight cyanosis of the extremities

119. Decreases in FHR during labor are called:
    1 Accelerations
    2 Decelerations
    3 Baseline rate
    4 Variability

120. Which of the following is an incorrect statement comparing the differences between true and false labor?
    1 True labor discomfort is usually felt in the lower back and lower abdomen.
    2 In false labor, walking tends to relieve or decrease contractions.
    3 In false labor, bloody show is often present.
    4 In true labor, contractions gradually develop a regular pattern.

121. Early decelerations are noted on the external fetal monitoring strip of a patient in active labor. The first nursing action is:
    1 No intervention is required; this is a reassuring pattern.
    2 Reposition the patient on her left side.
    3 Give the patient 2 L of oxygen.
    4 Notify the physician to obtain an order for an IV.

122. A woman in labor asks the nurse why she and her partner have to keep walking around the hall. All of the following reasons are appropriate, except:
    1 Walking helps to use gravity in the baby's descent.
    2 Walking decreases back pain.
    3 Walking will help the membranes rupture.
    4 Walking will stimulate contractions.

123. A nurse is teaching a student how to palpate contractions. The correct position of the examiner's hand is:
    1 On the symphysis pubis
    2 In the vagina
    3 On the fundus of the uterus
    4 On the woman's umbilicus

124. A primigravida calls the physician's office and gives the nurse the following information. She is having regular contractions every 8 minutes, and her membranes have not ruptured. The most appropriate intervention for the nurse would be:
    1 Walk around in her house and come to the hospital when her contractions are 5 minutes apart.
    2 Call an ambulance and come to the hospital immediately.
    3 Have someone drive her to the hospital quickly and safely.
    4 Come to the physician's office for a further assessment.

125. A student nurse asks the physician if a white blood cell count of 18,000/mm³ is of concern in a postpartum patient. The physician replies:
    1 "Yes, we need to get blood and urine cultures."
    2 "No, this is within the normal range."
    3 "Postpartum women are vulnerable to infection."
    4 "Postpartum women often have an elevated white blood cell count."

126. A woman who has just given birth is complaining of shaking and chills. The most appropriate nursing intervention is:
    1 Provide a warm blanket.
    2 Contact the physician.
    3 Monitor vital signs.
    4 Offer her a warm drink.

127. Which of the following assessments would be of most concern 24 hours after birth?
    1 A moderate amount of lochia with a dime-size clot
    2 A firm fundus deviated to the right
    3 A severely bruised perineum
    4 An intact slightly reddened perineum

128. A woman in labor states she feels like she has to push. The initial intervention by the nurse would be:
    1 Reassure the woman that this is a normal sensation in labor.
    2 Monitor the contractions to assess the duration.
    3 Assess the perineum for signs of bulging.
    4 Call the physician in preparation for delivery.

129. Spinal headache is best relieved by:
    1 Positioning the patient on her left side
    2 Using relaxed, calm breathing
    3 Injecting a blood patch into the epidural space
    4 Avoiding ambulation for 12 hours

130. A newborn is diagnosed with caput succedaneum. During an assessment, the nurse would expect to see:
    1 Depressed fontanels
    2 Swelling of the scalp
    3 A swelling on one side of the scalp
    4 Bulging fontanels

131. Cephalohematoma is most likely seen in:
    1 A baby delivered with forceps
    2 A baby delivered precipitously
    3 A baby delivered via CS
    4 A baby delivered in a breech position

132. What treatment is required for a cephalohematoma?
    1 No treatment is required; it disappears in 3 to 4 days.
    2 Gentle massage twice a day
    3 No treatment is required and disappears in 3 to 6 weeks.
    4 Careful monitoring to be certain it does not get larger

133. A major concern for women with PROM is:
    1 Dystocia
    2 Hemorrhage
    3 Infection
    4 Hypertension

134. During a prenatal visit, the woman is diagnosed with oligohydramnios. This condition is defined as:
    1 Excessive amniotic fluid
    2 Meconium stained amniotic fluid
    3 Scant amniotic fluid
    4 Leaking amniotic fluid

135. Oligohydramnios may indicate which anomaly in the newborn?
    1 Abnormalities of the gastrointestinal tract
    2 Cardiac abnormalities
    3 Neurological abnormalities
    4 Urinary tract abnormalities

136. A nurse reports the following assessments concerning an infant: noisy respirations on inspiration, mild intercostal retractions, cyanosis, and dyspnea. The physician

determines a diagnosis of:
1 Choanal atresia
2 Cleft lip
3 Congenital laryngeal stridor
4 Diaphragmatic hernia

137. A nurse is instructing a mother whose newborn is diagnosed with laryngeal stridor. The nurse knows the mother understands the instruction when the mother makes which of the following statements?
1 "My baby needs to be fed on a regular schedule."
2 "My baby needs to be fed in an upright position."
3 "My baby needs to be fed a nonlactose formula."
4 "My baby needs to be kept warm and dry."

138. The definition of polydactyl is:
1 Missing fingers and toes
2 Extra fingers and toes
3 Webbed fingers and toes
4 A missing extremity

139. Macrosomia is defined as:
1 An underweight baby
2 A baby with a smaller than average brain
3 An oversized baby
4 A baby with a larger than average brain

140. HELLP is defined as:
1 A severe form of anemia that needs to be treated in pregnancy
2 A mild form of PIH that needs close monitoring
3 A severe syndrome that occurs with PIH
4 A condition that occurs with hyperemesis gravidarum

141. The hormone that is responsible for positive pregnancy test is:
1 Estrogen
2 HCG
3 Progesterone
4 Testosterone

142. Which of the following mothers are at the highest risk for postpartum infection?
1 A woman who delivered a baby precipitously
2 A woman who delivered via CS
3 A woman with PROM
4 A woman with a prolonged labor

143. The key difference between true and false labor is:
1 The characteristics of the contractions
2 The dilation and effacement of the cervix
3 The location of the contractions
4 The degree of engagement of the presenting part

144. Engagement means:
1 The presenting part of the fetus has entered into the pelvis.
2 The position of the presenting part in relationship to the mother's ischial spines
3 The fetal part that enters the maternal pelvis first
4 The membranes have ruptured.

145. An infant is in the ninetieth percentile for weight. This would classify the baby as:
1 Appropriate for gestational age
2 Overweight
3 SGA
4 LGA

146. Women with diabetes are more prone to urinary tract infections because:
1 They have to limit their fluid intake.
2 They have increased amounts of glucose in their urine.
3 Their babies tend to be larger and put more pressure on the bladder.
4 Their insulin requirements fluctuate in pregnancy.

147. A primigravida in her thirty-eighth week tells her health care provider that she is breathing easier but has to go to the bathroom a lot more frequently. The nurse explains to the patient that this is called:
1 Ballottement
2 Molding
3 Lightening
4 Quickening

148. A woman and her partner are embarrassed about being sent home because of false labor. The best response of the nurse would be:
1 "Don't be upset; it happens all the time."
2 "Next time, wait until your contractions are 5 minutes apart."
3 "Do not hesitate to come to the hospital with any concern."
4 "Wait until your membranes rupture."

149. The duration of the contraction is defined as:
1 The time from the beginning of one contraction to the beginning of another
2 The length of the contraction measured from the beginning to its completion
3 The amount of indentation of the uterus
4 The time labor started

150. A woman is admitted in labor. Her mother and her husband are with her. The woman wants her mother to be with her, and the husband states he will wait in the waiting room. The most appropriate intervention for the nurse is:
1 Tell the husband that he will regret not being present at his baby's birth.
2 Explore the reasons behind the couple's request.
3 Explain to the husband that he will be at the mother's head and will not have to see any blood.
4 Respect the woman's wishes.

151. The primary reason for having a Foley catheter inserted before a CS is:
1 To make certain that the urinary output is adequate during surgery
2 To prevent infection
3 To keep the bladder empty so that it does not interfere with surgery
4 To eliminate the need for early ambulation after surgery

152. A patient asks what kind of exercise is safe during pregnancy? The best reply by the nurse is:
1 "It depends on your previous exercise pattern."
2 "Avoid anything that might be jarring to the baby."
3 "Start slowly and do plenty of stretching."
4 "Slow walking is really your only choice."

153. A primigravida in her second trimester is planning a long driving vacation with her partner. The most pertinent advice for the nurse to give is:
1 "Bring plenty of nutritious snacks so you won't get hungry."
2 "Elevate your legs at night to decrease edema."
3 "Let your partner do most of the driving to avoid leg cramps."
4 "Stop at least every 3 hours and elevate your legs."

154. A woman has given birth 3 hours ago. The nurse observes the patient trying to care for the baby. The woman states, "I am just too tired." She returns to bed. The best action for the nurse at this point is:
    1 Complete the newborn's care quietly and allow the mother to rest.
    2 Encourage the mother to complete the care.
    3 Complete the care but put in a consult to social services.
    4 Instruct the mother on completing the care while she is resting.

155. During a postpartum examination, the nurse assesses a small hematoma on the vulva. The most appropriate intervention (with a standing order) would be:
    1 Ice pack
    2 Bath
    3 Spray
    4 Lamp

156. A young couple wants to know when the sex of the fetus is determined. The correct answer is:
    1 At birth
    2 At conception
    3 During an amniocentesis
    4 From results of blood work after first prenatal visit

157. The physician is concerned because the baby has a nuchal cord. The nurse knows that this means:
    1 The cord is coming out before the head.
    2 The cord is too long.
    3 The cord is around the baby's neck.
    4 The cord is too high.

158. The hormone that stimulates uterine contractions and helps keep the uterus contracted after birth is:
    1 Prolactin
    2 Oxytocin
    3 Estrogen
    4 Progesterone

159. A patient tells the nurse that she is interested in using herbal medicines to ease some of the common discomforts of pregnancy. The best response for the nurse would be:
    1 "Most herbal medicines are natural and safe."
    2 "Check with the physician before taking any medicine."
    3 "Just be certain to watch your dose."
    4 "The safety of most of these medicines has not been determined for pregnancy."

160. After examination, a woman is determined to be 5 cm dilated and 50% effaced. The nurse knows that she is in the:
    1 Second stage
    2 First stage—latent phase
    3 First stage—transition phase
    4 First stage—active phase

161. Which of the following contraction patterns would be characteristic of the transition phase of labor?
    1 8:00 AM and end 8:00 AM and 30 seconds
      8:05 AM and end 8:05 AM and 30 seconds
    2 8:00 AM and end 8:01 AM
      8:03 AM and end 8:04 AM
    3 8:00 AM and end 8:00 AM and 20 seconds
      8:15 AM and end 8:15 AM and 20 seconds
    4 Irregular contractions lasting 45 to 60 seconds with no spaced pattern

162. Which of the following pregnant women might find working until full term the most difficult?
    1 A self-employed accountant
    2 A hair stylist
    3 A book editor
    4 A real estate agent

163. A woman in her third trimester is complaining of dyspnea. What is the most appropriate intervention for the nurse to suggest?
    1 "Move slowly when changing positions."
    2 "Eat several small meals daily."
    3 "Sleep with several pillows under your head."
    4 "Elevate your legs when sitting."

164. Which of the following measures should a mother be taught to decrease the discomfort of mastitis?
    1 Breast-feed the baby only on the unaffected side.
    2 Limit the amount of time on each breast.
    3 Empty the breasts completely at each feeding.
    4 Apply ice and a well-fitting bra until lactation ceases.

165. What advice should be given to relieve constipation?
    1 Increase fluid intake to eight glasses of water a day.
    2 Obtain a prescription for a stool softener.
    3 Exercise increases peristalsis.
    4 Use a natural laxative.

166. Which of the following snacks for a pregnant patient would be of most concern to the nurse?
    1 Caffe latte at 3:00 PM
    2 Ice cream at 9:00 PM
    3 Low-fat yogurt at 11:00 AM
    4 Gelatin for dessert

167. A new mother asks why her newborn's breasts are swollen. The nurse replies:
    1 "This happens because of the hormone from mother to baby."
    2 "Do not be concerned; it will disappear."
    3 "Warm compresses will relieve the swelling."
    4 "The pediatrician will examine the baby soon."

168. The mother asks when she can give her baby a tub bath? The nurse replies:
    1 Anytime, as long as you keep your hand on the baby at all times.
    2 When the baby can hold up its head.
    3 When the umbilical cord falls off.
    4 As soon as his circumcision heals.

169. A Native-American family asks permission to do a ceremony blessing their newborn. What further information is needed before an answer can be given?
    1 Is the woman in a private room?
    2 What exactly is involved in the ceremony?
    3 What supplies need to be provided by the hospital?
    4 Will hospital staff be permitted to attend the ceremony?

170. A patient is in the transitional phase of labor. Which of the following would best describe her behavioral pattern?
    1 Happy and talkative
    2 Anxious and uncomfortable
    3 Irritable and introverted
    4 Relaxed and receptive

171. The nurse evaluates her patient teaching concerning sibling rivalry as successful when her patient states the following:
    1 "I need to make sure I spend special time with each of my children."

2 "My oldest can help with baby-sitting chores."

3 "They need to understand that the baby will occupy a great deal of my time."

4 "Thank goodness that my 5 year old is starting kindergarten in the fall."

172. The second trimester is most commonly noted for which behavior in the woman?
1 Introversion—questioning her role as a mother
2 Separating the fetus from herself and making concrete plans
3 Acceptance of the fetus as part of her body image
4 Ambivalent feelings concerning being a mother

173. Late decelerations during labor:
1 Are of concern because they may indicate the fetus is not getting enough oxygen
2 Expected and not of any concern
3 Indicate that the fetus is tolerating the stress of labor
4 Are of concern because they indicate that the labor is progressing faster than expected

174. Which of the following statements by a primigravida indicates the need for further teaching?
1 "Fast food is OK as long as I make healthy choices."
2 "I am really nervous about the pain of childbirth."
3 "I know the signs of impending labor and when to call the doctor."
4 "I had a miscarriage 2 years ago."

175. A nurse is teaching a 14-year-old primigravida how to bathe her baby. Which of the following statements would be of most concern?
1 "I will make sure I bathe the baby after I feed her."
2 "The baby does not have to be on any special schedule."
3 "Sometimes I get so frustrated when she cries and cries and cries."
4 "My boyfriend said he will help me sometimes."

176. A couple has just had a diagnostic test to determine if their baby has trisomy 21 (Down syndrome). This type of test is called:
1 Ultrasound
2 Chorionic villi test
3 Amniocentesis
4 AFP test

177. Which of the following statements by a new mother best indicates that she understands the needs of a newborn during bath time?
1 "Sometimes my partner can help me with the bath."
2 "I don't have to be on a rigid schedule."
3 "I must never take my hands off the baby during bath time."
4 "I will feed my baby after I bathe him."

178. Which is the best suggestion to give new parents to prevent postpartum baby blues?
1 "You have to be strong and take responsibility for your baby."
2 "Keep your strength up with plenty of nutritious snacks."
3 "Be certain to spend time with each other and communicate your feelings."
4 "Call your physician if you are feeling sad and depressed."

179. Which of the following vitamin injections are given to the newborn very soon after birth?
1 B_{12}
2 C

3 B_6
4 K

180. The first nursing intervention immediately after the membranes rupture would be:
1 Assessing the maternal BP
2 Assessing the maternal pulse
3 Assessing the FHR
4 Assessing the interval between contractions

181. When the baby's head is visible in the birth canal, this is called:
1 Crowning
2 Station
3 Engagement
4 Effacement

182. The most appropriate instruction that should be given to help prevent a UTI would be:
1 Limit fluid intake to between meals.
2 Drink at least eight glasses of water a day.
3 Try to avoid emptying your bladder until you really have to.
4 Drink cranberry juice at least once a day.

183. If the nurse is uncertain whether the fluid is amniotic fluid, the proper intervention is to:
1 Send a sample to the laboratory.
2 Consult with the physician.
3 Arrange for a stress test.
4 Test the fluid with nitrazine paper.

184. Which of the following is a sign of illness in a newborn?
1 Refusing a feeding
2 A pulse rate of 120 bpm
3 Temperature over 100.2° F
4 Six voidings per day

185. A new mother is concerned when she sees the bulb syringe in her newborn's crib. The best reply for the nurse would be:
1 "Your baby has been a little congested. We use it to keep his nose clear."
2 "Do you want me to show you how to use it?"
3 "We put it there for all babies in case they get a little congested."
4 "New mothers worry about everything!"

186. A postpartum patient calls the maternity unit with a question about feeding. Her bottle-fed infant has only had two stools in the last 24 hours. The nurse advises her to call the physician and also gives her the following suggestion:
1 Try switching to a formula with increased iron.
2 Feed the infant on a strict schedule.
3 Increase the amount of fluid in the infant's diet.
4 Two stools per day is not unusual for a newborn.

187. One of the dangers of cold stress in a newborn is:
1 The newborn is prone to reverse peristalsis.
2 The newborn is prone to swallowing air and crying during feeding.
3 The newborn is at risk for hypoglycemia.
4 The newborn is at risk for infection.

188. Which of the following conditions would be an example of heat loss by evaporation?
1 Cold hands
2 A draft from an open door
3 Wet diapers
4 Contact with crib walls

189. One benefit of breast-feeding over bottle-feeding is:
    1 The infant receives passive immunity for some viral and bacterial infections.
    2 The infant receives a supply of vitamin K
    3 The infant receives a supply of iron.
    4 The infant is less likely to have problems with constipation.

190. Which of the following reflexes is most important in encouraging the newborn to eat?
    1 Gag
    2 Moro's
    3 Pupillary
    4 Rooting

191. A positive Babinski response in a full-term infant:
    1 Is abnormal and may indicate a spinal cord abnormality
    2 Is normal and indicates an intact CNS
    3 Is unusual but occurs as a genetic trait in some nationalities
    4 Occurs when an object is placed in the infant's hand

192. A key difference that distinguishes baby blues from postpartum depression would be:
    1 The woman cannot distinguish reality from fantasy.
    2 The woman is unable to care for her baby or the rest of her family.
    3 The woman has crying spells for no apparent reason.
    4 Feelings of sadness are more transient.

193. One reason why adolescents have a special need for nutritional counseling is because:
    1 They are influenced by their peers to eat the wrong food.
    2 They like to eat a lot of fast food because of their busy lifestyle.
    3 Their food may not include enough choices of healthy nutrients.
    4 They will tend to eat too few calories to avoid gaining a lot of weight.

194. Postpartum hemorrhage can cause which of the following types of shock?
    1 Hypovolemic
    2 Anaphylactic shock
    3 Septic
    4 Physiological

195. A pregnant woman is classified as nonimmune to rubella. The appropriate action at this point is:
    1 Counsel the patient that an abortion may need to be considered.

2 Advise the patient to avoid situations in which she may be exposed.
    3 Arrange for appropriate diagnostic tests to detect possible fetal abnormalities.
    4 Arrange for the vaccine to be administered immediately.

196. A patient is being cared for in a prenatal clinic. She tells the nurse that she is a vegetarian. What follow up information is required at this point?
    1 To what degree is the woman a vegetarian?
    2 How long has she been a vegetarian?
    3 Is the baby going to be a vegetarian?
    4 Is she going to eat meat during the pregnancy?

197. A gravida II, para I patient asks her physician about the possibility of a VBAC for her second child. Which of the following reasons would rule out this possibility?
    1 Her first baby was a breech.
    2 A transverse lower-abdominal incision
    3 A current diagnosis of placenta previa
    4 A history of maternal heart disease

198. Which of the following interventions is required for a cesarean birth mother and not for a mother who had a vaginal delivery?
    1 Checking vaginal bleeding
    2 Checking the abdominal dressing
    3 Checking the episiotomy
    4 Checking voiding

199. Which of these conditions would be a contraindication for discontinuing an IV line in a cesarean patient?
    1 The patient is afebrile.
    2 The patient has faint bowel sounds.
    3 The patient is complaining of nausea.
    4 The patient is tolerating clear liquids.

200. The physician has determined that an amniotomy is required for a woman in labor. The primary reason for this is:
    1 Fetal decelerations late in contractions
    2 To assess the fetal status
    3 To stimulate uterine contractions
    4 To protect against the possibility of infection.

201. The first nursing measure after an amniotomy is:
    1 Change the pad under the patient.
    2 Observe the patient for signs and symptoms of infection.
    3 Assess the character, odor, and amount of amniotic fluid.
    4 Assess the FHR.

ANSWERS AND RATIONALES

1. Comprehension, assessment, health promotion and maintenance (b).
   4 Quickening is the first movements of the fetus felt by the mother; this normally occurs at approximately 16 weeks.
   1 If this occurs prematurely in a pregnancy, it is an emergency situation.
   2 This occurs at approximately 10 weeks but is not used as an indicator for EDD.
   3 This occurs during the last 2 weeks (earlier for multigravidas) and is not a reliable indicator.

2. Comprehension, assessment, health promotion and maintenance (b).
   2 Most tests are accurate at this time.
   1 It will be accurate; it is not generally necessary to wait that long.
   3 Urine is used for home pregnancy tests.
   4 A sterile specimen is not needed.

3. Comprehension, assessment, health promotion and maintenance (a).
   3 The patient has been pregnant twice and has one child.
   1 This means pregnant once, one child.
   2 This means pregnant twice, two children.
   4 This means twice pregnant, no children.

4. Knowledge, assessment, health promotion and maintenance (a).
   2 This is the first sign that will usually cause a woman to seek medical attention.
   1 This is a probable sign at approximately the sixth week.
   3 Debate is ongoing about whether this is presumptive or probable; it occurs late in first trimester.
   4 This is a probable sign.

5. Comprehension, assessment, health promotion and maintenance (a).
   2 This is the correct time.
   1 This is too early.
   3, 4 At this point, the heart rate should be audible with a fetoscope.

6. Knowledge, implementation, health promotion and maintenance (a).
   3 These are the correct instructions.
   1 This is acceptable for a routine urinalysis.
   2 Pregnancy tests do not require a sterile specimen.
   4 This is untrue.

7. Application, planning, health promotion and maintenance (b).
   3 Further information is required; how long a woman works depends on the degree and type of activities that her job requires.
   1 This is not necessarily true.
   2 This is true, but more information is required to give advice.
   4 This is not necessarily true.

8. Application, evaluation, psychosocial integrity (b).
   2 An 8 year old is capable of helping with the baby under supervision.
   1 The fact that it is said does not mean it will be reality.
   3 This is also normal; however, circumstances may or may not allow it in the immediate future.

4 Three year olds do not like to share toys or their mom and dad.

9. Knowledge, assessment, health promotion and maintenance (a).
   2 German measles have a devastating effect on fetal growth: physical abnormalities, mental retardation, hearing impairment or deafness, blindness.
   1 Chickenpox may have a more severe action on the mother but will not cause fetal physiological defects or problems.
   3 This is a synonym for chickenpox.
   4 This is regular measles; it does not affect the unborn.

10. Knowledge, planning, health promotion and maintenance (b).
    1 This is the correct path.
    2 Blood leaves the heart through the pulmonary arteries bypassing the lungs.
    3 The chambers are developed before birth.
    4 Blood goes to the aorta.

11. Knowledge, planning, health promotion and maintenance (a).
    3 This is the correct answer.
    1 The ovum carries two X chromosomes.
    2 This is not true.
    4 This is true, but it does not answer the question.

12. Knowledge, planning, health promotion and maintenance (b).
    2 Increased thyroid hormones cause an increase in Basal metabolic rate (BMR).
    1 This is true but is not specific enough.
    3 This is true; however, it does not respond to the question.
    4 Increased caloric energy is needed, but this is not the cause for the increased BMR.

13. Application, evaluation, psychosocial integrity (b).
    2 This shows more reality in her planning.
    1 This is fine, but the baby is still her responsibility.
    3, 4 These are fine, but the acceptance of responsibility is not shown.

14. Application, planning, health promotion and maintenance (a).
    1 Smoking causes vasoconstriction and decreased oxygenation.
    2 Women who smoke actually tend to have smaller babies.
    3, 4 No documented connection exists.

15. Knowledge, planning, health promotion and maintenance (a).
    2 An inherited neurodegenerative disease of lipid metabolism.
    1 This is an anemia that is more common in African Americans.
    3 This is an anemia common in people from the Mediterranean area.
    4 This is more common in Caucasians, a disorder of fat metabolism.

16. Application, planning, psychosocial integrity (b).
    1 In the first trimester, the mother generally thinks more about herself and how the pregnancy will affect her life.
    2 This is fine, but it does not answer her concerns.
    3 This is judgmental and does not offer therapeutic communication.
    4 This is what is hoped for; however, it is not guaranteed.

17. Comprehension, assessment, health promotion and maintenance (b).
    1 Albumin is a protein; protein in the urine is a possible sign of pulmonary induced hypertension.
    2 Frequency or burning would be a sign of cystitis.
    3 Glucose is the urine would be a sign of diabetes.
    4 This is not an indication of heart disease.

18. Application, implementation, physiological integrity (b).
    3 This is the correct use of Kegel exercises.
    1 They are not dangerous to the heart.
    2 This is not a correct statement.
    4 Range-of-motion exercises will help with leg cramps.

19. Application, planning, physiological integrity (b).
    3 This is a factual statement.
    1 This is incorrect information.
    2 Pregnant women should not douche unless ordered by a physician.
    4 This is not a factual statement.

20. Application, planning, physiological integrity (b).
    1 The growing uterus leaves less space for the stomach; therefore food will sometimes remain there longer.
    2 This does not cause heartburn; it is sometimes recommended to decrease symptoms.
    3 This does not cause heartburn.
    4 These symptoms are not common in this trimester, and if present, may be indicative of hyperemesis gravidarum.

21. Application, implementation, physiological integrity (b).
    3 This is correct information and advice; decreased use of carbonated beverage will also assist in decreasing phosphorus.
    1 This does not alleviate leg cramps.
    2 This is for relief from the discomfort of varicose veins.
    3 This is not incorrect, but it is not the best answer.

22. Comprehension, implementation, physiological integrity (c).
    4 Within 72 hours, danger of seizure passes.
    1, 2 Danger of seizure lasts longer; normal recovery may be 1 to 2 hours or more.
    3 Danger of seizure lasts longer than 24 hours.

23. Knowledge, planning, physiological integrity (c).
    3 Third-trimester bleeding conditions are indicated particularly because physician orders include no vaginal or rectal examinations.
    1 The bleeding, pain, or contractions would not be as acute.
    2 The pregnancy in itself would not necessitate these nursing measures unless the mother had symptoms.
    3 This is fetal death without expulsion of products of conception; symptoms include slight bleeding, brownish discharge, no cramping; treatment is D&C.

24. Comprehension, planning, health promotion and maintenance (b).
    4 Estriol levels are usually tested for placental functioning in the third trimester; a level of 12 mg is good, but below 12 mg in 24 hours may place the fetus in jeopardy.
    1 Fetal age is determined by uterine height, a calculation of EDC.
    2 Amniocentesis procedure may reveal surfactant L/S ratio and help determine lung maturity.
    3 Human gonadotropin hormonal levels in the urine are tested early on in pregnancy, but the term uterine nomenclature is not related to the question.

25. Application, planning, psychosocial integrity (b).
    4 This is the correct answer.
    1 These are all true, but it is not a good answer to a pregnant mother.
    2 This is also true but is not the best answer.
    3 This is too vague; it is not the best answer.

26. Comprehension, planning, health promotion and maintenance (a).
    3 This is the correct answer.
    1 This is ballottement or locating of fetal parts; it is not a part of an NST.
    2 Sex of an infant may be seen on a screen during a sonogram, but not by a fetal monitoring device, which only measures FHT—strength of contractions and fetal movements through the FHT response.
    4 This is wrong; the mother is given orange juice for an NST; for the stress test, she is given oxytocin IV.

27. Comprehension, planning, health promotion and maintenance (a).
    2 This is the correct answer; elevated levels of AFP indicate up to 5% to 10% of a neural defect but must be followed by two consecutive AFP tests, ultrasound readings, and an amniocentesis.
    1 Fetal maturity is tested by an L/S ratio that determines lung maturity by measuring the ratio of the two components of surfactant (lecithin and sphingomyelin); an amniocentesis done after the thirty-fifth week of pregnancy should show an increase in the amount of lecithin and a decrease in sphingomyelin.
    3 Genetic work-up, including family history and a series of blood tests, can evaluate risk of disease in offspring.
    4 RDS is most likely to occur in low–birth-weight babies, premature babies, and babies known to be at risk for immature lung development following delivery.

28. Comprehension, planning, physiological integrity (a).
    1 This is the correct answer; the sooner the mother is seen and evaluated, the better.
    2 If the opportunity to see the high-risk mother was not before this time (20 to 24 weeks' gestation), by all means, see her. It is never too late.
    3 Although scheduled evaluation should occur even before this time, it is never too late to schedule continuing evaluations.
    4 Evaluation scheduling should have been started as early as possible and continue at appropriate times throughout pregnancy.

29. Comprehension, assessment, health promotion and maintenance (b).
    3 This is the correct answer; early, frequent, and continual testing of urine and BP would signal early signs that can be addressed rapidly and appropriately.
    1 This is usually a third-trimester complication and would not be considered a preventable condition.
    2 This is not exactly preventable but can be helped by easing discomfort, teaching, and advising on care.
    4 Abortions—spontaneous ones might have some early signs and symptoms that alert pending conditions, but this is not the best answer.

30. Knowledge, assessment, physiological integrity (b).
    2 This is the significant symptom of an impending convulsion.
    1 This is a sign of change in BP, preeclampsia.

3   Eye changes would not be noticed by the mother.
4   This is not necessarily a sign of impending convulsions; rather of fluid retention.

31. Application, planning, psychosocial integrity (c).
    3   The nurse is explaining procedure and giving reassurance.
    1   This response is rude, curt, and did not answer the question.
    2   The physician was in the room, but he asked the nurse.
    4   This answer creates unnecessary anxiety, with no explanation.

32. Application, assessment, physiological integrity (b).
    3   Megadoses of vitamins can be teratogenic.
    1   This is OK as long as the diet is balanced.
    2   This is OK as long as healthy choices can be made.
    4   Alternatives can be offered for milk.

33. Application, planning, health promotion and maintenance (a).
    3   This answers the question most accurately.
    1   Certain medications are passed to the fetus; however, this is not a function.
    2, 4   These are not true.

34. Knowledge, assessment, health promotion and maintenance (a).
    3   Fetal movement is normally felt at approximately 16 weeks.
    1   The cervix thickens and softens; this is normally felt by 6 weeks.
    2   This is normal during the first trimester.
    4   This is normal.

35. Application, planning, health promotion and maintenance (a).
    3   This is correct, and the cord generally does fall off in 10 to 14 days.
    1   Babies should always be held carefully, with the head supported.
    2   This is partially correct, but the cord does not fall off in 3 to 5 days.
    4   This is not a requirement for a tub bath.

36. Comprehension, assessment, health promotion and maintenance (b).
    3   The physician or nurse midwife will want to know the status of the fetus. This is an emergency situation, and the health care provider must be notified to prepare for a possible premature delivery.
    1   Test is not indicated at this point; it may have been done before this.
    2   This would be done second.
    4   This is not indicated and can be dangerous at this time.

37. Application, assessment, health promotion and maintenance (b).
    3   This is one sign of true labor.
    1   This is a normal range for FHR.
    2   Contractions relieved by walking are Braxton-Hicks contractions.
    4   This is normal in the beginning of the third trimester, caused by a growing baby putting pressure on the diaphragm.

38. Comprehension, planning, health promotion and maintenance (b).
    4   A combination of types of insulin with different durations allows for a steadier therapeutic level of insulin in the body.

1   Oral hypoglycemics are contraindicated during pregnancy because their effect on the fetus is uncertain.
2   Regular insulin is short acting and therefore would not act on a long-term basis.
3   The question has no mention of infection.

39. Application, implementation, physiological integrity (b).
    1   A pregnant woman with active disease needs effective treatment to protect her and her unborn fetus.
    2   Preventive therapy can be postponed until after pregnancy; the risk of doing nothing in active disease is too great.
    3   Treatment for active disease includes a minimum of two to three drugs.
    4   Risk to the mother and fetus is too great to wait until the third trimester.

40. Application, implementation, physiological integrity (b).
    4   Folic acid has been shown to be a benefit in preventing neurological conditions.
    1   This is given to newborns to prevent hemorrhaging.
    2   A B-complex vitamin involved in carbohydrate metabolism.
    3   This is useful in preventing certain forms of anemia in newborns.

41. Comprehension, implementation, physiological integrity (b).
    2   Treatment before birth of the infant is preferred; it decreases the chance of the infant's exposure to the organism.
    1   This has already been done.
    3   This is an option for high-risk women; however, treatment should not wait if a diagnosis has been made.
    4   This is also important; treatment takes priority.

42. Application, implementation, physiological integrity (b).
    2   Monitoring IV and urinary output is the priority.
    1   Patients need quiet; pain is not usually present.
    3   A baseline is important, but this is not a priority.
    4   Small meals may be provided after the intestinal tract has had the opportunity to rest.

43. Knowledge, planning, health promotion and maintenance (a).
    2   Postterm infants' skin is very dry and cracked in appearance.
    1   These are genetic anomalies not caused by an overdue date.
    3   These are characteristics of preterm infants.
    4   These are normal.

44. Comprehension, assessment, health promotion and maintenance (b).
    1   This is a priority and should be reported to the physician.
    2   This is normal.
    3   This is normal and called meconium.
    4   For newborns to sleep many hours is not unusual.

45. Application, assessment, safe, effective care environment (b).
    3   This may be the way that they were brought up in their culture. The father may be very proud of the infant and shows it privately.
    1   This is fine, but further information is needed first.
    2   This is not appropriate.
    4   This is very premature until a great deal of further information is gathered.

46. Application, implementation, health promotion and maintenance (b).
    1 This is factual information.
    2 This is the opposite.
    3 This is not true.
    4 She did not say she was worried, and this does not completely answer the question.
47. Application, implementation, health promotion and maintenance (b).
    3 This provides accurate information without inducing undue anxiety.
    1 This is true but does not answer the question.
    2 This is not necessary.
    4 This is also true; however, it does not answer the question.
48. Application, implementation, health promotion and maintenance (b).
    2 This is a generally recommended procedure in most cases, depending on the type of method used.
    1 Recording only the first voiding is generally necessary after the procedure.
    3 This is true; however, it does not answer the question.
    4 This is false and may actually increase the child's discomfort.
49. Application, evaluation, health promotion and maintenance (a).
    3 This is factual without causing undue alarm.
    1 This is true, but it may be insulting.
    2 This is true; however, it does not answer the question.
    4 This causes undue alarm.
50. Application, implementation, physiological integrity (b).
    1 Cold stress is dangerous for infants; this is the appropriate action.
    2 This can be done after the infant has spent time in the warmer.
    3 This should also be done after the first two interventions are completed.
    4 This is incorrect.
51. Application, evaluation, physiological integrity (b).
    1 These are signs of respiratory distress.
    2 This is a possible complication of RDS.
    3, 4 These are normal characteristics of an infant.
52. Knowledge, evaluation, physiological integrity (b).
    1 These are indicative of diaphragmatic hernia.
    2 This is indicative of a cleft lip or palate.
    3 This is an indication of spina bifida.
    4 This is not a sign; it may occur if patient chokes while feeding.
53. Comprehension, evaluation, health promotion and maintenance (b).
    3 This is a neurological symptom.
    1 These are normal, particularly with darker-skinned infants.
    2 This is called Klumpke's syndrome, indicative of neurological injury.
    4 This is normal.
54. Application, evaluation, health promotion and maintenance (b).
    1 This is correct, reassuring information.
    2 This is not necessary and alarming.
    3 This is incorrect information.
    4 This is a demeaning statement.

55. Application, evaluation, physiological integrity (c).
    2 This is a sign of fluid buildup.
    1 This is normal and resolves without treatment in approximately 5 days, caused by increased intracranial pressure during the birth process.
    3 This is normal; cephalhematoma disappears without treatment in 3 to 4 days.
    4 This is a sign of a cleft palate.
56. Comprehension, evaluation, psychosocial integrity (c).
    1 This is the correct answer. Because all newborns have an immature liver, putting a drug into the system jeopardizes the infant.
    2 Prolonged use of a drug by the mother just before conception does not necessarily cause newborn addiction unless the mother continues the habit from conception throughout pregnancy to term.
    3 This answer in itself is not correct; usage must be continued during pregnancy.
    4 Drugs may affect uterine growth because the addictive mother seldom has good nutritional habits; however, if carried through term, the infant does not necessarily have RDS.
57. Comprehension, assessment, health promotion and maintenance (a).
    2 This is the correct answer; the Apgar score is 6.
    Heart rate = 1
    Respiratory effort = 1
    Muscle tone = 1
    Reflex response = 2
    Color = 1
    1, 3, 4 These are incorrect.
58. Application, planning, physiological integrity (a).
    2 This is the best response; preparation is started; so if the procedure is ordered, time is not lost.
    1 Responsibility is not assumed until order is given by physician.
    3 Unless a standing order is in place, this would not be appropriate.
    4 Alarming the family without proper teaching or preparation is inadvisable.
59. Comprehension, planning, health promotion and maintenance (b).
    2 Hospitals normally have protocols in place that include additional observations for signs of infection.
    1 The maternity nurse can perform this after the baby's temperature has stabilized.
    3 The baby and the mother are normally not separated and are transferred to the maternity department as quickly as possible.
    4 This can be completed by the maternity nurse later.
60. Application, implementation, health promotion and maintenance (b).
    4 This is the definition for engagement.
    1 This would be station 0.
    2 This means that the baby is high in the pelvis.
    3 This would mean that the presenting part is visible to the health care provider.
61. Knowledge, evaluation, health promotion and maintenance (a).
    3 Stage 2 is from full dilation of the cervix until birth of the fetus.
    1 Pushing before full dilation can be dangerous to the fetus and exhausting to the mother.

2 This is still too high.

4 This is stage 3.

62. Comprehension, implementation, physiological integrity (c).

2 The heart may be under stress if the rate is above 100 bpm.

1 The use of epidural anesthesia is normal.

3 This should be done with all women; a full bladder may impede labor.

4 This should be done with all women.

63. Comprehension, evaluation, health promotion and maintenance (b).

1 This is the normal pattern.

2, 3, 4 Any deviations may be indicative of fetal anomalies.

64. Knowledge, evaluation, physiological integrity (a).

3 This is a problem with the passenger (fetus), which is one of many causes of dystocia.

1 This is normal as labor progresses.

2, 4 These are complications, not causes.

65. Application, evaluation, health promotion and maintenance (c).

3 A pattern of decelerations late in the contraction may indicate uteroplacental insufficiency.

1 Accelerations typically occur in response to fetal movement, uterine contractions, or maternal abdominal contractions.

2 This deceleration is generally benign and is a result of the fetal head pressing on the perineum.

4 If these are repetitive and worsen as labor progresses, they may be indicative of cord compression.

66. Comprehension, evaluation, health promotion and maintenance (a).

2 This is a normal finding at the fourth stage of labor.

1 It should not be soft; the patient may need Pitocin in her IV infusion.

3 It should be midline; deviation may mean a full bladder.

4 Soft may be an indication of uterine atony and is a cause for hemorrhage.

67. Knowledge, implementation, physiological integrity (b).

3 This is correct, simply relieving pressure by changing positions.

1 The symptoms are pallor, light-headedness, dizziness, and slight nausea; rubbing the legs does not correct the syndrome.

2 This is incorrect; it is caused by the heavy uterus exerting pressure on the aorta and hampering good circulation; determine the cause and effect first, then plan the intervention.

4 Know the cause and effect; because the patient is dizzy, the nurse would not recommend walking.

68. Comprehension, planning, health promotion and maintenance (a).

1 This is the correct answer.

2 These are nursing responsibilities for the second stage of labor.

3 These are major nursing interventions for the third stage of labor.

4 These are nursing care measures for the fourth stage of labor, or 1 hour after delivery, usually in the recovery room.

69. Knowledge, planning, physiological integrity (b).

1 This is the correct answer.

2 This does not explain the physiological dynamics.

3 Pitocin is an oxytocic that acts on the uterus.

4 This does not explain the physiological dynamics of immediate postpartum phenomenon.

70. Comprehension, assessment, physiological integrity (a).

3 Symptoms are indicative of abruptio placentae.

1 This would give rise to painless bleeding.

2 Onset is gradual, accompanied by nausea, possibly vomiting, and gradual shock; abdomen is tender but not boardlike.

4 This would not cause a rigid, boardlike abdomen.

71. Knowledge, assessment, health promotion and maintenance (a).

3 False labor is generally relieved by activity.

1 True labor will have a regular interval between contractions, and progress is shown in effacement and dilation of cervix.

2 True labor does progress differently; however, this is not true labor.

4 No way is known to determine when true labor will occur after an episode of false labor.

72. Comprehension, implementation, health promotion and maintenance (b).

2 First priority is to establish patent airway so that the baby can breathe, cry, and fill her lungs with oxygen.

1 This is not first priority.

3 Umbilical cord can be left attached; no danger exists in delaying the cutting of the cord while tasks with a higher priority are performed.

4 The delivery of the placenta may take from 5 to 20 minutes because it must separate from the walls of the uterus; therefore this is not the top priority.

73. Comprehension, evaluation, physiological integrity (b).

2 DTRs are absent; respiratory effort may quickly be impaired.

1 BP is not affected by the drug; as a result of CNS depression, BP will decrease.

3 It is being given to decrease the DTRs.

4 Proteinuria (1 to 2) is a classic sign of preeclampsia; proteinuria (3) is extremely high, which may indicate use of medication in a closely monitored setting.

74. Comprehension, planning, health promotion and maintenance (a).

4 According to Nagele's formula, this is correct.

1, 2, 3 These are wrong according to Nagele's formula.

75. Comprehension, planning, health promotion and maintenance (a).

1 These are reportable signs and symptoms that should be taught to the patient.

2 These are usual signs and symptoms and are normal.

3 These are nonemergency signs and symptoms, which can be addressed during regular visits.

4 These are later signs and symptoms and is a nonemergency.

76. Knowledge, assessment, physiological integrity (c).

2 This is the correct answer; signs and symptoms are bright-red clots first, then light, painless bleeding.

1 In abruptio placentae, pain is present, and bleeding may or may not occur; if bleeding is present, it is dark red and usually not clotted.

3 Bleeding would be bright red in variable amounts with pain.

4 The patient would experience painless vaginal bleeding with bloody amniotic fluid.

77. Comprehension, assessment, physiological integrity (b).

2 This is the correct statement and correct answer.

1 The nurse would consider doing follow-up tests to determine precise findings, and the physician would consider what medical treatment is needed.

3 This is a false assumption.

4 Making this kind of determination is not a part of the nursing process.

78. Comprehension, implementation, physiological integrity (a).

3 Prevent convulsions; be able to respond immediately.

1 A mother who is severely eclamptic should not be in a semi-private room and certainly not in a sunny room with visitors.

2 The room must be quiet, with absolutely no visitors.

4 Bright sunshine will aggravate the CNS, and being far from the nurses' station will hamper emergency nursing care.

79. Application, implementation, physiological integrity (b).

1 Exercise is generally safe during pregnancy if the woman has exercised previously; otherwise, beginning slowly may be necessary.

2, 3 These are true; however, they do not completely answer the question.

4 A physician should be consulted before starting exercise. A patient should not wait until pain is experienced.

80. Application, implementation, physiological integrity (a).

1 This will reduce perineal swelling and edema.

2 This is the normal location of the fundus a few hours after delivery.

3 A natural reaction is to be happy over an apparently successful birthing experience.

4 One pad saturated with red lochia several hours after delivery is normal and not a sign of hemorrhage.

81. Application, implementation, physiological integrity (b).

4 Return of lochia rubra after its initial cessation may be indicative of uterine subinvolution or hemorrhage.

1 At 10 days postpartum, the fundus has returned to its position as a pelvic organ and is no longer palpable.

2 Mothers commonly experience constipation; simple interventions can be suggested.

3 Postpartum blues occur most commonly during the third to tenth day postpartum.

82. Comprehension, implementation, health promotion and maintenance (b).

4 RhoGAM prevents the development of antibodies when given either prenatally or within 72 hours of delivery.

1, 2 These are compatible.

3 A negative blood type would not have caused the development of antibodies.

83. Comprehension, planning, physiological integrity (b).

2 In many cultures, drinking hot liquids after childbirth is important to restore the balance of nature.

1 A clear liquid diet is fairly self-explanatory; a dietician can basically offer the same items as the nurse can.

3 The patient is able to decide what she will drink or not drink according to her likes and desires.

4 This is not true and is judgmental.

84. Comprehension, implementation, safe, effective care environment (b).

3 Bonding and breast-feeding can continue with minimal exposure to other patients and staff.

1 Standard precautions and gown and gloves for direct care are appropriate.

2 If the baby is breast-feeding well, there is no reason to discontinue; there is also no reason to expose other babies in the nursery to potential infection.

4 Diagnosis is important, but precautions can start before that.

85. Comprehension, evaluation, physiological integrity (b).

2 In addition, she has to be able to support herself.

1 It takes time for sensation to return after the catheter is removed.

3 Further assessments need to be made other than these.

4 It is helpful for the patient to eat something, but it is not the only criteria.

86. Knowledge, planning, physiological integrity (b).

3 This procedure attempts to form a small clot to stop the leaking fluid.

1 This is done before childbirth and involves invading the epidural space.

2 This is done for chronic pain.

4 Infection is not a cause.

87. Application, evaluation, health promotion and maintenance (a).

3 This would indicate a healthy involution.

1 This would be normal for the 2 to 3 days after birth.

2 If the uterus is deviated to the right, the bladder needs to be emptied.

4 This is healthy immediately after birth.

88. Application, evaluation, physiological integrity (b).

3 This evaluation is the most accurate way of ensuring that the baby is receiving adequate nourishment and is not becoming dehydrated.

1 Many babies will fall asleep part way through a feeding and need to be stimulated to feed a little longer.

2 Time is no longer considered relevant for nourishment or to prevent complications.

4 This is a measurement but not on a short-term basis.

89. Comprehension, assessment, health promotion and maintenance (a).

2 This may be indicative of urinary infection.

1, 3, 4 These are normal at this time.

90. Application, evaluation, physiological integrity (c).

1 These are classic signs of postpartum hemorrhage.

2, 3, 4 These are not typical signs; further evaluation is needed to determine the cause.

91. Application, evaluation, physiological integrity (b).

2 This needs to be evaluated; complaints of severe perineal pain are abnormal.

1 This is a risk factor, not an assessment.

3 Hematomas may or may not be visible.

4 This is more indicative of infection.

92. Application, implementation, psychosocial integrity (b).

3 This answer allows for communication that will encourage the couple to deal with their pain as a family unit and allows for more effective coping with grief.

1 The patient is an adult who cannot have her rights for appropriate standards of care taken away from her.

2 Nurses should implement therapeutic methods of communication as an appropriate standard of care.

4 Patients exist as part of a family unit; family members' needs should be considered.

93. Application, implementation, health promotion and maintenance (a).

4 This provides 3 months of protection without daily attention.

1 This would be ideal, but it is not realistic.

2 This requires at least weekly attention.

3 Condoms rely on the partner's attention.

94. Application, implementation, health promotion and maintenance (b).

1 This is accurate information without producing undo anxiety.

2 This is true; however, it produces anxiety in the patient.

3 This is also true but does not answer the question.

4 This is also true, but this intervention was for assessment purposes.

95. Comprehension, implementation, health promotion and maintenance (b).

3 Medications may cause harm to the fetus when they cross the placental barrier.

1 Certain medications are given to delay the labor process (e.g., Brethine); however, this is not routine.

2 Certain medications are given to trigger labor (e.g., Pitocin); however, this is not routine.

4 This is true; however, it does not answer the question.

96. Knowledge, implementation, physiological integrity (a).

3 This will allow for greater expansion of the diaphragm and easier breathing.

1 This is important to do but will not ease the shortness of breath.

2 This will improve circulation but will not decrease shortness of breath.

4 Unless the meals are unusually large, this will not improve shortness of breath.

97. Knowledge, assessment, physiological integrity (a).

2 This sign marks the approximate midpoint of gestation.

1 The heartbeat can be heard with a Doppler transducer by the tenth week.

3 This is too early.

4 This is too late.

98. Knowledge, assessment, physiological integrity (b).

1 Placenta previa is characterized by painless bleeding in the third trimester. Abruptio placenta has characteristics of uterine or back pain.

2 Both are characterized by vaginal bleeding.

3 The position of the fetus is not a factor in these conditions.

4 Both have potential for fetal compromise.

99. Knowledge, assessment, physiological integrity (a).

4 Fallopian tube abnormalities cause ectopic pregnancies.

1, 2, 3 These are all potential causes of ectopic pregnancy.

100. Knowledge, assessment, physiological integrity (a).

3 This is the first part of the first stage. It is from 0 to 4 cm dilated and takes approximately 4 to 6 hours in a primigravida.

1 This is 4 to 7 cm and is the second part of the first stage.

2 This is the last part of the first stage and last from 7 to 10 cm.

4 This is 1 to 4 hours postpartum.

101. Knowledge, assessment, physiological integrity (a).

2 This stage is from full dilation until the birth of the baby.

1 This is from the start of dilation until 10 cm.

3 This is after the birth of the baby until the birth of the placenta.

4 This is the first 1 to 4 hours postpartum.

102. Knowledge, assessment, physiological integrity (b).

2 PIH occurs before the twentieth week.

1 No movement of the baby would be felt at all.

3 A period may be missed, but spotting is common as well.

4 The uterus is large for its gestational age.

103. Application, implementation, health promotion and maintenance (b).

1 The infant's immune system does take time to produce antibodies fully.

2 The portals of infection are the same for an infant as they are for an adult.

3 This is true; however, it does not answer the question.

4 This is also true; however, these antibodies do not fully protect breast-fed infants from infection.

104. Application, implementation, health promotion and maintenance (b).

2 This will relieve pressure on the vena cava by the uterus.

1 Having the patient sit will not relieve uterine pressure on the venacava.

3 This will improve circulation.

4 See #2.

105. Application, implementation, health promotion and maintenance (b).

3 This position or Trendelenburg's position would push the presenting part away from the cord by gravity.

1 This will not use gravity to help the presenting part.

2 Compressing or manipulating the cord can cause further distress to the fetus.

4 This should, of course, be done on a continual basis.

106. Comprehension, planning, physiological integrity (b).

3 Magnesium sulfate is given to lower BP and as an anticonvulsant.

1, 2 These have not been shown to be effective in PIH.

4 Calcium gluconate is the antidote for magnesium therapy and should be available if magnesium levels become toxic.

107. Knowledge, assessment, health promotion and maintenance (a).

4 This is the normal rate for a newborn.

1 Although the rate may occasionally be above 60 if the newborn is excited, above 60 on a regular basis is not normal.

2 See # 1.

3 This is normal for an adult.

108. Comprehension, planning, physiological integrity (b).

1 Phototherapy is used to reduce serum bilirubin levels.

2 Although an exchange transfusion is sometimes needed, routine IV therapy is not. The infant should always be monitored for signs of dehydration.

3 Although infants should always be kept warm, a radiant warmer is not necessary unless the temperature is below 97° F.

4 Antibiotics would be indicated in the treatment of infection.

109. Comprehension, assessment, health promotion and maintenance (b).

1 A high bilirubin within the first 24 hours of life is indicative of pathological jaundice, which is not normal and needs to be reported.

2 This may be a sign of drug withdrawal.

3 Elevated bilirubin is not an indication of infection in an infant.

4 A weak cry may be an indication of respiratory distress.

110. Comprehension, implementation, health promotion and maintenance (a).

3 A cross-eyed appearance is common in newborns. Muscle control will correct the problem without any special intervention.

1 The pediatrician will always assess eyesight; however, it is not necessary for him or her to evaluate this appearance in particular.

2 No evidence exists that this is caused by genetics.

4 Infants respond to contrasting colors. Correcting this problem is not necessary.

111. Knowledge, implementation, physiological integrity (a).

3 This is not needed and extremely painful.

1 This is necessary with any operative site.

2 This is for protection and comfort.

4 This is necessary with any operative site.

112. Comprehension, assessment, physiological integrity (b).

3 This answers concerns and gives information.

1 This does not answer the question.

2 This is inaccurate information.

4 Pediatrician will assess and note on the record.

113. Application, planning, physiological integrity (b).

4 Knowing what happened is important because feelings might differ if the pregnancies were voluntarily terminated or spontaneously terminated.

1 The para of this patient indicates that additional support may be required.

2 All women require careful assessments to determine their feelings about the pregnancy.

3 An assessment of anxiety must be made before an intervention can be effective.

114. Comprehension, application, health promotion and maintenance (a).

1 This is the correct amount of stool for a breast-fed infant.

2 For an infant to lose 5% to 10% of birth weight by the third to fourth day and regain it by the tenth day is normal.

3 This is true, but it does not answer the question.

4 Solid stools are characteristic of bottle-fed infants.

115. Comprehension, implementation, physiological integrity (a).

4 These are called milia and will disappear spontaneously.

1 No antibiotic cream is needed.

2 Extra washing is not needed.

3 This is anxiety producing and does not answer the question.

116. Comprehension, application, health promotion and maintenance (b).

2 This gives reassurance without dismissing anxieties.

1 This is true, but it does not address concerns.

3 This also may be true; feelings normally improve in the second trimester; it does not address concerns.

4 This also may be true, but the partner has concerns of his own. They will hopefully work out their feelings together.

117. Application, implementation, health promotion and maintenance (a).

3 This can be an indication of infection.

1 This is not necessarily needed unless advised by physician.

2 This is helpful and would promote comfort. It would not cure any infection.

4 Douching is not usually recommended in pregnancy.

118. Knowledge, assessment, health promotion and maintenance (a).

4 For extremities to be slightly cyanotic at birth is not unusual.

1, 2, 3 These are acceptable findings and would receive scores of 2.

119. Comprehension, assessment, physiological integrity (a).

2 Decelerations are rate decreases during contractions.

1 Accelerations are rate increases during contractions.

3 This is the rate between contractions.

4 This describes fluctuations in the heart rate from baseline.

120. Comprehension, application, physiological integrity (b).

3 In true labor, bloody show is often present.

1 In false labor, discomfort is often felt in the abdomen and groin.

2 In true labor, walking increases contractions.

4 In false labor, contractions are irregular.

121. Application, implementation, health promotion and maintenance (c).

1 This pattern indicates the fetus is receiving adequate oxygenation.

2 This would be appropriate for late decelerations caused by supine hypotension.

3 This would be appropriate for late decelerations and supine hypotension.

4 This may be needed for late decelerations.

122. Comprehension, application, physiological integrity (b).

3 No evidence exists that this helps the membranes rupture.

1, 2, 4 These are benefits of walking.

123. Application, implementation, physiological integrity (b).

3 This is the proper position.

1, 2, 4 These are inappropriate positions for accurate assessment.

124. Comprehension, application, health promotion and maintenance (b).

3 Regular contractions 8 minutes apart indicate the end of the latent phase of labor; she needs to be assessed.

1 Five minutes apart is the beginning of the active phase of labor. Walking can be done in the hospital.

2 An ambulance is not required at this point.

4 The hospital is appropriate at this point.

125. Comprehension, planning, health promotion and maintenance (c).

4 This is true and is related to the stress and inflammation response. Further evaluation of any symptoms of infection is needed.

1 This is not required. Assessing for other symptoms is required.

2 This value is not within normal range.

3 This is true; however, it does not answer the question.

126. Application, implementation, physiological integrity (b).

1 Experiencing chills is very common and thought to be a result of hormonal and system changes.

2 This is not necessary.

3 An elevated temperature and chills after 24 hours may be indicative of infection.

4 Fluids are usually offered but will not help as well as a blanket will.

127. Application, assessment, physiological integrity (b).

3 Slight bruising is normal. Ice is used for 12 to 24 hours; after that, heat may be comforting.

1 This is normal.

2 That is a concern. However, have the mother void and reassess.

4 The episiotomy should be intact. A slight redness related to the inflammatory process is normal.

128. Comprehension, assessment, physiological integrity (b).

3 Bulging indicates that the woman may be fully dilated and ready to push.

1 The urge to bear down usually indicates that the first stage is ending and the birth of the baby is imminent.

2 These should be done through out the labor process.

4 This should be done, but the assessment is required first in # 3.

129. Application, implementation, physiological integrity (b).

3 The anesthesiologist injects a blood specimen that seals the leak of the spinal fluid.

1 This is appropriate for supine hypotensive syndrome.

2 This would be beneficial during labor.

4 The woman may be advised to remain flat for several hours; however, no evidence exists that this helps prevent headaches.

130. Comprehension, assessment, physiological integrity (b).

2 Caput succedaneum is a swelling of the soft tissues of the head.

1 This would indicate dehydration.

3 This would be indicative of cephalohematoma.

4 Bulging fontanels indicate increased intracranial pressure, which can be caused by a variety of conditions.

131. Comprehension, assessment, physiological integrity (b).

1 Cephalohematomas are frequently caused by forceps.

2 Precipitous deliveries are quick. Cephalohematomas are more likely caused by prolonged labors.

3 Cesarean babies are not exposed to pressure in the birth canal.

4 The baby's head does not experience pressure in a breech delivery.

132. Knowledge, assessment, health promotion and maintenance (b).

3 This will disappear spontaneously in this time frame.

1 This is the time frame for caput succedaneum.

2 This is not required.

4 Of course it should be monitored, but this does not answer the question.

133. Comprehension, assessment, health promotion and maintenance (a).

3 Infection is a possibility once the membranes have ruptured.

1 Dystocia can increase the chances of infection.

2 The possibility of hemorrhage does not increase with PROM.

4 The possibility of hypertension does not increase with PROM.

134. Knowledge, assessment, health promotion and maintenance (a).

3 This is the correct definition.

1 The term for this is polyhydramnios and may indicate congenital anomalies.

2 Unless the baby is breech, this may indicate that the fetus is under distress.

4 This may occur before complete rupture of the membranes.

135. Knowledge, assessment, physiological integrity (b).

4 This is an indication of urinary or renal anomalies.

1, 2, 3 These assessments would be made postnatally.

136. Knowledge, assessment, physiological integrity (b).

3 This is an abnormal condition around the larynx that causes noisy respiration, including a crowing on inspiration.

1 This is an abnormal opening between the nose and throat. These symptoms are not typical.

2 This is a bilateral or unilateral opening into the upper lip.

4 This is herniation of the abdominal viscera into the thoracic cavity. Review symptoms of 1, 2, and 4 in the text.

137. Application, implementation, health promotion and maintenance (b).

2 Babies should be fed in this position to avoid aspiration.

1 Babies do not necessarily need to be on a special schedule.

3 This would be appropriate for an allergic baby.

4 All babies should be kept warm and dry.

138. Knowledge, assessment, physiological integrity (a).

2 This is the correct definition; heredity may be a factor.

1, 3, 4 These are not the correct definitions.

139. Knowledge, assessment, physiological integrity (a).

3 Oversized means fetal weight above the ninetieth percentile for gestational age as a birth weight greater than 4000 g.

1 Underweight is low birth weight caused by being born premature or because of intrauterine growth retardation.

2 This is called microcephaly, which is a congenital anomaly characterized by abnormal smallness of the head in relation to the rest of the body and underdevelopment of the brain.

4 This is called macrocephaly, which is a congenital anomaly characterized by abnormal largeness of the head and brain in relation to the rest of the body.

140. Knowledge, assessment, health promotion and maintenance (b).

3 This is a severe form of PIH.

1 This is not an anemic condition.

2 This is not a mild form of PIH.

4 This is not specifically associated with *Hyperemesis gravidarum*.

141. Knowledge, planning, physiological integrity (b).

2 This is the hormone that shows positive in the urine and blood of a pregnant woman.

1 Stimulates uterine growth and helps prepare breasts for lactation.

3 This helps prepare the glands of the breasts for lactation.

4 This is responsible for the development of male secondary characteristics.

142. Knowledge, planning, health promotion and maintenance (a).

3 **PROM leaves the birth canal and the newborn more vulnerable to infection.**

1 A quick delivery does not predispose to infection.

2 This does not increase the chances of infection.

4 Exhaustion is common but does not increase risk of infection.

143. Comprehension, assessment, physiological integrity (b).

2 **The cervix dilates and effaces only in true labor.**

1 In true labor, contractions tend to be progressive and in a pattern. However, this is not the major difference.

3 In true labor, contractions are lower in the abdomen.

4 Engagement does not occur until true labor.

144. Knowledge, assessment, physiological integrity (b).

1 **For example, the leading edge of the fetal head is at the level of the ischial spines of the mother.**

2 This is the definition of station.

3 This is the definition of presentation.

4 This is an incorrect definition.

145. Knowledge, assessment, health promotion and maintenance (a).

4 **This is the correct classification.**

1 Newborns within a certain weight range are *appropriate for gestational age*. This is incorrect.

2 No such classification exists.

3 Newborns under 2500 g are termed SGA.

146. Comprehension, assessment, health promotion and maintenance (b).

2 **Glucose provides an environment conducive to infection.**

1 This is not true.

3 Their babies do tend to be larger, but this is not the primary reason for infection.

4 This is true, but it does not answer the question.

147. Knowledge, assessment, physiological integrity (a).

3 **Lightening is movement of the fetus into the pelvis (engagement).**

1 Ballottement is a probable sign of pregnancy. Rebounding of the fetus in the amniotic fluid is felt by the examiner.

2 Molding is the shape that the head becomes as it passes through the birth canal.

4 This is the movement of the fetus felt in utero.

148. Application, implementation, physiological integrity (b).

3 **This is the safest comment and is reassuring to the couple.**

1 This does not answer their concern.

2 This is very late in labor.

4 This is late in labor and may predispose her to infection.

149. Knowledge, assessment, physiological integrity (a).

2 **This is the correct definition.**

1 This would be the interval or the frequency.

3 This is the definition for the intensity of the contractions.

4 This is an important part of the history.

150. Application, implementation, physiological integrity (b).

4 **This may be a cultural belief and should be respected.**

1 This may or may not be true, but it is judgmental.

2 This may be appropriate, but their rights need to be respected.

3 This may or may not be true, but the nurse does not know that this is the reason.

151. Application, implementation, physiological integrity (b).

3 **This is the correct reason. A full bladder may impede the surgery.**

1 No need exists to monitor the output of a healthy patient. In an emergency situation, a catheter would be inserted.

2 Catheterizations are a major source of infection.

4 Ambulation is vital after surgery.

152. Comprehension, implementation, health promotion and maintenance (b).

2 **This is the most specific instruction for a woman who is pregnant.**

1 This is true; however, if her previous pattern included potentially dangerous sports, this would be contraindicated.

3 This instruction would apply to anyone who is starting an exercise program.

4 Slow walking is not the only choice if her previous pattern involved running or swimming.

153. Comprehension, implementation. health promotion and maintenance (b).

4 **This is important in the prevention of thrombophlebitis.**

1 This is valuable advice anytime, not just when driving.

2 This is true; however, it does not help during driving.

3 Stretching legs will help with cramps anytime.

154. Analysis, implementation, health promotion and maintenance (a).

1 **The mother needs time to rest after birth.**

2 Anxiety producing and not appropriate at this time.

3 This is premature at this point.

4 This is generally not effective at this time. The mother needs time to rest.

155. Comprehension, implementation. physiological integrity (a).

1 **This is usually the treatment of choice for small hematomas. Surgical excision may be needed for larger hematomas.**

2 Baths help with episiotomy discomfort and hemorrhoids.

3 Sprays assist with episiotomy discomforts.

4 Lamps may be used for generalized perineal discomfort.

156. Knowledge, application, physiological integrity (a).

2 **The sex of the child depends on whether the X chromosome from the woman joins with an X or a Y chromosome from the man.**

1 May be first known at birth, but it is determined at conception.

3 This is learned during an amniocentesis.

4 Blood work does not determine sex.

157. Knowledge, assessment, health promotion and maintenance (b).

3 **This is the correct definition for nuchal cord. This can lead to lack of oxygen for the fetus.**

1 This is the correct definition for prolapsed cord.

2, 4 These are not correct definitions.

158. Knowledge, planning, physiological integrity (a).

2 **This is produced by the posterior pituitary gland and also stimulates milk ejection during breast-feeding.**

1 This prepares the breasts for lactation.

3 This is responsible for enlargement of the uterus, breasts, and genitals, among many other functions.

4 This promotes development of the breasts for lactation, among other functions.

159. Application, implementation, health promotion and maintenance (b).
4 This is true, and many commonly used herbs have been shown to be harmful in pregnancy.
1 This is not true, particularly in pregnancy.
2 This is always a wise precaution, but further information is needed in this case.
3 Herbs do not have doses and can be toxic with minimal or normal amounts.

160. Knowledge, assessment, physiological integrity (a).
4 First stage, active phase— 4-7 cm
1 Second stage— 10 cm to birth of the baby
2 First stage, latent phase— 0-4 cm dilation
3 First stage, transition phase 7-10 cm

161. Comprehension, assessment, physiological integrity (b).
2 In transition, contractions last 60 to 90 seconds and come every 2 to 3 minutes.
1 Active: every 5 minutes, lasting 30 to 45 seconds
3 Latent: every 10 to 15 minutes, lasting 15 to 20 seconds
4 These would be Braxton-Hicks contractions.

162. Application, planning, health promotion and maintenance (b).
2 This requires a great deal of time standing on your feet.
1, 3, 4 These allow for more rest periods and flexibility of hours.

163. Application, implementation, physiological integrity (a).
3 This will allow for greater expansion of the diaphragm and deeper breaths.
1 This will help with dizziness or hypotension, or both.
2 This will help prevent dizziness caused by hypoglycemia.
4 This will help ease edema and improve blood circulation.

164. Comprehension, implementation, physiological integrity (b).
3 Emptying the breasts completely prevents milk stasis. Milk stasis provides and environment for bacterial growth.
1 Starting on the unaffected side may ease discomfort, but any milk remaining in the affected breast should be expressed.
2 The amount of time does not matter with an infection. The baby must use correct technique when latching on.
4 Many women may decide to quit breast-feeding because they are discouraged. They do not necessarily have to quit because of an infection.

165. Knowledge, implementation, physiological integrity (a).
1 Fluids (with the exception of caffeine and carbonated beverages) increase the amount of fluids in stools, leading to easier passage.
2 This may be needed, but dietary changes should be made first.
3 Assessment of exercise pattern is needed first.
4 No laxative should be given without a physician's permission.

166. Application, implementation, health promotion and maintenance (b).
1 Caffe latte contains caffeine.
2 Unless weight control is a concern, this snack would be appropriate.
3 This is an appropriate snack.
4 This does not give any nutrients; however, it is not a danger. Fruit may be a better choice.

167. Comprehension, implementation, physiological integrity (b).
1 This answers the question without causing anxiety.
2 This does not answer the question.
3 This intervention is not necessary.
4 The physician will of course be examining the baby, but this response implies that something is wrong.

168. Comprehension, implementation, physiological integrity (b).
3 This is correct so as to minimize chances of infection.
1 Safety is always most important; however, the baby should be given a sponge bath until the cord falls off in 7 to 10 days.
2 This is incorrect and does not answer the question.
4 The circumcision heals in a few days; the cord falls off later.

169. Comprehension, planning, physiological integrity (b).
2 As long as no potential for danger exists, cultural ceremonies should be allowed.
1 A private room might be preferable, but this is not the primary information.
3 This is not a primary concern.
4 This might be educational, but it is not a primary concern.

170. Comprehension, assessment, physiological integrity (b).
3 This transitional phase is the last phase of the first stage of labor. The woman needs to use all of her energy to cope with labor.
1 This is characteristic of the latent phase of labor (0 to 4 cm).
2 This is from 4 to 7 cm and is characteristic of anxiety and discomfort.
4 In the third stage after the birth of the baby, the woman is usually relaxed and receptive to care.

171. Comprehension, evaluation, psychological integrity (b).
1 Each child needs to know that they are special and equally loved.
2 This may or may not be true, depending on the child's age, but being taken for granted may cause problems.
3 Depending on developmental level, this may or may not be possible.
4 A 5 year old still needs special attention.

172. Knowledge, assessment, psychological integrity (b).
3 This is the developmental task in the second trimester.
1 This is most common in the first trimester.
2 This would be characteristic of the third trimester.
4 This is most common in the first trimester.

173. Knowledge, assessment, health promotion and maintenance (b).
1 Decreased oxygen from the placenta is the most common cause of late decelerations.
2 Late decelerations are always of concern.
3 Early decelerations, which return to baseline, would indicate this.
4 No relationship exists between length of labor and decelerations.

174. Application, implementation, psychological integrity (b).
2 The person may benefit from learning breathing techniques and nonpharmacological methods of pain relief to increase her feelings of control.

1 This is true.

3 This is important for her to know. The nurse should review these with her.

4 This would require further assessment not necessarily teaching.

175. Application, implementation, psychological integrity (b).

3 This may indicate ineffective coping.

1 Feeding is preferable after bathing, but this is easily corrected with teaching.

2 This is a true statement.

4 This is fine; a father should be involved with his baby's care.

176. Knowledge, assessment, health promotion and maintenance (b).

3 Amniocentesis involves taking a small sample of genetic fluid for genetic testing.

1 This is done to detect any major anomalies and the fetus's sex can be detected.

2 This is rarely done. It can be used to detect chromosomal abnormalities, but it is much more dangerous for the fetus.

4 This is checking for neural tube defects.

177. Application, implementation, physiological integrity (b).

3 Safety comes first. Even young babies can roll off a platform.

1 This is a good way for a partner to help.

2 This is also true; babies do not tell time.

4 This is the preferred method because the bath provides stimulation and exercise, and the feeding promotes sleep.

178. Analysis, implementation, psychosocial integrity (b).

3 Communication and spending time with your partner allows for emotional support and reassurance.

1 This is true, but the parents' feelings need to be recognized as well.

2 Nutritious food is always important as a part of overall good health.

4 Depression is a serious medical condition that needs physician intervention. Depression lasts much longer than baby blues, which tend to have more of a transient nature.

179. Knowledge, planning, health promotion and maintenance (a).

4 This is given to prevent hemorrhage until the bacteria in the newborn's intestine mature in approximately 3 days.

1, 2, 3 These medications are not given to the newborn.

180. Comprehension, implementation, health promotion and maintenance (b).

3 This is the priority action because the danger of a prolapsed cord is greatest at this point.

1, 2 These can be done at the regular intervals required by hospital protocol.

4 This is also done on an ongoing basis.

181. Knowledge, assessment, physiological integrity (a).

1 This is the correct definition.

2 Station is the relationship of the presenting part to the mother's ischial spines.

3 Engagement is the presenting of the fetal part to a zero station, which is at the level of the mother's ischial spines.

4 Effacement is the thinning of the cervix during labor.

182. Knowledge, implementation, health promotion and maintenance (b).

2 Adequate fluids are important to prevent urinary stasis.

1 This is unnecessary.

3 Keeping the bladder as empty as possible prevents urinary stasis and allows the bladder to rest.

4 Cranberry juice is healthy, but water is the most vital.

183. Knowledge, assessment, physiological integrity (b).

4 Nitrazine paper is used to assess the fluid for a pattern called "ferning," which is a positive indication for amniotic fluid.

1 This is not required.

2 The physician should be notified when membranes have ruptured.

3 Stress tests are done before labor to assess the status of the fetus.

184. Knowledge, assessment, health promotion and maintenance (b).

3 This may be an indication of infection.

1 Refusal of two or more feedings is an indication to call.

2 The normal rate for a newborn is 120 to 160 bpm.

4 The infant should have a minimum of six voidings per day.

185. Knowledge, implementation, health promotion and maintenance (b).

3 This is correct information and the least anxiety producing.

1 This is anxiety producing. Many babies are a little congested after birth.

2 Of course, the mother needs to be shown how to use it.

4 This is degrading and does not answer the question.

186. Comprehension, implementation, health promotion and maintenance (b).

3 Less than two stools a day indicates possible constipation, and fluid intake needs to be increased.

1 Iron can cause constipation.

2 Infants do not need a strict schedule, and this has nothing to do with constipation.

4 A bottle-fed infant should have three to four stools each day.

187. Comprehension, planning, health promotion and maintenance (c).

3 Cold stress can decrease stores of glycogen in the liver.

1 Weak abdominal muscles make newborns prone to reverse peristalsis.

2 Babies need to be burped frequently to eliminate swallowed air.

4 Newborns are susceptible to infection for a variety of reasons.

188. Comprehension, implementation, health promotion and maintenance (b).

3 Evaporation comes from contact with wet linens or clothes and insensible water loss.

1 Cold hands would be conduction. This is when the infant comes in contact with cold surfaces.

2 This is an example of convection.

4 Radiation is contact with cold surfaces.

189. Knowledge, planning, health promotion and maintenance (a).

   1 The infant receives passive (3 to 5 months) immunity for any condition for which the mother has developed antibodies.
   2 The infant receives a vitamin-K injection to take the infant over until bacterial synthesis begins.
   3 Some iron may be stored in the baby's liver, but this is present at birth.
   4 No relationship exists between breast- or bottle-feeding and constipation.

190. Knowledge, implementation, health promotion and maintenance (a).

   4 Rooting is elicited by touching the cheek or lips causing the mouth to turn the head toward the stimulus.
   1 This is caused by stimulation of the uvula, causing reverse peristalsis.
   2 This is caused by sudden jarring or movement (startle).
   3 This is constriction of the pupil if stimulated by bright light.

191. Knowledge, assessment, health promotion and maintenance (b).

   2 The Babinski reflex is elicited when the sole of the foot is stroked and the toes are hyperextended and fanned out. It disappears at approximately 1 year.
   1 Absence is abnormal in a newborn.
   3 This is not true.
   4 This would be characteristic of the palmar reflex.

192. Knowledge, assessment, psychosocial integrity (a).

   2 If the feelings are interfering with her life, medical intervention is needed to help relieve the depression.
   1 This would be characteristic of postpartum psychosis.
   3 This is characteristic of baby blues.
   4 This is also characteristic of baby blues.

193. Comprehension, implementation, health promotion and maintenance (b).

   1 Adolescents are highly influenced by their peers.
   2 Women of all ages have busy lifestyles. Correct choices can be made in fast food restaurants.
   3, 4 These can be true of woman of any age.

194. Knowledge, assessment, health promotion and maintenance (a).

   1 This is the type of shock caused by a tremendous loss of blood.
   2 This shock is a severe allergic reaction.
   3 This shock is related to infection.
   4 This is a term not specifically related to shock.

195. Comprehension, implementation, health promotion and maintenance (b).

   2 This is appropriate at this time. A history of possible exposure may be needed.
   1 No evidence of exposure exists; this choice is very premature.
   3 This may be needed at a later time if evidence of exposure exists.
   4 The vaccine is contraindicated during pregnancy.

196. Analysis, planning, health promotion and maintenance (b).

   1 Some vegetarians will eat eggs, cheese, fish, or any combination. These are adequate sources of complete protein.
   2 This is not relevant.
   3 Babies need complete sources of protein. Education may be needed at a later point to ensure that the baby has adequate nutrition.
   4 If she is a strict vegan, alternative sources of complete protein are available.

197. Comprehension, planning, physiological integrity (b).

   3 Placenta previa is a placenta implanted in the lower third of the uterus, and a vaginal birth is contraindicated.
   1 The position of the second child needs to be determined.
   2 A transverse incision poses a decreased risk for uterine rupture.
   4 This is an indication for a CS because of the potential stress of labor on the heart.

198. Knowledge, implementation, health promotion and maintenance (a).

   2 Vaginal birth mothers do not have an abdominal dressing.
   1 Cesarean mothers may have less vaginal discharge, but it still needs to be checked.
   3 Cesarean mothers do not have an episiotomy.
   4 Voiding needs to be checked with both mothers.

199. Knowledge, assessment, health promotion and maintenance (a).

   3 IV lines should be maintained until the patient is tolerating fluids well.
   1 Being without a fever is a positive sign.
   2 Bowel sounds mean peristalsis is returning.
   4 This is a positive sign. See # 3.

200. Knowledge, planning, health promotion and maintenance (b).

   3 An amniotomy is the artificial rupture of membranes. This procedure should initiate contractions.
   1 This is an indication of fetal distress and may indicate the need for a CS.
   2 The status of the fetus is determined by other means.
   4 Once the membranes are ruptured, the woman is more prone to infection.

201. Comprehension, assessment, health promotion and maintenance (b).

   4 Any potentially dangerous patterns need to be reported. In addition, this procedure increases the chances of a prolapsed cord.
   1 This, of course, is done for patient comfort and to decrease the chances of bacteria growing; it does not have to be first.
   2 This needs to be done on an ongoing basis.
   3 The fluid should be clear. Meconium may indicate fetal distress. This should be done second after fetal heart assessment.

CHAPTER 8 Pediatric Nursing

Pediatric nursing includes the care of both well and sick children and covers both preventive health care and restorative nursing care. This chapter is divided into the following age groups: infancy, toddlerhood, preschool, school age, and adolescence. The areas covered include normal growth and development, psychosocial development, health promotion, and health problems specific to each age group. Other topics discussed include the battered child syndrome, hospitalization and the child, and nursing care of the hospitalized child. The information provided in this chapter presents both the physical and psychosocial aspects of care necessary in providing pediatric nursing care.

ASSESSMENT OF CHILD AND FAMILY

A. Functions and structure of family
  1. The functions and structure of the family are vital to the normal growth and development of the child
  2. Three primary functions of the family
    a. Providing physical care, such as food, clothing, shelter, safety; illness prevention; and care during illness
    b. Educating and training: language, values, morals, and formal education
    c. Protecting psychological and emotional health
B. Physical assessment of child
  1. Performing a health history, including the child's history and current complaints or problems, is done by the nurse, physician, or nurse practitioner
  2. Assessment of child's physical growth and development level is done by the physician or nurse practitioner
C. Concepts of child development (Table 8-1)
  1. Freud's theory of development is based on the child's psychosexual development
  2. Erikson's theory of development is based on psychosocial development as a series of developmental tasks
  3. Piaget's theory of development is based on intellectual (cognitive) development: how the child learns and develops his or her intelligence
  4. Kohlberg's theory of moral development is based on the concept that the acceptance of values and rules of society shapes a child's behavior

INFANCY (AGES 4 WEEKS TO 1 YEAR)

Normal Growth and Development
Physical Development*

A. 1 month
  1. Physical
    a. Weight: gains approximately 150 to 210 g (5 to 7 oz) weekly during the first 6 months of life

    b. Height: gains approximately 2.5 cm (1 inch) a month for the first 6 months of life
  2. Motor
    a. May lift the head temporarily; but generally, the head must be supported
    b. Holds the head parallel with the body when placed prone
    c. Can turn the head from side to side when prone or supine
    d. Asymmetrical posture dominates, such as tonic neck reflex
    e. Primitive reflexes are still present and strong (grasp, Moro, tonic neck)
  3. Sensory
    a. Follows a light to midline
    b. Eye movements coordinated most of the time
    c. Visual acuity: 20/100 to 20/50
    d. Quiet when hears a voice
  4. Socialization and vocalization
    a. Smiles indiscriminately
    b. Makes small throaty sounds
    c. Watches parent's face when he or she talks to infant
B. 2 to 3 months
  1. Physical: posterior fontanel closed
  2. Motor
    a. Holds the head erect for a short time and can raise chest supported on the forearms
    b. Can carry hand or an object to the mouth at will
    c. Reaches for attractive objects but misjudges distances
    d. Grasp, tonic neck, and Moro reflexes are fading
    e. Can sit when the back is supported; knees will be flexed and back rounded
    f. Step or dance reflex disappears
    g. Plays with fingers and hands
  3. Sensory
    a. Follows a light to the periphery
    b. Has binocular coordination (vertical and horizontal vision)
    c. Locates sounds by turning head in direction of the sound
  4. Socialization and vocalization
    a. Smiles in response to a person or object
    b. Coos and gurgles; shows pleasure in making sounds
    c. Stops crying when parent enters the room
C. 4 to 5 months
  1. Physical: drooling begins because salivary glands are functioning, but the child does not have sufficient coordination to swallow saliva
  2. Motor
    a. Balances the head well in a sitting position
    b. Sits with little support; holds the back straight when pulled to a sitting position

---

*From Saxton DF, Nugent PM, Pelikan PK: *Mosby's Comprehensive Review of Nursing,* ed 12, St Louis, 2002, Mosby.

TABLE 8-1	Concepts of Child Development				
Age	Developmental Stage	Freud's Theory	Erikson's Theory	Piaget's Theory	Kohlberg's Theory (Morality)
4 wk–1 yr	Infancy	Oral stage	Trust vs. mistrust	Sensorimotor phase	Preconventional morality (stage 0)
1-3 yr	Toddlerhood	Anal stage	Autonomy vs. shame and doubt	Preoperational phase	Preconventional morality (stage 1)
3-5 yr	Preschool age	Oedipal stage Latency stage	Initiative vs. guilt	Preoperational phase continued	Preconventional morality (stage 1-2)
6-12 yr	School age	Latency stage continued Genital stage	Industry vs. inferiority	Concrete operational phase Formal operational phase	Conventional morality (stage 3-4)
13-18 yr	Adolescence	Genital stage continued	Identity vs. identify confusion	Formal operational phase continued	Morality of self-accepted moral principles

c. Symmetrical body position predominates

d. Can sustain a portion of own weight when held in a standing position

e. Reaches for and grasps an object with the whole hand

f. Can roll over from back to side

g. Lifts the head and shoulders at a 90-degree angle when prone

h. Primitive reflexes (e.g., grasp, tonic neck, Moro) have disappeared

3. Sensory

a. Recognizes familiar objects and people

b. Beginning eye-hand coordination

4. Socialization and vocalization

a. Laughs aloud

b. Definitely enjoys social interaction with people

c. Vocalizes displeasure when an object is taken away

D. 6 to 7 months

1. Physical

a. Weight: gains approximately 90 to 150 g (3 to 5 oz) weekly during second 6 months of life; weight doubles by 6 months

b. Height: gains approximately 1.25 cm (1/2 inch) a month

c. Teething may begin with eruption of two lower central incisors, followed by upper incisors (Figure 8-1)

2. Motor

a. Can turn over equally well from stomach or back

b. Sits fairly well unsupported, especially if placed in a forward-leaning position

c. Hitches or moves backward when in a sitting position

d. Can transfer a toy from one hand to the other

e. Can approach toy and grasp it with one hand

f. Plays with feet and puts them in mouth

g. When lying down, lifts head as if trying to sit up

h. Transfers everything from hand to mouth

3. Sensory

a. Has taste preferences; will spit out disliked foods

b. Responds to own name

4. Socialization and vocalization

a. Begins to differentiate between strange and familiar faces and shows "stranger anxiety"

b. Makes polysyllabic vowel sounds (baba, dada)

c. Plays peek-a-boo

d. Responds to word no

E. 8 to 9 months

1. Motor

a. Sits steadily alone

b. Has good hand-to-mouth coordination

c. Develops pincer grasp, with preference for use of one hand over the other

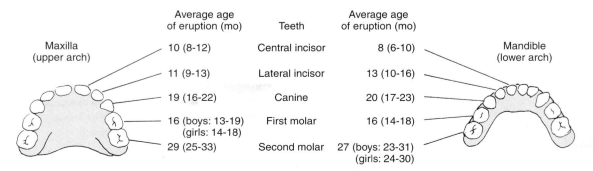

FIGURE 8-1. Sequence of eruption of primary teeth. Range represents ± 1 standard deviation or 67% of subjects studied. (Data from McDonald RE, Avery DR: Dentistry for the child and adolescent, ed 6, St Louis, 1994, Mosby.)

d. Crawls and then creeps (creeping is more advanced because the abdomen is supported off the floor)

e. Can raise self to a sitting position but may require help to pull self to feet

2. Sensory

a. Depth perception beginning to develop

b. Displays interest in small objects

3. Socialization and vocalization

a. Shows anxiety with strangers by turning or pushing away and crying

b. Definite social attachment is evident: stretches out arms to loved ones

c. Is voluntarily separating self from mother by desire to act on own

d. Reacts to adult anger: cries when scolded

e. Dislikes dressing, diaper change

f. No true words as yet, but comprehends words such as bye-bye, no-no

F. 10 to 12 months

1. Physical

a. Has tripled birth weight by 1 year

b. Upper and lower lateral incisors usually have erupted for total of 6 to 8 teeth

c. Head and chest circumferences are equal

d. Lumbar curve develops; lordosis is evident when walking

2. Motor

a. Stands alone for short times

b. Walks with help; moves around by holding onto furniture

c. Can sit down from a standing position without help

d. Can eat from a spoon and drink from a cup but needs help; prefers using fingers

e. Can play pat-a-cake

f. Can hold a crayon to make a mark on paper

g. Helps in dressing, such as putting arm through sleeve

3. Sensory

a. Visual acuity: 20/50

b. Amblyopia may develop with lack of binocularity

c. Discriminates simple geometric forms

4. Socialization and vocalization

a. Shows emotions such as jealousy, affection, anger

b. Enjoys familiar surroundings and will explore away from mother

c. Fearful in strange situation or with strangers; clings to mother

d. May develop habit of "security" blanket

e. Can say three to five words besides "dada" or "mama"

f. Understands simple verbal requests, such as, "Give it to me"

g. Knows own name

Psychosocial Development

A. Infants are in Erikson's stage of "trust vs. mistrust"; infants will develop a sense of trust or mistrust depending on how their needs are met by their parents (or other caregivers)

B. As infants grow, they slowly realize that they are separate from their environment and that they influence their environment with their actions

C. Infants' early activities are mostly reflexes: crying, sucking, kicking, and so on; as the months progress, they learn to move in certain ways, follow with their eyes, and smile in response to a smile and soft words

Health Promotion

A. Immunizations should be given on schedule (Figure 8-2)

B. Nutrition appropriate to the age and needs of the infant should be provided

1. Human milk is the most desirable complete diet for the first 6 months of life

2. Introduction of strained foods may begin at 6 months of age, starting with strained fruits

3. Solid foods should be introduced slowly, in small amounts, and one at a time, to determine the infant's likes and dislikes; this also helps detect possible allergies to certain foods; allow 4 to 7 days between introduction of each new food; honey should be avoided during the first 12 months because of the risk of botulism

4. Weaning from breast or bottle to a cup can begin between 5 and 6 months of age, although the infant cannot be weaned completely until between 12 and 24 months of age

C. Safety and accident prevention includes a safe home environment, safe toys, use of car seats, and close attention to the infant who is crawling or walking

Health Problems
Nutritional Disorders

Failure to Thrive (FTT)

A. Definition: a state of inadequate growth resulting from inability to obtain or use calories; leads to malnutrition

B. Symptoms: below normal weight and height (below fifth percentile for age), listlessness, poor feeding habits, unresponsive to holding and attention, voluntary regurgitation, prolonged periods of sleep

C. Diagnosis

1. Based on symptoms and a continued deviation from an established growth curve

2. Three general categories of FTT

a. Organic: result of a physical cause such as congenital defects of gastrointestinal (GI) system or heart

b. Nonorganic: unrelated to a disease; usually caused by psychosocial factors

c. Idiopathic: unexplained cause; may be grouped with nonorganic FTT

D. Treatment and nursing interventions (directed at correcting the malnutrition)

1. Correction of organic causes if possible

2. Development of a structured routine

3. Sensory stimulation

4. Adequate food for weight gain; this may include nasogastric (NG) feedings, as well as bottle feedings, during early treatment

5. Tender loving care; holding and cuddling, talking to the infant

6. Teaching and encouraging the mother and father regarding feeding, infant care, and parenting skills

7. Family counseling when needed

Colic

A. Definition: paroxysmal abdominal pain or cramping that is exhibited by crying and drawing the legs up to the abdomen; colic is most commonly seen in infants under the age of 3 months

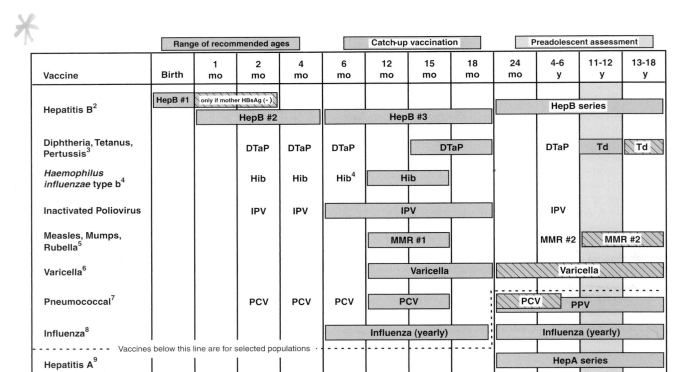

		Range of recommended ages				Catch-up vaccination				Preadolescent assessment		
Vaccine	Birth	1 mo	2 mo	4 mo	6 mo	12 mo	15 mo	18 mo	24 mo	4-6 y	11-12 y	13-18 y
Hepatitis B[2]	HepB #1 only if mother HBsAg (-)		HepB #2			HepB #3					HepB series	
Diphtheria, Tetanus, Pertussis[3]			DTaP	DTaP	DTaP		DTaP			DTaP	Td	Td
Haemophilus influenzae type b[4]			Hib	Hib	Hib[4]	Hib						
Inactivated Poliovirus			IPV	IPV		IPV				IPV		
Measles, Mumps, Rubella[5]						MMR #1				MMR #2	MMR #2	
Varicella[6]						Varicella					Varicella	
Pneumococcal[7]			PCV	PCV	PCV	PCV				PCV	PPV	
Influenza[8]						Influenza (yearly)				Influenza (yearly)		
Hepatitis A[9]						Vaccines below this line are for selected populations				HepA series		

1. Indicates the recommended ages for routine administration of currently licensed childhood vaccines, as of April 1, 2004, for children through age 18 years. Any dose not given at the recommended age should be given at any subsequent visit when indicated and feasible. ▨▨▨ Indicates age groups that warrant special effort to administer those vaccines not given previously. Additional vaccines may be licensed and recommended during the year. Licensed combination vaccines may be used whenever any components of the combination are indicated and the vaccine's other components are not contraindicated. Providers should consult the manufacturers' package inserts for detailed recommendations. Clinically significant adverse events that follow vaccination should be reported to the Vaccine Adverse Event Reporting System (VAERS). Guidance about how to obtain and complete a VAERS form is available at http://www.vaers.org/ or by telephone, 800-822-7967.

2. **Hepatitis B vaccine (HepB).** All infants should receive the first dose of HepB vaccine soon after birth and before hospital discharge; the first dose also may be given by age 2 months if the infant's mother is HBsAg-negative. Only monovalent HepB vaccine can be used for the birth dose. Monovalent or combination vaccine containing HepB may be used to complete the series; 4 doses of vaccine may be administered when a birth dose is given. The second dose should be given at least 4 weeks after the first dose except for combination vaccines, which cannot be administered before age 6 weeks. The third dose should be given at least 16 weeks after the first dose and at least 8 weeks after the second dose. The last dose in the vaccination series (third or fourth dose) should not be administered before age 24 weeks. Infants born to HBsAg-positive mothers should receive HepB vaccine and 0.5 mL hepatitis B immune globulin (HBIG) within 12 hours of birth at separate sites. The second dose is recommended at age 1–2 months. The last dose in the vaccination series should not be administered before age 24 weeks. These infants should be tested for HBsAg and anti-HBs at age 9–15 months. Infants born to mothers whose HBsAg status is unknown should receive the first dose of the HepB vaccine series within 12 hours of birth. Maternal blood should be drawn as soon as possible to determine the mother's HBsAg status; if the HBsAg test is positive, the infant should receive HBIG as soon as possible (no later than age 1 week). The second dose is recommended at age 1–2 months. The last dose in the vaccination series should not be administered before age 24 weeks.

3. **Diphtheria and tetanus toxoids and acellular pertussis vaccine (DTaP).** The fourth dose of DTaP may be administered at age 12 months provided that 6 months have elapsed since the third dose and the child is unlikely to return at age 15–18 months. The final dose in the series should be given at age ≥4 years. **Tetanus and diphtheria toxoids (Td)** is recommended at age 11–12 years if at least 5 years have elapsed since the last dose of tetanus and diphtheria toxoid-containing vaccine. Subsequent routine Td boosters are recommended every 10 years.

4. **Haemophilus influenzae type b (Hib) conjugate vaccine.** Three Hib conjugate vaccines are licensed for infant use. If PRP-OMP (PedvaxHIB® or ComVax® [Merck]) is administered at ages 2 and 4 months, a dose at age 6 months is not required. DTaP/Hib combination products should not be used for primary vaccination in infants at ages 2, 4, or 6 months but can be used as boosters after any Hib vaccine. The final dose in the series should be given at age ≥12 months.

5. **Measles, mumps, and rubella vaccine (MMR).** The second dose of MMR is recommended routinely at age 4–6 years but may be administered during any visit, provided at least 4 weeks have elapsed since the first dose and both doses are administered beginning at or after age 12 months. Those who have not received the second dose previously should complete the schedule by the visit at age 11–12 years.

6. **Varicella vaccine (VAR).** Varicella vaccine is recommended at any visit at or after age 12 months for susceptible children (i.e., those who lack a reliable history of chickenpox). Susceptible persons aged ≥13 years should receive 2 doses given at least 4 weeks apart.

7. **Pneumococcal vaccine.** The heptavalent **pneumococcal conjugate vaccine (PCV)** is recommended for all children aged 2–23 months and for certain children aged 24–59 months. The final dose in the series should be given at age ≥12 months. **Pneumococcal polysaccharide vaccine (PPV)** is recommended in addition to PCV for certain high-risk groups. See *MMWR* 2000;49(No. RR-9):1–35.

8. **Influenza vaccine.** Influenza vaccine is recommended annually for children aged ≥6 months with certain risk factors (including but not limited to asthma, cardiac disease, sickle cell disease, HIV, and diabetes), health care workers, and other persons (including household members) in close contact with persons in groups at high risk (see *MMWR* 2004;53;[RR][in press]) and can be administered to all others wishing to obtain immunity. In addition, healthy children aged 6–23 months and close contacts of healthy children aged 0–23 months are recommended to receive influenza vaccine, because children in this age group are at substantially increased risk for influenza-related hospitalizations. For healthy persons aged 5–49 years, the intranasally administered live, attenuated influenza vaccine (LAIV) is an acceptable alternative to the intramuscular trivalent inactivated influenza vaccine (TIV). See *MMWR* 2003;52(No. RR-13):1–8. Children receiving TIV should be administered a dosage appropriate for their age (0.25 mL if 6–35 months or 0.5 mL if ≥3 years). Children aged <8 years who are receiving influenza vaccine for the first time should receive 2 doses (separated by at least 4 weeks for TIV and at least 6 weeks for LAIV).

9. **Hepatitis A vaccine.** Hepatitis A vaccine is recommended for children and adolescents in selected states and regions and for certain high-risk groups. Consult your local public health authority and *MMWR* 1999;48(No.RR-12):1–37. Children and adolescents in these states, regions, and high-risk groups who have not been immunized against hepatitis A can begin the hepatitis A vaccination series during any visit. The 2 doses in the series should be administered at least 6 months apart.

Additional information about vaccines, including precautions and contraindications for vaccination and vaccine shortages is available at http://www.cdc.gov/nip or from the National Immunization Information Hotline, 800-232-2522 (English) or 800-232-0233 (Spanish). Approved by the **Advisory Committee on Immunization Practices** (http://www.cdc.gov/nip/acip), the **American Academy of Pediatrics** (http://www.aap.org), and the **American Academy of Family Physicians** (http://www.aafp.org).

FIGURE 8-2.   Recommended childhood and adolescent immunization schedule, United States, July-December 2004. Updated on a semi-annual basis. *From Centers for Disease Control and Prevention (2004). Recommended childhood and adolescent immunization schedule. United States, July-December 2004. MMWR 2004, 53(16).*

B. Symptoms: episodes of loud crying accompanied by abdominal cramping; despite obvious indications of pain, the infant usually tolerates feedings well and gains weight

C. Diagnosis: based on symptoms reported by parents or caregivers

D. Treatment and nursing interventions
1. Take a through history of the infant's daily activities, including the infant's diet, the diet of the breast-feeding mother, time of day when colic occurs, characteristics of crying, and activity before, during and after crying
2. If child is bottle-fed, investigate possibility of cow's milk allergy; substitution of another formula (such as casein hydrosylate [Nutramigen]) may be tried
3. Comfort measures that can be used by the parents and caregivers
   a. Place infant prone over a covered hot-water bottle or covered heating pad (ensure that hot water bottle is warm, not hot)
   b. Massage infant's abdomen
   c. Change infant's position frequently
   d. Provide smaller, frequent feedings; burp infant during and after feedings, and place infant in an upright seat after feeding
   e. Introduce pacifier for added sucking
4. Pharmacological agents such as sedatives, antispasmodics, antihistamines, and antiflatulents are sometimes recommended

Respiratory Disorders

Upper Respiratory Infection (URI)

A. Definition: viral or bacterial infection affecting the upper respiratory tract; nasopharyngitis or the "common cold" is particularly common in children of all ages

B. Symptoms: fever, sore throat, sneezing, nasal congestion, occasional cough, irritability, anorexia

C. Diagnosis: based on the symptoms

D. Treatment and nursing interventions
1. Bed rest until free of fever
2. Encouraging oral fluids
3. Antipyretics for fever (acetaminophen, ibuprofen; not aspirin)
4. Nose drops to relieve nasal congestion
5. Oral decongestants as ordered
6. Adequate nutrition for age; infants and young children can better tolerate high-calorie fluids and soft foods
7. Cool-air humidifier for moistened air (to assist in decreasing congestion)

Acute Otitis Media

A. Definition: infection and effusion in the middle ear; frequently caused by nasopharyngeal infections that travel through the infant's shortened, widened eustachian tubes; causative organisms include *Streptococcus pneumoniae* and *Haemophilus influenzae*

B. Symptoms: fever, irritability, restlessness, pulling or rubbing of the ears, loss of appetite, and purulent drainage if the tympanic membrane is perforated; otoscopic examination reveals a bright red, bulging tympanic membrane

C. Diagnosis: based on the symptoms and history of recent URI

D. Treatment and nursing interventions
1. Antipyretics for fever
2. Analgesics or antipyretics for discomfort (acetaminophen, ibuprofen)
3. Encourage oral fluids
4. Promote rest and quiet environment
5. Antibiotics may be ordered if symptoms do not subside or if infant is at high risk for infection because of immunosuppression; amoxicillin is usually the antibiotic of choice
6. Myringotomy and insertion of polyethylene tubes by the physician to allow for drainage of fluid
7. Observe for drainage; keep ears clean

Lower Respiratory Infections
Respiratory Syncytial Virus (RSV), Bronchiolitis

A. Definition
1. Bronchiolitis is an acute viral infection that occurs primarily in winter and spring and is most common in infants and children up to 2 years of age; it causes the bronchioles to become plugged with mucus, and the bronchiole mucosa to swell; the mucus traps the air in the lungs, making it difficult for the infant to expel the air
2. RSV is related to the parainfluenza virus; it is responsible for at least 50% of the diagnosed cases of bronchiolitis; the peak incidence for RSV infection is 2 to 5 months of age; it is transmitted predominantly through direct contact with respiratory secretions; RSV has been known to survive for hours on countertops, gloves, and cloth, and for 30 minutes on skin

B. Symptoms
1. Usually begins with a URI; symptoms include rhinorrhea, coughing, sneezing, pharyngitis, wheezing, and intermittent fever
2. With progression of the disease, increases in coughing and wheezing, air hunger, tachypnea, retractions, and cyanosis occur
3. Symptoms of severe illness include tachypnea of more than 70 breaths per minute, listlessness, poor air exchange, apneic spells, oxygen saturation less than 95%

C. Diagnosis
1. Based on clinical symptoms
2. RSV can be identified by various tests done on nasal or nasopharyngeal secretions to detect RSV antigen

D. Treatment and nursing interventions
1. Provide humidified oxygen inhalation (to relieve dyspnea and hypoxia)
2. Elevate head of crib
3. Monitor vital signs and oxygen saturation (via pulse oximeter)
4. Provide adequate fluid intake, including IV fluids as needed for hydration
5. Allow infant to rest as much as possible
6. Medical therapy for bronchiolitis has not proved to be effective; however, ribavirin, an antiviral agent, may be used specifically for RSV infection
   a. Ribavirin is administered by nebulization via an oxygen hood, tent, or mask for 12 to 20 hours per day, for 1 to 7 days
   b. Ribavirin is most commonly used in children with RSV infection who are at high risk for complications caused by other conditions, including chronic lung conditions, immunodeficiency, and certain neurologic diseases (such as severe cerebral palsy)

E. Prophylactic treatment
1. Synagis, a monoclonal antibody, has been used successfully in reducing hospitalizations caused by RSV
2. Monthly injections of Synagis are recommended for infants and children under 2 years of age with chronic lung disease; these injections are given throughout the RSV "season" (October through April)

Viral Pneumonia
A. Definition: inflammation of the lung, characterized by interstitial pneumonitis with inflammation of the mucosa and walls of bronchi and bronchioles
B. Symptoms: fever, cough, rapid respiratory rate, listlessness
C. Diagnosis: based on the symptoms and results of chest x-ray examination
D. Treatment and nursing interventions
1. Elevate the head of the crib
2. Croup tent for humidified oxygen inhalation
3. Chest physiotherapy and postural drainage
4. Antibiotics as ordered (for bacterial pneumonia)
5. Antipyretics for fever
6. Monitor vital signs frequently
7. Encourage clear fluids by mouth
8. Allow infant to rest to prevent dyspnea

Gastrointestinal Disorders

Infectious Gastroenteritis
A. Definition: diarrhea and vomiting that may be caused by viral or bacterial infections
B. Symptoms: frequent, loose stools, irritability, vomiting, abdominal distention; serious symptoms include dehydration, sunken fontanel, poor skin turgor, weak, rapid pulse
C. Diagnosis: based on the symptoms; specific bacterial cause can be isolated in a stool culture (most commonly *Escherichia coli* or rotavirus in the infant), and a stool for ova and parasites may also be done
D. Treatment and nursing interventions
1. Oral rehydration therapy (with commercially prepared solutions such as Pedialyte); amount is based on infant's weight and percentage of dehydration

2. Intravenous (IV) fluids with electrolytes as ordered, if oral rehydration therapy is not effective (or if dehydration is severe), take special care to maintain the infant's IV line
3. Return to normal diet (including formula, cow's milk, and age-appropriate solids) should be started as soon as they are tolerated; the "BRAT" diet (bananas, rice cereal, applesauce, tea/toast) is contraindicated for the infant with acute diarrhea because it has little nutritional value
4. Note amount, color, and consistency of stools and emesis
5. Keep accurate intake and output (I&O) record (if necessary, weigh diapers to measure urine output)
6. Maintain proper isolation technique (enteric precautions)
7. Provide good skin care to buttocks and perineum after each diaper change; cleanse well; leave area open to air when possible; apply ointments as ordered
8. Provide time for stimulation, holding, and cuddling
9. Antidiarrheal drug therapy is contraindicated in infants and young children because of possible adverse side effects and toxicity

Hypertrophic Pyloric Stenosis
A. Definition: hypertrophy of the pyloric muscle fibers and narrowing of the pylorus, which is at distal end of the stomach (Figure 8-3)
B. Symptoms: usually appear between 3 and 8 weeks of age; projectile vomiting of formula and mucus, irritability, weight loss, and dehydration; the physician can often palpate the olive-size pyloric mass in the abdomen
C. Diagnosis: based on the symptoms, physical examination, and, if necessary, upper GI radiographic or ultrasound studies
D. Treatment and nursing interventions
1. Preoperative
a. IV fluids with electrolytes as ordered
b. Nothing by mouth (NPO) unless ordered to feed
c. NG tube is often inserted to remove excess stomach contents immediately before surgery (pyloromyotomy)

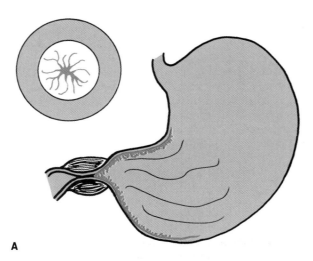
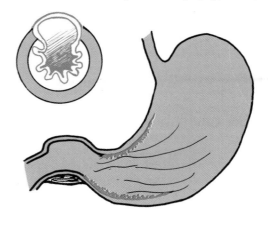

A   **B**

FIGURE 8-3. Hypertrophic pyloric stenosis. **A,** Enlarged muscular tumor nearly obliterates pyloric channel. **B,** Longitudinal surgical division of muscle down to submucosa establishes adequate passageway. *(From Hockenberry MJ et al: Wong's nursing care of infants and children, ed 7, St Louis, 2003, Mosby.)*

2. Postoperative
   a. Position the infant on right side or abdomen or in infant seat to prevent aspiration
   b. Maintain NPO status; first feeding begins within the first 24 hours after surgery (clear liquids with glucose and electrolytes); amounts are increased slowly, to administer small frequent feedings as ordered; formula is started 24 hours postoperatively if clear fluids are retained
   c. NG tube may remain in place for several hours
   d. General postoperative nursing care

Nervous System Disorders

Febrile Seizures

A. Definition: seizures caused by high fever (102° to 105° F; 38.8° to 40.5° C); most often seen between 6 months and 3 years of age
B. Symptoms: seizures characterized by stiffening of the body, with jerking movements of the extremities and face, ending with a lapse of consciousness
C. Diagnosis: based on evidence of seizure activity preceded by high fever
   1. Simple febrile seizures are brief and generalized
   2. Complex febrile seizures are prolonged and may have focal features
D. Treatment and nursing interventions
   1. Anticonvulsant (phenobarbital) and antianxiety (diazepam) medications to control the seizures; antipyretics (ibuprofen or acetaminophen) to control fever (see Chapter 3)
   2. Padded side rails
   3. Airway and suction equipment at bedside
   4. During seizure, do not restrain the infant; turn his or her head to the side to allow saliva to drain out of the mouth; do not try to insert a seizure stick or airway in the infant's mouth during a seizure; observe the seizure and protect the infant from harm
   5. Documentation: note the kinds of movements, behavior before the seizure (if known), duration of the seizure, skin color and vital signs during and after the seizure, and medications given during the seizure, including the infant or toddler's reaction to the medications
   6. Parent teaching should include care of the infant during a seizure

Meningitis

A. Definition: infection of the meninges and fluid; caused by several viruses and bacteria, including *H. influenzae* type B, *Neisseria meningitidis,* and *S. pneumoniae;* it may also occur secondary to other infections or as a complication of trauma and neurosurgery
B. Symptoms: elevated temperature, irritability, poor feeding, high-pitched cry, nuchal rigidity, seizures, bulging fontanel
C. Diagnosis: based on the symptoms and the presence of cloudy spinal fluid when lumbar puncture is performed (increased white blood cell [WBC] count; decreased glucose level and increased protein level in the spinal fluid; increased cerebrospinal fluid [CSF] pressure) (Figure 8-4)
D. Treatment and nursing interventions
   1. Acute bacterial meningitis is a medical emergency; early recognition and immediate treatment is required to avoid residual complications and to prevent death; therefore treatment is started before the causative agent is identified

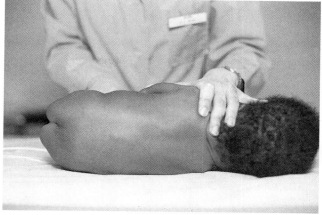

A

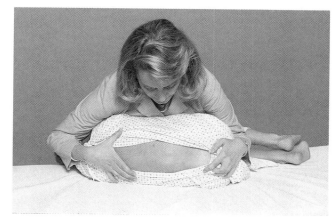

B

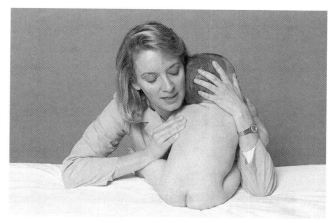

C

FIGURE 8-4. **A,** Modified side-lying position for lumbar puncture. **B,** Older child in side-lying position. **C,** Infant in sitting position allows for flexion of lumbar spine. *(From Hockenberry MJ et al:* Wong's nursing care of infants and children, ed 7, *St Louis, 2003, Mosby.)*

   2. Isolation from other children (for bacterial meningitis) for at least 24 hours after antibiotics started
   3. IV antibiotics as ordered for bacterial meningitis
   4. Monitoring vital signs, neurologic status, and level of consciousness frequently

5. IV fluids as ordered
6. Diet: infant may be NPO at first, until liquids can be tolerated
7. Antipyretics to reduce elevated temperature
8. Handle the infant as little as possible when the infant is irritable and uncomfortable; keep room quiet
9. Seizure precautions (padded side rails)
10. IV dexamethasone for management of increased intracranial pressure (recommended for treatment of *H. influenzae* type B meningitis)
11. Treatment for viral meningitis is symptomatic and supportive

Integumentary Disorders

Infantile Eczema
A. Definition: atopic dermatitis caused by an allergic reaction to some irritant; usually begins between 2 and 6 months of age and undergoes spontaneous remission around age 3
B. Symptoms: reddened, raised rash starting on cheeks and spreading to arms and legs; itching, oozing of vesicles
C. Diagnosis: based on the story and symptoms; the cause of the eczema (the allergen) must also be determined to control further episodes
D. Treatment and nursing interventions
   1. Good skin care; keep affected areas clean
   2. Provide tub baths with tepid water, baking soda, and cornstarch to relieve the itching
   3. Keep skin well hydrated; various lubricants or moisturizing lotions may be ordered
   4. Antihistamines and topical steroids as ordered to control itching
   5. "Mittens" to prevent scratching
   6. Elbow restraints to prevent scratching (only if necessary)
   7. Provide for sensory stimulation, holding, and cuddling at frequent intervals

Impetigo
A. Definition: infection of the skin caused by *Streptococcus* or *Staphylococcus* bacteria; occurs in nurseries when strict hand-washing technique is not followed (impetigo neonatorum); also occurs in preschool and school-age children, often occurring when recovering from an URI
B. Symptoms: reddened, vesicular lesions (pustules) with honey-colored crusts
C. Diagnosis: based on the symptoms; specific bacterial cause can be determined by culture of the draining lesions
D. Treatment and nursing interventions
   1. Isolation of infant (child) for 24 to 48 hours after treatment started
   2. Strict hand-washing technique by all persons coming in contact with the infant
   3. Warm saline compresses to lesions, followed by a gentle cleansing and topical antibiotic ointment
   4. Systemic antibiotics may be ordered for infants or children with widespread lesions

Congenital Defects and Hereditary Disorders

Gastrointestinal System
Cleft Lip and Palate
A. Definition: abnormal openings in the lip or palate; the defects may occur unilaterally or bilaterally
B. Symptoms: a cleft lip has a notched vermilion border, which may involve the alveolar ridge and dental abnormalities; a cleft palate includes a midline or bilateral cleft with variable extension from the uvula, soft and hard palates, exposed nasal cavities, and nasal distortion
C. Diagnosis: based on observation and examination at birth; may also be diagnosed by in utero ultrasound
D. Treatment and nursing interventions: based on the severity of the defect
   1. Modified techniques for feeding are used to promote adequate nutrition and growth
   2. Surgery to repair the cleft lip is done as early as possible, usually at age 3 to 6 months
   3. Surgery to repair the cleft palate depends on the deformity and size of the child, usually done by 1 year of age
   4. Treatment of recurrent otitis media as needed
   5. Promotion of parent-child bonding, emotional support for parents throughout the process
   6. Other disciplines involved in the care of these children may include ear, nose and throat specialist; speech and occupational therapists; psychologist; audiologist; orthodontic surgeon and dentist

Gastroesophageal Reflux (GER)
A. Definition: regurgitation of gastric contents into the esophagus; it can be physiologic (infrequent emesis), functional (frequent emesis after meals), or pathological (FTT, aspiration pneumonia, coughing, choking, dyspnea, frequent emesis)
B. Symptoms: emesis after meals, hiccups, and recurrent otitis media from secretions pooled in the nasopharynx are common to all types of GER; other manifestations include FTT, respiratory infections, weight loss, and irritability
C. Diagnosis: after other illnesses have been ruled out, GER may be confirmed by barium swallow, upper GI study, ultrasound, or endoscopy
D. Treatment and nursing interventions: based on symptoms
   1. Small frequent feedings of predigested infant formula (Nutramigen, Pregestimil)
   2. Position infant in prone position with head slightly elevated, or in right side-lying position (these positions are considered appropriate for infants with GER)
   3. For infants with pathological reflux, antacids, H2-receptor antagonists, mucosal protectants, and other medications may be used (see Chapter 3)
   4. Surgery (fundoplication) to prevent future reflux may be done in up to 15% of infants with GER

Hirschspring's Disease
A. Definition: distention of a portion of the lower colon caused by a congenital lack of nerve cells in the wall of the colon just below the distended section (Figure 8-5)
B. Symptoms: constipation (including a lack of meconium stool in the newborn in the first 24 hours), abdominal distention, bile-stained mucus and emesis, inadequate weight gain
C. Diagnosis: based on the symptoms, results of barium enema, rectal biopsy, anorectal manometry, or any combination
D. Treatment and nursing interventions: based on the type of surgery done (bowel resection, sometimes with temporary colostomy); surgery is done in two or three stages
   1. Preoperative
      a. Observation of stools: color, amount, and consistency
      b. IV fluids and electrolytes as ordered; if infant is malnourished, total parenteral nutrition (TPN) may be given before surgery

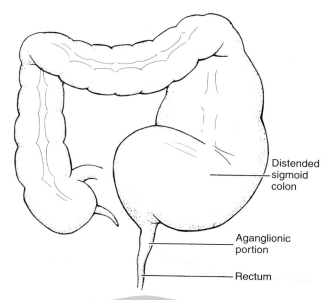

FIGURE 8-5.   **Hirschsprung's disease.** *(From Hockenberry MJ et al:* Wong's nursing care of infants and children, ed 7, *St Louis, 2003, Mosby.)*

2. Postoperative
   a. NG tube to low-suction or gravity drainage
   b. General postoperative care
   c. Routine colostomy care as necessary (PRN)
   d. Monitor vital signs as ordered; axillary temperatures should be taken
   e. IV fluids as ordered
   f. Maintain NPO status; resume diet as ordered
   g. Record I&O every shift (Foley catheter may be necessary)
   h. Observe stools and record amount and characteristics
   i. Observe for rectal bleeding and abdominal distention
   j. Provide parent teaching for providing care at home (colostomy care, dressing changes, skin care)

Omphalocele
A. Definition: the abdominal organs protrude through an abnormal opening in the abdominal wall and form a sac lying on the abdomen
B. Diagnosis: based on symptoms and physical examination

C. Treatment and nursing interventions
   1. Preoperative
      a. Keep the omphalocele covered with sterile gauze, moistened with normal saline and a plastic drape until surgery can be performed; minimize movement of the infant and the intestines
      b. Maintain sterile technique as much as possible in caring for the omphalocele
      c. Maintain proper body temperature; a warmer or an isolette may be used
   2. Postoperative
      a. Surgery: the organs are returned to the abdominal cavity, and the abdominal wall is closed
      b. General postoperative care, including mechanical ventilation for several days; care of NG tube; pain management
      c. Parenteral nutrition for several days
      d. Observe stools and record amount and characteristics

Imperforate Anus
A. Definition: the rectal pouch ends blindly at a distance above the anus; in some cases, no anal opening is present; various forms of this defect have been found
B. Symptoms: no stools in the first 24 hours after birth; rectal thermometer cannot be inserted properly
C. Diagnosis: made by digital rectal examination, intestinal x-ray examination, and endoscopy
D. Treatment and nursing interventions
   1. Surgical procedure to reconnect the ends of the rectum and form an anal opening
   2. General postoperative nursing care

Esophageal Atresia, Tracheoesophageal Fistula
A. Definition: the upper end of the esophagus ends in a blind pouch; the lower end may also end in a blind pouch or may be connected to the trachea by fistula defect (tracheoesophageal fistula) (Figure 8-6)
B. Symptoms: excessive salivation and drooling, coughing and choking during feedings, regurgitation of all feedings
C. Diagnosis: based on symptoms and passage of an NG tube or catheter down the esophagus to test for patency; exact anomaly is determined by x-ray studies
D. Treatment and nursing interventions
   1. Maintaining NPO status, with administration of IV fluids as ordered

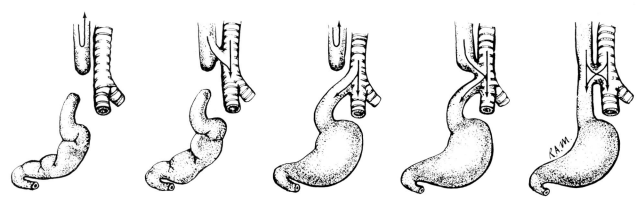

FIGURE 8-6.   **The five most common types of esophageal atresia and tracheoesophageal fistula.** *(From Hockenberry MJ et al:* Wong's nursing care of infants and children, ed 7, *St Louis, 2003, Mosby.)*

2. Suctioning of nose and mouth as needed
3. Insertion of an NG tube to drain mucus and fluid from the blind pouch
4. Antibiotic therapy as ordered (for probable aspiration pneumonia)
5. Surgical repair to correct the defects and reconnect the ends of the esophagus
6. Emotional support for the family; parent or caregiver teaching for home care

Intussusception   RED CURRENT Jelly STOOLS

A. Definition; telescoping of one portion of the bowel into a distal portion; the most common site is at the ileocecal valve; usually occurs between 3 and 12 months of age
B. Symptoms: appear suddenly; pallor, sharp colicky pain causes infant to draw up legs and cry out (this occurs every 5 to 10 minutes), vomiting, stools with blood and mucus ("red currant jelly" stools), signs of shock
C. Diagnosis: based on symptoms; definitive diagnosis can be made radiographically with barium enema
D. Treatment and nursing interventions: this is an emergency that requires immediate treatment; the initial treatment of choice is hydrostatic reduction by enema with water-soluble contrast or barium, and air pressure; if this is not effective, surgery is necessary
  1. Preoperative
    a. Careful observation and recording of vital signs frequently
    b. IV fluids with electrolytes as ordered
    c. Maintaining NPO status
    d. NG tube to remove gastric contents
    e. Emotional support for parents; explain all procedures; answer questions
    f. Observe for passage of abnormal brown stool (indicates the intussusception has reduced itself); report to physician immediately
  2. Postoperative

a. General postoperative care
b. IV fluids as ordered; maintain NPO status
c. Record I&O
d. Auscultate for return of bowel sounds
e. Observe all stools and record
f. Resume feedings slowly as ordered

Nervous System

Hydrocephalus

A. Definition: disorder caused by an obstruction of cerebrospinal fluid (CSF) drainage or by impaired absorption of CSF in the subarachnoid space; characterized by an excess of CSF within the cranial cavity, which causes an enlarged head and potential brain damage or retardation; it occurs in association with several other anomalies (developmental defects; complication of meningitis, tumor, or hemorrhage) (Figure 8-7)
B. Symptoms: bulging of the anterior fontanel, enlargement of the head, irritability, lethargy, opisthotonos, "setting-sun" sign (sclera can be seen above the iris because of increased intracranial pressure), lower extremity spasticity
C. Diagnosis: based on the symptoms, frequent measurements of head circumference, computed tomography (CT), and magnetic resonance imaging (MRI)
D. Treatment and nursing interventions
  1. Surgical repair is necessary to relieve the obstruction or to shunt the CSF from the ventricles of the brain into the abdomen (ventriculoperitoneal shunt)
  2. Postoperative care includes frequent position changes to prevent pressure on the head, care of the shunt, general postoperative care, and observation for complications (infection, shunt malfunction, return of increased intracranial pressure)
  3. Measure head circumference daily

Down Syndrome (DS)

A. Definition: an abnormality caused by extra chromosome 21 (trisomy 21); children with DS are born to women of all

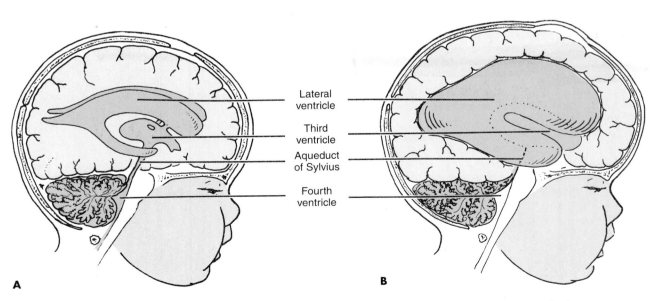

A   **B**

Lateral ventricle

Third ventricle

Aqueduct of Sylvius

Fourth ventricle

FIGURE 8-7.   Hydrocephalus: a block in flow of cerebrospinal fluid. A, Patent cerebrospinal fluid circulation. **B,** Enlarged lateral and third ventricles caused by obstruction of circulation—stenosis of aqueduct of Sylvius. *(From Hockenberry MJ et al:* Wong's nursing care of infants and children, *ed 7, St Louis, 2003, Mosby.)*

ages; the risk is higher in women over age 35, but infants with DS are born to women under age 35, although the risk is much lower; the incidence of DS in women age 40 is approximately 1 in 100

B. Symptoms: hypotonia; small, low-set ears; slanted eyes; protruding tongue; small, flattened nose; short, broad neck; single transverse palmar (simian) crease; dry, cracked skin; congenital heart defects; and mental retardation

C. Diagnosis: based on the physical defects; chromosomal studies are done to determine specific defects

D. Treatment and nursing interventions
1. Emotional support for parents; they expected a "normal" infant without defects
2. Assist family in preventing physical problems (respiratory, integumentary, nutrition)
3. Promote the child's developmental progress, and help parents set realistic goals for the child
4. Encourage activity and intellectual stimulation for the child through early intervention programs and school
5. Genetic counseling for the parents

Genitourinary System
Epispadias and Hypospadias
A. Definition: congenital conditions in male infants in which the urethra ends on the under side (hypospadias) or the top side (epispadias) of the penis, rather than at the end

B. Symptoms: obvious physical defects evident on physical examination; abnormal stream of urine

C. Diagnosis: based on physical examination

D. Treatment and nursing interventions
1. The surgery to extend the urethra to the end of the penis is usually done in several stages when the child is 6 to 18 months of age; the infant should not be circumcised because foreskin may be needed for later surgery
2. Postoperative care includes inspection of the operative site for bleeding, catheter care, and emotional support for the child and parents, as well as general postoperative care

Cryptorchidism
A. Definition: failure of one or both testes to descend into the scrotal sac; sterility may result if not treated

B. Symptoms: testes not palpable in the scrotal sac on physical examination

C. Diagnosis: based on symptoms

D. Treatment and nursing interventions
1. The testes usually descend by 1 year of age (in 75% of affected infants)
2. Hormonal therapy (human chorionic gonadotropin [HCG]) may be used at an early age to promote descent of the testes into the scrotum
3. Surgical intervention (orchiopexy), usually done between 6 and 24 months of age, often necessary to bring the testes down the inguinal canal and into the scrotum; routine postoperative care

Wilms' Tumor (Nephroblastoma)
A. Definition: tumor in the kidney region

B. Symptoms: sometimes asymptomatic, discovered on routine examination; occasional occurrence of hematuria and elevated blood pressure; swelling or mass in the abdomen

C. Diagnosis: the tumor is often palpable through the abdominal wall; occurs most often in children under 2 years of age

and is usually found by the caregiver before the child reaches the age of 3 years

D. Treatment and nursing interventions
1. Surgery to remove the tumor is performed within 48 hours of diagnosis; routine postoperative care is given
2. Radiation therapy is given postoperatively as ordered (for children with large tumors, metastasis, or recurrence)
3. Chemotherapy as ordered; most effective agents are actinomycin D and vincristine
4. Provide emotional support and education for parents

E. Prognosis is good with early diagnosis and treatment for children under 2 years of age

Musculoskeletal System
Congenital Clubfoot (Talipes Equinovarus)
A. Definition: defect in which the entire foot is inverted, heel is drawn up, and front of the foot is adducted; can affect one or both feet (Figure 8-8)

B. Symptoms: obvious physical defect evident on physical examination

C. Diagnosis: based on the presence of the physical defect on examination

D. Treatment and nursing interventions
1. The deformity is usually repaired in stages; the type of treatment depends on the severity of the defect
2. Various methods of treatment include manipulation and serial casting, splints, and surgery when necessary to repair the deformities; nursing care depends on method chosen

Developmental Dysplasia of the Hip (DDH) DDH
A. Definition: DDH describes a group of disorders related to abnormal development of the hip in which a shallow acetabulum, subluxation, or dislocation is present; DDH may result from laxity of the supporting capsule or an abnormality of the acetabulum

B. Symptoms: limited hip abduction, apparent shortening of femur, asymmetry of gluteal and thigh folds (Figure 8-9)

C. Diagnosis: symptoms found on physical examination by the physician or nurse practitioner

D. Treatment and nursing interventions
1. Treatment is started as soon as the defect is diagnosed; the hip is manipulated into proper position and an abduction device (Pavlik harness, Figure 8-10) or hip spica cast is applied; Bryant's traction, modified Bryant's traction, or modified Buck's extension may also be used
2. Nursing care includes parent teaching regarding application of the harness and cast care

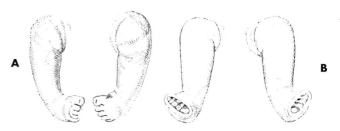

FIGURE 8-8. Feet casted for correction of bilateral congenital talipes equinovarus. A, Before correction. B, Undergoing correction in plaster casts. (*From Brashear HR Jr, Raney RB: Shands' handbook of orthopaedic surgery, ed 10, St Louis, 1986, Mosby.*)

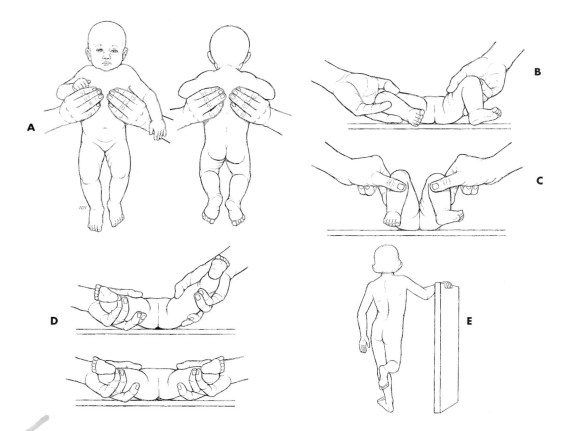

FIGURE 8-9.   Signs of developmental dysplasia of the hip. A, Asymmetry of gluteal and thigh folds. **B,** Limited hip abduction, as seen in flexion. **C,** Apparent shortening of the femur, as indicated by the level of the knees in flexion. **D,** Ortolani click (if infant is under 4 weeks of age). **E,** Positive Trendelenburg sign or gait (if child is weight bearing). *(From Hockenberry MJ et al:* Wong's nursing care of infants and children, ed 7, *St Louis, 2003, Mosby.)*

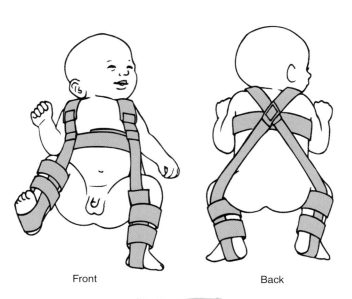

Front   Back

FIGURE 8-10.   Child in Pavlik harness. *(From Ball JW:* Mosby's pediatric patient teaching guides, *St Louis, 1998, Mosby.)*

Cardiovascular System
Congenital Heart Defects (Cyanotic and Acyanotic)
A. Atrial septal defect (ASD): abnormal opening in the septum between the two atria, or a patent foramen ovale, that causes left-to-right shunting of the blood (acyanotic)
B. Ventricular septal defect (VSD): abnormal opening in the septum between the two ventricles that causes left-to-right shunting of the blood (acyanotic)
C. Patent ductus arteriosus (PDA): the ductus arteriosus remains open after birth instead of closing off as normal, causing an overload of the left heart and a slight murmur (acyanotic)
D. Coarctation of the aorta: constriction of the aortic arch, causing hypertension in the upper body and hypotension in the lower body (acyanotic)
E. Tetralogy of Fallot: consists of four congenital defects—pulmonary stenosis, VSD, overriding of the aorta, and right ventricular hypertrophy (cyanotic)
F. Classic symptoms of congenital heart defects: dyspnea, difficulty with feeding, clubbing of fingers, cyanosis (in certain defects), heart murmurs, rapid pulse, recurrent respiratory infections, edema
G. Diagnosis: based on the symptoms, electrocardiograms, echocardiograms, cardiac catheterizations, and chest x-ray examinations

H. Treatment and nursing interventions
   1. Most defects must be corrected by surgical intervention, often in stages; some symptoms can be treated with medications as ordered
   2. Nursing care measures depend on the type of treatment or surgery; most often, immediate postoperative care is given in intensive care units
   3. Patient and parent teaching should include instructing parents to help the child conserve energy, without being overprotective

Sickle Cell Anemia

A. Definition: autosomal disease occurring mainly in blacks, but also occurs on occasion in whites of Mediterranean descent; causes breakdown of red blood cells (RBCs) carrying an abnormal hemoglobin S, which leads to a severe hemolytic anemia; the disease may not be recognized until the toddler or preschool period
B. Symptoms: appear only in children who inherit the trait from both parents; fatigue, anorexia, decreased hemoglobin; sickle cell crisis may occur, causing severe joint pain, abdominal pain, fever, and firm, distended abdomen (Figure 8-11); because children with sickle cell disease do not have a properly functioning spleen, they are more susceptible to infection and sepsis

C. Diagnosis: based on the symptoms, family history of the disease, and specific blood tests, including the sickle-cell slide preparation, sickle-turbidity test (Sickledex), and hemoglobin electrophoresis (Fingerprinting)
D. Treatment and nursing interventions
   1. IV fluids and fluids by mouth (PO) as ordered
   2. Oxygen therapy, especially during sickle cell crisis
   3. Bed rest
   4. Electrolyte replacement
   5. Analgesics for pain as ordered
   6. Blood transfusions as ordered (packed RBCs)
   7. Prophylactic antibiotic therapy as needed
   8. Education and genetic counseling for parents
   9. Proper nutrition, as tolerated
   10. Avoiding exposure to people with colds and infections

Endocrine System

Hypopituitarism (Dwarfism)

A. Definition; growth retardation resulting from deficiency of the growth hormone (GH)
B. Symptoms: short stature, well-nourished appearance, delayed physical development
C. Diagnosis: based on the family history, child's growth patterns, physical examination, x-ray studies, and endocrine studies

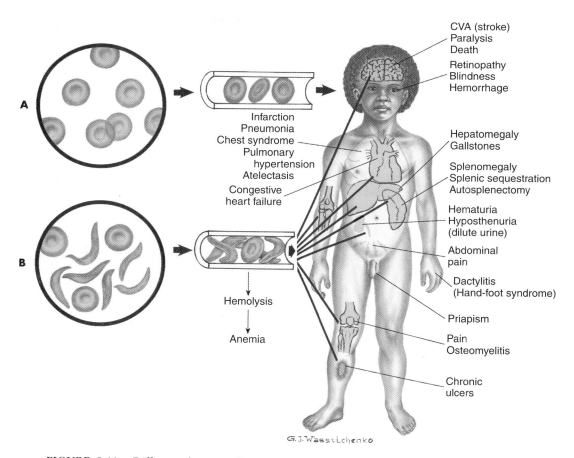

FIGURE 8-11. Differences between effects of **A**, normal, and **B**, sickled RBCs on circulation with selected consequences in a child. *(From Hockenberry MJ et al: Wong's nursing care of infants and children, ed 7, St Louis, 2003, Mosby.)*

D. Treatment and nursing interventions
1. Replacement of the GH by subcutaneous injections
2. Early diagnosis and treatment to help prevent many physical and emotional problems that occur later in childhood
3. Providing emotional support for the child and parents during diagnostic procedures and early stages of treatment (even after GH therapy is started, growth will be slower than normal)

Congenital Hypothyroidism (Cretinism)

A. Definition: lack of thyroid function resulting from a failure of the embryonic development of the thyroid gland
B. Symptoms: usually do not appear until 6 to 12 weeks of age in bottle-fed infants and after weaning in breast-fed infants; included are feeding problems, inactivity, anemia, thick, dry, mottled skin, bradycardia, relaxation of the abdominal muscles, and delayed development of the nervous system, which leads to mental retardation
C. Diagnosis: based on the symptoms and tests of thyroid function, such as initial measurement of the newborn's T4 (thyroxin) and thyroid-stimulating hormone (TSH) level
D. Treatment and nursing interventions
1. Early diagnosis and treatment are essential in preventing retardation and other severe physiological symptoms
2. Treatment is lifelong replacement therapy of the thyroid hormone
3. Parent teaching concerning administration of the thyroid hormone, including signs and symptoms of thyroid overdose

Sudden Infant Death Syndrome (SIDS)

A. Definition: sudden death of an infant under 1 year of age that remains unexplained after a complete postmortem examination, including an investigation of the death scene and a review of the infant's clinical history; the third leading cause of death in children between 1 and 12 months of age; the peak age for SIDS is 2 to 4 months; 95% of cases occur by the age of 6 months
B. Research: numerous theories have been proposed regarding the cause of SIDS, but the exact cause is unknown; many researchers believe that it may be related to a brain stem abnormality in the regulation of cardiorespiratory control; other studies have demonstrated that infants sleeping in the prone position are at an increased risk for SIDS; because of these findings, the American Academy of Pediatrics recommends that healthy infants up to 6 months of age sleep on their back
C. Infants at risk for SIDS include those with a history of apnea requiring vigorous stimulation or cardiopulmonary resuscitation (CPR), preterm infants who continue to have apnea after hospital discharge, siblings of two or more SIDS victims
D. Emotional support for the parents
1. Parents always feel guilty and must be reassured that SIDS is not their fault
2. Encourage them to allow an autopsy to try to determine a specific cause of death, which helps allay their guilt and feelings that they might have prevented it
3. Allow parents to spend some time with the child to say good-bye
4. Refer the parents to the SIDS Foundation for counseling and support

5. After the parents return home from the hospital, emotional support should continue to be provided for them by qualified health care professionals

TODDLERHOOD (AGES 1 TO 3)

Normal Growth and Development
Physical Development

A. Toddlerhood shows a decrease in the rate of growth but an increase in the rate of development
B. Toddlers gain approximately 4 to 6 lb (1.8 to 2.7 kg) each year and add 3 in (7.5 cm) in height per year
C. They have learned, and continue to learn, to walk between 1 and 2 years of age
D. Visual acuity of 20/20 is achieved during the toddler years
E. Anterior fontanel closes between 18 and 24 months of age
F. Toddlers continue to learn to talk, learning new words and phrases; their favorite word is "no!"

Psychosocial Development

A. Behavior in the toddler is characterized by several aspects
1. Negativism: toddlers say "no!" to almost everything; this is part of their becoming an individual person who is separate from his or her parents
2. Ritualism: developing and following certain patterns of behavior to develop their own security
3. Temper tantrums: toddlers like to do everything for themselves; when they cannot do certain things, they are frustrated, and this frustration leads to temper tantrums; tantrums should be ignored as much as possible, and the child should be dealt with after the "storm" is over
B. Toddlers are in Erikson's stage of "autonomy vs. shame and doubt"; they need to develop a sense of autonomy and self-control; to do so, toddlers must be able to make some choices, as well as learn to function, within the limits set for them; they are in Kohlberg's stage 1 of preconventional morality; they obey rules to avoid punishment
C. Discipline and limit setting must be consistent to be effective; it is important to remember to criticize the behavior, not the child
D. Toilet training is an important part of the socialization process in toddlers; they should be praised when they use the potty-chair or toilet properly, rather than being punished for not using it; toilet training should begin only when the toddler is physically capable of controlling bowel and bladder (18 to 24 months)

Health Promotion

A. Nutrition needs change because of change in growth rate; toddlers need less food, and their appetites decrease (18 months of age)
1. Teach parents that the decrease in food intake is normal
2. The child is more autonomous now; should be allowed to feed himself or herself as much as possible; "finger foods" are ideal
3. Snacks should be nutritious; cheese, fruits, and crackers are good choices
4. Desserts should not be used as rewards; this practice gets the toddler into a habit of expecting something sweet whenever doing something good

B. Prevention of accidents is a major responsibility with toddlers; keep dangerous items (sharp objects, medications, cleaning supplies) out of their reach; toddlers should not be left unattended near a bathtub, swimming pool, whirlpool bath, or hot objects, such as pans on the stove or open flames

C. Teaching the toddler good oral hygiene habits is necessary to prevent early tooth decay and problems with gums
   1. Brushing the teeth should begin between 12 and 18 months of age
   2. Dental checkups with the dental hygienist or dentist should begin at approximately 1 year of age
   3. Proper nutrition helps prevent a large amount of early dental caries

Health Problems
Respiratory Disorders

Epiglottitis
A. Definition: a severely inflamed epiglottis, which begins abruptly and progresses rapidly into severe respiratory distress; usually caused by *H. influenzae* bacteria (unlike croup, which is viral and progresses more slowly than epiglottitis)

B. Symptoms: fever, sore throat, difficulty swallowing; child insists on sitting up, leaning forward with chin thrust out, mouth open, and tongue protruding; drooling is common

C. Diagnosis: based on the symptoms and visualization of enlarged reddened epiglottis on careful throat examination and enlarged epiglottis on lateral neck x-ray examination

D. Treatment and nursing interventions
   1. Do not examine throat unless immediate intubation can be performed if necessary
   2. Keep child as quiet as possible; allow child to sit up in bed or on lap of parent
   3. Keep emergency tracheostomy tray (and intubation tray) with patient at all times
   4. Administer IV fluids and antibiotics as ordered
   5. Monitor child closely

Cystic Fibrosis (CF)
A. Definition: an autosomal recessive hereditary disease affecting the exocrine glands; the lungs, pancreas, liver and small intestine produce abnormal mucus secretions and become obstructed

B. Symptoms
   1. In newborns: meconium ileus, bile-stained emesis, distended abdomen, no stools, salty "taste" to the skin resulting from increased sodium in the perspiration
   2. In infants and children: harsh, dry cough, frequent bronchial infections, malnutrition, distended abdomen, barrel chest, clubbed fingers, also bulky, greasy, foul-smelling stools (steatorrhea)

C. Diagnosis: based on family history, a history of FTT, the symptoms, lung changes revealed by chest x-ray films, an elevated sweat chloride level (increased sodium in the perspiration), and stool analysis for fat and enzymes

D. Treatment and nursing interventions
   1. Pancreatic enzymes given as ordered with food to improve digestion of fats and proteins
   2. High-carbohydrate, high-protein, low-fat diet
   3. Increased amounts of salt and water-soluble vitamins
   4. Inhalation therapy: nebulizer treatments of bronchodilators (see Chapter 3) and recombinant human deoxyribonuclease (DNase) to decrease the viscosity of the mucus
   5. Daily routine of chest physiotherapy and postural drainage to help in expectoration of mucus
   6. Physical exercise to stimulate mucus secretion
   7. Antibiotics for all pulmonary infections
   8. Parent teaching regarding diet, medications, and inhalation therapy for proper home care after discharge
   9. Referral to the Cystic Fibrosis Foundation for education and financial or emotional support
   10. Genetic counseling for parents

Cardiovascular Disorder: Kawasaki Disease (KD) (Mucocutaneous Lymph Node Syndrome)

A. Definition: an acute inflammation of the vascular system; cause unknown; most common in children under age 5, with peak incidence seen in the toddler age group; diagnosed in every racial group, but is most common in Japanese children; most cases diagnosed in late winter and early spring; with proper treatment, 25% of children develop cardiac complications, including damage to the cardiac blood vessels and the heart muscle itself

B. Symptoms and diagnosis: child must exhibit five of the following six criteria, including fever:
   1. Fever for 5 or more days
   2. Bilateral conjunctival inflammation
   3. Changes in the oral mucus membranes, including dryness and erythema
   4. Changes in the extremities, such as erythema and peeling of the palms and soles, and peripheral edema
   5. Cervical lymphadenopathy
   6. Polymorphous rash

C. Treatment and nursing interventions
   1. High dose IV immune globulin (IVIG) to decrease the fever and incidence of coronary artery damage
   2. Salicylate therapy to control fever and symptoms of inflammation
   3. I&O, daily weight (to assess for signs of congestive heart failure)
   4. Mouth care
   5. Careful observation of the IV site
   6. Quiet environment and proper rest
   7. Emotional support for the child and family
   8. Long-term follow-up should include monitoring of heart disease risk factors (abnormal blood pressure and cholesterol levels) and promotion of a heart-healthy lifestyle (proper nutrition, exercise, and avoidance of smoking)

Gastrointestinal Disorder: Celiac Disease (Gluten Enteropathy)

A. Definition: a defect of metabolism precipitated by the ingestion of wheat or rye gluten, leading to impaired fat absorption; exact cause unknown

B. Symptoms: usually appear between 1 and 5 years of age; chronic diarrhea with bulky, greasy, foul-smelling stools; malnutrition; anorexia; unhappy disposition; retardation of growth; distended abdomen; muscle wasting especially of extremities and buttocks

C. Diagnosis: laboratory tests, including stool analysis for fecal fat; blood studies for anemia, hypoproteinemia, and serum iron; definitive diagnosis is based on these tests, the symptoms, and a jejunal biopsy to demonstrate changes in the jejunal mucosa

D. Treatment and nursing interventions
1. Gluten-free, low-fat diet; rice cereal for infants; children with celiac disease may also be lactose intolerant
2. Parent teaching regarding diet and specific foods to avoid
3. The child should be protected from respiratory infections, which may lead to exacerbations of the disease known as celiac crisis (characterized by severe vomiting and diarrhea, dehydration, and acidosis)

Neurosensory Disorders

Eye Disorders

Strabismus   Cross eye

A. Definition: failure of the eyes to direct and focus on the same object at the same time
B. Symptoms: deviation of one eye to the center (esotropia) or to the other corner (exotropia)
C. Diagnosis: based on the symptoms
D. Treatment and nursing interventions
1. Patching of unaffected eye to increase visual stimulation of weaker eye
2. Eyeglasses and exercise to help improve vision
3. Surgery to correct the muscle defects; often necessary when conservative treatment is ineffective
4. Preoperative and postoperative nursing care as indicated

Amblyopia ("Lazy Eye")

A. Definition: reduced visual acuity in one eye, usually caused by strabismus; the eyes are unable to focus and work together, and blindness may occur in the weaker eye if left untreated
B. Symptoms: blurred vision, double vision, development of a "blind spot"
C. Diagnosis: based on results of Snellen's eye test and the symptoms
D. Treatment and nursing interventions: patching of the unaffected eye so that the child is forced to use and focus the weaker eye; the best time for treatment is during early childhood

Cerebral Palsy

A. Definition: a group of nonprogressive disorders caused by a malfunction of the motor centers of the brain; oxygen deprivation (anoxia) damages the brain's motor centers prenatally, during or immediately after delivery, or during childhood after an accident or disease
B. Symptoms: abnormal muscle tone and coordination, delays in development, hearing and vision impairment, seizures, mental retardation (in some cases)
C. Diagnosis: based on the mother's prenatal history, birth history, history of an accident or disease, presence of delays in growth and development, abnormal neurological examination (Table 8-2)
D. Types of cerebral palsy
1. Spastic: hypertonicity with poor control of posture, balance, and coordination; impaired motor skills; hypertonicity of muscles and tendon reflexes lead to development of contractures
2. Dyskinetic: abnormal involuntary movement; athetosis, characterized by slow, writhing movements that involve extremities, trunk, neck, facial muscles, and the tongue

TABLE 8-2	Cerebral Palsy: Predisposing Factors and Known Causes
Risk Factors	**Associated Causes**
Prenatal	
Maternal	Metabolic diseases
	Nutritional deficiencies (e.g., anemia)
	Twin or multiple births
	Bleeding
	Toxemia
	Blood incompatibilities
	Exposure to radiation
	Infection (e.g., rubella, toxoplasmosis, cytomegalic inclusion disease)
	Premature labor
Prematurity	Asphyxia leading to cerebral hemorrhage
Genetic factors	Absence of corpus callosum, aqueductal stenosis, cerebellar hypoplasia
Congenital anomalies of the brain	Unknown causes not evident on clinical examination
Perinatal	Anesthesia or analgesia during labor and delivery
	Mechanical trauma during delivery
	Immaturity at birth
	Metabolic disorders (e.g., hyperbilirubinemia, hypoglycemia, amino acid disorders, hyperosmolality)
	Electrolyte disturbances (e.g., hypernatremia, hypoglycemia)
Postnatal	Head trauma
	Infections (e.g., meningitis, encephalitis)
	Cerebrovascular accidents
	Toxicosis
	Environmental toxins (e.g., lead ingestion, methyl mercury ingestion from contaminated fish)

From McCance KL, Huether SE: *Pathophysiology: the biologic basis for disease in adults and children,* ed 4, St Louis, 2003, Mosby.

3. Ataxic: wide-based gait; disintegration of movements of the upper extremities when the child reaches for objects
4. Mixed type: combination of spasticity and athetosis
E. Treatment and nursing interventions
1. Treatment and care are supportive to ensure optimal level of development for the child
2. Physical and occupational therapy to help the child learn some control over muscle movements
3. Braces or splints as needed to hold extremities in correct positions of function
4. Use of wheelchairs, walkers, and crutches as needed for ambulation and locomotion

5. Speech therapy or assistance with feeding as needed
6. Treatment for respiratory problems, seizures, contractures as needed
7. Emotional support for the family and child; most often, children with cerebral palsy are of normal intelligence and have only physical disabilities
8. Encourage the child to live as normal a life as possible; refer the family to supportive groups such as the Easter Seal Society

Accidents

A. Accidents are the major cause of death in children between 1 and 14 years of age, chiefly because of their ability to walk and move more freely than they do during infancy, along with their unawareness of danger within the environment
B. Accident prevention during toddlerhood is a major task that requires the involvement of both parents and other family members; following are several basic suggestions for accident prevention
   1. Supervise play, especially around dangerous areas such, as, cars, swimming pools, and open flames or hot appliances
   2. Use well-designed, safe car seats or restraints (use rear-facing car seat in the middle of the back sear for infants)
   3. Turn all handles of pots and pans in toward the stove, away from the child's reach
   4. Cover electrical outlets with protective plastic caps
   5. Do not allow the child to play with the bathtub faucets; do not leave the child unattended in the bathroom
   6. Keep all medications and poisonous substances out of the child's reach (preferably in a locked cabinet)
   7. Know the number and location of the nearest poison control center and hospital
   8. Put up gates at the top and bottom of stairwells
   9. Choose well-made toys appropriate for the child's age, without sharp edges or small removable pieces
   10. Store all guns and dangerous tools and equipment in a locked cabinet
   11. Teach the toddler about common dangers such as "hot" items, looking "both ways" before crossing the street, and water safety
   12. Provide bicycle helmets for toddlers to wear every time they ride a bike

PRESCHOOL AGE (AGES 3 TO 5)

Normal Growth and Development
Physical Development

A. Growth is slow during the preschool years; children gain approximately 5 lb (2.3 kg) and 2 to 3 in (5 to 7.5 cm) in height each year
B. Deciduous teeth are being replaced by permanent teeth; proper dental hygiene and regular dental checkups are definitely needed at this age level and throughout childhood
C. Language development of preschoolers is rapid; 3 year olds talk to themselves and their toys; 4 year olds begin to talk and communicate more with other people

Psychosocial Development

A. Preschoolers are in Erikson's stage of "initiative vs. guilt"; at this age level, they learn how to interact with other children and adults; they also learn the difference between proper and improper behavior, as well as the rewards and disciplines associated with each; without proper adult guidance, preschoolers can learn improper behavior and develop a sense of guilt and inferiority rather than a sense of initiative and accomplishment
B. Preschoolers begin to develop their imaginations; they use "magical thinking" and have difficulty distinguishing fantasy from reality
C. Preschoolers become acutely aware of their sexuality, including their roles as boys or girls and their sex organs; parents must work with their children in a positive way to help them develop healthy attitudes toward themselves and their bodies
D. Preschoolers continue to learn through play; they still use parallel play but also begin to use associative play (play with other children) and imitative play (play by imitating the actions of adults or other children)
E. Preschoolers are in stage 2 (preconventional morality) of Kohlberg's "Theory of Moral Development"; they conform to rules to obtain rewards

Health Promotion

A. Immunizations started in infancy and toddlerhood should continue according to schedule (see Figure 8-2)
B. Nutrition should be appropriate to age, keeping in mind that growth is slow during this period; preschoolers should be eating foods from all four basic food groups

Health Problems
Communicable Diseases

See Appendix F

Respiratory Disorders: Tonsillitis and Adenoiditis

A. Definition: inflammation of the tonsils and adenoids caused by chronic URI
B. Symptoms: sore throat, difficulty in swallowing and breathing ("mouth breathers"), hoarseness, harsh cough
C. Diagnosis: based on the symptoms and the presence of swelling and redness of the tonsils and adenoids on examination
D. Treatment and nursing interventions
   1. Acute infections are treated with antibiotics as ordered, increased oral fluids, and warm saltwater gargles
   2. If chronic infections continue after antibiotic treatment, surgery is often indicated (tonsillectomy and adenoidectomy); however, surgery is less common today than it was in the past
   3. Postoperative nursing care measures include keeping the child in a prone position with head to the side until fully awake; monitoring vital signs frequently; checking the throat and nares for active bleeding; keeping the suction equipment at the bedside for emergency use; observing the child for frequent swallowing (this may indicate oozing of blood in the nasopharynx or pharynx); providing analgesic and antipyretic drugs for discomfort; and encouraging cool clear oral fluids after the nausea subsides (synthetic juices less irritating than natural juices);

warm saltwater gargles may be used beginning 1 week after the surgery

4. Teach the child not to cough, clear the throat, or blow the nose, to help decrease risk of bleeding; provide written instructions to parents regarding postoperative care and possible complications

Genitourinary Disorders

Nephrotic Syndrome

A. Definition: massive proteinuria, hypoalbuminemia, hyperlipemia, and edema; is the most common glomerular injury in children; it can be classified as primary (restricted to glomerular injury) or secondary (when it develops as part of a systemic illness)

B. Symptoms: edema of the face, extremities, and abdomen; proteinuria, hypoalbuminemia, respiratory distress; malnutrition; irritability; increased susceptibility to infection

C. Diagnosis: based on decreased serum protein levels and increased proteinuria, edema, and hypocholesterolemia, and on results of a renal biopsy

D. Treatment and nursing interventions
1. Nephrotic syndrome is a chronic disorder, with remissions and exacerbations, usually lasting 12 to 18 months; treatment measures continue for an extended period
2. Corticosteroids ordered to reduce the edema
3. An oral alkylating agent, usually Cytoxan, alternating with prednisone, ordered to reduce the relapse rate and induce long-term remission
4. Frequent urine testing for protein and albumin
5. Recording of I&O
6. Daily weights
7. Diuretics as ordered (not always effective)
8. Low-salt diet during exacerbations
9. Antibiotics as ordered during exacerbations
10. Proper care of the skin to avoid breakdown caused by the edema
11. Parent teaching for home care regarding medications, diet, and follow-up

Acute Glomerulonephritis

A. Definition: inflammation of the glomeruli and nephrons of the kidney; it may occur as a primary event, or as a reaction to an infection (most often streptococcal, pneumococcal, or viral)

B. Symptoms: edema of the face and eyes, anorexia, dark-colored ("tea") urine, oliguria, listlessness, irritability, headache, abdominal discomfort, vomiting, slightly elevated blood pressure, proteinuria; if the disease occurs as a result of a systemic infection, the symptoms occur approximately 10 days after the infection

C. Diagnosis: based on the symptoms and a positive recent history of streptococcal or other infection

D. Treatment and nursing interventions
1. Regular activity with rest periods as needed
2. Antibiotics as ordered (see Chapter 3)
3. Regular, low-salt diet
4. Measurement of I&O, observation of color of urine
5. Frequent checking and recording of blood pressure
6. Urine testing for protein and specific gravity
7. Daily weights
8. Antihypertensives and diuretics for elevated blood pressure as ordered

Circulatory Disorders

Hemophilia

A. Definition: a group of bleeding disorders resulting from a congenital deficiency of certain coagulation proteins; X-linked recessive in nature; hemophilia is typed according to which clotting factor is affected

B. Symptoms: prolonged bleeding and clotting times; easy bruising and bleeding into tissues and joints; joint pain

C. Diagnosis: based on the symptoms, as well as family health history, and a prolonged clotting time

D. Treatment and nursing interventions
1. Observations for any signs of internal bleeding and shock
2. Transfusions as ordered with the missing clotting factor
3. Frequent laboratory tests, such as partial thromboplastin time (PTT), clotting time, complete blood count (CBC); screening for human immunodeficiency virus (HIV) and hepatitis (from receiving contaminated transfusions or clotting factors)
4. Corticosteroids and nonsteroidal antiinflammatory drugs as ordered
5. Exercise and physical therapy to strengthen muscles around joints
6. Protection of the child from injuries as much as possible
7. Emotional support and counseling for the child and parents
8. Parent teaching regarding follow-up physical examinations, protecting the child from physical harm, the need for immediate care if any injury occurs, and administering the clotting factor to the child
9. Referrals to community resources, such as the National Hemophilia Foundation
10. Genetic counseling for parents

Leukemia

A. Definition: a broad term given to a group of malignant diseases of the bone marrow and lymphatic system; an unrestricted proliferation of immature WBCs in the blood-forming tissues of the body; classified according to its predominant cell type and level of maturity, acute lymphocytic leukemia (ALL) is the most common childhood leukemia

B. Symptoms: the three main consequences of bone marrow dysfunction are anemia, infection, and bleeding; other symptoms include lethargy, pallor, anorexia, fever, pain in the bones and joints; petechiae, easy bruising, and sores in the mouth; also decreased RBCs and WBCs

C. Diagnosis: made on the basis of history, symptoms, an elevated WBC count, and presence of immature leukocytes and blast cells in a bone marrow biopsy or aspiration

D. Treatment and nursing interventions
1. Leukemia is a chronic, sometimes fatal, disease with remissions and exacerbations; the child and family need a great deal of emotional support from the physician and nursing staff
2. Chemotherapy drugs and corticosteroids as ordered (see Chapter 3)
3. IV fluids and blood transfusions as ordered
4. Administration of pain medications as ordered; joint pain during exacerbations may be severe, especially in

the more advanced stages; higher-than-normal doses are often required

5. Proper skin and mouth care
6. Providing proper nutrition as the child's condition allows
7. Prevention of infections whenever possible; chemotherapy drugs lower the WBC count, which, in turn, decreases the child's resistance to infection
8. Observation for possible side effects of chemotherapy drugs
9. Bone marrow transplants may be ordered in certain types of leukemia to replace unhealthy bone marrow; an exact *match* is often difficult to find

Musculoskeletal Disorder: Muscular Dystrophy (MD)

A. Definition: a group of hereditary muscle diseases (recessive trait) characterized by gradual degeneration of muscle fibers, which is evidenced by muscle wasting and weakness and increasing disability and deformity
B. Symptoms: gradual muscle weakness, including difficulty walking, standing up, a "waddle" gait, and mild mental retardation; most symptoms appear in children between 3 and 5 years of age
C. Diagnosis: based on the history of the symptoms, family history, muscle biopsy to determine muscle degeneration, electromyography (EMG), and serum enzyme (creatine phosphokinase [CPK]) measurement
D. Treatment and nursing interventions
   1. No cure has been discovered for MD; thus treatment is supportive; the primary goal is to maintain function in the unaffected muscles for as long as possible
   2. Encourage the child to be as active and to lead as normal a life as possible
   3. Range-of-motion exercises and physical therapy as ordered to prevent contractures
   4. Use of walkers, crutches, braces, and wheelchairs as needed
   5. Emotional support for the parents and child; this is a progressive disease, and the family requires ongoing support by the health care team
   6. Frequent medical checkups to observe for progressive symptoms such as respiratory distress
   7. Genetic counseling for the parents; referral to Muscular Dystrophy Association for education and community services

Psychosocial Disorders: Attention-Deficit Hyperactivity Disorder (ADHD)

A. Definition: ADHD is the most common chronic behavioral disorder of children; it is associated with problems in attention and concentration, impulse control, and overactivity
B. Symptoms: behaviors in the categories of inattention (e.g., carelessness, difficulty attending to work and play, easily distracted, does not listen) and of impulsivity and hyperactivity (e.g., fidgeting with hands, feet or hair, difficulty concentrating on quiet activities, excessive talking, unable to remain seated for long periods)
C. Diagnosis: based on the reports of the child, parent, and teacher or teachers; the behavior or symptoms must be present in two out of three areas (home, school, social situations) to support the diagnosis; the American Psychiatric Association requires that a child must exhibit six or more of the common behaviors to be diagnosed with ADHD

D. Treatment and nursing interventions: the goal of treatment of ADHD is to decrease the frequency and intensity of negative behaviors
   1. Setting realistic expectations for the child when attempting to change behaviors
   2. Working with the parents to adapt the environment and develop strategies that will support positive behaviors
   3. Behavioral and psychotherapy for the child and family
   4. Psychostimulant medications (such as Ritalin, Dexedrine, and Adderall) as a possible part of the treatment plan
   5. Parent or caregiver education about the disorder and treatment methods

SCHOOL AGE (AGES 6 TO 12)

Normal Growth and Development
Physical Development

A. Growth is slow in children between the ages of 6 and 10 years; the child gains 4 1/2 to 6 1/2 lb (2 to 3 kg) and 2 in (5 cm) per year
B. Bone growth is slow; the cartilage is replaced by bone at the bone epiphyses
C. Middle childhood (ages 6 to 12) is the stage of development when deciduous teeth are shed

Psychosocial Development

A. School-age children are in Erikson's stage of "industry vs. inferiority"; an eagerness to develop new skills and interests, and the processes of cooperating and competing with other children are characteristics of this age that engender a sense of accomplishment rather than a sense of inferiority and poor self-worth
B. School-age children are in Kohlberg's stage of conventional morality (level 2); the child conforms to rules to please others
C. Children ages 7 to 10 start to become more influenced by their peer group than by their parents; they develop "best friends" and start to separate into boy and girl groups
D. The most significant skill acquired during the school-age period is the ability to read

Health Promotion

A. Communicable disease prevention is accomplished by timely immunizations, proper rest and diet, and frequent medical and dental checkups
B. Accident prevention remains a major factor at this age level; safety measures should include rules for bicycle and skateboard safety (helmets and pads for safety in competitive sports such as baseball, football, and soccer)
C. Sex education should begin at this age level and should be presented by the parents in simple, honest terms; audiovisual aids such as books and pictures are available to assist parents in presenting the information on the child's level
D. Education about the dangers of drug and alcohol abuse should begin at this age level
E. Promotion of a balanced diet continues to be important at this age level; high-calorie, low-nutrition snacks are

popular with school-age children but often lead to excess weight gain

Health Problems
Respiratory Disorders: Allergic Conditions

Asthma

A. Definition: a chronic inflammatory disorder of the airways, associated with airflow limitation or obstruction caused by edema of the bronchial mucosa, increased mucus production, and bronchial muscle contraction; it is often caused by an allergic response to allergens ("triggers") such as pollen, animal fur, food, or irritants, such as tobacco smoke, exercise, cold air, respiratory infections, and changes in the weather; it is the most common chronic disease of childhood

B. Symptoms: irritability; restlessness; tightness in the chest; hacking, nonproductive cough; dyspnea; and wheezing; asthma is classified into four categories—mild intermittent, mild persistent, moderate persistent, and severe persistent

C. Diagnosis: based on the symptoms, physical examination, the child's history, family history, chest x-ray examination that rule out other respiratory diseases, and pulmonary function studies (including peak expiration flow rate)

D. Treatment and nursing interventions
1. Pharmacological therapy is used in a step-wise approach, based on the child's asthma severity classification; medications are categorized as long-term control (preventive) and quick relief
2. Bronchodilator medications as ordered (administered by inhalation, by mouth, or by injection) (see Chapter 3)
3. Antiinflammatory medications, either corticosteroids (prednisone) or nonsteroidal agents (cromolyn sodium) administered by inhalation, by mouth, or by injection
4. Chest physiotherapy
5. IV fluids as ordered
6. Liquid diet, progressing to a regular diet
7. Identification and removal of the allergens if possible
8. Parent and child teaching regarding home care, including medications, use of nebulizer or metered-dose inhaler (MDI), removal of any potential "triggers," use of peak flow meter to measure peak expiratory flow rate, and follow-up examinations

Allergic Rhinitis (Hay Fever)

A. Cause: an allergy to some pollen, dust, or animal fur
B. Symptoms: sneezing, runny nose, postnasal drip, and watery, itchy eyes
C. Diagnosis: based on the symptoms and results of allergy testing done to discover specific allergen
D. Treatment and nursing interventions
1. Find and remove the allergen if possible
2. Provide antihistamines or decongestants as ordered
3. Immunotherapy may be necessary if symptoms cannot be controlled

Gastrointestinal Disorders

Appendicitis

A. Definition: inflammation of the appendix, often following an infection elsewhere in the body
B. Symptoms: localized abdominal tenderness in the right lower quadrant (increased on rebound during palpation),

abdominal rigidity, decreased bowel sounds, fever, nausea and vomiting, constipation

C. Diagnosis: based on the symptoms, physical examination, and WBC count (usually elevated); abdominal ultrasound and CT scan may also be used

D. Treatment and nursing interventions
1. Removal of the inflamed appendix (appendectomy), preferably before it ruptures and spreads the infection throughout the abdomen, causing peritonitis
2. Routine postoperative care, including monitoring vital signs, frequently observing the incision or dressing for bleeding, careful recording of I&O, and administering IV fluids as ordered
3. Antibiotics may be ordered owing to the possibility of infection or a ruptured appendix
4. Pain medication as ordered

Pinworms

A. Definition: worms that affect the intestine; the worms or eggs are swallowed and are spread easily from person to person by the hands, linen, or food
B. Symptoms: itching around the anus (especially at night), sleeplessness, anorexia, and diarrhea
C. Diagnosis: made by the cellophane tape test; the eggs are captured from the anal area during the night or early morning hours by placing a tongue blade covered with cellophane tape at the anal opening; the worms come out of the intestine at night to lay their eggs, and the eggs are picked up on the tape
D. Treatment and nursing interventions
1. Good hand-washing technique to prevent spread of the worms and reinfection; keep fingernails short
2. Frequent changes of underwear and linen
3. Medication of choice is mebendazole (see Chapter 3) for children over 2 years of age
4. Examination and treatment of all family members because pinworms are easily transmitted

Nervous System Disorder: Epilepsy

A. Definition: chronic seizure disorder with recurrent and unprovoked seizures; although many causes can be found for seizures, most are idiopathic
B. Symptoms: classification of seizures (Box 8-1)
C. Diagnosis: based on the evidence of seizures; differentiation of the type of seizure by physical examination, neurological assessment, patient history, and changes in the electroencephalogram (EEG) (changes in the brain wave patterns)
D. Treatment and nursing interventions
1. Anticonvulsant medications as ordered (see Chapter 3)
2. Parent and child education regarding medications and the necessity of taking them as prescribed, safety factors, actions to take if the child has a seizure at home, and the importance of follow-up physical examinations and laboratory work (to measure blood levels of anticonvulsants)
3. In children with poorly controlled seizures, a ketogenic diet (either with or without the use of anticonvulsants) has been tried with moderate success in some children; children on this strict diet must be followed closely by a dietitian, neurologist, and pediatrician; the length of time of the diet ranges from 1 to 3 years
4. Community referrals to support groups such as the National Epilepsy Foundation

BOX 8-1 Classification of Seizures and Epilepsy Syndromes

Partial Seizures

Simple Partial Seizures with Motor Signs
Characterized by:
  Localized motor symptoms
  Somatosensory, psychic, autonomic symptoms
  Combination of these
  Abnormal discharges remain unilateral
Manifestations:
Aversive seizure (most common motor seizure in children)
  Eye or eyes and head turn away from the side of the focus
  Awareness of movement or loss of consciousness
Rolandic (Sylvan) seizure
  Tonic-clonic movements involving the face
  Salivation
  Arrested speech
  Most common during sleep
Jacksonian march (rare in children)
  Orderly, sequential progression of clonic movements
    beginning in a foot, hand, or face and moving or
    "marching" to adjacent body parts

Simple Partial Seizures with Sensory Signs
Characterized by various sensations, including:
  Numbness, tingling, prickling, paresthesias, or pain
    originating in one area (e.g., face, extremities) and
    spreading to other parts of the body
  Visual sensations or formed images
  Motor phenomena such as posturing or hypertonia
  Uncommon in children under 8 years of age

Complex Partial Seizures (Psychomotor Seizures)
Observed more often in children from 3 years through
  adolescence
Characterized by:
  Period of altered behavior
  Amnesia for event (no recollection of behavior)
  Inability to respond to environment
  Impaired consciousness during event
  Drowsiness or sleep usually following seizure
  Possible prolonged confusion and amnesia
  Complex sensory phenomena (aura)
    Most frequent sensation: strange feeling in the pit of the
      stomach that rises toward the throat
  Often accompanied by:
    Odd or unpleasant odors or tastes
    Complex auditory or visual hallucinations
    Ill-defined feelings of elation or strangeness (e.g., déjà vu,
      a feeling of familiarity)
  May be strong feelings of fear and anxiety, distorted sense
    of time and self
  Small children may emit a cry or attempt to run for help
  Patterns of motor behavior:
  Stereotypic
  Similar with each subsequent seizure
  May suddenly cease activity, appear dazed, stare into space,
    become confused and apathetic, and become limp or stiff
    or display some form of posturing
  May be confused
  May perform purposeless, complicated activities in a repetitive
    manner (automatisms), such as walking, running, kicking,

laughing, or speaking incoherently, most often followed by
postictal confusion or sleep; may exhibit oropharyngeal
activities, such as smacking, chewing, drooling, swallowing,
and nausea or abdominal pain followed by stiffness, a fall,
and postictal sleep; rage or temper tantrums rare; aggressive
acts uncommon during seizure

Generalized Seizures

Tonic-Clonic Seizures
(formerly known as grand mal)
Most common and most dramatic of all seizure manifestations
Occur without warning
Tonic phase: lasts approximately 10 to 20 seconds
Manifestations:
  Eyes rolling upward
  Immediate loss of consciousness
  If standing, falls to floor or ground
  Stiffens in generalized, symmetric tonic contraction of
    entire body musculature
  Arms usually flexed
  Legs, head, and neck extended
  May utter a peculiar piercing cry
  Apneic; may become cyanotic
  Increased salivation and loss of swallowing reflex
Manifestations:
  Violent jerking movements as the trunk and extremities
    undergo rhythmic contraction and relaxation
  May foam at the mouth
  May be incontinent of urine and feces
As event ends, movements become less intense, occur at
  longer intervals, then cease entirely
Status epilepticus: series of seizures at intervals too brief to
  allow the child to regain consciousness between the time
  one event ends and the next begins
  Requires emergency intervention
  Can lead to exhaustion, respiratory failure, and death
Postictal state:
  Appears to relax
  May remain semiconscious and difficult to arouse
  May awaken in a few minutes
  Remains confused for several hours
  Poor coordination
  Mild impairment of fine motor movements
  May have visual and speech difficulties
  May vomit or complain of severe headache
  When left alone, usually sleeps for several hours
  On awakening, is fully conscious
  Usually feels tired and complains of sore muscles and headache
  No recollection of entire event

Absence Seizures
(formerly called petit mal or lapses)
Characterized by:
  Onset usually between 4 and 12 years of age
  More common in girls than they are in boys
  Usually cease at puberty
  Brief loss of consciousness
  Minimal or no alteration in muscle tone
  May go unrecognized because of little change in child's
    behavior

Continued

| BOX 8-1 | Classification of Seizures and Epilepsy Syndromes—cont'd |

Abrupt onset; suddenly develops 20 or more attacks daily

Event often mistaken for inattentiveness or daydreaming

Events can be precipitated by hyperventilation, hypoglycemia, stresses (emotional and physiologic), fatigue, or sleeplessness

Manifestations:

Brief loss of consciousness

Appear without warning or aura

Usually last approximately 5 to 10 seconds

Slight loss of muscle tone that may cause child to drop objects

Able to maintain postural control; seldom fails

Minor movements such as lip smacking, twitches of eyelids or face, or slight hand movements

Not accompanied by incontinence

Amnesia for episode

May need to reorient self to previous activity

Atonic and Akinetic Seizures

(also known as drop attacks)

Characterized by:

Onset of usually between 2 and 5 years of age

Sudden, momentary loss of muscle tone and postural control

Events recurring frequently during the day, particularly in the morning hours and shortly after awakening

Manifestations:

Loss of tone causes child to fall to the floor violently

Unable to break fall by putting out hand

May incur a serious injury to the face, head, or shoulder

Loss of consciousness only momentary

Myoclonic Seizures

A variety of seizure episodes

May be isolated as benign essential myoclonus

May occur in association with other seizure forms

Characterizations by:

Sudden, brief contractures off a muscle or group of muscles

Occur singly or repetitively

No postictal state

May or may not be symmetric

May or may not be loss of consciousness

Infantile Spasms

Also called infantile myoclonus, massive spasms, hypsarrhythmia, salaam episodes, or infantile myoclonic spasms

Most commonly occur during the first 6 to 8 months of life

Twice as common in male infants as they are in female infants

Child may have numerous seizures during the day without postictal drowsiness or sleep

Outlook for normal intelligence poor

Manifestations:

Possible series of sudden, brief, symmetric, muscular contractions

Head flexed, arms extended, and legs drawn up

Eyes may roll upward or inward

May be preceded or followed by a cry or giggling

May or may not be loss of consciousness

Sometimes flushing, pallor, or cyanosis

Infants who are able to sit but not stand:

Sudden dropping forward of the head and neck with trunk flexed forward and knees drawn up—the "salaam" or "jack-knife" seizure

Less often: alternate clinical forms observed

Extensor spasms rather than flexion of arms, legs, and trunk and head nodding

Lightning events involving a single, momentary, shocklike contraction of the entire body

From Wong DL et al: *Wong's essentials of pediatric nursing,* ed 6, St. Louis, 2001, Mosby

Musculoskeletal Disorder: Scoliosis

A. Definition: a lateral S-shaped curvature of the spine; it can be congenital or caused by a variety of conditions but most often has no known cause (idiopathic); most often seen in young girls and is most noticeable at the time of the preadolescent growth spurt

B. Symptoms: poor posture; uneven length of legs; asymmetry of shoulder and hip height; pelvic obliquity

C. Diagnosis: based on symptoms, x-ray examination, and physical examination

D. Treatment and nursing interventions
   1. A brace (Milwaukee brace or Boston brace) or splint is often used along with exercises to prevent an increase in the degree of curvature; this may be the only treatment, or it may be used before surgery
   2. Spinal fusion may be necessary to correct severe scoliosis; provide postoperative care as indicated

Integumentary Disorders

Ringworm

A. Definition: a fungal infection transferred from person to person or from animal to person; it can occur on the scalp (tinea capitis), the body (tinea corporis), and the feet (tinea pedis) (Figure 8-12)

B. Symptoms: small papules that have a distinct red ring with a clear center, dry, scaly skin, and itching on the affected part

C. Diagnosis: based on the symptoms

D. Treatment and nursing interventions
   1. Washing the affected areas with soap and water and removal of crusts
   2. Antifungal ointment to affected areas as ordered
   3. Antifungal oral medication as ordered (see Chapter 3); tinea capitis is treated orally for 1 month

Pediculosis

A. Definition: infestation by lice of the scalp and hairy areas of the body

B. Symptoms: severe itching in the affected area, appearance of lice on the hair or clothing

C. Diagnosis: based on the symptoms

D. Treatment and nursing interventions
   1. Pediculicide shampoo to hair or scalp as ordered; remaining nits are removed with an extra-fine-tooth comb
   2. Resistant head lice may be treated successfully with systemic trimethoprim-sulfamethoxazole (Bactrim)
   3. Washing of all linens and clothing in hot water to destroy the nits (small lice) and eggs of the lice
   4. Emphasis on importance of follow-up treatment to prevent reinfestation

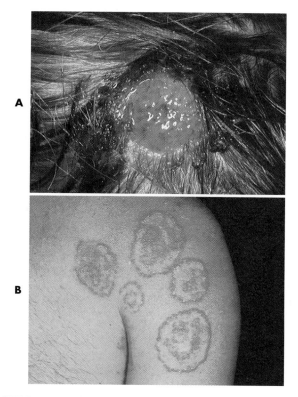

FIGURE 8-12. **A,** Tinea capitis. **B,** Tinea corporis. Both infections are caused by *Microsporum canis,* the "kitten" or "puppy" fungus. *(From Habif TP:* Clinical dermatology: a color guide to diagnosis and therapy, ed 3, *St Louis, 1996, Mosby.)*

5. Examination and treatment of other family members (if affected)
6. Report to school or day-care facility

Hives (Urticaria)

A. Definition: an allergic reaction on the skin, usually caused by an allergy to food or drugs
B. Symptoms: bright red, raised wheals on the skin and itching of the affected areas
C. Diagnosis: based on the symptoms; allergy testing may be done to determine the specific allergen
D. Treatment and nursing interventions
   1. Determination and removal of the allergen
   2. Antihistamines as ordered to decrease the swelling and inflammation
   3. Cool-water soaks to the affected areas to decrease the itching
   4. Local soothing antipruritic lotions to affected areas as ordered
   5. Keeping the child's nails short to avoid itching and possible infection

Rheumatic Fever

A. Definition: autoimmune reaction to a group A beta hemolytic streptococcal pharyngitis (strep throat); involves the joints, skin, brain, and heart

B. Symptoms: begin 2 to 6 weeks after the initial streptococcal infection; lethargy, anorexia, muscle and joint pain, fever, polyarthritis, chorea (muscle tremors and emotional upset), and carditis (Figure 8-13)
C. Diagnosis: based on the symptoms; specific diagnosis is based on the Jones criteria (Box 8-2, p. 481)
D. Treatment and nursing interventions
   1. Bed rest to decrease the workload on the heart and help prevent or ease the carditis
   2. Feeding meals to the child during strict bed rest
   3. Medications as ordered, including salicylates for pain, steroids to decrease inflammation of the muscle and connective tissue, and antibiotics to fight infection (penicillin is the drug of choice) (see Chapter 3)
   4. Emotional support and nonstressful diversion for the child during bed rest
   5. Monitoring of frequent laboratory tests, including the WBC count and the erythrocyte sedimentation rate (ESR) (elevated in inflammatory diseases)
   6. Parent and child teaching for home care, including the need for rest, proper nutrition, proper administration of medications, and the need for prophylactic antibiotic therapy before dental work and invasive procedures

Diabetes Mellitus

A. Definition: in type 1 diabetes, the beta cells of the pancreas stop producing insulin, which is necessary for the metabolism of fats, carbohydrates, and proteins; peak incidence is 10 to 15 years of age
B. Symptoms: rapid onset of symptoms, including easy fatigability, polydipsia (excessive thirst), polyphagia (increased appetite), polyuria (increased urine output), glycosuria (glucose in the urine), and weight loss
C. Diagnosis: based on the symptoms, blood glucose levels, and the presence of glucose and ketones in the urine
D. Treatment and nursing interventions
   1. Daily insulin administration by subcutaneous injections (usually twice a day) or by a means of a portable insulin pump (see Chapter 3)
   2. Meal plan that includes three meals and between-meal snacks as planned by a dietitian, based on the child's age, weight, blood sugars, and normal eating pattern
   3. Routine blood sugar monitoring; Chemstrips, Accu-check, or one-touch glucometers are commonly used for this purpose
   4. Routine urine testing for glucose and ketones may be done
   5. Child and parent teaching regarding insulin injection technique, diet, exercise, urine testing, blood glucose monitoring, signs of hypoglycemia and hyperglycemia, sick day rules, long-term complications, and need for regular follow-up visits to the pediatrician
   6. Support group for parents and child

ADOLESCENCE (AGES 13 TO 19)

Normal Growth and Development
Physical Development

A. During the adolescent period, a growth spurt takes place; this accelerated growth includes an increase in both height and weight; in girls, this occurs between 10 and

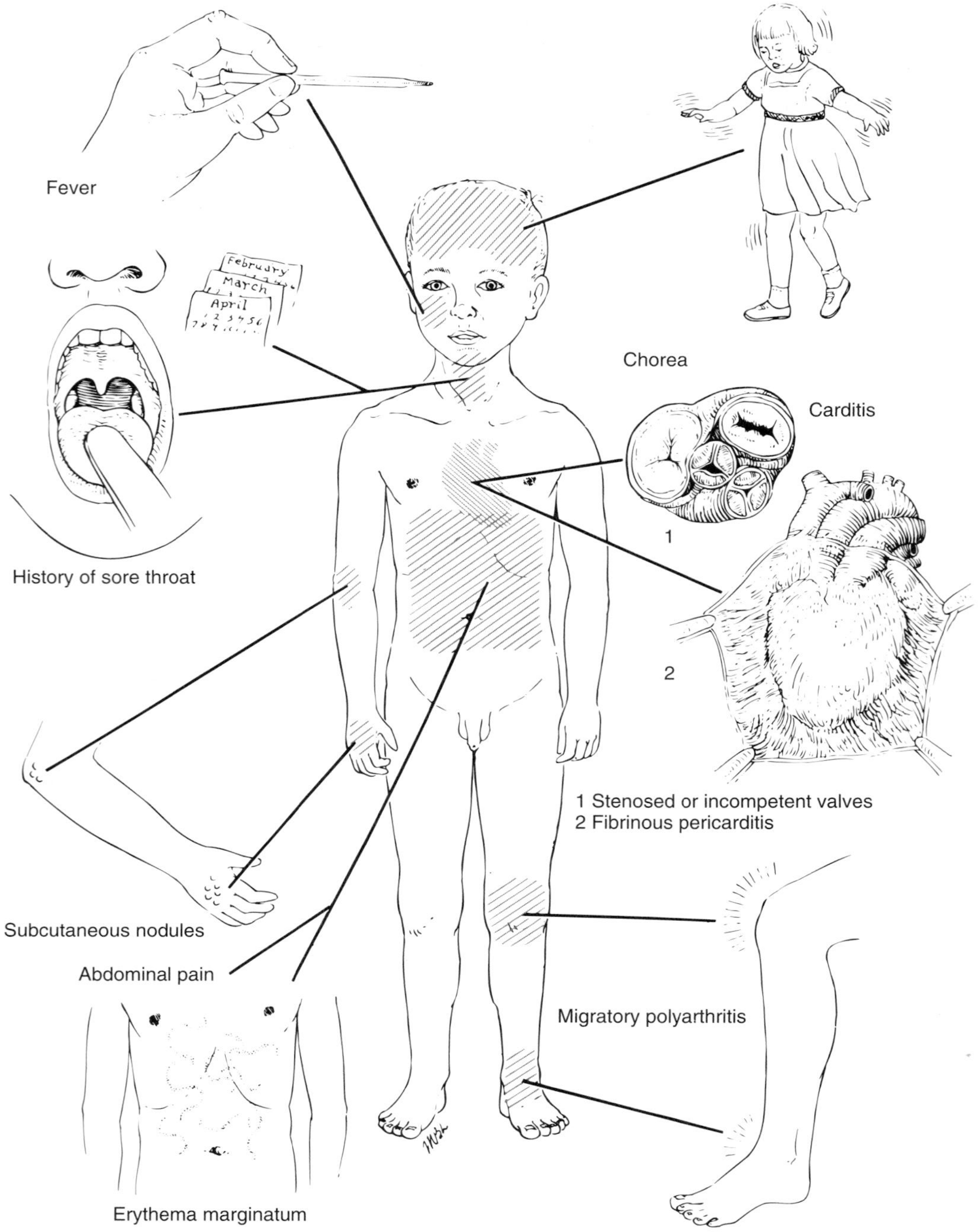

FIGURE 8-13.   Signs and symptoms of rheumatic fever. *(From Novak JC, Broom BL: Ingalls & Salerno's maternal and child health nursing, ed 9, St Louis, 1999, Mosby.)*

12 years of age; in boys it occurs between 12 and 14 years of age

B. Secondary sex characteristics also develop during early adolescence
   1. In girls, the pelvis widens, the breasts develop and enlarge, and body hair starts to appear
   2. In boys, the penis and scrotum enlarge, and pubic and facial hair start to appear; puberty in boys officially begins with the first nocturnal emission

Psychological and Emotional Development

A. Adolescence is the time of transition from childhood to adulthood; adolescents are in Erikson's stage of "identity vs. role confusion"; they are in the process of developing a self-image or a sense of identity about who they are and what they want in life; if they do not develop a positive self-image and identity, they may develop a sense of inferiority, or a negative self-image

B. Adolescents are in Kohlberg's stage of morality known as self-accepted moral principles (level 3); the focus in on

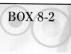

| BOX 8-2 | Guidelines for the Diagnosis of Initial Attack of Rheumatic Fever (Jones Criteria, 1992 Update)* |

Major Manifestations
Carditis
Polyarthritis
Chorea
Erythema marginatum
Subcutaneous nodules

Minor Manifestations
Clinical findings
• Previous rheumatic fever or rheumatic heart disease
• Arthralgia
• Fever
Laboratory findings
• Acute phase reactants
   ▪ Erythrocyte sedimentation rate
   ▪ C-reactive protein, leukocytosis
• Prolonged PR interval

Supporting Evidence of Streptococcal Infection
Increased titer of streptococcal antibodies
• Antistreptolysin O (ASO)
• Other antibodies
Positive throat culture for group A Streptococcus
Recent scarlet fever

From Guidelines for the Diagnosis of Rheumatic Fever, *JAMA* 268:2070, 1992. Copyright©1992, American Medical Association.
*The presence of two major criteria or of one major and two minor criteria indicates a high probability of the presence of rheumatic fever. Evidence of a preceding streptococcal infection greatly strengthens the possibility of acute rheumatic fever; its absence should make the diagnosis doubtful (except in Sydenham's chorea or long-standing carditis).

individual rights and principles of conscience, with a concern for what is best for all
C. Development of a positive self-image and healthy personality depends a great deal on the adolescents' relationships with their peer group, as well as with their family
D. Body image is the major part of adolescents' self-concept; sexuality and sexual feelings are a new part of their body images; physical appearance is important to how they perceive themselves as being accepted by their peer group
  1. Boys' responses to puberty include pleasure at becoming a "man" as evidenced by enlargement of the sex organs, being able to shave, and the sexual feelings they begin to have during this stage; because of their strong sex drive, they often masturbate to relieve themselves of strong sexual tension
  2. Girls' responses to puberty include a developing awareness of their bodily changes, both internal and external (e.g., hormonal changes, menstruation); the sex drive in girls is usually not as strong as it is in boys

Health Promotion

A. Immunizations and physical examinations should continue according to schedule
B. Counseling and sex education, especially concerning acquired immunodeficiency syndrome (AIDS), venereal disease, and birth control should continue to be made available to all adolescents
C. Counseling regarding drug and alcohol abuse should continue to be presented and readily available to all adolescents who are in need of it
D. Emotional stress is high during adolescence; psychiatric counseling is necessary for some adolescents to work through their stresses and fears
E. Proper nutrition needs may not be met because of increased snacking, especially on high-calorie, high-fat foods; nutritional counseling may be helpful

Health Problems
Substance Abuse (Drugs, Alcohol)

A. Definition: abuse of alcohol or mood-altering drugs, usually because of peer pressure or increased tension and stress
B. Signs of abuse: increased school absences, poor academic performance, changes in behavior patterns, wearing dark glasses inside, wearing long-sleeved shirts or blouses every day, and a sloppy, unclean appearance; signs often depend on the drug being used
C. Diagnosis: based on the symptoms (signs of abuse)
D. Substances abused
  1. Alcohol
  2. Narcotics
  3. Psychedelic drugs (lysergic acid diethylamide [LSD], marijuana, phencyclidine [PCP])
  4. Depressants (barbiturates, methaqualone [Quaalude])
  5. Minor tranquilizers (Valium)
  6. Hallucinogens (marijuana, LSD, PCP)
  7. Analgesics (codeine)
  8. Opiates (heroin, morphine, methadone)
  9. Valium
  10. Organic solvents (e.g., glue, cleaning fluids)
  11. Stimulants (amphetamines ["speed"], cocaine, Ecstasy [3,4-methylenedioxy-n-methylamphetamine (MDMA) —"date rape" drug])
  12. Inhalants
  13. Tobacco
E. Treatment and nursing interventions
  1. Prevention of the problem is of course the best treatment
  2. Emergency measures when necessary (such as CPR and gastric lavage)
  3. Psychiatric counseling as needed for the adolescent and family; identify reason or reasons for drug abuse
  4. Follow-up health care; group support and counseling as needed for adolescent and family

Suicide

A. Definition: the act of taking one's own life voluntarily
B. Etiology: suicide usually does not occur without warning; the adolescent usually has a history of emotional problems, difficult relationships, and emotional upsets, including factors such as divorce in the family, death of a family member or friend, or a self-identity crisis
C. Treatment and nursing interventions
  1. Prevention is the best treatment; listen for verbal clues, such as, "After tomorrow, it won't matter anymore"; watch for warning signs, such as giving away favorite possessions
  2. Psychiatric counseling to determine the reasons for the adolescent's actions; this should also include the family members

3. Follow-up medical care as needed
4. Emotional support and counseling for the family members, especially during the crisis stages

Anorexia Nervosa and Bulimia

A. Definition (eating disorders can occur together or separately)
   1. Anorexia nervosa: an eating disorder characterized by a refusal to maintain a minimally normal body weight; most often seen in female adolescents
   2. Bulimia: an eating disorder characterized by repeated episodes of "binge eating," followed by inappropriate compensatory measures, such as self-induced vomiting; misuse of laxatives, diuretics, or other medications; fasting; or excessive exercise
B. Symptoms
   1. With anorexia nervosa, three basic psychological disturbances occur: the inability to correctly perceive body size, the absence of hunger or inability to perceive hunger, and feelings of inadequacy or lack of self-esteem; other symptoms include amenorrhea, constipation, dry skin, low blood pressure, anemia, lanugo (fine, soft hair) on the back and arms
   2. With bulimia, as the disease increases, the frequency of binges increases; the adolescent loses control over the binge-purge cycle; other symptoms include loss of tooth enamel, dental caries, esophageal varices
C. Diagnosis: based on the symptoms, family history, and psychologic evaluation
D. Treatment and nursing interventions
   1. The adolescent is usually hospitalized to correct the malnutrition and to identify and treat the psychological cause
   2. Behavior-modification techniques are often used to assist in changing the adolescent's behavior; for example, privileges or visitors are withdrawn until the adolescent begins to gain weight
   3. Psychological counseling for the adolescent and family members to determine the cause

Crohn's Disease

A. Definition: a chronic, recurrent inflammatory disorder of the intestines; occurs most often in upper-middle-class men and women, ages 15 to 35 years
B. Symptoms: regional ileitis causing acute low abdominal pain, fever, chronic diarrhea, weight loss, abdominal tenderness and distention, anemia, and failure to grow
C. Diagnosis based on the symptoms, x-ray films of the intestine (barium enema), endoscopy, and mucosal biopsy of the intestines
D. Treatment and nursing interventions
   1. The goal of treatment is to relieve the symptoms and discomfort
   2. Adequate rest and relaxation to alleviate stress
   3. High protein, high calorie, low-fiber diet
   4. Corticosteroids as ordered to decrease inflammation of the intestines
   5. Sulfasalazine as ordered (because this interferes with the absorption of folic acid, folic acid may be ordered)
   6. Antidiarrheal drugs as ordered
   7. Antispasmodic drugs as ordered to relieve intestinal spasms
   8. Emotional support and psychological counseling as needed to decrease the stress level

Mononucleosis

A. Definition: an acute infectious viral disease, causing an increase in mononuclear WBCs and signs of general infection; usually thought to be only mildly contagious and is spread by oral contact; the Epstein-Barr virus is the principal cause
B. Symptoms: general malaise, sore throat, fever, enlarged lymph glands, lack of energy, headache, red, flat rash on the body, tonsillitis
C. Diagnosis: based on the symptoms, an elevated WBC count, and a positive Monospot blood test, which indicates increased agglutinins in the blood count
D. Treatment and nursing interventions
   1. Antibiotics as ordered
   2. Antipyretics to relieve fever and discomfort
   3. Increased oral fluids; IV fluids may be ordered for severe dehydration
   4. Gargles or lozenges as ordered for sore throat
   5. Adequate rest and sleep
   6. Diet as tolerated; if the patient can only tolerate fluids, high-calorie fluids should be provided
   7. Patient teaching regarding follow-up care, including the need for adequate rest and sleep

Acne Vulgaris

A. Definition: a disorder of the sebaceous glands; the glands become irritated with the secretion of sebum and the interaction of the sebum with the hormones; the glands become impacted with sebum and form comedones (noninflamed) and papules and pustules (inflamed)
B. Symptoms: the appearance of the comedones, papules, and pustules on the face; they can also appear on other places on the body such as the chest and back
C. Diagnosis: based on the symptoms
D. Treatment and nursing interventions
   1. Cleaning the affected areas with soap or soap substitute and water daily
   2. A diet low in greasy foods, chocolate, and nuts to help decrease the amount of oil in the skin while avoiding other foods that tend to exacerbate the condition
   3. Nonprescription topical creams and lotions (such as benzoyl peroxide and Retin-A) have limited effectiveness; retinoic acid (Accutane) is reserved for severe acne that has not responded to other treatments; a pregnancy test should be done before beginning Accutane
   4. Encouraging the adolescent to keep stress levels to a minimum when possible may help in keeping acne to a minimum
   5. Provide patient teaching: papules and pustules should not be squeezed; they can become infected and spread
   6. Provide counseling for the adolescent to maintain a positive body image

Acquired Immunodeficiency Syndrome (AIDS)

A. Definition: an immune disorder caused by a retrovirus, The human immunodeficiency virus (HIV)
   1. The AIDS virus is known to be transmitted by blood and other body fluids containing blood (semen; saliva) (see Chapter 5, Chapter 7)
   2. Three primary modes of transmission of the AIDS virus in children are prenatal exposure to infected mothers, blood transfusion, and engaging in high-risk

activities (sexual or IV drug use, specifically with adolescents)

3. As of June 2000, more than 8800 children under 13 years of age with AIDS had been reported to the Centers for Disease Control and Prevention (CDC); however, estimates suggest that 1.4 million children under 15 years of age are living with HIV/AIDS; the majority of children with HIV are under 7 years of age; the number of adolescents with HIV continues to increase; AIDS is the ninth leading cause of death in the United States for people ages 15 to 24 years

B. Symptoms: recurrent or chronic infections (because of decreased number of CD-4 T cells), including meningitis, pneumonia, and urinary tract infections; other symptoms include fever, weight loss, FTT, anemia, hepatospleno-megaly, persistent lymphadenopathy

C. Diagnosis: abnormal laboratory values, including abnormal T-cell ratio, decreased T lymphocytes and hypergamma-globulinemia; history of possible exposure to AIDS virus; positive HIV test; and history of recurrent infections

D. Treatment and nursing interventions
   1. No cure has been discover for AIDS; thus treatment and nursing care measures are supportive and designed to prevent and alleviate opportunistic infections
   2. Antiretroviral drugs work to prevent reproduction of new virus particles and delay the progression of the disease (see Chapter 3)
   3. Antibiotics and antifungal drugs as ordered (see Chapter 3)
   4. IV gamma globulin may be helpful in compensating for the deficiency of B lymphocytes
   5. Adequate nutrition and fluid intake
   6. Use of standard precautions when caring for the child in the hospital, clinic, or home
   7. Maintaining an environment as free from infection as possible
   8. Immunizations against childhood diseases (as well as the pneumococcal and influenza vaccines) should be given; however, inactivated poliovirus should be given rather than the oral poliovirus
   9. Promotion of normal development of the child
   10. Education and emotional support for the child and family

E. Prognosis: poor, especially in children with AIDS who are under 1 year of age

BATTERED CHILD SYNDROME

A. Definition: abuse of children by parents or other caregivers; the abuse can be physical, sexual, nutritional, or emotional and can occur at any age

B. Characteristics of battered children
   1. They are often from a unplanned pregnancy
   2. Many of them were premature, had a low birth weight, or had major birth defects
   3. They sometimes resemble a person that the parents disliked

C. Characteristics of abusive parents
   1. One parent often has a previous emotional problem
   2. The abuse is usually done by one parent; the other parent knows about the abuse but usually does not report it

3. Abusive parents often have very high expectations of their children; if they do not *perform* up to these expecta-tions, they are *punished*
4. Abusive parents are often substance abusers
5. The most common characteristic of abusive parents is that often they were abused themselves as children; however, this is not always true
6. Abusive parents come from all socioeconomic levels

D. Identifying the battered child
   1. The child has many scars, bruises, and injuries that are not consistent with the explanation of the injuries; many of these markings are characteristic of abuse (Figure 8-14)
   2. Bone fractures may be seen on x-ray examination at various stages of healing
   3. The child exhibits signs of physical neglect: malnourish-ment or improper or dirty clothing
   4. The parents' explanations of the child's injury are incon-sistent; one parent's explanation differs from the other parent's, or it changes from one time to the next
   5. The child withdraws when approached by the parents, nurse, or physician
   6. The parents' emotional reaction is consistent with the extent of the child's injury

E. Nursing interventions for the battered child and parents
   1. Interview the parents calmly regarding the history of the incident; document all information carefully
   2. Nursing personnel must control their own feelings and attitudes toward the parents so as to work effectively with the family
   3. Provide physical care for the child as needed
   4. Emotional care for the child should include providing a safe environment, explaining all procedures, providing toys and familiar belongings while the child is hospital-ized, and provide physical cuddling and holding when appropriate
   5. Referrals should be made to the hospital social worker, the local department of children and family services, the police, and the psychologist as needed; nurses are considered "mandated reporters" and must report all suspected and confirmed cases of abuse and neglect

POISONINGS

A. The most common age for poisoning deaths in young chil-dren in the United States is 1 to 4 years of age; most poi-sonings occur as a result of oral ingestion; children are poisoned by plants, insecticides, household and personal care products, medicines, vitamins, lead, and carbon monoxide

B. Assessment and treatment begin with an accurate history of the ingestion; laboratory tests are performed to assess serum levels of the substance involved; other laboratory tests and x-ray examinations are performed as needed

C. When a child who has ingested a poison arrives at the hospital, the first step in treatment is to assess the airway, breathing, and circulation (ABC); when the child is stabi-lized, the main goal is to remove the poison, prevent further absorption of the poison, and limit complications

D. Treatment is specific to the type of poison ingested (see Table 8-3, p. 485)

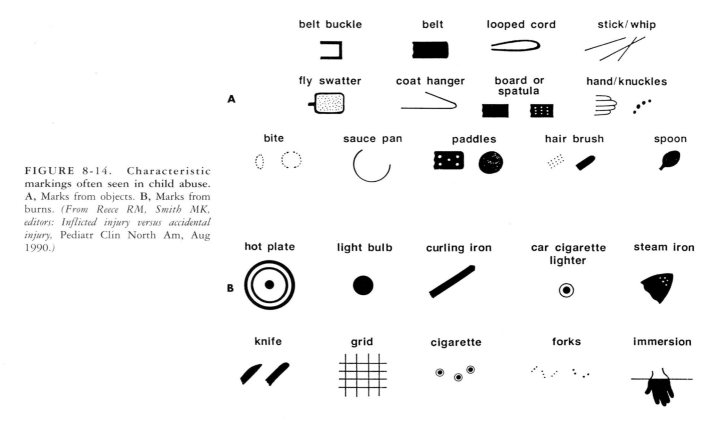

FIGURE 8-14. Characteristic markings often seen in child abuse. A, Marks from objects. B, Marks from burns. *(From Reece RM, Smith MK, editors: Inflicted injury versus accidental injury,* Pediatr Clin North Am, Aug 1990.)*

HOSPITALIZATION AND THE CHILD

A. Preparation for hospitalization
   1. The rationale for preparing children for hospitalization is based on the theory that fear of the unknown is more severe than fear of the known
   2. Preadmission preparation can be done by both parents and professionals (nurses and physicians) honestly at a level the child can understand
   3. Hospital admission procedures include the admission history, blood tests, chest x-ray studies when necessary, physical examination, and placement in the child's room and bed; these procedures should be explained to the child during preadmission preparation
   4. Establish a good working relationship with the parents by answering their questions honestly; in preparing the child for any hospital procedure, the nurse or parent should include all necessary information regarding the procedure and any necessary preparation; time should be allowed for questions from the child and parents
B. Hospitalization as a crisis
   1. Children are more vulnerable to the crisis of illness and hospitalization because stress is a change from their usual state of health and routine, and children have a limited number of coping mechanisms to deal with stressful events
   2. Their reactions to stress differ in each developmental age group
      a. Infants and toddlers: major stress is separation anxiety (fear of being separated from their parents and family)
      b. Preschoolers: major stresses are separation anxiety and fear of loss of body control and of bodily injury and pain
      c. School-age children: major stresses are fear of separation (sometimes more from peers than from family), of loss of body control, and of bodily injury, mutilation, pain, and death
      d. Adolescents: major stresses are fear of separation from their peer group; of loss of body control, independence and identity; and of bodily injury and pain, especially concerning sexual changes
   3. Nursing measures can be used to minimize the hospitalized child's fears and stresses
      a. Provide open visiting for parents and siblings; visiting by peers in the school-age and adolescent groups should be encouraged
      b. Explain procedures or preparation for procedures at the child's age level (medical play)
      c. Allow the child to have favorite toys and games from home
      d. Nursing personnel should not lie to the child about the parents' visits; the visits should not be used as rewards or as something to be withheld if the child does not cooperate or behave
      e. Allow the child as much physical freedom as his or her condition will allow
      f. Allow the child to participate in decision making as much as possible, especially regarding treatments and procedures; this allows the child some control in the situation
      g. Encourage the parents to visit as much as possible; explain all procedures to them, and encourage them to assist in their child's care if they are comfortable in doing so

TABLE 8-3   Common Poisonous Substances

Substance	Pathophysiology	Clinical Manifestations	Treatment
Acetaminophen (Tylenol, Many Over-the-Counter Products)			
Toxic dose: uncertain; do not exceed recommended levels. Seriousness of ingestion determined by amount ingested and length of time before intervention, and if it is an acute or accumulative toxicity. Other factors, such as decreased oral intake have been linked with hepatotoxicity.	Metabolic by-products deplete liver glutathione and cause damage to hepatic cells. Children younger than 6 yr seem to be more resistant to development of hepatotoxicity than do older children and adults.	*First stage* (first 24 hr): malaise, nausea, vomiting, sweating, pallor, weakness *Second stage* (24-48 hr): latent period, with a rise in liver enzymes (aspartate and alanine aminotransferase) and bilirubin, right upper quadrant pain, prolonged prothrombin time *Third stage* (3-7 days): jaundice, liver necrosis, signs of hepatic failure *Fourth stage* (5-7 days): recovery or progression to death	Induce vomiting or gastric lavage within 1 hr of ingestion, depending on amount ingested. Administer antidote: N-acetylcysteine (Mucomyst) as ordered. IV fluids Sodium-restricted, high-calorie, high-protein diet
Salicylates (Aspirin, Many Over-the-Counter Products, Oil of Wintergreen)			
Toxic dose: single dose exceeding 200-280 mg/kg Peak gastric absorption occurs within 2 hr of ingestion.	*First stage:* stimulation of respiratory center, leading to respiratory alkalosis *Second stage:* loss of potassium; increase in metabolic rate; accumulation of ketones, leading to metabolic acidosis, hypokalemia, and dehydration Inhibition of prothrombin formation, decreased platelet levels and adhesiveness, capillary fragility (chronic poisoning)	GI effects: nausea, vomiting, thirst CNS effects: hyperventilation, tinnitus, confusion, seizures, coma, respiratory failure, circulatory collapse Renal effect: oliguria Hematopoietic effects: bleeding tendencies Metabolic effects: sweating, dehydration, fever, hyponatremia, hypokalemia, dehydration, hypoglycemia	Induce vomiting with syrup of ipecac or perform gastric lavage; administer activated charcoal to decrease absorption. IV fluids, sodium bicarbonate (enhances excretion), potassium replacement; volume expanders as needed to support circulation Vitamin K for bleeding tendencies (chronic poisoning) Glucose for hypoglycemia Hemodialysis in severe cases if child unresponsive to therapy
Corrosives (Toilet and Drain Cleaners, Bleach, Ammonia)			
Extent of damage depends on causticity of substance and amount ingested.	Severe chemical burns of mouth, throat, esophagus; "splash" burns of eyes and skin Alkali substances can continue to cause damage after initial contact. If damage is severe, long-term care is needed, including gastric button or tube, repeated esophageal dilations, and surgical repair of esophagus, sometimes with colon tissue transplant (done when child is older).	Whitish burns of mouth and pharynx, color darkens (red, swollen, oozing as ulcerations form and tissue erodes) Edema, difficulty swallowing, drooling Respiratory distress, pain Difficulty swallowing; subsequent healing of burns can produce esophageal strictures Severe burns causing perforation, which can lead to vascular collapse and shock	All medical personnel wear protective equipment; corrosives continue to burn. Do not induce vomiting; do not lavage. Activated charcoal may be given. Dilute with small amounts of water or milk (take care not to stimulate vomiting). Flood external areas with large amount of water. Endoscopy to diagnose esophageal burns

IV, Intravenous; *GI,* gastrointestinal; *CNS,* central nervous system; *NPO,* nothing by mouth; *EDTA,* ethylenediaminetetraacetic acid.
From James SR, Ashwill JW, Droske SC: *Nursing care of children: principles and practice,* ed 2, Philadelphia, 2002, WB Saunders.

Continued

TABLE 8-3   Common Poisonous Substances—cont'd

Substance	Pathophysiology	Clinical Manifestations	Treatment
			Possible gastrostomy, possible esophageal dilations to prevent strictures and to maintain patency of esophagus IV fluids while NPO Analgesics, steroids, antibiotics, nasogastric tube feedings

Hydrocarbons (Gasoline, Kerosene, Paint Thinner, Lighter Fluid, Turpentine, Furniture Polish)

Substance	Pathophysiology	Clinical Manifestations	Treatment
Extent of damage depends on amount of substance ingested	Chemical pneumonitis from aspiration of hydrocarbon Pneumonia and acute hemorrhagic necrotizing disease, usually in 24 hr	Burning sensation in mouth and pharynx Characteristic petroleum breath odor Nausea, vomiting, anorexia, CNS depression, fever Respiratory distress, wheezing	Do not induce vomiting. Support ventilation; administer oxygen. IV fluids

Lead (Paint Chips from Older Homes, Soil Contaminated with Lead, Lead Solder Used in Plumbing, Vinyl Mini-Blinds, Improperly Glazed Pottery)

Substance	Pathophysiology	Clinical Manifestations	Treatment
Diet high in fat and low in iron and calcium increases lead absorption. Serum lead level >10 μg/dl: considered harmful; 10-15 μg/dl: more frequent screening indicated; 15-20 μg/dl: nutritional and educational interventions and environmental investigation; >20 μg/dl: possible removal and treatment	GI tract is a major route of absorption. Lead is deposited in blood, bone, and soft tissue. Major toxic effects occur in bone marrow, nervous system, and kidney. Amount of lead ingested, size of the particle, and repeated ingestion over time contribute to severity of lead poisoning.	Symptoms may be vague with insidious onset. CNS effects: irritability, lethargy, hyperactivity, cognitive and perceptual-motor difficulties, clumsiness, seizures, coma, and death (associated with blood level of 100 μg/dl) Hematopoietic effect: anemia GI effects: anorexia, nausea, vomiting, constipation, lead line along gums Skeletal effects: increased density of long bones, lead line in long bones Renal effects: glycosuria, proteinuria, possible acute or chronic renal failure; although kidney damage is reversible early in the disease, with continued lead exposure, permanent kidney damage may occur.	>25 μg/dl: remove child from lead source, hospitalize if level is significantly higher. Administer chelating agents: succimer orally for lead level of 35-45 μg/dl; EDTA for level >70 μg/dl given IV over several hours for 5 days (causes lead to be deposited in bone and excreted by kidneys); bronchoalveolar lavage every 4 hr for six doses for level >70 μg/dl. Monitor kidney function because EDTA is nephrotoxic; monitor calcium levels because EDTA enhances excretion of calcium. Provide adequate hydration. Calcium, phosphorus, and vitamins C and D Anticonvulsants Oral or intramuscular iron for anemia Follow-up lead levels to monitor progress (lead is excreted more slowly than it accumulates in the body).

TABLE 8-3	Common Poisonous Substances—cont'd		
Substance	Pathophysiology	Clinical Manifestations	Treatment
Carbon Monoxide			
Most often from improperly ventilated heaters; also from poorly ventilated vehicles. Cause of the exposure should be determined and eliminated.	An odorless, colorless gas that binds to receptors on hemoglobin more effectively than does oxygen, thereby causing hypoxia	Headache, visual disturbances. Altered level of consciousness, cherry-red lips and cheeks, nausea, and vomiting	100% oxygen by rebreathing mask. Serum carboxyhemoglobin levels; hyperbaric chamber treatment may be necessary for patients with high carboxyhemoglobin levels. Other interventions based on signs and symptoms

h. Instruct the parents not to lie to the child; lying only sets up a sense of mistrust among the child, the parents, and the hospital staff
i. Administer pain medications as ordered whenever necessary; a child's pain response is affected by developmental level
j. Expect some regressive behavior during the child's hospital stay; tell the parents that this is normal during stressful periods

C. Use of play during hospitalization
1. Play in the hospital helps relieve tension and anxiety, lessens the stress of separation and feelings of homesickness, and helps the child relax and feel more secure
2. The play activities should be based on the child's age, interests, and limitations
3. Play can be used for diversion, for recreation, and to play out the child's fears and anxieties over his illness and treatment
4. Toys can come from home or from the hospital play area; they can even be adapted from hospital "stock" supplies
5. Play therapy can be used to teach the child about procedures and surgery, as well as to help the child work through fears and anxieties about hospitalization

D. Preparation and teaching for discharge
1. Preparation for discharge should begin during the admission by setting long-term goals concerning discharge
2. Discharge planning should include several areas
   a. Parent-child teaching regarding home-care procedures and medication regimen
   b. Follow-up care, including physician appointments and the importance of keeping them
   c. Referrals to community agencies, public health nurses, and other resources as needed

Nursing Care of the Hospitalized Child

A. Safety factors
1. Side rails should be kept up at all times when the child is in bed; if the bed is adjustable, it should be kept in the low position
2. When restraints are used, they should be applied securely to the child; extremities should be checked frequently for impaired circulation caused by tight restraints; appropriate charting should be done

3. Small toys, game pieces, and other small objects should be kept away from infants and toddlers who may swallow them
4. Toddlers and young children should not be left unattended in their rooms or hallways; if they are out of bed, they should be observed continuously to avoid accidents and injuries
5. Medications, needles, and syringes should be kept out of the reach of all children

B. Medication administration
1. General guidelines in giving medications to children
   a. Approach the child with a cheerful, positive attitude, and explain what you are going to do
   b. Be honest when talking to the child; tell the child it is medicine, not "juice" or "candy."
   c. When necessary, use foods or liquids to disguise the taste of bad-tasting medications
   d. Oral syringes or syringes without needles may be used to deliver oral medications to infants and young children
   e. Allow the child some control in the situation; make sure the question you ask the child is appropriate to the child's age level and the situation
   f. Intramuscular (IM) injections are safer and easier to give to a young child if a second person helps restrain the child
   g. Tell the child that it is all right to cry if the shot "hurts"; offer a bandage strip
   h. Teach the child to "say NO" to street drugs but that the medicines received in the hospital are okay to take
2. Safe IM injection technique includes the same steps used for IM injections in adults
   a. In infants, the lateral thigh (vastus lateralis muscle) should be used
   b. In toddlers and preschoolers, the ventrogluteal area is the preferred site (lateral thigh can also be used)
   c. In older children and adolescents, other regularly used injection sites may be used (ventrogluteal muscle is the safest; deltoid and dorsogluteal muscles may also be used) (Figure 8-15)

C. Assisting with treatments and procedures
1. All tests and procedures should be explained to the child in an honest, simple manner; older children and

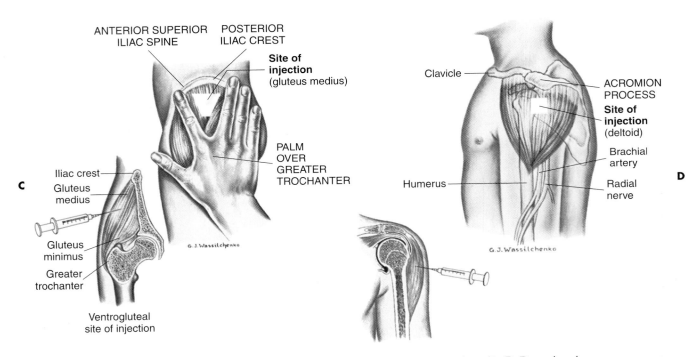

FIGURE 8-15.   Acceptable intramuscular sites in children. A, Vastus lateralis. **B,** Dorsogluteal.
C, Ventrogluteal. **D,** Deltoid. *(From Hockenberry MJ et al: Wong's nursing care of infants and children,*
ed 7, St Louis, 2003, Mosby.)

adolescents should be allowed to ask questions and receive answers,
2. All children should be allowed to say "ouch" or to cry if the procedure is a painful one; rewards are often given after a painful procedure (a reward sticker, toy, or special food treat)
3. The child may need to be held or restrained in certain positions for procedures; all equipment should be assembled before the procedure is started so that the nurse can stay with the child as much as possible

D. Preoperative teaching
1. Patient teaching in pediatrics should include the child (preschool age and older) and the parents; both should be involved in the teaching and preparation for surgery
2. Use words that the child can understand; audiovisual aids (pictures, dolls, puppets, and bandages) are extremely useful in helping the child understand the procedure or surgery
3. Be honest with the child, especially regarding procedures or treatments that may be uncomfortable or painful

4. Tell the child that he or she will not feel any pain during the surgery because of the "special sleep" of anesthesia and that he or she will wake up after surgery is over in the recovery room

5. Include details specific to the child's surgery such as dressings, tubes, IV fluids, medications, the specific site of the pain or discomfort, and the diet restrictions before and after surgery

E. General postoperative care
  1. Basic postoperative care is similar to nursing care of adult postoperative patients
    a. Frequent vital signs; pulse oximetry, as needed
    b. Observation of the incision or dressings
    c. Level of consciousness
    d. I&O, IV fluids, Foley catheter, NG tube
    e. Administering pain medications as needed (IV, PO, epidurals; IM may be used but should be avoided)
  2. Allow the child's parents to assist in the child's care if they desire to do so
  3. Explain all postoperative procedures before doing them

F. Care of the child in a cast
  1. The child should be repositioned every 2 hours to allow the cast to dry completely
  2. Observe and record the condition of the skin at the edges of the cast for color, warmth, irritation, sensation, and edema; cast should be handled lightly with open palms while it is still damp to avoid indentations

3. Check the color of the nail beds below the cast; check the pulse in the area below the cast if it is in an accessible area (radial or pedal pulse)

4. Teach the child not to put anything inside the cast or to "scratch" the skin beneath the cast

5. Check the cast for drainage or discoloration; any drainage should be marked, timed, dated, and documented

6. Observe for signs of osteomyelitis (most commonly seen after injury, surgery to a long bone): pain, tenderness at site of infection, fever, irritability; osteomyelitis is most often caused by *Staphylococcus aureus* organism

7. Protect the cast from water, urine, and stool

8. "Petal" the edges of the cast before the patient goes home. (If cast is damp, teach parents the proper way to do it.)

9. Before discharge, talk to the parents regarding a safe method for restraining the child with a cast while in the car; infants and children in long leg and hip spica casts will need adapted car seats or safety belts, or both

G. Care of the child in traction
  1. Types of traction
    a. Skeletal: uses pins, wires, and tongs
    b. Skin: uses tapes, plastic, and bandages attached to the skin

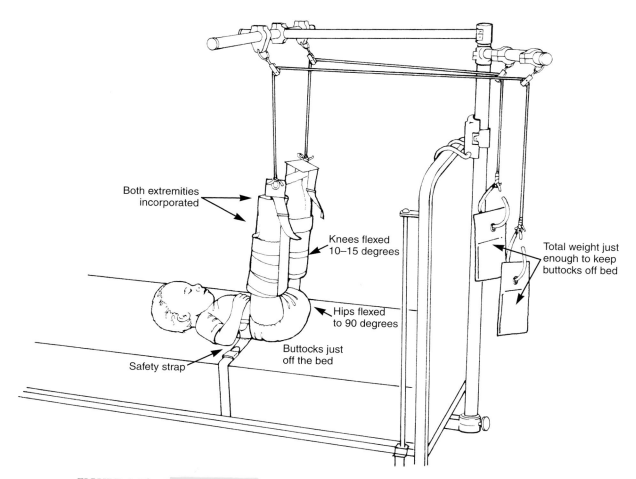

Both extremities incorporated

Knees flexed 10–15 degrees

Hips flexed to 90 degrees

Total weight just enough to keep buttocks off bed

Buttocks just off the bed

Safety strap

FIGURE 8-16. Bryant's traction is used with children under 3 years of age and weighing less than 35 lb (15.9 kg) who have developmental dysplasia of the hip. (*From Folcik MA, Carina-Garcia G, Birmingham JJ: Traction: assessment and management, St Louis, 1994, Mosby.*)

c. Bryant's, modified Bryant's: a type of skin traction; most commonly used in infants and toddlers for treatment of a fractured femur and congenital hip dislocation (Figure 8-16)

2. Nursing care measures for the child in traction

a. Explain the traction apparatus to the child; allow the child to participate in his or her care as much as possible

b. Maintain traction alignment; be sure that all ropes are in the center tracks of the pulleys and that the weights are hanging freely

c. Provide proper skin care; observe for reddened, irritated areas at the edges of the tape and elastic bandages, as well as at other pressure sites

d. Observe skeletal pin sites for bleeding, inflammation, and signs of infection; provide pin-site care as ordered

e. Observe affected extremity for skin color, nail bed color, and changes in sensation and mobility

f. Administer pain medications as ordered, and keep the child as comfortable as possible

g. Provide range-of-motion exercises to the unaffected body parts to help prevent contractures and muscle atrophy

h. Provide toys and activities appropriate to the child's age level and limited mobility

SUGGESTED READINGS

Ball JW: *Mosby's pediatric patient teaching guides,* St Louis, 1998, Mosby.

Jackson PL, Vessey JA: *Primary care of the child with a chronic condition,* ed 2, St Louis, 1996, Mosby.

James SR, Ashwell JW, Droske SC: *Nursing care of children: principles and practice,* ed 2, Philadelphia, 2002, WB Saunders.

James SR, Ashwell JW, Droske SC: *Study guide for nursing care of children: principles and practice,* ed 2, Philadelphia, 2002, WB Saunders.

McCance KL, Huether SE: *Pathophysiology: the biologic basis for disease in adults and children,* ed 3, St Louis, 1999, Mosby.

Wong DL et al: *Whaley & Wong's nursing care of infants and children,* ed 7, St Louis, 2003, Mosby.

Wong DL: *Clinical manual of pediatric nursing,* ed 5, St Louis, 2003, Mosby.

REVIEW QUESTIONS

1. Infancy is the period from:
   1 Birth to 6 weeks of age
   2 Birth to 1 year of age
   3 4 weeks to 1 year of age
   4 4 weeks to 2 years of age

2. Hospitalized adolescents have the most difficulty with:
   1 Dependence vs. independence
   2 Trust vs. autonomy
   3 Reality vs. fantasy
   4 Initiative vs. guilt

3. The best way for the pediatric nurse to establish a good working relationship with parents is to:
   1 Avoid contact whenever possible
   2 Answer their questions honestly
   3 Refer all questions to the physician
   4 Keep them out of their child's room as much as possible

4. Which of the following pathophysiological mechanisms is responsible for respiratory alterations seen in children with Cystic fibrosis (CF)?
   1 Decreased ciliary action, causing stasis of mucus in lungs
   2 Edema of the epiglottis, causing upper airway occlusion
   3 Excessive production of thick mucus, leading to airway obstruction
   4 Laryngeal stricture, leading to bronchospasm

5. The child with Cystic fibrosis (CF) takes pancreatic enzymes with each meal. The purpose of this therapy is to facilitate:
   1 Absorption of vitamins A, C, and K
   2 Increased carbohydrate metabolism for growth
   3 Digestions and absorption of fats and proteins
   4 Sodium excretion and electrolyte balance

6. In caring for a child with Down syndrome (DS), the nurse should be aware that a frequent accompanying defect is:
   1 Congenital heart disease
   2 Congenital hip dysplasia
   3 Central auditory imperception
   4 Pyloric stenosis

7. The safest place to give an infant an IM injection is the:
   1 Deltoid muscle
   2 Vastus lateralis muscle
   3 Ventrogluteal muscle
   4 Dorsogluteal muscle

8. The best, most reliable method of assessing for pinworms in a child is by:
   1 The history, symptoms, and a stool culture
   2 A blood culture
   3 Capturing the eggs from the anal edge on cellophane tape
   4 Sending a stool culture to the laboratory

9. The lateral S-shaped curvature of the spine that most often occurs in school-age girls is:
   1 Scoliosis
   2 Nephrosis
   3 Lordosis
   4 Kyphosis

10. A 2-year-old female patient has a complex febrile seizure in her crib while the nurse is caring for her. What is the most important nursing activity at this time?
    1 Place a seizure stick between her jaws
    2 Prepare the suction equipment
    3 Observe the seizure and protect her from harm
    4 Restrain her to prevent injury

11. Which of the following is responsible for the airway narrowing characteristic of an asthma episode?
    1 Laryngeal edema, dehydration, anxiety
    2 Bronchospasm, edema, increased accumulation of mucus
    3 Increased negative pleural pressure, laryngospasm, mucus plugging
    4 Carbon dioxide retention, pharyngeal hyperemia, alveolar collapse

12. Bulimia is an eating disorder characterized by:
    1 Anorexia with severe weight loss
    2 Binge eating followed by induced vomiting
    3 Sudden weight gain
    4 Chronic diarrhea

13. A 3-month-old infant is admitted to the pediatric unit for treatment of bronchiolitis. Oxygen therapy is ordered for the infant primarily to:
    1 Reduce fever
    2 Allay anxiety and restlessness
    3 Liquefy secretions
    4 Relieve dyspnea and hypoxemia

14. The stage of development where parallel play takes place is:
    1 Infancy
    2 Toddler
    3 Preschool age
    4 School age

15. Which of the following statements about pain in children is true?
    1 A child's behavioral response to pain is affected by his or her age and developmental stage
    2 Recovery from a painful experience occurs at a faster rate in children than it does in adults
    3 Narcotic use in children is dangerous because of the increased risk of addiction and respiratory depression
    4 Immaturity of the nervous system in young children provides them with increased thresholds for pain

16. The first immunizations an infant receives at 2 months of age are:
    1 DPT only
    2 PPD, IPV, first hepatitis B vaccines
    3 DTP, IPV, MMR
    4 DTP, IPV, Hib, second hepatitis B vaccine

17. The leading cause of death in children between 1 year and 14 years of age is:
    1 Meningitis
    2 Leukemia
    3 Accidents
    4 AIDS

18. In caring for a child in a full leg cast, which of the following findings should the nurse report to the physician immediately?
    1 The cast is still damp after 4 hours
    2 The child's pedal pulse is 80 beats per minute (bpm)
    3 The child complains of pain in his leg
    4 The child is unable to move his toes

19. Of the following, the most important criterion on which to base the decision to report suspected child abuse is:
    1 Inappropriate parental concern for the degree of injury
    2 Absence of the parents for questioning about the child's injuries
    3 A complaint other than the one associated with the signs of abuse
    4 Incompatibility between the history given and the injury observed

20. By the end of the school-age years, a child should have developed a sense of:
    1 Initiative, purpose
    2 Industry, competence
    3 Identity, role
    4 Intimacy, fidelity
21. The patient is 2 years of age and her favorite word is "No!" She is in Erikson's developmental stage of:
    1 Trust vs. mistrust
    2 Initiative vs. guilt
    3 Autonomy vs. shame and doubt
    4 Industry vs. inferiority
22. A 12-month-old girl with sickle cell anemia is admitted in sickle cell crisis. Her symptoms might include:
    1 Fever, seizures, coma
    2 Abdominal pain, swollen painful joints
    3 Polycythemia, tachycardia
    4 Severe itching, vomiting
23. The treatment of a child with nephrotic syndrome includes administration of corticosteroids to:
    1 Decrease the amount of proteinuria
    2 Increase the amount of albumin in the blood
    3 Help control hypertension
    4 Reduce edema of the face, extremities, and abdomen
24. A child with asthma would most likely present with which of the following symptoms?
    1 Laryngitis, sore throat, productive cough
    2 Fever, rhinorrhea, coarse breath sounds
    3 Tightness in the chest, nonproductive cough, wheezing
    4 Rapid respiratory rate, difficulty swallowing, fever
25. The two main types of medication used to treat asthma are:
    1 Antiinflammatory agents, immunosuppressants
    2 Bronchodilators, antiinflammatory agents
    3 Antibiotics, bronchodilators
    4 Decongestants, antihistamines
26. The hepatitis B vaccine series should begin at what age?
    1 Newborn
    2 2 months
    3 6 months
    4 12 months
27. A 5-month-old infant with chronic lung disease is admitted with a severe case of respiratory syncytial virus (RSV). Treatment for this child will include:
    1 Cromolyn (Intal) nebulizer treatments, IV fluids
    2 Ribavirin (Virazole), humidified oxygen
    3 Antibiotics, IV fluids
    4 Prednisone (LiquiPred), oxygen
28. Which of the following statements about respiratory syncytial virus (RSV) or bronchiolitis is true?
    1 It occurs primarily in fall and winter
    2 Peak incidence for RSV infection is 6 to 18 months of age
    3 RSV can survive for hours on gloves, countertops, and skin
    4 RSV causes the bronchioles to plug with mucus, trapping air in the lungs
29. At the time of delivery, an infant is born with its abdominal organs, covered by a sac, protruding through an abnormal opening in the umbilical ring. This condition is known as:
    1 Intussusception
    2 Diaphragmatic hernia
    3 Omphalocele
    4 Gastroschisis

30. The nurse is about to give an oral medication to an uncooperative 2-year-old toddler. Which of the following actions would be the best way to give the child the medication?
    1 Get an order to change the medication to an injectable form
    2 Sedate the child
    3 Allow a parent to assist
    4 Use wrist and ankle restraints
31. The treatment of choice for children with infectious gastroenteritis is:
    1 Oral rehydration therapy
    2 IV fluids, antibiotics
    3 The "BRAT" diet
    4 Low-fiber diet, skim milk
32. The symptoms of croup are caused by: *aka Spasmodic laryngitis*
    1 A bacterial infection of the larynx
    2 Inflammation of the trachea and esophagus
    3 Spasms of the larynx
    4 Inflammation of the lungs
33. Discharge planning and preparation for home care of the hospitalized child should begin:
    1 On the day of the discharge
    2 As soon as the discharge order is written
    3 During the admission, by setting long-term goals
    4 Only if the child will need home care and treatment
34. Down syndrome (DS) is:
    1 A chromosomal abnormality
    2 Caused by a bacterial infection
    3 Caused by a viral infection
    4 A result of a lack of oxygen to the brain at birth
35. The most common method of treatment for an infant with a fractured femur is:
    1 Surgery and placement of a pin to set the fracture
    2 Putting the child in skeletal traction
    3 Immediate setting and casting of the fractured leg
    4 Putting the child in Bryant's or modified Bryant's traction
36. Sickle cell disease is caused by:
    1 A virus
    2 An abnormal hereditary trait
    3 Streptococcus bacteria
    4 A mismatched blood transfusion
37. A fungal infection of the skin that can occur on the scalp, body, and feet is:
    1 Ringworm
    2 Pediculosis
    3 Herpes type 2
    4 Urticaria
38. The total number of deciduous teeth is:
    1 18
    2 20
    3 22
    4 24
39. The pediatrician ordered aspirin gr. v PO. The nurse has aspirin 300 mg tablets on hand. The nurse should give:
    1 ½ tablet
    2 1 tablet
    3 1½ tablets
    4 2 tablets
40. A 4-year-old boy is admitted with a diagnosis of nephrotic syndrome. Treatment for this child will include:
    1 High-Fowler's position
    2 Regular diet

3 Diuretics as ordered

4 Sodium and potassium supplements

41. Nursing care for the child with eczema includes:
    1 Keeping the child in the same position
    2 Keeping the child fully clothed
    3 Keeping the skin clean and dry
    4 Warm, moist dressings to relieve the itching

42. The nurse needs to instill eardrops into a 2-year-old toddler's left ear. The correct way to position her ear for administration of the eardrops is to:
    1 Pull the outer ear up and toward the back of the head
    2 Pull the outer ear down and toward the back of the head
    3 Pull the ear lobe down and toward the chin
    4 Pull the ear lobe up and toward the nose

43. Treatment of the preschooler with Kawasaki disease (KD) includes the administration of high-dose IV immuno-globin. This is used to:
    1 Treat the infection causing the Kawasaki disease (KD)
    2 Relax the child and allow the child to get the appropriate rest they need
    3 Maintain proper hydration and blood pressure levels
    4 Decrease the fever and incidence of coronary artery damage

44. The nurse completes her nursing assessment of a normal 18-month-old boy and begins to document her findings. An expected characteristic of a normal 18-month-old child is:
    1 Moving slowly and carefully
    2 "Getting into everything"
    3 Playing quietly and cooperatively with other children
    4 Preferring toys that can be played while sitting still

45. A mother of an otherwise healthy 18 month old tells the nurse that the child has had two diarrhea stools. When she asks what fluids and foods she can safely give the child, the nurse tells her to:
    1 Keep the child NPO until 24 hours after the diarrhea stops
    2 Continue to offer normal diet items, but substitute foods the child especially likes
    3 Encourage fluids (diluted juice, soda, Pedialyte) and offer small crackers
    4 Offer constipating foods, such as cheese, with each meal, and decrease fluid intake

46. The nurse is assigned to care for a 3-year-old boy on the pediatric unit that has a Wilms' tumor. Which nursing intervention is appropriate?
    1 Encourage the child to choose his own activities, but tell him he must accept responsibility for his own safety
    2 Avoid manipulation or pressure on the child's abdomen that can increase the possibility of metastasis
    3 Palpate the tumor each shift to determine any change in size or configuration
    4 At regular intervals, position the child appropriately and perform postural drainage techniques

47. The nurse is caring for a child in acute respiratory distress from bronchitis. One appropriate nursing intervention is to provide a cool moist environment, because it:
    1 Relieves symptoms immediately
    2 Prevents drug toxicity by liquid dispersion in the lungs
    3 Promotes adequate hydration and fever reduction
    4 Reduces inflammation and keeps secretions thin

48. A teenage girl at the pediatrician's office has been diagnosed with infectious mononucleosis. When her mother asks how her daughter might have gotten the disease, the nurse explains to her that it is caused by:
    1 Kissing
    2 Poor health habits
    3 A virus
    4 Bacteria

49. When talking to a mother of a 6-month-old girl who has just been diagnosed as having an intussusception, she asks what intussusception means. The nurse's best response is:
    1 "A hole has developed between two parts of her intestine, the duodenum, and the ileum."
    2 "The lower segment of her bowel has no anal opening."
    3 "One portion of her intestine has telescoped into another portion of the intestine."
    4 "A portion of her bowel has twisted around itself, causing a blockage."

50. A preschooler visiting the pediatrician is diagnosed with eczema. His father asks what can be causing the disease, and the nurse tells him that a likely cause is:
    1 A metabolic disorder
    2 An allergic disorder
    3 An infectious disorder
    4 A nutritional disorder

51. Which child is most likely to develop osteomyelitis?
    1 A child that has experienced a traumatic birth experience
    2 A child that inherited the gene for osteomyelitis
    3 A child that had trauma to a long bone in an extremity
    4 A child that experienced protein loss as a result of inadequate calcium intake

52. Which organism is the major cause of osteomyelitis?
    1 Beta-hemolytic Streptococcus
    2 Haemophilus influenzae
    3 Escherichia coli
    4 Staphylococcus aureus

53. The desired clinical outcome for a child experiencing respiratory distress from epiglottitis is:
    1 The child remains asleep for 8 hours a night
    2 The child is in no pain or discomfort
    3 The airway remains patent
    4 Oral mucus membranes remain moist and pink

54. A 6-year-old child with a 3-year history of celiac disease is brought into the clinic for a checkup. If the child and his family have been in compliance with the necessary diet regimen, the nurse should expect to see:
    1 Slow, steady weight loss
    2 Increase in appetite
    3 Hemoglobin level above 12.0 g/dL
    4 Decrease in steatorrhea

55. During a physical assessment of a young infant, the nurse palpates his suture lines and fontanels. The nurse should expect the anterior fontanel of a normal child to be completely closed at age:
    1 3 to 4 months
    2 6 months
    3 9 to 17 months
    4 18 to 24 months

56. In a 6-month-old infant who is teething, which teeth would the nurse expect to erupt first?
    1 Two lower lateral incisors
    2 Two lower central incisors
    3 Four first molars
    4 Four upper molars

57. During the physical assessment of a child with glomeru-lonephritis, the nurse's priorities should be:
    1 Color, motion, and sensation of lower extremities
    2 Severity of abdominal pain, bowel sounds
    3 Blood pressure, observation for dependent edema
    4 Neurological checks, level of consciousness
58. The posterior fontanel of an infant is expected to be closed:
    1 At the time of birth
    2 Within hours after birth
    3 By the end of the first month of life
    4 By the age of 2 to 3 months
59. What is the legal responsibility of a nurse regarding the reporting of suspected child abuse or neglect?
    1 None; nurses can be sued if they report suspected child abuse or neglect
    2 Nurses must report abuse and neglect to the child's pediatrician before calling a child abuse center
    3 Only physicians are legally required to report abuse or neglect
    4 Nurses must report all suspected and confirmed abuse or neglect
60. A 3-month-old infant is receiving continuous IV fluids because of dehydration. In providing nursing care for her, the nurse's priority should be to:
    1 Help the infant adjust to restricted activities
    2 Relieve the infant's anxiety
    3 Promote fluid elimination
    4 Prevent interference with the IV therapy
61. The theory of child development that is based on psychosocial development as a series of developmental tasks is known as:
    1 Freud's theory
    2 Erikson's theory
    3 Masterson's theory
    4 Piaget's theory
62. Piaget's theory of child development is based on:
    1 Intellectual (cognitive) development
    2 Psychosexual development
    3 Psychosocial development
    4 Social and physical development
63. Normal physical development characteristics for a 1-month-old infant include:
    1 Closed posterior fontanel
    2 Can raise chest supported on forearms
    3 Can turn head from side to side when prone or supine
    4 Can carry hand or an object to the mouth
64. Teething usually begins at the age of:
    1 3 to 4 months
    2 5 months
    3 6 to 7 months
    4 8 months
65. "Stranger anxiety," fear of strangers demonstrated by pushing away and crying, usually begins at age:
    1 4 to 5 months
    2 6 to 7 months
    3 8 to 9 months
    4 10 to 11 months
66. Erikson's theory of development states that the develop-mental task of infancy is:
    1 Autonomy
    2 Trust
    3 Initiative
    4 Gratification

67. An infant with a congenital heart defect that is not eating or growing normally may also be diagnosed with which type of Failure to thrive (FTT)?
    1 Organic Failure to thrive (FTT)
    2 Systemic Failure to thrive (FTT)
    3 Nonorganic Failure to thrive (FTT)
    4 Idiopathic Failure to thrive (FTT)
68. When asked to explain the pathophysiology of Respiratory syncytial virus (RSV) to an infant's caregiver, the nurse should tell her that Respiratory syncytial virus (RSV) is:
    1 A bacterial infection of the lungs, similar to pneumonia
    2 A viral infection of the lungs and trachea that causes inflammation
    3 An inflammation of the pleural cavity that can be prevented with ribavirin
    4 A viral infection that causes the bronchioles to become plugged with mucus
69. Ribavirin, an antiviral agent given in the treatment of RSV, is administered:
    1 Via slow IV infusion
    2 Via an oxygen hood or mask
    3 Via IM injection
    4 Orally; can be given with juice or formula
70. A newborn with Hirschsprung's disease will often exhibit classic signs and symptoms including:
    1 Respiratory distress, wheezing
    2 Pallor, bruising, low hemoglobin
    3 An olive-shaped mass in the abdomen, projectile vomiting
    4 Lack of meconium stool, bile-stained emesis
71. Treatment for an infant newly diagnosed with esophageal atresia should include:
    1 Liquid diet, monitoring of vital signs, accurate I&O
    2 NPO, IV fluids, suctioning of mouth and nose as needed
    3 Oxygen via nasal cannula, bronchodilators
    4 Half-strength formula in small, frequent amounts, IV fluids
72. The failure of one or both testes to descend into the scrotal sac is known as:
    1 Epispadias
    2 Hypospadias
    3 Cryptorchidism
    4 Nephrotic syndrome
73. A drug that is sometimes given to promote the descent of the testes into the scrotum is:
    1 Dexamethasone
    2 Human chorionic gonadotropin (HCG)
    3 Growth Hormone (GH)
    4 Recombinant human DNA
74. Tetralogy of Fallot consists of four separate cardiac defects:
    1 Atrial septal defect (ASD), Ventricular septal defect (VSD), coarctation of the aorta, Patent ductus arteriosus (PDA)
    2 Ventricular septal defect (VSD), pulmonary stenosis, overriding of the aorta, right ventricular hypertrophy
    3 Coarctation of the aorta, pulmonary stenosis, Atrial septal defect (ASD), right ventricular hypertrophy
    4 Ventricular septal defect (VSD), left ventricular hypertrophy, PDA, overriding of the aorta
75. Treatment for a child in sickle cell crisis includes:
    1 IV fluids, oxygen, analgesics for pain
    2 NPO, NG tube to suction, bed rest

3 Bone marrow transplant, IV fluids, oxygen
4 Analgesics for pain, pancreatic enzymes, bed rest
76. To promote healthy psychosocial development in the toddler, it is important to remember to:
1 Attempt to quiet and reason with a toddler during a temper tantrum
2 Criticize the child's bad behavior, not the child
3 Help him or her to develop a strong sense of initiative, not a sense of guilt
4 Make every attempt to have them potty trained by age 2 years
77. The condition in which a child's eyes are unable to focus and work together and visual acuity is reduced in one eye is called:
1 Strabismus
2 Esotropia
3 Amblyopia
4 Exotropia
78. Spastic cerebral palsy is characterized by:
1 Mental retardation, wide-based gait, flexion contractures, and involuntary movements
2 Disintegration of movements of the upper extremities, hypertonicity of the lower extremities
3 Abnormal involuntary movement, athetosis, and slow, writhing movements
4 Hypertonicity of muscles and tendon reflexes, poor coordination, contractures
79. Suggestions to parents to help avoid accidents in children include:
1 Allow the preschool child to ride his or her bike without a helmet, as long as an adult is nearby
2 Keep all medications and poisonous substances in the back of a low cabinet in the kitchen
3 Turn all handles of pots and pans outward so that the child can see them and learn not to touch them
4 Supervise play, especially around dangerous areas such as cars, pools, and open flames
80. The age level in which children begin to learn the difference between proper and improper behavior is part of Erikson's developmental task of "initiative vs. guilt." The age level for this task is:
1 Toddler
2 Preschool
3 School-age
4 Adolescent
81. A normal part of the development of preschoolers is:
1 Developing their imagination using "magical thinking"
2 Developing a sense of trust, depending on how their caregivers treat them
3 Developing "best friends" and beginning to be influenced by their peer group
4 Developing and following certain regular patterns of behavior
82. Immediate postoperative care of the child after a tonsillectomy includes:
1 Supine position, with head of bed slightly elevated
2 Offering the child cold fluids and ice cream when awake
3 Placing the child in an oxygen tent with cool mist
4 Observing the child for frequent swallowing and active bleeding
83. Treatment of nephrotic syndrome includes frequent urine testing for protein and albumin, measurement of I&O, low

salt diet, and several medications, including:
1 Corticosteroids, oral alkylating agents
2 Diuretics, antibiotics
3 Antihypertensives, diuretics
4 Antibiotics, corticosteroids
84. The mother of a school-age child with hemophilia asks the nurse what sport would be safest in which her child can participate during gym: football, basketball, swimming, or archery. An appropriate response by the nurse would be:
1 Football
2 Basketball
3 Swimming
4 Archery
85. In leukemia, the three main consequences of bone marrow dysfunction are:
1 Anemia, increased blood clotting, infection
2 Infection, anemia, bleeding
3 Decreased clotting, increased hemoglobin, sickling of the RBCs
4 Prolonged bleeding time, decreased WBCs, increased coagulation
86. Treatment of leukemia includes administration of chemotherapy agents to lower the WBC count. This decrease in the WBC count may:
1 Lower the child's resistance to infection
2 Cause joint pain and sores in the mouth
3 Lead to a decrease in hemoglobin and increased anemia
4 Lead to lethargy, petechiae, and bruising
87. At which age level is cartilage replaced by bone at the bone epiphyses?
1 Toddler
2 Preschool
3 School-age
4 Adolescent
88. According to the International Classification of Epileptic Seizures, tonic-clonic (grand-mal) seizures are classified as:
1 Simple partial seizures
2 Complex partial seizures
3 Unilateral seizures
4 Generalized seizures
89. Care of the child with pediculosis includes:
1 Antifungal oral medication, pediculicide shampoo
2 Corticosteroids, antifungal ointment
3 Pediculicide shampoo, removal of eggs with comb
4 Antibiotic shampoo, ointment and destruction of linens
90. Which of the following is an important concept to teach parents and a school-age child that has recently been diagnosed with insulin-dependent diabetes?
1 Blood sugar monitoring will be required every 1 to 2 days
2 Symptoms of hypoglycemia include glycosuria, blood sugar over 120 mg/dL, and dizziness
3 Insulin injections will be required, and the child and the parents should be taught how to do injections
4 The child's diet will remain the same, as long as the child exercises daily
91. The growth spurt in adolescent boys occurs:
1 Earlier than girls, at age 10 to 12
2 Later than girls, at age 14 to 16
3 At the same time as girls, at age 10 to 12
4 Later than girls, at age 12 to 14

92. Antiretroviral agents are used to treat a child with AIDS to slow progression of the disease by:
    1 Killing the bacteria that lead to the development of AIDS
    2 Working to prevent the reproduction of new virus particles
    3 Decreasing inflammation and promoting formation of healthy T cells
    4 Compensating for the deficiency of B lymphocytes in the body

93. The rationale for preparing children for hospitalization is based on the theory that:
    1 Children have a right to know what is going to happen to them
    2 Leaving their child in the hospital overnight will then be easier for the parents
    3 Fear of the unknown is more severe than fear of the known
    4 If they are well prepared, parents will not have to visit as often

94. Which of the following promotes age-specific care and safety of the child in the hospital?
    1 Allow a toddler to keep her "Candyland" game in her bed at all times
    2 Keep one side rail down at night, so the child can get out of bed to go to the bathroom
    3 If using a restraint, it should be applied securely, and the extremity's circulation checked frequently
    4 Allow the adolescent to keep her medication from home in her bedside table

95. Bryant's traction, used with infants for the treatment of fractured femur, is a type of:
    1 Skin traction
    2 Skeletal traction
    3 Wire traction
    4 Pelvic traction

96. When providing care for a child with an extremity in a new cast, the nurse should:
    1 Use a hairdryer to circulate the air and speed up the drying time of the cast
    2 Handle the cast using your fingertips to prevent pressure areas under the cast
    3 Turn or reposition the child every 2 hours to ensure that the cast dries evenly
    4 Keep the casted extremity covered with a sheet or blanket

97. Of the following antibiotics, which one is usually ordered for the treatment of acute otitis media?
    1 Vancomycin
    2 Amoxicillin
    3 Gentamycin
    4 Ribavirin

98. An adolescent presents at the pediatrician's office with symptoms of mononucleosis: malaise, sore throat, fever, and lack of energy. Which of the following is another common symptom in the early stages of mononucleosis?
    1 Acute otitis media
    2 Red, flat rash on the body
    3 Cardiac enlargement
    4 Edema in the lower extremities

99. The age that salivary glands begin to function and drooling begins is:
    1 6 weeks
    2 3 months

3 4 months
4 6 months

100. The infant begins to demonstrate eye-hand coordination at age:
    1 2 to 3 months
    2 4 to 5 months
    3 6 to 7 months
    4 9 to 10 months

101. Ingestion of honey should be avoided during the first 12 months of life because of the risk of:
    1 Allergy
    2 Constipation
    3 Malnutrition
    4 Botulism

102. A Wilms' tumor is a type of adenosarcoma that is found in the Kidney .

103. Adolescence begins when:
    1 The child starts to be attracted to the opposite sex
    2 The growth rate increases rapidly
    3 The child reaches age 13
    4 Secondary sex characteristics appear

104. Treatment of an infant with symptoms of colic includes:
    1 Changing from formula to regular milk
    2 Taking a thorough history of the infant's diet and activities
    3 Feeding the infant large amounts of formula every 4 hours
    4 Following each feeding with a small mount of rice cereal

105. In bronchiolitis, swelling of the bronchiole mucosa traps air in the lungs and leads to:
    1 Difficulty in expelling air
    2 A loose, congested cough
    3 Bradycardia
    4 Inflammation of the epiglottis

106. Synagis, the drug used for prophylactic treatment of Respiratory syncytial virus (RSV), is classified as a:
    1 Long-term antibiotic
    2 Decongestant
    3 Monoclonal antibody
    4 Immunosuppressant

107. A nurse's daughter, age 8 years, has developed a red raised rash on her face, neck, and trunk. She also has a temperature of 101.6° F (38.5° C) and whitish spots on the back of her throat. From these symptoms the nurse knows that the child has:
    1 Chickenpox
    2 Measles (rubeola)
    3 Eczema
    4 German measles (rubella)

108. The patient, age 3 years, has an order for sulfisoxazole (Gantrisin) 600 mg PO every morning. The nurse has sulfisoxazole 0.5 g/5 ml on hand. The nurse should give the patient _____ 6 ml.

109. One type of treatment that is contraindicated for infants and young children with gastroenteritis is:
    1 IV fluids with electrolytes
    2 Oral rehydration with Pedialyte
    3 Age appropriate solid foods when tolerated
    4 Antidiarrheal drug therapy

110. The patient, age 3 years, was admitted with a diagnosis of possible epiglottitis. If the nurse suspects the patient

has epiglottitis, the nurse should:
1 Check her throat carefully with a flashlight
2 Increase her oral intake
3 Have the child lay flat in bed
4 Have emergency tracheostomy equipment immediately available

111. High fever that may lead to febrile seizures is most effectively and safely treated with:
1 Cool water sponge baths
2 Aspirin
3 Ice packs to arm pits and groin
4 Ibuprofen

112. Acute bacterial meningitis is:
1 Easily treated with oral antibiotics
2 More common in adults than it is in children
3 A medical emergency requiring immediate treatment
4 Diagnosed by blood culture and CT scan

113. According to Erikson's theory of psychosocial development, preschoolers are in the stage of ___Initative___ vs. ___guilt___.

114. Rheumatic fever is caused by:
1 A virus
2 Streptococcus bacteria
3 Escherichia coli bacteria
4 A fungus

115. Celiac disease is characterized by a disturbance in the absorption of:
1 Proteins
2 Fiber
3 Vitamins
4 Fats

116. Before surgery, an infant with Hirschsprung's disease may require:
1 TPN for malnutrition   Rt malabsorption
2 Small, frequent NG feedings
3 Diagnostic ultrasound of the stomach
4 IV antibiotics

117. The congenital malformation in which the rectal pouch ends blindly at a distance above the anus is known as ___Imperforated Anus___

118. Symptoms of celiac disease include which of the following?
1 Constipation, anorexia, malnutrition
2 Malnutrition, severe thirst, weight loss
3 Distended abdomen, constipation, anorexia
4 Bulky, greasy stools, distended abdomen; malnutrition

119. The initial treatment of choice for an intussusception is:
1 Reduction by manual abdominal pressure
2 Surgical bowel resection
3 Temporary colostomy
4 Hydrostatic reduction with water-soluble contrast

120. The most common signs and symptoms of leukemia related to bone marrow involvement are:
1 Headache, papilledema, irritability
2 Muscle wasting, weight loss, fatigue
3 Decreased intracranial pressure, seizures, confusion
4 Anemia, infection, bleeding

121. The most common symptoms the nurse would observe in a 16-month-old child with meningitis would be:
1 Weak or absent cry, coma
2 Bulging fontanel, irritability
3 Absent reflexes, rigid digits
4 Dilated and fixed pupils

122. Although children with Down syndrome (DS) are born to women of all ages, the incidence of DS in women age 40 is:
1 No higher than in women in their mid-30s
2 1 in 100 live births
3 1 in 500 live births
4 1 in 1000 live births

123. An 18 month-old patient is admitted to day surgery for a bilateral myringotomy because of frequent occurrences of otitis media. Otitis media occurs more frequently in young children than it does in older children because of the different position and shape of the young child's:
1 Epiglottis
2 Tympanic membranes
3 External ear canals
4 Eustachian tubes

124. Surgical repair of cryptorchidism is known as:
1 Epispadias
2 Cystotomy
3 Orchiopexy
4 Removal of the testicles

125. The nurse is caring for a child who weighs 45 lb. The usual dose for ampicillin for children is 100 mg/kg/day. Which of the following would be an appropriate dose for this child?
1 Ampicillin 250 mg every 4 hours
2 Ampicillin 500 mg four times daily
3 Ampicillin 200 mg every 6 hours
4 Ampicillin 300 mg four times daily

126. The most effective chemotherapy agents for the treatment of nephroblastoma are: →CA
1 Vancomycin, methotrexate   ↓
2 Actinomycin D, vincristine   Chemo drugs
3 Cytoxan, dexamethasone
4 Adriamycin, cytoxan

127. The childhood disease that exhibits symptoms of lethargy, muscle pain, polyarthritis, and chorea and is diagnosed by using the Jones criteria is:
1 Leukemia
2 Muscular dystrophy (MD)
3 Cystic fibrosis (CF)
4 Rheumatic fever

128. During a physical examination, a 1-month-old infant has limited abduction of the hip and asymmetrical gluteal folds. These are classic signs of:
1 Talipes equinovarus
2 Osteosarcoma
3 Cerebral palsy
4 Hip dysplasia

129. Fluids by mouth are initially contraindicated for an infant with bronchiolitis because of feeding difficulty caused by:
1 Tachypnea   Fast breathing
2 Nausea
3 Irritability
4 Fever

130. The disorder characterized by a malfunction of the motor centers of the brain (because of lack of oxygen to the brain) is:
1 Down syndrome
2 Hydrocephalus
3 Osteomyelitis
4 Cerebral palsy

131. Treatment of congenital hypothyroidism (cretinism) includes:
    1 Subcutaneous injections of growth hormone
    2 Blood transfusions and pain medication as needed
    3 Lifelong thyroid replacement therapy
    4 Monthly Synagis injections

132. A disorder caused by an obstruction of Cerebrospinal fluid (CSF) drainage is:
    1 Opisthotonos
    2 Hirschsprung's disease
    3 Hydrocephalus
    4 Meningitis

133. Normal annual weight gain for toddlers should be approximately:
    1 4 to 6 lb
    2 8 to 9 lb
    3 11 to 12 lb
    4 13 to 14 lb

134. At age 2, toddlers are in Kohlberg's stage 2 of pre-conventional morality. They obey the rules to
    Avoid punishment

135. Characteristics of an infant diagnosed as Failure to thrive (FTT) include:
    1 Sociable smile at 2 months
    2 Weight below fifth percentile
    3 Distrust of human contact
    4 Interested in playing with toys

136. Symptoms that are typically seen in infants with cystic fibrosis include:
    1 Abdominal pain
    2 Loose, congested cough
    3 Greasy, foul-smelling stools
    4 Hypertension, dyspnea

137. A 4-week-old infant is brought to the pediatrician's office with symptoms of weight loss, irritability, and projectile vomiting. On physical examination, the infant appears dehydrated. From these symptoms, you know that the infant probably has:
    1 Tetralogy of Fallot
    2 Pyloric stenosis
    3 Esophageal atresia
    4 Intussusception

138. Mucocutaneous lymph node syndrome, a cardiovascular disorder seen most often in toddlers, is also known as
    _KD_ .

139. An 18-month-old infant with developmental dysplasia of her right hip is being hospitalized for surgery and application of a hip spika cast. Which of the following measures will be necessary in caring for her?
    1 Avoid giving her pain medication as much as possible to prevent addiction
    2 Limit fluids so she will be less likely to get the cast wet when she voids
    3 Instruct the parents that they can take her home in the car propped up on pillows, with her legs down
    4 Assess sensation, circulation, and motion of her feet and toes

140. The appropriate dosing schedule for the administration of Synagis is:
    1 Daily injections for 4 weeks in October
    2 Weekly injections from October through December
    3 Monthly injections from October through April
    4 Daily oral doses for 2 weeks when symptoms begin

141. Research has shown that SIDS may be related to a brain stem abnormality in the regulation of cardiorespiratory control. Recent studies have demonstrated that the risk of SIDS is increased in infants who:
    1 Breast-feed rather than bottle-feed
    2 Have a history of apnea requiring vigorous stimulation
    3 Are more than 10 months of age
    4 Use a pacifier while they sleep on their back

142. The medication used to decrease fever and the incidence of coronary artery damage in Kawasaki disease (KD) is:
    1 Dexamethasone
    2 Ibuprofen
    3 IV Immune globulin
    4 Sulfasalazine

143. A ketogenic diet is sometimes used in the treatment of:
    1 Epilepsy
    2 Crohn's disease
    3 Hirschsprung's disease
    4 Acute glomerulonephritis

144. Children diagnosed with celiac disease are also often diagnosed with:
    1 Lactose intolerance
    2 Type 2 diabetes
    3 Hirschsprung's disease
    4 Hypothyroidism

145. A 2-month-old male infant presents at the pediatrician's office with a 2-week history of paroxysmal abdominal cramping. The mother states that he is "very fussy," and cries as if he is in pain. He is tolerating his normal amounts of formula well and has gained weight since his last visit. These signs and symptoms indicate that he most likely has:
    1 Intussusception
    2 Colic
    3 Pyloric stenosis
    4 Gastroenteritis

146. The safest place in a vehicle to place an infant in a car seat is the:
    1 Front seat passenger side, facing the rear of the car
    2 Back seat passenger side, facing the front
    3 Middle of the back seat, facing the rear of the car
    4 Back seat, driver side, facing the front

147. Which of the following statements about Respiratory syncytial virus (RSV) and bronchiolitis is true?
    1 RSV causes the bronchioles to plug with mucus, trapping air in the lungs
    2 Peak incident for RSV infection is 6 to 18 months of age
    3 RSV occurs primarily in fall and winter
    4 RSV can survive for hours on gloves, countertops, and skin

148. According to Kohlberg's Theory of Moral Development, preschoolers conform to rules to:
    1 Obtain rewards
    2 Avoid punishment
    3 Please others
    4 Avoid disapproval

149. After a tonsillectomy, an early sign of postoperative bleeding is:
    1 Brown-tinged mucus
    2 Low blood pressure
    3 Fever
    4 Frequent swallowing

150. The nurse receives an order for a preoperative injection: meperidine (Demerol) 40 mg and atropine 0.1 mg IM. The meperidine is supplied at 50 mg/ml and the atropine at 0.2 mg/ml. What volume of meperidine and the volume of atropine should the nurse give?
    1 Meperidine 0.35 ml, atropine 0.5 ml
    2 Meperidine 0.6 ml, atropine 0.4 ml
    3 Meperidine 0.8 ml, atropine 0.5 ml
    4 Meperidine 0.85 ml, atropine 0.1 ml

151. If nephrotic syndrome is classified as primary in nature, the disease is caused by:
    1 Streptococcal infection
    2 Glomerular injury
    3 A systemic illness
    4 Urinary tract infection

152. The nurse has an order to administer ampicillin 600 mg IVPB. Ampicillin is supplied as 1 g/4 ml. What volume of ampicillin should the nurse draw from the vial?
    1 1.25 ml
    2 1.7 ml
    3 1.9 ml
    4 2.4 ml

153. Symptoms of acute glomerulonephritis include:
    1 Frequent, painful urination
    2 Respiratory distress
    3 Edema in the extremities
    4 Dark, tea-colored urine

154. Treatment measures for the child with acute glomerulonephritis includes:
    1 Regular activity with rest periods as needed
    2 Cytoxan and prednisone
    3 Corticosteroids and antibiotics
    4 Frequent urine checks for albumin

155. Because no cure has been discovered for muscular dystrophy (MD), the primary goal of treatment is to:
    1 Prevent involvement of the respiratory system
    2 Maintain function in unaffected muscles as long as possible
    3 Limit the child's food intake to avoid weight gain
    4 Avoid physical activity whenever possible

156. A child has an order for an IV of D 5% in 0.25% NS to be infused at 50 ml/hr. If the IV tubing delivers 10 gtt/ml, at what rate should the nurse infuse the IV fluid?
    1 8 gtt/min
    2 13 gtt/min
    3 16 gtt/min
    4 21 gtt/min

157. The foul-smelling, frothy stools seen in children with CF results from the presence of large amounts of:
    1 Proteins and enzymes
    2 Bacteria and mucus
    3 Sodium and glucose
    4 Undigested fats   *r+ lack of lipase*

158. The organ of the digestive system most commonly involved in Cystic fibrosis (CF) is the:
    1 Pancreas
    2 Small intestine
    3 Esophagus
    4 Stomach

159. School-age children are in Kohlberg's stage of conventional morality (level 2). In this stage, the child conforms to rules:
    1 To avoid punishment
    2 To obtain rewards
    3 To please others
    4 Out of concern for others

160. Of the following foods, which is contraindicated in the diet of the child with celiac disease?
    1 Rye breads
    2 Lean meats
    3 Fresh fruits
    4 Broccoli

161. An 18-year-old girl is seen in the clinic and is diagnosed with anorexia nervosa. Her symptoms would most likely include:
    1 Diarrhea
    2 Dysmenorrhea
    3 Abdominal distention
    4 Tachycardia

162. A chronic respiratory disorder associated with airflow limitation caused by edema of the bronchial mucosa, increased mucus production, and bronchial muscle contraction is *Asthma*

163. A 2-week-old newborn has been admitted to the hospital with a diagnosis of possible hydrocephalus. Which assessment would be most important for the nurse to make?
    1 Fasting blood sugar checks each morning
    2 Frequent neurovascular checks
    3 Specific gravity on all urine output
    4 Daily head circumference measurement

164. The medication of choice for treatment of school-age children with pinworms is:
    1 Mebendazole
    2 Antifungal ointment
    3 Pediculicide cream
    4 Ribavirin

165. The nurse is admitting a child with a diagnosis of trisomy 21. Another term for this genetic problem is:
    1 Marfan syndrome
    2 Cri du chat syndrome
    3 Turner's syndrome
    4 Down syndrome (DS)

166. An infant is expected to triple his birth weight at what age?
    1 9 months
    2 12 months
    3 18 months
    4 24 months

167. Hirschsprung's disease is caused by:
    1 An autoimmune reaction causing damage to the muscles of the large intestine
    2 Damage to the bowel from a birth injury or accident
    3 A congenital absence of the ganglion nerve cells in the lower colon
    4 An infectious organism that causes inflammation and swelling in the lower bowel

168. A diagnostic test frequently used when diagnosing asthma is the:
    1 Chest x-ray examination
    2 Peak expiratory flow rate
    3 Sweat chloride test
    4 Sputum culture

169. Ringworm is a skin disorder caused by:
    1 A bacteria
    2 A fungus
    3 A virus
    4 An allergy

170. A 9-year old boy is admitted to the pediatric unit complaining of localized abdominal tenderness, rigidity, and a fever. He has rebound abdominal tenderness, and decreased bowel sounds. These are characteristic signs of:
    1 Meckel's diverticulum
    2 Acute appendicitis
    3 Bulimia
    4 Ulcerative colitis

171. During the initial assessment of a 7-year-old boy with nephrotic syndrome, the nurse should expect to see:
    1 Absence of tears
    2 Increased urine output
    3 Jaundice
    4 Scrotal edema

172. The blood test that is often elevated in inflammatory diseases such as rheumatic fever is:
    1 RBC count
    2 Clotting time
    3 Erythrocyted sedimentation rate (ESR)
    4 Blood urea nitrogen

173. A 12-year-old has just been diagnosed with type 1 diabetes. The following are classic symptoms of the onset of this disease:
    1 Hypoglycemic episodes throughout the day
    2 Excessive thirst and frequent urination
    3 Nausea before meals
    4 History of increased appetite and weight gain

174. Prednisone is often used in the treatment of rheumatic fever because it:
    1 Prevents cardiac damage
    2 Cures the disease
    3 Suppresses inflammation
    4 Takes the place on antibiotic prophylaxis

175. Primitive newborn reflexes disappear at:
    1 6 to 8 weeks
    2 3 month
    3 5 months
    4 8 months

176. An adolescent asks his physician what is required to keep his type 1 diabetes under control. The physician tells him he will be required to:
    1 Limit his activity, eat a regular diet, and take insulin
    2 Check his blood sugar regularly, and take an oral hypoglycemic drug
    3 Exercise regularly, take insulin, and limit his carbohydrates
    4 Take insulin three times a day, and limit his diet to 1000 calories a day

177. According to the 2002 revision to the immunization schedule, clinicians were advised that the last dose of the hepatitis B series should not be administered before:
    1 6 months of age
    2 9 months of age
    3 12 months of age
    4 18 months of age

178. Kohlberg's Theory of Moral Development states that adolescents are at the stage where their focus is on:
    1 Following the rules to please others
    2 Seeking rewards for a job well done
    3 Behaving in a manner that does not displease others
    4 Individual rights and principles of conscience

179. Infectious gastroenteritis in the infant is most often caused by:
    1 Rotavirus infection
    2 Respiratory syncytial virus (RSV) infection
    3 E. coli infection
    4 Staphylococcal infection

180. The nurse is providing postoperative care for an infant that has had a pyloromyotomy for pyloric stenosis. The first feeding of glucose water will most likely be given:
    1 Immediately after surgery
    2 Within the first 24 hours after surgery
    3 Via NG tube 12 hours after surgery
    4 On the second day after surgery

181. Abuse of the drug ecstasy (MDMA) has increased in adolescents. This drug is a:
    1 Stimulant
    2 Opiate
    3 Hallucinogen
    4 Depressant

182. A child with H. influenzae type B meningitis is usually treated with IV fluids, antibiotics, and:
    1 IV dexamethasone
    2 IM Synagis
    3 PO Benadryl
    4 IV Lasix

183. Symptoms of Crohn's disease include:
    1 Hypertension, headache, nausea
    2 Abdominal pain, diarrhea, weight loss
    3 Sore throat, swollen joints, fever
    4 Bronchial infections, malnutrition, peripheral edema

184. The principle cause of mononucleosis is:
    1 The Epstein-Barr virus
    2 A streptococcal infection
    3 An allergy to certain medications
    4 Malnutrition and insufficient sleep

185. Daily head circumference measurements are important nursing interventions postoperatively for the child with:
    1 A Wilms' tumor
    2 An omphalocele
    3 A ventriculoperitoneal shunt
    4 A spinal cord injury

186. Adolescents with severe cases of acne vulgaris are often treated with:
    1 Cortisone ointment
    2 Retinoic acid (Accutane)
    3 Sulfasalazine
    4 Cromolyn sodium

187. Diagnosis of nephrotic syndrome in a child is based on:
    1 Symptoms of edema, hyperalbuminemia, orange urine
    2 Results of renal ultrasound, proteinuria, increased levels of protein in the blood
    3 Increased proteinuria edema, decreased serum protein, renal biopsy

4 Edema of face abdomen, positive renal CT scan, increased serum protein

188. Antiretroviral drugs are used in the treatment of HIV infection to:
1 Compensate for the deficiency of B lymphocytes
2 Decrease joint pain and fever
3 Prevent reproduction of new virus particles
4 Promote an increase in T cells

189. A bleeding disorder resulting from a congenital deficiency in certain coagulation proteins is:
1 Sickle cell anemia
2 Thalassemia major
3 Hemophilia
4 Leukemia

190. A hereditary musculoskeletal disorder that exhibits symptoms of gradual muscle weakness, a "waddle gait," and difficulty standing and sitting is known as:
1 Multiple sclerosis
2 Cerebral palsy
3 Talipes equinovarus
4 Muscular dystrophy

191. When a teenage girl is hospitalized, one of the major stresses she faces is:
1 Separation from family
2 Fear of death
3 Loss of control, independence, and identity
4 Worry about missing classes and getting behind in school

192. An adolescent who exhibits changes in behavior patterns, an increase in school absences, a decrease in academic performance, and starts to spend time with people other than his regular friends, may be showing signs of:
1 Manic-depression
2 Schizophrenia
3 Drug abuse
4 Obsessive-compulsive disorder

193. The cancer that is seen most often in children is:
1 Lymphoma
2 Leukemia
3 Wilms' tumor
4 Osteosarcoma

194. The diagnosis of Hirschsprung's disease is usually confirmed by:
1 A rectal biopsy
2 An upper GI series
3 An abdominal ultrasound
4 A gastroscopy

195. Projectile vomiting in an infant is a classic sign of:
1 Intussusception
2 Viral gastroenteritis
3 Tracheoesophageal fistula
4 Pyloric stenosis

196. An example of a cyanotic congenital heart defect is:
1 Tetralogy of Fallot
2 Coarctation of the aorta
3 Atrial septal defect (ASD)
4 Patent ductus arteriosus (PDA)

197. An infant weighing 15 lb has been ordered to receive morphine sulfate 0.7 mg subcutaneously for postoperative pain. The normal dose of morphine is 0.1 mg/kg. The ordered dose of IV morphine is:
1 Too low, based on the weight of the infant

2 Twice the appropriate dose, based on the weight of the infant
3 Inappropriate; morphine should be not be given subcutaneously
4 Correct, based on the weight of the infant

198. A Ventral septal defect (VSD) causes shunting of blood from the _Left_ side to the _Right_ side of the heart.

199. The following is a diagram of a common obstructive disorder that develops in the first few weeks of life. This obstruction is known as _hypertrophic_.
Pyloric Stenosis

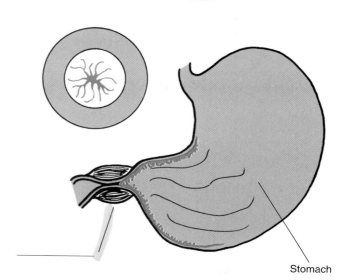

Stomach

200. A complication that commonly occurs in the child with cleft palate is:
1 Chronic otitis media
2 Failure to thrive
3 Inability to taste formula and foods
4 Gastroenteritis

201. Providing nutrition for the infant with Gastroesophageal reflux (GER) normally includes:
1 Infusion of TPN
2 Gastrostomy feedings of regular infant formula
3 Giving the infant formula every 4 hours while on their back
4 Small frequent feedings of predigested formula (Pregestimil, Nutramigen)

202. Children with sickle cell disease are more prone to infection and sepsis because:
1 They have poor eating habits and often develop malnutrition
2 They do not have a properly functioning spleen
3 They are frequently on antibiotics, which makes them resistant to treatment of infection
4 The side effects of the Sickledex medication that they often take decreases their resistance to infection

203. Acetaminophen poisoning is treated by gastric lavage and:
1 A dose of activated charcoal
2 Administration of acetylcysteine (Mucomyst)
3 Several doses of a chelating agent
4 Administration of vitamin K for bleeding tendencies

204. To confirm the diagnosis of Attention deficit hyperactivity disorder (ADHD):
    1 Symptoms must be relieved by administering an antianxiety medication
    2 A CT scan is necessary to confirm an abnormal development of the brain
    3 Negative behaviors must decrease after removing high levels of sugar from the diet
    4 The behaviors of inattention and hyperactivity must be present in more than one environment

ANSWERS AND RATIONALES

1. Knowledge, assessment, health promotion and maintenance (b).

   3 This is the period of life known as infancy.

   1 Birth to 4 weeks is the newborn period; birth to 6 weeks includes newborn and part of infancy.

   2 Birth to 4 weeks is the newborn and is not considered part of the infancy period.

   4 After 1 year of age until 3 years of age is considered the toddler period.

2. Knowledge, assessment, health promotion and maintenance (a).

   1 Adolescents are at the stage when they are constantly struggling to develop a positive self-image and their own identity and independence.

   2 These are the developmental skills developed during infancy and toddlerhood.

   3, 4 These occur during the preschool stage.

3. Comprehension, implementation, safe, effective care environment (a).

   2 The parents will deal best with a nurse who is open and honest with them.

   1 This will put a strain on the relationship between the parents and the nurse.

   3 The nurse should answer as many questions as possible and refer only questions that she cannot answer to the physician.

   4 The parents should be involved as much as possible in their child's care recovery, and this should be encouraged by the nurse.

4. Comprehension, assessment, physiological integrity (a).

   3 Large amounts of abnormally thick mucus are produced in the lungs, as well as the pancreas and liver.

   1, 4 These do not occur in CF.

   2 This occurs in epiglottitis.

5. Knowledge, assessment, physiological integrity (b).

   3 Pancreatic enzymes are given regularly with food to improve the digestions and absorption of proteins and fats in the small intestine.

   1 Pancreatic enzymes do not directly affect vitamin absorption.

   2 Pancreatic enzymes do not affect carbohydrate metabolism.

   4 Although sodium levels are a problem in the child with CF, pancreatic enzymes do not affect them.

6. Comprehension, assessment, physiological integrity (a).

   1 Some form of congenital heart defect is often seen in children with DS.

   2, 3, 4 These are not frequently seen in children with DS.

7. Knowledge, implementation, physiological integrity (b).

   2 This is the best-developed muscle in infants and is therefore the safest for IM injections.

   1 This muscle is not well developed in infants, toddlers, and or young children.

   3, 4 These muscles are not well developed in infants and toddlers.

8. Knowledge, assessment, health promotion and maintenance (a).

   3 The cellophane tape test is used in diagnosing pinworms.

1 The child's history and symptoms are not enough to definitely diagnose pinworms; a stool culture will not diagnose pinworms.

2 A blood culture would not be helpful in diagnosing pinworms.

4 A stool culture will not diagnose pinworms.

9. Knowledge, assessment, physiological integrity (a).

   1 Scoliosis of the spine often occurs because of rapid growth and is seen most often in girls.

   2 Nephrosis is a disease of the kidneys, causing edema and proteinuria.

   3 Lordosis is a concave curvature of the spine, called swayback.

   4 Kyphosis is a convex curvature of the spine, called hunchback.

10. Application, implementation, safe, effective care environment (b).

    3 Observing the length and type of seizure is important, as is preventing the child from injuring herself.

    1 This can injure the child's mouth.

    2 Suctioning may be needed, but it would not be feasible until the seizure was over.

    4 Restraints can lead to severe injury.

11. Comprehension, assessment, physiological integrity (b).

    2 These changes in the respiratory system lead to narrowing of the child's airway.

    1, 3, 4 These do not occur in asthma.

12. Knowledge, assessment, physiological integrity (a).

    2 Binge eating followed by induced vomiting is the classic symptom of bulimia.

    1 This is a symptom of anorexia nervosa.

    3, 4 These are not symptoms of bulimia.

13. Comprehension, assessment, physiological integrity (b).

    4 The infant with bronchiolitis needs oxygen to relieve his extreme dyspnea and resultant hypoxemia.

    1 Oxygen would not reduce a fever.

    2 This is not the primary reason for oxygen therapy.

    3 Oxygen would not liquefy secretions.

14. Knowledge, assessment, health promotion and maintenance (b).

    2 Toddlers use parallel play when playing with other children.

    1 Infants usually play alone or with an adult.

    3 Preschoolers use associative play.

    4 School-age children use associative play.

15. Comprehension, assessment, physiological integrity (a).

    1 This statement is true.

    2 Recovery from a painful experience does not occur faster in children.

    3 Narcotics are both safe and often necessary in managing children's pain.

    4 Children do not have increased pain thresholds.

16. Knowledge, assessment, health promotion and maintenance (a).

    4 These are the immunizations normally given at 2 months of age.

    1 The IPV is also given.

    2 The PPD is not given.

    3 The MMR vaccine is not given.

17. Comprehension, assessment, health promotion and maintenance (b).

    3 Accidents of all types are the leading cause of death in this age level.

1 Meningitis is not always fatal.
2 Leukemia occurs less often than do accidents.
4 AIDS occurs less often than do accidents.

18. Comprehension, implementation, physiological integrity (b).
    4 This may indicate nerve damage at the fracture site or pressure from a tight cast and should be reported immediately.
    1, 2 These are normal findings.
    3 This is usually a normal finding; any sudden increase in pain or severe muscle spasms should be reported to the physician.

19. Knowledge, assessment, psychosocial integrity (b).
    4 In cases of child abuse, the history given by the caregiver does not fit with the severity or type of injury.
    1 This may occur with other types of injury, as well as child abuse.
    2, 3 These are not indications of abuse.

20. Knowledge, assessment, health promotion and maintenance (a).
    2 School-age children are in the stage of industry vs. inferiority.
    1 This is the developmental task in the preschool child.
    3 This is the developmental task in the adolescent.
    4 This is the developmental task in the young adult.

21. Knowledge, assessment, health promotion and maintenance (b).
    3 Toddlers (age 1 to 3 years) are in the stage of autonomy vs. shame and doubt.
    1 Infants are in the stage of trust vs. mistrust.
    2 Preschool children are in the stage of initiative vs. guilt.
    4 School-age children are in the stage of industry vs. inferiority.

22. Knowledge, assessment, physiological integrity (a).
    2 A child in sickle cell crisis often experiences abdominal pain, swollen, painful joints, and fever.
    1 These do not occur in sickle cell crisis.
    3, 4 These are not symptoms of sickle cell crisis.

23. Comprehension, planning, physiological integrity (b).
    4 The antiinflammatory effects of corticosteroids will decrease the edema commonly seen with nephrotic syndrome.
    1 Steroids have no effect on proteinuria.
    2 Steroids have no effect on increased albumin levels.
    3 Steroids are not antihypertensive drugs.

24. Comprehension, application, physiological integrity (c).
    3 The bronchoconstriction and inflammation of the airways seen in asthma cause these symptoms.
    1 These are symptoms of a cold; a child with asthma has a nonproductive cough.
    2 Asthma does not produce a fever or rhinorrhea.
    4 These are symptoms of epiglottitis.

25. Comprehension, planning, physiological integrity (c).
    2 Bronchodilators (to relieve bronchial constriction) and antiinflammatory agents (to relieve inflammation of bronchial mucosa) are most often used together to treat asthma.
    1 Immunosuppressants are not regularly used to treat asthma.
    3 Antibiotics are not used to treat asthma.
    4 Decongestants and antihistamines are not effective in relieving the bronchoconstriction and inflammation seen in asthma.

26. Knowledge, planning, health promotion and maintenance (b).
    1 The first hepatitis B vaccine is given to the newborn infant, usually within the first 24 to 48 hours after delivery.
    2 At 2 months, the infant receives the DTP, OPV, Hib, and the second dose of hepatitis B vaccine.
    3 At 6 months, the infant receives the DTP, OPV, and the third dose of hepatitis B vaccine.
    4 At 12 months, the infant receives the MMR, the varicella zoster vaccine, and the DTP.

27. Application, planning, physiological integrity (c).
    2 Ribavirin (Virazole), an antiviral agent, is used specifically for an RSV infection, especially in children with chronic conditions; humidified oxygen relieves the dyspnea and hypoxia seen with RSV disease.
    1 Cromolyn (Intal), a nonsteroidal antiinflammatory agent, is used in the treatment of asthma.
    3 Antibiotics are not used for RSV infection.
    4 Prednisone (LiquiPred) is not used for RSV infection.

28. Knowledge, assessment, physiological integrity (c).
    4 This is the pathophysiology of RSV bronchiolitis.
    1 RSV occurs primarily in the winter and spring.
    2 Peak incidence for RSV infection is 2 to 5 months of age.
    3 RSV can survive for hours on many surfaces, but for only 30 minutes on skin.

29. Knowledge, assessment, physiological integrity (b).
    3 An omphalocele is a defect in which the abdominal contents protrude through the abdominal wall in an intact sac.
    1 Intussusception is a telescoping of the bowel and occurs within the abdomen.
    2 A diaphragmatic hernia is a congenital defect in the diaphragm that allows the abdominal contents to enter the thoracic cavity.
    4 Gastroschisis is a herniation of the abdominal contents, not covered by a peritoneal sac, that herniates lateral to the umbilical ring.

30. Application, planning, safe, effective care environment (b).
    3 Having a parent assist in procedures such as these often helps calm the child, making it easier to give the medication.
    1 Giving a medication orally is much less traumatic and more preferable than giving it via an injection.
    2 Sedation is used only as a last resort for traumatic procedures, not for administering medications.
    4 Restraints should be used only if no parent or other nurse is available to assist.

31. Comprehension, planning, physiological integrity (b).
    1 This is the preferred method of treatment for infectious gastroenteritis.
    2 IV fluids may be used if oral therapy does not work, but it is not the preferred method.
    3, 4 These are incorrect treatments for this disease.

32. Comprehension, analysis, physiological integrity (c).
    3 Croup is also known as spasmodic laryngitis.
    1 Croup is usually of viral origin.
    2 The esophagus is not involved in croup.
    4 This would be pneumonia or pneumonitis.

33. Application, planning, safe, effective care environment (b).
    3 This is the best time to begin planning for the child's discharge.
    1, 2 These are much too late to begin discharge planning.

4 All children need to have some form of discharge planning to make the transition from hospital to home go smoothly.

34. Knowledge, analysis, physiological integrity (a).

1 DS is a chromosomal abnormality (trisomy 21).

2, 3 DS is not caused by an infection.

4 DS is not caused by a lack of oxygen at birth.

35. Comprehension, analysis, physiological integrity (b). 59

4 Bryant's, or modified Bryant's, traction is the usual method of treatment for an infant with a fractured femur.

1 This is more extensive treatment than is usually needed.

2 Skeletal traction is not usually used for infants with fractured femurs, although it is often used for older children.

3 Traction is usually necessary before casting can be done if the fracture is to heal properly.

36. Knowledge, analysis, physiological integrity (a).

2 Sickle cell disease is caused by a hereditary trait that occurs primarily among African Americans.

1 It is not a viral disease.

3 It is not a bacterial disease.

4 It is not caused by a mismatched blood transfusion.

37. Comprehension, assessment, physiological integrity (a).

1 Ringworm is caused by a fungus and can occur on the scalp (tinea capitis), body (tinea corporis), or feet (tinea pedis).

2 This is an infestation of lice.

3 This is caused by a virus.

4 This is hives, often caused by allergies to foods or animal fur.

38. Knowledge, assessment, health promotion and maintenance (b).

2 This is the total number of deciduous (baby) teeth.

1 This figure is too low.

3, 4 These figures are too high.

39. Application, implementation, physiological integrity (b).

2 gr. v = 300 mg; one tablet is the correct answer.

1, 3, 4 These are not the correct answer.

40. Analysis, implementation, physiological integrity (b).

3 Use of diuretics is necessary because of the patient's edema.

1 Semi-Fowler's position in the most comfortable position to facilitate respiration.

2 The normal diet for a child with nephrotic syndrome is a high-protein diet.

4 Sodium and potassium supplements are not usually given; sodium is limited.

41. Application, implementation, physiological integrity (b).

3 This aids in the prevention of infection.

1 The child's position should be changed frequently to avoid pressure areas and severe itching.

2 To reduce itching and subsequent scratching, a minimum amount of clothing is recommended.

4 Warm, moist dressings would increase the itching; cool, moist dressings should be used.

42. Application, implementation, physiological integrity (b).

2 In a 2 year old, pulling the outer ear down and back straightens the ear canal so that the drops can be properly instilled.

1 This is the correct position for children over 3 years of age.

3, 4 These are not the correct positions.

43. Application, planning, physiological integrity (c).

4 IVIG is given to help decrease the fever and to decrease the incidence of coronary artery damage commonly seen as a complication of KD.

1 The cause of KD is unknown.

2 IVIG does not promote rest or sleep.

3 IVIG does not regulate fluid levels or blood pressure.

44. Knowledge, assessment, health promotion and maintenance (b).

2 This is normal behavior for toddlers at this age level.

1 Toddlers do not move carefully; they tend to run and bump into objects and people.

3 Toddlers are noisy; typical play at this age is known as "parallel play," in which the toddler plays next to another toddler but not with them.

4 Toddlers like to move when they play.

45. Application, implementation, physiological integrity (b).

3 These are appropriate fluids and food for a child with mild diarrhea.

1 This can lead to dehydration.

2, 4 These are inappropriate choices for a child with diarrhea.

46. Application, planning, physiological integrity (b).

2 Palpation of the tumor is to be avoided to decrease the chance of cancer metastasis.

1 A 3 year old cannot be held responsible for his or her own safety.

3, 4 These are not part of the care of a child with Wilms' tumor.

47. Application, planning, physiological integrity (c).

4 The cool, moist air helps reduce inflammation in the airway and helps keep secretions moist.

1 Symptoms are relieved over a period.

2 The cool, moist air does not prevent drug toxicity.

3 The cool, moist air may assist in reducing fever but does not promote hydration.

48. Comprehension, implementation, physiological integrity (b).

3 The Epstein-Barr virus is the principal cause of mononucleosis.

1 Kissing is one of the methods that this virus can be passed.

2 This is not a cause of mononucleosis.

4 Mononucleosis is a viral, not a bacterial, disease.

49. Comprehension, implementation, physiological integrity (b).

3 An intussusception occurs when one part of the intestine telescopes into another part of the intestine.

1, 2, 4 These are not what happens with an intussusception.

50. Comprehension, implementation, physiological integrity (b).

2 Eczema (atopic dermatitis) is usually associated with an allergy, along with a family history of the disease.

1 Eczema is not a metabolic disorder.

3 Eczema is not an infectious disorder, but a secondary infection may result without proper treatment.

4 Eczema is not a nutritional disorder, but it can be a result of a food allergy.

51. Comprehension, assessment, health promotion and maintenance (c).

3 Osteomyelitis most often occurs after an injury to a long bone.

1, 4 These do not lead to the development of osteomyelitis.

2 No gene exists for osteomyelitis.

52. Knowledge, assessment, health promotion and maintenance (b).
    4 S. aureus is the main organism that causes osteomyelitis.
    1, 2, 3 These organisms do not normally cause osteomyelitis.

53. Comprehension, evaluation, physiological integrity (c).
    3 The most important clinical outcome for a child in respiratory distress is that the airway remains patent.
    1, 2 These are not appropriate clinical outcomes for a child in respiratory distress.
    4 Although this is a positive outcome, it is not the most important clinical outcome for a child in respiratory distress.

54. Comprehension, evaluation, physiological integrity (c).
    4 A child who follows the appropriate diet should have less fat in their stools.
    1 The goal should be a slow, steady weight gain.
    2, 3 These are not related to a child with celiac disease following their diet.

55. Knowledge, assessment, health promotion and maintenance (b).
    4 The anterior fontanel begins to close throughout infancy but is not completely closed until 18 to 24 months of age.
    1, 2, 3 The anterior fontanel is still open at these ages.

56. Knowledge, assessment, health promotion and maintenance (b).
    2 The two lower central incisors erupt first, between 6 and 8 months of age.
    1 These teeth erupt at the age of 12 to 13 months.
    3, 4 These teeth erupt at the age of 16 months.

57. Application, assessment, physiological integrity, (b).
    3 Blood pressure measurement and observation for edema are assessment priorities when caring for a child with glomerulonephritis.
    1, 2, 4 These parts of the assessment are not appropriate for a child with glomerulonephritis.

58. Knowledge, assessment, health promotion and maintenance (b).
    4 The posterior fontanel is closed between 2 to 3 months of age.
    1, 2, 3 The posterior fontanel remains open at these ages.

59. Application, implementation, psychosocial integrity (b).
    4 Nurses are considered mandated reporters of actual and suspected child abuse and neglect.
    1 Because nurses are mandated reporters, they are legally bound to report abuse and neglect, regardless of possible legal consequences.
    2 Nurses are not required to report abuse to a physician before calling a child abuse center.
    3 Nurses are also required to report abuse.

60. Application, planning, physiological integrity (b).
    4 In an infant receiving IV therapy, special attention should be paid to maintaining the IV line and infusion of IV fluids.
    1, 2 These are part of the infant's care but are not a priority.
    3 This is not generally a necessary part of the infant's care.

61. Knowledge, assessment, health promotion and maintenance (c).
    2 This is Erikson's theory of child development.
    1 Freud's theory is based on psychosexual development.
    3 No theory of child development by this name exists.
    4 Piaget's theory is based on intellectual (cognitive) development.

62. Comprehension, assessment, health promotion and maintenance (c).
    1 This is the basis of Piaget's theory of child development.
    2 This is the basis of Freud's theory of child development.
    3 This is the basis of Erikson's theory of child development.
    4 This is not a theory of child development.

63. Knowledge, assessment, health promotion and maintenance (c).
    3 This is a normal characteristic for a healthy 1-month-old infant.
    1, 2, 4 These are normal characteristics for a healthy 2- to 3-month-old infant.

64. Knowledge, assessment, health promotion and maintenance (b).
    3 Teething normally begins at this age.
    1, 2 These are earlier than the time teething normally begins.
    4 Infants usually have 4 to 6 teeth by this age.

65. Comprehension, evaluation, health promotion and maintenance (c).
    3 Infants at this age first begin to demonstrate fear of strangers consistently.
    1, 2 Fear of strangers has not developed at this age.
    4 The infant continues to be fearful of strangers; demonstration of anxiety begins earlier.

66. Knowledge, assessment, health promotion and maintenance (b).
    2 Trust is Erikson's developmental task of infancy and is developed depending on how their needs are met by their parents or caregivers.
    1 This is the developmental task of toddlers.
    3 This is the developmental task of preschoolers.
    4 This is not a developmental task.

67. Comprehension, evaluation, physiological integrity (c).
    1 Organic FTT occurs as a result of a physical cause, such as congenital heart disease.
    2 This is not a classification of FTT.
    3 Nonorganic FTT is unrelated to a disease.
    4 Idiopathic FTT has no explained cause.

68. Comprehension, assessment, physiological integrity (c).
    4 RSV bronchiolitis is a viral infection that causes the bronchioles to swell and become plugged with mucus. The trapped mucus makes expelling air difficult for the infant.
    1, 2, 3 These are not the pathophysiology of RSV.

69. Application, implementation, physiological integrity (b).
    2 Ribavirin is administered by nebulization via an oxygen hood, tent, or mask for 12 to 20 hours per day for 1 to 7 days.
    1, 3, 4 These are inappropriate ways to administer ribavirin.

70. Knowledge, assessment, physiological integrity (b).
    4 Hirschsprung's disease, caused by a congenital lack of nerve cells in the wall of the colon, will exhibit these symptoms during the first several hours of life.
    1, 2 These are not signs of Hirschsprung's disease.
    3 These are symptoms of pyloric stenosis.

71. Comprehension, planning, physiological integrity (c).
    2 The infant with esophageal atresia must be kept NPO and on IV fluids until after surgery is completed to correct the defects. Suctioning of excess mucus is often necessary.
    1, 4 The infant must be NPO.
    3 This is not the treatment for esophageal atresia.

72. Knowledge, assessment, physiological integrity (b).
    3 This is the term for the condition when one or both of the testes fail to descend into the scrotal sac.
    1 Epispadias is a congenital condition in which the urethra ends on the top side of the penis.
    2 Hypospadias is a congenital condition in which the urethra ends on the bottom side of the penis.
    4 Nephrotic syndrome is a kidney disorder.

73. Comprehension, implementation, physiological integrity (b).
    2 This drug (HCG) is sometimes given to young men with cryptorchidism.
    1, 3 These drugs are not given for cryptorchidism.
    4 This drug is given in the treatment of CF.

74. Comprehension, assessment, physiological integrity (c).
    2 These are the four separate cardiac defects known as tetralogy of Fallot.
    1, 3, 4 These conditions do not make up the condition tetralogy of Fallot.

75. Comprehension, planning, physiological integrity (c).
    1 Treatment for sickle cell crisis includes IV fluids, oxygen as needed, bed rest, analgesics for pain, blood transfusions as needed, proper nutrition, oral fluids, antibiotic therapy as needed.
    2 Children in sickle cell crisis need increased fluids and do not need an NG tube.
    3 Children with sickle cell disease do not require bone marrow transplants.
    4 Pancreatic enzymes are used in the treatment of CF.

76. Application, planning, psychosocial integrity, (c).
    2 Bad behavior should be criticized, and limits set; criticizing the child only leads to development of shame and self-doubt.
    1 Reasoning with a toddler should be attempted after the temper tantrum.
    3 This is the developmental task of a preschooler.
    4 Many toddlers are not *ready* to be potty trained at age 2 years.

77. Knowledge, assessment, physiological integrity (b).
    3 These are the symptoms of amblyopia, or "lazy eye."
    1 Strabismus is a condition in which the eyes fail to direct and focus on the same object at the same time.
    2, 4 These are types of strabismus.

78. Comprehension, assessment, physiological integrity (c).
    4 These are characteristic signs of the spastic type of cerebral palsy.
    1, 2 This is the mixed type of cerebral palsy.
    3 These are signs of ataxic cerebral palsy.

79. Application, planning, health promotion and maintenance (a).
    4 This type of advice will help prevent childhood accidents.
    1 Children of all ages should wear bicycle helmets every time they ride a bike.
    2 Medications and poisonous substances should be placed in a high, locked cabinet.
    3 Handles of pots and pans should be turned inward, away from the reach of children.

80. Comprehension, assessment, health promotion and maintenance (b).
    2 Preschool (3 to 5 years of age) is the age level of children developing this task.
    1 The developmental task of toddlers is autonomy vs. shame and doubt.

3 The developmental task of school-age children is industry vs. inferiority.
    4 The developmental task of adolescents is identity vs. role confusion.

81. Comprehension, assessment, health promotion and maintenance (b).
    1 This is a normal developmental stage in preschoolers.
    2 This is a normal developmental stage in infants.
    3 This is a normal developmental stage in school-age children.
    4 This is a normal developmental stage in toddlers.

82. Application, implementation, physiological integrity (c).
    4 Postoperative care for the child after a tonsillectomy includes these nursing interventions.
    1 The child should be kept prone, with the head to the side, until fully awake.
    2 Clear, cool fluids should be given to the child after the nausea subsides.
    3 This is not usual postoperative care for a child after tonsillectomy.

83. Comprehension, implementation, physiological integrity (b).
    1 Nephrotic syndrome is treated with corticosteroids to decrease the edema and oral alkylating agents to reduce the relapse rate and induce long-term remission.
    2, 4 Antibiotics are not used to treat nephrotic syndrome.
    3 Antihypertensives are not used to treat nephrotic syndrome.

84. Application, implementation, health promotion and maintenance (b).
    3 Swimming is the safest of the four sports listed for a child with hemophilia.
    1, 2, 4 These are not safe sports for a child with hemophilia.

85. Comprehension, assessment, physiological integrity (c).
    2 These are the three main consequences of bone marrow dysfunction seen in leukemia.
    1, 3, 4 Blood clotting function is not a consequence of bone marrow dysfunction in leukemia.

86. Comprehension, evaluation, physiological integrity (b).
    1 A decreased WBC count often lowers a child's resistance to infection.
    2, 4 These symptoms of leukemia are not all caused by a decrease in WBCs.
    3 This is not caused by a decreased WBC count.

87. Knowledge, assessment, health promotion and maintenance (b).
    3 This is the age when bone growth slows, and cartilage is replaced by bone at the epiphyses.
    1, 2 These ages are too young for cartilage to be replaced.
    4 At this age, most of the cartilage has already been replaced by bone at the epiphyses.

88. Comprehension, assessment, physiological integrity (b).
    4 Generalized seizures are bilaterally symmetrical and accompanied by impaired consciousness; grand mal seizures are one type of generalized seizure.
    1, 2, 3 Grand mal seizures are not classified as this type of seizure because of their characteristics.

89. Application, planning, physiological integrity (a).
    3 This is the appropriate treatment for pediculosis.
    1 Corticosteroids are not used in the treatment of pediculosis.
    2, 4 These are not used in the treatment for pediculosis.

90. Application, implementation, psychosocial integrity (c).
    3 The child with insulin-dependent diabetes, along with his or her parents (or other caregivers), should be taught how to do insulin injections.
    1 Blood sugar (glucose) monitoring will most likely be required more than once a day.
    2 Symptoms of hypoglycemia include low blood sugar and a normal glucose in the urine.
    4 The child's diet will be different than before the diagnosis; he or she will also be required to exercise to help maintain a regular blood sugar.

91. Knowledge, assessment, health promotion and maintenance (b).
    4 The growth spurt in adolescent boys is later than it is in girls and usually occurs between 12 and 14 year of age.
    1, 2, 3 These are not the time that the growth spurt occurs in adolescent boys.

92. Comprehension, planning, physiological integrity (c).
    2 This is the action of antiretroviral agents in the treatment of HIV.
    1, 3, 4 These are not the actions of antiretroviral agents.

93. Application, implementation, psychosocial integrity (b).
    3 This is the rationale for preparing children for hospitalization.
    1 This is true, but it is not the rationale for preparing children for hospitalization.
    2, 4 These are not the rationales for preparing children for hospitalization.

94. Application, implementation, safe, effective care environment (b).
    3 Restraints may be necessary; if used, they should be on securely, and circulation should be checked regularly and documented.
    1 "Candyland" has small pieces that a toddler can choke on or swallow.
    2 A child's side rails should always be up when he or she is in bed.
    4 No medications should be left with children of any age.

95. Comprehension, implementation, physiological integrity (b).
    1 Bryant's traction is a type of skin traction.
    2, 3 Bryant's traction is not these types of traction.
    4 Pelvic traction is another type of skin traction, but it is not the same as Bryant's traction.

96. Application, implementation, physiological integrity (b).
    3 For the entire cast to dry, all areas must be open to the air.
    1 Hairdryers should not be used to dry the cast.
    2 The cast should be handled using open palms, not fingertips, to avoid denting the cast.
    4 The cast should remain open to the air to dry.

97. Application, implementation, physiological integrity (c).
    2 Amoxicillin is most commonly ordered for treatment of otitis media.
    1, 3 These antibiotics are not usually used in the treatment of otitis media.
    4 This is not an antibiotic.

98. Knowledge, assessment, physiological integrity (b).
    2 A red, flat rash is normally seen on the body of an adolescent with mononucleosis.
    1, 3, 4 These are not common symptoms of mononucleosis.

99. Knowledge, assessment, health promotion and maintenance (b).
    3 This is the age at which salivary glands begin to produce saliva.
    1, 2 Salivary glands are not functioning at this age.
    4 Salivary glands are already functioning, and drooling began at an earlier age.

100. Knowledge, assessment, health promotion and maintenance (b).
    2 This is the age when eye-hand coordination has developed and can be observed.
    1 The infant has not developed eye-hand coordination.
    3, 4 Eye-hand coordination has already developed and been observed at an earlier age.

101. Comprehension, implementation, safe, effective care environment (b).
    3 Ingestion of C botulinum spores or vegetative cells in honey may cause infant botulism.
    1 Allergy to honey is not commonly seen in infants and young children.
    2 Honey is not constipating.
    3 Ingestion of honey does not lead to malnutrition.

102. Knowledge, assessment, physiological integrity (b).
    The answer is kidney.

103. Comprehension, assessment, health promotion and maintenance (b).
    4 This is when adolescence is considered to begin in each child's life.
    1 This occurs more than once in childhood.
    2 Developing a self-image is part of adolescence, but it may be positive or negative during the teenage years.
    3 Adolescence often begins before the start of the teenage years.

104. Application, implementation, physiological integrity (b).
    2 Treatment of colic begins with identifying potential causes of the symptoms.
    1 This will not relieve colic and may worsen symptoms.
    2 Large amounts of formula may increase symptoms.
    3 Ingestion of rice cereal may or may not relieve symptoms of colic.

105. Analysis, assessment, physiological integrity (b)
    1 The swelling of bronchiole mucosa leads to difficult expiration and expiratory wheezing.
    2 An infant with bronchiolitis has a tight cough.
    3 Bronchiolitis usually causes tachycardia and tachypnea.
    4 The epiglottis is not affected by bronchiolitis.

106. Comprehension, implementation, physiological integrity (c).
    4 Synagis is classified as a monoclonal antibody and is used to prevent RSV.
    1 Synagis is not an antibody.
    2 Synagis is not a decongestant.
    3 Synagis is not an immunosuppressant.

107. Comprehension, assessment, physiological integrity (c).
    2 These are symptoms of rubeola.
    1, 3, 4 These are not all symptoms of this disease.

108. Application, implementation, physiological integrity (b).
    The answer is 6 ml.

109. Comprehension, implementation, physiological integrity (c).
    4 These medications are contraindicated because of possible adverse side effects and toxicity.

1 This may be used to treat severe gastroenteritis.
2 Pedialyte is often used for rehydrating infants and children.
3 Solids as appropriate should be given to the infant or child as soon as they can be tolerated.
110. Application, implementation, physiological integrity (a).
   4 This equipment may be necessary if the enlarged epiglottis completely obstructs the airway.
   1 Any examination of the throat can lead to laryngospasm.
   2 The child with epiglottitis has difficulty swallowing.
   3 The child should be upright, in a position of comfort.
111. Comprehension, implementation, physiological integrity (a).
   4 Oral ibuprofen is the safest, most effective way to decrease a fever.
   1 Cool-water baths may lead to chills, shivering, and increased fever.
   2 Aspirin should not be given to infants and children.
   3 Ice packs should never be used; they often increases the body's core temperature, raise the fever, and may lead to febrile seizures.
112. Comprehension, planning, physiological integrity (b).
   3 Prompt diagnosis and treatment is required to prevent serious side effects and death.
   2 Bacterial meningitis is treated with IV antibiotics.
   1 This disease is more commonly seen in children.
   4 Diagnosis is made by analysis of spinal fluid and symptoms.
113. Knowledge, assessment, health promotion and maintenance (a).
   The answer is initiative vs. guilt.
114. Knowledge, assessment, physiological integrity (b).
   2 Rheumatic fever is a chronic disease caused by a streptococcal infection.
   1 It is not caused by a virus.
   2 It is not caused by the *E. coli* bacteria.
   3 It is not caused by a fungus.
115. Knowledge, assessment, physiological integrity (a)
   4 Celiac disease is a basic defect of metabolism, leading to impaired fat absorption.
   1 Celiac disease does not affect absorption of proteins.
   2 Celiac disease does not affect absorption of fiber.
   3 Celiac disease does not affect absorption of vitamins.
116. Application, implementation, physiological integrity (c).
   1 Because of malabsorption, an infant with Hirschsprung's disease often needs TPN before surgery.
   2 This is not appropriate treatment before surgery.
   3 Hirschsprung's disease affects the intestine, not the stomach.
   4 IV antibiotics are not necessary for a child with Hirschsprung's disease before surgery.
117. Knowledge, application, physiological integrity (b).
   The answer is imperforate anus.
118. Knowledge, assessment, physiological integrity (b).
   4 These are all common symptoms of celiac disease.
   1, 2, 3 These are not common symptoms of this disease.
119. Application, implementation, physiological integrity (b).
   4 This is the safest, most effective method for reducing an intussusception.
   1 This will not reduce an intussusception.
   2 Surgery may be necessary if hydrostatic reduction is not successful.

3 This is not necessary for reducing an intussusception.
120. Comprehension, assessment, physiological integrity (b).
   4 These symptoms of leukemia result directly from changes in the bone marrow.
   1 These symptoms are caused by leukemic effects on the nervous system that lead to increased intracranial pressure.
   2 These symptoms result from the body's increasing need to meet the metabolic needs of the leukemic cells.
   3 These are not symptoms of leukemia.
121. Comprehension, assessment, physiological integrity (b).
   2 These signs are the most notable because these symptoms are caused by increased intracranial pressure, a serious complication in meningitis.
   1 The child's cry would be shrill and high-pitched.
   3, 4 These are not symptoms seen in meningitis.
122. Knowledge, assessment, health promotion and maintenance (b).
   2 This is the correct incidence of DS in women at age 40.
   1 Women in their 30s have a lesser incidence.
   3, 4 This is incorrect; the incidence is higher.
123. Comprehension, assessment, health promotion and maintenance (b).
   4 Eustachian tubes are shorter and wider in the young child than they are in the older child, which allows for easier introduction of bacteria.
   1, 2 The shape and position of these do not affect otitis media.
   3 The external ear canals are basically the same shape and in the same position as they are in young and older children.
124. Knowledge, implementation, physiological integrity (a).
   3 This is the correct term for this surgery.
   1 Epispadias is an opening of the urethral meatus on the top of the penis.
   2 Cystotomy is a surgical opening in the bladder.
   4 Removal of the testicles is an orchiectomy.
125. Application, implementation, physiological integrity (b).
   2 45 lb = 20.4 kg
   100 mg × 20.4 kg/day = 2040 mg/day
   2040 mg ÷ 4 doses = 510 mg
   Appropriate order is 500 mg four times daily
   1, 3, 4 These are not appropriate order for this child.
126. Application, implementation, physiological integrity (c).
   2 These two chemotherapy drugs are used in effective treating of nephroblastoma.
   1, 3, 4 These two drugs are not commonly used in treating nephroblastoma.
127. Comprehension, assessment, physiological integrity (a).
   4 The Jones criteria are used only to diagnose rheumatic fever.
   1 Leukemia is diagnosed by evaluation blood count levels and physical symptoms.
   2, 3 These are hereditary diseases.
128. Comprehension, assessment, physiological integrity (b).
   4 These are symptoms commonly seen in DDH.
   1 These are not classic signs of clubfoot.
   2 These are not classic signs of bone cancer.
   3 These are not classic signs of cerebral palsy.
129. Comprehension, assessment, physiological integrity (b).
   1 Severe tachypnea seen in bronchiolitis is a contraindication for oral feedings.

2 An infant with bronchiolitis cannot verbalize complaints of nausea.

3, 4 These are not contraindications for oral fluids.

130. Comprehension, assessment, physiological integrity (b).

4 Cerebral palsy is a disorder that affects the motor centers of the brain; it is usually caused by birth trauma or head trauma.

1 This is a chromosomal abnormality.

2 This is excess CSF around the brain.

3 This is an infection in a bone.

131. Comprehension, implementation, physiological integrity (b).

3 This is the treatment for congenital hypothyroidism.

1 This is used in children lacking GH (dwarfism).

2 These are commonly used in treatment of sickle cell anemia and leukemia.

4 Synagis is used to prevent RSV.

132. Knowledge, assessment, physiological integrity (a).

3 Hydrocephalus occurs when an obstruction of the CSF drainage pathways is present.

1 Opisthotonos is a sign of increased intracranial pressure.

2 It does not cause Hirschsprung's disease.

3 It does not cause meningitis.

133. Knowledge, assessment, health promotion and maintenance (b).

1 This is the amount of weight a toddler should gain each year.

2, 3, 4 These amounts are higher than the normal annual weight gain for toddlers.

134. Knowledge, assessment, health promotion and maintenance (c).

The answer is to avoid punishment.

135. Knowledge, assessment, physiological integrity (b).

2 This is diagnostic of an infant with FTT.

1 This is a characteristic of a healthy infant.

3 The infant with FTT is distrustful of people and often does not like being held.

4 The infant with FTT usually does not play with toys.

136. Knowledge, assessment, physiological integrity (b).

3 Physiological changes in the child with CF cause this symptom.

1, 2, 4 These are not commonly seen in children with CF.

137. Comprehension, assessment, physiological integrity (b).

2 These are classic symptoms of an infant with pyloric stenosis.

1 These are not symptoms of tetralogy of Fallot

3 These are not symptoms of esophageal atresia.

4 These are not symptoms of intussusception.

138. Comprehension, assessment, physiological integrity (b).

The answer is Kawasaki disease (KD).

139. Application, planning, physiological integrity (b).

4 Assessing sensation, circulation, and motion in affected extremities is necessary for all children in a cast.

1 Children should be medicated for pain as needed.

2 Fluids should be encouraged; the cast can be kept dry by careful diapering and padding of the cast.

3 The child will need an adapted car seat to take her home safely.

140. Application, implementation, physiological integrity (c).

3 This is the correct dosing schedule, monthly injections during the RSV season (October through April).

1, 2, 4 These are incorrect dosing schedules for Synagis.

141. Knowledge, evaluation, physiological integrity (b).

2 Several studies have demonstrated that infants with this history are at a greater risk of SIDS.

1 This is not applicable to SIDS.

3 The peak age for SIDS is 2 to 4 months.

4 This is not applicable to SIDS.

142. Application, implementation, physiological integrity (c).

3 This medication is used in the treatment of these symptoms of KD.

1, 2, 4 These medications are not used in treating KD.

143. Application, planning, physiological integrity (b).

1 In epileptic children with poorly controlled seizures, a ketogenic diet is often suggested as a method of treatment.

2 Children with Crohn's disease are usually on a soft, low-fiber diet.

3 Children with Hirschsprung's disease are not placed on a ketogenic diet.

4 Children with acute glomerulonephritis are usually on a low-sodium diet.

144. Analysis, evaluation, physiological integrity (c).

1 This is commonly seen in children with celiac disease.

2, 3, 4 These diseases are not commonly seen in children with celiac disease.

145. Comprehension, assessment, physiological integrity (b).

2 The infant with colic demonstrates these signs and symptoms.

1 Signs and symptoms of intussusception begin suddenly and include vomiting and bloody stools.

3 Signs and symptoms of pyloric stenosis include projectile vomiting and weight loss.

4 Signs and symptoms of gastroenteritis include dehydration, irritability, vomiting, and weight loss.

146. Application, implementation, physiological integrity (b).

3 According to several studies, this is the safest place to position an infant in a car seat.

1, 2, 4 These car seat positions are more dangerous than the correct answer.

147. Knowledge, assessment, physiological integrity (b).

4 This is the pathophysiology of RSV bronchiolitis.

1 RSV occurs primarily in the winter and spring.

2 Peak incidence for RSV infection is 2 to 5 months of age.

3 RSV can survive for hours on many surfaces but for only 30 minutes on skin.

148. Knowledge, assessment, health promotion and maintenance (c).

1 Kohlberg's theory states that preschoolers conform to rules to obtain rewards.

2 Toddlers follow rules to avoid punishment.

3, 4 School-age children follow rules to please others and avoid disapproval.

149. Application, evaluation, physiological integrity (b).

4 This is a common sign of bleeding in the early postoperative period.

1 This is normally seen posttonsillectomy.

2 This is a late sign of blood loss and hypovolemic shock.

3 This is not a sign of early bleeding.

150. Application, implementation, physiological integrity (c).

3 Meperidine: DD = 40 mg

DH = 50 mg, V = 1 ml

DD/DH = 40 mg/50 mg $\times$ 1 ml = 0.8 ml

Atropine: DD = 0.1 mg

DH = 0.2 mg, V = 1 ml

DD/DH = 0.1 mg/0.2 mg × 1 ml = 0.5 ml

1, 2, 4 These are not the correct doses

151. Comprehension, assessment, physiological integrity (c).

2 Glomerular injury is the cause of primary nephrotic syndrome.

1 This might be a cause of secondary nephrotic syndrome.

3 Some types of systemic illnesses can lead to secondary nephrotic syndrome.

4 This is not a cause of primary nephrotic syndrome.

152. Application, implementation, physiological integrity (b).

4 DD = 600 mg

DH = 1 g (1000 mg), V = 4 ml

DD/DH = 600 mg/1000 mg × 4 ml = 2.4 ml

1, 2, 3 These are not correct doses.

153. Knowledge, assessment, physiological integrity (b).

4 This is commonly seen in acute glomerulonephritis.

1, 2, 3 These are not symptoms of glomerulonephritis.

154. Application, implementation, physiological integrity (c).

1 The child should follow a regular schedule of activity accompanied by rest period when necessary.

2, 3 These medications are not used in treating this disease.

4 Checking the urine for albumin is unnecessary in the child with acute glomerulonephritis.

155. Comprehension, planning, psychosocial integrity (b).

2 This is the main treatment goal for children with MD.

1 The respiratory system is usually not involved in early stages of MD.

3 This is not a goal of MD treatment.

4 Physical activity should be encouraged to promote muscular function.

156. Knowledge, implementation, physiological integrity (b).

1 This is the correct rate of infusion.

2, 3, 4 These rates are too fast.

157. Comprehension, analysis, physiological integrity (a).

4 Fats are not completely digested in a child with CF because of the lack of the enzyme lipase. These fats are excreted with the stool, making it frothy and foul smelling.

1, 2, 3 These do not cause the abnormal stools seen in CF.

158. Knowledge, analysis, physiological integrity (b).

1 The pancreas is the organ most severely affected by CF.

2, 3, 4 These organs are not directly affected by CF.

159. Knowledge, assessment, health promotion and maintenance (c).

3 Kohlberg's theory states that school-age children follow rules to please others.

1 Toddlers follow rules to avoid punishment.

2 Preschoolers follow rules to obtain rewards.

4 Adolescents follow rules out of concern for others.

160. Comprehension, analysis, physiological integrity (b).

1 Celiac syndrome is a metabolic defect precipitated by the ingestion of rye or wheat gluten.

2, 3, 4 These are not contraindicated for children with celiac disease.

161. Comprehension, assessment, physiological integrity (b).

1 This is a symptom of anorexia nervosa.

2 Abdominal distention is not often seen in these patients.

3 Bradycardia and hypotension are common, probably because of the state of starvation.

4 Constipation, not diarrhea, is a symptom of anorexia nervosa.

162. Analysis, assessment, physiological integrity (b).

The answer is asthma.

163. Application, assessment, physiological integrity (b).

4 This is the most important assessment to make on a child with hydrocephalus.

1, 3 These are not important assessments to make on this child.

2 Frequent neurological checks may be necessary but not neurovascular checks.

164. Application, implementation, physiological integrity (b).

1 This is the medication used to treat pinworms effectively.

2, 3, 4 These are not used to treat pinworms.

165. Knowledge, assessment, physiological integrity (a).

4 This is another name for trisomy 21.

1, 2, 3 These are other types of genetic syndromes.

166. Knowledge, assessment, health promotion and maintenance (b).

2 An infant normally triples his or her birth weight at 12 months of age.

1 This is too early of an age to expect tripling of birth weight.

3, 4 By this age, the birth weight of the infant should be more than tripled.

167. Knowledge, assessment, physiological integrity (b).

3 Hirschsprung's disease is a congenital anomaly (absence of the ganglion nerve cells) that results in a mechanical obstruction of the colon.

1, 2, 4 These are not the causes of Hirschsprung's disease.

168. Comprehension, assessment, health promotion and maintenance (b).

2 This is the test most commonly used is diagnosing asthma.

1 A chest x-ray examination may be ordered, but it alone cannot diagnose asthma.

3 This test is used to diagnose CF.

4 This test is not used in the diagnosis of asthma.

169. Comprehension, assessment, health promotion and maintenance (b).

2 Ringworm is a fungus.

1 Ringworm is not caused by a bacteria.

3 Ringworm is not caused by a virus.

4 Ringworm is not an allergy.

170. Comprehension, assessment, physiological integrity (b).

2 These are classic symptoms of acute appendicitis.

1, 3, 4 These are not signs of this disease.

171. Comprehension, assessment, physiological integrity (b).

4 Scrotal edema, along with edema to the face, extremities, and abdomen, are common signs of nephrotic syndrome.

1 This is a sign of severe dehydration.

2 Urinary output is decreased in a child with nephrotic syndrome.

3 The child with nephrotic syndrome is not jaundiced.

172. Comprehension, assessment, health promotion and maintenance (b).

3 Inflammation causes the ESR to be elevated.

1, 2, 4 These levels are not usually affected by inflammation caused by rheumatic fever.

173. Comprehension, assessment, physiological integrity (b).

    2 The elevated blood glucose and ketones cause thirst and frequency in urination.

    1 A newly diagnosed, untreated person with diabetes will be hyperglycemic.

    3 This is not a common symptom of type 1 diabetes.

    4 A child with newly diagnosed diabetes may be hungry but experiences weight loss.

174. Comprehension, evaluation, physiological integrity (c).

    3 Prednisone is given to decrease inflammation.

    1, 2, 4 Prednisone is not used for this reason in the treatment for rheumatic fever.

175. Knowledge, assessment, health promotion and maintenance (c).

    3 Primitive reflexes (grasp, tonic neck) disappear by 5 months of age.

    1, 2 Primitive reflexes remain strong at these ages.

    4 Primitive reflexes have disappeared earlier than they do at this age.

176. Application, implementation, physiological integrity (c).

    3 These are required for the adolescent to maintain control of his diabetes.

    1 Activity should not be limited.

    2 Oral hypoglycemics are not effective for type 1 diabetes.

    4 This would be too few calories and probably too much insulin for the adolescent.

177. Knowledge, implementation, health promotion and maintenance (c).

    1 The American Academy of Pediatrics advised that the last dose should not be administered before 6 months of age.

    2, 3, 4 The third dose might be given before these ages.

178 Knowledge, assessment, health promotion and maintenance (b).

    4 Adolescents are guided by their conscience and focused on their rights as a person.

    1 School-age children follow rules to please others.

    2 Preschoolers follow rules to obtain rewards.

    3 Avoiding punishment is the reason that toddlers follow rules.

179. Comprehension, assessment, physiological integrity (b).

    1 The most common cause for infectious gastroenteritis in infants is the rotavirus.

    2, 4 These are not common causes for infectious gastroenteritis.

    3 *E. coli* is normally found in the stool and is usually not a cause for infectious gastroenteritis in infants.

180. Application, planning, physiological integrity (b).

    2 Normally, the first glucose-water feeding will be given within the first 24-hour postoperative period.

    1 This is too early for oral feedings to begin.

    3 NG feedings are not used after this surgery.

    4 This is usually when formula is started after surgery.

181. Knowledge, assessment, physiological integrity (b).

    1 Ecstasy is classified as a stimulant.

    2, 3, 4 These are incorrect classifications for ecstasy.

182. Application, implementation, physiological integrity (b).

    1 This steroidal medication is usually used for this specific type of meningitis.

    2, 3, 4 These drugs are not used for the treatment of *H. influenzae* type B meningitis.

183. Knowledge, assessment, physiological integrity (a).

    2 These are commonly seen in children with Crohn's disease.

    1, 3, 4 These are not symptoms of Crohn's disease.

184. Comprehension, assessment, physiological integrity (b).

    1 This is the virus that causes mononucleosis.

    2, 3, 4 These do not cause mononucleosis.

185. Application, implementation, physiological integrity (b).

    3 Nursing care of the child after ventriculoperitoneal shunt should include head circumference measurements to help determine if the shunt is draining CSF properly.

    1, 2, 4 This is not a necessary postoperative nursing intervention for this disorder.

186. Application, implementation, physiological integrity (c).

    2 Severe acne can often be successfully treated with application of Retinoic acid.

    1, 3, 4 These medications are not used in treating severe acne.

187. Comprehension, assessment, physiological integrity (c).

    3 These are signs and symptoms of nephrotic syndrome.

    1 Nephrotic syndrome includes hypoalbuminemia.

    2, 4 Nephrotic syndrome is diagnosed via renal biopsy; levels of protein in the blood are decreased.

188. Analysis, implementation, physiological integrity (c).

    3 These drugs help to prevent the development of AIDS in patients who are HIV positive.

    1, 2, 4 These are not the actions of antiretroviral drugs.

189. Knowledge, assessment, physiological integrity (b).

    3 This bleeding disorder is known as hemophilia.

    1, 2, 4 These are not the definitions for this bleeding disorder.

190. Knowledge, assessment, physiological integrity (b).

    4 These are all characteristic signs of MD.

    1, 2, 3 These are not characteristic signs of this disease.

191. Application, evaluation, health promotion and maintenance (b).

    3 Along with separation from peers, these are the major issues that hospitalized adolescents face.

    1 This is a major stressor for toddlers.

    2 This is a major stressor for preschoolers.

    4 This is usually not a major stressor for most adolescents.

192. Comprehension, assessment, health promotion and maintenance (b).

    3 These are typical signs of an adolescent that is abusing drugs or alcohol.

    1, 2, 4 These are not all typical signs of this disorder.

193. Knowledge, assessment, physiological integrity (b).

    2 Leukemia is the most common cancer seen in children.

    1, 3, 4 This type of cancer is seen in children but is not as common as leukemia.

194. Comprehension, implementation, health promotion and maintenance (b).

    1 This test, along with a barium enema, is used to confirm Hirschsprung's disease.

    2, 3, 4 These tests are not used to confirm Hirschsprung's disease.

195. Knowledge, assessment, physiological integrity (b).

    4 Projectile vomiting is a classic sign of pyloric stenosis.

    1, 2, 3 This is not a classic sign of this disease.

196. Analysis, assessment, physiological integrity (c).

    1 Tetralogy of Fallot is a cyanotic heart defect consisting of four separate congenital defects.

    2, 3, 4 This is an acyanotic congenital heart defect.

197. Application, intervention, physiological integrity (c).

   4 This is the correct dose
   2.2 lb = 1 kg; 15 lb ÷ 2.2 lb = 6.8 kg
   DD = 0.1 mg/kg
   6.8 kg × 0.1 mg = 0.68 mg (rounded to 0.7 mg)

   1, 2 These are not correct doses.

   3 Morphine can be given via subcutaneously, IM, IV, and epidural routes.

198. Analysis, assessment, physiological integrity (b).

   The answer is left to right.

199. Comprehension, assessment, physiological integrity (c), Figure 8-3

   The answer is hypertrophic pyloric stenosis.

200. Analysis, assessment, physiological integrity (c).

   1 The opening in the palate allows formula to enter the nose, airway, and ear canal.

   2, 3, 4 These are not common complications of cleft palate.

201. Application, intervention, physiological integrity (b).

   4 The safest, most appropriate method for providing nutrition in infants with GER is by small, frequent feedings of one of these types of formulas.

   1 TPN is not used for infants with GER.

   2 Infants with GER do not have gastrostomies.

   3 Infants with GER should be fed while being held and then positioned prone with their head slightly elevated.

202. Analysis, planning, safe, effective care environment (c).

   2 A malfunctioning spleen causes the child with sickle cell disease to be immunocompromised.

   1 Malnutrition is not a common characteristic of children with sickle cell disease.

   3 These children are only on antibiotics if an infection develops.

   4 Sickledex is a laboratory test, not a medication.

203. Application, implementation, physiological integrity (b).

   2 The antidote for acetaminophen poisoning is acetyl-cysteine (Mucomyst).

   1 Activated charcoal is given for corrosive poisoning.

   3 Chelating agents are used to treat lead poisoning.

   4 Vitamin K would be given for bleeding tendencies in chronic poisoning.

204. Comprehension, assessment, health promotion and maintenance (b).

   4 The behaviors of inattention and hyperactivity must be present in at least two settings (home, school, social situations) to support the diagnosis of ADHD.

   1 Psychostimulant medications are used in the treatment of ADHD.

   2, 3 Diagnosis of ADHD is made by observation of behaviors.

CHAPTER 9   Nursing Care of the Aging Adult

The percentage of the American population over age 65 is rapidly passing 13% and continues to constitute our fastest-growing age group. As the life expectancy of Americans continues to lengthen, the year 2010 will see the first baby boomers retiring. By the year 2030, we will be challenged to care for an aging adult population that constitutes 22% of the total population. Minority populations are expected to increase to 25.4% of the elderly population in 2030. Maintenance of health and wellness, and caring for increasingly older adults, will be the emphasis in future years. How we address these future trends will be reflected in history as a measure of our civility.

The nursing challenge is to meet the care needs of our older adults, who are vulnerable to the biases of our fast-paced, youth-oriented society. As nurses, we have an opportunity to play a significant role in determining whether these will be years of continued growth and development, years of happiness and accomplishment, or years of forced shame, illness, and neglect.

This chapter focuses on aging as a normal process and strives to increase the practitioner's knowledge of and understanding for a stage of life through which we will all pass.

"For age is opportunity no less than youth itself, though in another dress."

—Henry Wadsworth Longfellow

GOVERNMENT RESOURCES FOR THE OLDER ADULT

Income

A. Social Security (Federal Old-Age, Survivors, and Disability Insurance [FOASDI]); first adopted in 1935
   1. Funded by employee and employer payroll taxes
   2. Entitlement is determined by United States Social Security Administration; benefits are granted in accordance with:
      a. Age
      b. Lifetime earnings record; retirement age is steadily increasing
      c. Free earnings credits for active military service
      d. Whether the required number of work credits has been earned (work credits are measured in quarters)
   3. Specific maximum benefit amount with cost-of-living protection against inflation
   4. Minimum retirement benefits begin at age 62
   5. Railroad workers have a separate retirement system; workers who have less than 10 years of railroad service may transfer earnings to Social Security to be counted toward Social Security benefits
   6. Federal employees are covered under the Civil Service Retirement System, the Federal Employees Retirement System, and the Thrift Savings Plan
   7. Social Security benefits are reduced according to monies earned over a stated maximum annual allowable income
   8. Social Security benefits are not reduced for full-time employees over the age of 70
   9. Payments are indexed according to inflation rate
B. Supplemental Security Income (SSI); established in 1972
   1. Funded from general tax revenues
   2. Cash-assistance program
   3. Administered by the Social Security Administration
   4. Designed to provide for disabled, blind, or aged with limited incomes and resources
   5. Medicaid eligibility in many states is based on SSI eligibility

Health

A. Medicare (Title XVIII of Social Security Act); established in 1965
   1. Administered by Health Care Finance Administration of U.S. Department of Health and Human Services
   2. Designed to help people over 65 years of age and certain disabled people under 65, who are eligible under Social Security, to meet medical care costs regardless of income, and people of any age with permanent kidney failure
   3. Major insurance companies in each state handle claims (e.g., Travelers Insurance Company in New York)
   4. Pays for only limited time in long-term care
   5. Do not have to be retired to receive benefits
   6. Financed by employer and employee payroll taxes and by self-employment tax monies
   7. Everyone over age 65 who is entitled to Social Security benefits receives hospital insurance without paying premium charges
   8. Automatic hospital insurance is provided to disabled persons who have been entitled to Social Security disability benefits for 24 consecutive months
   9. Initial enrollment period begins 3 months before the month that the individual will become 65 years of age and continues for 4 months after individual turns 65 years of age
   10. Annual enrollment periods: January 1 through March 31
   11. Premiums generally increase if people do not apply when they are eligible
   12. Deductible is applied to each benefit period
   13. Two parts
      a. Part A is designed as hospital insurance that has certain exclusions
      b. Part B covers physician services and outpatient services
      c. If subscribing to part A, the person is automatically enrolled in part B unless it is declined

B. Medicaid (Title XIX of Social Security Act); established in 1965
1. Purposes
   a. To cover specific expenses not provided for by Medicare
   b. To reduce expenses of individuals who have exhausted their Medicare benefits
   c. To defray medical expenses of persons who cannot afford Medicare premiums
2. Funded by federal and state contributions
3. State-operated programs
4. Funds the majority of long-term care after Medicare and personal funds are depleted
5. Other programs
   a. Qualified Medicare Beneficiary (QMB) Program
      (1) Annual income must be at or below the national poverty level; 12% of older adults fall below the poverty line
      (2) Functions similar to a Medigap policy
      (3) State Medicaid program helps pay
      (4) Pays Medicare Part B premium
      (5) Pays Medicare Part A premiums for eligible older adults and disabled persons, Medicare deductible, and co-insurance fees
   b. Specified Low-Income Medicare Beneficiary (SLMB)
      (1) Income cannot be more than 20% above the 'national poverty level
      (2) The person must be eligible for Medicare Part A
      (3) The state will pay Medicare Part B premiums
      (4) Medicare co-insurance or deductibles are not paid
C. Private health insurance
1. Medigap
   a. Medicare supplement insurance
   b. Regulated by state and federal law
   c. Ten standard plans
   d. Lifetime maximums are established
   e. Not government sponsored
   f. Policies of choice may be purchased from any insurer providing Medigap policies in the state of residency for a 6-month period from date enrolled in Medicare Part B; and for those age 65 or older
   g. Plans pay all or most medical co-insurance amounts; some policies pay for Medicare deductibles
2. Medicare Select
   a. Medicare Select Plan is Medigap insurance
   b. Supplements Medicare's benefits
   c. Sold by insurance companies and health maintenance organizations (HMOs)
   d. Difference between Medicare Select and Medigap is that specific physicians and certain hospitals must be used for nonemergent care to qualify for full benefits
   e. Federally approved through 1998 in all states

Housing

A. U.S. Department of Housing and Urban Development
1. Rent Supplement Program: rent-subsidized apartments for older adults, disabled individuals, or low-income families
   a. Utility and rent costs in existing buildings
   b. Renovations of existing units
   c. Building of new units
2. Provides home improvement loans

3. Provides mortgage insurance
4. Has age, asset, income eligibility requirements
B. Older adult and handicapped housing (Housing Act of 1959)
1. Provides funding to private, nonprofit organizations for renovation or building of units for the older adult and handicapped
2. Provides low-interest federal loans for same
C. National Housing Act (Housing and Urban Development Act, 1968): provides funding to private corporations for construction of low- and middle-income housing
D. National Housing Act of 1952: provides funding to private, profit, or nonprofit groups for nursing home construction or renovation

Title XX of the Social Security Act

A. Federal monies for social programs that are available and appropriate for the older adult
B. State administered
C. Individual must be eligible for SSI

Food Stamp Program

A. Administered by U.S. Department of Agriculture
B. The recipient must meet income requirements
C. Each state's welfare department determines eligibility
D. Components
1. Home-delivered meals
2. Grocery store food purchases

Administration on Aging

A. State, regional, area, and local units: area units are responsible for providing program coordination and development expertise
B. Major services
1. Nutritional programs
   a. On-site meals
   b. Home-delivered meals
2. Senior centers
   a. Services
   b. Programs
3. Home care
   a. Homemaker
   b. Home health aide
   c. Home visits
   d. Telephone calls
   e. Chore maintenance
4. Information and referral
5. Transportation
   a. Urban Mass Transit Act
   b. Area agencies on aging

LEGISLATION AFFECTING THE OLDER ADULT

A. Social Security; established in 1935 by Theodore Roosevelt; legislators predict benefits may be depleted by the year 2015
B. Medicare and Medicaid programs; developed in 1965; programs have been through many reforms
C. Older Americans Act; first initiated in 1987 and revised in 1992; established standards for safeguarding the rights of the older adult

D. The Omnibus Budget Reconciliation Act (OBRA) of 1991; established to improve the lives of those individuals residing in nursing homes; attached stringent guidelines for the use of physical and chemical restraints

E. The Patient Self Determination Act; established in 1991; developed in an effort to allow individuals to control end-of-life care

  1. Living wills: completed while the individual is well and outlines what the individual may or may not want done if unable to make decisions regarding end-of-life care

  2. Health care proxy: the individual designates a person to make end-of-life care decisions for them should they become incapacitated

NURSING ROLES AND THE CARE OF THE OLDER ADULT

A. Care provider: nurses are in the unique position to meet the health care needs of the older adult

  1. Nursing's goal in the care of the older adult is to assist the individual in attaining their optimal state of health

  2. Nursing care focuses on prevention of acute and chronic health problems, promotion of a healthy lifestyle, and management of the symptoms of chronic health problems

B. Educator

  1. Nurses educate the older adult concerning health promotion and maintenance of acute and chronic health problems

  2. Nurses increase public awareness of problems affecting the older adult

C. Data collection

  1. Nurses must assess the older adult's need for services

  2. Area agencies on aging are the best resource regarding services for older adults in the community

D. Patient advocate

  1. Nurses act as patient advocates to ensure that the rights of the older adult are preserved in regards to health care practices, treatment modalities, and end-of-life care

  2. The American Nurses' Association's Council on Gerontological Nursing has established Nursing Standards of Gerontological Practice

  3. Nurses recognize the older adult as a unique individual, molded by life experience, family, society, religion, and culture (Box 9-1)

THEORIES OF AGING

Sociological Theories

A. Disengagement

  1. Controversial

  2. Mutual withdrawal from social interaction by aged individual and society

  3. Describes engagement as active occupation and devotion

  4. Supports leisure as a form of activity

  5. Respects individual-initiated withdrawal

B. Activity

  1. Remains active and interacts with society's events

  2. Pursues new interests, friends, and roles to substitute for lost roles

---

BOX 9-1   Cultural Considerations

Chinese: achieving old age is a blessing; the family is expected to take care of the older adult. Use alternative medicine such as herbs, acupressure, and acupuncture. May be hesitant to seek out services for the older adult.

Japanese: the older adults are viewed with respect; close family bonds are established. Many Japanese men would wed younger wives—the proportion of widows is higher. May reject modern medicine in favor of traditional practices.

Hispanic: describes individuals from Spain, Cuba, Mexico, and Puerto Rico; view illness as an act of God. Old age is viewed as a positive time. Families avoid long-term care; and this ethnic group has the lowest rate of institutionalization.

Native American: the older adults are respected as leaders in the community. Illness and health are viewed as good and evil, and evil actions are punished by illness. Many elders believe that the questions used by nurses are too probing and inappropriate.

African American: many African Americans never reach old age; therefore old age is viewed as a goal. The rate of institutionalization among this ethnic group is low. Older adults look to family members for advice and care before contacting service agencies.

Jewish Americans: although not actually a particular culture, the Jewish religion dictates the customs and practices of these people. Illness typically draws the family together; and this group, with its normally highly educated members, does not hesitate to seek out modern medicine as needed.

---

  3. Supports social activity as beneficial to life satisfaction, morale, and mental health

C. Continuity or development

  1. Lifelong personality characteristics and coping strategies continue

  2. Sense of inferiority develops when continuity disrupted

  3. Supportive network of relationships is established

D. Passages: life cycle changes can be identified, predicted, planned for, and managed

Biological Theories

A. Wear and tear

  1. Stress and use deplete the body cells of repair ability; aging results from accumulated stress and damage, not chronological age

  2. Coping mechanisms decline because of the decrease in available energy

B. Collagen

  1. Most abundant body protein

  2. Collagen molecules are held together by bonds

  3. Chemical reactions cause a switching of bonds between collagen molecules, resulting in structural changes characteristic of the aging process

C. Lipofuscin accumulation

  1. Lipofuscin granules or age pigments are insoluble end products of cell metabolism

2. Lipofuscins accumulate in the cell, altering the cell's ability to function normally

D. Immunologic responses
   1. Aging is an autoimmune disease process
   2. Cells change, and the body does not recognize its own cells
   3. Autoimmune responses damage the cells, causing cell death

E. Cell death of genetic programming
   1. Cell reproduction is programmed
   2. Programming determines the rate and time a given species ages and dies

F. Free radical
   1. Molecules that have an extra electron are free radicals
   2. Free radicals attach to other molecules, altering function or structure, causing damage and aging
   3. Free radicals come from internal and external sources
   4. The belief holds that the free radicals damage membrane function and structure (vitamins A, C, and E are thought to reduce free-radical activity)

G. Mutation and error
   1. Cell division errors occur progressively over time; radiation is cited as a contributing factor
   2. Mutated cells are altered in their function and effectiveness
   3. Error theory expands mutation theory to include errors in interpretation of cell messages

Psychological Theories

A. Freud: did not recommend psychoanalysis for the aged population (see Chapter 6)
B. Sullivan: see Chapter 6
C. Maslow: see Chapter 2
D. Erikson: see Chapter 6
   1. Eighth stage (65 to 100 years of age) identified as "integrity vs. despair" (Figure 9-1)
   2. The older adult who views his or her own life as having no meaning ends life's stages in despair; the older adult who can review his or her accomplishments and errors derives a sense of integrity

E. Peck
   1. Expanded Erikson's developmental theory of the eighth stage of humankind
   2. Focuses on alternatives to preoccupation with body changes and illness, thereby achieving life satisfaction (Figure 9-2)

ROLE CHANGES

A. Types
   1. Crisis
      a. Sudden, unplanned, stress producing
      b. No readily available substitute
   2. Gradual
      a. Develops slowly
      b. Time available for preparation, which eases transition
      c. Control over whether to develop a substitute

B. Sufficient preparation and adequate support determine adjustment success or failure

C. Role changes that occur to the older adult are predominantly crisis oriented, both sudden and gradual
   1. Forced retirement
   2. Alteration in income
   3. Loss of spouse
   4. Illness
   5. Friends who move away or die
   6. Family members who relocate, assume new roles, have increasingly less time for relationships
   7. Society's assigned role of decreased psychological and physiological functioning

D. Role losses
   1. Work
      a. Income

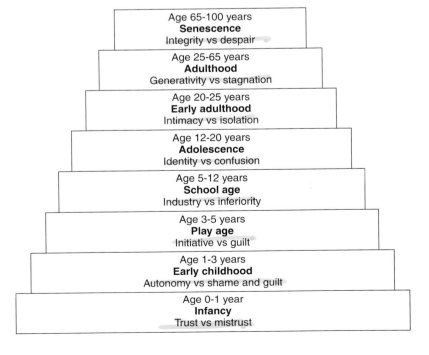

FIGURE 9-1 Erikson: eight stages of man. (*From Forbes ES, Fitzsimmons VM:* The older adult: a process for wellness, *St. Louis, 1981, Mosby.*)

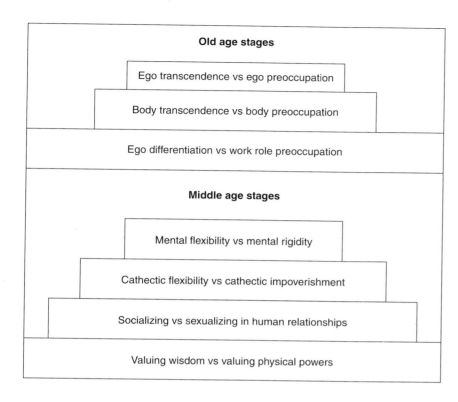

FIGURE 9-2 Peck: stages of middle age and old age. *(From Forbes ES, Fitzsimmons VM:* The older adult: a process for wellness, *St. Louis, 1981, Mosby.)*

b. Job-related companionship
c. Usefulness, competence, identity
d. Sense of purpose
e. Self-esteem

2. Family
   a May no longer be the decision maker
   b. May not be held in the same esteem
   c. Loss of independence; reversal of roles with children

E. Role gains
   1. Grandparenthood or great-grandparenthood
   2. Family support roles assumed
      a. Economic
      b. Child care
      c. Caring role in illness
      d. Care of the home
   3. Community activities
   4. Religious activities
   5. Recreational activities
   6. Clubs, organizations, and associations
   7. Advisory roles
   8. New friends
   9. Adult education
   10. Volunteerism

ALTERATIONS IN LIFESTYLE

Employment

A. Society emphasizes the employed as valuable and the unemployed as useless
B. The number of older women working has increased
C. The number of older men working has decreased
D. Part-time employment is more common
E. The trend is toward early retirement
F. Serial careers are emerging in keeping with interest changes
G. More women are joining the workforce at a time when men are winding down their working lives
H. The older worker possesses involuntary limitations
   1. Health problems
   2. Sensory or perceptual alterations, for example, in vision and auditory acuity
   3. Decline in physical strength, endurance, and speed
I. Older workers possess innumerable strengths
   1. Reliability
   2. Dependability
   3. Knowledge
   4. Expertise
   5. Experience

Retirement

A. Mandatory retirement in federal employment has been eliminated
B. Mandatory retirement age is raised to 70 years of age in private employment
C. Changes in the economy is leading to forced retirements
D. More people are taking advantage of early retirement because of incentives by companies to retire older workers, replacing them with younger workers
E. Health problems are the primary reason for voluntary retirement
F. Leisure time is increased
G. Tremendous anxiety may be created for some older adults
H. Some older adults derive an initial feeling of relief; however, for most, it is a loss that comes at a time of meaningful productivity

I. Adjustment depends on previously established patterns of adjustment, degree of financial security, state of health, and future outlook

J. For most older adults, retirement creates an additional series of losses and problems at a time in life when coping and problem-solving abilities are fragile

K. Job loss
1. Loss of daily routine
   a. Alters household routine
   b. Alters lifestyle
   c. Creates discouragement, depression, and loneliness
   d. Alters family relationships, may increase marital stress
   e. May result in alcohol abuse from drinking as a reaction to a loss
2. Loss of income
   a. Relocation
   b. Daily decision making determined by economics
   c. Decreases self-esteem
   d. Increases fear and anxiety
   e. Increases insecurity

L. Welcome changes can result if retired adult remains socially engaged
1. New friends
2. New activities
3. New interests and time to devote to established interests
4. Renewal of marriage
5. Seeking new and different employment
6. Finding purpose and opportunity
7. Rest and relaxation

Economic Changes

A. Most older adults live on fixed incomes

B. Of older adult persons, 1 out of 10 lives below the nation's poverty level

C. Independence declines as costs increase and buying power decreases

D. For many older adults, Social Security is the sole source of income

E. Many older adults are not receiving the assistance to which they are entitled
1. Lack of resource knowledge
2. Inability to find out about resources
   a. Lack of mobility
   b. Health problems

F. Supplemental Social Security: may qualify for in addition to or instead of Social Security benefits

G. Economic penalties: limit on the amount a Social Security beneficiary can earn annually without losing some monthly payments

H. Income tax reforms: for example a once-in-a-lifetime capital gains tax exemption on sale of personal residence for person over 55 years of age

I. Income sources
1. Public
   a. Social Security (Federal Old-Age Survivors and Disability Insurance [FOASDI])
   b. Supplemental Social Security Income
2. Private (e.g., pensions, investments)
3. Other (e.g., Railroad Retirement System, Federal Employee's Retirement System, Civil Service Retirement System)

Health

A. Most older adults have more than one chronic disease

B. Health care needs increase with age

C. Cost of health care is increasing as financial income is either decreasing or fixed

D. Older adults account for one third of the nation's health care costs

Housing

A. Most older adults prefer to remain independent as long as family and friends live nearby

B. Most older adults live with spouse, alone, or with family

C. A large percentage of older adults continue to own their home and prefer this lifestyle as it provides:
1. Security
2. Privacy
3. Independence
4. Sense of purpose
5. Familiarity
6. Household activities
7. Pride
8. Socialization

D. Other housing alternatives
1. Mobile homes
   a. Convenient
   b. Economical
2. Retirement communities
   a. Minimum age requirement
   b. Different cost levels, for example, houses, apartments, and condominiums
3. Foster home
4. Life care facilities: living, recreational, medical facilities on the premises
5. Nursing homes: 5% of individuals ages 65 to 85 live in nursing homes; after the age of 85, 25% live in nursing homes; the typical nursing home resident is a woman and over 80 years of age; the terms extended care facility (ECF) and long-term care facility may be used interchangeably with the term nursing home
6. Assisted living facilities are increasing to meet the needs of older adults with minor to moderate health care problems
7. House sharing
8. Public housing
9. Rooming houses
10. Hotels: single room occupancy (SRO)

E. Special assistance needs of older adults enable them to remain in their own homes longer
1. Transportation
   a. Reliable
   b. Nearby
   c. Inexpensive
   d. Safe
2. Meals are available in the event of illness or disability
3. Health hotlines: most older adults are institutionalized because of health needs and lack of convenient community health services
4. Housecleaning services
5. Homemaker services
6. Social services
7. Home care services
8. Neighborhood safety programs

Recreation

A. Although older adults have more time for recreation, deterring factors exist
1. Cost
   a. Transportation
   b. Special equipment
   c. Special clothing
   d. Fees for membership and use of facilities
2. Health problems
3. Diminished energy level
4. Lack of incentive
5. Sensory losses
6. Lack of environmental aids
7. Lack of conveniently located facilities, for example, restrooms
8. Lack of handicapped facilities
B. Most older adults depend on a family as the major source of activity and interaction
C. Alternatives
1. Religious activities
2. Community activities, for example, volunteerism
3. Adult day care
4. Senior citizen centers
5. Clubs, organizations, and associations
6. Recreation centers
7. Adult education
8. Shopping
9. Cultural events
10. Elder hostel

SOCIAL ISOLATION

A. Four classifications (Ebersole and Hess, 1985)
B. Attitudinal: that which is self-imposed and those imposed by society
1. Self-imposed aloneness, loneliness
2. Society imposes myths about the aged, perceptions of aging
C. Presentational: set apart or sets one apart
D. Behavioral: exhibits behaviors that are not acceptable to a youth-oriented society, for example, confusion, eccentricity
E. Geographic
1. Lack of resources to relocate
2. Psychological safety and security at present location
3. Fear of being victims of crime
4. Distance from family and friends who have moved away
F. Rural areas have a higher proportion of older people

Drug Use

A. The largest users of prescription medications are those over the age of 65
B. The tendency is to self-medicate; use of over-the-counter remedies and supplements is common
C. The frequency of hospital admissions that are drug-related is higher than that for other age groups
D. Self-administration errors are common
E. Absorption of the drug into the system is slower as a result of a decline in gastric acid secretion and decreased gastric motility
F. Circulatory alterations affect drug distribution to body tissues

G. Drug metabolism is altered by factors such as a diminished rate of body metabolism
H. Drug excretion time is delayed by illness, disease, and the aging process, especially decreased renal blood flow
I. Management
1. Patient education
2. Medication administration times that are more compatible with lifestyle
3. Color coding
4. Larger print on labels
5. Easily removable bottle and vial caps
6. Monitoring of drug effectiveness and compatibility
7. Drug holidays
8. Daily or weekly medication containers
9. Cost of medications is frequently the reason for noncompliance, either not taking the medication or not taking it as ordered

Alcohol Abuse

A. High-risk group for alcoholism
1. A significant number of alcohol abusers are over age 60
2. Adult men have a higher incidence of abuse than do adult women
3. Statistics are inaccurate because of protection by family members
B. Tolerance to alcohol decreases with age because the body systems do not excrete and detoxify as rapidly as those of a younger adult
C. Substitution for unmet psychological needs and untreated physiological problems; drinking frequently increases after a loss, such as the death of a spouse or retirement
D. Alcohol abuse is the cause of accidents, nutritional deficiencies, drug incompatibilities, self-neglect, alterations in self-esteem, psychosocial and physiological health care problems

Elder Abuse

A. Physical (Box 9-2)
1. Battering
2. Neglect
3. Sexual abuse
4. Confinement or restraint
B. Psychological: threatened or forced
1. Relinquishment of assets
2. Institutionalization
3. Loss of control over independent functioning
4. Social isolation
5. Sensory deprivation
C. Prevention
1. Acquire knowledge of family abuse and patterns of violence
2. Identify predisposing factors
3. Incorporate assessment tools into interviewing and counseling strategies; if abuse is suspected, interview alone
4. Increase public awareness and education
5. Identify actual and potential sources of emergency protection
6. Acquire knowledge of community resources

BOX 9-2	Physical Indicators of Actual or Potential Elder Abuse or Neglect

General Appearance
Anxious, fearful, passive
Poor eye contact
Looks to caregiver for answers
Poor hygiene, inappropriate dress
Underweight or malnourished
Physically handicapped
No glasses, false teeth, or hearing aid despite need

Skin
Contusions, abrasions, burns, scars in various stages of healing
Decubitus ulcers, urine burns
Rope marks

Abdominal and Rectal
Distended
Internal bleeding
Fecal impactions

Musculoskeletal Fractures
Evidence of old healed fractures
Current fractures and sprains
Limited range of motion
Contractures

Genital and Urinary
Vaginal lacerations, bruises, and infections
Urinary tract infections

Neurological
Slurred speech
Confusion

From Fortinash KM, Holoday-Worret PA: *Psychiatric-mental health nursing,* ed 2, St Louis, 1999, Mosby.

HEALTHY OLDER ADULT

A. Although older adults are sometimes plagued by chronic health problems, most live in the community
B. The focus of education for the older adult regarding healthy living include:
1. Disease prevention: prevention of acute or chronic health problems
a. Self-maintenance: taking responsibility for own health practices
b. Maintenance of activity: engaging in moderate physical activity at least three times every week
c. Dietary practices: eating a varied diet that includes adequate amounts of carbohydrates, proteins, and fats
d. Diagnostic testing: regularly undergoing examinations for the detection and early treatment of disease (mammograms, prostate examination, colorectal screening)
e. Influenza and pneumonia vaccines: as recommended by a physician
f. Management of stress

2. Health promotion: maintenance for chronic health problems
a. Regularly visiting physician for examinations
b. Engaging in healthy lifestyle practices
c. Taking prescribed medications

Physiological Alterations (Normal Aging Process) and Selected Disorders (Abnormal)

A. Normal aging changes are gradual and begin in early middle age
B. Specific changes of aging do not alter the older adult's ability to cope on a day-to-day basis
C. Because of specific changes of aging, the older adult has a decreased capacity to *bounce back* from stress or illness, known as a deceased physiological reserve

Integumentary System

A. Alterations
1. Moisture loss, dryness
2. Epithelial layer thinning; fragility
3. Shrinkage and rigidity of elastic collagen fibers: sagging and wrinkling
4. Sweat glands decrease in number, activity, and size: less efficient body cooling system
5. Subcutaneous fat loss, deepening of hollows, and more prominent contours
6. Loss of capillaries and melanocytes: skin sallowness
7. Skin pigmentation increases: keratoses (scaly, raised areas), senile lentigines (liver spots—brown or yellow spots)
8. Changes in hair color (gray, white), changes in texture (becomes fine or coarse), and thinning (balding)
9. Appearance of facial hair for women; decrease in facial hair for men
B. Factors contributing to problems of the integumentary system
1. Peripheral circulation diminishes, causing thick brittle nails
2. Cardiovascular changes cause decreased healing of wounds
3. Immune system decreases ability to overcome disease
C. Resulting problems
1. Skin tears
2. Decubitus ulcers
D. Nursing management of the dependent older adult
1. Use extra lotions or creams on dry skin
2. Gentle handling when moving; position to prevent pressure, reposition every 2 hours
3. Use extra care when performing venipunctures
4. Assess and document condition of skin; intervene to prevent the development of decubitus ulcers; document new lesions or changes in existing lesions; older adults are at risk for basal cell carcinoma

Musculoskeletal System

A. Alterations
1. Loss of lean muscle mass and muscle cells: decreased muscle strength, size, and tone
2. Loss of elastic fibers in muscle tissue: increased stiffness and decreased flexibility
3. Thinning of long bones: brittle, porous bones
4. Thinning of intervertebral disks: height loss and changes in posture
B. Factors contributing to general musculoskeletal problems
1. Poor nutritional patterns

2. Endocrine system changes: decreased estrogen and testosterone
3. Gastrointestinal system changes: decreased absorption of vitamins and minerals
4. Cardiovascular system changes: poor circulation
5. Neurological deficits that cause safety hazards
6. Decreased level of activity and periods of prolonged bed rest
7. Side effects of medications; for example, steroids

C. Resulting problems
1. Susceptibility to fractures is increased, especially in the postmenopausal woman who develops osteoporosis
2. Risk factors for osteoporosis include: early menopause, white or Asian heritage, thin, sedentary lifestyle, cigarette smoking, caffeine usage, low calcium intake
3. Altered body image
4. Pain and discomfort
5. Decreased mobility
6. Impaired ability to perform activities of daily living (ADL)
7. Increasing feelings of dependency
8. Calcium deposits in blood vessels and renal structures
9. Weakened muscles affecting other systems
   a. Diaphragm
   b. Bladder
   c. Myocardium
   d. Abdominal wall

D. Nursing management of the dependent older adult
1. Handle patient gently
2. Reduce environmental safety hazards
3. Encourage mobility and exercise; weight-bearing and weight-lifting exercises are effective in reducing the progression of bone and muscle loss
4. Allow extra time for performing activities
5. Assist with ADL and exercises as needed
6. Provide encouragement and support for accomplishments
7. Prevent deformities
   a. Proper positioning
   b. Range-of-motion (ROM) exercises
8. Alleviate pain
   a. Rest periods
   b. Positioning
9. Encourage liberal fluid intake

Respiratory System

A. Alterations
1. Structural alterations (scoliosis, kyphosis, osteoporosis): decrease in lung expansion
2. Alveoli enlarge and thin out: decreased oxygen and carbon dioxide diffusion
3. Loss of bronchiole elasticity: decreased breathing capacity, increased residual air
4. Diaphragm becomes fibrotic and weakened; diminished efficiency
5. Respiratory muscle structure and function decrease: diminished strength for breathing and coughing
6. Changes in larynx: weaker, higher-pitched voice
7. Decrease in ciliary function: increased susceptibility to upper respiratory tract infection

B. Factors contributing to respiratory problems
1. Decreased resistance to infection
2. Musculoskeletal system changes: weakened muscles and postural changes
3. Long history of smoking and exposure to pollutants
4. Periods of prolonged bed rest
5. Cardiovascular system changes
6. Side effects of medications, for example, sedatives and hypnotics

C. Resulting problems
1. Dyspnea
2. Chronic cough
3. Fatigue and debilitation
4. Cerebral hypoxia
   a. Confusion
   b. Restlessness
   c. Behavioral changes
5. Decreased activity tolerance
6. Cardiovascular problems, for example, congestive heart failure
7. Anorexia

D. Nursing management of the dependent older adult
1. Assist with ADL as necessary
2. Encourage breathing exercises; activities such as singing and those that create laughter are excellent for increasing air exchange
3. Administer oxygen therapy
4. Change position frequently
5. Encourage liberal fluid intake
6. Discourage smoking
7. Position for maximum comfort and efficiency of respiration, for example, extra pillows, Fowler's position
8. Allow rest periods
9. Assess pulmonary status when assessing behavioral changes

Cardiovascular System

A. Alterations
1. Decrease in enzymatic stimulation: longer and less forceful contractions
2. Increase in fat and collagen amounts: decline in cardiac output
3. Increase in oxygen demands of coronary arteries and brain: decreased peripheral circulation
4. Loss of elasticity of vessel walls; decrease in contraction and recoiling responses; heart develops collateral circulation to compensate for coronary artery
5. Reduced or unaltered heart rate at rest
6. Mild tachycardia on activity
7. Slow increase in serum cholesterol

B. Factors contributing to problems of the cardiovascular system
1. Poor nutritional patterns
2. Anxiety and stress
3. Decreased activity level
4. Arteriosclerosis, hypertension
5. Pulmonary system changes
6. Side effects of medications

C. Resulting problems
1. Fatigue and decreased activity tolerance
2. Increased anxiety
3. Edema
4. Hypertension: increased risk of cerebrovascular accident (CVA)
5. Behavioral changes
6. Poor circulation to other systems and extremities: delayed healing, decreased efficiency of kidneys
7. Potential risk for coronary artery disease, heart failure

D. Nursing management of the dependent older adult
   1. Assist with ADL as necessary
   2. Encourage moderate activity and exercise
   3. Provide patient teaching considerations regarding:
      a. Confusion
      b. Forgetfulness
      c. Resistance to change
   4. Avoid excess pressure on the skin
   5. Assess cardiovascular status when assessing behavioral changes
   6. Avoid tight, constrictive clothing and shoes
   7. Provide special foot care
      a. Prevent trauma
      b. Prevent infection

Gastrointestinal System

A. Alterations
   1. Muscle atrophy in the tongue, cheeks, mouth
   2. Esophageal wall thinning, increase incidence of gastroesophageal reflux disorder (GERD)
   3. Decrease in ptyalin and amylase secretion by salivary gland: alkaline saliva
   4. Decrease in saliva secretion: thicker mucus and dryness
   5. Oral sensitivity loss, loss of taste discrimination
   6. Ill-fitting dentures, periodontal disease, lack of teeth: nutritional deficiencies
   7. Shrinkage of bony structures of mouth
   8. Gastric mucosa shrinks: decline in digestive enzyme secretion leads to delayed digestion
   9. Decrease in lipase secretion: fat intolerance
   10. Decrease in gastric acid: diminished ability to use calcium
   11. Decrease in intrinsic factor: pernicious anemia
   12. Decrease in iron absorption: iron-deficiency anemia
   13. Internal sphincter muscle tone loss: alterations in bowel evacuation
B. Factors contributing to problems of the gastrointestinal system
   1. Decreased level of activity
   2. Dental problems
   3. Poor nutritional patterns
   4. Weakened muscles
   5. Nervous system changes
   6. Overuse of laxative and enemas
   7. Anorexia, which may be related to depression
   8. Side effects of medications; for example, opiates and steroids
C. Resulting problems
   1. Discomfort; for example, heartburn and bloating
   2. Constipation and impaction
   3. Fecal incontinence
   4. Anorexia
   5. Increased risk of aspiration
D. Nursing management of the dependent older adult
   1. Promote nutritional intake
      a. Consistency of food
      b. Ability to manage utensils
      c. Extra time for feeding (oral and tube)
   2. Provide good oral hygiene
   3. Encourage mobility and exercise
   4. Provide adequate fluid intake
   5. Educate patient regarding constipation and laxative abuse

6. Check bowel habits regularly
7. Give prompt assistance to bathroom or with bedpan
8. Prevent skin and mucosal breakdown
   a. Prompt, thorough cleansing of anal area
   b. Extra gentleness when inserting rectal and feeding tubes

Renal System

A. Alterations
   1. Decrease in kidney size
   2. Decline in renal blood flow
   3. Reduced ability of nephron to filter urine: decreased clearance
   4. Reduced ability of tubule cells to selectively secrete and reabsorb: fluid and electrolyte alterations
   5. Decreased bladder capacity: frequency and urgency
   6. Loss of muscle tone of bladder and uterus
   7. Loss of pelvic muscle tone
   8. Decreased urine concentration ability
   9. Prostate gland enlargement
B. Factors contributing to problems of the renal system
   1. Periods of prolonged bed rest
      a. Increased urinary stasis, increased urinary tract infections
      b. Renal calculi formation
   2. Cardiovascular system changes, for example, decreased renal perfusion
   3. Nervous system changes
   4. Decreased fluid intake
   5. Muscle weakness
   6. Social withdrawal and apathy, for example, sensory deprivation
   7. Side effects of medication, for example, diuretics, antiparkinsonian drugs
C. Resulting problems
   1. Hyperglycemia
   2. Behavioral changes, for example, confusion, elevated blood urea nitrogen (BUN), electrolyte imbalance
   3. Interference with sleep and recreational patterns
      a. Urinary frequency
      b. Urinary urgency
      c. Nocturia
   4. Increased chance of skin breakdown; for example, incontinence
   5. Feelings of embarrassment, rejection, and withdrawal
D. Nursing management of the dependent older adult
   1. Prevent urinary stasis
      a. Encourage liberal fluid intake
      b. Encourage frequent change of position
      c. Encourage ambulation
   2. Prevent skin breakdown: prompt and thorough cleansing
   3. Bladder retraining
   4. Promptly respond to call for bathroom or bedpan
   5. Leave night light on if patient experiencing nocturia
   6. Assess renal status when assessing behavior changes
   7. Early recognition of urinary tract infection; first sign may be a change in mental status

Neurological System

A. Alterations
   1. Decrease in weight and size of brain
   2. Decline in number of neurons

3. Diminished nerve conduction speed
   a. Voluntary movement slower
   b. Decreased reaction time
   c. Delayed decisions
4. Alterations in sleep-wake cycle
   a. Less rapid-eye-movement (REM) sleep
   b. Less deep sleep: tendency to catnap
   c. Easily awakened
   d. Difficulty falling asleep
   e. Average 5 to 7 hours sleep at night
   f. Need less sleep but require more rest periods
5. Brain tissue atrophy and meningeal thickening: short-term memory loss

B. Factors contributing to problems of the neurological system
1. Poor nutrition patterns
2. Cardiovascular system changes, for example, decreased circulation
3. Pulmonary system changes, for example, cerebral hypoxia
4. Sensory deprivation; may be physiological or environmental
5. Side effects of medications, for example, sedatives

C. Resulting problems
1. Safety hazards
   a. Impaired senses, for example, vision, hearing, pain, and temperature
   b. Forgetfulness and confusion
2. Anorexia, for example, decreased taste buds
3. Social isolation and rejection
4. Impaired ability to perform ADL
   a. Decreased coordination
   b. Decreased concentration
   c. Safety hazards
5. Increased sense of dependency
6. Incontinence
7. Altered self-image and declining confidence
8. Behavioral changes, for example, forgetfulness and confusion

D. Nursing management of the dependent older adult
1. Provide for safety
2. Establish means of communication if patient has hearing impairment
3. Assess all systems when assessing behavioral changes
4. Maintain sense of independence when possible
5. Assist with ADL only when necessary; allow extra time
6. Encourage socialization
7. Provide sensory stimulation
8. Consider forgetfulness and confusion when teaching
   a. Be consistent
   b. Provide repetition when necessary
   c. Be patient
   d. Provide positive reinforcement and encouragement
9. Assess other symptoms carefully when assessing for infection and trauma: decreased temperature control and pain perception mask these symptoms
10. Carefully check temperature of bath water and forms of heat therapy to avoid burns: discrepancy in sensation of heat and cold
11. Maximize use of environmental aids

Endocrine System

A. Alterations
1. Decline in growth hormone secretion
2. Diminished estrogen secretion
3. Decreased size of the uterus
4. Decreased size and motility of fallopian tubes
5. Loss of elasticity of vagina
6. Shrinking vulva and external genitalia with loss of subcutaneous fat
7. Diminished vaginal secretions
8. Increased time required in response to sexual stimulation
9. Reduced elasticity of breast tissue
10. Decreased testosterone secretion
11. Decreased size and firmness of testes
12. Decreased production of sperm
13. Increased time required to achieve an erection and subsides more rapidly
14. Development of drug, Viagra, treats erectile dysfunction in some men
15. Shorter and less forceful ejaculation
16. Increasing time between erection and orgasm
17. Decreased basal metabolic rate
18. Diminished glucose metabolism
19. Decreased pancreatic secretions

B. Factors contributing to problems of the endocrine system: Related changes in other body systems

C. Resulting problems
1. Adult-onset diabetes mellitus
2. Musculoskeletal system changes
3. Hypothyroidism
4. Sexual dysfunction

D. Nursing management of diabetes mellitus: special considerations
1. Poor vision: diabetic retinopathy a common complication
2. Lack of coordination
3. Poor nutritional patterns
4. Forgetfulness and confusion
5. Resistance to change
6. Masking of symptoms by physiological changes of aging and disease
7. Decreased activity level can increase insulin requirements; exercise will decrease the amount of insulin needed
8. Stress and anxiety
9. Increased susceptibility to complications, including nephropathy, neuropathy, peripheral vascular disease, coronary artery disease, diabetic foot ulcers
10. Proper management of blood sugar helps reduce the development of complications

Immune System

A. Alterations
1. Diminished immunoglobulin production
2. Weakened antibody response
3. Atypical signs and symptoms frequently a response to infection, for example, subnormal temperature, behavior changes, and decreased pain sensation

B. Factors contributing to problems in the immune system
1. Weakened antibody response
2. Reduced immunoglobulin production
   a. Thymus gland wasting
   b. Reticuloendothelial system alterations

C. Resulting problems
1. Self-destructive autoaggressive phenomenon
2. Increased susceptibility to infection; for example, herpes zoster (shingles), a reactivation of the chicken pox virus along the nerve route occurs after the age of 50

3. Increased susceptibility to disease
4. Misdiagnosis
D. Nursing management of the dependent older adult
  1. Be careful in observation and assessment; knowing what is normal for each older adult is especially important; any change is suspect
  2. Be aware that atypical symptoms of infection are common among the older adult; for example, with otitis media, difficulty in hearing is too often dismissed as a typical aging problem
  3. Use early nursing intervention
  4. Educate regarding available vaccines; the use of the influenza and pneumococcal vaccines is recommended for the high-risk older adult and all adults residing in group living facilities

Sense Organs

A. Vision
  1. Alterations
    a. Diminished pupil size: loss of responsiveness to light
    b. Decline in peripheral vision
    c. Decreased accommodation ability, causing presbyopia (farsightedness)
    d. Decreased tear production
    e. Decrease in lens transparency and elasticity
    f. Decline in ability to focus quickly
    g. Decline in color discrimination
    h. Difficulty in adjusting to dark-light changes
    i. Altered depth perception
  2. Selected disorders
    a. Cataracts affect 70% of adults over age 75; appears to be related to metabolic changes in the eye and exposure to ultraviolet light and radiation; can be accelerated by chronic diseases and steroid use; intake of antioxidants may help reduce their development; primary symptoms are a gradual loss of vision and seeing halos around objects; treatment is surgical
    b. Glaucoma has been described as a thief in the night because symptoms are subtle until vision is lost; open-angle glaucoma is the most common type; intraocular pressure is increased, leading to damage of the optic nerve and irreversible blindness; age, family history, persons of African-American and Chinese backgrounds, and female gender are risk factors; intraocular pressure and visual field assessments are the primary monitoring tools; loss of peripheral vision is the primary symptom; treatment for glaucoma begins with ophthalmic medications to lower intraocular pressure; if medications are unsuccessful, surgical intervention may be an option
    c. Senile macular degeneration is the leading cause of blindness in older adults; the retina and the layers below the retina are affected which leads to a loss of central vision; tasks requiring close focus become difficult, and objects, especially lines, may appear wavy and distorted; treatment options are limited; laser surgery may reduce the amount of distortion
B. Auditory alterations
  1. Progressive loss of hearing, starting with high-frequency tones
    a. Presbycusis (loss of sound perception): a type of sensorineural hearing loss; the primary cause is aging
    b. Otosclerosis (bone cell overgrowth): a form of conductive hearing loss that results from the reduction in sound passage to the cochlea
    c. Cerumen accumulation is a cause of conductive hearing loss; older adults are at risk for cerumen impaction because of the thicker cerumen produced by the aging glands; the use of hearing aids is an additional factor for cerumen impaction; cerumen build up can be viewed with an otoscope; the older adult may experience dizziness, pain, pruritus, and pressure in the ear, as well as a decrease in hearing
  2. Thickened and more opaque eardrum
C. Taste bud alterations
  1. Declining number of taste buds
  2. Declining taste sensation
D. Olfactory alterations
  1. Decrease in olfactory nerve fibers
  2. Diminished sense of smell
E. Tactile alterations
  1. Dulled sense of touch
  2. Higher pain threshold
  3. Diminished sense of vibration
  4. Declining heat or cold discrimination
F. Vestibular or kinesthetic alterations
  1. Diminished proprioception
  2. Decrease in coordination
  3. Decline in equilibrium

SPECIAL CONSIDERATIONS

Nutrition

A. Diet
  1. Nutritional needs of older adults are the same as those of other adults
  2. The need for calories decreases
  3. Older adults need adequate protein to prevent muscle wasting and weakness
  4. Older adults need adequate fats for padding, insulation, and energy; low saturated–fat intake is recommended by physicians
  5. Older adults need adequate carbohydrates from unprocessed foods for energy: the tendency is to buy high-carbohydrate, empty-calorie foods because they:
    a. Are less costly
    b. Are filling
    c. Are easy to chew
    d. Require minimal preparation
  6. Ethnic, cultural, and lifestyle preferences should be encouraged for identity reinforcement and appetite stimulation
  7. Fluid intake should be 1500 to 2000 ml per day: the tendency is to reduce intake because of urinary frequency, urgency, and incontinence
  8. Older adults need vitamin supplements to prevent deficiencies: women should continue with increased intake of calcium supplements
  9. Lactose deficiency is common: calcium can be obtained from other sources, for example, spinach, asparagus, broccoli, and sardines
  10. Older adults need fiber, roughage, and bulk to aid elimination

11. Consistency and preparation is needed in accordance with chewing, swallowing, and digestive abilities
12. Small, frequent meals are easier to digest and conserve energy
13. Older adults need to pay attention to cholesterol and fat intakes
14. Older adults need to be aware of food-drug and food-food interactions, for example, Coumadin and foods high in vitamin K, antibiotics and antacids, levodopa and vitamin B_6, monoamine oxidase inhibitors (MAOIs) and aged cheese

B. Provide unhurried atmosphere to increase appetite and incentive to eat
C. Caution against food fads and megavitamin therapy
D. Assess facilities for appropriateness
   1. Storage
   2. Cooking
   3. Refrigeration
E. Encourage financial assistance and planning
F. Arrange for transportation to and from grocery store
G. Provide assistance with packages because of weakness and physical disabilities or limitations
H. Provide mealtime socialization
I. Provide assistance for the confused, forgetful, and ill person
J. Encourage regular meals; older adults have a tendency to skip meals
K. Provide education classes on purchasing healthful foods on limited income
L. Identify factors that increase risk of nutritional problems in the older adult (Box 9-3)

Hygiene

A. Skin
   1. Water temperature 100° to 105° F (37.7° to 40.5° C)
   2. Daily baths are not necessary
   3. Oil-base or emollient lotion
   4. Alcohol and dusting powder are not appropriate because they dry out the skin (dusting powder can be inhaled)
   5. Avoid friction
   6. Avoid pressure
   7. Neutral-reaction or oil-based soap
   8. Susceptible to bruising and skin tears
B. Nose: blunt-end scissors to trim nasal hairs that extend beyond nares
C. Oral hygiene
   1. Dentures
      a. Take out dentures at night, and reinsert the next morning to prevent tissue swelling, unless contraindicated by dentist
      b. Provide frequent cleaning
      c. Encourage proper storage
      d. If patient is institutionalized, make sure dentures are labeled
   2. Soft nylon toothbrush, electric toothbrush, or adaptive toothbrush
   3. Mouthwash (optional)
   4. Lanolin to lips
   5. Semiannual dental visits
   6. Frequent mouth inspection for food accumulation, injury, disease, and infection (tendency to pocket food can lead to infection)

BOX 9-3 Factors That Increase Risk of Nutritional Problems in the Older Adult

Physiological Factors
Decreased secretion of enzymes; indigestion, gastric reflux common
Decreased absorption of nutrients and minerals
Reduced mobility of stomach; slowing of peristalsis
Restricted intake of nutrients caused by problems with teeth and dentures (e.g., ill-fitting dentures, periodontal disease, missing teeth)
Decreased production of saliva
Reduced sensitivity to sweet and salty flavors
Low activity level
Disease-related symptoms that can reduce appetite, energy, or ability to ingest food
Side effects of medications

Psychosocial Factors
Limited finances that prohibit purchase of proper food
Lack of knowledge regarding nutritional needs, nutritional value of foods
Inability to shop, store foods, or cook (e.g., lack of transportation, no kitchen facilities, dementia)
Personal preferences that violate principles of good nutritional intake
Loneliness or eating alone
Mood disturbances (e.g., depression, anxiety)

From Eliopoulos C: *Manual of gerontologic nursing,* ed 2, St Louis, 1999, Mosby.

D. Ears
   1. Clean with warm, soapy water and dry with towel
   2. Do not use cotton swabs because they force cerumen back against the tympanum
   3. Trim ear hair growth in men
   4. Provide hearing aid maintenance
      a. Wash mold and receiver with mild soap and warm water
      b. Check cannula for patency, and clean and dry with pipe cleaner
      c. Remove batteries when aid is not in use
      d. Store batteries in refrigerator to retain freshness
      e. Turn aid to off position when inserting in patient's ear
      f. Turn aid on to adjust volume
      g. Store aid in its original box away from cold, heat, and sunlight
      h. Components, styles, nursing care (Box 9-4)
E. Eyes
   1. Decreased tear production may necessitate use of artificial tears
   2. Provide eyeglass care
      a. More frequent cleaning of eyeglasses is required
      b. Use warm water to clean eyeglasses
      c. Store only in eyeglass case
      d. If patient is institutionalized, make sure glasses are labeled
F. Nails
   1. Provide daily care
   2. Use moisturizer on nails and cuticles
   3. Encourage circulation with buffing of nails

BOX 9-4   Hearing Aids

Components
Microphone: converts sounds into electric energy
Amplifier: increases energy
Receiver: converts energy back into sound waves
Volume control
On-off switch

Styles
Behind the ear: limited amplification
In the ear: entire unit worn in the ear; limited amplification
Eyeglass attached: unit built in the frame of the eyeglass; limited amplification
Body aided: amplifier housed in a case worn on body; offers most amplification of all

Nursing Care
Encourage client to obtain hearing aid from a reputable dealer after a full audiometric examination has been done.
Ensure that batteries are functioning before the aid is applied; it is recommended that batteries be changed weekly.
Identify common hearing aid problems:
- Whistling sound: bad connection between earpiece and amplifier; excessively high volume
- Insufficient amplification: volume set too low; weak or dead battery; blockage from cerumen; disconnected tubing or wiring
- Periodic loss of amplification: loose connection; poor battery contact; dirt in switch; cracked case.
Recognize that adjustment to a hearing aid is difficult and may take time, and reassure the client that this is not unusual.

Adapted from Eliopoulos C: *Manual of gerontologic nursing*, ed 2, St Louis, 1999, Mosby.

4. File with emery board (cutting makes them more brittle and risks injury)
G. Hair
   1. Use mild shampoo that is not irritating to the eyes
   2. Remove facial hair from women with tweezers or waxing
   3. Use of a shaving brush is recommended for men
   4. Moisturizers are beneficial for men's facial hair
H. Feet: the older adult is often unable to care for the feet adequately because of limitation of movement or visual difficulties
   1. Give daily care (washing, inspection, skin care)
   2. Inspect between and under toes for abrasions, cracking, lacerations, scaling
   3. Clip toenails straight across
   4. Pumice stone should be used to remove dry, hard skin
   5. Discourage use of irritants
   6. Avoid elastic-top socks or knee-high stockings
   7. Emphasize the danger of roll garters
   8. Recommend properly fitting shoes with low, broad, rubber heels for safety, comfort, fatigue reduction
   9. Persons with diabetes need especially attentive assessment of feet; a person with newly diagnosed diabetes should be initially evaluated by podiatrist and as necessary thereafter

Safety

A. Susceptibility to accidents is increased by:
   1. Decline in sensory acuity
   2. Decreased ability to interpret environment
   3. Increased reflex time
   4. Postural change sensitivity
   5. Gait disturbances
   6. Muscular weakness
   7. Urinary urgency and frequency
   8. Confusion
   9. Judgment alterations
   10. Forgetfulness
   11. Proprioceptive inadequacies
   12. Improper footwear
   13. Depression
   14. Environmental hazards
   15. Medications that cause drowsiness
B. Accident prevention
   1. Attire
      a. Provide short or three-quarter–length sleeves rather than long, loose-fitting sleeves
      b. Avoid long garments
      c. Provide Velcro closures
   2. Furniture
      a. Proper height
      b. Chairs with arms
   3. Floors
      a. No-slip wax
      b. No scatter rugs or deep-pile carpeting
      c. Avoiding clutter
      d. Rubber tips on ambulation aids
   4. Kitchen
      a. Tong reachers instead of footstools, chairs, and stepladders
      b. Temperature-controlled faucets
      c. Electric rather than gas stoves
      d. Stoves with controls on the front
      e. Shelves within comfortable reach
      f. Wall cabinets at comfortable height instead of floor-based cabinets to avoid bending and stooping
      g. Avoiding trash accumulation
      h. Easy-grip utensils
   5. Bathroom
      a. Nonskid strips or rubber mats in tub and shower
      b. Temperature-controlled faucets
      c. Good soap containers
      d. Tub and toilet handrails
      e. Bathtub seats
      f. Shower chairs
      g. High toilet seats
      h. Colored toilet seats
      i. Night light
   6. Bedroom
      a. Bedside commode
      b. Side rails
      c. Night light
      d. Telephone next to bed (amplifier; dial enlarger)
   7. General
      a. Proper lighting
      b. Railings on stairways
      c. Safe electric appliances
      d. No overloading of electric outlets

e. No frayed wiring or extension cords
f. Securely taped cords
g. Emergency telephone numbers readily available at telephone
h. Smoke detectors
i. Crime-prevention assessment and implementation
j. Medications
   (1) Separated from those of other household members
   (2) Internal and external medications in different locations
   (3) Large print labels
   (4) Color-coded labels
   (5) Daily supply containers
   (6) Calendar or alarm clock reminders
   (7) Discard outdated medications and prescriptions
k. Medical emergency alarm system
8. Mobility aids (Table 9-1)

Vision

A. Bright, diffused light is best
B. Place items on better-vision side
C. Avoid glare
D. Strips on stairs improve depth perception
E. Eyeglasses should be kept clean (older adults frequently forget or ignore this)
F. Use colors that increase visual acuity, for example, red, orange, and yellow
G. Avoid night driving
H. Use resources and aids for visually handicapped
I. Preserve independence
J. Visual losses increase susceptibility to illusions, disorientation, confusion, isolation
K. Place objects directly in front of individual with decreased peripheral vision
L. Stimulate other senses

Hearing

A. Older adults usually do poorly on hearing tests because of their cautious responsiveness
B. Reduce distractions
C. Do not fatigue with unnecessary noise and talk
D. Speak in a normal tone of voice; shouting is misinterpreted by persons who have normal hearing
E. Observe for signs of developing hearing loss
   1. Leaning forward
   2. Inappropriate responses
   3. Cupping ear when listening
   4. Loud speaking voice
   5. Requests to repeat what has been said
F. Reduce background noise before speaking, for example, television and radio
G. Hearing deficits increase social isolation, suspiciousness, fears
H. Speak toward the better ear
I. Be sure to have the person's attention before speaking
J. Use resources and aids for the hearing impaired, for example, television and telephone amplifiers, sound lamps, and alarm clocks that shake the bed
K. Keep hands and objects away from mouth when speaking

Activities of Daily Living

A. Older adults may ignore appearance because of fatigue, unawareness, or lack of incentive

B. Clean clothing is essential for maintaining pride and dignity
C. Choosing what to wear provides a source of control over one's life, fosters independence, and increases self-confidence and self-esteem
D. Lifelong sleeping attire or lack of attire should be encouraged
   1. Reinforces individuality
   2. Reduces sleep interference
E. Standard clothing sizes no longer fit; loose-fitting, comfortable clothing should be encouraged
F. Front closures are more easily managed
G. Cotton socks absorb perspiration
H. Zippers, Velcro, and large buttons make dressing easier
I. Layering and sweat suits provide warmth in cold weather
J. Daily exercise should be encouraged and paced
K. Increase self-awareness with mirrors
L. Use daily living resources and aids
   1. Zipper aids
   2. Extra-long shoehorns
   3. Shoelace tiers, Velcro fasteners
   4. Adaptive utensils
M. Functional independence: ability to perform ADL and instrumental activities of daily living (IADL); examples of IADLs include shopping, using the telephone, ability to pay bills, obtaining meals, obtaining transportation

Sexuality

A. Cultural stereotypes deny freedom of sexual expression for the older adult
B. Lifelong sexual adjustment will determine how the older adult deals with sexual needs
C. Partner availability is made difficult
   1. Older adult women outnumber men
   2. Social and business roles change
D. Physiological alterations affect self-image and foster nonparticipation
E. Families of older adult persons tend to discourage sexual relationships because of stereotypes and inheritance threats
F. Sexual focus shifts to companionship
G. Older persons continue to enjoy sexual activity; decrease is primarily a result of declining health or lack of available partner (Box 9-5)

Speech

A. Older adults tend to rely more on speech than they do on action
B. Speak slowly and clearly
C. Allow sufficient time for comprehension and response
D. Speak to and treat the individual as an adult
E. Explanations will reduce fear
F. Recovery of speech is influenced by multiple impairments and dependency

NEUROLOGICAL SYSTEM (SELECTED DISORDERS)

Organic Mental Syndromes (Box 9-6)

A. Onset may be rapid or progressive
B. Cognitive function alterations
   1. Judgment
   2. Memory

TABLE 9-1	Mobility Aids		
Aid	**Characteristics**	**Fit**	**Use**
Cane	Assists balance by widening base of support; not intended for weight bearing Comes in a variety of styles: • Regular (straight): provides minimal assistance with balance • Three- and four-point (quad): broader base of support, more cumbersome	Length should approximate distance between greater trochanter and floor. Elbow should be flexed slightly when cane rests 6 in from side of foot.	Use on unaffected side Advance when affected limb advances (i.e., if right leg is weak, the cane is held on the left and moved forward as the right leg steps). Hold close to body; do not move forward beyond toes of affected foot. All canes should have suction grips to prevent slippage on floor.
Walker	Broader base of support; more stability than a cane Comes in a variety of styles: • Pickup: assists with weight bearing • Rolling: pushed on wheels rather than lifted; reduces physical strain; often have seats to allow rest after several steps or propulsion from a sitting position	Height equivalent to distance between greater trochanter and floor Elbows slightly flexed when hands on sides of walker	When weight bearing is allowed, advance walker and step normally. When partial or no weight can be borne on one limb, thrust weight forward, then lift walker and replace all four legs on floor. Always use both hands when transferring from chair or commode; back walker to seat, and use arms of chair or commode to assist in standing.
Wheelchair	Used when patient's disability prohibits other walking aids Should not be used for convenience or speed of patient or staff	Individually prescribed based on height, weight, limb use, arm strength, and self-propulsion capacity	Prepare environment for wheelchair use: widen doorways and toilet stalls; plan a functional furniture layout with no rugs; lower mirrors, telephones, drinking fountains, counters; install ramps. Use special pads and cushions to reduce pressure damage; shift weight and reposition frequently. Lock wheels and remove footrests when transferring to and from chair.
Crutches	Frequently difficult for older person to use because of inadequate upper body strength, arthritic hands, and balance problems Not as stable as other mobility aids	Individually sized Length should be equivalent to 2 inches below axilla to point on floor 6 inches in front of client Hand bars placement crucial because hands should bear total weight. Elbow should be flexed, wrist slightly hyperextended Axillary pressure can cause radial nerve paralysis	Tailor gait to patient's needs; consult with physical therapist. Use good posture and pay particular attention to foot position on affected side (walking exclusively on ball of foot or toes can cause footdrop). General rule when climbing stairs: stronger foot goes up first, down last. Upstairs: step up with stronger foot; bring crutches to that step; raise affected foot. Downstairs: crutches to lower step; lower affected foot; follow with stronger foot. Eliminate obstacles: • Waxed floors • Throw rugs • Extension cords • Uneven surfaces • Clutter

Adapted from Eliopoulos C: *Manual of gerontologic nursing,* ed 2, St Louis, 1999, Mosby.

BOX 9-5   Encouraging Intimacy in the Older Adult

Educate others, including family members, concerning need for intimacy in old age.

If sexual intimacy is not possible, promote expression of intimacy in other ways (hugging, cuddling, spending time together).

Avoid belittling the older person's desire for intimacy.

Provide education for the older adult concerning intimacy because it is not always comfortable for the older adult to inquire about this subject.

Older adults may need detailed instruction after life-altering events such as myocardial infarction, cerebrovascular accident, or other acute or chronic illness.

3. Intellect
4. Orientation
5. Affect
C. Associated factors (Table 9-2)
D. Cognitive dysfunction dementia

DEMENTIA

A. Alzheimer's disease: progressive, deteriorating, chronic dementia is the most common form of dementia; incidence increases with age; cause is unknown, but theories include acetylcholine decrease, beta-amyloid protein accumulation, genetic factors, and viruses
  1. Types
     a. Senile dementia Alzheimer's type (SDAT): onset over age 65
     b. Presenile dementia: onset between ages 40 and 60
  2. Cerebral pathophysiology
     a. Senile plaques
     b. Neurofibrillary tangles
     c. Neurotransmitter abnormalities
     d. Atrophy
  3. Diagnosis confirmed by above findings on autopsy
  4. Assessment: Mini-Mental State Examination (MMSE) is used as assessment tool; scores below 24 generally indicates dementia
     a. Personality changes
     b. Memory changes
     c. Aphasia (language difficulties), apraxia (impaired ability to perform purposeful tasks), and agnosia (impaired ability to recognize persons or objects)
     d. Behavioral changes
     e. Impaired cognition
     f. Late-stage physical alterations affecting mobility and swallowing
  5. Nursing intervention and management
     a. Support independence with ADL: do not rush; focus on one task at a time
     b. Provide structured, consistent environment
     c. Facilitate sleep-activity balance; plan quiet, nonstimulating events in the evening
     d. Promote bowel and bladder continence: toilet every 2 hours, reduce fluid intake after evening meal, and encourage fluids before noon

BOX 9-6   Organic Mental Syndromes

Delirium: a reduced ability to maintain attention to external stimuli and to shift attention to new external stimuli appropriately; disorganized thinking, as manifested by rambling, irrelevant, or incoherent speech; reduced level of consciousness; sensory misperceptions; disturbances of the sleep-wake cycle and level of psychomotor activity; disorientation to time, place, or person; memory impairment

Dementia: impairment of short- and long-term memory; changes in abstract thinking; impaired judgment

Amnestic syndrome: impairment in short- and long-term memory that is attributed to a specific organic factor; immediate memory is not impaired

Organic delusional syndrome: delusions resulting from specific organic factor such as amphetamine use or cerebral lesions of the right hemisphere

Organic hallucinosis: hallucinations that are persistent or recurrent and caused by a specific organic factor such as use of hallucinogens, which produce visual hallucinations, or alcohol, which induces auditory hallucinations

Organic mood syndrome: persistent depressed, elevated, or expansive mood caused by a specific organic factor such as a toxic effect of substances, including reserpine or methyldopa, an endocrine disorder such as hyperthyroidism, or structural brain disease that results from hemispheric strokes

Organic anxiety syndrome: recurrent panic attacks or generalized anxiety caused by a specific organic factor such as endocrine disorder, use of psychoactive substances, brain tumors in the vicinity of the third ventricle, vitamin-B_{12} deficiency, aspirin intolerance, or heavy metal intoxication

Organic personality syndrome: persistent personality disturbance caused by a specific organic factor such as structural damage to the brain caused by neoplasms, head trauma, or cerebrovascular disease

Intoxication: maladaptive behavior and a substance-specific syndrome caused by the recent ingestion of a psychoactive substance such as alcohol, cannabis, amphetamine, or cocaine

Withdrawal: development of a substance-specific syndrome that follows the cessation of, or reduction in, intake of a psychoactive substance that the person previously used regularly

Adapted from Haber J et al: *Comprehensive psychiatric nursing,* ed 5, St Louis, 1998, Mosby.

     e. Provide reality orientation, remotivation, reminiscence
     f. Provide patient safety: reduce environmental dangers; use *visual barriers* such as half doors, red lines, stop signs
        (1) At risk for wandering
        (2) Becomes lost easily
        (3) Fails to recognize environmental hazards
     g. Encourage socialization because withdrawal and social isolation are common
     h. Reduce anxiety-provoking situations: do not argue or try to reason

TABLE 9-2	Factors Associated with Organic Mental Syndromes and Disorders
Influential Factors	**Examples**
Volatile agents	Gasoline, aerosols, glues, paint removers, solvents, lacquers, varnishes, dry-cleaning agents, home cleaning products alone or when mixed
Heavy metals	Lead paints, ceramic glazes, moonshine whiskey, mercury, arsenic, manganese
Insecticides	Dichlorodiphenyltrichloroethane (DDT), parathion, malathion, diazine
Brain trauma	Concussion, contusion, hemorrhage, thrombosis, penetrating wounds, blast effects, electrical trauma; exposure to repeated courses of electroconvulsive therapy; oxygen deprivation
Drugs	Alcohol, barbiturates, opioids, cocaine, amphetamines, cannabis, hallucinogens such as lysergic acid diethylamide (LSD) and phencyclidine (PCP)
Infections	Tuberculous and fungal meningitis, viral encephalitis, neurosyphilis (tabes dorsalis), Jakob-Creutzfeldt disease, human immunodeficiency virus (HIV) related disorders (AIDS, ARC)
Neoplasms, tumors	Astrocytoma, medulloblastoma, meningioma
Metabolic and endocrine disorders	Hepatic disease, uremic encephalopathy, porphyria; thyroid, parathyroid, and adrenal dysfunction; Wernicke-Korsakoff syndrome
Nutritional deficiencies	Lack of protein; deficiencies in vitamin C and the B vitamins (folic acid, niacin, pyridoxine, riboflavin, thiamine, B_{12}); fluid and electrolyte imbalance
Seizures	Petit mal, grand mal, focal seizures, psychic seizures
Hypoxia-ischemia	Anoxia related to delayed or prolonged cardiopulmonary resuscitation
Neurological disease (possible genetic influence)	Huntington chorea, multiple sclerosis, Pick's disease, cerebral degeneration, Parkinson's disease
Cerebral changes associated with Alzheimer's disease	Loss of neurons, plaques, neurofibrillary degeneration, tangles, amyloid deposits, loss of dendritic tree, choline acetyl transferase (CAT) defects, degeneration of basal forebrain, elevated platelet fluidity, inherited genetic factor

From Haber et al: *Comprehensive psychiatric nursing,* ed 5, St Louis, 1998, Mosby.

   i. Provide nutritional needs; high-calorie, easily managed finger food can be offered to the wandering, restless patient
   j. Recognize self-concept needs
   k. Encourage verbal communications; use validation techniques to focus
   l. Monitor effectiveness of medications; cholinesterase inhibitors such as tacrine (Cognex), donepezil (Aricept), and rivastigmine (Exelon) will slow the progression of symptoms of Alzheimer's disease
B. Multiinfarct dementia: cognitive impairment caused by cerebrovascular disease is the second leading cause of dementia in older adults; often a history of transient ischemic attacks (TIAs) and hypertension symptoms are often similar to Alzheimer's disease, but onset is more abrupt; changes in functioning fluctuate rather than progress slowly as in Alzheimer's disease; treatment is aimed at the vascular cause
C. Psychoactive substance-induced mental disorders: chemically induced organic disease; delirium frequently accompanies these disorders; in many cases, delirium can be reversed

PARKINSONIAN SYNDROME

Progressive neurological movement disorder
A. Primary
   1. Parkinson's disease
   2. Paralysis agitans
B. Secondary
   1. Tumors

   2. Drugs
   3. Infection
C. Assessment
   1. Slowness of movement
   2. Waxlike rigidity of extremities
   3. Facial masking
   4. Tremors while at rest; characteristic pill-rolling motion
   5. Muscular weakness
   6. Shuffling gait
   7. Stature alterations
   8. Drooling; swallowing difficulties
   9. Cognitive impairment
   10. Mood swings
D. Nursing intervention and management
   1. Foster independence with ADL
   2. Maintain physical mobility
   3. Provide adequate nutrition
      a. Keep swallowing difficulties in mind
      b. Person may require suction and is prone to aspiration
      c. Monitor weight weekly
      d. Provide adaptive eating devices
      e. Provide thick liquids
   4. Prevent constipation
   5. Encourage communication
      a. Be attentive: speech is soft and low pitched
      b. Allow time: speech is slow and monotonous
   6. Enhance self-concept
      a. Focus on patient's strengths
      b. Encourage activities that foster success
      c. Give positive feedback
      d. Establish realistic goals

e. Encourage verbalization of feelings

f. Maintain intellectual activity stimulation

7. Monitor effectiveness of medications in controlling tremors and rigidity and alleviating characteristic depression

    a. Tricyclic antidepressants; MAOIs

    b. Antihistamines

    c. Anticholinergics

    d. Levodopa (eliminate vitamin B_6 from diet)

    e. Catechol-O-methyltransferase (COMT) (e.g. Tolcapone inhibitors)

    f. Non-ergot dopamine agonists

8. Provide safety

9. Decrease stress

PSYCHOLOGICAL CHANGES (NORMAL AGING PROCESS)

Self-Image

A. Physiological alterations

B. Youth-oriented society

C. Retirement

D. Income alterations

E. Role changes

F. Sexual expression alterations

Intelligence

A. Verbal ability and retained information remain unchanged

B. Abstract thinking and performance response decline

C. Performance of activities involving neuromuscular learning decline

D. Attention span shortens

E. Literal approach to problem solving affects ability

F. Fluid intelligence declines after adolescence

G. Crystallized intelligence continues to increase throughout life

H. Learning capacity continues

Memory

A. Short term: concentration and retention decline

B. Long term: minimal impairment occurs

C. Remote

    1. Remote memory is better than short-term memory

    2. Remote memory is involved in reminiscence

Motivation

A. Not risk takers

B. Do not actively seek change

C. Possess fear of failure

D. Self-fulfilling prophecies

E. Competitiveness declines

F. Energy levels decline

Attitudes, Beliefs, Interests

A. General attitude realignment

B. Interests either narrow or expand

C. Tend to keep lifelong beliefs amid rapidly changing society

Personality

A. Personality is basically unchanged

B. Some exaggeration of behavioral responses is evident

C. Adaptive capacities are diminished

D. The ability to handle stress is reduced

PSYCHOLOGICAL DISORDERS (ABNORMAL)

Depression

A. Reaction to loss of:

    1. Independence

    2. Status

    3. Spouse, relatives, friends

    4. Possessions

    5. Income

    6. Mobility

B. Many commonly prescribed medications can cause depression (e.g., digitalis, propranolol, levodopa, oxycodone, zolpidem)

C. Physical illness and changes can be intensified by existing depression or can be a contributing factor to depression, or both

    1. Lowered self-esteem

    2. Self-concept alterations

    3. Feelings of hopelessness and worthlessness

D. Types

    1. Exogenous

        a. Referred to as neurotic; external; caused by outside events

        b. Common in the older adult

        c. Usually a reaction to losses

    2. Endogenous

        a. Referred to as psychotic; caused by internal events

        b. Characterized by:

            (1) Guilt

            (2) Reduced self-regard

            (3) Early morning awakening

            (4) Slowing of thought, verbalization, and level of activity

        c. Classifications

            (1) Unipolar: life history of depression

            (2) Bipolar (manic-depressive psychosis)

                (a) Mood swings from depression to euphoria

                (b) More likely to have hallucinations and delusions

E. Symptoms of depression (Box 9-7)

F. Nursing intervention

    1. Encourage self-expression; increase self-esteem

    2. Improve appearance

    3. Provide structure, routine

    4. Assist with maintaining or regaining control

    5. Have kind, understanding attitude

    6. Provide physical care as needed; encourage independence

    7. Provide safety, security

    8. Reduce environmental stimuli and stress

    9. Continuously test reality perception

    10. Ascertain emotional support network

    11. Prevent isolation and avoidance

    12. Realize potential for suicide exists

        a. Suicide is an act that stems from depression

        b. Approximately 25% of suicides occur in persons over age 65

        c. White men over age 75 have the highest rate

        d. Refer to Chapter 6 for suicidal risk assessment, crisis intervention, and nursing intervention

    13. Teach about medications, evaluate understanding

BOX 9-7	Symptoms of Depression as Observed in Cognitive, Affective, and Somatic Changes

Cognitive
Indecisiveness
Confusion*
Impaired thinking*
Poverty of thought
Hopelessness/emptiness
Suicidal ideation*
Guilt
Inability to concentrate
Worry
Believes self a failure*
Believes self causing harm to others*
Believes self going crazy*
Believes self deserving of punishment*

Affective
Fear*
Anxiety
Sadness
Irritability
Anger*
Feels distant from others*
Depersonalized

Somatic
Tearful
Crying spells
Agitation*
Anorexia
Weight loss
Constipation
Palpitations
Fatigue/weakness
Insomnia
Restlessness*

Data from Morris J, Wolf R, Kerman L: *J Gerontol* 30:209, 1975; Zung W: *Arch Gen Psychiatry* 29:328, 1973.
*Presence of clinically significant depression.

Aggressive Behavior

A. Abnormal anger, rage, or hostility, which, if turned inward, would lead to depression and, if turned outward, would lead to aggressiveness
B. Response to:
  1. Anxiety
  2. Stress
  3. Guilt
  4. Insecurity
  5. Loss of self-esteem
  6. Loss of control of destiny
  7. Forced dependency
C. Clinical manifestations
  1. Lack of cooperation
  2. Irritability
  3. Demanding
  4. Hostility

5. Demonstration of coping mechanisms characteristically used to decrease stress, for example, rationalization and repression
  6. Altered interpersonal relationships
  7. Altered reality testing
D. Nursing intervention
  1. Reduce stress source and sensory overload
  2. Encourage verbalization
  3. Set realistic, reachable goals
  4. Respond to questions directly and briefly
  5. Allow ample time for task completion
  6. Meet physical needs as necessary
  7. Encourage environmental participation and activity involvement
  8. Positively recognize attainments
  9. Set limits on activities
  10. Anticipate hostile, demanding behavior
  11. Allow only the degree of independence that can be successfully handled
  12. Avoid responses and action that might lead to guilt, feelings of rejection, bother, dislike
  13. Increase feeling of self-worth
  14. Medication
  15. Provide therapy if indicated

Regression

The display of regressive behavior, an ego defense mechanism, is not an uncommon response in the older adult to external stressors; this return to an earlier behavioral stage (e.g., temper tantrums, rocking, incontinence) requires prevention, early detection, and prompt intervention (remove source of stress and reverse the behavior).

Paranoid Behavior

A. Inappropriate attempt of coping with stress
B. Response to:
  1. Physical impairments
  2. Sensory deprivation
  3. Loss
  4. Loneliness
  5. Medications
  6. Environmental changes
  7. Isolation
  8. Vision alterations
  9. Auditory alterations
C. Clinical manifestations
  1. Secretiveness
  2. Mistrust
  3. Mood disturbances
  4. Oversensitivity
  5. Insecurity
  6. Superiority attitude
  7. Alterations in behavior
  8. Delusions
  9. Withdrawal
  10. Fearfulness
  11. Aloofness
  12. Refusal to take medications, eat, or carry out normal self-care activities
D. Nursing intervention
  1. Attempt to allay anxiety
  2. Allow patient to refuse treatments

3. Do not argue with patient
4. Try not to take patient's anger personally
5. Administer medication
6. Do not make promises to patient
7. Look for alterations in ADL as cues to whether the patient's verbalizations are of real concern or are for attention
8. Be aware of events precipitated by environment
9. Use stress-management techniques
10. Bring patient-predicted events that do not occur to patient's attention
11. Encourage independence
12. Monitor impact on hygiene and nutrition
13. Encourage socialization

REHABILITATION/MAINTENANCE OF COGNITIVE FUNCTION

Reality Orientation (Table 9-3)

A. A total approach to keeping individuals oriented; small groups that emphasize time, place, and person; weather; holidays, and so forth
B. First used with disoriented, confused older adults at Veterans Administration Hospital in Tuscaloosa, Alabama, in 1965
C. Orientation boards may be used to provide contact with reality
D. Program success depends on total staff commitment and 24-hour implementation
E. Many facilities that care for the older adult have implemented modified programs

F. Program implementation is not limited to an institutional setting
G. Components
1. Small groups
2. Formal classroom sessions
a. 20 to 30 minutes
b. Morning sessions recommended (older adults are more alert in the morning)
c. Reality orientation board, calendars, clocks, and other materials used according to instructor plan
d. Positive verbal feedback emphasized
e. Confusion never reinforced
H. All personnel who come in contact with patients participating in the program are expected to use reality orientation
1. Address patient by name and title
2. Orient patient to time, place, and person
3. Give positive verbal feedback
4. Do not reinforce confusion

Remotivation

A. Similar to reality orientation
B. Normal behavior is reinforced through structured group program
C. Stimulating participation and interest in the environment are key components
D. Sessions average 20 to 60 minutes
E. Visual aids are used, for example, items that stimulate sensory responses
F. Patient behavior is recorded
G. Staff support and involvement is essential

TABLE 9-3 Differences Between Remotivation and Reality Orientation	
Reality Orientation	**Remotivation**
Correct position or relation with the existing situation in a community; maximum use of assets	Orientation to reality for community living; present oriented
Called reality orientation and classroom reality orientation program	Called remotivation
Structured	Definite structure
Refreshments or food may be served for identification	Refreshments not served
Appreciation of the work of the world; constantly reminded of who they are, where they are, why they are here, and what is expected of them	Appreciation of the work of the group stimulates the desire to return to function in society
Classes range from 3 to 5 patients, depending on degree/level of confusion or disorientation from any cause	Group size: 5 to 12 patients
Meeting 1/2 hr daily at same time in same place	Meeting once to twice weekly for 1 hr
Planned procedures: reality-centered objects	Preselected and reality-centered objects
Consistence of approach response of resident responsibility of teacher	No exploration of feelings
Periodic reality orientation test pertaining to residents' level of confusion or disorientation	Progress ratings
Emphasis on time, place, person orientation	Topic: no discussion of religion, politics, or death
Use of portion of mind function still intact	Untouched areas of the mind
Residents greeted by name, thanked for coming, and extended handshake or physical contact (or both) according to attitude approach in group	No physical contact permitted; acceptance and acknowledgment of everyone's contribution
Conducted by trained aides and activity assistants	Conducted by trained psychiatric aides

From Barns E, Sack A, Shore H: Guidelines to treatment approaches. Modalities and methods for use with the aged, *Gerontologist* 13:513, 1973.

Reminiscence

A. Small-group sessions
B. Based on life-review process
C. Older adults with cognitive dysfunction retain long-term memory and through reminiscence can adapt to the aging process
D. Purposes
   1. Resolving conflict
   2. Sharing memories
   3. Achieving sense of identity and self-importance
   4. Focusing on a life that has meaning rather than a life viewed as a waste of time
   5. Reminiscence is natural for older adults
      a. They feel comfortable
      b. They are good at it
      c. Reinforces sense of belonging (everyone talks about life's trials and tribulations)
   6. Therapeutic relationship with leader is more likely to develop as patients realize that their memories are important and valued
   7. Depressed patients find a caring listener and an opportunity to externalize their anger
   8. Psychologically disturbed patients receive acceptance, group validation, and a forum for expression: encourage active exploration of past strengths
   9. Strive to change outlook on the past rather than establishing new future directions
   10. Reminiscence is a psychological assessment tool (e.g., insight into past coping mechanisms)
   11. Reminiscence reduces isolation, insecurity, and negative self-esteem
   12. Confused patients can be assisted in exploring a memory that will stimulate latent thoughts, become more oriented, and improve ability to focus
   13. Current circumstances are often reflected through memories
E. If patients have difficulty focusing their thoughts, assist by selecting a specific memory
F. Stimulation of dormant thoughts to the surface decreases disorientation
G. Patients who are reluctant to talk can usually be stimulated with topics of food, movies, or music
H. Program implementation is not limited to institutional settings

Cognitive Training

A. Consists of memory exercises, problem-solving situations, and memory training
B. Leader must be familiar with the patient's past leisure time utilization, hobbies, and occupations
C. Individual, small, or large groups are used
D. The purpose is to maintain mental activity

Pet Therapy

A. Carefully chosen pets as part of a pet therapy program for a facility or personal pets
B. Benefits: decreases tension, stimulates interests in surroundings, provides emotional support, and encourages activity and comforts by touch

Music Therapy

A. May reach patients when other methods fail
B. Uses

   1. Calms and reduces agitation in patients with Alzheimer's disease
   2. Promotes attention span and expression of feelings
   3. Provides motivation for exercise and socialization
   4. Sing-a-longs can enhance cognitive function and foster contact with reality

Relaxation Therapy

A. Promotes sense of physical well being, reduces stress, releases tension
B. Uses small groups
C. Involves rhythmic breathing, tension-relaxation exercises, and altered state of consciousness

Validation Therapy

A. Useful for persons with permanent cognitive loss
B. The nurse accepts the patient's feeling to give him or her a sense of dignity and self worth
C. Validation therapy provides comfort to patient and enables nurse to find meaning in patient's behavior

BLADDER RETRAINING: URINARY INCONTINENCE

A. Causes
   1. Physiological changes
      a. Decline in muscle support of pelvis
      b. Reduction in bladder's capacity to hold urine
      c. Sphincter weakness
   2. Behavioral alterations
      a. Regression
      b. Insecurity
      c. Rebellion
      d. Attention seeking
      e. Dependency
      f. Sensory deprivation
   3. Drugs
   4. Consciousness alterations
   5. Disease
   6. Obstruction
   7. Trauma
   8. Immobility
   9. Bedpans and urinals
   10. Lack of privacy
   11. Lack of time
B. Types
   1. Stress or passive
      a. Bladder outlet weakness
      b. Involuntary
      c. Frequency when sneezing, coughing, laughing, lifting
   2. Paradoxical or overflow
      a. Uncontrollable contraction waves
      b. Bladder does not empty
      c. Frequency accompanied by retention
      d. At risk for urinary tract infection
   3. Total
      a. Constant dribbling
      b. Storage problem
C. Older adults susceptible to:
   1. Urinary tract infections
   2. Urgency
   3. Frequency

D. Patient reactions to incontinence
   1. Insecurity
      a. Social withdrawal
      b. Isolation
      c. Sensory deprivation
      d. Avoidance of previously developed relationships
   2. Depression
      a. Embarrassment
      b. Guilt
      c. Shame
E. Intervention
   1. Pelvic exercises
      a. Bearing down
      b. Push-ups from a chair
   2. Indwelling catheter as a last resort if skin integrity is threatened
   3. Condom drainage
   4. Absorbent, waterproof underpants
   5. Keep patient clean and dry
   6. Skin care
   7. Retraining
      a. Assess and record voiding pattern for minimum of 72 hours
         (1) Time
         (2) Place
         (3) Quantity
         (4) Activity
         (5) Patient awareness
         (6) Significant medications
         (7) Character of urine
         (8) Presence or absence of constipation or discharge
         (9) Problems: for example, clothing and ambulation hindrances
      b. Reestablish voiding pattern
         (1) First scheduled voiding of the day should be attempted immediately after awakening in the morning even if bed is wet
         (2) Voiding should be attempted at intervals determined from the assessment period (usually at 1-, 2-, or 3-hour periods; goal is every 4 hours)
         (3) Patient takes one or two 8-oz (240-ml) glasses of fluid 1 hour before attempting to urinate
         (4) No fluids should be taken between 6:00 PM and 6:00 AM if no urinating is desired
         (5) Fluid intake should be at least 2000 ml per day
         (6) Alcoholic drinks are contraindicated
         (7) Soft drinks, tea, and coffee should be avoided
         (8) All fluid intake should be measured and recorded
         (9) All urine output should be measured and recorded

BOWEL RETRAINING: FECAL INCONTINENCE

A. Causes
   1. Physiological changes
      a. External anal sphincter relaxation
      b. Perineal relaxation
      c. Muscle atony
   2. Behavioral alterations
      a. Regression
      b. Rebellion

      c. Dependency
      d. Sensory deprivation
   3. Central nervous system injury
   4. Obstruction
   5. Impaction
   6. Consciousness alterations
   7. Immobility
   8. Trauma
B. Intervention
   1. Keep patient clean and dry
   2. Provide absorbent, waterproof underpants
   3. Provide skin care
   4. Provide retraining
      a. Bowel retraining is easier than bladder retraining; if patient is incontinent of urine and stool, start a bowel-retraining program first
      b. Use no laxatives
      c. Ensure adequate fluid intake (2 L per day)
      d. Fluids and solids that promote patient's bowel movements (e.g., bran, orange juice) and roughage should be included in the diet
      e. Encourage physical activity
      f. Obtain bowel history
      g. Procedure
         (1) Establish regular day and time to assist patient to the toilet for evacuation, preferably after a meal
         (2) After 20 minutes, if patient has not had a bowel movement, insert a lubricated glycerin suppository
            (a) Do not use directly from refrigerator
            (b) Do not insert into a bolus of stool (ineffective)
            (c) After ascertaining that patient requires the suppository for training, it can be inserted 1 to 2 hours before the scheduled training time and after a meal
         (3) Digital stimulation is recommended after 48 hours if the previously mentioned procedure is not successful
         (4) Take the patient to the bathroom at the scheduled time daily, even if he or she has had a bowel movement between scheduled times

SUGGESTED READINGS

Eliopoulos C: *Manual of gerontologic nursing,* ed 2, St Louis, 1999, Mosby.

Eliopoulos C: *Gerontological nursing,* ed 4, Philadelphia, 1997, Lippincott-Raven.

Feldman RS: *Development across the life span,* Englewood Cliffs, NJ, 1999, Prentice Hall.

Hamdy RC, Edwards J, Turnbull JM: *Alzheimer's disease: a handbook for caregivers,* ed 3, St Louis, 1998, Mosby.

Hogstel MO: *Clinical manual of gerontological nursing,* St Louis, 1992, Mosby.

Hogstel MO: *Geropsychiatric nursing,* ed 2, St. Louis, 1995, Mosby.

Morice SV: *Geriatric nursing,* Aurora, 1996, Skidmore-Roth Publishing.

Polan E, Taylor DC: *Journey across the life span,* 1998, FA Davis.

REVIEW QUESTIONS

1. A patient with Parkinson's disease has difficulty swallowing. The patient will be able to meet dietary requirements when he can:
   1. Eat solid food
   2. Drink thin liquids
   3. Eat a meal in 20 minutes
   4. Swallow without choking
2. Routine nursing care following a total knee replacement in an older adult should include which of the following?
   1. Keeping the affected leg in abduction
   2. Elevating the affected knee when the patient is out of bed
   3. Using wedge pillows between the patient's legs
   4. Keeping the head of the bed elevated to 45 degrees
3. Which of the following statements is accurate regarding ice application to the affected knee following a total knee replacement?
   1. Reduces edema and bleeding
   2. Reduces the chance of infection
   3. Increases circulation and movement
   4. Reduces fluid accumulation in the joint
4. A 67-year-old patient is admitted to a nursing home with a diagnosis of Senile dementia Alzheimer's type (SDAT). The nurse observes the resident moving toward the exit door. The nurse meets the resident at the door and volunteers assistance. The resident responds, "You can leave me alone. I'm going home." Which of the following nursing actions is most appropriate?
   1. Go with the resident
   2. Engage him in an activity
   3. Call the security department
   4. Physically prevent him from leaving
5. An older adult with Alzheimer's disease is restless and agitated. Which of the following activities is most appropriate for the patient?
   1. Taking a nap
   2. Taking a walk
   3. Listening to music
   4. Watching television
6. A patient with Alzheimer's disease demonstrates progressive personality changes. The patient begins to show signs of hostility and combativeness. The nurse should include which of the following in the plan of care?
   1. Use memory aids
   2. Simplify daily activity
   3. Decrease environmental stimuli
   4. Secure doors leading from the house
7. When caring for older adults, the nurse must know that the most common and easily reversed cause of dementia is:
   1. Pick's disease
   2. Drug toxicity
   3. Parkinson's disease
   4. Alcoholism
8. An 89-year-old nursing home resident with a history of poor nutritional intake eats a few mouthfuls of dinner and then gets up and leaves the table. Which of the following nursing approaches is most appropriate?
   1. Apply a vest restraint during meals
   2. Offer five to six small feedings daily
   3. Have a staff member feed him his meals
   4. Provide him with a variety of finger foods
9. The physician orders a restraint chair to be used in accordance with agency policy when a nursing home resident becomes overly agitated and combative. Which of the following statements by the nurse indicates the best understanding of the resident's response to the chair?
   1. The use of a restraint chair causes decubitus ulcers
   2. The use of a restraint chair fosters incontinence
   3. The use of the chair can increase a patient's agitation level
   4. All agitated patients should be restrained for their own safety
10. A patient diagnosed with Parkinson's disease is placed on Sinemet 10/100 orally three times daily by his physician. As he is leaving the physician's office, he asks the nurse what the drug will do. Which of the following explanations by the nurse is most correct?
    1. "You'll have to discuss that with the physician."
    2. "It can decrease your tremors and improve your gait."
    3. "It's the carbidopa-levodopa content ratio of the drug."
    4. "It's really very complicated and not necessary for you to know."
11. Which of the following assessments of a patient on Sinemet should indicate possible drug toxicity to the nurse?
    1. Akinesia, drooling
    2. Muscle stiffness, rigidity
    3. Muscle and eyelid twitching
    4. Slow movements, handwriting changes
12. A patient on Sinemet reports to the nurse that he really does not want to eat and occasionally vomits when he does eat. To reduce the gastrointestinal side effects of Sinemet and enhance its absorption, which of the following instructions should the nurse give the patient?
    1. Take the medication after meals
    2. Take the medication before meals
    3. Crush the medication and mix it with his food
    4. If any problems exist, call the physician to lower the dosage
13. An older nursing home resident has a history of paranoid behavior. When planning care for the patient, which of the following demonstrated behaviors should the staff identify as unusual?
    1. Verbalized hallucination
    2. Demonstrated superiority
    3. Verbalized oversensitivity
    4. Refused meals and treatments
14. A 73-year-old nursing home resident reports that the staff ignores her needs but takes care of all the other patients. The nurse knows this report to be inaccurate and understands that the patient is:
    1. Looking to cause trouble
    2. Experiencing active hallucinations
    3. Attempting to manipulate the staff
    4. Demonstrating manifestations of paranoia
15. An 80-year-old widower lives with his four cats in a two-bedroom, fourth-floor walkup. His children want him to move to a smaller apartment on the ground floor. He refuses and says he will stay where he is until he dies. His children must recognize that their father is:
    1. Afraid to move
    2. Becoming paranoid
    3. Displaying eccentricity
    4. Feeling secure where he is

16. A 78-year-old widow is brought to the local emergency room by the police, who found her wandering aimlessly about the street. She is confused, disoriented, and hospitalized for pneumonia. The nurse should recognize that the cause of her confusion and disorientation is:
    1 Infection
    2 Unknown
    3 Arteriosclerosis
    4 Organic brain syndrome

17. An elderly man is hospitalized with pneumonia and has a poor nutritional intake. The patient's appetite may improve if:
    1 His food is blenderized
    2 All liquids are served warm
    3 A roll is served with each meal
    4 He is served small meals frequently

18. An elderly patient hospitalized with pneumonia asks the time of each staff member who enters his room. The nurse knows that this behavior is characteristic of:
    1 Confusion
    2 Disorientation
    3 Memory deficit
    4 Impaired judgment

19. The night staff in a nursing home expresses concern about an elderly resident who is awake most of the night. Which of the following would be the most appropriate response by the nurse?
    1 "We'll increase his daytime activities."
    2 "I'll get a physician's order for a sedative."
    3 "As people get older, they require less sleep."
    4 "Older adults require less sleep at night, and more rest periods."

20. An elderly stroke survivor is being followed in the outpatient clinic. He is on sodium warfarin (Coumadin) daily. His prothrombin times have been unstable, and the physician requests the nurse to review the patient's dietary intake for indications of possible food-drug interactions. The nurse ascertains that the patient eats large quantities of the following foods. Which foods high in vitamin K should he avoid ingesting in large quantities?
    1 Rice and beans
    2 Chicken and rice
    3 Spaghetti and meatballs
    4 Broccoli and turnip greens

21. Which of the following patient concerns would result from the age-related change of loss of subcutaneous tissue?
    1 Foot pain
    2 Muscle cramps
    3 Increased urination at night
    4 Increased susceptibility to infection

22. Given the normal aging changes in the sensory system, which of the following colors would be most effective when color coding the door to the room of an elderly nursing home resident?
    1 Red
    2 Pink
    3 Blue
    4 Green

23. To evaluate the judgment of a patient in the early stages of Alzheimer's disease, the nurse should pay particular attention to the patient's ability to:
    1 Set the dining room table

2 Cooperate with caregivers
    3 Manage personal finances
    4 Navigate in familiar surroundings

24. An 80-year-old patient with diabetes mellitus is hospitalized and scheduled for a right below-the-knee amputation (BKA). On the fifth postoperative day, the nurse notices that the residual limb is edematous. The nurse should plan to:
    1 Elevate the limb on a pillow
    2 See if the patient has an order for a diuretic
    3 Instruct the patient to sit on the edge of the bed and dangle
    4 Ensure proper application of the Ace bandage to the residual limb

25. Aging causes respiratory changes that may result in:
    1 A lower-toned, frailer voice and dyspnea
    2 A much higher-pitched, stronger, resonant voice
    3 Decreased activity tolerance, dyspnea, fatigue
    4 Decreased activity tolerance, orthopnea, fatigue

26. Which of the following activities would an individual with presbyopia have the most difficulty completing?
    1 Walking, gardening
    2 Needlepoint, knitting
    3 Playing bingo, shopping
    4 Seeing road signs while driving

27. The nurse suggests to an older adult that she wear some makeup and a pretty robe when she goes to physical therapy. The nurse's suggestion is:
    1 Inappropriate because it infantilizes her
    2 Appropriate because it may increase her self-esteem
    3 Appropriate because she needs encouragement to bathe
    4 Inappropriate because she is unaware of her surroundings

28. When attempting to teach a patient with dementia, an important point for the nurse to remember is to:
    1 Speak quickly and repeat several times in succession
    2 Talk in a very animated, loud voice so the patient can hear you
    3 Eliminate background noise by shutting doors and turning off the television
    4 Talk to the patient when she is stress free, such as while she is watching television

29. The nurse is caring for a 72-year-old patient who has no known organic disease. The patient often calls the nurse by her daughter's name. The best course of action would be to:
    1 Tell her that her daughter will be visiting soon
    2 Go along with it because she is unlikely to reorient well
    3 Tell her the nurse's name and explain what the nurse will be doing for her
    4 Tell her that the daughter went home for a rest and will be back soon

30. The nurse is administering medications via a small-bore feeding tube to a 68-year-old individual. Which of the following is the correct sequence of administration?
    1 Check residual, give medication, flush with at least 150 ml of water
    2 Check tube placement, flush with water, give medication, check residual
    3 Flush tube with water, check residual, give medication, flush with water again
    4 Check tube placement, flush with water, give medication, flush with water again

31. When assessing the functional status of the older adult, the nurse must remember that:
    1 Older adults should be assessed on more than one occasion
    2 The best setting for a functional assessment is in a hospital setting
    3 Older adults will usually verbalize they are having difficulty with their ADL
    4 Assistive aids such as walkers and wheelchairs should not be included in the functional assessment

32. In which of the following facilities would the resident most likely receive skilled nursing care?
    1 Nursing home
    2 Adult day care
    3 Personal care home
    4 Senior citizen center

33. One day after open reduction internal fixation (ORIF) of the right hip, an 80-year-old patient is exhibiting extremely restless behavior. What is the first nursing action at this time?
    1 Medicate him for pain
    2 Ask his wife what is wrong with him
    3 Assess his cardiac and respiratory status
    4 Call the physician from the nurse's station to see him

34. A nurse is instructing an older adult concerning the Patient Self-Determination Act. Which of the following statements by the nurse accurately describes a health care proxy or durable power of attorney?
    1 The health care proxy makes financial decisions for the patient
    2 The state appoints a guardian who is given the power to make health care decisions for the patient
    3 The patient forms a list of activities that he does not want done if he should become incapacitated
    4 The patient appoints an individual who is given power of attorney to make medical decisions for the patient

35. A nurse is presenting a seminar on culture to a group of nursing assistants. The nurse relates that the culture most likely to use traditional or alternative therapies before accessing health care is:
    1 African Americans
    2 Jewish Americans
    3 Chinese Americans
    4 Hispanic Americans

36. Which of the following culture(s) boasts the lowest rate of nursing home use?
    1 Caucasians
    2 Asian Americans
    3 Jewish Americans
    4 Hispanic Americans

37. Which of the following provides income for the majority of retired older adult's income?
    1 Medicare
    2 Medicaid
    3 Social Security
    4 Tax-sheltered annuities

38. The nurses in a long-term care facility are attending a meeting by a noted gerontologist who is sharing his theories of aging. The gerontologist believes that by consuming vitamins A, C, and E, individuals can slow the aging process. The gerontologist most likely adheres to the:
    1 Free-radical theory of aging
    2 Collagen-fiber theory of aging
    3 Immunologic-response theory of aging
    4 Lipofuscin-accumulation theory of aging

39. The primary focus in the care of the older adult is on:
    1 Prevention of acute illness
    2 Prevention of chronic illness
    3 Health maintenance of acute illnesses
    4 Symptom management of chronic illnesses

40. An 81-year-old patient presents to the physician's office with a fractured right ankle. A family member states that the individual fell down the stairs. Which of the following additional assessments most strongly suggests elder abuse?
    1 Anorexia, ill-fitting dentures
    2 Chronic cough, shortness of breath
    3 Confusion, abrasions in various stages of healing
    4 Fatigue, extreme pain on palpation of the right ankle

41. A 69-year-old patient is admitted with an accidental drug overdose. The patient states that she is unable to read the number of pills to take because the print on the bottle is too small. The nurse should:
    1 Call for a psychiatric consult
    2 Call the patient's pharmacist to request large-print bottles
    3 Advise the family that they need to fill pillboxes for the patient
    4 Consult a home health nurse to go to the patient's home to give medications

42. A 77-year-old individual is brought to the emergency department after a neighbor found him lying in the street. The neighbor states that the man's apartment is filthy and no food is in the cupboards or refrigerator. The patient appears to be intoxicated. Which of the following questions should the nurse ask during her data collection?
    1 "Do you drink too much?"
    2 "Do you eat three meals a day?"
    3 "How much alcohol did you drink today?"
    4 "Do you have any family members living near you?"

43. The physician explains to the family of a patient with newly diagnosed Alzheimer's disease that he is to begin taking the drug Cognex as part of his medication regime. Which of the following statements made by the son would indicate understanding of the purpose of the drug?
    1 "He should be cured in about 3 months."
    2 "The progression of Alzheimer's should slow down."
    3 "The drug should be stopped if we don't see any improvement."
    4 "I should start to see improvement in my dad's memory in 3 to 4 weeks."

44. A caretaker for an older adult expresses concern that the person frequently goes to the bathroom at night without contacting her. The nurse advises the caretaker that she should:
    1 Buy side rails for his bed
    2 Give him a sedative at night
    3 Provide a clear path to the bathroom
    4 Restrain him if he gets up more than once

45. An older patient asks the nurse if the new drug, Viagra, would be something that would help him resume sexual relations with his wife. The most correct response by the nurse would be:
    1 "Viagra allows for a more intimate sexual experience."
    2 "It is best that you put that part of your life behind you."

3 "Viagra assists some individuals in achieving an erection."

4 "Viagra helps some people become more sexually excited."

46. A nursing assistant asks the nurse why some older residents fail to fill in all the responses to a multiple-choice survey concerning nutrition. The nurse responds that older adults:
    1 Have brain atrophy that affects intelligence
    2 Do not care about surveys concerning nutrition
    3 May be afraid to take the risk of answering "wrong"
    4 Were probably unable to see the small circles on the paper

47. The nurse is instructing a nursing assistant to put in a patient's hearing aid. The nurse instructs the assistant to turn the hearing aid on:
    1 Before placing it in the ear
    2 While inserting it in the ear canal
    3 Only after the aid is in the ear canal
    4 When the person decides to turn it on

48. A family member complains that his father, who has a hearing aid, no longer seems able to hear him speak. Which of the following is the best suggestion by the nurse?
    1 "Let's check the batteries on his hearing aid."
    2 "I'll have his physician come in and check him out."
    3 "Maybe he is just tired and doesn't want to listen now."
    4 "Let's make him an appointment at the hearing aid clinic."

49. The nurse is evaluating the best possible mobility aid for a patient with vertigo. Which of the following mobility aids would be the most stable for this patient?
    1 Cane
    2 Walker
    3 Crutches
    4 Wheelchair

50. A 79-year-old woman states that she needs respite care for her husband, who has dementia, while she undergoes a diagnostic procedure in an outpatient clinic. To which of the following types of facilities should the nurse refer the couple?
    1 Nursing home
    2 Personal care home
    3 Local area agency on aging
    4 Social Security Administration

51. The minimum data set (MDS) is used to:
    1 Assess mental status
    2 Determine roommate assignment
    3 Order daily medications
    4 Collect essential information

52. The completed MDS must be signed by:
    1 Nursing home resident
    2 Registered nurse assessment coordinator
    3 Attending physician
    4 Medication nurse

53. One factor that is considered when determining if negligence has occurred is the:
    1 Policy and procedure of the facility
    2 Age of the nurse
    3 Sex of the resident
    4 Severity of the injury

54. Reminder devices that are used to help prevent falls include:
    1 Wheeled walkers, quad canes
    2 Roll belts, vest restraints
    3 Wedge cushions, lap trays
    4 Side rails, overhead trapezes

55. After knocking on the resident's door, the nurse enters the room and observes a male resident masturbating. The most appropriate action by the nurse is to:
    1 Distract the resident in a conversation about the weather
    2 Get the resident out of bed and walk with him to the day room
    3 Quietly leave the room, making sure to close the door
    4 Tell the resident to stop

56. In planning a resident's first day at a long-term care facility, the schedule that keeps relocation trauma to a minimum is:
    1 Breakfast in group dining area, morning exercise group, interdisciplinary meeting
    2 Morning prayer meeting, breakfast in group dining area, interdisciplinary meeting
    3 Breakfast in resident's room, one-on-one admissions interview in room, interdisciplinary meeting
    4 Breakfast in room, free time until lunch, lunch in group dining area, interdisciplinary meeting

57. The best way to help the resident of an Alzheimer's unit identify their room is to:
    1 Put the resident's name on the door
    2 Post a picture of the resident taken 15 to 20 years earlier on the door of the resident's room
    3 Post a very recent picture of the resident on the door of the resident's room
    4 Color code the door of the room to match the resident's identification bracelet

58. A nurse observes a resident with a diagnosis of senile dementia buttering her napkin and using it to soak up sauce from her dinner plate. This resident is exhibiting symptoms of:
    1 Aphasia
    2 Agnosia
    3 Vertigo
    4 Akinesia

59. Reminiscence is a therapy based on:
    1 Life review
    2 Memory training
    3 Tension release
    4 Reorientation

60. The term tunnel vision describes the vision changes that occur with:
    1 Cataracts
    2 Night blindness
    3 Glaucoma
    4 Macular degeneration

61. The nurse knows that additional medical assessment is needed when a 65-year-old woman reports:
    1 "I just can't get enough to drink."
    2 "My knees are a little stiff in the morning."
    3 "It's easier for me to read when I sit by the window in the daytime."
    4 "It's taking me longer to reach orgasm lately."

62. An elderly person with non–insulin-dependent diabetes who develops pneumonia is at the greatest risk for developing:
    1 Diabetic coma
    2 Hyperglycemic hyperosmolar nonketotic coma
    3 Urinary tract infection
    4 Hypoglycemia

63. An appropriate intervention for a resident who is at risk for falls is:
 1 A 2-hour toileting schedule while the resident is awake
 2 Keeping side rails up at all times while the resident is in bed
 3 Obtaining an order for a vest restraint as needed
 4 Dressing the resident in heavy clothing

64. An 88-year-old resident of a dementia unit tells the nurse that she and her mother will be baking apple pies today. The of the following responses by the nurse is the most appropriate?
 1 "Your mother has been dead for 25 years."
 2 "Tell me about your mother."
 3 "You know you're not going to do that today."
 4 "What kind of apples do you use in your pies?"

65. A patient's wife died 4 years ago. The patient has kept all of her personal belongings and cries every time he speaks of her. The patient is exhibiting symptoms of:
 1 Dysfunctional grief
 2 Depression
 3 Anticipatory grief
 4 Paranoia

66. A 68-year-old female patient is 3 days postoperative open-reduction internal fixation (ORIF) of the left hip. The procedure was performed under general anesthesia. Before her surgery, the patient was oriented in all spheres and verbalized appropriately. She is now oriented only to self and tells the nurse that bugs are crawling on the walls. She is showing signs of:
 1 Sepsis
 2 Dementia
 3 Delirium
 4 Depression

67. Validation therapy is best described as:
 1 A way to reorient demented individuals
 2 A communication technique that accepts feelings and provides comfort
 3 Maintaining mental activity
 4 Life review

68. A useful technique for involving a patient in reminiscence therapy is to encourage:
 1 Reading the daily newspaper
 2 Writing a journal
 3 Compiling a family photo album
 4 Talking with family everyday

69. Some of the common manifestations of hypothyroidism in older adults include:
 1 Periorbital edema, weight loss, pale skin
 2 Moon face, edema, hypotension
 3 Slurred speech, increased perspiration, weight loss
 4 Fatigue, forgetfulness, dry skin

70. Mr. Smith, age 81, tells the nurse "I don't know why I bother; life just isn't worth living anymore." The most appropriate response by the nurse is:
 1 "Life is good, Mr. Smith; smile."
 2 "You sound upset; let's sit down and talk."
 3 "Don't be silly; you have a lot of friends."
 4 "Surely you're not thinking about killing yourself."

71. Senile macular degeneration results in:
 1 Loss of central vision
 2 Loss of peripheral vision
 3 Hemianopsia
 4 Aphakia

72. Glaucoma can be a contributing factor to the development of:
 1 Cataracts
 2 Blepharitis
 3 Vitreal hemorrhage
 4 Optic nerve damage

73. The development of cataracts is related to:
 1 Vitamin-B_6 deficiency
 2 Exposure to ultraviolet light
 3 Alcohol abuse
 4 Male gender

74. The effects of warfarin sodium (Coumadin) are enhanced by:
 1 Ginkgo biloba
 2 Chamomile
 3 Basil
 4 Saw palmetto

75. Compounds that block the action of free radicals are known as:
 1 Antiradicals
 2 Radical blocker
 3 Oxidizers
 4 Antioxidants

76. An appropriate nursing intervention for a patient with a diagnosis of global aphasia is:
 1 Keeping head of bed elevated
 2 Offering thickened liquids, gradually progressing diet
 3 Using a magic slate or tablet for communication
 4 Using a picture board for communication

77. The nurse knows that a patient needs additional teaching regarding alendronate sodium (Fosamax) when she says:
 1 "I'll take this with water right before bed."
 2 "I'll sit up for at least 30 minutes after I take it."
 3 "I'll take it with water in the morning."
 4 "If I forget to take it in the morning, I'll just skip it for that day."

78. When teaching a patient to use calcitonin-salmon (Miacalcin), the nurse must:
 1 Establish the patient's baseline bone density
 2 Instruct the patient to wear a medic alert tag
 3 Instruct the patient to alternate nostrils for administration
 4 Instruct her to sit up for at least 20 minutes after using it

79. The risk factors for osteoporosis are best described by:
 1 Late menopause, 10 lbs under ideal body weight, square dances three times a week
 2 Early menopause, coffee drinker, sedentary lifestyle
 3 Late menopause, vegetarian diet, walks 2 miles daily
 4 Late menopause, 25 lbs above ideal body weight, employed as a housekeeper

80. The assessment finding that requires immediate intervention is:
 1 Pedal pulses + 1 bilaterally
 2 Bilateral ankle edema, + 2 pitting
 3 Pedal pulse rate of 60 beats per minute
 4 Nonblanchable erythema of both heels

81. An important point to include in developing a teaching plan for a patient with gout is:
 1 Diet teaching about concentrated sweets
 2 Pain management techniques for chronic pain
 3 Proper use of cane
 4 Medications, dosage, side effects, therapeutic effects, signs of toxicity

82. A recently retired older person who lives alone and has started to drink heavily is most accurately described as being:
   1 A reactive drinker
   2 Depressed
   3 An alcoholic
   4 A substance abuser

83. Alcohol use in older adults is most likely to increase after:
   1 The holiday season
   2 Moving to a new home
   3 The death of a spouse
   4 Retirement from a job

84. The most significant factor contributing to decreased alcohol tolerance in older adults is:
   1 Age
   2 Gender
   3 Metabolic rate
   4 Ethnic background

85. Wernicke's encephalopathy and Korsakoff's syndrome are associated with a deficiency of:
   1 Vitamin C
   2 Vitamin B_{12}
   3 Vitamin K
   4 Vitamin B_1

86. Pill-rolling is a movement sometimes seen in:
   1 Huntington's chorea
   2 Tardive dyskinesia
   3 Parkinson's disease
   4 Diabetic retinopathy

87. The most common form of skin cancer in older adults is:
   1 Basal cell carcinoma
   2 Malignant melanoma
   3 Squamous cell carcinoma
   4 Malignant psoriasis

88. Excessive dryness of the skin sometimes seen in older adults is termed:
   1 Intertrigo
   2 Stasis dermatitis
   3 Xerosis
   4 Eczema

89. Herpes zoster is characterized by:
   1 Red welts that ooze serous fluid
   2 Vesicular eruption along a nerve route
   3 Dry scaly skin on one side of the body
   4 Redness and pruritus in the axillary folds

90. Aphasia, apraxia, and agnosia characterize:
   1 Depression
   2 Dementia
   3 Delirium
   4 Paranoia

91. The nurse knows that the caregiver understands an important aspect of caring for the family member with Alzheimer's dementia when the caregiver says:
   1 "I will avoid arguing or trying to reason with him."
   2 "I'll keep him busy all evening."
   3 "He can listen to radio talk shows."
   4 "It's important that he wear incontinent products at all times."

92. The most significant changes in the aging heart occur in the:
   1 Left ventricle
   2 Mitral valve
   3 Myocardium
   4 Pericardium

93. A physiological adaptation to atherosclerosis is:
   1 Increased cardiac output
   2 Collateral circulation
   3 Coronary artery disease
   4 Coronary artery bypass

94. The most prominent symptom of coronary artery disease is:
   1 Dyspnea
   2 Edema
   3 Pain
   4 Vomiting

95. Right-sided neglect or right-sided body blindness is related to:
   1 Seizure disorders
   2 Myocardial infarctions
   3 A CVA affecting the right side of the brain
   4 A CVA affecting the left side of the brain

96. The most common reason for decreased sexual activity among elderly women is:
   1 Decreased estrogen
   2 Cultural attitudes
   3 Lack of a partner
   4 Disability

97. The most appropriate way to enhance sexuality in a long-term care facility is to:
   1 Routinely assign men and women as roommates
   2 Provide sexually explicit reading materials
   3 Plan group activities that encourage socialization
   4 Serve alcoholic beverages with the evening meal

98. A resident is showing changes in behavior, including confusion. The nurse should first:
   1 Review the medications orders of the resident
   2 Obtain a urine specimen for culture and sensitivity
   3 Administer the ordered analgesic
   4 Assess the resident completely

99. A 78-year-old resident wanders from room to room looking for Dora, his deceased wife. The nurse says to the resident, "You loved your wife very much." This response is an example of:
   1 Reality orientation
   2 Validation
   3 Reminiscence
   4 Life review

100. Decreased cardiac output is most directly responsible for:
   1 Mitral regurgitation
   2 Cardiac enlargement
   3 Deceased coronary circulation
   4 Reduced renal blood flow

101. Reality therapy is most useful for the resident experiencing:
   1 Dementia
   2 Depression
   3 Delirium
   4 Disorientation

102. When music therapy is used with a restless resident exhibiting acting out behaviors, a successful outcome is the:
   1 Resident is comforted; behavior is calm
   2 Resident is reoriented to self
   3 Resident is free of injury
   4 Resident's functional level improves

103. An 80-year-old resident has frequent complaints of a dry mouth despite adequate fluid intake. The nurse should:
    1 Check resident's blood sugar
    2 Request a dental consult
    3 Review the medication orders
    4 Apply petroleum jelly to his lips

104. Longevity in men is most closely related to:
    1 Red wine consumption
    2 Marital status
    3 Occupation
    4 Religion

105. When preparing a room for a patient with a nasogastric feeding, the nurse should be sure to include a:
    1 Suction set up
    2 Scale
    3 Syringe
    4 Communication board

106. The nurse visits an 84-year-old home care patient on a sunny 78° day. The patient is wearing a sweater and is wrapped in an afghan. The nurse knows that:
    1 The patient needs a complete assessment for diabetes
    2 This is an unsafe situation
    3 The patient is lonely and afraid
    4 Older adults are frequently cold because of reduced heat production

107. A family is planning a surprise birthday party for their father's eighty-sixth birthday. The music that would best encourage socialization in this age group is:
    1 Big bands of the 1940s
    2 Classical piano concertos
    3 Gospel hymns
    4 Folk ballads

108. An open house for prospective residents of a new personal care home is planned. The food service that would be best suited and also encourage socialization is:
    1 A help-yourself buffet
    2 A sit-down meal with assigned seating
    3 A variety of snack foods
    4 A selection of small sandwiches and cookies

109. A home care patient, who is 80 years of age, needs a new doorbell. The best sound selection is:
    1 Chimes
    2 Music
    3 Bird calls
    4 Low-pitched buzz

110. One advantage of employing the older worker is that he or she:
    1 Increases employee morale
    2 Can orient new employees
    3 Has a better memory than young employees have
    4 Has an established work ethic

111. Assessing for pain in the older adult is important because older adults:
    1 Have lower pain thresholds
    2 Exhibit more pain behaviors than younger people do
    3 Are easily addicted to pain medications
    4 Have a higher pain threshold

112. A 70-year-old Jewish woman is scheduled for a bowel resection. The best time to schedule this procedure would be:
    1 8:00 AM Friday
    2 8:00 AM Thursday

    3 4:00 PM Friday
    4 8:00 AM Saturday

113. The most accurate description of a nursing home resident is:
    1 Female, age 70
    2 Male, age 70
    3 Female, age 82
    4 Male, age 82

114. A thin elderly woman of Asian heritage is at risk for:
    1 Hashimoto's disease
    2 Osteoporosis
    3 Herpes zoster
    4 Glaucoma

115. An older adult tells the nurse that she is sometimes unable to remember if she took her morning medication. The nurse should first:
    1 Set up a daily pillbox system for the patient
    2 Contact the patient's family
    3 Refer the patient to her physician
    4 Ask the patient about her usual morning routine

116. An older adult woman with osteoarthritis of her hands is compliant with her medication regime. She asks the nurse for suggestions to help relieve the morning stiffness of her hands. An appropriate response by the nurse is:
    1 "Gentle range-of-motion exercises of your hands and fingers can be useful."
    2 "Try using ice packs on your hands."
    3 "Soak your hands in Epsom salt water."
    4 "Massage your hands with cortisone cream."

117. While interviewing an older patient, the nurse observes that he squints his eyes and leans forward as she is talking. The nurse should suspect that the patient:
    1 Has a hearing loss
    2 Is legally blind
    3 Is anxious
    4 Is confused

118. A 70-year-old patient will be discharged to her daughter's home to recover after her hip replacement. The nurse knows that the daughter may need additional teaching when she says:
    1 "I had grab bars installed in the bathroom."
    2 "I took all the throw rugs up off the floors."
    3 "I brought your favorite little chair over for your bedroom."
    4 "I rented a bedside commode for you to use for a while."

119. Which of the following older adults would most likely have a diagnosis of hypertension?
    1 A 60-year-old African-American man
    2 A 60-year-old Puerto Rican woman
    3 A 60-year-old Asian-American man
    4 A 60-year-old Native-American woman

120. An older adult tells the nurse, "Having grandchildren is like getting extra interest on your savings account." This response is an example of Erikson's stage of:
    1 Ego transcendence vs. ego preoccupation
    2 Generativity vs. stagnation
    3 Integrity vs. despair
    4 Identity vs. role confusion

121. Check all that apply to the aging adult's eyes.
    1 _____ Pupils get smaller
    2 _____ Lens loses elasticity

3 _____ Tear production increases
4 _____ Color of iris lightens

122. Check all that may be related to a sudden onset of confusion.
    1 _____ Age
    2 _____ Medication
    3 _____ Infection
    4 _____ Environment

123. The most common cause of conductive hearing loss in the older adult is:
    1 Otosclerosis
    2 Cerumen impaction
    3 Otitis media
    4 Mastoiditis

124. A mentally stimulating activity for older adults that uses remote memory is:
    1 Reality orientation
    2 Reminiscence
    3 Spelling bee competition
    4 Scrabble

125. A 75-year-old male patient has been diagnosed with inoperable pancreatic cancer. The nurse observes that his wife is melancholy and is devoting much of her time scrap-booking and compiling family photo albums. The wife's behavior is best described as:
    1 Situational depression
    2 Denial
    3 Anticipatory grieving
    4 Social withdrawal

126. A 75-year-old female patient has diagnoses of bilateral cataracts, hypertension, and generalized anxiety disorder. The nurse observes that the patient is wearing one green sock and one blue sock. The nurse knows that:
    1 The patient is exhibiting decisional conflict related to her anxiety
    2 The patient is experiencing retinal changes related to her hypertension
    3 The patient is experiencing visual changes related to her cataracts
    4 The patient is colorblind

127. An older patient is complaining of inability to sleep through the night. He says he is restless and tosses and turns. Interventions that are helpful in promoting restful sleep include:
    1 Wearing earplugs, exercising 1 hour before bedtime
    2 Drinking 8 ounces of red wine 1 hour before bedtime, practicing controlled relaxation
    3 Maintaining a regular bedtime, wearing an herbal sleep mask
    4 Using a fan for white noise, limiting fluids in the evening

128. A 65-year-old woman has the diagnoses of osteoporosis and arthritis of her knees and hips. The nurse should encourage which of the following exercise programs?
    1 Aerobic dancing, swimming
    2 Walking, water aerobics
    3 Weight training, square dancing
    4 Bicycling, bowling

129. When a patient has a known diagnosis of decreased cardiac output, the nurse must assess:
    1 Blood sugar control, edema
    2 Appetite, urinary output

3 Weight, sleeping position
4 Bowel function, urinary output

130. A 72-year-old patient is admitted with an acute exacerbation of chronic obstructive pulmonary disease (COPD). The most appropriate nursing diagnosis for this patient is:
    1 Deficient knowledge of treatment regimen
    2 Anxiety
    3 Risk for infection
    4 Ineffective breathing pattern

131. An older patient tells the nurse that constipation has become a real problem and asks for suggestions that might help. The most appropriate response by the nurse is:
    1 "Most people have trouble with their bowels as they get older; you should talk to your doctor about it."
    2 "Changes in what you eat and drink can often help. Tell me what kinds of foods you usually eat."
    3 "Many medications are available that can help. What have you tried so far?"
    4 "That can be serious; how are you feeling? Have you had any blood from your rectum or abdominal pain?"

132. An 80-year-old patient tells that nurse, "I feel like my life has been wasted. My friends are all dying and I'm a burden on my family. I can't see, I can't hear, the golden years are a farce." This exemplifies Erikson's stage of:
    1 Trust vs. mistrust
    2 Identity vs. role confusion
    3 Integrity vs. despair
    4 Generativity vs. stagnation

133. An older adult receives a prescription for metronidazole (Flagyl). Which of the following complementary therapies would be contraindicated with this medication?
    1 St. John's wort
    2 Gin-soaked raisins
    3 Chamomile tea
    4 Acupuncture

134. An 82-year-old female resident of an assisted care facility insists on wearing the same set of clothes every day. An appropriate intervention is:
    1 Asking the family to take the clothes home
    2 Washing the clothes every day
    3 Hiding the clothing
    4 Asking the family to buy several identical sets of clothes

135. A 70-year-old man has a diagnosis of tuberculosis. The nurse knows that the result that will be positive is the:
    1 Venereal Disease Research Laboratory (VDRL)
    2 Purified protein derivative (PPD)
    3 Erythrocyte sedimentation rate (ESR)
    4 Human chorionic gonadotropin (HCG)

136. An older adult has a PPD (Mantoux) test result of 12-mm induration at 48 hours. The nurse should anticipate that the follow-up will be:
    1 Second step PPD in 4 weeks
    2 Bronchoscopy
    3 Computed tomographic (CT) scan of the chest
    4 Chest x-ray examination

137. Dr. Kübler-Ross identified the five stages of grief as:
    1 Denial, anger, resolution, peace, joy
    2 Denial, anger, bargaining, depression, acceptance
    3 Denial, pain, bartering, depression, acceptance
    4 Denial, anger, pain, bartering, resolution

138. An older adult develops symptoms of constipation, fatigue, ankle edema, and forgetfulness. These symptoms are consistent with an elevated:
    1 Blood glucose level
    2 White blood cell count
    3 Thyroid-stimulating hormone
    4 Systolic blood pressure

139. A 72-year-old man who has recently experienced a cerebral vascular accident affecting his right hemisphere is most likely to exhibit:
    1 Emotional lability
    2 Impotence
    3 Aphasia
    4 Right-sided paralysis

140. Factors that contribute to the increase in HIV/AIDS in older adults include (check all that apply):
    1 Past blood transfusions
    2 Lack of concern regarding birth control
    3 Increase in the number of sexual partners
    4 Aging immune system

141. The best way for a charge nurse to communicate a procedure change to nursing assistants is to:
    1 E-mail them on their home computers
    2 Post a notice at the time clock
    3 Tell the nursing assistant who arrives first about the change; have her tell the other assistants
    4 Have a brief meeting with everyone involved at the start of the shift to explain the change

142. A 70-year-old Chinese woman is hesitant to undress for an examination. The nurse should have the patient:
    1 Write a detailed description of her symptoms
    2 Draw a picture of her symptoms
    3 Point out the symptoms on the nurse
    4 Point out the symptoms on a model doll

143. A 65-year-old man has been placed on vitamin B_{12} injections for pernicious anemia. The nurse knows that the patient understands the therapy when he says:
    1 "This will give me more energy and improve my appetite."
    2 "I will have these injections for a year, then I can take pills."
    3 "I'll have these shots for my blood for the rest of my life."
    4 "These are my iron shots."

144. The nurse knows that a patient understands the low-sodium diet instructions when he makes the following choices from the lunch menu:
    1 Grilled cheese sandwich, tomato soup, ice cream
    2 Hot dog with sauerkraut, macaroni salad, chocolate cake
    3 Bacon, lettuce and tomato club sandwich, potato salad, an apple
    4 Baked chicken sandwich, fruit salad, orange sherbet

145. A nurse has the following responsibilities before breakfast (prioritize these tasks from one through four):
    1 _____ Neurological checks on a resident who fell during the night
    2 _____ Insulin administration for two residents
    3 _____ Routine vital signs for three residents
    4 _____ Eye drops for four residents

146. A resident is ordered a diet of 2400 calories via continuous tube feeding. The feeding formula has a concentration of 1.3 calories/ml. The nurse should set the feeding pump for _____ ml/hr.

147. As part of preoperative teaching, a 72-year-old patient scheduled for a total knee replacement should be taught about:
    1 Buck's traction
    2 Spica casts
    3 Continuous passive motion device (CPM)
    4 Patient-controlled analgesia (PCA)

148. Elderly female relatives are highly esteemed and frequently consulted for advice by:
    1 African Americans
    2 Italian Americans
    3 Native Americans
    4 Chinese Americans

149. A resident of a nursing home has a new medication order for ceftriaxone sodium (Rocephin). This order should be questioned if the resident is allergic to:
    1 Penicillin
    2 Sulfa
    3 Aspirin
    4 Shellfish

150. A nursing assistant asks the charge nurse what to do with the religious-looking object that a resident is wearing around his neck. The best response by the nurse is:
    1 "Call the family and ask them."
    2 "Put it in the bedside stand for now."
    3 "Take it off and I'll lock it in the medication cart."
    4 "Leave it on unless the resident asks for it to be removed."

ANSWERS AND RATIONALES

1. Application, evaluation, physiological integrity (b).
   - **4 When the patient swallows without choking and takes his time eating, he is safely able to meet dietary requirements.**
   - 1 Feeding a patient who has difficulty swallowing any type of solid food is inappropriate.
   - 2 Thin liquids are very difficult to swallow for individuals who have dysphagia.
   - 3 This patient may take much longer to eat because special precautions must be taken.

2. Application, implementation, physiological integrity (b).
   - **2 This is routine postoperative total knee replacement care to control edema and bleeding.**
   - 1 Abduction is used postoperative for total hip replacement to prevent hip flexion.
   - 3 Wedge pillows are used to abduct the leg postoperatively for total hip replacements.
   - 4 This is not appropriate for a total knee replacement.

3. Application, assessment, physiological integrity (b).
   - **1 The cold will cause vasoconstriction, which will control bleeding and edema.**
   - 2 Cold will not reduce the incidence of infection.
   - 3 CPM machines will increase circulation and movement.
   - 4 Drains should reduce fluid accumulation.

4. Application, implementation, safe, effective care environment (b).
   - **2 The nurse uses the short-term memory loss to her advantage; this produces little anxiety in the resident.**
   - 1 Accompanying the resident may be appropriate if diversion does not work.
   - 3 Show of force will only further agitate the resident.
   - 4 Agitation will increase if the resident is confronted.

5. Application, implementation, psychosocial integrity (c).
   - **2 Agitation is best reduced by an active diversion, such as walking.**
   - 1 Although this choice appears calming, it will not calm an agitated patient.
   - 3 Listening to music is a passive exercise that will not reduce agitation.
   - 4 This passive activity will not reduce restlessness or agitation.

6. Comprehension, planning, psychosocial integrity (b).
   - **3 Agitated and hostile individuals should remain in as non-stimulating, calm an environment as possible to defuse aggressiveness.**
   - 1 Memory aids will serve to preserve the patient's memory, but this does not address the hostility issue.
   - 2 This also helps the patient's memory, but it does not decrease hostile tendencies.
   - 4 This will preserve the patient's safety.

7. Knowledge, assessment, health promotion and maintenance (b).
   - **2 Drug toxicity is the only reversible cause of dementia listed.**
   - 1 Pick's disease is a progressive neurological disease that is not reversible.
   - 3 Parkinson's disease is progressive and results in dementia, and it is not reversible.
   - 4 The effects of alcoholism may be reversed but not quite as easily as the effects of drug toxicity.

8. Application, implementation, physiological integrity (b).
   - **4 This is the best choice for the resident who does not sit at mealtime; it ensures proper nutritional intake.**
   - 1 Restraints should be used for resident safety only.
   - 2 Normally, this would be a good choice; however, the resident does not sit at the table.
   - 3 This is inappropriate because it promotes dependence.

9. Comprehension, planning, psychosocial integrity (b).
   - **3 Physically restraining a resident will increase the agitation level of the resident.**
   - 1 The chair itself does not cause decubitus ulcers.
   - 2 If the resident is toileted by the staff, the chair itself should not foster incontinence.
   - 4 This is a sweeping statement that does not demonstrate knowledge of agitated patients.

10. Application, implementation, physiological integrity (b).
    - **2 This is the only response that answers the patient's question.**
    - 1 This does not acknowledge the patient's question.
    - 3 This response does not answer the patient's question.
    - 4 This is demeaning to the patient.

11. Application, assessment, physiological integrity (b).
    - **3 These are toxic effects of Sinemet.**
    - 1, 2 These are symptoms of Parkinson's disease.
    - 4 Patients with Parkinson's disease have these changes.

12. Application, implementation, physiological integrity (b).
    - **2 Administering the drug before meals with enhance absorption and decrease gastrointestinal irritation.**
    - 1 This will diminish absorption of the drug.
    - 3 This is inappropriate; medications should not be mixed with the patient's food.
    - 4 No indication exists that this may be necessary; the physician determines this.

13. Application, assessment, psychosocial integrity (b).
    - **1 Hallucinations are not usually characteristic of paranoid behavior in older adults.**
    - 2 This is an expected characteristic of paranoid behavior.
    - 3 Oversensitivity is also a characteristic of paranoia.
    - 4 Many paranoid individuals refuse meals and treatments.

14. Comprehension, evaluation, psychosocial integrity (c).
    - **4 These actions are characteristic of paranoia.**
    - 1 This is judgmental and does not correctly describe the behavior.
    - 2 The resident is not displaying hallucinations.
    - 3 Although this may be the outcome of her actions, the resident is displaying paranoid behavior.

15. Comprehension, assessment, health promotion and maintenance (b).
    - **4 The patient most likely feels secure, and moving at this time would contribute further to his losses.**
    - 1 The patient may not be afraid to move but wishes to lessen his losses.
    - 2 These actions do not indicate paranoid behavior.
    - 3 This situation does not indicate eccentric behavior.

16. Comprehension, assessment, physiological integrity (b).
    - **2 Not enough information is given to arrive at a diagnosis.**
    - 1 This may be the cause; however, further evaluation is necessary.
    - 3 No indication exists that this may be the cause of the episode.
    - 4 Further testing is required before this diagnosis can be made.

17. Comprehension, planning, physiological integrity (b).
    4 Frequent small meals are easier to digest and not as overwhelming to the patient.
    1 No indication exists for blenderized foods.
    2 No reason to believe exists that warm liquids would increase his appetite.
    3 Rolls would most likely not stimulate his appetite.

18. Comprehension, assessment, psychosocial integrity (b).
    2 This situation is presented as an impairment in orientation to time, place, and person.
    1 Manifestation of a physiological problem and may be present; however, the patient is specifically having difficulty with time orientation.
    3 Although memory deficit may be present, the situation describes time disorientation.
    4 No evidence exists that impaired judgment is present.

19. Comprehension, planning, health promotion and maintenance (b).
    4 This is a normal aging change.
    1 This would not be compatible with the rest needs of the patient.
    2 A more thorough assessment is needed before medication is given.
    3 The quality and continuity of sleep patterns change.

20. Application, assessment, physiological integrity (c).
    4 Broccoli and turnip greens are high in vitamin K.
    1 These are not vitamin K–rich foods.
    2 These are important to the diet and not high in vitamin K.
    3 This is not an especially rich source of vitamin K.

21. Comprehension, assessment, physiological integrity (c).
    1 Loss of fat tissue on the soles of the feet, coupled with the trauma of walking, places the patient at risk for foot problems.
    2 With the decrease in muscle mass, tendons shrink and sclerose.
    3 Changes in the kidney predispose the patient to nocturia.
    4 Respiratory system changes alter the body's ability to handle foreign particles and secretions, which increases susceptibility to infection.

22. Application, planning, safe, effective care environment (b).
    1 Because of the yellowing of the lens of the eye, older adults can see reds, oranges, and yellows best.
    2 This is a lower color tone, which is not seen well by older adults.
    3 Blue is difficult for older adults to differentiate.
    4 Green is difficult for older adults to distinguish from other colors.

23. Comprehension, evaluation, psychosocial integrity (b).
    3 Difficulty managing personal finances indicates impaired cognition. Because of poor judgment, the patient may make unwise financial decisions and have difficulty with bill paying and checkbook balancing.
    1 Although the patient may have a decreased ability to do this, it does not demonstrate a cognitive function; it is most likely caused by deficits in the sensory and motor system.
    2 Resistance to care is an abnormal behavior pattern, not a cognitive deficit.
    4 This is a visual-spatial impairment.

24. Application, planning, physiological integrity (c).
    4 A properly applied Ace wrap will reduce edema and shape the limb in preparation for prosthesis application.
    1 The stump is elevated for the first 24 hours postoperatively; after that, it is not elevated to prevent hip flexion contractures.
    2 A diuretic is not indicated in this situation.
    3 This will not decrease the amount of edema in the stump; it will create further edema.

25. Comprehension, assessment, health promotion and maintenance (b).
    3 Changes in the respiratory system can cause decreased tolerance in activity, dyspnea, and fatigue.
    1 These changes cause a higher-pitched, frailer voice; dyspnea is a common complaint.
    2 The voice is not stronger or more resonant.
    4 Aging changes do cause a decrease in activity tolerance, but they do not cause orthopnea.

26. Comprehension, evaluation, safe, effective care environment (b).
    2 Individuals with presbyopia have difficulty with near vision; activities that require near vision such as needlepoint and knitting will be the most difficult for them to complete.
    1 These activities should not be difficult for individuals with presbyopia.
    3 Bingo and shopping require very little near vision and should not pose a problem.
    4 Driving requires far vision, and viewing road signs should not be a problem.

27. Comprehension, assessment, psychosocial integrity (c).
    2 Applying makeup and wearing appealing clothing may increase the patient's self-worth.
    1 This suggestion, as it is presented, does not appear to demean the individual.
    3 No indication exists that the patient has not bathed.
    4 As presented, the situation does not involve a patient who is unaware of her surroundings.

28. Application, implementation, psychosocial integrity (b).
    3 This will be the best way to get the patient's attention.
    1 Speaking too quickly will confuse the patient.
    2 Talking loudly may agitate the individual.
    4 Watching the television would provide too much distraction.

29. Application, implementation, psychosocial integrity (b).
    3 Given that the patient has no known organic disease, she may be confused and would most likely reorient well to the situation.
    1 This may not be true and gives false reassurance.
    2 No indication exists that this patient will not reorient to time, place, and person.
    4 This may not be true and will give false reassurance to the patient.

30. Application, implementation, physiological integrity (c).
    4 This is the proper sequence to administer medications through a small-bore feeding tube.
    1 The tube should be flushed with a small amount of water (unless specified by physician) before and after the medication.
    2 Checking residual after giving the medication will result in withdrawing some of the medication from the tube; the nurse will not get a true residual amount.
    3 Residual amounts should be checked before flushing with water.

31. Application, assessment, health promotion and maintenance (b).
    1 Older adults have both good and bad days and should be assessed on more than one occasion to gather the most correct data.
    2 The best setting for a functional assessment is in the patient's own environment.
    3 Older adults have difficulty relating any problems with ADL.
    4 Any assistive aids that are used on a day-to-day basis should be included in the functional assessment.

32. Knowledge, evaluation, safe, effective care environment (b).
    1 This is the only choice where skilled nursing care is performed.
    2 Adult day care provides a structured environment for individuals for less than a 24-hour basis.
    3 Personal care homes assist residents in the ADL and basic care.
    4 Senior citizen centers provide recreational programs for seniors.

33. Application, planning, physiological integrity (c).
    3 Any restless and confused behavior necessitates a cardiac and respiratory assessment; the patient may be hypoxic.
    1 The patient is not complaining of pain; a thorough assessment must be made before any intervention can be done.
    2 The spouse may provide valuable information about her husband's former cognitive status; however, the nurse needs to perform an assessment.
    4 This may be appropriate if an emergency problem is found with the patient, but the nurse should first assess the patient.

34. Comprehension, implementation, safe, effective care environment (b).
    4 The patient appoints an individual to make medical decisions for the patient should the patient become incapacitated.
    1 The health care proxy makes medical decisions for the patient.
    2 The patient usually chooses the individual; if the state makes the decision, a family member may or may not be chosen.
    3 This more accurately describes a living will.

35. Comprehension, implementation, health promotion and maintenance (b).
    3 Chinese Americans are most likely to access alternative or traditional therapies before contacting the modern medical establishment.
    1 African Americans use community and family resources readily and are likely to access health care in a short period.
    2 Jewish Americans are likely to readily access modern health care.
    4 Hispanic Americans tend to access health care after consulting community and family relations.

36. Knowledge, planning, health promotion and maintenance (b).
    4 The Hispanic culture values assisting older adults at home; families are expected to care for the ill or elderly individuals.
    1 Caucasians have the highest rate of nursing home use.
    2 Asian Americans have a low rate of nursing home use.
    3 Jewish Americans tend to readily use long-term care.

37. Knowledge, assessment, safe, effective care environment (b).
    3 Social Security provides the majority of the retired older adult's income.
    1 Medicare is a program that provides health coverage for older adults.
    2 Medicaid is a program that provides health coverage for low-income individuals.
    4 Tax-sheltered annuities may provide some of the older adult's income.

38. Comprehension, assessment, health promotion and maintenance (b).
    1 The free-radical theory of aging postulates that free molecules eventually damage cells. The intake of vitamins A, C, and E (antioxidants) can decrease the damage done to the cells.
    2 This theory states that the structure of the collagen fibers in the body causes aging to begin.
    3 This states that the body does not recognize changed cells and attacks them as foreign particles, initiating the aging process.
    4 Lipofuscin granules are age pigments that accumulate in the cell, which may initiate the aging process.

39. Knowledge, implementation, health promotion and maintenance (b).
    4 The focus of care for the majority of the older adult population encompasses the management of the symptoms of chronic illness.
    1 Although prevention is important, older adults have many chronic illnesses that must be managed.
    2 Prevention is always important; however, older adults have many chronic illnesses that need symptom management.
    3 Health maintenance is not usually associated with acute illnesses.

40. Application, assessment, safe, effective care environment (b).
    3 These assessment data most strongly indicates that elder abuse may be a problem. The confusion might be caused by excessive stress, and individuals who have had repeated abuse may have wounds in various stages of healing.
    1 These assessment data indicate changes in the patient's gastrointestinal system and can signify weight loss.
    2 Chronic cough and shortness of breath are symptoms associated with aging changes in the respiratory system.
    4 Fatigue can be caused by a variety of factors; pain on movement and palpation of the ankle is to be expected with a fracture.

41. Application, planning, safe, effective care environment (c).
    2 This is the best response because it solves the patient's problem while preserving independence.
    1 This may not be necessary given that the overdose has already been determined to be accidental.
    3 This may alleviate the patient's problem; however, it does cause dependency.
    4 This is an unnecessary expense and promotes dependency.

42. Application, assessment, psychosocial integrity (b).
    3 This is the only question that does not ask for a yes or no answer. By asking how much alcohol the patient drank that day, the nurse is more likely to get an accurate response.
    1 This is judgmental and is a yes or no question.
    2 This is important to know, but it is a yes or no question.

4 This may be relevant, but it closes communication because it is a yes or no question.

43. Application, implementation, physiological integrity (b).
    2 Cognex is a drug given to patients in early Alzheimer's disease to slow the progression of the disease.
    1 No cure has been found for Alzheimer's disease.
    3 No visible improvement may occur.
    4 A noticeable improvement will not occur; the progression of the disease is slow.

44. Application, implementation, safe, effective care environment (b).
    3 This limits the chance for the patient to fall trying to get to the bathroom.
    1 This promotes dependence and incontinence.
    2 If the patient does not request a sedative, it should not be given for this reason.
    4 A patient should not be restrained; this is inappropriate and fosters dependence.

45. Comprehension, implementation, physiological integrity (b).
    3 This is the most correct statement. Viagra is used to treat erectile dysfunction.
    1 This may not be true; Viagra does not promote a more intimate experience.
    2 This is judgmental; the individual obviously wishes to resume sex with his wife.
    4 This is not a true statement.

46. Application, implementation, health promotion and maintenance (b).
    3 Older adults do not take risks and will not fill in answers to multiple-choice tests if they think they will get them "wrong."
    1 The slight brain shrinkage that older adults experience does not result in loss of intelligence.
    2 The nurse cannot generalize that all older adults do not care about nutrition.
    4 This assumes that all older adults have a profound loss of vision.

47. Comprehension, implementation, physiological integrity (b).
    3 The hearing aid should be turned on only when it is in the ear canal to decrease unpleasant noise from the aid.
    1 This will result in squealing and pain as it is inserted.
    2 Air flow will cause a high-pitched squeal, which is annoying and painful to the patient.
    4 The patient should be encouraged to turn the aid on when it is safely in the ear canal so that the nursing assistant can help adjust the volume.

48. Application, implementation, physiological integrity (b).
    1 This is the simplest and easiest way to ascertain if the aid is functioning.
    2 This may be necessary if the aid is working and the patient is still unable to hear.
    3 This is an inappropriate response; the nurse should investigate the family's concern.
    4 This may be necessary after checking the aid out and contacting the physician.

49. Knowledge, planning, safe, effective care environment (b).
    2 A walker would provide a stable mobility aid while fostering as much independent movement as possible.
    1 A cane is not as stable as a walker.
    3 Crutches are a very dangerous mobility aid for a patient with vertigo.

4 Although a wheelchair is very stable, this patient needs to have as much independent movement as possible.

50. Application, assessment, safe, effective care environment (b).
    3 This agency would most likely have a respite care program.
    1 Nursing homes provide skilled nursing care.
    2 Personal care homes provide care for individuals who live in the facility.
    4 This agency is concerned with providing monetary benefits to older adults and others who qualify.

51. Knowledge, assessment, safe, effective care environment (b).
    4 The MDS is the required assessment tool.
    1 This is a small component of the MDS.
    2 This is determined by other factors, including client preference.
    3 The MDS is not an order form.

52. Knowledge, assessment, safe, effective care environment (b).
    2 This is a requirement of the MDS collection.
    1 The information relates to the resident, but no signature is required.
    3 The physician's plan of care is involved, but the physician's signature is not necessary.
    4 The medication nurse may contribute valuable information and complete portions of the form, but the signature is not required.

53. Comprehensive, implementation, safe, effective care environment (b).
    1 This is the guideline for employee actions.
    2 This is not a factor; all nurses, regardless of age, must comply with faculty policies and procedures.
    3 Gender of the client is not an issue in providing safe care.
    4 Although this may impact on the final outcome, the severity of the injury is purely incidental.

54. Comprehension, implementation, safe, effective care environment (b).
    3 These devices can be removed by the patient and fit the definition of reminder devices.
    1 These are ambulatory aids.
    2 These are restraints.
    4 Side rails may be either a restraint or a positioning device; a trapeze is a positioning device.

55. Application, implementation, health promotion and maintenance (b).
    3 The sexual self-gratification of the resident is a private matter and should be respected.
    1 This denies the resident's needs.
    2 This infringes on resident's rights.
    4 This is judgmental and disrespectful.

56. Comprehension, planning, psychosocial integrity (b).
    3 This reduces over-stimulation and permits the resident time to adjust and absorb information regarding the facility
    1 This is too stimulating
    2 This assumes the resident would participate in prayer
    4 The interdisciplinary meeting should be earlier in the day- mental alertness is usually better in the morning

57. Comprehension, implementation, psychosocial integrity (a).
    2 Person's with Alzheimer's disease relate to themselves at an earlier stage in their life.
    1 The ability to read and understand is frequently impaired.

3 Frequently the person with Alzheimer's disease is unable to recognize himself.

4 This is too complicated for the resident to understand.

58. Comprehension, assessment, psychosocial integrity (a).

2 The resident is not recognizing the napkin as a napkin.

1 This is a disturbance in speaking or understanding speech.

3 This is dizziness.

4 This is inability to sit still.

59. Knowledge, implementation, psychosocial integrity (a).

1 This is the proper description.

2 This is cognitive therapy.

3 This describes relaxation therapy.

4 This is reality oriented or remotivation.

60. Knowledge, application, physiological integrity (a).

3 Glaucoma results in narrowing of the visual field.

1 Cataracts result in decreased visual acuity.

2 This is decreased ability to see at night.

4 Macular degeneration results in central vision loss.

61. Analysis, assessment, physiological integrity (a).

1 Polydipsia is symptom of diabetes.

2 Decreased flexibility is normal with aging.

3 The older adult requires more light to see clearly.

4 This is a normal change of aging.

62. Knowledge, application, physiological integrity (a).

2 The stress of infection is a major precipitating factor for hyperosmolar hyperglycemic nonketotic coma.

1 This is more likely to occur in the person with insulin-dependent diabetes.

3 Other factors not included would be necessary for this to occur.

4 Low blood sugar is unlikely with the stress of an infection.

63. Application, implementation, safe, effective care environment (b).

1 This avoids a sudden need for the resident to ambulate to the bathroom or impatiently attempting to manage for themselves.

2 Side rails are very ineffective in preventing a fall.

3 This is an inappropriate order for a vest restraint.

4 This might help prevent injury but not the fall itself.

64. Application, implementation, psychosocial integrity (b).

2 This encourages life review and exploration of feelings.

1 This may create an adversarial situation.

3 This is a negative response and is demeaning to the resident.

4 Although this may be helpful in encouraging conversation, it does not address the most important topic for the resident.

65. Analysis, assessment, psychosocial integrity (c).

1 The extended time frame and the inability to let go and move on with their life are characteristic of dysfunctional grief.

2 This may be a component but does not directly answer the question.

3 This occurs before the loss.

4 No indication exists of the client feeling suspicious or persecuted.

66. Analysis, assessment, physiological integrity (c).

3 The acute onset related to anesthesia is characteristic of delirium.

1 Although the client is at risk for sepsis, the determining symptoms are not present.

2 Dementia is not an acute event.

4 Depression is not characterized by disorientation.

67. Knowledge, implementation, psychosocial integrity (a).

2 Validation therapy identifies and focuses on the feelings and meaning of the behavior.

1 This describes reality orientation.

3 This is the function of cognitive training.

4 This describes reminiscence.

68. Application, planning, psychosocial integrity (b).

3 This actively encourages reflection and life review.

1 This is an example of reality orientation.

2 This technique assists in identifying and validating feelings.

4 This is useful but is not any particular technique.

69. Comprehension, assessment, physiological integrity (c).

4 These are all hypothyroid symptoms.

1, 2, 3 None of the other answers are any specific syndrome when they occur simultaneously.

70. Application, planning, psychosocial integrity (b).

2 This response provides opportunity to explore client's feelings.

1 This denies the client's feelings.

3 This offers false reassurance and denies feelings.

4 This is a negative response and shuts down communication.

71. Knowledge, assessment, physiological integrity (b).

1 This describes the usual visual field loss with macular degeneration.

2 This occurs with glaucoma.

3 This describes loss of one half of the usual field.

4 This is the absence of the lens of the eye.

72. Comprehension, implementation, physiological integrity (b).

4 Increased eye pressure may be a contributing factor.

1 Cataracts and cataract surgery may contribute to glaucoma.

2 This describes inflammation of the eyelids.

3 This is usually associated with cataract surgery.

73. Knowledge, evaluation, physiological integrity (a).

2 Ultraviolet light contributes to the crystallization, clouding and decreased flexibility of the lens of the eye.

1, 3, 4 These are not related to cataract development.

74. Comprehension, application, physiological integrity (b).

1 Ginkgo biloba increases the anticoagulant effect of Coumadin.

2, 3, 4 These have no effect on Coumadin.

75. Knowledge, application, physiological integrity (b).

4 This is the proper descriptive term.

1, 2, 3 These do not apply.

76. Application, implementation, physiological integrity (c).

4 A picture board would enable a client to understand.

1 This is appropriate for aspiration prevention.

2 This is pertinent to dysphagia.

3 This is not useful because the client cannot understand written or spoken language.

77. Analysis, implementation, physiological integrity (b).

1 She must remain upright for at least 30 minutes after taking Fosamax.

2, 3, 4 These are correct instructions.

78. Application, implementation, physiological integrity (b).

3 This is the proper method for administering Miacalcin.

1 Bone density studies are nice but not a necessity.

2 This is not necessary.

4 This does not affect the absorption or utilization.

79. Knowledge, assessment, health promotion and maintenance (c).
    2 These are risk factors.
    1 Square dancing is weight-bearing exercise, which is not a risk factor.
    3 None of these are risk factors.
    4 None of these are risk factors.

80. Application, implementation, physiological integrity (a).
    4 This describes a stage-1 pressure ulcer and requires immediate attention.
    1 This is within normal.
    2 This needs further assessment before proceeding.
    3 This is within normal.

81. Comprehension, implementation, physiological integrity (c).
    4 Gout is treated with medications that require careful monitoring.
    1 Reduction in proteins and alcohol is required in gout.
    2 Gout pain is considered acute pain.
    3 This is useful but is not the most important; gout may affect any joint.

82. Analysis, assessment, psychosocial integrity (c).
    1 For an increase in drinking after a stressful event, this is the correct description.
    2, 3, 4 These may also be correct, but not enough information is given to make this determination.

83. Knowledge, assessment, health promotion and maintenance (b).
    3 This is considered the most stressful life event of those listed.
    1, 2, 4 These are also life stressors.

84. Knowledge, assessment, physiological integrity (b).
    3 The slowing of metabolic rate that occurs with aging is most responsible for the older adults' increased response to smaller amounts of alcohol.
    1 A related factor, but chronological age is not the determinant.
    2 In general, women have less tolerance for alcohol throughout their life span.
    4 Some ethnic groups have a greater percentage of genetic metabolic conditions that interfere with the tolerance to alcohol.

85. Knowledge, physiological integrity (b).
    4 Vitamin-B$_1$, thiamine deficiency is typically seen in chronic alcoholism and is associated with these neurological disturbances.
    1 Vitamin-C deficiency results in scurvy.
    2 Vitamin-B$_{12}$ deficiency results in anemia.
    3 Vitamin-K deficiency results in bleeding disorders.

86. Knowledge, evaluation, physiological integrity (a).
    3 The repetitive grasping, rolling movements of the fingers is most often seen with Parkinson's disease.
    1 Movements associated with Huntington's disease are related to disturbances in large muscle groups and are generally "jerky" in nature.
    2 Tardive dyskinesia movements are usually with side effects of antipsychotic medications.
    4 Diabetic retinopathy is a vision disorder.

87. Knowledge, assessment, physiological integrity (b).
    1 Basal cell carcinoma is the most common form of skin cancer in all age groups.
    2 Malignant melanoma is the least common skin cancer.
    3 Squamous cell is less common.
    4 Malignant psoriasis is not an accepted diagnosis.

88. Knowledge, assessment, health promotion and maintenance (b).
    3 This is the correct definition.
    1 Intertrigo is a fungal condition frequently found in persons with diabetes.
    2 Stasis dermatitis is a skin condition frequently found in lower extremities with peripheral vascular disease.
    4 Eczema is a specific skin condition associated with food allergy responses found more in infants and children.

89. Application, assessment, physiological integrity (b).
    2 This describes the typical herpes zoster outbreak.
    1 This describes a large number of conditions.
    3 This is not indicative of any particular process.
    4 This may describe an allergic response.

90. Comprehension, assessment, physiological integrity (c).
    2 These are the classic symptoms of dementia.
    1 Depression is a mood disorder.
    3 Delirium is most often characterized be disorientation.
    4 Paranoia describes a type of altered thought process.

91. Comprehension, evaluation, psychosocial integrity (b).
    1 This response reduces the confrontation and stress and permits redirection.
    2 Excessive evening activity will increase agitation and sleeping disturbances.
    3 Radio talk shows may contribute to disorientation.
    4 Incontinence is not always a problem; a toileting schedule may delay its onset.

92. Knowledge, implementation, health promotion and maintenance (b).
    3 The muscle is most affected.
    1 Enlargement may occur for compensation.
    2 Changes are not directly related to aging.
    4 This is not as significantly affected.

93. Knowledge, implementation, physiological integrity (c).
    2 Additional blood vessels develop to compensate for loss of flow because of the atherosclerotic process.
    1 Cardiac output may decrease.
    3 Coronary artery disease may result but is not an adaptation.
    4 This is a surgical treatment.

94. Knowledge, assessment, physiological integrity (b).
    3 Chest pain caused by reduced oxygen to the myocardium is the most prominent.
    1 Breathing difficulty may be a secondary symptom.
    2 Edema indicates a decreased cardiac output.
    4 Vomiting is not a prominent symptom of coronary artery disease, although nausea is frequently reported.

95. Application, implementation, physiological integrity (a).
    4 Left-sided brain damage will result in disturbance of the right side of the body.
    1 Seizure disorders may result from CVAs.
    2 This is not a factor.
    3 This might result in left-sided neglect.

96. Knowledge, evaluation, physiological integrity (b).
    3 Women outlive men; the ratio of women to men increases as age increases.
    1, 2, 4 These are contributing factors.

97. Application, implementation, psychosocial integrity (b).
    3 Mixer activities that encourage interaction enhance sexuality.
    1 This is contraindicated unless mutually acceptable to both roommates.
    2 This may be offensive to some residents.

4 Alcohol metabolism is slowed in older adults; routine serving of alcoholic beverages is contraindicated. Alcohol may be ordered on an individual basis.

98. Analysis, assessment, health promotion and maintenance (b).

4 All pertinent data regarding the resident needs to be collected before proceeding.

1 This is important but is not the first thing that should be completed.

2 This may be indicated after the assessment.

3 The assessment needs to be completed before making this determination.

99. Comprehension, implementation, psychosocial integrity (b).

2 Validation affirms and accepts the resident's feelings.

1 Reality orientation focuses on the present.

3 Reminiscence focuses on life review and its meaning.

4 This is part of reminiscence therapy.

100. Application, evaluation, physiological integrity (b).

4 Cardiac output is directly related to renal blood perfusion.

1 This may be a cause of decreased cardiac output.

2 This may be a physiological integrity to reduced cardiac output.

3 This is a cause of angina.

101. Comprehension, implementation, psychosocial integrity (c).

4 The goal of reality orientation is to assist the individual who is not aware of proper person, place, or time to be correctly oriented.

1 Reality therapy has limited usefulness with dementia because of the short-term memory loss that is associated with dementia.

2 Disorientation is not usually a problem with depression.

3 Depending on the extent and type of delirium, reality therapy may be useful.

102. Analysis, evaluation, psychosocial integrity (c).

1 This is the most appropriate goal for this therapy with this specific behavior.

2 No indication exists that this resident is not oriented to self.

3 This is an ongoing goal for all residents.

4 This is not specific for the targeted behavior described.

103. Application, planning, physiological integrity (c).

3 Dry mouth is a frequent side effect of many medications; this may be the cause of the resident's discomfort.

1 No indication exists that the resident is diabetic. Elevated blood sugar may cause increased thirst; it is not usually described as dry mouth.

2 This may be an appropriate intervention but is not the first intervention.

4 Dry lips do not necessarily accompany dry mouth; further assessment is necessary to determine if this intervention is appropriate.

104. Comprehension, evaluation, psychosocial integrity (b).

2 Married men live longer than men who are widowed or bachelors.

1, 3, 4 These influence longevity but not as much as marital status.

105. Application, implementation, physiological integrity (a).

1 Aspiration is a high risk for patients who are receiving nasogastric feedings, the nurse should anticipate the risk and be prepared.

2 A weight will be necessary but not the priority of aspiration prevention.

3 This may or may not be required.

4 This may or may not be required.

106. Comprehension, evaluation, health promotion and maintenance (a).

4 This is the correct explanation, related to reduced metabolism and activity level.

1 This situation is not indicative of diabetes.

2 No indication of a safety problem exists.

3 The information provided does not validate loneliness and fear.

107. Analysis, implementation, psychosocial integrity (b).

1 This music was popular dance music of their young adult years and will help the social feelings associated with life at that time.

2, 3, 4 These are specific music types that may work for other groups.

108. Comprehension, implementation, psychosocial integrity (c).

4 This permits socialization and mingling and is an appropriate food selection, being easily physically managed.

1 Buffet service is frequently difficult for older adults to handle because of mobility and coordination impairments.

2 Assigned seating may discourage socialization.

3 Snack foods are typically high in fat, sodium, and empty calories. Nutritious food choices should be offered.

109. Application, implementation, physiological integrity (a).

4 Older adults hear low-pitched sounds best.

1, 2, 3 These are high pitched and less easily distinguishable from other sounds.

110. Knowledge, implementation, psychosocial integrity (c).

4 The older adult has a known work history.

1 No evidence exists of this effect on morale.

2 Being older does no necessarily mean that the employee will be good at orientation.

3 Memory is not better or worse.

111. Comprehension, implementation, health promotion and maintenance (b).

4 Research has shown this to be true; and older adults are less likely to offer complaints of pain.

1, 2, 3 These are misconceptions.

112. Application, implementation, psychosocial integrity (b).

2 Of the choices available, 8:00 AM Thursday is the least likely to cause interference with the Jewish Sabbath, which lasts from sundown Friday through sunset Saturday.

1 This would be the second choice.

3, 4 These interfere with the Sabbath.

113. Knowledge, assessment, safe, effective care environment (a).

3 This most accurately describes the nursing home population regarding age and sex.

1, 2, 4 These are not accurate, given the options available.

114. Application, assessment, health promotion and maintenance (b).

2 All four descriptions are risk factors for osteoporosis.

1 This is a thyroid condition more common in women.

3 Herpes zoster is most common in older adults.

4 Not related to the other factors listed.

115. Analysis, implementation, physiological integrity (b).

4 This provides information necessary for the nurse to obtain before identifying the problem and helping the client with a solution.

1 This is a possible solution, after more information is gathered.

2 The client may wish to do this; it is not the nurse's first action.

3 After further assessment, this may be advised.

116. Application, planning, physiological integrity (b).

1 Morning pain and stiffness is common with arthritis. Gently moving the involved joints helps to prevent further restriction and relieve pain.

2 Although cold reduces inflammation, it may aggravate the restriction of movement associated with arthritis.

3 This may be effective, but Epsom salt might be irritating for some skin types.

4 Cortisone cream should not be used over large areas and is not effective for arthritis pain relief.

117. Analysis, assessment, psychosocial integrity (a).

1 The client is attempting to read lips and listen closely.

2 Squinting may indicate a visual disturbance, but the combination of the two behaviors is most suggestive of a hearing loss.

3, 4 These behaviors are not associated with anxiety or confusion.

118. Application, implementation, physiological integrity (a).

3 The little chair may permit too much hip flexion. The size and type of chair should be determined and if unsuitable, the daughter should be reinstructed in her mother's restrictions.

1, 2, 4 These are appropriate safety interventions for recovery after a hip replacement.

119. Comprehension, assessment, health promotion and maintenance (b).

1 Hypertension is most common in African-American men.

2 Puerto Rican women have an increased incidence of diabetes.

3 Asian-American men have a greater incidence of stomach cancer.

4 Native-American women have a greater incidence of diabetes.

120. Comprehension, assessment, psychosocial integrity (c).

2 This statement reflects the contributions and accomplishments of the adult's person's life, not only with their children, but also with the "extra" of the grandchildren.

1 This is an old-age stage according to Peck.

3 This is the eighth stage described by Erikson and has more to do with acceptance and satisfaction than it does generativity.

4 Identity vs. confusion is the stage typically faced in adolescence.

121. Knowledge, assessment, health promotion and maintenance (b).

1, 2, 4 These are all normal changes of aging.

3 Tear production decreases with age.

122. Comprehension, evaluation, physiological integrity (a).

2, 3, 4 These may be responsible for sudden confusion.

1 Age alone is not a cause of sudden confusion.

123. Knowledge, evaluation, physiological integrity (b).

2 Frequently associated with the use of hearing aids and hygiene, cerumen impaction is the most frequent cause.

1, 3, 4 These are less common causes of conductive hearing loss.

124. Comprehension, implementation, psychosocial integrity (b).

3 The spelling bee uses information and social interaction patterns learned during grade school years.

1 Reality therapy focuses on the present.

2 Reminiscence is a life-review process, not necessarily using remote memory.

4 Scrabble is mentally challenging but does not use remote memory to the extent of a spelling bee.

125. Comprehension, assessment, psychosocial integrity (b).

3 The wife is preparing for the loss of her spouse and has started the grieving and remembering process.

1 No indication of depression exists.

2 The wife is working on accepting, not denial.

4 No indication exists that she has withdrawn from social contacts.

126. Comprehension, assessment, physiological integrity (b).

3 Cataract formation frequently impairs green and blue color discrimination.

1 This is possible but not the best explanation.

2 Hypertension does not usually affect color discrimination.

4 Color blindness affects red and green color discrimination.

127. Application, implementation, physiological integrity (c).

4 These interventions can be helpful in promoting restful sleep by eliminating distractions.

1 Exercising close to bedtime can raise metabolic rate, which makes sleeping peacefully more difficult.

2 Alcohol may make falling asleep easier but frequently interferes with sleep patterns.

3 Herbal sleep masks may be distracting and uncomfortable.

128. Application, implementation, health promotion and maintenance (a).

2 Walking provides weight-bearing exercise that may lessen the progression of osteoporosis; water aerobics provides ROM with support.

1 Aerobic dancing would be too high impact for her joints.

3 Weight training may put too much stress on her joints.

4 Bicycling requires extensive ROM of hips and knees, which can aggravate arthritis.

129. Application, implementation, physiological integrity (b).

3 Weight changes indicate changes in fluid balances; sleeping positions, especially use of two or more pillows to sleeping or sleeping in a chair, is suggestive of increasing congestive failure.

1 Blood sugar will not be affected by cardiac output.

2 Appetite will not be directly affected by cardiac output.

4 Bowel function will not be directly affected by cardiac output.

130. Analysis, assessment, physiological integrity (a).

4 An exacerbation of COPD by its very definition is an ineffective breathing pattern.

1, 2, 3 These may be correct but are not the priority.

131. Application, assessment, physiological integrity (c).
    2 This gathers the information needed to make suggestions.
    1 This may be an appropriate response after additional information is gathered.
    3 Dietary habits must be assessed first.
    4 This is an overreaction to the situation.

132. Comprehension, assessment, psychosocial integrity (b).
    3 This statement of futility is an example of Erikson's eighth stage of senescence.
    1 This is Erikson's infancy stage.
    2 This is Erikson's adolescence stage.
    4 This is Erikson's older adulthood stage.

133. Application, implementation, physiological integrity (b).
    2 The alcohol in this complementary arthritis therapy would cause a disulfiram-type reaction with the metronidazole.
    1 St. John's wort is noted for its photosensitization.
    3 No indication exists of drug interaction with chamomile.
    4 Acupuncture would not be herb contraindicated.

134. Application, implementation, psychosocial integrity (b).
    4 This respects the resident's preferences and provides for hygiene to be maintained.
    1 This does not respect the resident's right to choose.
    2 This is feasible but not the best option.
    3 This is an invasion of the resident's personal property.

135. Comprehension, assessment, physiological integrity (b).
    2 The PPD skin test will be reactive in tuberculosis.
    1 This is a test for the syphilis antibody.
    3 This is a blood test used for inflammatory conditions.
    4 This tests for the presence of HCG in pregnancy.

136. Comprehension, planning, physiological integrity (c).
    4 This is the next step after a significant reaction to a tuberculosis skin test.
    1 This is contraindicated after a significant positive reaction.
    2 This is not indicated at this time.
    3 After the results of the client x-ray examination are known, a CT may be ordered.

137. Knowledge, planning, psychosocial integrity (a).
    2 This is the correct order of stages described by Dr. Kübler-Ross.
    1, 3, 4 These are incorrect.

138. Comprehension, assessment, physiological integrity (c).
    3 These are symptoms of hypothyroidism indicated by an elevated thyroid-stimulating hormone.
    1 An elevated blood glucose is associated with diabetes.
    2 An elevated WBC count is associated with infection.
    4 An elevated systolic blood pressure indicates hypertension.

139. Comprehension, assessment, physiological integrity (c).
    1 Emotional instability is commonly associated with right-hemisphere CVAs.
    2 Impotence is not related to the hemispheric CVA.
    3, 4 These are seen with CVAs that affect the left hemisphere.

140. Knowledge, assessment, health promotion and maintenance (b).
    1, 2, 3, 4 All of these are factors in the increase in AIDS/HIV infection in the older adult.

141. Application, implementation, safe, effective care environment (b).
    4 This permits explanation and clarification of the change.
    1 E-mail is unreliable.
    2 This may breach confidentiality.
    3 This is not within the responsibility of a nursing assistant.

142. Comprehension, implementation, psychosocial integrity (c).
    4 This is a nonthreatening, neutral method of assessing symptoms for reluctant clients.
    1 You are not certain of this client's verbal ability.
    2 Many clients are reluctant and embarrassed to draw pictures.
    3 For the client to point at or touch the nurse may be inappropriate.

143. Comprehension, evaluation, physiological integrity (b).
    3 This shows a very basic understanding of vitamin-B12 deficiency.
    1 This is an expected outcome but not the best answer.
    2 Pernicious anemia is treated by injections.
    4 Vitamin B_{12} is not iron.

144. Comprehension, evaluation, health promotion and maintenance (a).
    4 These are all low-sodium foods.
    1 Canned soups are high in sodium.
    2 Hotdogs and sauerkraut are high in sodium.
    3 Bacon is high in sodium.

145. Application, implementation, physiological integrity (b).
    1 This is the most critical.
    2 Insulin needs to be given before breakfast and is a priority.
    4 Routine medication administration comes after giving the priority medications.
    3 Routine vital signs can be delegated to a nursing assistant.

146. Application, implementation, physiological integrity (b).
    2400 calories divided by 24 hours = 100 calories per hour.
    100 cal/hr ÷ 1.3 cal/ml = 77 ml/hr.

147. Application, planning, physiological integrity (b).
    3 Preoperative teaching should include the equipment that will be used postoperatively. CPM devices are used specifically after knee replacement.
    1 This is skin traction used after a fracture and before surgery.
    2 Spica casts are used to maintain abduction.
    3 PCA devices may or may not be used. They are not specific to knee surgery.

148. Knowledge, implementation, safe, effective care environment (b).
    1 Elderly women are highly regarded and frequently consulted in the primarily matriarchal group.
    2 Italian Americans are more patriarchal.
    3 Native Americans vary according to tribal origin.
    4 Chinese Americans are more patriarchal than they are matriarchal.

149. Knowledge, implementation, physiological integrity (b).
    1 Ceftriaxone sodium (Rocephin) is a third-generation cephalosporin; a degree of cross-sensitivity to penicillin exists.
    2, 3, 4 None of these allergies interfere with this medication being administered as ordered.

150. Application, implementation, safe, effective care environment (b).

   4 If unsure about a significant object, it is best not to disturb it unless directed by the resident; this respects the resident's rights.

   1 The family may not be of the same belief system, unless a specific designee has been appointed; this can confuse the issue.

   2 This may be disrespectful.

   3 The resident's belongings should not be locked in medication carts. Each facility has a policy for checking valuables that the resident does not want to keep in their possession.

This chapter emphasizes the nursing assessments and interventions that are essential to preserving the lives of victims of acute illness or injury. Rapid clinical assessment emphasizing airway, breathing, and circulation, establishment of care priorities, and implementation of lifesaving measures should be instituted until emergency medical care is available. The most serious and life-threatening injuries should be treated first, and all first-aid measures should be carried out before transporting the victim or victims.

Concurrent with emergency management of physical needs is the practitioner's recognition and understanding of the victim's emotional state. The feelings of the victim's significant others should also be acknowledged and responded to as realistically, gently, and expeditiously as possible.

Nurses should be familiar with the extent of protection and legal limitations of practice under the Nurse Practice Act and Good Samaritan Act, which vary from state to state.

The high incidence of acquired immunodeficiency syndrome (AIDS) and hepatitis B necessitates that nurses consider all patients to be potentially infected; have access to equipment that minimizes the need for mouth-to-mouth, mouth-to-nose, and mouth-to-stoma resuscitation; and implement universal infection control precautions.

BASIC LIFE SUPPORT

Artificial Respiration

A. Simultaneously shake victim and shout to establish unconsciousness
B. Activate the emergency medical system (EMS) (call 9-1-1)
  1. Do so immediately when the victim is an adult or a child (under 8 years of age) known to be at risk for ventricular fibrillation or ventricular tachycardia who experience sudden witnessed collapse
  2. Provide 1 minute of cardiopulmonary resuscitation (CPR) before activating EMS when the victim is an adult whose arrest may be the result of airway compromise, including:
    a. Submersion or near drowning (1 minute CPR, then activate EMS)
    b. Poisoning, drug overdose (1 minute CPR, then activate EMS)
    c. Trauma (1 minute CPR, then activate EMS)
    d. Respiratory arrest (1 minute CPR, then activate EMS)
  3. When the victim is an infant or child, call for help (even if you do not see anyone in the immediate vicinity), give 1 minute of CPR (20 cycles), check for pulse, and then activate EMS
C. Quickly place victim in supine position
D. Establish airway using the head tilt–chin lift maneuver (Figure 10-1) or head tilt–jaw thrust maneuver if additional forward displacement of the jaw is required; for patients with possible neck or spine injuries, use only jaw-thrust maneuver
  1. Infant: maintain neck in neutral position
  2. Child: maintain neck slightly further back than neutral position
  3. For patients with a stoma, use mouth-to-stoma breathing
E. Put your ear near the victim's mouth, and look, listen, and feel for breathing
F. Begin rescue breathing by delivering two breaths (1 1/2 to 2 seconds per breath) at the lowest possible pressure, using the bag-mask technique; if a mask or bag is not available, begin mouth-to-mouth, mouth-to-nose, or mouth-to-stoma resuscitation
G. Allow for victim's exhalation between breaths by removing your mouth
H. Check the carotid pulse (brachial pulse for infant) for 5 seconds
I. In the presence of a pulse, continue to deliver one breath every 5 seconds (12 breaths per minute) for the adult and every 3 seconds (20 breaths per minute) for the infant and for a child until breathing is restored (rescue breathing)

Cardiopulmonary Resuscitation

A. Follow the previously mentioned steps A to G; be sure victim is on a firm surface for the compression activities
B. In the absence of a pulse, place the heel of one hand on top of the other two fingerbreadths above the victim's xiphoid process (Figure 10-2)
  1. Child (age 1 to 8 years): place heel of one hand two fingerbreadths above the end of the sternum and deliver 100 compressions per minute
  2. Infant (less than 1 year): place two fingers one fingerbreadth below an imaginary line drawn between the nipples, and deliver compressions at the rate of 100 per minute for a single rescuer
  3. Infant when two rescuers are available: use the two thumb–encircling hand chest compression technique
C. Compress the adult sternum 1 1/2 to 2 inches for 15 compressions at the rate of 100 per minute; then deliver two breaths
D. Compress the sternum of the child 1 to 1 1/2 inches for five compressions; then deliver one breath
E. Compress the infant sternum 1/2 to 1 inch for five compressions; then deliver one breath
F. Continue the 15 compressions and two breaths sequence in the adult or five compressions and one breath sequence for infants and children for a single rescuer or for two rescuers
G. Check the carotid pulse:
  1. After four cycles of 15:2 (1 minute) in the adult
  2. After 20 cycles of 5:1 (1 minute) in the child

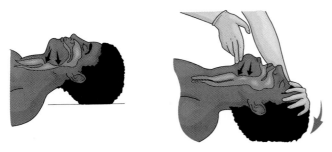

FIGURE 10-1. **Head tilt–chin lift maneuver.** One hand is on the person's forehead. Pressure is applied to tilt the head back. The chin is lifted with the fingers of the other hand. *(From Sorrentino SA: Mosby's textbook for nursing assistants, ed 6, St. Louis, 2004, Mosby.)*

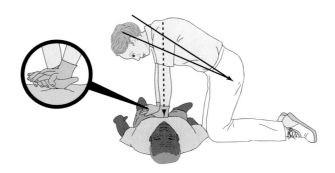

A

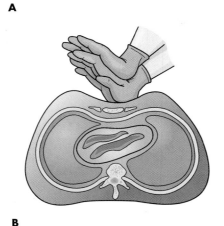

B

FIGURE 10-2. **Body and hand position for CPR. A,** The rescuer should be kneeling, with knees slightly separated and elbows in straight, locked position over the hands. **B,** The rescuer's fingers are extended or interlaced and kept off the chest. *(From Sorrentino SA: Mosby's textbook for nursing assistants, ed 6, St. Louis, 2004, Mosby.)*

H. Check the brachial pulse after 20 cycles of 5:1 (1 minute) in the infant
I. If no pulse, resume CPR; if a pulse is present but no breathing, resume artificial respiration (rescue breathing)

Heimlich Maneuver

The Heimlich maneuver is used for management of foreign body airway obstruction (FBAO). Do not interfere if the victim can cough, speak, or breathe.
A. Conscious adult victim
　1. Stand behind the victim, encircle his or her waist with your arms, place your fist above the umbilicus and below

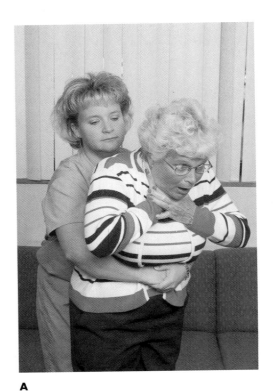

A

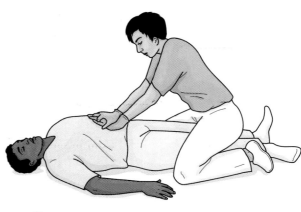

B

FIGURE 10-3. **Heimlich maneuver. A,** Abdominal thrusts with the person standing. **B,** Abdominal thrusts with the person lying down. The rescuer straddles the thighs. *(From Sorrentino SA: Mosby's textbook for nursing assistants, ed 6, St. Louis, 2004, Mosby.)*

the xiphoid process with your thumb against victim's abdomen; grasp your fist with your other hand, and apply pressure with an inward and quick upward motion (Figure 10-3, A)
　2. Repeat the thrusts until the obstruction is relieved, or switch to procedure for conscious victim who loses consciousness
B. Conscious adult victim who loses consciousness
　1. Place victim in supine position, call for help, and activate the EMS
　2. Perform tongue-jaw lift and carefully sweep your curved finger in one direction along the back of the victim's throat to retrieve object
　3. Establish airway using the head tilt–chin lift maneuver
　4. Deliver two breaths

5. Kneel at level of victim's hips or straddle victim to deliver five abdominal thrusts by placing the heel of one hand above the umbilicus and below the xiphoid process; place your second hand on top of the first hand and apply pressure with an inward and upward motion (see Figure 10-3, *B*)

6. Perform the tongue-jaw lift and carefully sweep curved finger in one direction along the back of the victim's throat to retrieve object

7. Establish airway using the head tilt–chin lift maneuver

8. Attempt to ventilate by delivering one breath

9. Continue repeating abdominal thrusts, finger sweeps, and breathing attempts in rapid sequence

C. Unconscious adult victim
1. Simultaneously shake victim and shout to establish unconsciousness
2. Activate EMS
3. Quickly place victim in supine position
4. Establish airway using the head tilt–chin lift maneuver
5. Put your ear near victim's mouth, and look, listen, and feel for breathing
6. Deliver two breaths
7. If unable to ventilate, reposition head and again attempt to deliver two breaths
8. Repeat steps 5 to 8 of conscious adult victim who loses consciousness until effective

D. Child
1. Same as adult, except:
2. Provide 1 minute of rescue support, then activate EMS
3. Do not perform finger sweeps; use tongue-jaw lift and remove object only if visualized

E. Obese victim and later stages of pregnancy
1. Conscious victim: deliver chest thrusts (place thumb side of fist on middle of breast bone) until foreign body is expelled or victim becomes unconscious
2. Unconscious victim
   a. Deliver chest thrusts with victim in supine position by placing heel of hand on lower half of sternum with other hand on top (CPR position)
   b. Follow Heimlich maneuver, finger sweep, ventilate sequence

F. Conscious infant
1. Supporting head and neck, position infant face down with head lower than trunk along rescuer's forearm
2. With heel of hand, administer five back blows between the shoulder blades
3. Continue to support head and turn infant over, keeping head lower than trunk
4. Compression location is directly below the point where the sternum is bisected by an imaginary line between the nipples
5. With the ring and middle fingers, administer five chest thrusts
6. Continue to administer back blows and chest thrusts until airway is cleared or infant becomes unconscious

G. Conscious infant who loses consciousness
1. Place in supine position, call for help, and activate EMS
2. Perform tongue-jaw lift and remove object only if you see it (DO NOT perform finger sweeps)
3. Establish airway using the head tilt–chin lift maneuver
4. Attempt to deliver two breaths; if unable to ventilate, reposition head and repeat
5. Administer five back blows

6. Administer five chest thrusts
7. Perform tongue-jaw lift and remove object only if you see it
8. Establish airway using head tilt–chin lift maneuver and deliver two breaths
9. Continue repeating back blows, chest thrusts, tongue-jaw lift, and breathing until effective

H. Unconscious infant
1. Simultaneously shake and tap victim to establish unconsciousness
2. Call for help, even if you do not see anyone in the immediate vicinity
3. Quickly place infant in supine position while supporting the head and neck
4. Establish airway using head tilt–chin lift maneuver but do not tilt too far
5. Put your ear near victim's mouth, and look, listen, and feel for breathing
6. Administer two breaths
7. If unable to ventilate, reposition head and again deliver two breaths
8. Activate EMS
9. Administer five back blows
10. Administer five chest thrusts
11. Perform tongue-jaw lift and remove object only if you see it
12. Attempt to ventilate
13. Repeat steps 9 through 12 until effective

HEMORRHAGE

A. Description: loss of a large amount of blood in a short period; may be externally or internally

B. Types
1. Venous: dark color; steady flow
2. Arterial: bright color; spurting flow
3. Capillary: red; oozing flow

C. Assessment for shock
1. Restlessness
2. Anxiety
3. Rapid, weak pulse
4. Cool, moist, pale skin
5. Rapid respirations
6. Thirst
7. Nausea and vomiting
8. Alteration in level of consciousness
9. Hypotension
10. If bleeding is internal (within a cavity or joint), pain will develop because the cavity is stretched by increasing blood volume

D. Intervention: external
1. Apply direct pressure with a clean cloth for at least 6 minutes (use gloves if available)
2. Elevate injured part above heart level
3. If arterial bleeding does not respond to direct pressure, attempt to control by applying direct pressure on supply artery (Figure 10-4)
4. Tourniquets are not recommended unless an extremity is amputated or severely mutilated
   a. Leave tourniquet exposed (visible)
   b. Tag or label victim with location of tourniquet
   c. Apply proximal to wound

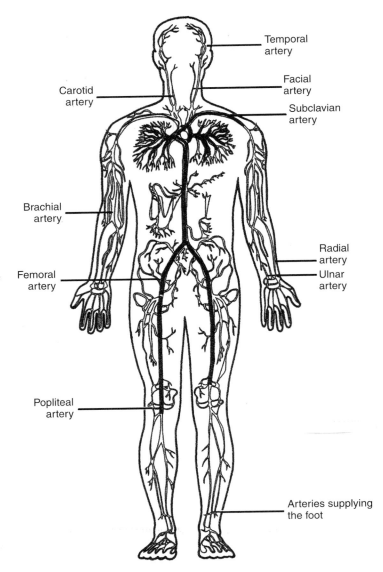

FIGURE 10-4.   Pressure points for bleeding control. *(From Kidd PS, Sturt P:* Mosby's emergency nursing reference, *ed 2, St Louis, 2000, Mosby.)*

d. Tourniquet should not be removed except by a physician

5. Cover victim to maintain body temperature; maintain supine position

6. Treat for shock and transport immediately

E. Intervention: internal

1. Cover victim to maintain body temperature

2. Keep victim in supine position

3. Monitor vital signs

4. Treat for shock and transport immediately

F. Usual medical care

1. Replacement of fluids intravenously to expand blood volume

2. Blood transfusions

3. Locate source of and stop hemorrhage

Epistaxis (Nosebleed)

A. Description: bleeding from the nose caused by trauma, local irritation, violent sneezing, or chronic conditions such as hypertension

B. Assessment: obvious bleeding from one or both nares (most often unilateral)

C. Intervention

1. Sit victim upright, head slightly forward to prevent aspiration of blood

2. Apply firm, continuous pressure by using thumb and forefinger to pinch nose

3. Apply ice compress to nose

4. Limit activity; restrict drinking of hot or cold liquids

5. Monitor vital signs

D. Usual medical care

1. Nasal pack soaked in a topical vasoconstrictor

2. Cauterization (silver nitrate or electrocautery)

SHOCK

A. Description: depressed state of vital body functions that, if untreated, can result in death

B. Types: (three basic types) (Box 10-1)

<table>
<tr><td>

BOX 10-1 Causes of Shock

Hypovolemic
External major bleeding
Hemothorax
Hemoperitoneum
Fractures
Gastrointestinal bleeding
Major vomiting
Major diarrhea
Major diaphoresis
Renal failure
Excessive diuretic use
Fluid loss from diabetes
Burns
Ascites

Cardiogenic
Myocardial infarction
Cardiomyopathy
Cardiac contusion
Dysrhythmia
Diseases of heart valve

Distributive
Sepsis
Anaphylaxis
Spinal cord injury
Overdose
Anoxia

</td></tr>
</table>

Modified from Emergency Nurses Association: *Sheehy's emergency nursing: principles and practice,* ed 5, St Louis, 2003, Mosby.

1. **Hypovolemic:** primarily a fluid problem caused by a loss of blood or fluid volume (e.g., hemorrhage, severe burns, trauma, dehydration)
2. **Cardiogenic:** reduced cardiac output (e.g., myocardial infarction, cardiomyopathy, diseases of the heart valves) that is the result of faulty pumping action
3. **Vasogenic or distributive:** a vascular problem or disturbance in tissue perfusion caused by alteration in circulating blood volumes (vascular dilation); may be one of three types
   a. **Septic:** massive bacterial infection resulting in release of endotoxin that causes vasodilation (e.g., gram-negative organisms)
   b. **Neurogenic or spinal:** disruption of arterioles and venules, resulting in a decrease of circulating blood volume (e.g., spinal cord injury)
   c. **Anaphylaxis:** severe sensitivity reaction resulting in histamine release, increased capillary permeability with eventual dilation of arterioles and venules
C. Assessment: determination of the exact cause is vital to patient survival
   1. Shallow, rapid respirations
   2. Cool, pale, clammy skin
   3. Thirst
   4. Tachycardia

5. Decreased blood pressure
6. Weak, thready pulse
7. Restlessness
8. Decreased urine output
9. Possible confusion or disorientation
D. Intervention: isolation of cause determines specific intervention strategies, which include the following:
   1. Ensure adequate airway and ventilation
   2. Control bleeding if present
   3. Place in supine position, with legs elevated unless contraindicated (e.g., head injuries)
   4. Insert urinary catheter
   5. Monitor vital signs
   6. Cover victim to conserve body heat
   7. Remain with victim if possible
E. Usual medical care
   1. Intravenous (IV) fluids
   2. Oxygen
   3. Medications specific to the type of shock

ANAPHYLACTIC REACTION

A. Description: a type of vasogenic or distributive shock (see previous section on Shock)
B. Assessment
   1. Pallor
   2. Diaphoresis
   3. Tachycardia or bradycardia
   4. Hypotension
   5. Wheezing, dyspnea
   6. Anxiety, restlessness
   7. Urticaria
   8. Edema
   9. Pruritus
   10. Rash
   11. Possible respiratory distress
   12. Diffuse erythema
C. Intervention
   1. Ensure adequate airway and ventilation
   2. Elevate feet slightly, unless contraindicated (e.g., head injuries)
D. Usual medical care
   1. Oxygen
   2. Epinephrine
   3. Antihistamines
   4. Steroids
   5. IV fluids
   6. Drug therapy for cardiovascular support
E. Preventive measures
   1. Allergy history
   2. Medical identification tag for high-risk persons
   3. Insect (sting) emergency medical kits
   4. Skin testing when possible
   5. Question previous allergic reactions before administering medications

HEAD INJURIES

Traumatic damage to the head from blunt or penetrating trauma resulting in scalp, skull, and brain injuries

Scalp Injury

TYPE	INTERVENTION
Abrasion	Wash with soap and water
Hematoma	Apply ice
Laceration	Stop bleeding by compression (only if no depression is present)
	Shave around laceration
	Cleanse wound
	Suture

Skull Fracture

A. Simple: linear crack in surface of skull with no displacement of bone
  1. Observation for alteration of respiration, vision, level of consciousness, pupils (dilated, fixed, pinpoint), motor strength, and speech
  2. X-ray examination
B. Depressed: skull fracture with depressed bone fragments resulting in a concave appearance
  1. Intervention
    a. Ensure adequate airway and ventilation
    b. Administer oxygen
    c. Control bleeding
    d. Treat for shock
    e. Observe for alteration of respiration, vision, level of consciousness, pupils (dilated, fixed, pinpoint), motor strength, and speech
    f. Maintain body temperature
    g. Protect cervical spine
    h. Monitor vital signs
  2. Usual medical care
    a. Surgical intervention
    b. Antibiotic therapy
    c. X-ray examination
C. Basilar: fracture located along base of skull
  1. Assessment
    a. Periorbital ecchymosis (black eyes)
    b. Cerebrospinal fluid (CSF) leak from nose or ear
    c. Ecchymosis behind ears (Battle's sign)
    d. Blood behind eardrum (hemotympanum)
  2. Intervention:
    a. Observe for alterations of respiration, vision, level of consciousness, pupils (dilated, fixed, pinpoint), motor strength, and speech; monitor vital signs
    b. If CSF leak is noted, do not attempt to stop; apply a loose bulky dressing over area; protect cervical spine
  3. Usual medical care
    a. X-ray examination (although usually not visible)
    b. Antibiotic therapy if CSF leak occurs

Brain Injury

A. Concussion: temporary alteration of neurological functioning caused by a blow to the head, which results in jarring of the brain
  1. Assessment
    a. Nausea and vomiting
    b. Headache
    c. Possible brief period of unconsciousness and memory loss

    d. Possible skull fracture
    e. Confusion
  2. Intervention
    a. Observe for alteration of respiration, vision, level of consciousness, pupils (dilated, fixed, pinpoint), and motor strength
    b. Administer nonnarcotic analgesics as ordered
    c. Maintain hydration
    d. Protect cervical spine
B. Contusion: brain surface bruise resulting in structural alteration
  1. Assessment
    a. Nausea and vomiting
    b. Visual alterations (diplopia)
    c. Neurological alterations (ataxia, confusion)
  2. Intervention
    a. Maintain adequate airway and ventilation
    b. Observe
    c. Protect cervical spine
    d. Monitor vital signs
  3. Usual medical care
    a. Hospitalization
    b. Antiemetics
C. Intracranial bleeding: hemorrhage or bleeding within the cranial vault
  1. Assessment
    a. Epidural (extradural) hematoma: bleeding between skull and dura mater; short period of unconsciousness followed by consciousness; severe headache, hemiparesis if conscious, bradycardia, increased blood pressure
    b. Subdural hematoma: bleeding between dura mater and arachnoid membrane; can be acute or chronic; loss of consciousness, fixed dilated pupils, hemiparesis, positive Babinski's sign
    c. Subarachnoid hematoma: bleeding between arachnoid membrane and the pia mater; severe headache, nausea and vomiting, delirium, syncope, or coma
  2. Intervention
    a. Maintain adequate airway and ventilation
    b. Administer oxygen
    c. Monitor vital signs
    d. Protect cervical spine
    e. Observe for alterations of respiration, vision, level of consciousness, pupils (dilated, fixed, pinpoint), and decreased motor strength (signs of increased intracranial pressure [ICP])
    f. Maintain body temperature
    g. Treat for shock
  3. Usual medical care
    a. Hospitalization
    b. Computed tomography (CT) scan
    c. Possible surgery

EYE INJURIES

Foreign Body In Eye

A. Evert eyelid (Figure 10-5)
B. Touch particle gently with sterile swab moistened in sterile saline solution or water (do not remove if particle is on the cornea or if eyeball penetration has occurred)
C. Apply an eye patch after ensuring that the eye is closed

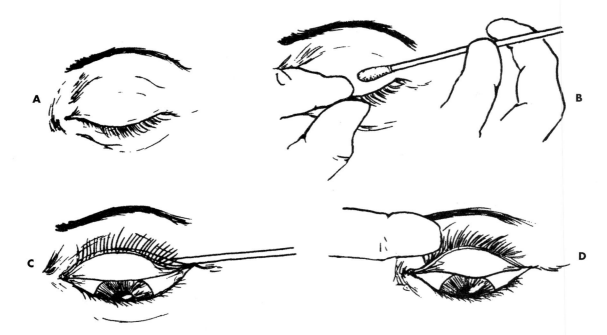

FIGURE 10-5. Steps in everting eyelid. **A,** Eyelid. **B,** Placement of cotton swab (eyelashes are pulled down and back over swab). **C,** Eyelid everted over swab. **D,** Examination of inside of eyelid and eye. *(From Emergency Nurses Association:* Sheehy's emergency nursing: principles and practice, *ed 5, St Louis, 2003, Mosby.)*

Foreign Body in Conjunctiva

A. Evert eyelid
B. Remove particle as previously described
C. Irrigate with saline solution or water
D. Eye patch may be applied

Eyelid Contusion (Black Eye)

A. Cold compresses or ice pack intermittently for the first 24 hours
B. Warm compresses after 48 hours
C. Bilateral eye patches if intraocular hemorrhage is present

Corneal Abrasion

A. Assessment
　1. Pain
　2. Photosensitivity
　3. Spasms of the eyelid
　4. Excessive tear production
B. Intervention: apply eye patch to injured eye
C. Usual medical care: local ophthalmic antibiotics

Burns

A. Chemical
　1. If the action of chemical is not enhanced by water, immediately flush area with copious amounts of normal saline solution or tap water for 15 minutes (damage increases with length of chemical contact)
　2. Usual medical care: topical application of antibiotics, administration of cycloplegic agents or corticosteroids (alkali burns)
　3. The following solutions will neutralize the following types of burns
　　a. Acid: sodium bicarbonate 2% solution
　　b. Lime: ammonium tartrate 5% solution
　　c. Alkali: boric or citric acid solution
B. Thermal (usually occurs with facial burns)
　1. Irrigate with normal saline solution or tap water
　2. Apply bilateral eye patches
　3. Usual medical care: analgesia, sedation, antibiotics, cycloplegics
C. Radiation
　1. Types
　　a. Ultraviolet (sun); severity depends on period of exposure
　　b. Infrared (x-rays); severity depends on wavelength and period of exposure (may cause loss of vision)
　2. Assessment
　　a. Excessive blinking
　　b. Excessive tear production
　　c. Feeling that something is in the eye
　　d. Pain
　3. Intervention
　　a. Cold compresses
　　b. Bilateral eye patches
　4. Usual medical care
　　a. Topical antibiotics
　　b. Cycloplegics
　　c. Analgesics

Penetrating Eye Injuries

A. Place a protective shield, such as a paper cup, over the eye to prevent further damage by pressure
B. Apply eye patch to the uninjured eye
C. See an ophthalmologist immediately

SPINAL CORD INJURIES (Table 10-1)

A. Assessment
   1. Pain, tenderness
   2. Numbness, tingling, paralysis
   3. Weakness of extremities
   4. Alterations of sensation and motor function below level of injury
   5. Possible signs and symptoms of shock
B. Intervention
   1. Ensure adequate airway and ventilation; if helmet is on victim, leave it in place if airway is accessible; never attempt to remove helmet alone
   2. Treat for shock
   3. Immobilization (movement may cause further damage)
   4. Maintain body temperature
   5. When help (EMS) arrives, place victim on board without flexing neck or back
   6. Transport immediately (via EMS)

SOFT-TISSUE NECK INJURIES

Fractured Larynx

A. Assessment
   1. Hoarse voice
   2. Cough with hemoptysis
   3. Difficulty breathing; respiratory distress
   4. Subcutaneous emphysema
B. Intervention
   1. Administer oxygen
   2. Observation

TABLE 10-1	Cervical Spine and Spinal Cord Lesions and Resultant Physiological Function
Lesion	**Resultant Function**
C3, C4, or above	Respiratory arrest; flaccid paralysis; quadriplegia (tetraplegia)
C5, C6	Reduced respiratory effort; almost total dependence; flaccid paralysis; quadriplegia (tetraplegia)
C7	Reduced respiratory effort; almost total dependence; splints necessary for functioning of forearms; quadriplegia (tetraplegia)
T1	Reduced respiratory effort; partial dependence; paraplegia
T1, T2	Reduced respiratory effort; complete independence; paraplegia
T7	Complete independence; walking with long-leg braces; paraplegia
L4	Complete independence; walking with foot braces; paraplegia

From Sheehy SB, Lenehan GB: *Manual of emergency care,* ed 5, St Louis, 1999, Mosby.

C. Usual medical care
   1. Emergency cricothyrotomy or tracheostomy
   2. Broad-spectrum antibiotics

Penetrating Neck Wounds

A. Assessment
   1. Noticeable penetrating wound
   2. Airway obstruction
   3. Signs and symptoms of hypovolemia, hemathorax, or shock
B. Intervention
   1. Ensure adequate airway and ventilation
   2. Control bleeding
   3. Surgery

CHEST INJURIES

Fractured Rib (Simple, Undisplaced)

A. Assessment
   1. Chest pain (increases on inspiration), tenderness
   2. Shortness of breath, shallow breathing
   3. Tachycardia
   4. Hypotension
   5. Ecchymosis
B. Intervention (individualized)
   1. Rest
   2. Intermittent ice for first 24 hours, then heat
   3. Observe for signs and symptoms of pneumothorax by monitoring breathing patterns and lung sounds
   4. Encourage deep breathing
   5. Administer analgesics sparingly

Flail Chest

A. Fracture of several ribs resulting in loss of chest wall stability; pulmonary or myocardial contusion may also be present because of force of injury; may be life threatening
B. Assessment
   1. Pain
   2. Difficulty breathing
   3. Shallow, rapid, noisy respirations
   4. Chest moves in opposite from normal direction: moves in on inspiration, out on expiration
   5. Tachycardia and cyanosis
   6. Possible bruising
C. Intervention
   1. Ensure adequate airway and ventilation
   2. Stabilization of chest wall
   3. Application of pressure dressing
   4. Position victim on affected side in semi-Fowler's position
   5. Monitor vital signs and lung sounds
D. Usual medical care
   1. Pain control
   2. Possible intubation and ventilation with severe flail
   3. Possible traction

Simple Pneumothorax

A. Description: air enters the pleural cavity; negative pressure is lost, resulting in partial or total lung collapse
B. Assessment
   1. Chest pain

2. Dyspnea, tachypnea
3. Decreased breath sounds
C. Intervention
   1. Ensure adequate airway and ventilation
   2. Place victim in semi-Fowler's position
   3. Administer oxygen
D. Usual medical care: possible chest tube placement

Tension Pneumothorax

A. Description: air enters the pleural cavity on inspiration and is trapped during exhalation, creating pressure that causes eventual collapse of the lung (same side) resulting in a life-threatening condition in which mediastinal shift occurs, which compresses the heart, great vessels, and trachea, as well as the opposite lung
B. Assessment
   1. Extreme shortness of breath
   2. Observed tracheal deviation
   3. Paradoxical movement of the chest
   4. Neck vein distention
   5. Hypotension
   6. Tachycardia
   7. Restlessness
   8. Cyanosis
   9. Distant breath sounds
   10. History of chest trauma
C. Intervention
   1. Ensure adequate airway, breathing, and circulation
   2. Administer oxygen
D. Usual medical care
   1. Needle thoracotomy
   2. Chest tube placement
   3. IV fluids

Open Pneumothorax (Sucking Chest Wound)

A. Description: presence of air in the chest resulting from an open wound in the chest wall
   1. One-way flap: air enters pleural space but cannot escape (tension pneumothorax)
   2. Two-way flap: air enters and leaves pleural space
B. Assessment
   1. Audible sucking noise
   2. Shortness of breath
   3. Chest pain
   4. Cyanosis
   5. Shock
   6. Possible signs and symptoms of tension pneumothorax
C. Intervention
   1. Ensure adequate airway, breathing, and circulation
   2. Cover wound with airtight dressing (depends on size of wound)
   3. Administer oxygen
   4. CPR may be necessary
D. Usual medical care
   1. Chest tube placement
   2. Antibiotic therapy
   3. Treat for shock

Spontaneous Pneumothorax

A. Description: presence of air in the intrapleural space resulting from rupture of lung tissue and visceral pleura with no evidence of trauma; can occur during periods of strenuous physical activity
B. Assessment
   1. Sudden, sharp chest pain
   2. Shortness of breath
   3. Diaphoresis
   4. Anxiety
   5. Hypotension
   6. Tachycardia
   7. Cessation of normal chest movement on affected side
C. Intervention
   1. Ensure adequate airway and ventilation
   2. Keep victim quiet
   3. Place in semi- or high-Fowler's position
D. Usual medical care
   1. Needle aspiration
   2. Chest tube
   3. IV fluids
   4. Oxygen

Hemothorax

A. Description: blood in the pleural space from traumatic injury (stabbing) or rupture of congenital blebs
B. Assessment
   1. Chest pain
   2. Shortness of breath
   3. Distant breath sounds
   4. Anxiety
   5. Shock
   6. Cyanosis
C. Intervention
   1. Ensure adequate airway and ventilation
   2. Treat for shock
D. Usual medical care: chest tube placement; thoracentesis

Pulmonary Embolism

A. Description: thrombus becomes detached and lodges in a branch of the pulmonary artery, causing a partial or total occlusion and resulting in a pulmonary infarct; commonly seen with trauma, surgery, or long-bone fractures
B. Assessment
   1. Sudden, sharp chest pain
   2. Shortness of breath
   3. Pallor, possible cyanosis
   4. Anxiety
   5. Tachycardia
   6. Rapid, shallow respirations (tachypnea)
   7. Possible hypotension, elevated temperature
   8. Possible cough, wheeze, hemoptysis
   9. Possible sudden death if large blood vessel is blocked
C. Intervention
   1. Ensure adequate airway, breathing, and circulation
   2. Treat for shock
   3. Administer oxygen
   4. Keep victim quiet
   5. Place patient in semi-Fowler's to high-Fowler's position if vital signs permit
D. Usual medical care
   1. Anticoagulant therapy
   2. IV fluids
   3. Surgical intervention in cases of profound shock or cardiovascular collapse

INTRAABDOMINAL INJURIES

Penetrating Wound

A. Description: wounds resulting from stabbings, shootings, impalement
B. Assessment
   1. Hypotension
   2. Shock
   3. Diminished bowel sounds
   4. Pain
   5. Tenderness
   6. Progressive abdominal distention
   7. Nausea or vomiting
C. Intervention
   1. Do not move victim
   2. Ensure adequate airway, breathing, and circulation
   3. Control bleeding
      a. Look for entrance and exit wounds
      b. Apply compression for external bleeding
      c. Look for chest injuries
   4. Cover wounds with wet, sterile, or nonadhesive dressings (e.g., saline or plastic wrap); leave impaled objects in place to control bleeding
   5. Monitor vital signs
   6. Treat for shock
   7. Administer nothing by mouth (NPO)
D. Usual medical care
   1. IV fluids
   2. Oxygen
   3. Tetanus prophylaxis
   4. Antibiotics
   5. Analgesics
   6. Indwelling catheter
   7. Nasogastric tube
   8. X-ray examination
   9. Possible surgery

Blunt Wound

A. Description: wounds resulting from a motor vehicle accident (MVA), contact-sport injury, falls, or physical abuse (e.g., domestic violence)
B. Assessment
   1. Observable bruises and abrasions
   2. Abdominal pain, rigidity, palpable masses, or distention
   3. Signs and symptoms of shock
   4. Guarding
   5. Diminished bowel sounds
C. Intervention
   1. Do not move victim
   2. Ensure adequate airway, breathing, and circulation

   3. Observe for hemorrhage
   4. Observe for chest injuries
   5. Monitor vital signs
   6. Treat for shock
D. Usual medical care
   1. Oxygen
   2. Nasogastric tube
   3. X-ray examination
   4. Peritoneal lavage
   5. Possible surgery

BURNS

A. Depth of classification (Table 10-2)
B. Surface area classification
   1. The greater the body surface area (BSA) affected, the more serious the damage
   2. Use rule of nines (Figure 10-6) to estimate the percentage of BSA affected

Major Burns

A. Burns are considered major or critical if they fulfill the following criteria:
   1. Deep partial-thickness burns: greater than 25% of BSA in adults or greater than 20% in children under age 10 and adults over age 40 years
   2. Full-thickness burns: greater than 10% of BSA in adults and children
   3. Electrical burns
   4. Burns involving face, eyes, ears, hands, feet, and perineum
   5. Burns in victims with preexisting chronic conditions (diabetes, cardiac conditions, renal failure)
B. Intervention
   1. Lay victim flat (standing forces him or her to breathe flames and smoke; running fans flames)
   2. Roll victim in carpet or blankets, or use water to extinguish fire
   3. Remove any smoldering clothing that is nonadherent
   4. Ensure adequate airway and ventilation
   5. Administer oxygen
   6. Assess for inhalation burns
   7. Remove nonadherent, tight-fitting clothing
   8. Remove tight jewelry
   9. Apply cold soaks
   10. Cover burns with moist, sterile dressings or clean cloth
   11. Elevate affected parts if possible
   12. Cover victim
   13. Insert indwelling catheter
   14. Treat burned areas as ordered by physician

TABLE 10-2	Burn Classification		
Depth		**Degree**	**Assessment**
Superficial, partial thickness (involves only the epidermis)		First	Pain; red; minimal or no edema
Deep partial thickness (involves epidermis and part of the dermis)		Second	Pain; mottled color; blistering; wet appearance
Full thickness (involves epidermis and damage to subcutaneous layer, muscle, and bone)		Third	Gray, white, brown, leathery, or charred appearance; edema; minor or no pain

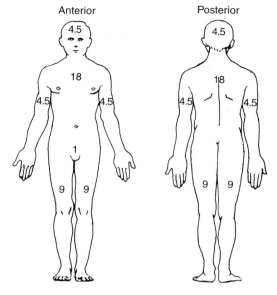

FIGURE 10-6. Rule of nines is used to estimate amount of skin surface burned. (*From Phipps WJ et al:* Medical-surgical nursing: health and illness perspectives, *ed 7, St Louis, 2003, Mosby.*)

C. Usual medical care
  1. Tetanus prophylaxis
  2. Central venous pressure line
  3. Pain management
  4. Nasogastric tube
  5. Standard Precautions
  6. IV therapy
  7. Antibiotic therapy
D. Warnings
  1. Do not use salves, ointments, or oils
  2. Do not soak large burns unless you can maintain body warmth
  3. Do not use ice or ice water on deep partial-thickness or full-thickness burns; causes further injury and promotes hypothermia
  4. Monitor urine for myoglobin, a sign of tissue damage especially common in electrical burns

Chemical Burns

A. Powdered chemicals: sweep off skin
B. Nonpowdered chemicals: irrigate with copious amounts of water or saline solution
C. Cover loosely with a clean cloth
D. Usual medical care: treated as thermal burns (cleanse wound, open blisters and remove outer layer, apply topical antibacterial agent)

Electrical Burns

A. Assessment
  1. Discoloration
  2. Edema
  3. Cardiac irregularities
  4. Entrance and exit sites of current visible
  5. Confusion
  6. Unconsciousness
  7. Respiratory distress

B. Intervention
  1. Do not touch the victim
  2. Remove electrical source with a nonconductor (i.e., non-metal object), or shut off current source, or both
  3. If victim has no pulse and is not breathing, begin CPR
  4. Extremities should be handled minimally and with extreme caution
  5. Check victim for other injuries
  6. Monitor cardiac and renal function

Radiation Burns

A. Intervention
  1. Remove contaminated clothing
  2. Apply cool, moist compresses
B. Usual medical care: possibly antipyretics

Smoke Inhalation

A. Assessment
  1. History of exposure
  2. Singed hair in nares
  3. Mouth burns
  4. Brassy cough
  5. Respiratory distress
  6. Rales, rhonchi, or wheezes
  7. Restlessness
  8. Cyanosis
B. Intervention
  1. Ensure adequate airway and ventilation
  2. Administer oxygen
  3. Be prepared to initiate CPR
C. Usual medical care
  1. Hospitalization for 24 to 48 hours
  2. IV fluids
  3. Chest physical therapy
  4. Possible endotracheal intubation or tracheostomy
  5. Bronchodilators, steroids
  6. Nasogastric tube

WOUNDS

A. Open (break in skin integrity)
  1. Laceration: jagged cut through the skin and underlying tissue
  2. Abrasion: skin scrape or "brush burn"
  3. Avulsion: flap of skin and subcutaneous tissue torn loose
  4. Puncture: tissue penetration by a sharp object
  5. Abscess: localized pus formation
B. Closed (no break in skin integrity; [e.g., contusion]): injury to underlying tissue by blunt object
C. General management
  1. Stop bleeding
    a. Apply pressure dressing
    b. Elevate affected part
    c. Use digital pressure on supply artery
    d. Apply tourniquet only as a lifesaving measure and leave tourniquet visible
  2. Treat for shock
  3. Control infection
    a. Wounds requiring medical care: generally recommended not to clean them until they are seen by a physician

b. Cover open wounds with a clean, nonadhesive dressing; use moist dressing if an evisceration is present

c. Apply ice during the first 24 to 48 hours for closed wounds

d. Minor wounds being treated at home: clean well with soap and water; thoroughly rinse; approximate wound edges with adhesive; cover with a clean dressing; seek medical care for signs of infection

4. Puncture wounds
   a. Impaled object should be stabilized and left in place
   b. Medical attention should be sought

D. Special wounds

1. Human bites
   a. May be self-inflicted or inflicted by another person; evidenced by teeth marks and often by knuckle lacerations (occurs when fist hits another person's teeth during a fight)
   b. Intervention
      (1) Clean with soap and water
      (2) Rinse thoroughly
      (3) Apply clean dressing
      (4) Keep injured part elevated
   c. Usual medical care
      (1) Tetanus prophylaxis
      (2) Antibiotic therapy
      (3) Observe closely for systemic responses to bite: toxic shock syndrome, hepatitis, human immunodeficiency virus (HIV), which can occur after the injury or during the healing process

2. Animal bites: potential for contracting rabies must be seriously considered with any animal bite
   a. Dog bites are most common, causing crushing injury to skin and underlying tissue or avulsion injuries, should the victim attempt to pull away
   b. Cat bites are more likely to cause puncture wounds
   c. Intervention
      (1) Obtain history of bite
      (2) Clean minor wounds with soap and water
      (3) Rinse thoroughly
      (4) Flush with povidone-iodine (Betadine) or other cleansing solutions (hydrogen peroxide) if victim is allergic to Betadine
      (5) Apply clean dressing

NOTE: major wounds (severe bleeding) require control of bleeding and medical attention.

   d. Usual medical care
      (1) Antibiotic therapy for large, contaminated bites
      (2) Tetanus prophylaxis
      (3) Rabies prophylaxis if necessary

3. Snakebites
   a. Assessment
      (1) Teeth marks; possibly fang marks
      (2) Edema
      (3) Pain
      (4) Ecchymosis
      (5) Bleeding
      (6) Numbness of affected part
   b. Intervention
      (1) Have victim lie quietly in shaded area
      (2) Clean wound
      (3) Suction
         (a) Do not use mouth suction if you have open sores in your mouth
         (b) Suction wound using snakebite kit
         (c) Use mouth suction only if no other means is available
      (4) Apply clean dressing
      (5) Immobilize affected limb
      (6) Affected limb should be in dependent position
   c. Usual medical care
      (1) Analgesics
      (2) IV fluids
      (3) Tetanus prophylaxis
      (4) Antivenin therapy

4. Insect (bees, wasps, hornets)
   a. Assessment
      (1) Obtain detailed medical and activity history
      (2) Pruritus
      (3) Burning
      (4) Swelling
   b. Intervention
      (1) Remove the stinger by scraping; do not pull out because this releases more toxin; do not squeeze
      (2) Clean with soap and water
      (3) Apply ice (DO NOT apply heat)
      (4) Apply ammonia diluted with warm water or a paste of baking soda and water
   c. Usual medical care
      (1) Epinephrine
      (2) Antihistamines
      (3) Steroids

5. Tick
   a. Attaches to host with its teeth
   b. Releases a toxin that may cause tick paralysis or Lyme disease
   c. Squeezing tick releases more toxin
   d. If paralysis progresses, respiratory failure and subsequent death may occur
   e. Paralysis will disappear after tick is removed
   f. Intervention
      (1) Grasp tick with tweezers and pull slowly and steadily to remove with head intact
      (2) Wash area with soap and water
      (3) Seek medical treatment

FRACTURE

A. Description: a complete or incomplete break in bone continuity
   1. Fracture without displacement presents normal alignment despite the fracture
   2. Fracture with displacement presents a separation of bone fragments at fracture site
   3. Compound or open: bone protrusion through skin
   4. Simple or closed: no bone protrusion through the skin
   5. Incomplete: part of bone is broken
   6. Complete: breakage produces two fragments
B. Types of fractures (Box 10-2)
C. Assessment
   1. Five Ps (pain, pallor, pulses, paresthesia, and paralysis)
   2. Discoloration; ecchymosis

BOX 10-2 Types of Fractures

Typical Complete Fractures

Closed (simple) fracture: noncommunicating wound between bone and skin

Open (compound) fracture: communicating wound between bone and skin

Comminuted fracture: multiple bone fragments

Linear fracture: fracture line parallel to long axis of bone

Oblique fracture: fracture line at 45-degree angle to long axis of bone

Spiral fracture: fracture line encircling bone

Transverse fracture: fracture line perpendicular to long axis of bone

Impacted fracture: fracture fragments are pushed into each other

Pathologic fracture: fracture occurs at a point in the bone weakened by disease, for example, with tumors or osteoporosis

Avulsion: a fragment of bone connected to a ligament breaks off from the main bone

Extracapsular: fracture is close to the joint but remains outside the joint capsule

Intracapsular: fracture is within the joint capsule

Typical Incomplete Fractures

Greenstick fracture: break on one cortex of bone with splintering of inner bone surface

Torus fracture: buckling of cortex

Bowing fracture: bending of bone

Stress fracture: microfracture

Transchondral fracture: separation of cartilaginous joint surface (articular cartilage) from main shaft of bone

From McCance KI, Huether SE: *Pathophysiology: the biological basis for disease in adults and children,* ed 4, St Louis, 2002, Mosby.

3. Swelling
4. Deformity, possible limb shortening and external rotation
5. Crepitus (characteristic grating sound)
6. Possible bone snap heard by victim
7. External bleeding from associated wounds
8. Tenderness (pain) relative to specific area of the body (sacrum, hip, symphysis pubis)

D. Intervention
1. Control bleeding if necessary
2. Treat for shock
3. Immobilize affected part
4. Apply splint above and below the fracture
5. Apply ice
6. Elevate affected part, if possible
7. Observe for changes in sensation, temperature, and color (indicate nerve injury or circulation interference)
8. Remove jewelry from extremities to reduce risk of further injury if swelling should occur

E. Usual medical care
1. X-ray examination
2. Possible cast application
3. Possible surgery
4. Analgesics
5. Traction

DISLOCATION

A. Description: joint injury and bone displacement
B. Assessment
1. Pain, tenderness
2. Swelling
3. Deformity
4. Alterations in function
5. Discoloration
C. Intervention
1. Control hemorrhage if present (not usually seen with a simple dislocation)
2. Immobilize the affected part
3. Apply sterile dressing to any open wounds
4. Apply splint above and below the site in the position found
5. Apply ice
6. Elevate affected part, if possible
7. Check for fractures
8. Monitor neurological status (check pulses distal to the injury)

SPRAIN

A. Description: stretched or ruptured ligaments; sprain should be considered a fracture until proven otherwise by x-ray examination
B. Assessment
1. Pain, tenderness
2. Discoloration
3. Swelling
4. Alterations in function
C. Intervention
1. Elevate affected part
2. Apply ice intermittently for 72 hours
3. Apply elastic (Ace) bandages
4. Immobilize affected part

STRAIN

A. Description: muscle or tendon damage caused by excessive physical use
B. Assessment
1. Pain
2. Discoloration
C. Intervention
1. Elevate affected part
2. Apply ice intermittently for 72 hours
3. Apply elastic (Ace) bandages
4. Immobilize affected part
5. Limit activity to no weight bearing

HYPERTHERMIA

Heat Stroke

A. Description: life-threatening emergency; body's mechanism for heat regulation breaks down, and excessive body heat is retained; occurs with overexposure to high environmental temperatures, especially those accompanied by high relative humidity and low wind

B. Assessment
   1. Hyperpyrexia to 106° or 107° F (41.1° to 41.6° C)
   2. Flushed, hot, dry skin or clammy and diaphoretic
   3. Dizziness
   4. Headache
   5. Confusion
   6. Nausea
   7. Tachycardia
   8. Hypotension
   9. Fixed and diluted pupils
   10. Seizures
   11. Possible altered level of consciousness
   12. Shallow, rapid breathing
   13. Delirium
C. Predisposing factors are:
   1. Age (older adults and infants)
   2. Obesity
   3. Alcoholism
   4. Preexisting illness (cardiovascular or neurological dysfunctions)
   5. Prescription medications that decrease perspiration (anticholinergics such as antihistamines and antispasmodics; diuretics and beta blockers such as propranolol)
   6. Excessive strenuous exercise
D. Intervention
   1. Ensure adequate airway, breathing, and circulation
   2. Move victim out of sun
   3. Loosen or remove clothing
   4. Provide rapid cooling, for example, immerse in cold water; apply towels soaked in cold water; use air conditioning, fanning, and cool-water sponge
   5. If conscious, provide cool water
   6. Control shivering (this causes body temperature to increase)
   7. Advise victim to avoid reexposure and warn of possible lowered tolerance to heat for a long time or possibly indefinitely
E. Usual medical care
   1. Oxygen
   2. IV therapy

Heat Exhaustion

A. Description: ineffective circulating blood volume caused by excessive fluid loss and exposure to heat without sufficient fluid and electrolyte replenishment
B. Assessment
   1. Headache
   2. Dizziness, faintness
   3. Nausea and vomiting
   4. Marked diaphoresis
   5. Cool, pale, damp skin
   6. Muscle cramps
   7. Possible temperature elevation
   8. Orthostatic hypotension
   9. Tachycardia
   10. Dehydration
   11. Anxiety
   12. Anorexia, thirst
C. Especially at risk are:
   1. Older adults

   2. Very young children
D. Intervention
   1. Move victim to cool, quiet area
   2. Loosen or remove constricting clothing
   3. Administer salted water if vomiting is absent
   4. Provide rest
   5. Relieve muscle cramps (firm pressure against muscle with palm of hand)
   6. Advise victim of preventive measures: drink plenty of fluids and curtail activity on hot days

COLD INJURIES

Frostbite

A. Classification
   1. Superficial: superficial tissue below the skin freezes
   2. Deep: deep subcutaneous tissue freezes, and temperature of affected part is lowered
B. Most frequently affected areas: ears, nose, cheeks, fingers, and toes
C. Assessment
   1. Superficial
      a. Numbness, tingling, burning
      b. Gray-white appearance of affected parts
   2. Deep
      a. Hyperemic skin
      b. Edema
      c. Blister formation
      d. Discoloration
      e. Numbness
D. Intervention
   1. Superficial
      a. Remove wet, constricting clothing
      b. Give warm-water soaks
      c. Advise victim of preventive measures
   2. Deep
      a. Remove wet, constricting clothing
      b. Give warm-water soaks only if continuously available; otherwise, keep area dry, place sterile gauze between affected fingers and toes, cover, and elevate frozen part
      c. If victim is conscious, give warm liquids
      d. Do not allow use of frostbitten part
   3. Usual medical care
      a. Tetanus prophylaxis
      b. Analgesics
      c. Antibiotic therapy
E. Warnings
   1. Do not rub area with snow or ice
   2. Do not massage

Immersion Foot

A. Cause: wet foot in continuous contact with cold temperatures
B. Assessment
   1. Foot is cold and damp
   2. Foot appears shriveled
   3. Gangrene (if conditions were prolonged and repeated)
C. Intervention
   1. Dry footwear
   2. Warm-water soaks

Chilblain

A. Description: localized redness and swelling of the skin resulting from excessive exposure to cold
B. Commonly affected areas: fingers, toes, and earlobes
C. Assessment: burning, itching, blistering, and ulceration (similar to thermal burn) are possible
D. Intervention
  1. Protect part from cold and further injury
  2. Gentle warming
  3. Avoid use of tobacco products

Hypothermia

A. Description: exposure to cold resulting in heat loss and reduction in body temperature below the average normal range
B. Assessment (Table 10-3)
C. Intervention
  1. Ensure adequate airway and ventilation
  2. Administer oxygen
  3. Remove wet clothing and cover victim
  4. Give warm beverages high in sugar content
  5. Warm body gradually
    a. Passive rewarming: warm room, blankets, and draft prevention (mild hypothermia)
    b. Active external rewarming: heat packs, warming blankets, and overhead radiant warmers (mild to moderate hypothermia)
D. Usual medical care: (moderate to severe hypothermia) active internal warming)
  1. Warmed humidified oxygen
  2. Warmed gastric and peritoneal lavage
  3. Warmed IV fluids
E. Warning: do not rub or massage the skin

POISONING

Food

A. Cause: pathogenic organisms transferred to victim from contaminated food; illness is caused by toxins produced by the organism
B. Botulism *(Clostridium botulinum)*
  1. Causes
    a. Improperly canned food
    b. Improperly cured food
  2. Assessment
    a. Headache
    b. Fatigue
    c. Nausea and vomiting
    d. Double vision (diplopia)
    e. Muscle incoordination
    f. Difficulty swallowing, talking, and breathing
  3. Intervention
    a. Ensure adequate airway and ventilation
    b. Be prepared to administer CPR
    c. Induce vomiting if consumption was recent, if victim has clinical and neurological symptoms, no seizure activity, and no alterations in level of consciousness
    d. Usual medical care: antitoxin
C. *Staphylococcus aureus*
  1. Causes
    a. Secretions from respiratory tract and skin of food handlers
    b. Unrefrigerated cream-filled foods
    c. Fish
    d. Meat
  2. Assessment
    a. Nausea and vomiting
    b. Diarrhea
    c. Abdominal cramps
    d. Weakness
  3. Intervention
    a. Fluids
    b. Bed rest
  4. Usual medical care
    a. Possible IV therapy
    b. Antiemetics
    c. Antidiarrheals
D. Salmonella
  1. Causes: inadequately cooked meat, poultry, and eggs
  2. Assessment
    a. Nausea and vomiting
    b. Diarrhea
    c. Weakness
    d. Abdominal pain
    e. Elevated temperature
    f. Chills
  3. Intervention
    a. Bed rest
    b. Fluids
  4. Usual medical care
    a. Possible IV therapy
    b. Antiemetics
    c. Antidiarrheals

TABLE 10-3	Stages, Signs, and Symptoms of Hypothermia	
Stage	**Core Temperature**	**Symptoms**
Mild	90°–95° F (32°–35° C)	Tachypnea, tachycardia, ataxia, shivering, lethargy, confusion, occasional atria fibrillation
Moderate	86°–90° F (30.0°–32.2° C)	Rigidity, hypoventilation, decreased level of consciousness, increased myocardial irritability, hypovolemia, blood sludging with metabolic acidosis, Osborne or J wave (positive deflection in the RT segment)
Severe	Under 86° F (30° C)	Loss of reflexes, coma, hypotension, acidosis, apnea, cyanosis, ventricular fibrillation, asystole

From Kidd PS, Sturt P: *Mosby's emergency nursing reference, ed 2,* St Louis, 2000, Mosby.

Accidental Poisoning

A. Description: ingestion, inhalation, or absorption of toxic substances or other substances such as drugs, which, when taken in large amounts, are toxic to the body
B. Assessment: signs and symptoms will vary according to cause
   1. General
      a. Nausea and vomiting
      b. Abdominal pain
      c. Convulsions
      d. Change in level of consciousness
      e. Decreased pulse and respirations
   2. Drug poisoning: coma; flaccid muscles; hypotension (symptoms vary depending on drug)
   3. Chemical poisoning
      a. Burns around lips and mouth
      b. Excessive salivation
      c. Difficulty swallowing
      d. Breath odor (from cleaning or petroleum products)
   4. Inhalation poisoning
      a. Coughing and choking
      b. Headache; bright red skin (carbon monoxide—late indicator)
   5. Absorption poisoning: localized itching and burning (poison)
C. Intervention (Box 10-3)
D. Usual medical care
   1. IV fluids (severe cases)
   2. Hyperbaric oxygenation (carbon monoxide poisoning)

BOX 10-3   Guidelines to Stop Absorption of Poisons

Inhaled Poison
Remove victim from source of toxic gas.
Assess cardiopulmonary status and give artificial ventilation if possible.
Give oxygen if available.

Contact Poison
Rinse skin with copious amounts of water.
Remove garments and rinse skin again.

Ingested Poison
If person is conscious, call physician or poison control center for assistance.
Substances other than caustics or hydrocarbons:
   Induce emesis by giving 15-30 ml syrup of ipecac; follow with full glass of warm water.
   Inactivate poison by giving activated charcoal (especially after drug ingestion).
Caustics or hydrocarbons (petroleum products):
   Give nothing by mouth.
   Seek immediate medical attention.
   Do not induce emesis.
If person is unconscious, transport without delay to medical facility.

From Phipps WJ et al: *Medical-surgical nursing: health and illness perspectives*, ed 7, St Louis, 2003, Mosby.

DIABETES MELLITUS AND HYPOGLYCEMIA

A. Ketoacidosis: acute insulin deficiency (develops over a period of 2 to 3 days); hyperglycemia
   1. Assessment
      a. Polydipsia
      b. Weak, rapid pulse
      c. Hypotension
      d. Dry, warm, flushed skin
      e. Pallor
      f. Diaphoresis
      g. Acetone odor on breath
      h. Kussmaul's respirations
      i. Nausea and vomiting
      j. Alterations in consciousness
      k. Dehydration
      l. Weakness
      m. Headache
      n. Abdominal tenderness
   2. Intervention
      a. Ensure adequate airway and ventilation
      b. Monitor vital signs, fluid intake and output, and level of consciousness
      c. Provide fluids if conscious, for example, broth
   3. Usual medical care
      a. Regular insulin
      b. IV therapy: normal saline solution or 0.45% saline solution
      c. Monitor blood sugar and serum potassium levels
B. Hypoglycemia (low blood sugar; insulin reaction)
   1. Assessment
      a. Sudden onset of symptoms
      b. Weakness
      c. Pallor
      d. Hunger
      e. Nervousness; irritability
      f. Cool, moist skin
      g. Tachycardia
      h. Tremors
      i. Dizziness, syncope
      j. Headache
      k. Visual disturbances
      l. Drowsiness
      m. Confusion
   2. Intervention
      a. Ensure adequate airway and ventilation
      b. Administer quick-acting carbohydrate, for example, orange juice with sugar, honey, lump sugar, cola beverage, hard candy
   3. Usual medical care, if unconscious
      a. IV therapy: 50% glucose
      b. Monitor blood sugar

DROWNING

A. Description: asphyxiation that results from aspiration of fluid into the lungs, which is inhaled as the individual panics or gasps for breath
B. Causes

1. Accidental, for example, exhaustion, inability to swim, panic, injury, medical incident such as a seizure
2. Intentional: suicide attempt
C. Intervention
   1. Remove victim from water
   2. If victim is not breathing, commence artificial respiration (may need to be instituted while victim is being removed from the water)
   3. If no carotid pulse is present, commence CPR
   4. Observe for pulmonary edema
D. Usual medical care
   1. IV fluids
   2. Oxygen under pressure

DRUG ABUSE

A. Description: use of a substance in a manner or in amounts or in situations in which the drug use causes problems or greatly increases the chance of problems occurring
B. Assessment
   1. Needle marks on the body along the veins (many addicts wear long-sleeved shirts to conceal mainlining)
   2. Anorexia
   3. Abdominal cramping
   4. Constipation
   5. Nutritional deficiencies
   6. Watery, reddened eyes
   7. Runny nose
   8. Dilated or constricted pupils
   9. Central nervous system (CNS) alterations (agitation, euphoria, seizures)
   10. Poor personal hygiene
   11. History of difficulty in school, on job, with interpersonal relationships
   12. Accident-prone
   13. History of personality change
   14. Possibly hepatitis
C. Clinical manifestations and treatment (Table 10-4)
D. Intervention
   1. Ensure airway, breathing, and circulation
   2. Administer oxygen
   3. Insert indwelling catheter
   4. Monitor vital functions and neurological status
   5. Take seizure precautions
E. Usual medical care
   1. Arterial blood gases
   2. Specific drug antagonist (e.g., naloxone hydrochloride [Narcan])
   3. IV therapy
   4. Central venous pressure line
   5. Possible dialysis
   6. High-protein, high-calorie diet
   7. Vitamin supplements
   8. Psychotherapy
   9. Withdrawal treatment: methadone hydrochloride (Dolophine); usually used for heroin addiction
      a. Legal synthetic drug addiction
      b. Supervised administration
   10. Rehabilitation

ACUTE ALCOHOLISM

A. Description: large alcohol intake in a short time
B. Assessment
   1. Alcohol on breath
   2. Slurring of speech
   3. Ataxia
   4. Agitation
   5. Belligerence
   6. Vomiting
   7. Drowsiness to stuporousness to unconsciousness
   8. Respiratory failure
   9. Death
C. Intervention
   1. Protect airway
   2. Observe for respiratory depression
   3. Monitor cardiac status
   4. Assess for head injury
D. Usual medical care
   1. Hydration
   2. Vitamin supplements
   3. High-protein diet
   4. Anticonvulsants to control or prevent seizures

Mild Alcohol Withdrawal

A. Assessment
   1. Nausea and vomiting
   2. Shaking
   3. Headache
   4. Ataxia
B. Intervention
   1. Rest
   2. Quiet environment
C. Usual medical care
   1. Analgesics
   2. Hydration

Delirium Tremens

A. Assessment
   1. Tachycardia
   2. Insomnia
   3. Hypertension
   4. Tremors
   5. Anxiety
   6. Hallucinations (auditory, visual, tactile, and [rarely] olfactory)
   7. Disorientation
   8. Amnesia
   9. Seizures
B. Intervention
   1. Ensure adequate airway and ventilation
   2. Treat for shock
   3. Hydration
   4. Monitor vital signs
   5. Provide crisis counseling
C. Usual medical care
   1. Treatment for seizures
   2. Anticonvulsant drugs
   3. IV therapy
   4. Sedation

TABLE 10-4	Clinical Manifestations and Treatment of Acute Intoxication and Withdrawal of Mind-Altering Drugs		
	Acute Intoxication		
Drug Group	Clinical Manifestations	Treatment	Clinical Manifestations of Withdrawal
Narcotics	Respiratory depression, bradycardia, hypotension, cold clammy skin, decreased body temperature; deep sleep, stupor or coma, pinpoint pupils	Maintain ventilation; provide oxygen Give narcotic antagonist: naloxone (Narcan) 0.4 mg IV Monitor vital signs every 15-30 min until patient is conscious Treat for shock	(Not life-threatening) Early: restlessness, irritability, drug craving, yawning, lacrimation, diaphoresis, rhinorrhea, followed by "yen" sleep (intense desire to sleep; sleeps restlessly) Later: awakens with more severe symptoms, nausea, vomiting, anorexia, abdominal cramps, bone and muscle pain, tremors, piloerection (goose flesh)
Other CNS depressants	Same as narcotics (above)	Lavage if recent oral ingestion with possible tremors, activated charcoal treatment Maintain ventilation; provide oxygen Monitor vital signs every 15-30 min until patient is conscious Position patient side-lying or prone, not supine Treat for shock Hemodialysis for renal shutdown	(May be life-threatening) Insomnia, restlessness, anorexia, followed by convulsions, and symptoms similar to DTs (confusion, visual and auditory hallucinations), fever, dehydration
CNS stimulants	Labile cardiovascular symptoms (flushing or pallor, pulse and blood pressure changes, dysrhythmias), hyperpyrexia, mental disturbances (agitation, paranoia, hallucinations), convulsions, circulatory collapse	Give chlorpromazine, 25-50 mg IM Provide a quiet environment Orient patient to reality Monitor vital signs until stable	(Withdrawal is not severe) Somnolence, apathy, irritability, depression, fatigue
Hallucinogens	Physiological toxicity low at doses that produce strong psychological effects Acute panic reaction (bad trip) may lead to suicide "Flashback" episodes Prolonged psychotic disorders (paranoia, depression) Phencyclidine: CNS depression or stimulation may lead to death	Provide quiet, supportive environment and constant attention Give diazepam (Valium) 2-10 mg IM or major tranquilizers (Thorazine IM), or both, for severe anxiety	No evidence of withdrawal symptoms
Cannabis	Adverse reactions infrequent Simple depression, paranoid ideation, confusion, disorientation, hallucinations	Provide support and reassurance Give tranquilizer for agitation	(Withdrawal symptoms rare) Insomnia, anorexia

IV, Intravenous; *IM,* intramuscular; *CNS,* central nervous system; *DTs,* delirium tremens.
From Phipps WJ et al: *Medical-surgical nursing: health and illness perspectives,* ed 7, St Louis, 2003, Mosby.

TABLE 10-4	Clinical Manifestations and Treatment of Acute Intoxication and Withdrawal of Mind-Altering Drugs—Cont'd		
Acute Intoxication			
Drug Group	Clinical Manifestations	Treatment	Clinical Manifestations of Withdrawal
Deliriants	Slowing of heart rate, brain activity, and breathing Slurred speech, blurred vision, inflamed mucous membranes, excessive tearing, nasal secretions With high doses, loss of consciousness and seizures may occur Brain damage may occur (memory loss, depression, paranoia, hostility) Feeling of stimulation and energy Death may occur from suffocation or cardiac arrest	Maintain respirations Provide quiet environment and support Monitor vital signs Orient patient to reality	Chills, hallucinations, pains, cramps, DTs

5. Vitamin therapy
6. High-protein diet

Disulfiram (Antabuse) Reactions

A. Assessment
1. Nausea and vomiting
2. Diaphoresis
3. Hypotension
4. Consciousness alterations
5. Tachycardia
6. Headache
7. Facial flushing
8. Reddened conjunctiva
B. Intervention
1. Ensure adequate airway, breathing, and circulation
2. Administer oxygen
C. Usual medical care
1. IV therapy
2. Diphenhydramine hydrochloride (Benadryl)
3. Chlorpheniramine maleate (Chlor-Trimeton)
4. Ascorbic acid

SEXUAL ASSAULT

A. Victim should be examined and treated as quickly as possible
B. Notify law enforcement
C. Victim should not be left alone
D. Victim should be asked who they wish to have stay with them; offer to call family member, friend, or rape crisis center advocate
E. Provide immediate privacy
F. Kindness and support are crucial
G. Obtain history

H. Assess acuteness of physical and psychological needs
I. Assess victim's readiness for physical examination
J. Explain all procedures and encourage questions
K. Obtain necessary written permissions, including consent to take photographs
L. Assist victim in undressing
M. Observe for and ask about other possible injuries
N. Assist with physician's examination
1. A water-moistened speculum is used
2. History will indicate the body orifices from which specimens for semen analysis will be required
3. Pubic hair is combed for foreign hairs
4. Clothing is usually saved for analysis, and replacement clothing will be necessary; save in paper bags rather than plastic bags, which retain moisture that can cause evidence to deteriorate
5. Follow protocol for collection of specimens that will be used as evidence
6. Testing done for sexually transmitted diseases (STDs), including HIV; follow-up testing done at appropriate intervals
7. STD prophylaxis
8. Pregnancy prophylaxis if contraception not in effect at time of attack: the "morning after" pill (norgestrel [Ovral]), a combination of estrogen and progesterone, given within 72 hours of sexual assault; treatment and side effects should be thoroughly explained
9. If possible and desired, offer accommodations for bathing and douching
10. Care for tissue trauma: immediate and follow-up
11. Care for psychological trauma: immediate and follow-up
12. If present, family and friends often require assistance and counseling

DISASTER

A. Definition: catastrophic event
   1. Natural, for example, flood, earthquake, hurricane
   2. Man-made, for example, riot, fire, train accident
B. May involve as few as 10 or more than 100 victims
C. Prevention
   1. Community planning
   2. Public education
D. Assessment
   1. Civilian triage: care priority to persons whose life is threatened
   2. Military triage: care priority to persons most likely to survive
E. Planning: the most capable person is designated to sort casualties
F. Intervention
   1. First aid should be rendered before victims are transported
   2. Care priorities
      a. Ensure airway, breathing, and circulation
      b. Control bleeding
      c. Treat for shock
   3. Intervention
      a. Whole blood
      b. IV fluids
      c. Parenteral medications
      d. Pain relief
      e. Emergency wound care
         (1) Preserve motor and sensory functioning
         (2) Provide psychologic support
         (3) Treat and transport

SUGGESTED READINGS

Anderson KN, Anderson LE, Glanze WD, editors: *Mosby's medical, nursing, and allied health dictionary,* ed 6, St Louis, 2002, Mosby.

Emergency Nurses Association: *Sheehy's emergency nursing: principles and practice,* ed 5, St Louis, 2003, Mosby.

Kidd PS, Sturt P, Fultz J: *Mosby's emergency nursing reference,* ed 2, St Louis, 2000, Mosby.

Phipps WJ: *Medical-surgical nursing: text and virtual clinical excursions package,* ed 7, St Louis, 2003, Mosby.

Skidmore-Roth L: *Mosby's 2003 nursing drug reference,* ed 3, St Louis, 2003, Mosby.

Spratto GR, Woods AL: *PDR nurse's drug handbook,* 2002 edition, Montvale, 2001, Delmar Learning.

REVIEW QUESTIONS

1. For chest compression of the newborn in CPR, the rescuer's hands are appropriately placed:
   1 One on top of the other, with the heel of the hand on the xiphoid process
   2 With fingers laced together over the upper one third of the sternum
   3 Encircling the torso with the thumbs on the sternum and the fingers under the body
   4 One hand underneath the body and the other hand palm down on the middle of the sternum

2. The nurse knows that a patient with epistaxis should be positioned:
   1 In a prone position with the head elevated
   2 Leaning forward with direct pressure on the nose
   3 Sitting straight up with the head tilted backward
   4 On the side with ice compresses to the back of the neck

3. The mother of a pediatric patient states that the child began to have difficulty breathing after eating a peanut butter sandwich. The child is now hypotensive, dyspneic, and restless. The nurse recognizes these as symptoms of:
   1 Folic acid deficiency
   2 Anaphylaxis
   3 Electrolyte imbalance
   4 Inborn error of metabolism

4. The patient who is being showered after exposure to a caustic substance on the job says that it is uncomfortable and he wants to stop the treatment. The nurse explains to him that the shower is necessary to:
   1 Reduce his body temperature and therefore slow down any chemical processes taking place with the chemical
   2 Stimulate circulation to the skin to enhance the detoxification process
   3 Remove debris and secretions from the skin so that topical medications can be applied
   4 Flush the chemical from the body to reduce the damage to his skin

5. A patient is brought to the emergency room after falling from a ladder and sustaining a fracture of the left leg. The nurse observes that the skin is broken and part of the bone fragment is visible. The appropriate intervention is to:
   1 Immobilize the leg and cover the open wound
   2 Apply traction to the leg to attempt to reduce the fracture
   3 Elevate the leg as high as possible with pillows
   4 Apply an adduction pillow between the patient's knees

6. The nurse receives a telephone call from a neighbor whose husband has collapsed while mowing the lawn. He is described as being dizzy, confused, clammy, and nauseated. The nurse should instruct the wife to:
   1 Encourage the patient to ambulate vigorously to stimulate circulation
   2 Have the patient drink salted water to replace fluids lost through vomiting and diaphoresis
   3 Leave the patient in the position in which he was found and apply blankets
   4 Move the patient to a cool, quiet area and loosen his clothing

7. A runner comes to the emergency room with pain and discoloration in his calf muscles. The nurse instructs him to treat this muscle strain by:
   1 Applying warm moist heat to the legs three times a day for 4 days
   2 Completing active range-of-motion exercises with the legs twice daily for 3 days
   3 Applying ice intermittently for 3 days and restrict weight bearing
   4 Ambulating for at least 20 minutes for 1 week to increase circulation to the legs

8. A man who was in a drowning has been resuscitated and brought to the emergency room for follow-up. The nurse should assess and observe for:
   1 Pulmonary edema
   2 Ketoacidosis
   3 Fluid and electrolyte imbalance
   4 Left shift

9. A patient who is being evaluated and treated for delirium tremens should have:
   1 Nutritional assessment
   2 Seizure precautions
   3 Range-of-motion activities
   4 Universal precautions

10. In addition to injuries related to entry and exit wounds from electrical shock, a patient who has been struck by lightening is at risk for injury to the:
    1 Liver
    2 Kidneys
    3 Lungs
    4 Spleen

11. A fireman who was brought to the emergency department for evaluation after an accident in a factory insists that he is not injured and wants to wait until other victims are treated before being seen by the physician. The nurse observes that he has singed nasal hair and a brassy cough and recognizes that he is at risk now for:
    1 Pulmonary edema as a result of smoke inhalation
    2 Respiratory infection caused by exposure to toxic chemicals
    3 Esophageal reflux as a result of irritation to the oropharynx
    4 Increased sputum production related to oxygen deprivation

12. As follow-up care for a patient with a human or animal bite, the nurse prepares to administer:
    1 Immune globulin
    2 Tetanus booster
    3 Erythropoietin
    4 Corticosteroids

13. A marathoner comes to the emergency department reporting the sudden onset of sharp chest pain and difficulty breathing during his usual daily workout. Chest excursion on the affected side is reduced. The nurse assesses him for:
    1 Muscle strain
    2 Respiratory infection
    3 Spontaneous pneumothorax
    4 Myocardial infarction

14. A patient is brought in by her roommate for suspected drug overdose. She is tachycardic, restless, hallucinating, and agitated. The nurse assesses the patient for use of:
    1 Cannabis
    2 Heroin
    3 Phencyclidine
    4 Alcohol

15. To preserve possible evidence, clothing from a sexual assault victim is stored in:
    1. Airtight plastic bags
    2. Cloth bags with drawstrings
    3. Nonconductive plastic bags
    4. Paper bags sealed with tape

16. In two-rescuer CPR of the adult victim, the standard ratio of compression to breaths is:
    1. 15:2
    2. 5:2
    3. 15:1
    4. 5:1

17. The appropriate analgesic to administer to a patient with a brain injury is:
    1. Acetaminophen (Tylenol)
    2. Meperidine hydrochloride (Demerol)
    3. Morphine sulfate (Morphine)
    4. Dextromethamphetamine sulfate (Dexedrine)

18. To remove a foreign body from the eye, the nurse should use:
    1. Forceps
    2. Gauze compress
    3. Saline moistened sterile swab
    4. Vacuum extraction

19. A patient who has been in a motorcycle accident states that he is experiencing pain in his neck, numbness and tingling in his legs, and weakness on his left side. The nurse should:
    1. Remove his helmet as quickly as possible
    2. Ask him to remove his helmet
    3. Leave his helmet in place until assistance is available to remove it
    4. Secure the helmet in place with adhesive tape

20. An elderly patient with diabetes is brought to the emergency department from a nursing home where she received scald burns to her perineum and feet in the bathtub. This injury is considered:
    1. Superficial
    2. Major
    3. Minor
    4. Minor with the potential to become moderate

21. A patient who has been burned in a factory accident tells the nurse that although his injured arm appears grey at the burn site, it does not hurt. He wants to return to work this afternoon. The nurse explains to him:
    1. "Since you are not having any pain, that should not be a problem."
    2. "This is a third-degree burn and will require admission to the hospital."
    3. "We need to observe you for at least an hour to make sure that you are OK."
    4. "You can leave now if you will agree to come to the clinic tomorrow for a follow-up visit."

22. A patient is brought to the emergency department after experiencing a sudden onset of sharp chest pain at home. He is now pale and tachycardic, and he is wheezing and coughing small amounts of blood. The nurse assesses him for:
    1. Myocardial infarction
    2. Pulmonary embolus
    3. Tension pneumothorax
    4. Pneumonia

23. A neighbor's child has been found in a field after the child was lost in a snowstorm for several hours. The nurse instructs the mother to offer:
    1. Commercial electrolyte solutions to correct fluid imbalance
    2. Hot tea or coffee to warm the child's body quickly
    3. Cocoa or orange juice to provide carbohydrates
    4. Cold soft drinks to allow gradual warming of the child's body

24. A nurse has fallen from a stepstool in the utility room and states that she believes she has dislocated her shoulder. What should be the first intervention?
    1. Apply heat
    2. Straighten the affected arm and splint it in a functional position
    3. Splint the affected arm in the position it was found
    4. Treat the patient for shock

25. A nurse sees a motorcycle rider struck by a car and stops at the scene. The patient is alert, complains of inability to move his legs, and has his helmet still in place. The nurse's next action should be to:
    1. Leave the patient and seek help
    2. Elevate his legs with his helmet after carefully removing it from his head
    3. Remain with the patient and continue ongoing assessment of his status
    4. Begin CPR

26. A patient comes to the emergency department after accidentally driving a nail into his hand while working in his garage. The nurse should first:
    1. Remove the nail and apply a sterile dressing
    2. Ask the patient when his last tetanus shot was
    3. Stabilize the nail until a physician is available to remove it
    4. Flush the wound with sterile saline after removing the nail

27. A patient on a medical unit complains of sudden chest pain. She has shortness of breath and a heart rate of 110 beats per minute (bpm). The nurse hears no breath sounds on the patient's right side. The patient, who appears to have a simple pneumothorax, should be placed:
    1. On her affected side with pillows to support her
    2. Supine with her feet elevated 30 degrees
    3. Prone with her arms raised over her head
    4. In semi-Fowler's position

28. The first priority for a patient who has splashed a caustic chemical into his eyes in a work setting is to:
    1. Flush the eyes with water for at least 10 to 15 minutes to remove the chemical
    2. Patch the eyes to prevent further chemical reactions
    3. Instill cycloplegic drops to facilitate ophthalmic examination of the injured eyes
    4. Obtain a medical history from the patient to determine any allergies that might worsen his condition

29. A motor vehicle accident (MVA) victim has a hoarse voice, subcutaneous emphysema, cough with hemoptysis, and respiratory distress. The nurse should prepare him for an immediate: Fx larynx
    1. Blood transfusion
    2. Computerized axial tomography (CAT) scan or magnetic resonance imaging (MRI)
    3. Cricothyrotomy or tracheostomy
    4. Intubation

30. Tourniquets are indicated for control of hemorrhage only when:
    1 Injuries are so diffuse that maintaining direct pressure is not a possibility
    2 An extremity is severely mutilated or amputated
    3 Application of ice and elevation has not stopped the bleeding
    4 The patient must be transported

31. Two nurses are performing CPR on a 3-year-old child who was found unresponsive in his hospital bed. They correctly perform the compressions and respirations in which ratio?
    1 15:2
    2 5:1
    3 15:1
    4 5:2

32. While shopping for groceries, the nurse witnesses another shopper fall to the ground. The patient is assessed and found to be without pulse or respirations. The nurse begins CPR by giving two breaths and then places his hands on the sternum to begin compressions at a depth of:
    1 ½ to 1 inch
    2 1 to 1½ inches
    3 1½ to 2 inches
    4 2 to 2½ inches

33. Assessment of a fracture of the right ulna should include:
    1 Determining limitations to range of motion
    2 Observing for alterations in sensation, temperature, and color of the extremity
    3 Ascertaining the patient's previous use of the extremity
    4 Measuring the length of the affected limb in comparison with the nonaffected one

34. A 36-six year old man is brought to the emergency department with a diagnosis of morphine overdose. The first medication to administer in his treatment should be:
    1 Disulfiram (Antabuse)
    2 Epinephrine (Adrenalin)
    3 Methylprednisolone (Solu-Medrol)
    4 Naloxone (Narcan)

35. A 23-year old patient is brought to the hospital in an agitated state and is hyperventilating. She has an elevated blood pressure and an elevated temperature of 100.1° F. She is hallucinating. The nurse should suspect that the patient has taken:
    1 Inhalants
    2 Stimulants
    3 Depressants
    4 Cannabis

36. While assessing a motor vehicle accident (MVA) victim, the nurse notes clear fluid leaking from the right ear. This symptom indicates:
    1 Concussion
    2 Contusion
    3 Basilar skull fracture
    4 Orbital fracture

37. An elderly woman with diabetes is brought to the hospital by a neighbor who is concerned about a change in her level of consciousness and activity. The patient admits that she does not remember when she last ate or took her insulin. In addition to measuring her blood glucose, the nurse should also check the patient's level of:
    1 Potassium
    2 Hemoglobin
    3 Protein
    4 Estrogen

38. A man who was mowing his lawn was stung by a bee and has been brought to the emergency room with swelling, burning, and pruritus at the site. The nurse should:
    1 Apply warm moist heat to the area to relieve pain
    2 Vigorously squeeze the site after removing the stinger to make sure the toxin is expressed from the wound
    3 Apply ice after cleaning the site with soap and water
    4 Pull out the stinger and apply direct pressure to the site

39. A man is brought to the hospital after being in a house fire. He is burned over all of his chest and his right leg. Using the rule of nines, the nurse estimates the burned percentage of his body is:
    1 25% to 30%
    2 1% to 5%
    3 0% to 15%
    4 75% to 80%

40. A patient arrives in the emergency department with a fractured left wrist. The complaint that is the most likely to indicate serious injury and must be addressed first is:
    1 Pain in the affected wrist
    2 Swelling in the fingers
    3 Bruising in the hand and arm
    4 Numbness in the fingers

41. On her regular jogging path, the nurse discovers a woman who has fallen into a shallow pond, face down. The nurse pulls her out of the water and observes that the woman is not breathing. The nurse should:
    1 Immediately activate EMS and then proceed to initiate CPR
    2 Complete 1 minute of CPR before activating EMS
    3 Give two breaths and then activate EMS
    4 Perform CPR for 5 minutes, then activate EMS

42. A firefighter is brought to the hospital by ambulance from the scene of a factory explosion where he was burned and also sustained a severe laceration to his lower right leg. His heart rate is 112 bpm, respirations 78 and shallow, and blood pressure is 72/40 mm Hg. The nurse recognizes that the patient is in:
    1 Hypovolemic shock
    2 Neurogenic shock
    3 Septic shock
    4 Cardiogenic shock

43. While dressing for the prom, the nurse's teenage daughter complains about having to wear a medical identification tag. The nurse's best response to this is:
    1 "You have to wear it so that people will know that you have diabetes."
    2 "If you promise to follow your diet you can leave it at home for tonight."
    3 "Why don't you just carry it in your purse instead?"
    4 "Let's see if you can wear it around your ankle."

44. The usual medical intervention for orally ingested drug overdose is:
    1 Lavage with normal saline
    2 Gavage with activated charcoal
    3 Emesis induced by paregoric
    4 IV normal saline by bolus

45. A patient with a history of alcohol abuse is brought to the emergency room with vomiting, hypotension, and facial flushing. The nurse prepares to administer:
   1 Diphenhydramine (Benadryl) to sedate the patient, who is having delirium tremens
   2 Naloxone (Narcan) to reverse the narcotic effect of ethanol ingestion
   3 Normal saline fluid challenge for this patient who is dehydrated from vomiting
   4 Chlorpheniramine maleate (Chlor-Trimeton) to counteract the reaction to disulfiram (Antabuse)

46. A surgical patient who has been in the hospital for 3 days begins to have symptoms of tremors, anxiety, and hallucinations. The nurse institutes precautions for:
   1 Aspiration of emesis
   2 Seizures related to alcohol withdrawal
   3 Falling caused by unstable gait
   4 Elopement caused by anxiety and disorientation

47. A patient with insulin-dependant diabetes is brought to the emergency department with a blood glucose of 680 mg/dl. The nurse prepares an IV infusion of:
   1 50% glucose
   2 Normal saline *BC-there is 0 dextrose*
   3 5% dextrose
   4 Mannitol

48. A group of family members is brought to the emergency department after becoming ill at a picnic. They are having symptoms of headache, fatigue, and muscle incoordination. The nurse asks them if they had eaten:
   1 Chicken that was not thoroughly cooked
   2 Unrefrigerated cream-filled foods
   3 Any foods canned or cured by someone at home *Botulism*
   4 Food prepared by someone who had a respiratory or skin infection

49. An elderly woman who wandered away from her home is brought to the emergency department after being found in a field wearing only her nightgown. She is shivering and her temperature is 94.5° F. The nurse prepares to administer:
   1 Hot beverages such as black coffee or tea
   2 Warmed gastric and peritoneal lavage
   3 Warmed IV fluids
   4 Heat packs and warming blankets

50. A hiker is brought to the emergency department after being bitten on his lower leg by a snake. The nurse immobilizes the affected limb and:
   1 Places it in a dependent position
   2 Elevates it on two pillows
   3 Places warm moist packs on it
   4 Cleans it vigorously with antimicrobial soap

51. A spill of powdered chemicals occurs at a factory, and one of the employees was contaminated with the substance. Before transporting him to the emergency department, the contaminant should be:
   1 Flushed from his skin with running water for at least 10 minutes *This ↑ # of contaminant*
   2 Contained by applying dry dressings to the affected skin
   3 Swept from the skin with a dry dressing
   4 Neutralized with petroleum jelly

52. A patient who had been burned with scalding soup is reluctant to remove her wedding rings. The nurse explains to her:
   1 "We can just tape your rings in place and they will be OK."
   2 "For now, we will leave your rings in place, but we will remove them if your fingers begin to swell."
   3 "I'll put your rings in a safe place."
   4 "Removing your rings now will ensure that they are kept in a safe place and that they will not injure your finger later if your hands start to swell."

53. A man who was involved in a motor vehicle accident (MVA) insists that he is "only bruised" and does not want to be admitted to the hospital for observation. The nurse observes that he has decreased chest wall stability caused by several fractured ribs. She tells him:
   1 "You can go home if you promise to come back if you start having trouble breathing."
   2 "You may have injuries to your lungs or your heart as a result of these rib fractures. Staying here means that we can make sure you get immediate treatment if you should develop further problems with pain or breathing."
   3 "You probably don't have anything really wrong, but it would be a good idea to stay anyway."
   4 "You will have to sign this form stating that you are leaving against medical advice."

54. A patient who was severely injured in a fall from a scaffold is concerned about how much of his independent function he will be able to regain. The nurse knows that his injury is at the T7 level. She tells him:
   1 "You may have to be on a ventilator for a while, but you will eventually be able to breathe without help."
   2 "You may need to wear long-leg braces to walk, but you will be able to function independently in activities of daily living."
   3 "You probably won't have any problems because your injury is so low on your spinal cord."
   4 "You will most likely have flaccid paralysis in all extremities and will need help with breathing and activities of daily living."

55. A patient with a myocardial infarction is clammy, tachycardic, and disoriented. The nurse recognizes that he has shock that is described as:
   1 Vasogenic
   2 Cardiogenic
   3 Distributive
   4 Hypovolemic

56. An 18-year-old woman fell during a rock-climbing expedition with some friends. She complains of severe pain in her left elbow, and deformity in the extremity is obvious. The nurse includes in ongoing monitoring an assessment of *@ risk for compromised circulation distal to injury site*:
   1 Presence of ecchymosis on the upper arm
   2 Ability to adduct the extremity
   3 Temperature and radial pulse in the extremity
   4 Orientation and level of consciousness

57. A 10-year-old boy is stabbed on the school playground. By the time the school nurse reaches him, he is pale, cyanotic, diaphoretic, and has a pulse of 120 bpm. The nurse's highest priority action is to:
   1 Administer fluid boluses to maintain blood pressure
   2 Cover him with a blanket or jacket to maintain his body temperature

3 Establish and maintain a patent airway
4 Elevate his feet on a folded jacket to promote venous return

58. A 3-year-old boy was bitten by another child at his day care center. In giving discharge instructions, the nurse includes information about:
1 Contacting an attorney
2 Administering the full dose of the prescribed antibiotic
3 Waking the child every hour through the night to make sure he is rousable
4 Making sure the child has a fluid intake of at least 700 ml over the next 24 hours

59. A 26-year-old woman is being examined for complaints of right lower quadrant abdominal pain. She is febrile and has a white blood cell count of 26,000/mm³ In responding to her request for something cold to drink, the nurse replies:
1 "It would be better for you to have a hot beverage right now."
2 "You can have plain water but no ice."
3 "Given that you may go to surgery in the very near future, you must refrain from drinking anything right now."
4 "How about a nice cold soft drink?"

60. A 26-year-old woman who has diabetes was found unconscious at home and transported to the emergency department. Her blood glucose was 46 mg/dl. The nurse prepares to administer:
1 10 units of regular insulin subcutaneously
2 500 ml 0.9% normal saline bolus IV
3 100 ml orange juice orally
4 50% dextrose bolus IV

61. A 36-year-old sexual assault survivor is brought to the emergency department for examination and treatment. For the prevention of pregnancy, the nurse prepares to administer:
1 Cefixime (Suprax)
2 Norethindrone-mestranol (Ortho-Novum)
3 Estrogen-progesterone (Orval)
4 Doxycycline (Vibramycin)

62. The police brought a 43-year-old man who is having tremors, intestinal cramps, chills and sweating to the emergency department. His eyes are watery and his nose is running. The nurse suspects:
1 Overdose of narcotics
2 Withdrawal from narcotics
3 Overdose of stimulants
4 Withdrawal of stimulants

63. A hunter is brought to the emergency department with feet that are cold, damp, and shriveled. The nurse recognizes this condition as:
1 Chilblain
2 Frostbite
3 Immersion foot   AT cont contact c̄ cold temp of wet feet
4 Hypothermia = Temp <95°

64. A 2-year-old boy is brought to the emergency department for treatment of a bee sting. He is wheezing, has urticaria, and diffuse erythema. The nurse's priority action is to:
1 Ensure adequate airway and ventilation
2 Apply cold packs to the affected area for comfort
3 Administer antibiotics to prevent infection
4 Administer steroids and antihistamines to counteract swelling

65. The burn patient at greatest risk for mortality related to second-degree burns is:
1 A 6-year-old child who has bitten an electric cord and has burns on his lips
2 An 84-year-old woman who has been splashed with very hot coffee
3 A 46-year-old factory worker who was contaminated with a caustic chemical
4 A 12-year-old girl who was caught in a house fire

66. A 46-year-old man diagnosed with a pulmonary embolus is waiting for treatment. The nurse should prepare to administer what type of medication?
1 Antiarrhythmic
2 Anticonvulsant
3 Anticoagulant
4 Antipsychotic

67. A 36-year-old woman on antibiotic therapy for a gram-negative infection comes to the emergency department complaining of weakness, restlessness, and thirst. The vital sign assessment reveals a temperature of 103.8° F. The nurse recognizes that this patient is likely experiencing:
1 Anaphylactic shock
2 Neurogenic shock
3 Septic shock
4 Anxiety reaction

68. Assessment of a trauma patient reveals that his chest moves inward with inhalation and outward with exhalation. The nurse recognizes this as a sign of:
1 Flail chest
2 Pulmonary embolus
3 Simple rib fracture
4 Tension pneumothorax

69. The nurse has succeeded in patient teaching with a man admitted for treatment of chilblain when the patient states:
1 "I should rub my toes and fingers until they warm up."
2 "I should avoid cigarettes because of the effects on circulation."
3 "This will spread to my whole body if I'm not careful."
4 "I inherited this tendency from my father."

70. During an intake interview with a patient, the nurse learns that he is taking methadone (Dolophine), which indicates that the patient is being treated for withdrawal from:
1 Alcohol
2 Barbiturates
3 Benzodiazepines
4 Heroin

71. A trauma patient with an abdominal stab wound is brought by ambulance to the emergency department. Inspection reveals that a loop of bowel is protruding from the wound. The nurse's priority action is to:
1 Administer oxygen by nasal mask
2 Administer tetanus toxoid injection
3 Apply wet dressings to the wound site
4 Apply pressure dressing to the wound after replacing the bowel

72. A burn patient's wife is alarmed that his urine appears reddish brown in the drainage bag. The nurse explains to her that this is most likely the result of damage to his:
1 Kidney
2 Muscle tissue
3 Skin
4 Urethra

73. A mother reports that she allowed her two small children to eat raw dough containing eggs when she was making cookies yesterday. Last night, they began to have severe stomach cramps, headaches, and fever. The nurse tells the mother:
    1 "This may be Salmonella poisoning from eating uncooked eggs."
    2 "This may be an allergic reaction to an ingredient in the recipe."
    3 "This is probably the flu that has been going around."
    4 "This sounds like Trichinosis poisoning from eating undercooked dough."

74. A day care supervisor telephones the emergency department to report that a 3-year-old child has swallowed an undetermined amount of drain cleaner from a bottle under a sink. The nurse should instruct the supervisor to:
    1 Have the child drink milk to dilute and neutralize the chemicals
    2 Induce vomiting with syrup of ipecac *will cause further burning to the esophagus*
    3 Keep the child NPO and transport immediately
    4 Call the poison control center for information on how to treat the ingestion

75. After an earthquake, the victim who would be triaged with the highest priority is a(an):
    1 Crying 4-year-old boy with bleeding head laceration
    2 Dazed 26-year-old woman with a broken right arm
    3 Unresponsive 48-year-old man with contusions of the head
    4 Alert 70-year-old woman with diabetes who has burns of both arms

76. While working out at the gym, a woman with diabetes tells her friend that she feels very weak and hungry. The friend's first action is to:
    1 Have her lie down and cover her with a blanket
    2 Give her some hard candy
    3 Begin CPR
    4 Give her an injection of regular insulin

77. A 52-year-old dockworker comes to the emergency department complaining of severe crushing chest pain radiating to his left arm. He is cool, pale, and diaphoretic. Recognizing that he may be having a myocardial infarction, the nurse first:
    1 Applies electrodes for the cardiac monitor
    2 Administers nitroglycerine sublingually
    3 Administers oxygen at 5 L/min by mask
    4 Inserts a large-bore IV and begins a normal saline infusion

78. A 29-year-old man who has been stressed at work came home and drank several beers "to relax." He took three of his wife's prescription temazepam (Restoril) tablets. She became concerned about his slurred speech and inability to walk in a straight line, so she brought him to the emergency department. The nurse should give priority to monitoring his:
    1 Respiratory rate
    2 Temperature
    3 Breath sounds
    4 Pupil size

79. A motor vehicle accident (MVA) victim is brought to the emergency department and diagnosed with an unstable fracture of the pelvis. The nurse should report to the physician the presence of:
    1 Nausea and vomiting
    2 External rotation of the lower extremities *already sx of pelvic ft.*
    3 Pain in the lower extremities
    4 Increasing tenderness over the symphysis pubis *pt hemorrhage*

80. A patient who has choked on a piece of steak at dinner is brought by his wife to the emergency department in some respiratory distress. The nurse recognizes that he has a partial airway obstruction by the presence of:
    1 Hacking cough and lethargy
    2 Absent respiratory effort
    3 Flaring of nostrils and deep cough
    4 Anxiety and use of accessory muscles to breathe

81. A construction worker without a hardhat on was injured when he was hit on the head by falling lumber. He is bleeding profusely from the laceration on his scalp. The nurse's priority is to:
    1 Flush the wound with normal saline until it appears to be free of debris
    2 Scrub the wound with 4 × 4 gauze dressings and antiseptic skin cleanser
    3 Cover the open wound with a clean, nonadhesive dressing until it is examined by a physician
    4 Apply antibiotic ointment to the wound and apply a pressure dressing

82. When performing adult mouth-to-mouth resuscitation, the rescuer should deliver breaths that are:
    1 Full and given every 3 seconds
    2 Forceful and given every 4 seconds
    3 Shallow and given every 5 seconds
    4 Full and given every 5 seconds

83. During initial management of a patient who was burned over 70% of the body with second- and third-degree injury, the nurse's priority action is to:
    1 Establish and maintain an airway
    2 Establish and maintain vascular access
    3 Establish and maintain a sterile environment
    4 Establish a medical history

84. In performing chest compressions for CPR, the hands are placed on the adult chest:
    1 Side by side over the entire sternum
    2 On top of one another, two finger-breadths above the xiphoid process
    3 Fisted, on either side of the manubrium
    4 On top of one another, two finger-breadths below the xiphoid process

85. A 21-year-old construction worker was found unconscious but breathing in a roadside ditch. He was transported to the emergency department where the priority for his care should be to:
    1 Stabilize his cervical spine
    2 Insert an endotracheal tube
    3 Use painful stimuli to rouse him
    4 Insert a large-bore IV line

86. A short-term goal for a rape survivor who is being treated in the emergency department would be to:
    1 Initiate social interaction with friends and co-workers
    2 Express feelings about the event
    3 Return to pretrauma level of functioning
    4 Verbalize two methods of stress management

87. A 32-year-old person with insulin-dependent diabetes comes to the emergency department with a blood glucose by finger stick of 46 mg/dl. The nurse expects to see which symptom?
    1 Fruity acetone breath
    2 Complaints of hunger *sx hypoglycemia*

3 Dry, warm skin

4 Kussmaul's respirations

88. Epinephrine (Adrenalin) is ordered for a patient in anaphylactic shock. This drug should not be administered intramuscularly because:

1 Gas gangrene may occur

2 Necrosis may occur

3 Hemolysis may occur

4 The medication is not rapidly absorbed by this route

89. On the way to work, a nurse comes across a motor vehicle accident (MVA) with multiple trauma victims. The priority care goes to the one with:

1 Hemorrhaging

2 Altered level of consciousness

3 Cyanosis of nail beds   *compromised O2*

4 Obvious fracture of the femur

90. A patient called 9-1-1 after collapsing with a headache, dizziness, and nausea. The ambulance personnel found him unconscious but breathing. They suspect that the victim was overcome by carbon monoxide from a faulty furnace. Initial treatment for this patient may include oxygen administration at:

1 2 L/min via nasal cannula

2 5 L/min via nasal cannula

3 40% by facemask

4 100% by facemask   *Need to saturate body c O2!*

91. A 30-year-old farmer has a crush injury to his lower left arm as a result of a tractor accident. The nurse at the scene is unable to palpate a radial pulse. The next action to take is to:

1 Begin CPR

2 Assess for pulse in another artery

3 Initiate transport immediately

4 Cover the wound with a pressure dressing

92. For the first 24 hours after sustaining an eyelid contusion (black eye), the patient should apply:

1 Continuous warm most packs

2 Intermittent cold packs

3 Continuous cold packs

4 Intermittent warm moist packs

93. If direct pressure and elevation do not stop bleeding from a laceration, the next intervention should be to apply:

1 A tourniquet

2 Pressure to the supply artery

3 Ice packs

4 Warm moist packs

94. The maneuver for removal of a foreign body in the airway is known as the:

1 Henderson maneuver

2 Hasselbach maneuver

3 Valsalva maneuver

4 Heimlich maneuver

95. To establish an airway in a patient with possible neck or spine injuries, the nurse uses the:

1 Head tilt–chin lift

2 Head tilt–jaw thrust   *∅ tilting of head!*

3 Chin-lift only

4 Jaw-thrust only

96. A patient who hit her head on the windshield in a motor vehicle accident (MVA) has fixed, dilated pupils and a positive Babinski's sign. The nurse recognizes that these signs indicate: *Subdural hematoma*

1 Intracranial bleeding

2 Internal bleeding

3 Spinal cord injury

4 Meningitis

97. A patient who fractured his larynx on the steering wheel in a motor vehicle accident (MVA) is unable to give consent for surgery. The nurse should explain to his wife that the surgery is a:

1 Laryngectomy

2 Laryngoscopy

3 Tracheostomy

4 Thyroidectomy

98. A lineman sustained electrical burns on both hands when he fell from a utility pole. His wife says that his burns do not appear to be too serious. The nurse should explain to her why these burns are considered to be:

1 Superficial

2 Minor

3 Moderate

4 Major

99. In addition to inspecting the site of a penetrating wound, the nurse should also assess for a(an):

1 Foreign body such as a bullet

2 Exit wound

3 Medical information tag

4 Concealed weapon

100. A college student is brought to the emergency department by some friends who report that he drank 1 gallon of whisky in a 2-hour period. He is agitated and belligerent. After conducting an initial assessment, the nurse should closely monitor the patient's:

1 Respiratory status

2 Blood sugar

3 Range of motion

4 Inappropriate behavior

101. A penetrating wound, such as might be caused by a nail, results in which type of injury?

1 Laceration

2 Contusion

3 Incision

4 Puncture

102. Which of the following are considered to be major or critical burns (select all that apply)?

1 Caused by electrical trauma   *tissue damage*

2 Full-thickness burns that are less than 10% of BSA

3 Occurring in cases with preexisting chronic conditions

4 Partial-thickness burns that are greater than 20% of BSA in children under age 10

5 Involving face, hands, or perineum   *more likely to have complications*

103. The nurse notes that the patient admitted with burns has the following areas indicated on "rules of nines" diagram:

Frontal aspect of the right arm   *4.5%*

Frontal aspect of the left arm   *4.5%*

Right anterior chest wall   *9%*

The approximate amount of body surface area (BSA) involved in this injury is _____ *36% 18%* .

104. In performing one-rescuer CPR on an adult, the rate of chest compressions per minute is:

1 80

2 100

3 120

4 72

105. A patient caught the sleeve of her robe on fire while cooking breakfast. She is a 45-year-old women with insulin-dependent diabetes. She has superficial burns over 5% of her arm. This injury is classified as:
    1 Minor
    2 Moderate   *R+ Age + Diabetes*
    3 Major
    4 Superficial

106. Among the medications reported by a patient who is seeking treatment for a severe laceration of his lower leg, the nurse notes disulfiram (Antabuse). This medication indicates that the patient might have a severe reaction from medications that contain:
    1 Phenylpropanolamine
    2 Thimerosal
    3 Alcohol
    4 Eggs

107. A young man has been diagnosed with a strain to his left ankle sustained when he tripped on a rock while he was jogging. The nurse should instruct him to:
    1 Place his foot on the floor to stabilize the ankle
    2 Soak his ankle in warm water with Epsom salts
    3 Use crutches to avoid weight bearing
    4 Exercise the foot to reduce the chance for stiffening of the joints

108. When assessing a recent fracture, the nurse will focus on which of the following (select all that apply)?
    1 Pain
    2 Purulence   *Sx of infection (not evident)*
    3 Pallor
    4 Pulses
    5 Paresthesia   *may result from compromised Function* — *Neurological*

109. A patient who has been hemorrhaging from a severe injury is becoming restless, anxious, and clammy. The nurse recognizes that this indicates possible progression to:
    1 Shock
    2 Sepsis
    3 Sedation
    4 Syndactyly

110. Symptoms of a concussion might include:
    1 Cerebrospinal fluid leaking from the nose or ear
    2 Blood behind the eardrum
    3 Blood leaking from the ear
    4 Severe headache

111. A patient who was in a motorcycle accident has a diagnosis of compound fracture of the lower left extremity. The nurse explains to him and his wife that this involves:
    1 Breakage of the bone, producing two fragments
    2 Fracture of the bone in more than one location   *Comminuted*
    3 Protrusion of bone through the skin
    4 Fracture complicated by tearing of tendons or ligaments

112. A 34-year-old man was working in his garage when he accidentally impaled his hand on a screwdriver. He was brought to the emergency room with a towel wrapped around his hand, and the towel is now soaked in blood. The nurse should treat the wound by:
    1 Removing the screwdriver immediately to prevent further tissue damage
    2 Removing the screwdriver after flushing the area with normal saline for 5 minutes
    3 Leaving the screwdriver in place to control bleeding
    4 Leaving the screwdriver in place as long as the patient is not in pain

113. Before notifying the EMS, the rescuer should perform CPR on infants and children up to 8 years of age for:
    1 5 minutes
    2 1 minute
    3 3 minutes
    4 10 minutes

114. A patient with a tension pneumothorax complains of increased pain and dyspnea; his heart rate has increased to 100 bpm. The nurse recognizes that this may be the result of:
    1 Coarctation of the aorta
    2 Cardiac tamponade
    3 Vasovagal response
    4 Mediastinal shift

115. An elderly woman who was brought to the emergency department from her nursing home experienced sudden, sharp chest pain with shortness of breath and pallor. She is very anxious; her heart rate is 112 bpm, and her respiratory rate is 28. The nurse should explain to her that, to confirm the physician's diagnosis of possible pulmonary embolism, she will have:
    1 A chest x-ray examination   *Not show pathology*
    2 A bronchoscopy
    3 A ventilation-perfusion (V/Q) scan
    4 A lung biopsy

116. A child is brought to the emergency department by his mother after lacerating his scalp in a fall. She is very anxious about the amount of blood that is oozing from his head. The nurse explains to the mother that bright red blood signals that this type of bleeding is:
    1 Capillary   *Bright red + oozes*
    2 Venous   *Dark + flows steady*
    3 Arterial   *Bright + spurts*
    4 Afferent

117. For a patient with a tracheostomy, CPR would entail which type of breathing?
    1 Mouth to mouth
    2 Mouth to nose
    3 Mouth to stoma
    4 Mouth to mouth and nose

118. In a conscious infant who loses consciousness, removing a foreign body from his airway should entail:
    1 Shining an examination light into the mouth to visualize the object
    2 Vigorous finger-sweeps to palpate the object
    3 Removing the object only if it is visible
    4 Applying pressure on the cricoid cartilage to expel the object

119. In triage of a disaster event, the civilian priority is to the victims who:
    1 Are most likely to survive
    2 Have children
    3 Have the least serious wounds and can be quickly cared for
    4 Have the most serious, life-threatening injuries

120. A 3-year-old child is brought to the emergency department after a motor vehicle accident (MVA). She has a scalp laceration that is oozing blood; pain, discoloration, and swelling of her right lower arm; and right-sided chest pain that increases on inspiration. The nursing actions with the highest priority are:
    1 Administration of analgesic medication and tetanus toxoid

2 Immobilization and elevation of the right arm

3 Assessing and maintaining airway and adequate ventilation

4 Application of ice packs and pressure dressings to the scalp laceration

121. A victim of domestic violence is brought to the emergency department by the police. She is complaining of abdominal pain where she was struck forcibly with a baseball bat. On examination, she is found to have guarding, diminished bowel sounds, and bruising on the abdomen. The nurse explains to her that she may undergo:

1 Peritoneal lavage *determines if intra abd wound exists + requires surgery*

2 Gastric lavage

3 Barium enema

4 Abdominal MRI *work yet lavage is more economical*

122. A nurse arrives at the scene of a motor vehicle accident (MVA) and quickly assesses the injured parties. The priority care should be given to the:

1 Driver with a head laceration and severe knee pain

2 Passenger with a bleeding nose who is complaining of a headache

3 Driver with a hoarse voice who is coughing blood

4 Passenger with an arm laceration who is crying hysterically

123. During afternoon rounds, the nurse discovers a 60-year-old patient with diabetes unconscious on the floor near his bed. The nurse's immediate action should be to:

1 Call the physician and prepare IV glucose

2 Establish an airway and assess for breathing and circulation

3 Check the blood glucose and administer regular insulin

4 Check for medical alert identification and call the family

124. A 79-year-old woman comes to the urgent care clinic complaining of nausea, headache, and muscle cramping. She reports that she was in the garden all afternoon weeding. She is anxious and pale. The nurse's first action should be to:

1 Move the patient to a cool, quiet room

2 Administer a bolus of normal saline IV

3 Encourage the patient to drink 1 liter of water with 2 tablespoons of table salt dissolved in it

4 Apply ice packs to facilitate rapid cooling

125. A 46-year-old man who was shoveling his driveway all morning is brought to the urgent care clinic by his wife. The nurse notes that his toes are numb, discolored, and blistered. She explains to them that these signs indicate:

1 Immersion foot

2 Chilblain

3 Frostbite

4 Hypothermia

ANSWERS AND RATIONALES

1. Knowledge, implementation, safe, effective care environment (a).

   3 The American Heart Association endorses this technique over previously used methods because it can provide better blood flow than the two-finger technique.

   1, 2, 4 These would apply too much pressure to the infant's body.

2. Knowledge, implementation, safe, effective care environment (a).

   2 This position reduces the risk of aspiration of blood.

   1, 3, 4 These positions would increase the risk of aspiration of blood from the nasal hemorrhage.

3. Comprehension, assessment, safe, effective care environment (b).

   2 This is characteristic of an anaphylactic reaction, which suggests an allergy to peanuts.

   1 This is characterized by weakness and confusion.

   3 This is characterized by weakness, confusion, and electrocardiograph changes.

   4 This condition is not characterized by the symptoms the child is having.

4. Comprehension, implementation, safe, effective care environment (b).

   4 As much of the chemical as possible must be removed from the skin to decrease the damage to the integumentary system.

   1 The chemical processes are better slowed by removing the chemical from the skin. Body temperature does not contribute to the process.

   2 Stimulating circulation is not a goal of the process; removing the substance from the skin is the desired outcome.

   3 The most important substance to remove is the caustic chemical. Medication may not be applied to the skin at all.

5. Comprehension, planning, physiological integrity (b).

   1 The bone ends may cause further injury to the surrounding tissue, and this patient has an increased risk for infection.

   2 Reduction of the fracture will be undertaken later, possibly in surgery.

   3 Moving the leg to elevate it can cause further injury.

   4 Proper immobilization would require the use of splints above and below the fracture site.

6. Comprehension, planning, safe, effective care environment (b).

   4 The patient should be removed from the heat and made as comfortable as possible to reduce further illness caused by heat and exertion.

   1, 3 The patient should not exert himself or be subjected to any more heat.

   2 If the patient is vomiting, nothing should be given by mouth so as to prevent aspiration or gastric distention.

7. Application, implementation, physiological integrity (a).

   3 The strained limbs should be iced, immobilized, and rested for 3 days.

   1, 2, 4 Further use of the affected areas increases the strain on the muscles and risks more permanent damage.

8. Analysis, evaluation, physiological integrity (c).

   1 The patient is at risk of developing pulmonary edema as a result of the trauma of the near drowning.

   2 Alteration in glucose metabolism is less likely to occur compared with the risk of respiratory distress and pulmonary edema.

   3 Alteration in fluid imbalance is less likely to occur compared with the risk of respiratory distress and pulmonary edema.

   4 Alterations in blood counts are less likely to occur compared with the risk of respiratory distress and pulmonary edema.

9. Application, implementation, safe, effective care environment (b).

   3 Seizures are an important risk for the patient in delirium tremens.

   1, 2, 4 These interventions have low priority for the patient in comparison with the need for safe, effective care environment.

10. Analysis, assessment, physiological integrity (b).

    2 The patient who has received electrical shock is at risk for renal involvement as a result of trauma to muscle tissue.

    1 The liver may be damaged by direct electrical shock but is not affected by tissue damage elsewhere in the body.

    3 The lungs may be damaged by direct electrical shock but are not affected by tissue damage elsewhere in the body.

    4 The spleen may be damaged by direct electrical shock but is not affected by tissue damage elsewhere in the body.

11. Comprehension, assessment, physiological integrity (c).

    1 Smoke inhalation, as evidenced by brassy cough, singed nasal hairs, and respiratory distress, is a serious complication that can lead to death if left untreated.

    2 Infection is not an immediate risk.

    3 Gastric distress is not an immediate risk.

    4 Sputum production is not related to oxygen deprivation.

12. Application, implementation, health promotion and maintenance (b).

    2 Because of the impairment in skin integrity and the fact that tetanus is transmitted by the saliva of infected humans or animals, the patient should be given prophylactic treatment with tetanus.

    1 Immune globulin does not provide prophylaxis against tetanus.

    3 Erythropoietin does not provide prophylaxis against tetanus.

    4 Corticosteroids do not provide prophylaxis against tetanus.

13. Comprehension, assessment, physiological integrity (b).

    3 Spontaneous pneumothorax can occur during periods of strenuous activity.

    1 Muscle strain does not commonly cause sudden pain in the chest.

    2 Infection does not commonly cause sudden pain in the chest.

    4 Myocardial infarction does not typically produce alterations in chest excursion.

14. Knowledge, assessment, physiological integrity (b).

    3 Phencyclidine is a hallucinogen that commonly causes agitation and stimulation.

    1 Cannabis tends to produce a more depressed effect on the patient and does not tend to be accompanied by hallucinations in cases of acute intoxication.

    2 Heroin tends to produce a more depressed effect on the patient and does not tend to be accompanied by hallucinations in cases of acute intoxication.

4   Alcohol tends to produce a more depressed effect on the patient and does not tend to be accompanied by hallucinations in cases of acute intoxication.

15. Knowledge, planning, psychosocial integrity (b).

4   Clothing is placed in paper bags, which will not retain moisture and subsequently cause evidence to deteriorate.

1   Plastic can cause moisture to be retained.

2   Cloth bags are not easy to write on for labeling purposes.

3   Plastic can cause moisture to be retained.

16. Knowledge, planning, physiological integrity (b).

1   Frequent interruptions in compressions reduce overall blood flow.

2   This produces too many interruptions in the process to produce adequate blood flow.

3   This does not provide adequate ventilation.

4   This produces too many interruptions and does not provide enough ventilation.

17. Comprehension, implementation, physiological integrity (b).

1   If the patient can take medication by mouth, acetaminophen is indicated for pain because it is a nonnarcotic and will not depress respirations. The medication is available in liquid form that can be administered via nasogastric tube.

2   Meperidine (Demerol) is a CNS depressant that can compromise respiration and level of consciousness.

3   Morphine is a CNS depressant and can mask symptoms of brain injury and compromise respiration.

4   Amphetamine, not an analgesic, is a CNS stimulant and can mask signs of brain trauma.

18. Knowledge, implementation, safe, effective care environment (b).

3   The particle should be touched gently with a sterile swab moistened with saline or water.

1, 2, 4   These risk further injury to the eye.

19. Comprehension, implementation, safe, effective care environment (b).

3   To reduce risk of further injury to the patient's cervical spine, the helmet should be removed only when assistance is available to stabilize his neck.

1, 2, 4   These actions would increase the risk of further injury to the patient.

20. Application; assessment, physiological integrity (b).

2   Because of the patient's age, chronic illness, and location of burns, this would be considered a major or critical injury.

1, 3, 4   In light of the patient's risk factors, the injury is considered to be major.

21. Comprehension, assessment, safe, effective care environment (b).

2   A burn that is grey and painless is full thickness and places the patient at risk for infection and fluid and electrolyte imbalance. This situation should be monitored in the hospital until the patient is stable.

1, 3, 4   The lack of pain is an indication that the injury has destroyed the pain receptors in the skin and signals a serious wound that should be closely monitored.

22. Knowledge, assessment, physiological integrity (b).

2   Pulmonary embolism is characterized by sudden chest pain, hemoptysis, and wheezing. The patient may proceed rapidly to shock and even death if a large blood vessel is blocked.

1   Myocardial infarction does not usually produce sharp chest pain and hemoptysis.

3   Pneumothorax usually produces pain on one side of the chest, unless bilateral involvement occurs; it does not usually produce hemoptysis.

4   Pneumonia usually features chest pain associated with coughing. Hemoptysis is not usually sudden in onset and is related to the trauma of coughing.

23. Comprehension, implementation, physiological integrity (b).

3   The child requires calories to accomplish the work of rewarming, and providing these in a warm beverage helps the process.

1   More than electrolytes, the child needs carbohydrates to support him as he warms.

2   Beverages that are too hot may cause thermal injury to the child's mouth and throat.

4   Cold drinks impede the warming.

24. Knowledge, implementation, physiological integrity (b).

3   The affected arm should be immobilized above and below the dislocation to prevent further injury.

1   Cold is applied to dislocations to reduce swelling and pain.

2   The affected arm should not be moved because it might cause further injury.

4   If the patient is verbalizing and awake, treatment for shock is a secondary intervention.

25. Application, planning, physiological integrity (b).

3   The nurse should remain with the patient and monitor him for a change in status.

1   The patient should not be left unattended. He may have more serious injuries than was detected on first assessment, and he needs to be protected from further injury.

2   The helmet should not be removed and the legs should not be moved until qualified medical assistance with proper equipment arrives on the scene.

4   If the patient is awake and talking, resuscitation is not a requirement.

26. Comprehension, planning, physiological integrity (b).

3   The nail should remain in place until a physician is available to remove it because it might be preventing hemorrhage, or the process of removing it might cause further injury.

1, 4   The nail should be left in place to reduce further risk of injury to the patient.

2   Tetanus immunization is a lesser consideration with respect to stabilizing the wound.

27. Application, implementation, physiological integrity (b).

4   The patient will have less difficulty breathing in a semi-Fowler's position. Oxygen should be administered as soon as possible.

1, 2, 3   These positions increase the difficulty of breathing for this patient.

28. Comprehension, implementation, physiological integrity (b).

1   The longer the chemical is in contact with the eye, the more damage may occur. Flushing with running water or saline should be implemented before any other action.

2, 3, 4   These delay the removal of the chemical substance and increase the risk of further injury.

29. Application, implementation, physiological integrity (b).

3   The patient with a fractured larynx must be prepared for immediate surgical intervention to establish an airway.

1 Blood loss is a secondary risk in comparison with the compromised airway.

2 Without a patent airway, the patient would likely have a respiratory arrest during a radiologic assessment examination.

4 Because of the injuries to the neck, establishing an airway through traditional vertical access will most likely not be possible.

30. Comprehension, planning, physiological integrity (b).

2 The use of tourniquets should be reserved only for extreme cases of injury because they increase the likelihood that the extremity will have to be amputated.

1 Direct pressure can be maintained on widely spread wounds.

4 The patient who is being transported may not be monitored closely enough to assess tissue damage during the process. Transport is not a justification for the use of tourniquets.

3 If ice and elevation have not controlled the bleeding, direct pressure should be applied.

31. Knowledge, implementation, physiological integrity (b).

2 The 5:1 ratio should be used in pediatric arrest by professional responders regardless of whether one or two rescuers are involved.

1, 3, 4 These ratios do not provide the optimum oxygenation and ventilation needed in children according to the American Heart Association guidelines.

32. Knowledge, implementation, physiological integrity (b).

3 This is the correct depth of compression for an adult victim according to the American Heart Association guidelines.

1 This is the appropriate depth for infant compressions.

2 This is the correct depth for compression for a child.

4 This is too deep for effective compressions in resuscitation efforts.

33. Knowledge, implementation, physiological integrity (b).

2 These are indices of adequate circulation in the extremity.

1, 4 Moving the affected limb may cause further damage to it.

3 Determining the patient's history is not an immediate need in the stabilization of a fracture or the process of observing it. This information is important for planning rehabilitation of the limb.

34. Knowledge, implementation, physiological integrity (b).

4 Naloxone is a narcotic antagonist and will reverse the adverse effects of an overdose.

1 Disulfiram is prescribed for alcohol dependency.

2 Epinephrine is not indicated for initial treatment of narcotic overdose.

3 Methylprednisolone is not indicated for initial treatment of narcotic overdose.

35. Comprehension, assessment, physiological integrity (b).

2 Effects of stimulant overdose include agitation, increased body temperature and blood pressure, hallucinations, and possibly death.

1 Inhalant overdose is characterized by anxiety; respirations will likely be depressed.

3 Depressants produce decreased heart rate and respirations, stupor, and coma.

4 Cannabis intoxication is characterized by confusion and disorientation but usually not agitation and increased heart and respiratory rates.

36. Comprehension, assessment, physiological integrity (a).

3 This is a characteristic of basilar skull fracture.

1, 2, 4 These conditions involves bleeding and do not produce clear fluid, especially in the ear.

37. Application, assessment, physiological integrity (b).

1 Because potassium is given along with glucose and insulin to patients with hypoglycemia, a baseline of this electrolyte is needed to monitor the effectiveness of treatment and to avoid causing cardiac problems for the patient.

2, 3, 4 These laboratory values do not play an important role in the management of hypoglycemia and ketoacidosis.

38. Comprehension, implementation, physiological integrity (b).

3 The application of ice to the site will decrease blood flow and reduce pain and the circulation of toxins.

1 Heat increases circulation and the spread of toxins; it will not relieve pain from an insect sting.

2 Squeezing increases circulation and the spread of toxins.

4 Removing the stinger increases the risk of releasing and circulating more toxin.

39. Knowledge, assessment, physiological integrity (a).

1 The chest is estimated at 18% of the body and the leg is estimated at 9%; therefore the combined area would be approximately 27%.

2 This percentage is equal to less than the area of one arm.

3 This percentage is approximately equal to the area of one arm.

4 This is a much larger area than is indicated on the patient's chart.

40. Application, assessment, physiological integrity (b).

4 Numbness in the fingers can signal nerve damage.

1 Pain is an expected symptom in a fracture.

2 Swelling is an expected symptom in a fracture.

3 Bruising is a common symptoms of a fracture.

41. Knowledge, implementation, physiological integrity (b).

2 Because near drowning is a special situation in which airway compromise may be the cause of arrest, the rescuer should provide 1 minute of CPR before notifying EMS.

1 CPR should be initiated first, then EMS is activated.

3 CPR should be given for 1 minute before EMS is activated.

4 Only 1 minute of CPR should be given before EMS is activated.

42. Knowledge, assessment, physiological integrity (b).

1 Hypovolemic shock is primarily a fluid problem caused by loss of blood or fluid volume.

2 Neurogenic shock results from widespread dilation of blood vessels caused by an imbalance in autonomic stimulation of the smooth muscles in vessel walls. It is usually associated with spinal cord injury.

3 Septic shock results from complications of massive bacterial infection in which toxins released into the blood cause vasodilation.

4 Cardiogenic shock is the result of faulty pumping action, an unlikely condition in a fireman in good physical condition.

43. Application, implementation, physiological integrity (b).

4 Moving the tag to a less conspicuous location offers a good compromise between not wearing it at all and having to wear it on her wrist or as a necklace.

1 This opens the door to discussion about privacy issues and does not further the cause of wearing the jewelry.

2 Medical identification should be worn at all times.

3 Medical identification tags need to be prominent enough so that rescuers and health care professionals can notice them and be aware of the indicated warnings.

44. Comprehension, implementation, physiological integrity (b).

2 Gavage with activated charcoal is implemented for substances other than caustics or hydrocarbons.

1 Lavage is useful only in limited circumstances, usually within 30 minutes of ingestion.

3 Emesis is induced with ipecac, not paregoric.

4 IV infusion has limited usefulness in diluting gastrointestinal contents.

45. Comprehension, implementation, physiological integrity (c).

4 The symptoms indicate a reaction to disulfiram (Antabuse), and the antihistamine is indicated to control the symptoms.

1 The patient is not having symptoms of delirium tremens. Diphenhydramine, though indicated in the treatment of disulfiram reactions, is not administered for its sedative effect but rather its antihistamine activity.

2 Narcan is indicated for the treatment of opioid ingestion, not ethanol or disulfiram.

3 Fluid challenges are administered for hypotension caused by hypovolemia.

46. Comprehension, planning, physiological integrity (c).

2 The patient is exhibiting symptoms of delirium tremens and is at risk for seizures.

1 Aspiration is a less likely complication compared with seizures.

3 Falling is a less likely and less serious complication compared with seizures.

4 The patient is not exhibiting signs of nausea or vomiting, ataxia, or risk of elopement.

47. Comprehension, planning, physiological integrity (b).

2 Normal saline contains no dextrose and is used as a maintenance fluid for the patient with hyperglycemia.

1, 3 These are contraindicated in a patient with hyperglycemia.

4 This would exacerbate the patient's hyperglycemia.

48. Application, assessment, safe, effective care environment (b).

3 The patients are exhibiting symptoms of botulism, which is often caused by eating food that was not properly canned or cured.

1 Improperly cooked poultry can cause Salmonella infections, which is characterized by fever and gastrointestinal symptoms.

2, 4 These often cause infections from *Staphylococcus aureus*, characterized by nausea, vomiting, and diarrhea.

49. Comprehension, implementation, physiological integrity (b).

4 This patient is having symptoms of mild hypothermia and should be offered active external rewarming, which might also include overhead radiant warmers.

1 Beverages that are offered to the conscious hypothermia patient should include a high sugar content to help metabolism in the rewarming process.

2, 3 These interventions are more suitable for a patient with severe hypothermia.

50. Comprehension, implementation, physiological integrity (b).

1 The affected limb is placed in a dependant position to minimize circulation of toxins.

2 Elevation would facilitate circulation of the toxin.

3 Heat and increased circulation would facilitate circulation of the toxin.

4 Cleaning and increased circulation would facilitate circulation of the toxin.

51. Knowledge, implementation, physiological integrity (b).

3 The powder should be carefully swept from the skin, making sure not to contaminate anyone else in the process.

1 Diluting with water increases the volume of the contaminant and increases the risk of tissue injury.

2 The contaminant should be removed from the skin immediately.

4 Petroleum jelly is ineffective in neutralizing powdered chemicals.

52. Application, implementation, physiological integrity (b).

4 The rings should be taken off as soon as possible to facilitate their removal and safe, effective care environment. If they remain in place and the fingers swell, they might have to be cut off, and they might cause tissue damage to the fingers.

1 Leaving the rings in place increases the risk of damage.

2 Jewelry should be removed as soon as possible and placed in a safe location.

3 To increase the patient's compliance, the nurse needs to explain the risks involved in leaving the rings in place.

53. Application, implementation, physiological integrity (c).

2 The patient has a flail chest and may have cardiorespiratory problems as a result. Explaining the risks to him increases his understanding of the situation and makes his compliance with admission more likely.

1 If the patient develops respiratory difficulty, he may not be able to return to the hospital in time to receive assistance.

3 The nurse should not dismiss the risks of complications and must inform the patient of the situation and its possible outcomes.

4 The nurse must inform the patient of the risks involved and not encourage him to leave against medical advice.

54. Application, evaluation, physiological integrity (b).

2 This injury is often characterized by paraplegia, but the individual may be able to rehabilitate to walk with support.

1 This outcome is characteristic of an injury at the cervical spine level.

3 Advising the patient that he will have no problems in the case of any spinal injury is unrealistic.

4 This outcome is characteristic of injury at higher levels (cervical and upper thoracic spine).

55. Comprehension, assessment, physiological integrity (b).

2 Cardiogenic shock is the result of faulty pumping action that results in reduced cardiac output.

1 Vasogenic is the result of sepsis, spinal cord injuries, or anaphylaxis.

3 Distributive shock is the result of sepsis, spinal cord injuries, or anaphylaxis.

4 Hypovolemic shock is the result of blood or fluid loss associated with thermal or other injury.

56. Application, assessment, physiological integrity (c).

3 The patient is at risk for compromised circulation distal to the injury.

1 Bruising is likely the result of the nature of the fall; its occurrence above the injury is not as significant as it would be below the injury.

2   Adduction is a function of muscles in the upper arm, not related to the elbow.

4   The patient is not likely to become disoriented or unconscious as a result of the elbow dislocation, although other injuries may produce these changes.

57. Application, implementation, physiological integrity (b).

   3   Establishing and maintaining an airway is the highest priority.

   1   Fluid balance is a lesser priority compared with maintaining the airway.

   2   Body temperature is a lesser priority compared with maintaining the airway.

   4   These interventions, though appropriate for treatment of shock, are lesser priorities compared with maintaining the airway.

58. Application, implementation, physiological integrity (b).

   2   To treat or prevent infection in the wound, all of the antibiotic must be administered as ordered.

   1   Discussing legal matters with the parents regarding the event is inappropriate for the nurse.

   3   Checking levels of consciousness is indicated for head injuries.

   4   Forcing fluids is not indicated for treatment of human bites.

59. Application, planning, safe, effective care environment (b).

   3   The patient should be NPO before surgery for appendicitis.

   1, 2, 4   The patient should have no oral intake before surgery.

60. Comprehension, implementation, physiological integrity (b).

   4   This is the treatment of choice for the unconscious person with diabetes in hypoglycemia.

   1   Insulin is contraindicated in hypoglycemia.

   2   This would be an appropriate intervention for hypotension, not hypoglycemia.

   3   Oral administration is contraindicated in the unconscious patient.

61. Application, implementation, physiological integrity (b).

   3   This medication is used after sexual contact to prevent pregnancy.

   2   This contraceptive is prescribed for administration on an ongoing basis before sexual contact.

   1, 4   These are antibiotics that have no contraceptive activity.

62. Comprehension, assessment, physiological integrity (b).

   2   Watery eyes and runny nose are characteristic of narcotic withdrawal.

   1   Overdose of narcotics does not produce chills, sweating, or intestinal cramps. In addition, the patient would most likely be comatose.

   3, 4   Stimulants do not produce the symptoms, either in overdose or withdrawal.

63. Comprehension, assessment, physiological integrity (a).

   3   This condition is caused by continuous contact with cold temperature of a wet foot.

   1   Chilblain is characterized by localized redness and swelling of the skin resulting from excessive exposure to cold.

   2   Frostbite is the traumatic effect of extreme cold on skin and subcutaneous tissue evidenced by pallor of exposed skin surfaces.

   4   Hypothermia is characterized by body temperature below 95° F.

64. Comprehension, implementation, physiological integrity (b).

   1   Anaphylactic shock can easily progress to respiratory arrest or compromised airway. The priority action is to establish and maintain the airway.

   2   Although the application of cold may provide comfort and decrease swelling, it is not a priority action.

   3   Administration of antibiotics is a lesser priority compared with establishing and maintaining an airway.

   4   Administration of medications is a lesser priority compared with establishing and maintaining an airway.

65. Comprehension, assessment, physiological integrity (b).

   2   The very young and the very old are at greater risk for complications from thermal injuries.

   1   Electrical burns to the lips are not likely to be life threatening.

   3   This patient's injury is less likely to be life threatening.

   4   A second-degree burn in a healthy child of 12 is less likely to be life threatening.

66. Comprehension, implementation, physiological integrity (b).

   3   Anticoagulant therapy is indicated to decrease clotting and control further embolization.

   1   This patient does not have a cardiac arrhythmia at this time.

   2   No indication exists that this patient is at risk for seizures.

   4   This medication is not indicated in the treatment of pulmonary embolus.

67. Comprehension, assessment, physiological integrity (c).

   3   Septic shock results from the release of endotoxin that causes vasodilation.

   1   Although the patient might be allergic to antibiotics, a reaction would not be characterized by these symptoms.

   2   Neurogenic shock is the result of a decrease in circulating blood volume caused by an injury such as spinal cord trauma.

   4   The patient's fever indicates that her experience is not psychogenic.

68. Comprehension, assessment, physiological integrity (b).

   1   Paradoxical breathing results from instability of the chest wall in flail chest.

   2   Pulmonary embolus is characterized by sudden chest pain, dyspnea, and cyanosis.

   3   Symptoms of a simple rib fracture include pain on inspiration and rapid, shallow breathing.

   4   Tension pneumothorax is characterized by neck vein distention, tracheal deviation, and distant breath sounds on the affected side, in addition to paradoxical breathing.

69. Application, evaluation, physiological integrity (b).

   2   Nicotine causes vasoconstriction that will worsen the symptoms of chilblain.

   1   Friction will worsen the symptoms of burning, itching, and blistering.

   3   Chilblain is a localized reaction to excessive exposure to cold.

   4   Although the patient may have underlying risks for compromised circulation in the extremities, such as Raynaud's disease or diabetes mellitus, chilblain is the result of excessive exposure to cold.

70. Knowledge, assessment, physiological integrity (b).

   4   Methadone (Dolophine) is indicated for use in the withdrawal of heroin.

1 Disulfiram (Antabuse) is used for treatment of withdrawal from alcohol.

2 Phenobarbital is often used in the treatment of barbiturate withdrawal.

3 Progressively smaller doses of the drug in question are used in the treatment of benzodiazepine withdrawal.

71. Application, implementation, physiological integrity (b).

3 Tissue death will take place if the exposed bowel dries.

1 This is not a priority action for exposed bowel tissue.

2 After ascertaining that the patient has had a primary tetanus immunization, the nurse should prepare to administer a booster. However, this is not a priority action for exposed bowel tissue.

4 The bowel should be replaced by a physician, possibly in a surgical procedure, and is not within the scope of the nurse's practice.

72. Application, assessment, physiological integrity (c).

2 The presence of myoglobin in the urine indicates muscle damage.

1 Renal tissue damage is not necessarily indicated by the color of urine.

3 Epithelial tissue damage is not demonstrated by urine color.

4 Internal injuries do usually occur with burns.

73. Application, assessment, safe, effective care environment (b).

1 Food poisoning such as this is caused by eating raw eggs that are contaminated with Salmonella bacteria.

2 Allergic reactions are not characterized by these symptoms.

3 This history of eating raw eggs points to another probable cause for the illness.

4 Trichinosis is caused by eating undercooked contaminated meat such as pork.

74. Application, implementation, physiological integrity (b).

3 The child needs immediate medical attention and should be kept NPO and moved to the emergency department as soon as possible.

1 Milk will not neutralize a caustic substance such as drain cleaner. The child should be NPO.

2 Vomiting should not be induced because it will cause further burning of the esophagus, throat, and mouth.

4 The child should be transported immediately. Delays in contacting a poison control center can cause further damage to his system.

75. Application, evaluation, physiological integrity (c).

3 The unconscious victim must be monitored for airway management.

1 The crying child appears to have superficial injuries and can be treated later.

2 The fractured arm is not as much of a treatment priority as is the head injury with loss of consciousness.

4 Although the age and underlying disease state of this patient makes her a high risk for complications, this is not as high a priority as is the head injury with loss of consciousness.

76. Application, implementation, physiological integrity (b).

2 A conscious person with diabetes who is having symptoms of hypoglycemia should be given a fast-acting carbohydrate.

1 This intervention would be appropriate for treating shock.

3 No indication exists that the patient requires CPR.

4 Insulin is contraindicated in cases of hypoglycemia.

77. Comprehension, implementation, physiological integrity (b).

3 Immediate administration of oxygen may prevent more severe pain and tissue damage.

1 Comfort and preservation of tissue integrity are a higher priority.

2 Further assessment must be done before administering medication.

4 Comfort and preservation of tissue integrity are a higher priority.

78. Comprehension, assessment, physiological integrity (b).

1 Sedatives combined with alcohol produce respiratory depression.

2 Body temperature is not affected by sedatives or alcohol.

3 Although auscultation of the chest is part of the baseline assessment, no indication exists that the patient might have alterations of respiration, other than rate.

4 Pupil size and reactivity are part of the initial baseline assessment.

79. Comprehension, assessment, physiological integrity (c).

4 Hemorrhage related to internal injuries can produce life-threatening complications in the patient with a pelvic fracture.

1 Nausea and vomiting are common in patients who have pain and injury.

2 External rotation is characteristic of pelvic fracture.

3 Pain in the back and lower extremities is common in patients with pelvic fracture.

80. Comprehension, assessment, physiological integrity (b).

4 The patient is still able to have some air exchange but shows signs of hypoxia.

1 Lethargy is not a symptom of partial airway obstruction.

2 The lack of respirations may be caused by complete occlusion of the airway.

3 Coughing deeply requires more air than would be possible with a partial obstruction.

81. Comprehension, implementation, safe, effective care environment (b).

3 The wound should not be cleaned until after it is examined by a physician.

1 Flushing the wound can cause alterations in its appearance or damage tissue by dislodging clots that have formed.

2 Scrubbing would change the appearance of the wound and might cause tissue damage and further bleeding.

4 Applying ointment would change the appearance of the wound.

82. Application, implementation, physiological integrity (b).

4 The breaths should be every 5 seconds and full enough to cause chest excursion.

1 This rate is too rapid to allow the lungs to deflate between breaths.

2 Forceful breaths tend to cause gastric distention.

3 Shallow breaths do not allow enough air to enter into the lungs.

83. Application, implementation, physiological integrity (b).

1 Establishing and maintaining an airway is always a priority for the burn patient. Because of the possible complications of smoke inhalation, the respiratory status must be continually monitored.

2   Although this is a very important aspect of burn care, it is a priority secondary to maintaining an airway.

3   This is not as high a priority as is maintaining an airway.

4   This has the lowest priority of all the interventions mentioned.

84. Knowledge, implementation, safe, effective care environment (a).

   2   Placing the hands higher than the xiphoid process prevents further damage to the chest and facilitates the compression of the heart between the sternum and the spine.

   1   This might cause injury to internal organs from the xiphoid process.

   3   This does not facilitate pressure from compression and might cause injury.

   4   This would cause injury and not facilitate compression between the sternum and the spine.

85. Comprehension, implementation, physiological integrity (b).

   1   Because the nature of the injury is unknown, the cervical spine must be protected.

   2   Given that the patient is breathing on his own, intubation is not indicated.

   3   Determining level of consciousness is secondary to preserving function.

   4   Stabilizing the cervical spine is a priority over establishing venous access. If the patient should awaken during the procedure because of the painful stimulus, he might move and risk spinal cord injury.

86. Comprehension, planning, psychosocial integrity (b).

   2   This is the only appropriate short-term goal for this situation. All of the other options are long-term goals.

   1   This goal may take weeks to months to achieve.

   3   This long-term goal may take months to achieve.

   4   The patient may not be able to achieve this goal for days or weeks.

87. Knowledge, assessment, physiological integrity (a).

   2   This is a symptom of hypoglycemia.

   1   This symptom of ketoacidosis is the result of the insulin deficiency.

   3   The patient with hypoglycemia is likely to have cool, moist skin.

   4   Air hunger is a symptom of ketoacidosis or severe hyperglycemia.

88. Knowledge, implementation, physiological integrity (c).

   1   Vasoconstrictive agents may cause gas gangrene if administered intramuscularly because of resulting reduced oxygen tension, which provides a suitable growing atmosphere for *Clostridium* microbes that may have colonized on the patient's skin.

   2   Tissue damage is more likely to occur with repeated injections at the same site.

   3   Hemolysis is not likely to occur from the medication.

   4   Absorption may be more rapid with intramuscular injection because it is going into a more vascular site.

89. Application, planning, physiological integrity (b).

   3   Cyanosis is a distinct sign of compromised oxygenation and is the highest priority of the situations listed.

   1   Hemorrhage may produce compromised oxygenation but is a lesser priority compared with cyanosis.

   2   Altered level of consciousness is less life threatening compared with cyanosis or hemorrhage.

4   This fracture is not a life-threatening emergency.

90. Application, implementation, physiological integrity (b).

   4   Saturating the blood with oxygen may allow the body's tissues to remain oxygenated.

   1   This rate of flow would not provide adequate oxygenation.

   2   This rate of flow will allow carboxyhemoglobin to remain in place.

   3   This rate of flow would not break the affinity of hemoglobin for carbon monoxide.

91. Application, assessment, physiological integrity (b).

   2   Assessment for adequate circulation should be done at the carotid artery. The radial artery may have been compromised in the accident.

   1   If the patient is breathing and has evidence of circulation, no indication for CPR exists.

   3   Further assessment is indicated before any transportation.

   4   Further assessment is indicated before any interventions.

92. Knowledge, implementation, physiological integrity (a).

   2   Intermittent cold packs will help reduce swelling and discoloration.

   1   Warm packs cause vasodilation and would increase swelling and discoloration.

   3   Continuous application of cold packs would be uncomfortable and possibly cause tissue damage resulting from prolonged vasoconstriction.

   4   Warm compresses would be appropriate after the first 48 hours.

93. Knowledge, implementation, physiological integrity (a).

   2   Decreasing the blood flow above the injury may help stop the hemorrhage.

   1   Tourniquets are used only as a last resort to control bleeding.

   3   Ice packs will not produce enough vasoconstriction to stop severe bleeding.

   4   Warm packs will cause vasodilation, which will increase the bleeding.

94. Knowledge, implementation, physiological integrity (a).

   4   The method was introduced in 1974 by Henry Heimlich.

   1   This is not the name of any well-known technique in emergency medicine.

   2   The Henderson-Hesselbach equation is used to determine acid-base balance.

   3   The Valsalva maneuver is performed by attempting to forcibly exhale while keeping the mouth and nose closed. It is used as a diagnostic tool to evaluate the condition of the heart and is sometimes done as a treatment to correct abnormal heart rhythms or relieve chest pain.

95. Knowledge, implementation, physiological integrity (a).

   4   Tilting the head may cause further injury if the patient has trauma to the neck or spine.

   1   This is the first method to be used in the case of a patient who does not have suspected neck or spine injury.

   2   This is the method to use in the case of a patient who does not have suspected neck or spine injury if additional displacement of the jaw is required.

   3   Lifting only the chin will not open the airway; it is likely to further occlude it.

96. Comprehension, assessment, physiological integrity (b).

   1   These are signs of a subdural hematoma.

   2   Internal bleeding refers to the abdominal organs and would not produce these symptoms.

3 Spinal cord injuries do not produce these symptoms.

4 Meningitis, which would take several days to develop, does not produce these symptoms.

97. Application, planning, safe, effective care environment (a).

3 The patient will need to have an airway surgically created to maintain ventilation.

1 No indication exists at this point that the larynx will need to be removed.

2 Examination of the laryngeal area is of secondary priority to creating and maintaining an airway.

4 No indication exists at this point that the thyroid will need to be removed.

98. Application, assessment, physiological integrity (a).

4 All electrical burns are considered to be major because of the possibility of internal damage to tissue.

1 Superficial burns involve only the epidermal layer of tissue.

2 Minor burns involve 15% or less of BSA.

3 Moderate burns involve 15% to 25% of BSA.

99. Comprehension, assessment, physiological integrity (a).

2 Penetrating wounds often have an entrance and an exit and must be inspected thoroughly to assess the extent of the trauma.

1 Internal inspection of a wound should be conducted by the physician.

3 Information about conditions is a lesser priority compared with determining the extent of the injury.

4 Although the patient may be armed, this information is a lesser priority compared with determining the extent of the injury.

100. Comprehension, assessment, physiological integrity (a).

1 The patient with acute alcoholism is at risk for respiratory depression and aspiration from vomiting.

2 The patient's nutritional status is a lesser priority compared with his respiratory status.

3 No indication exists that the patient's range of motion is altered.

4 As long as the patient is not a danger to himself or others, his behavior is a low priority for monitoring.

101. Knowledge, assessment, safe, effective care environment (b).

4 Puncture wounds are caused by sharp instruments that penetrate deeply into the tissues.

1 A laceration is a jagged cut through the skin and underlying tissue.

2 A contusion is a mechanical injury (usually caused by a blow), resulting in hemorrhage beneath unbroken skin.

3 An incision is a division of soft tissue made by a sharp instrument, such as a knife.

102. Knowledge, assessment, safe, effective care environment (b).

1 Electrical burns can produce tissue damaged based on conductivity through the body.

3 Chronic conditions such as diabetes or renal failure can cause life-threatening complications for burn patients.

4 Because of the ratio of body mass to BSA, the amount of involvement for partial-thickness burns in children (20%) is less for children than it is for adults (25%).

5 Burns of the face, hands, or perineum are more likely to produce complications compared with other areas of the body and are always considered as major injuries.

2 Full-thickness burns are considered major when they involve greater than 10% of BSA.

103. Application, assessment, safe, effective care environment (c).

The correct answer is 18%. Each aspect of the arm is estimated at 4.5%, and the right anterior chest is approximately 9%.

104. Knowledge, implementation, physiological integrity (b).

2 This rate of compressions promotes optimum blood flow and blood pressure.

1 Although this was the previously recommended rate, it has been revised by the American Heart Association to a more rapid rate to provide better circulation of blood.

3 This rate is too rapid to allow adequate blood flow and blood pressure.

4 Although this rate is the normal heart rate of the average adult, it is not rapid enough to promote adequate blood flow and blood pressure in resuscitation.

105. Application, assessment, physiological integrity (b).

3 Because of the age of the patient and her underlying chronic condition, this burn is considered as a major injury.

1, 2, 4 Although the burn is superficial, her age and underlying condition escalate the classification of the burn.

106. Knowledge, planning, physiological integrity (b).

3 Because disulfiram is given for the treatment of alcoholism, it can produce strong reactions when given in combination with medications that contain alcohol.

1 Phenylpropanolamine has been associated with an increased risk of hemorrhagic stroke.

2 Thimerosal is a mercurial compound used as a preservative in parenteral injections. Although it can cause sensitivity reactions, it is not likely to react in combination with disulfiram.

4 Patients who have a sensitivity to eggs may react to medications that have been prepared with egg, such as certain vaccines.

107. Application, implementation, physiological integrity (b).

3 Treatment for sprains includes immobilization and limited weight bearing.

1 The extremity should be elevated to reduce swelling.

2 Ice is recommended to reduce pain and swelling. Warm packs or soaks will increase swelling.

4 The foot should be immobilized until it has recovered from the damage resulting from excessive physical use.

108. Knowledge, assessment, physiological integrity (b).

1 The periosteum is richly supplied with nerve endings, producing significant pain in a fractured bone.

3 Compromised circulation may be evidenced by pallor resulting from impaired blood flow to the injured tissue.

4 Vascular compromise may result from compression by bone fragments, swelling, or other tissue injury. Assessing for pulses on an ongoing basis is necessary to detect changes as early as possible.

5 Paresthesia may result from compromise to the neurological function of the injured tissue.

2 Purulence is a sign of infection, which would not be evident in the early stages of recovery from a fracture.

109. Knowledge, assessment, physiological integrity (b).

1 Restlessness, anxiety, and clammy skin are signs of shock in the bleeding patient.

2 Although sepsis may produce shock in a bleeding patient, these are not symptoms of infection.

3 Sedation is produced by the administration of medications.

4 Syndactyly is a congenital webbing of fingers or toes.

110. Comprehension, assessment, physiological integrity (b).

4 Pain may result from concussion, the jarring of the brain that results from a blow to the head.

1 Leaking CSF is an indication of skull fracture.

2 Hemotympanum is a sign of skull fracture.

3 Blood leaking from the ear would most likely be the result of local trauma.

111. Knowledge, assessment, physiological integrity (a).

3 A compound or open fracture is characterized by bone protrusion through the skin.

1 A complete fracture results in two fragments of bone.

2 A comminuted fracture is one resulting in several pieces of broken bone.

4 Fractures are not classified by the collateral damage but strictly by the type of damage to the bone.

112. Application, implementation, physiological integrity (b).

3 An impaled object should be left in place to control possible bleeding and to avoid further injury to the tissue.

1 Removing the screwdriver can cause further trauma to the hand and cause severe bleeding.

2 Cleaning the surrounding area would not diminish the possible damage that removing the screwdriver might cause.

4 The patient is likely to experience pain either way, but removing the screwdriver can cause further complications.

113. Knowledge, implementation, physiological integrity (a).

2 American Heart Association guidelines recommend that rescuers should provide approximately 1 minute of CPR on children before activating EMS.

1, 3, 4 These intervals are too long to wait before summoning help.

114. Comprehension, assessment, physiological integrity (b).

4 Mediastinal shift is a life-threatening condition that occurs when pressure within the intrapleural space increases and the heart and mediastinal structures are pushed to the contralateral side.

1 Coarctation of the aorta is a congenital condition characterized by stenosis of the vessel.

2 Cardiac tamponade results from the accumulation of fluid in the pericardium.

3 When the vagus nerve is activated, heart rate and blood pressure decrease.

115. Comprehension, planning, physiological integrity (b).

3 Nuclear scintigraphic V/Q scanning of the lung is the diagnostic modality for detecting pulmonary thromboembolism.

1 A chest x-ray examination would not necessarily demonstrate the pathology of a pulmonary embolism.

2 A bronchoscopy is used to evaluate tissue within the bronchial tubes.

4 A biopsy would be contraindicated for a patient with a diagnosis related to blood clotting.

116. Application, assessment, safe, effective care environment (a).

1 Capillary blood is bright red and oozes from a wound.

2 Venous bleeding is dark in color and flows steadily.

3 Arterial blood is bright, but it spurts.

4 Afferent describes the direction that blood is flowing in a vessel and can be used in reference to both arteries and veins, depending on their function.

117. Knowledge, implementation, physiological integrity (b).

3 Given that the patient's airway is altered, any breathing other than to the stoma would likely be ineffective.

1 Mouth-to-mouth breathing would not ventilate this patient because of the changes in his upper airway.

2 Mouth-to-nose breathing would not ventilate this patient because of the changes in his upper airway.

4 Mouth-to-mouth-and-nose breathing would not ventilate this patient because of the changes in his upper airway.

118. Comprehension, implementation, physiological integrity (b).

3 The object should be removed only if it is clearly visible and can be grasped.

1 If the object is not readily visible, no further efforts towards examination should be made because they will delay the rescue.

2 Finger sweeps may force the object further into the airway.

4 Locating this anatomical landmark on the neck of an infant would be difficult, and pressure on the neck or throat area would not facilitate removal of a foreign body in the airway.

119. Comprehension, assessment, physiological integrity (a).

4 The civilian priority is for the care of patients whose lives are threatened.

1 The military priority is for those who are most likely to survive.

2 Triage is done on the basis of risk to the patient, not to survivors or family members.

3 This choice would place persons already at the greatest risk in further danger of morbidity or mortality.

120. Application, assessment, physiological integrity (b).

3 Maintaining an airway and adequate ventilation is always the highest priority.

1 Administering medication is not as high a priority compared with maintaining an airway and ventilation.

2 A fractured arm is a lesser priority compared with airway and ventilation.

4 Given that the scalp laceration is oozing and not bleeding freely, it is not as great a priority compared with airway and ventilation.

121. Application, planning, physiological integrity (b).

1 Diagnostic peritoneal lavage helps determine whether an intraabdominal injury exists and whether surgery is required.

2 Gastric lavage is indicated in cases of ingestion of drugs or poisons.

3 As a radiologic examination of the lower intestine, the barium enema would not be the best way to obtain information about possible internal injuries to the abdomen.

4 Although an abdominal MRI would show information about abdominal trauma, peritoneal lavage provides a method of intervention and treatment as well, and it is much more economical.

122. Application, evaluation, physiological integrity (c).

   3 The victim who is hoarse and coughing blood may have serious injuries to the throat that can compromise the airway.

   1 This victim has no apparent injuries that would compromise his airway or circulation.

   2 This victim should be leaned forward to avoid aspiration of blood but is not a treatment priority.

   4 This victim may have the least serious injury and is not the greatest priority.

123. Application, implementation, physiological integrity (c).

   2 The priority for any unconscious victim is to establish an airway and assess for breathing and circulation.

   1 This assumes that the patient is unconscious because of insulin shock.

   3 This assumes that the patient is unconscious because of hypoglycemia.

   4 Notification of the family is a lower priority compared with interventions with the patient.

124. Application, implementation, physiological integrity (b).

   1 Removing one of the causes of heat exhaustion is important in preventing the progression of the condition.

   2 Fluid replacement is a lesser priority compared with controlling the progression of the condition.

   3 The patient is nauseated and might vomit if she drinks large quantities of salted water.

   4 Rapid cooling is an appropriate treatment for heat stroke.

125. Comprehension, assessment, physiological integrity (b).

   3 Deep frostbite is characterized by hyperemic skin, numbness, blister formation, and edema.

   1 Immersion foot gives the extremity a shriveled appearance.

   2 Burning, itching, and ulcerations characterize chilblain.

   4 Hypothermia is a generalized condition characterized by tachypnea, tachycardia, and confusion. Frostbite is a localized condition.

Chapter 10 Answers and Rationales

Part 1

This examination contains individual questions, the majority of which relate to clinical situations. Read all questions carefully. Each question has only *one best answer*.

Test time allotment (Part 1): approximately 2 hours

Answers and Rationales begin on p. 615.

1. Fluid and electrolytes are carefully monitored in patients with renal disease. A priority concern would be an increase in which of the following electrolytes?
   1 Calcium
   2 Chloride
   3 Sodium
   4 Potassium

2. A dark-skinned patient is at high risk for a pressure ulcer. The nurse assesses the patient's pressure points for blanching. The color that describes blanching in patients with dark skin is:
   1 Pale, as in someone who is anemic
   2 Grayish, as in ashes in a fireplace
   3 Hyperemic, as in the color of a plum
   4 Pinkish, as in circles of red blush makeup

3. Celiac disease is characterized by disturbance in the absorption of:
   1 Proteins
   2 Carbohydrates
   3 Vitamins
   4 Fats

4. A patient who has diabetes mellitus fell on the ice and sustained a skin abrasion. She asks the nurse to apply an ice wrap to her ankle. The nurse hesitates based on the understanding that:
   1 The open area will become infected
   2 She will first have to get an x-ray examination of her ankle
   3 Rebound swelling may occur once the ice is removed
   4 People with diabetes have a greater potential for injury related to cold

5. The nurse is preparing to ambulate a postoperative patient for the first time. Which of the following actions should the nurse take to maintain patient safety?
   1 Use one person to assist
   2 Use two persons to assist
   3 Give a narcotic 15 minutes before ambulation
   4 Encourage the patient to dangle alone for 1 hour before ambulation

6. Fluids by mouth are initially contraindicated for an infant with bronchiolitis because of feeding difficulty caused by:
   1 Tachypnea
   2 Bradycardia
   3 Irritability
   4 Fever

7. The reason for recommending that a patient stop smoking when he has peripheral vascular disease is:
   1 Smoke causes hypotension
   2 Nicotine constricts blood vessels
   3 Smoke irritates the lungs
   4 The tars in smoke decrease the red blood cell (RBC) count

8. When assessing a patient who is in kidney failure, the nurse suspects electrolyte imbalance, based on the patient's symptoms. Which of the following are signs of electrolyte imbalance and should be reported to the physician?
   1 Nausea, vomiting, increased depth of respirations
   2 Anxiety, irregular heartbeat, abdominal cramps
   3 Crackles, nausea, excessive thirst
   4 Dry lips, loss of weight, dark-amber urine

9. The nurse is caring for a patient who has had a subtotal thyroidectomy. The nurse is aware that accidental removal of the parathyroid glands can occur and will closely monitor the patient for:
   1 Tetany
   2 Seizures
   3 Renal shutdown
   4 Loss of the gag reflex

10. During a patient's annual physical, the physician notes an enlarged boggy prostate. Based on this information, which of the following data is most important?
    1 Hesitancy, change in urine stream
    2 Color and odor of urine
    3 Constipation, smoking history
    4 Type and amount of fluids taken daily

11. During routine morning rounds, the nurse notes that a patient with chronic pulmonary disease is more forgetful today. The nurse also notes an unusual odor on the patient's breath while assessing lung sounds. The nurse must evaluate the patient within the hour because the patient:
    1 May need to be oriented to her environment more today
    2 May be developing a respiratory infection
    3 May need more encouragement to eat today
    4 Is at risk for developing acidosis

12. A patient scheduled for an open reduction and internal fixation of the left hip resulting from a fracture should be taught that the immediate expected postoperative outcome of this surgery relative to activity is:
    1 Bed rest only
    2 Pivoting into a chair
    3 Ambulating with full weight bearing
    4 Confinement in bed with skeletal traction

13. A patient with severe degenerative joint disease has been scheduled for an arthroscopy of the left knee. The patient asks the nurse what to expect after the surgery. Which of the following is the nurse's best response?
    1 "You may need to ask your surgeon that question."
    2 "You should not need a knee replacement in the future."
    3 "You should have less pain and improved joint function."
    4 "The procedure will virtually cure your degenerative joint disease."

14. After a thyroidectomy, a patient develops carpopedal spasms and tingling of the lips. Which of the following complications would the nurse consider as the most likely to occur?
    1 Hyperglycemia
    2 Hypocalcemia
    3 Hyperkalemia
    4 Thyroid storm

15. A nurse is caring for an overweight patient with osteoarthritis. Which of the following would the nurse suggest to the patient to help control joint strain?
    1 Exercising the involved joint
    2 Reducing and maintaining weight
    3 Applying intermittent heat
    4 Taking medication at the onset of pain

16. The nurse assesses a patient in an emergency situation in which of the following sequences?
    1 Breathing, airway, circulation
    2 Airway, breathing, circulation
    3 Circulation, airway, breathing
    4 Breathing, circulation, airway

17. The nursing assistant asks the nurse about the turning schedule for a patient who had a right pneumonectomy yesterday. The nurse explains that the patient should be turned every hour from:
    1 Back to left side to right side
    2 Back to left side to back
    3 Left side to right side to left side
    4 Back to right side to back

18. Other than assessing baseline vital signs, an important nursing intervention to perform the morning of dialysis is to:
    1 Administer Benadryl
    2 Weigh the patient
    3 Do a urinalysis
    4 Keep the patient NPO

19. The disorder characterized by a malfunction of the motor centers of the brain caused by a lack of oxygen to the brain is:
    1 Down syndrome
    2 Scoliosis
    3 Osteomyelitis
    4 Cerebral palsy

20. When caring for a comatose patient, the nurse knows that discussing the patient's condition with the family at the patient's bedside is inappropriate because:
    1 It may confuse the patient
    2 It may upset the family
    3 It may speed up the dying process
    4 Hearing is one of the last senses lost

21. The nurse knows that family members assisting in the care of a dying loved one is beneficial because this:
    1 Prolongs the dying process
    2 Lessens the nurse's workload
    3 Helps prevent the family from feeling helpless
    4 Causes too much work for a grieving family

22. Which of the following is a normal assessment finding in the urine?
    1 Lack of odor
    2 Clear, yellow liquid
    3 Presence of a high specific gravity
    4 Presence of RBCs in the urine

23. When caring for a patient with a tracheostomy, the nurse observes that the tube appears to be filled with dry mucus. Which of the following actions is appropriate for the nurse to implement at this time?
    1 Remove the inner cannula and clean with alcohol-soaked Q-tips
    2 Remove the inner cannula and clean with hydrogen peroxide
    3 Remove the outer cannula and clean with hot water
    4 Remove the outer cannula and suction the trachea

24. The child of a nurse's neighbor, age 7 years, has developed a red, raised rash on her face, neck, and trunk. She also has a temperature of 101.4° F (38.5° C) and whitish spots on the back of her throat. From these symptoms, the nurse knows that the child has:
    1 Chickenpox
    2 Measles (rubeola)
    3 Mumps
    4 German measles (rubella)

25. A patient is being discharged following a suprapubic prostatic resection. He had an intravenous (IV) and a three-way Foley with continuous bladder irrigation, which was discontinued last evening. Which of the following is an appropriate discharge instruction for this patient?
    1 "Use daily laxatives to avoid straining to have a bowel movement."
    2 "Limit fluid intake to what you had in the hospital to prevent stretching the bladder."
    3 "If dribbling or incontinence occurs, use the Kegel exercises 10 to 20 times an hour."
    4 "Don't worry if your urine turns a bright red because that is caused by passing clots."

26. An elderly patient who states that she has "always been healthy" is being treated for a respiratory tract infection. The nurse observes that the patient uses her diaphragm during inspiration and plans to teach her pursed-lip breathing, based on the understanding that:
    1 Older persons need to consciously think about taking deep breaths
    2 The older a person becomes, the more likely he or she will develop chronic obstructive pulmonary disease (COPD)
    3 Age-related changes of loss of elastic recoil of the lungs occur
    4 Older people lose the use of their intercostals muscles

27. A Wilms' tumor is an adenosarcoma found in the
    _____.

28. A nurse obtains a positive Hemoccult test on a patient's stool. Which of the following statements made by the patient would lead the nurse to question the validity of the test results?
    1 "I love my coffee. I drink four or five cups a day."
    2 "I wish they would stop giving me that blue gelatin, I am sick of it!"
    3 "I really enjoyed the steaks I've had on my tray the past two evenings."
    4 "The hospital must have its own garden, judging by the amount of vegetables they feed you."

29. A newly admitted clinic patient complains of extreme fatigue, weight loss, and anorexia. One of her nursing diagnoses is altered nutrition: less than body requirements. Which of the following nursing interventions is most appropriate for this patient?
    1 Suggest use of hard candy, chewing gum, or artificial saliva to increase moisture in the mouth
    2 Discuss benefits of adequate moisture in the environment
    3 Keep a dietary record of amount, type, and frequency of food intake
    4 Plan low-calorie snacks into daily routine

30. A 5-week-old infant is brought to the pediatrician's office with symptoms of irritability, weight loss, and projectile vomiting. On physical examination, the infant appears dehydrated. From these symptoms, you know that the infant probably has:
    1 Hirschsprung's disease
    2 Pyloric stenosis
    3 Esophageal atresia
    4 Intussusception

31. While collecting a 24-hour urine specimen, the nurse should:
    1 Discard every other voided specimen
    2 Save all urine that the patient voids
    3 Insert a retention catheter for 24 hours
    4 Send each void to the laboratory separately

32. A nurse is caring for a patient who has a diagnosis of dysphagia. Which of the following should be included in the patient's plan of care?
    1 Facial exercises
    2 Special feeding precautions
    3 Allowing extra time for formation of words
    4 Referral to an occupational therapist for assessment

33. The nurse makes a diagnosis of altered sensory perceptions related to hemianopsia. Which of the following nursing interventions is appropriate?
    1 Cover the eyes with a blindfold
    2 Approach the patient on the right side
    3 Teach the patient to scan the environment
    4 Use artificial tears to prevent drying of the corneas

34. Which of the following nursing activities occurs during the assessment phase of the nursing process?
    1 Observing the patient's skin integrity
    2 Teaching the patient deep-breathing exercises
    3 Determining the priority patient care problem
    4 Collaborating with the patient to determine a realistic diet plan

35. A patient has a "straight cath, prn" order. Which of the following observations by the nurse might indicate that the order needs to be implemented?
    1 The patient has not voided in 4 hours
    2 The patient has consumed 2000 ml of fluid in 6 hours
    3 The patient had an incontinent episode 30 minutes ago
    4 The patient voids 5 to 10 ml of amber-colored urine every hour

36. Which of the following would the nurse expect the drug of choice to be for treating a hypertensive crisis?
    1 Propranolol hydrochloride (Inderal)
    2 Enalapril maleate (Vasotec)
    3 Nifedipine (Procardia)
    4 Nitroprusside (Nipride)

37. A nurse is caring for a patient with a hearing impairment. Which of the following measures should the nurse do *first?*
    1 Call the hospital's American Sign Language practitioner
    2 Ask significant others how the patient communicates at home
    3 Arrange for a family member to stay with the patient continually
    4 Arrange for a social worker to visit with patient and family members

38. A patient asks the nurse why his eyes water and his nose runs during episodes of hay fever. Which of the following responses by the nurse best describes the reason?
    1 The body is attempting to flush out the irritant
    2 The hay fever response is an autoimmune reaction
    3 These are normal reflexes that the body uses in times of stress
    4 The hay fever is actually an allergic response to grass and tree pollen

39. The physician orders diazepam (Valium) 7.5 mg IV. Diazepam is supplied in a 10-mg/2-ml Bristoject container. How many ml should be administered? _____ ml

40. A patient has decided to decrease her intake of red meat, but she is concerned that she will also be decreasing her intake of iron. The nurse suggests that she can increase her intake of iron by eating additional:
    1 Milk and dairy products
    2 Refined cereal products
    3 Dried fruits, such as apricots
    4 Yellow vegetables, such as carrots

41. Which of the following drugs would the nurse expect to be the drug of choice for treating left ventricular heart failure?
    1 Dopamine hydrochloride (Intropin)
    2 Furosemide (Lasix)
    3 Nitroprusside sodium (Nipride)
    4 Dobutamine hydrochloride (Dobutrex)

42. A patient has been diagnosed with a peptic ulcer and has been placed on medication therapy. Which of the following instructions would be most beneficial concerning diet therapy?
    1 "Include a lot of dairy products in your diet."
    2 "Eat a very bland diet, eliminating all caffeine and spicy foods."
    3 "Eat a well-balanced diet while taking your medications."
    4 "Eat six small meals a day to decrease your stomach discomfort."

43. A patient is admitted to the rehabilitation unit following a cerebrovascular accident (CVA). He has been experiencing dysphagia as a result of his brain infarct. To assist him, the nurse should put him in which of the following positions?
    1 Sitting in an upright position with head slightly forward
    2 Standing with legs abducted for 2 minutes then adducted for 1 minute
    3 Sitting in a comfortable position to promote speaking
    4 Turning him every 2 hours to a different position

44. Which of the following arrhythmias is the most dangerous and life threatening?
    1 A sinus arrhythmia
    2 An atrial arrhythmia
    3 An atrioventricular (AV) nodal arrhythmia
    4 A ventricular arrhythmia

45. An outbreak of *Escherichia coli*–related illness in the community. When providing information to the public, the nurse is knowledgeable that *E. coli*–related illness can be prevented by:
    1 Properly home canning of food
    2 Ensuring that red meats are well done
    3 Heating food to at least 140° F for 10 minutes
    4 Making sure that eggs are used quickly after purchase

46. Following a seizure, the nurse knows to place the patient in which of the following positions?
    1 Side lying
    2 Prone
    3 Supine
    4 High-Fowler's

47. A patient tells the nurse that she is going on a strict vegetarian diet, which includes no meat or dairy products. What nutrient would this patient be particularly deficient in if she continues on this diet?
    1 Iron
    2 Protein
    3 B-complex vitamins
    4 Fat-soluble vitamins

48. The patient with Parkinson's disease experiences posture and gait changes. Which of the following statements best reflects how gait is affected in this disease?
    1 Patient displays muscle rigidity and brief, jerky motor movements
    2 Patient displays limp, fidgeting movement of legs when walking
    3 Tremors cause the patient's ambulation to appear spastic
    4 Patient is bedridden; ambulation is not possible

49. A patient asks the nurse what information is available concerning omega-3 fatty acids. Which of the following statements by the nurse is most correct?
    1 "No fatty acids are good for you."
    2 "Why don't I make an appointment for you with the dietician?"
    3 "Physicians believe that omega-3 fatty acids may actually prevent cancer."
    4 "Some research suggests that these fatty acids may help prevent heart disease."

50. A patient tells the nurse that she uses mineral oil as a base for her salad dressing. The nurse's best response to this statement should be:
    1 "That's a good idea! It even fits into your mother's bland diet."
    2 "That's a good idea! Mineral oil doesn't add calories to your diet."
    3 "I would use another type of oil. Mineral oil is high in calories with very few vitamins."
    4 "I would suggest using vegetable oil because mineral oil hinders absorption of important vitamins."

51. A 76-year-old woman is admitted to the surgical unit following hip replacement surgery. The nurse administers meperidine (Demerol) 20 mg IV, as ordered for pain. The patient sleeps for 3 hours and awakens confused, drowsy, and lethargic. The nurse should:
    1 Call the physician and report the patient's condition
    2 Not call the physician but chart the patient's response to the medication
    3 Keep reminding the patient of where she is, the day, and the time
    4 Observe the patient because older adults metabolize drugs at a slower rate

52. The patient, age 4, was admitted with a diagnosis of positive epiglottitis. The nurse caring for this patient should include which of the following in her plan of care?
    1 Check the patient's throat with a flashlight
    2 Increase the patient's oral intake
    3 Direct warm steam toward the patient
    4 Have tracheostomy equipment available

53. A nurse is counseling a 23-year-old woman who is trying to eat a healthier diet. She says she is trying to quit smoking, but is having a hard time doing so. Which of the following vitamins should the nurse recommend as a supplement?
    1 Vitamin A
    2 Vitamin K
    3 Vitamin C
    4 Vitamin B

54. A woman brings her father in to the clinic because he has been lost and was unable to remember his address. Which of the following questions should the nurse ask first to identify a possible cause of the problem?
    1 "What medications are you taking?"
    2 "When did you move to this address?"
    3 "Have you had trouble sleeping lately?"
    4 "Are you eating balanced meals daily?"

55. A 30-year-old patient has been admitted to the neurosurgical unit following surgery for a brain tumor. She reports to the nurse that she is seeing zigzag lines in front of her face and hears voices singing. The nurse should *first*:
    1 Note her comments in the chart and refer them to her psychiatrist
    2 Have the patient lie down
    3 Start an IV and administer IV Valium
    4 Call the patient's physician

56. Which of the following statements should indicate to the nurse that a mother understands the dietary needs of her teenage daughter with diabetes?
    1 "Lots of fruit is good because fruit has natural sugar."
    2 "She can eat my baked goods if I use a sugar substitute."
    3 "I am definitely going to start serving more pasta and whole grains."
    4 "I am definitely not going to let her go with her friends to fast-food places."

57. A home health care nurse is interviewing and assessing a family with a newborn. Two toddlers are also living in the household. Which of the following foods on the kitchen counter would be of most concern to the nurse?
    1 Apples
    2 Whole milk
    3 Chocolate cake
    4 Bag of popcorn

58. A patient who underwent a transurethral resection of the prostate has had his catheter removed and is placed on the four-bottle technique. He has just voided for the fifth time today. The nurse knows to discard the:
    1 Bottle contents on the left and place the newest specimen bottle to the right
    2 Bottle contents on the right and place the newest specimen bottle to the left
    3 #2 bottle contents and place the newest specimen bottle to the right
    4 #3 bottle contents and place the newest specimen bottle to the left

59. To foster feelings that bolster a patient's self-esteem, the nurse must:
    1 Constantly criticize the patient's behavior
    2 Accept and give positive reinforcement for appropriate behavior
    3 Enforce behavior modification, ignoring all previous unacceptable behavior
    4 Remain strict with unacceptable behavior and structure precise patient expectations

60. A 19-year-old patient who has type 1 diabetes mellitus is taking Ortho-Novum for birth control. She comes to the physician's office complaining of an upper respiratory infection and is subsequently prescribed ampicillin for 1 week. The nurse should instruct her to:
    1 Use another means of birth control

2 Perform a urine test to check her blood sugar
3 Take ampicillin until she feels better
4 Expect a rash from the ampicillin

61. Which of the following would be the most therapeutic response for the nurse to make to a patient who complains of feeling "blue?"
1 "You have been so successful."
2 "Don't be blue; put this out of your mind."
3 "Don't let your feelings get the best of you."
4 "Is there something in particular that is worrying you?"

62. The nurse is caring for a patient recently diagnosed with breast cancer. While discussing the new diagnosis with her, the patient tells the nurse, "You must have me confused with someone else, I have polycystic disease." What defense mechanism is the patient using?
1 Repression
2 Denial
3 Fantasy
4 Rationalization

63. The nurse assigned to a neurology floor is to assess a 21-year-old male patient admitted with facial trauma. The nurse then asks the patient to occlude each nostril separately and close his eyes while she presents sources of familiar odors. The nurse is assessing which of the following cranial nerves?
1 I
2 II
3 III
4 VII

64. The nurse just received a call from the emergency room that a patient diagnosed with acquired immunodeficiency syndrome (AIDS) is coming to the unit. Which of the following actions should the nurse take first?
1 Prepare the patient's room for isolation
2 Confront her own feelings about AIDS
3 Orient the patient to his room
4 Explain unit policies to the patient

65. A 16-year-old patient is admitted to the neurology floor after being involved in an automobile accident. His head hit the windshield, and he is being admitted for observation. During the afternoon, he begins to complain of a headache, has two episodes of vomiting, and is more difficult to arouse. The initial nursing intervention is to:
1 Do nothing; he needs his rest
2 Place him in a recumbent position, administer oxygen, and notify the physician immediately
3 Prepare him for emergency surgery
4 Assess his neurological status, elevate the head of the bed slightly, and notify the physician immediately

66. A nurse who is providing discharge teaching for a patient on antidepressant therapy should tell the patient that he can expect to feel better in what length of time?
1 2 to 3 days
2 5 to 7 days
3 2 to 4 weeks
4 4 to 6 weeks

67. Prednisone is often used in the treatment of rheumatic fever because it:
1 Prevents infection
2 Cures the disease

3 Suppresses inflammation
4 Takes the place of antibiotic prophylaxis

68. An infant can be expected to triple his or her birth weight at _____ months of age.

69. An individual with a seizure disorder is being evaluated in the primary care center. Appropriate assessment data would include questioning the patient regarding:
1 Events that occurred before or after the seizure
2 Diet and exercise history
3 Social and educational levels
4 Work history

70. A priority teaching strategy for the nurse to include for the individual diagnosed with epilepsy is to:
1 Control seizure activity and prevent injury
2 Wear a Medic-Alert bracelet, and avoid situations known to trigger seizures
3 Follow up with the primary care physician on an annual basis
4 Refrain from going into crowded areas

71. The nurse is admitting a patient who is delusional and knows a priority nursing measure should be to:
1 Encourage the patient to talk about the delusions
2 Explain the delusion to the patient
3 Place the patient in seclusion
4 Explain to the patient that he is wrong and the delusion is not real

72. A nurse has just received a laboratory report on a patient with a bipolar disorder. The patient's lithium level is 1.9 mEq/L. What should the nurse do first?
1 Administer the next dose of lithium
2 Hold the lithium and call the physician
3 Double the lithium dose
4 Hold the lithium and administer Xanax

73. A nurse is caring for a patient who is receiving total parenteral nutrition (TPN). Appropriate nursing interventions for this patient include:
1 Weigh daily, monitor blood glucose levels, and wean from TPN gradually
2 Assess for degree of hunger every shift
3 Monitor liver function, renal function, and cardiovascular function
4 Weigh every week, monitor for glycosuria, and discontinue TPN on the third day

74. A nurse is preparing a patient for discharge. Because the patient is on a monoamine oxidase inhibitor (MAOI), the nurse will emphasize which of the following instructions?
1 "Avoid aged cheeses."
2 "Take the medication with food."
3 "Take the medication at bedtime."
4 "Limit caffeine intake."

75. A patient with a personality disorder is brought to the outpatient clinic by her mother, who states her daughter is out of control. The nurse should begin to foster trust with the patient by:
1 Telling her that she is available regardless of the patient's behavior
2 Telling her that she cares about her but may not always approve of the patient's behavior
3 Avoiding the establishment of trust because the relationship will eventually be terminated
4 Letting the patient know that she can call the nurse day or night

76. The patient tells the nurse to leave her alone; she says, "I'm no good to anyone. Why don't you attend to someone else?" Which response by the nurse would be the most therapeutic?
    1 "I will stay with you for 15 minutes."
    2 "I am responsible for you, so I will stay with you."
    3 "You are a good person."
    4 "Why do you say you are no good to anyone?"

77. A 12-year-old patient presents to the emergency department with a dislocated shoulder following a playground accident. The physician orders midazolam (Versed), 0.5 mg IV, before reducing the shoulder. Which of the following nursing diagnoses is appropriate for this patient?
    1 Risk for ineffective breathing patterns
    2 The patient will have a normal respiratory pattern
    3 Position head to allow for maximum ventilation
    4 Stable respiratory pattern

78. During the termination phase of the nurse-patient relationship, the patient abruptly gets up and leaves. The most appropriate nursing action should be to:
    1 Go after the patient and bring him back
    2 Remain at the interaction site until the end of the contracted time
    3 Resume the patient's regularly scheduled activities
    4 Speak with the head nurse about assigning another nurse to the patient

79. The patient was admitted 3 days ago for depression and attempted suicide. Her depression seems to have lifted. The nurse knows that this means her risk for suicide:
    1 Is less than it was when she was severely depressed
    2 Is more than it was when she was severely depressed
    3 Does not exist anymore because she is no longer depressed
    4 Needs to be reevaluated

80. The average 2- to 3-month-old infant:
    1 Babbles
    2 Has a crude pincer grasp
    3 Has a closed posterior fontanel
    4 Has one lower incisor

81. A patient's injuries sustained in a car accident have resulted in cerebral edema. Which of the following positions is the most appropriate for this patient?
    1 Supine
    2 Prone
    3 Low- to mid-Fowler's
    4 Mid- to high-Fowler's

82. Following a myocardial infarction, a patient receives warfarin (Coumadin). Which of the following symptoms would alert the nurse to a possible adverse effect to the Coumadin?
    1 Vomiting
    2 Epistaxis
    3 Back pain
    4 Blurred vision

83. A 72-year-old patient is taking diuretics for congestive heart failure. As part of his home care directions, the nurse should instruct him to weigh himself:
    1 Each morning on arising
    2 1 hour after taking his medication
    3 If he notices an increase in pedal edema
    4 Whenever he develops shortness of breath

84. Which instruction is most appropriate for a patient with chronic obstructive pulmonary disease (COPD) who has copious bronchial secretions?
    1 "Decrease your fluid intake to solidify bronchial secretions."
    2 "Tracheal suctioning is the best method for removing heavy secretions."
    3 "Try to drink several glasses of juice or water daily to loosen secretions."
    4 "You'll find it easier to breathe if you sit up straight during postural drainage treatments."

85. A patient, diagnosed with a seizure disorder, is being treated with phenytoin (Dilantin) and valproic acid (Depakene). Which of the following statements should the nurse consider the priority teaching need for this patient?
    1 Must use good oral hygiene
    2 Must increase intake of green, leafy vegetables
    3 Must carry a padded tongue blade at all times
    4 Must sleep 6 to 8 hours each night

86. A patient is being transferred to the unit where he is to be observed following a 2-day stay in coronary care for a possible myocardial infarction. The patient is receiving several medications and is complaining of a headache. Which of the following medications taken by the patient commonly causes the side effect of headache?
    1 Tylenol
    2 Lanoxin
    3 Nitroglycerin
    4 Potassium chloride

87. Following a thoracentesis, the patient is monitored closely for which of the following?
    1 Increased respiratory rate, chest tightness, hypoxemia
    2 Decreased respiratory rate, low blood pressure, decreased pulse rate
    3 Bradycardia, dry hacking cough, hypotension
    4 Normal sinus rhythm, normotension, ventilation

88. A concern for a patient having experienced a recent myocardial infarction is the development of cardiogenic shock. Which of the following are signs of cardiogenic shock?
    1 Bounding pulses, clammy skin, fever
    2 Hypotension, weak pulses, clammy skin
    3 Hypertension, shallow respirations, chest pain
    4 Hot, dry skin, rapid respirations, mental confusion

89. A nurse happens on the scene of an accident and finds a man lying on the ground with his eyes closed. The nurse's first action should be to:
    1 Notify emergency personnel
    2 Open the airway with the head tilt–chin lift maneuver
    3 Attempt to arouse the person
    4 Start cardiopulmonary resuscitation (CPR)

90. A 36-year-old woman has been experiencing intermittent episodes of mild chest pain and shortness of breath, particularly with exertion but also at rest. The physician wants to assess if the symptoms are aggravated or precipitated by activity. The nurse will anticipate counseling the patient in the use of:
    1 A glucometer
    2 Urine collection equipment
    3 A Holter monitor
    4 A Doppler flow study

91. A patient sustained an injury to his spinal cord to the C5 level. Based on a spinal cord injury at this level, the would most likely expect the patient to have loss of:
    1 Emotions
    2 Movement of all extremities
    3 Sexual desires
    4 Speaking ability

92. A child with *Haemophilus influenzae* type B meningitis is usually treated with IV fluids, antibiotics, and:
    1 IV dexamethasone
    2 Intramuscular (IM) ribavirin
    3 Oral (PO) Benadryl
    4 IV Lasix

93. In planning care for a patient with arteriosclerosis obliterans, the nurse would consider which of the following?
    1 Direct application of heat to improve circulation to the affected area
    2 Giving instructions in avoiding injury and maintaining circulation
    3 Elevating the foot of the bed to increase arterial circulation
    4 Massaging the extremities several times a day to improve circulation

94. A competitive racer had a near-drowning accident when the canoe she was paddling tipped over and struck her on the head. Her lips and nails are cyanotic. Immediate emergency care for this patient's hypoxia includes:
    1 Inserting chest tubes to drain the water
    2 Cricothyroid puncture to ensure a patent airway
    3 Placing her in Trendelenburg position to facilitate fluid drainage
    4 Bag-valve-mask resuscitation

95. In a patient with chronic bronchitis, for which of the following early signs of hypoxemia should the nurse watch?
    1 Dyspnea, hypotension, bradycardia
    2 Bradycardia, wheezing, confusion
    3 Capillary refill greater that 3 seconds, shortness of breath, confusion
    4 Restlessness, tachycardia, yawning

96. The nurse needs to obtain a sterile urine specimen for culture and sensitivity. The best way to obtain this specimen in a patient with an indwelling Foley catheter is to:
    1 Disconnect the catheter from the drainage tubing and let the urine drip into a sterile bottle
    2 Use a needle and syringe to withdraw urine from the tubing port and inject the specimen into a sterile tube
    3 Place a towel under the bag and open the drainage valve at the bottom of the drainage bag
    4 Remove the old Foley and recatheterize with a straight catheter

97. The patient is to receive acetyl salicylic acid (ASA) 600 mg. The label reads, "gr V." How many tablets should be given? _____ tablets

98. The patient's wife is concerned because her husband, who suffered a CVA 3 days ago, laughs and cries inappropriately. The nurse's best reply is:
    1 "This is a normal healing sign for someone who has had a stroke."
    2 "I would ignore him when he starts acting like that."

3 "He has what is call 'emotional lability,' which may occur after a stroke."
    4 "Men your husband's age like to tease us by acting this way."

99. A patient who grows her own fruits and vegetables is concerned that her urine, which is red in color, indicates that she is bleeding. The most appropriate response from the nurse is:
    1 "You must increase your milk intake to about 8 to 10 glasses a day."
    2 "This is nothing to be concerned about. Let me know if it is still happening next week."
    3 "Tell me, do you feel any pain or pass flatus when you urinate?"
    4 "Tell me, what types of vegetables and fruits have you been eating?"

100. A nurse instructs a nursing assistant not to fully bathe a resident with extremely dry skin every day. Which of the following is the best reason why older adults do not need to have a complete bath every day?
    1 Body odor is diminished
    2 Activity level is decreased
    3 Interest in hygiene is diminished
    4 Sweat and oil glands are less active

101. A patient entered the clinic with symptoms of nervousness and weight loss. A tentative diagnosis of hyperthyroidism was made. Which of the following additional assessment data would support the diagnosis?
    1 Constipation, depression, brittle hair
    2 Increased sweating, hand tremors, palpitations
    3 Urinary frequency, blurred vision, frequent infections
    4 Dry skin, intolerance to cold, slowed response time

102. A patient has a radioactive device implanted to treat carcinoma of the bladder. Of the following approaches, which would best address the safety of the nurse in performing daily care?
    1 Perform nursing measures as quickly and completely as possible
    2 Enter the patient's room frequently to assess the implanted device
    3 Perform skills slowly to facilitate discussion of the patient's disease
    4 Spend as much time with the patient as possible to decrease feelings of loneliness in the patient

103. The nurse is to administer eye medications for a group of six patients, all of whom have glaucoma and are receiving cholinergic agents (miotics) such as pilocarpine (salagen). The nurse knows that these medications must be given as ordered, which is based on the understanding that:
    1 Giving medications on time is part of the nurse's job
    2 These medications keep the pupil constricted to permit better aqueous humor drainage
    3 Glaucoma is a leading cause of blindness
    4 The patient will experience severe eye pain if a dose is late

104. While bathing a patient, the nurse notices a reddened area on the right hip. The appropriate nursing action is to:
    1 Massage the area every 2 hours and keep him off his right side
    2 Clean with alcohol and apply a sterile dressing
    3 Apply warm, moist compresses intermittently
    4 Apply lotion and powder before turning him on his right side

105. Which of the following foods should be suggested to combat constipation in older adults?
    1 Fruit juices and dairy products
    2 Meats, cheeses, and poultry products
    3 Processed carbohydrates and milk products
    4 Whole-grain cereals, fresh vegetables, and water

106. The presence of human immunodeficiency virus (HIV) infection is increasing. Which of the following measures is essential for the nurse to incorporate into care?
    1 Ask the patient his or her HIV status
    2 Have an HIV-positive health care worker care for the patient
    3 Adhere strictly to Standard Precautions
    4 Observe Standard Precautions only if exposure to blood or body fluids is obvious

107. Rheumatic fever is caused by:
    1 A fungus
    2 Staphylococcus bacteria
    3 A virus
    4 Streptococcus bacteria

108. A 42-year-old man has ingested 18 Valium (diazepam) tablets and 18 unidentified capsules. He is in the emergency department and is now alert after gastric lavage. He is calling his son to come and take him home. He is exhibiting which of the following defenses:
    1 Sublimation
    2 Projection
    3 Denial
    4 Regression

109. A 78-year-old man is returning home with his daughter. The daughter is concerned that her home is not safe for her father. Which of the following may indicate a possible safety hazard?
    1 Electric stoves
    2 Hardwood floors
    3 Nonglare lighting
    4 Elevated toilet seats

110. Which of the following is a reason that adverse drug reactions occur in the older adult?
    1 Older adults excrete drugs more effectively
    2 Older adults have a higher percentage of muscle tissue
    3 Older adults have altered drug distribution caused by circulatory changes
    4 Increased gastric motility causes changes in the absorption of drugs

111. A patient who has been receiving antipsychotic drugs reports that he has a dry mouth, tight throat, and mouth movements. The nurse should consider that:
    1 These may be somatic delusions
    2 The patient is probably manipulating for more medication
    3 These are transitory reactions that will disappear
    4 These may be extrapyramidal reactions that require intervention

112. A 21-year-old unconscious man is brought to the emergency department by a friend. His breath smells of alcohol, and the friend reports that they were at a fraternity party where everyone was drinking quite heavily. The nurse should:
    1 Treat the patient for shock
    2 Ensure adequate airway and ventilation
    3 Recommend rest in a quiet environment
    4 Administer disulfiram (Antabuse) immediately

113. Which of the following nursing interventions would be appropriate when giving an older adult oral medications?
    1 Elevate head of bed 15 degrees
    2 Give fluids before and after medications
    3 Give all medications at one time to enhance absorption
    4 Crush the medications and mix them with the patient's food

114. An 80-year-old patient asks the nurse what is included in an advance directive. Which of the following contains accurate information concerning advanced directives?
    1 Guardianships and living wills
    2 Organ procurement and donation
    3 Living wills and health care proxies
    4 Active and passive acts of euthanasia

115. CPR recommendations for calling for help suggest "phone first" for an adult and "phone fast" for a child. The best explanation for this rule is:
    1 Children can go longer without oxygen
    2 An arrest in a child is usually caused by an obstructed airway
    3 An arrest in an adult is usually caused by cardiac arrhythmias
    4 It is usually too late by the time the first responder finds an adult

116. An 18-month-old infant is to have a long-acting antibiotic given IM. The nurse selects the best muscle or site to use, which is:
    1 Deltoid
    2 Gluteus maximus
    3 Vastus lateralis
    4 Ventrogluteal area

117. Which of the following eye conditions is the most common reason for blindness in the older adult?
    1 Glaucoma
    2 Cataracts
    3 Presbyopia
    4 Macular degeneration

118. The nurse should anticipate that a patient with early Alzheimer's disease would have difficulty:
    1 Remembering how to operate an automobile
    2 Remembering that she has put a meal in the oven
    3 Remembering where she put the house keys the evening before
    4 Recalling a telephone conversation right after hanging up the telephone

119. A patient has sustained burns on the front and back of both her legs and her right arm. What percentage of her body would the nurse estimate is involved?
    1 45%
    2 54%
    3 72%
    4 18%

120. The normal inflammatory response is not always a reliable indicator of disease in the older adult because:
    1 Aging changes heighten the older adult's pain perception
    2 Cardiovascular changes heighten the erythema that develops around infection sites

3 Changes in the hypothalamus diminish the ability of the older adult to produce a fever

4 Changes in the hypothalamus grossly elevate temperature changes in the older adult

121. Within the first few hours after treating a severe burn patient, the nurse should observe for which of the following?

1 Laryngeal and tracheal edema

2 Eschar formation

3 Absence of pain

4 Leathery appearance to skin

122. The nurse is the first to arrive on the scene of a motorcycle accident and observes that the bone is protruding through the skin of the victim's leg. The nurse's *first* action would be to:

1 Apply a splint to the victim's leg

2 Apply antibiotic ointment to the skin

3 Cover the area with a dressing

4 Push the bone back through the skin

123. A confused, demented patient should bring personal items along to a long-term care facility. The purpose of doing this is to:

1 Increase attention span

2 Decrease dementia behaviors

3 Facilitate short-term memory

4 Foster recognition in the environment

124. A patient complains of tenderness at her IV puncture site. On assessment, the nurse notes redness and swelling. The nurse should first:

1 Stop the flow of the IV fluids, and report this to the head nurse

2 Notify the physician, and fill out an incident report

3 Elevate the arm, and apply warm compresses to the puncture site

4 Change the dressing over the puncture site using sterile technique

125. While the nurse's 14-year-old neighbor boy is mowing her lawn, he is stung by a bee. He starts wheezing and complaining of difficulty breathing. The nurse takes him to the emergency room where he is diagnosed as having:

1 Anaphylaxis

2 Asthma

3 Hay fever

4 Pneumonia

Part 2

This examination contains individual questions, the majority of which relate to clinical situations. Read all questions carefully. Each question has only *one best answer*.

Test time allotment (Part 2): approximately 2 hours

Answers and Rationales begin on p. 624.

1. A patient who has had frequent bouts of pneumonia spends most of her time in bed, insisting that the head of the bed remain at 90 degrees. Because she has reddened areas on her coccyx, the nurse teaches her that:
   1 She needs to stay off her back for the next 24 hours
   2 The head of the bed should be kept at 15 to 30 degrees
   3 She keeps getting pneumonia because of the moisture that forms on her skin
   4 Her buttocks hurt because the skin over the bones is dying

2. The nurse has taught the elderly patient with type 2 diabetes mellitus the importance of maintaining good glucose control. The nurse knows learning has occurred when the patient states:
   1 "My fasting blood sugar should be 100 to 140 mg/dl and between 120 and 180 mg/dl after eating."
   2 "My fasting blood sugar should be 180 to 240 mg/dl and between 250 and 300 mg/dl after eating."
   3 "My fasting blood sugar should be between 75 and 100 mg/dl and 150 and 275 mg/dl after eating."
   4 "My fasting blood sugar should be between 225 and 275 mg/dl and 276 and 375 mg/dl after eating."

3. Symptoms of hypertension are vague and subtle. When assessing hypertensive patients, the nurse may observe symptoms of:
   1 Nausea, vomiting, nosebleeds
   2 Increased urination, fatigue, blurred vision
   3 Chest pain, shortness of breath, nervousness
   4 Blurred vision, irritability, occipital headaches

4. A patient who has had lung surgery is having difficulty doing deep-breathing and productive-coughing exercises, even with the use of an incentive spirometer. Nursing notes indicate that the patient's cough is weak and dry and that he tires easily. The most appropriate plan of action the nurse should consider is to:
   1 Encourage the patient to drink 8 to 10 glasses of water a day
   2 Ask the physician for as needed (PRN) throat lozenges and cough demulcent orders
   3 Report to the physician and ask if aerosol treatments may help
   4 Increase the room temperature to 70° F and humidity to 70%

5. Digoxin, a water-soluble drug, should be administered cautiously in the older adult for which of the following reasons?
   1 Digoxin is distributed in larger compartments in older adults
   2 Digoxin is less likely to accumulate to toxic levels
   3 Digoxin dosing is the same in the older adult as it is in the younger adult
   4 Digoxin is distributed in smaller compartments in older adults

6. A patient is admitted with a diagnosis of mitral stenosis or mitral insufficiency. Which of the following symptoms would be found in either of these conditions?
   1 Angina
   2 Murmur
   3 Syncope
   4 High blood pressure

7. A patient's sputum has suddenly become pink and frothy. The nurse has gathered the following data during her assessment. Which of the data is significant and needs to be reported and documented?
   1 Decreased appetite
   2 Respirations 16, regular, easy
   3 Complaints of dull headache
   4 Coughing when supine

8. Uncontrolled hypertension over time can affect the heart, brain, kidneys, and eyes. The patient wants the nurse to tell him the name of the recommended annual eye examination he is to have. The best response by the nurse would be to explain the examination called a:
   1 Vision screen
   2 Tonometer test
   3 Funduscopic examination
   4 Visual fields examination

9. When performing external cardiac compression, the victim must be positioned on a firm surface because:
   1 This position enables the rescuer to deliver more compressions
   2 The heart is compressed between sternum and spine
   3 The risk of breaking the xyphoid process is reduced
   4 Palpation of landmarks is easier

10. A patient confides to a nurse that she is desperate to lose 10 pounds before going to her class reunion in 2 weeks. She tells the nurse she plans to eat strictly fruits and drink a lot of water. The most appropriate response by the nurse should be:
    1 "All nutrients are needed in a healthy diet."
    2 "It is all right for a short period, but be sure to take plenty of vitamins."
    3 "The fruit will supply you with energy, and the water will help circulation."
    4 "Eat a variety of foods from all levels of the food guide pyramid and increase exercise."

11. The nutritional requirements of older adults differ from those of younger people. In particular, they will require:
    1 Increased fats
    2 Fewer calories
    3 Decreased fluid intake
    4 Fewer vitamins and minerals

12. A 75-year-old patient is recovering from a right total hip replacement. The nurse has identified a diagnosis of impaired physical mobility related to decreased muscle strength and should plan to:
    1 Keep the right leg in extension and abduction
    2 Provide passive range of motion (ROM) to the right ankle
    3 Provide active ROM to the right ankle
    4 Encourage quadriceps-setting exercises

13. A patient is known to be lactose intolerant. When discussing dietary adjustments with the patient, the nurse advises her to avoid which of the following?
    1 Citrus fruits
    2 Highly seasoned foods
    3 Milk and milk products
    4 Foods containing seeds and nuts

14. When cleansing an open wound, the nurse should:
   1 Apply constant pressure
   2 Forcefully irrigate all wound areas
   3 Scrub encrusted areas thoroughly
   4 Work from cleanest to dirtiest areas

15. The nurse established a nursing diagnosis of fluid volume excess related to decreased glomerular filtration caused by acute glomerulonephritis. Clinical data that support this nursing diagnosis include which of the following?
   1 Fever
   2 Thirst
   3 Polyuria
   4 Periorbital edema

16. A patient, receiving an initial dose of IV ampicillin, begins complaining of itching after infusion of the drug. The nurse notes that her back and abdomen are covered by red wheals. The nurse's next course of action is to:
   1 Discontinue the IV immediately and notify the physician
   2 Discontinue the IV and set up for a restart in the opposite arm
   3 Discontinue the piggyback unit, restart original fluid, and notify the physician
   4 Reassure her regarding this normal reaction and apply ointment to the rash

17. A patient has undergone complicated abdominal surgery and is now receiving TPN via a central venous catheter. During the morning bath, the patient suddenly becomes dyspneic, anxious, and cyanotic. The nurse finds that the TPN is disconnected from the central line. The nurse should first:
   1 Initiate the hospital's protocol for respiratory emergency
   2 Reconnect the TPN ports after swabbing them with alcohol
   3 Place the patient on his left side with his head below chest level
   4 Place the patient in high-Fowler's position to assist respiratory efforts

18. When preparing to administer oxygen via nasal cannula, the nurse attaches the oxygen flowmeter to a container of sterile distilled water to:
   1 Decrease the danger of oxygen combustion
   2 Increase the patient's level of oxygen absorption
   3 Remove any particle contaminants from the tubing
   4 Prevent drying the patient's nasooropharyngeal mucosa

19. The best criteria for evaluating the care given based on the nursing diagnosis of altered nutrition: less than body requirements related to anorexia, nausea, and vomiting includes which of the following?
   1 Moist mucous membranes
   2 Absence of diarrhea
   3 Stable body weight
   4 Normal body temperature

20. When preparing a feeding pump for a patient's tube feeding, the nurse knows that the pump should be filled with:
   1 The full day's supply of formula
   2 One full can of formula each time
   3 8 hours' worth of feeding each time
   4 No more than a 2-hour supply each time

21. Which of the following is a critical nursing measure when caring for patients undergoing nasogastric suctioning?
   1 Mouth care every 2 hours
   2 Thorough skin care to the nares
   3 Turn and position every 2 hours
   4 Maintain accurate intake and output record

22. A patient has been taking a diuretic for the last 3 months. Of the following statements made by the patient, which would alert the nurse to a possible dietary deficiency caused by the diuretic?
   1 "I seem to bruise so easily these days."
   2 "My eyes seem especially sensitive to light."
   3 "Every once in a while, my heart feels like it's skipping beats."
   4 "I feel so terribly nervous. Do you think I need a tranquilizer?"

23. The physician has determined that a patient has increased intracranial pressure. The nurse will position her in which of the following positions?
   1 Elevation of the head of the bed to 20 degrees
   2 Elevation of the head of the bed to 30 degrees
   3 Elevation of the head of the bed to 60 degrees
   4 Elevation of the head of the bed to 90 degrees

24. An 84-year old woman is in the health care provider's office complaining of fatigue, anorexia, and indigestion. Which of the following groups of vitamins might be prescribed if the health care provider suspects a deficiency?
   1 C and B_{12}
   2 B_6 and B_{12}
   3 A, D, and E
   4 C and B complex

25. When monitoring a patient receiving IV therapy, which of the following observations may indicate infiltration?
   1 Poor skin turgor
   2 Redness at insertion site
   3 Warmth at insertion site
   4 Swollen area above the catheter

26. According to the history of maternity care in the United States, the single greatest deterrent to maternal complications, particularly pregnancy-induced hypertension (PIH), has been:
   1 Discovery and use of antihypertensive drugs
   2 Good prenatal care
   3 A salt-free diet
   4 The age of the mother

27. A patient is concerned with edema that develops in her feet throughout the day. Which of the following food choices made by the individual can contribute to the edema formation?
   1 Eggs and toast
   2 Tuna fish and cantaloupe
   3 Hamburger and French fries
   4 Salami sandwich and potato chips

28. The nurse is gathering data related to the growth and development of a 3-week-old infant. The nurse should expect to observe which of the following behaviors in the infant?
   1 Moro "startle" reflex
   2 Cooing and babbling
   3 Recognizing a familiar face
   4 Holding head erect

29. A patient in her sixth month of pregnancy is complaining of insomnia. The intervention that the nurse might suggest includes:
   1 Keeping legs uncrossed
   2 Elevate hips
   3 Warm milk at bedtime
   4 A balanced diet

30. A patient with cancer is experiencing anorexia. Which of the following recommendations made by the nurse should assist the client in increasing oral intake?
   1 "Try to eat three large meals every day."
   2 "Take pain medication after your meals."
   3 "Try to supplement your meals with nutritious milk-shakes."
   4 "Eat as many fruits and vegetables as you can instead of protein foods."

31. A prenatal patient is complaining of low back pains. The clinic nurse might suggest which of the following for some relief of the discomfort the patient is experiencing?
   1 Sitz baths
   2 Heating pads to the back
   3 Pelvic rock-tilt exercise
   4 Visits to the chiropractor

32. Which of the following is the most appropriate nursing action when caring for a patient with meningitis?
   1 Strict isolation precautions
   2 Judicious hand washing
   3 Wound precautions
   4 Respiratory precautions

33. Which of the following assessments would be of most concern to the nurse during examination of a 2-week-old newborn?
   1 The Babinski reflex is present
   2 A cephalhematoma is present
   3 A small red pin dot present in the white of the sclera
   4 The infant is waking up twice during the night

34. The nurse should explain to the patient that the contraction stress test (CST) is an invasive test because medication is given in the veins and it:
   1 Is uncomfortable for a short while
   2 Is not painful at all
   3 Will take a few minutes to complete
   4 Is a routine procedure for all pregnant women

35. When discussing nutrition with a patient who is a 3-month pregnant gravida 1, para 0, the nurse explains that the most important consideration in her prenatal diet is to provide:
   1 An adequate diet to ensure optimum nutrition for mother and fetus
   2 A low-calorie diet to maintain the mother's weight
   3 Limited fluid intake to prevent edema in the body tissues of both the mother and the fetus
   4 A diet high in protein for nourishment of the fetus

36. Because of her history of diabetes, a patient is classified as a high-risk pregnancy. The health care provider knows that her prenatal visits will be scheduled approximately as follows:
   1 Two times a month for the first 28 weeks
   2 Every 2 weeks after the thirty-eighth week
   3 Every week from the thirty-sixth week and thereafter
   4 Scheduled on a week-to-week basis

37. A patient who drinks alcohol while taking chlorpropamide (Diabinese) can expect what specific type of reaction?
   1 Disulfiram (Antabuse)-type reaction
   2 Anaphylactic reaction
   3 Reverse reaction
   4 Antigen-antibody reaction

38. A gravida 2, para 1 goes into labor at 24 weeks and gives birth prematurely. Physically, the infant's appearance would most closely resemble which of the following descriptions?
   1 12 inches long, 1-$\frac{1}{2}$ pounds, and covered with vernix caseosa
   2 19 inches long, 7 pounds, and small amount of vernix caseosa
   3 7 inches long, 6 ounces, and covered with lanugo
   4 10 inches long, 1 pound, and covered with vernix caseosa

39. The nurse in a local nursing home assigns a nursing assistant to an 87-year-old resident. The nurse will instruct the certified nursing assistant to help the resident with his total bath:
   1 Three times a week and to bathe with tepid water
   2 Once a week and to bathe with hot water
   3 Every other week and to bathe with tepid water
   4 Every other day and to bathe with cold water

40. A charge nurse has the following tasks to perform at 9:00 AM: monitor vital signs on two residents, administer medications for four residents, attend an interdisciplinary care team meeting, and document on four residents. Which of the previous tasks would be most appropriate to assign to a nursing assistant?
   1 The documentation
   2 Administering medications
   3 Monitoring the vital signs
   4 Attending the care planning meeting

41. The physician prescribes oral acyclovir (Zovirax) for a patient with genital herpes lesions. The nurse should include which of the following statements when teaching the patient about this medication?
   1 "Once the lesions disappear, you will be cured of genital herpes."
   2 "You may stop taking this drug once the pain and itching subside."
   3 "You should drink at least 3 quarts of water every day while you are taking this medication."
   4 "As long as you are taking the medication, your sexual partner will be protected from contracting the virus."

42. Which of the following nursing interventions should be the priority after a fall has occurred?
   1 Move the patient to a bed or stretcher
   2 Check the extremities for symmetry and alignment
   3 Assess for skin intactness and any bruises or swelling
   4 Assess the patient's airway and any difficulty breathing

43. The physician prescribes propranolol (Inderal), a nonselective beta-adrenergic blocking agent, to treat a patient's hypertension. The nurse should monitor the patient for which side effect?
   1 Nervousness
   2 Photophobia
   3 Tachycardia
   4 Dyspnea

44. A patient states that he has difficulty climbing stairs. Which of the following would be the best way for the nurse to validate this claim?
    1 Ask a family member if it is true
    2 Watch the patient as he climbs the stairs
    3 Ask for a physical therapy referral for the patient
    4 Ask the patient what happens when he climbs the stairs

45. In caring for an unconscious victim who is suspected of having an airway obstruction, the nurse should take which of the following actions first?
    1 Immediately start CPR
    2 Open the airway using the head tilt–chin lift maneuver
    3 Place victim in supine position on a firm, flat surface
    4 Remove any foreign object obstructing the airway

46. A licensed practical nurse is assisting a registered nurse in counseling an older couple concerning finances and long-term care. The couple indicates that they thought that Medicare would cover nursing homes. The nurse advises the couple that:
    1 Medicare should cover all of the expenses of long-term care
    2 Medicare covers only 1 or 2 years of long-term care expenses
    3 Social Security will cover the expenses incurred during nursing home stays
    4 Medicare covers the majority of the expenses incurred in nursing home care

47. To best assist a patient who has been on bed rest to prepare for ambulation, the nurse should:
    1 Dangle the patient's legs and swing them back and forth daily
    2 Have him push his popliteal space against the bed to the count of five, several times daily
    3 Perform passive ROM exercises three times daily
    4 Have him perform push-ups and use the bed trapeze bar as much as possible

48. A conscious person with diabetes arrives at the emergency room with blood glucose of 378 mg/dl. The treatment of choice is to:
    1 Administer regular insulin
    2 Administer 50% glucose IV
    3 Initiate a dextrose IV infusion
    4 Monitor the potassium level

49. When a patient in diabetic ketoacidosis comes to the emergency room, blood electrolyte levels should be monitored. The nurse is aware that the most important electrolyte to monitor in this patient is:
    1 Calcium
    2 Chloride
    3 Potassium
    4 Sodium

50. Which of the following would be a priority nursing concern for a victim with severe burns?
    1 Administering CPR
    2 Relieving pain
    3 Stopping the burning process
    4 Tetanus prophylaxis

51. A 36-year-old woman has had a total hip replacement. The postoperative orders include aspirin, 5 grains (325 mg), PO, daily. The nurse is aware that the rationale for this treatment is to:
    1 Prevent joint inflammation
    2 Produce a mild anticoagulant effect
    3 Provide better pain control
    4 Maintain normal body temperature

52. The nurse is caring for a rape trauma survivor. The initial assessment indicates that the patient appears calm and very much in control. Which characteristic psychological reaction best describes the patient's behavior?
    1 Denial
    2 Disorganization
    3 Hyperalertness
    4 Reorganization

53. When performing passive ROM for a patient, the nurse should:
    1 Exercise the joint just past the point of stiffness to gradually increase joint motion
    2 Perform no more than five repetitions for each exercise to avoid tiring the patient
    3 Watch the patient's nonverbal communication to help evaluate the response to the exercise
    4 Vary the order in which the exercises are performed so that the patient does not become bored

54. A patient is in the clinic waiting room awaiting results of the biopsy of his prostate gland. He is laughing and cracking jokes. The nurse should:
    1 Ask the patient to be quiet
    2 Recognize the patient is manifesting anxiety
    3 Ignore the patient's behavior
    4 Overlook the patient's different behavior

55. A patient is admitted for possible obstructive urinary retention caused by an enlarged prostate gland. During the assessment the nurse would expect the patient to complain of:
    1 Hematuria
    2 Hesitancy in initiating voiding
    3 Burning on urination
    4 Nausea

56. The nurse is caring for a patient with bipolar disorder who is currently in the manic phase and is trying to get the patient involved in a diversional activity. Which of the following would be the most appropriate activity?
    1 Bridge
    2 Jigsaw puzzle
    3 Ping-pong
    4 Exercise class

57. When receiving physician's orders by telephone, the nurse must:
    1 Repeat the orders, then write the orders on the physician's order sheet
    2 Write the physician's name on the order sheet
    3 Write the patient's name, next of kin, and date on the order sheet
    4 Write the order as the physician gives the order, and repeat the order back to the physician for immediate verification

58. The nurse is interacting with a patient with obsessive compulsive disorder. What statement by the patient may validate that certain activities help her to deal with her anxiety?
    1 "I worry about dirt and germs, and I clean a lot."
    2 "I worry about the health of my aging parents."
    3 "I have a stupid problem, don't I?"
    4 "I am willing to take medication if necessary."

59. When caring for a patient with COPD, the nurse notes that the patient is more comfortable after:
    1 Being placed in low-Fowler's position
    2 Having postural drainage
    3 Fluids are restricted
    4 He has provided all his own care

60. A nurse is caring for a patient taking haloperidol (Haldol). What is a common side effect the nurse should observe for in this patient?
    1 Sedation
    2 Weight loss
    3 Dry mouth
    4 Anxiety

61. Frequent assessment of a patient with a fractured left leg would include maintaining proper alignment and:
    1 Checking sensation and circulation in the leg
    2 Increasing the weight of traction as necessary to maintain countertraction
    3 Taking the apical pulse every 2 hours
    4 Checking temperature and performing ROM in his right leg

62. A patient is admitted for possible obstructive urinary retention possibly because of an enlarged prostate gland. In planning his care, the nurse would expect him to have which of the following complaints?
    1 Dysuria
    2 Nocturia
    3 Increased thirst
    4 Diminished force of urinary stream

63. A nurse is assigned to administer medications to 20 patients. The gold standard for administering medications is to adhere to:
    1 The five rights of medication administration: right drug, dose, route, patient, time
    2 The six rights of medication administration: right drug, dose, route, patient, time, documentation
    3 The five rights of medication administration: right drug, hospital policy, dose, patient, route
    4 Computerized guidelines as defined by the pharmacist

64. A patient is hearing voices that are telling him to do harmful things to himself. Which of the following nursing diagnoses should be included on this patient's plan of care?
    1 Potential for violence
    2 Self-care deficit
    3 Sensory perception alteration
    4 Impaired communication

65. The nurse is gathering objective data about her patient who is experiencing "kidney problems." The nurse looks at the laboratory results, knowing that the glomerular filtration rate (GFR) can be measured by evaluating the:
    1 Hemoglobin
    2 Blood urea nitrogen
    3 White blood cells
    4 Creatinine clearance

66. An individual known to be taking lithium and currently under psychiatric care has taken cocaine. She telephones the hospital with abdominal cramps and extreme anxiety. The nurse's best response would be to:
    1 Have her come to the emergency room immediately
    2 Refer her to her psychiatrist
    3 Give her the cocaine hotline number
    4 Put her on hold and get another nurse to take the call

67. Autonomic hyperreflexia may occur after a spinal cord injury. Which of the following is the most common stimuli that can cause the manifestation of autonomic hyperreflexia?
    1 Visitors
    2 Full bladder
    3 Taking tympanic temperatures
    4 Taking an apical pulse

68. A patient has shallow respirations at 8 to 10 times per minute. This hypoventilation results in acidosis by:
    1 The retention of carbon dioxide (CO_2)
    2 Excreting needed CO_2
    3 Excreting oxygen (O_2)
    4 Retaining too much O_2

69. A 32-year-old patient is being admitted to the medical floor with a diagnosis of bronchiectasis. She has a chronic cough with expectoration of copious amounts of purulent sputum and hemoptysis. An appropriate outcome criteria is that:
    1 The patient will demonstrate improved ventilation and adequate oxygenation
    2 The nurse will encourage alternating rest and activity
    3 The patient may have activity intolerance related to fatigue
    4 The patient's arterial blood gases are improved

70. When two rescuers are performing CPR, the ratio of compressions to respirations is:
    1 15:2
    2 5:2
    3 15:1
    4 5:1

71. Assessment of motor function in a patient who has had a stroke includes assessing:
    1 Cranial nerves VIII through XII
    2 Body position, level of consciousness, and mental status
    3 Muscle movement, strength, and coordination
    4 Intellectual function and speech pattern

72. A patient with diabetes mellitus is going to engage in a strenuous activity. Which of the following snacks would the nurse suggest that the patient consume before engaging in the activity?
    1 An orange
    2 A candy bar
    3 A can of soda
    4 Cheese and crackers

73. A 60-year-old patient is being discharged after undergoing cardiac catheterization. Which of the following important instructions should the nurse include at the time of discharge?
    1 Do not change the bandage for 48 hours, and report site soreness to the physician
    2 Rest for 3 days and avoid heavy lifting or strenuous activity
    3 Take a tub bath after the puncture site is healed
    4 Drive a car that has an automatic transmission

74. A resident in long-term care has a diagnosis of elevated ammonia levels related to cirrhosis. Which of the following foods would the nurse advise the nursing assistant to eliminate as a possible snack for the resident?
    1 Pretzels
    2 Crackers and cheese
    3 Chicken salad sandwich
    4 A bowl of vanilla ice cream

75. A 72-year-old patient is admitted to the cardiac floor with a diagnosis of acute myocardial infarction. The most reliable blood test to detect damage of heart muscle is:
    1 Complete blood cell count
    2 Creatinine kinase myoglobin (CK-MB)
    3 Fibrin split products
    4 Lactic dehydrogenase (LDH)
76. In which of the following positions should a nurse assist the patient after a thyroidectomy?
    1 Supine
    2 Left Sims'
    3 Trendelenberg's
    4 Semi-Fowler's
77. A patient is 2 days post myocardial infarction. Which of the following data might suggest that the patient may be experiencing left-sided heart failure?
    1 Nausea
    2 Heart murmur
    3 Crackles in the lungs
    4 Edema in feet and legs
78. The nurse is aware that oral hypoglycemic agents may be used for patients with diabetes mellitus who have:
    1 Obesity
    2 Liver disease
    3 Type 1 diabetes
    4 Some insulin production
79. A new mother asks the nurse at what age is it best to hang a new, colorful mobile for her newborn baby boy. The nurse can answer that newborns can follow bright and colorful objects at:
    1 1 year of age
    2 First week of life
    3 9 to 10 months of life
    4 2 or 3 weeks of life
80. Patients with sensory dysfunction, such as persons with paraplegia, have many teaching needs. Which one of the following is a high-priority teaching need?
    1 Importance of doing 5-minute weight shifts every hour
    2 Importance of decreasing calcium intake
    3 Importance of avoiding cold or very hot foods
    4 Importance of adequate fluid intake of 2000 ml/day
81. In a patient receiving continuous bladder irrigations following a transurethral prostatectomy, the nurse assesses that the catheter may be blocked. The most appropriate instruction the nurse should give the patient is to:
    1 Try to void around the catheter
    2 Deep breath, cough, and remain still until the physician arrives
    3 Notify the nurse if he notices a change in the color of the drainage in the bag
    4 Increase fluid intake to 4000 ml/day
82. A patient receiving chlorpromazine (Thorazine) should be instructed to:
    1 Avoid certain foods containing tyramine
    2 Use a sunscreen when outdoors
    3 Take medication with milk
    4 Use prophylactic antacid
83. The nurse on the previous shift charted that the patient was drowsy. Which of the following behaviors would support this description of the patient's level of consciousness?
    1 Appropriate response when aroused
    2 Absence of response even to painful stimuli

3 Incomplete arousal to painful stimuli
4 Response to verbal command is inconsistent and vague
84. When preparing a patient for a bowel-retraining program, the nurse should understand that the most important factor for a successful retraining program is:
    1 Establishing regular day or days and time to assist the patient to the toilet
    2 Making sure the patient understands the purpose of the program
    3 Regular administration of a mild laxative
    4 Skipping a day in the program if the patient has had more than one bowel movement the day before
85. A patient is being observed for increased intracranial pressure. Which classification of medications, other than anticonvulsants and corticosteroids, would you expect to be ordered?
    1 Narcotic analgesics
    2 Antiemetics
    3 Osmotic diuretics
    4 Antibiotics
86. In a patient with head trauma being treated for increased intracranial pressure, which of the following would be least likely to cause complications?
    1 Isometric exercises
    2 Aerobic exercises
    3 Passive ROM exercises
    4 High-Fowler's position
87. Which of the following nursing actions is the most appropriate to stop the bleeding from an occipital laceration?
    1 Applying pressure to the site
    2 Applying ice to the site
    3 Elevating the head of the bed
    4 Elevating the extremities
88. A nurse is working in the newborn nursery when a baby that one of his colleagues is feeding begins to choke on the formula. Immediately, he assesses the situation and begins the procedure for obstructed airway on a conscious infant. To perform the procedure correctly, the nurse knows that he has to administer:
    1 Eight back blows and eight chest thrusts
    2 Six back blows and six chest thrusts
    3 Five back blows and five chest thrusts
    4 Four back blows and four chest thrusts
89. A patient is being instructed on post lumbar puncture care and is apprehensive about getting "sick with a terrible headache like her neighbor did when she had that test done." The nurse's most appropriate response is:
    1 "Moving about after the test is the best way to prevent a headache."
    2 "You will need to remain flat on your stomach after the test. This will prevent getting a headache."
    3 "You will be able to drink fluids after the test. This, as well as lying flat, helps most people."
    4 "With all the advances in medicine, these types of headaches are not common anymore."
90. Which one of the following special precautions will the nurse incorporate into the plan of care for an 82-year-old patient who has undergone an open reduction and internal fixation (ORIF) of the hip?
    1 Monitor for nutritional problems
    2 Maintain proper alignment of the extremity

3 Keep the side rails in an elevated position

4 Observe linen and dressings for drainage

91. Immediate physical observations of a burn patient would most importantly include:
1 Physical development
2 Head circumference
3 Height and weight
4 Quality of respirations

92. The nurse is determining an asthmatic patient's achievement of the goals for the nursing diagnosis: activity intolerance related to imbalance between oxygen supply and demand. Which of the following expected outcomes is appropriate?
1 No evidence of anxiety
2 Demonstrated knowledge of disease process
3 Able to perform activities of daily living
4 Clear breath sounds

93. During a major snowstorm, a 51-year-old man suffers from frostbite of both hands. Because continuous warm water soaks are not available, the nurse would:
1 Rub the hands with snow
2 Massage the hands vigorously
3 Do aggressive ROM to both hands
4 Apply a dry dressing with gauze between the fingers

94. The nurse's neighbor fell from a ladder and is complaining of pain in his right arm. The nurse notes deformity between the wrist and the elbow. The first action for the nurse would be to:
1 Check for a patent airway
2 Observe for bleeding from the site
3 Apply a split from the wrist to the elbow
4 Have him lie flat with his right arm elevated

95. A nurse witnesses a motorcycle accident in which the victim is thrown forcefully from the vehicle to the pavement. On initial assessment of the patient, the nurse notes a crack in the helmet. When administering care to this accident victim, which of the following should receive priority?
1 Maintaining an open airway
2 Maintaining normal body temperature
3 Minimizing movement of the individual's head
4 Monitoring pulse and respiratory rate every 15 minutes

96. A 70-year-old woman has been hospitalized several times in the last year with complications from chemotherapy for metastatic breast cancer. She is placed on an antidepressant medication the day of her discharge. Discharge teaching for the patient should include which of the following?
1 Fluids should be limited to three glasses a day while taking the antidepressant
2 Call the physician immediately if dry mouth or orthostatic hypotension occurs
3 3 or more (even up to 12) weeks may be required before symptoms improve
4 If this antidepressant fails to control depression, others would not be effective either

97. A patient who wears a hearing aid in her left ear has sensory perceptual alteration: auditory, related to decreased hearing secondary to cerumen buildup. The most appropriate plan is to encourage:
1 Chewing motions and daily washing of the external parts of the ears
2 Periodic ear washing in the clinic
3 Increasing fluid intake to 2000 ml/day
4 Cleaning the hearing aid with hydrogen peroxide

98. The nurse must recognize which of the following as a recommendation made by the U.S. Food and Drug Administration (FDA) and the Joint Commission on Accreditation of Healthcare Organizations (JCAHO) about restraints?
1 Restraints can be used indefinitely once the need for them has been documented
2 Alternatives to restraints should be developed and implemented before using restraints
3 Restraints should be removed every 4 hours to allow for activities of daily living
4 Restraints should be tied with a square knot to the immovable part of the bed

99. One important complication to avoid following a cesarean section is a pelvic thrombosis. The nursing care plan would therefore include:
1 Teaching good perineal care
2 Encouraging early ambulation
3 Splinting the lower abdomen when coughing
4 Keeping the urinary and bowel tracts emptied by forcing fluids and offering stool softeners

100. In planning preoperative care for a patient who is about to undergo a below-the-knee amputation, the nurse may focus on postoperative care by explaining:
1 Elements of the exercise program
2 Postoperative measures to control pain
3 Visiting hours immediately after surgery
4 Turning, coughing, and deep-breathing maneuvers

101. If the amniotic sac is to be ruptured by the physician, what is the priority nursing responsibility?
1 Time and check contractions afterward and report
2 Note time and instrument used and check fetal heart tone after the procedure
3 Note the amount and characteristics of fluid, test with Nitrazine, and report
4 Note the time and amount and place pad on perineum

102. A patient with diabetes is being treated for pneumonia. She received 22 units of regular insulin at 6:30 AM and was unable to eat her breakfast. The nurse should be alert for signs of:
1 Polydipsia
2 Somnolence
3 Diaphoresis
4 Increased urine output

103. A patient with a diagnosis of myocardial infarction has been admitted to the coronary care unit. The nurse assesses the patient's breath sounds and hears fine crackles in the lower lung bases. This symptom may indicate:
1 Pneumonia
2 Dysrhythmias
3 Lung congestion from heart failure
4 An extension of the myocardial infarction

104. A nurse who is observing a 2-day-old, full-term infant girl in the nursery notices that her hands and feet are cyanotic but that her body and cheeks are pink. She has passed greenish-black stool and has lost several ounces since birth. This baby is:
1 Premature
2 Immature
3 Normal
4 Slightly abnormal

105. A patient has chronic respiratory disease and is newly diagnosed with Alzheimer's disease. In planning his care, the nurse should prioritize his care as:
    1 Safety, physiological assessment, comfort
    2 Psychological care, personal integrity, comfort
    3 Safety, pain relief, cueing
    4 Physiological assessment, reorientation, cueing

106. A 9-year-old child was admitted to the hospital in sickle cell anemia crisis. Symptoms of sickle cell crisis include all of the following *except*:
    1 Severe abdominal pain
    2 Elevated temperature
    3 Joint pain
    4 Elevated hemoglobin

107. A patient has started receiving bronchodilators (theophylline). When checking for toxic and side effects, the nurse should observe for:
    1 Hypotension, abdominal cramping, diarrhea
    2 Urticaria, nausea and vomiting, dehydration
    3 Restlessness, tachycardia, insomnia
    4 Anorexia, blurred vision, cramps

108. While the nurse is visiting a patient's home, the wife of an elderly man with diabetes tells the nurse that he has been "crankier than usual" the last few days. He is also "moody and hungry as a horse." Which of the next following statements tells the nurse that she needs to check his blood sugar?
    1 He refuses to take a bath and stinks
    2 He has had a cough the last 3 or 4 days
    3 He had diarrhea once last week in the middle of the night
    4 He has been in the bathroom off and on all morning urinating

109. A patient is being evaluated because of complaints of cervical neck pain. As part of the evaluation, the intent is to rule out the possibility of a ruptured disk. Which of the following is a common symptom of cervical disk involvement?
    1 Stiff neck
    2 Difficulty walking
    3 Numbness of the lower extremities
    4 Atrophy of the gastrocnemius muscle group

110. A patient with a diagnosis of heart failure is being treated with furosemide (Lasix). The patient has begun to experience tinnitus. The nurse advises her that:
    1 She will not be able to drive
    2 The sounds she hears are normal
    3 This symptom is caused by nerve deafness
    4 This may be related to her diuretic medication

111. A patient with multiple sclerosis has a neurogenic bladder. When evaluating the patient's response to medical therapy, the nurse would expect which of the following medications to be therapeutic for this bladder condition?
    1 Oxybutynin (Ditropan)
    2 Bethanechol (Urecholine)
    3 Propantheline bromide (Pro-Banthine)
    4 Trimethoprim sulfamethoxazole (Bactrim, Septra)

112. An elderly patient who is going to have gastrointestinal testing done has hematuria. The nurse needs to take a complete medication history because this condition can be caused by:
    1 Diuretics
    2 Pyridium
    3 Macrodantin
    4 Anticoagulants

113. While sitting in the park in the middle of the afternoon, the nurse hears cries for help from a young mother. The infant is not breathing and has no pulse. To commence CPR, the nurse places two fingers:
    1 At the nipple level
    2 On the top half of the sternum
    3 One finger width below the nipple level
    4 Two finger widths above the xiphoid process

114. A patient is admitted with the diagnosis of ruptured appendix. The nurse is alert for the development of the complication of peritonitis. Which of the following assessment findings would support the diagnosis of peritonitis?
    1 Fever, nervousness
    2 Fever, reduced urine output
    3 Increased bowel motility accompanied by fever
    4 Abdominal muscular rigidity accompanied by fever

115. A retired schoolteacher whose husband is on a low-cholesterol diet following a heart attack says that she is totally confused about cholesterol and its importance in the diet. Of the following statements about cholesterol, which should the nurse know to be true?
    1 It is best to be totally eliminated from the diet
    2 It is a normal component of blood and all body cells
    3 It is not necessary for normal body functions
    4 It is found in increased amounts in grain products

116. When a patient returns from dialysis, the nurse notes that she is diaphoretic, restless, vomiting, and has tachycardia. Which of the following actions by the nurse is most appropriate initially?
    1 Apply a cool washcloth to the patient's forehead and monitor vital signs
    2 Encourage frequent sips of water and elevate foot of the bed
    3 Lower head or elevate foot of bed and turn the patient on her side
    4 Decrease the temperature in the room and turn the patient on her side

117. A 14-year-old girl had spina bifida corrected at birth. She has since developed a marked scoliosis and is now admitted to the hospital for spinal fusion and instrumentation. During her admission procedure, the primary goal is to provide:
    1 Privacy
    2 Orientation to the ward
    3 Her mother's presence
    4 Introduction to her roommates

118. A patient presents to the emergency room following an automobile accident. Which of the following problems would the nurse consider the most emergent?
    1 The blood glucose level is high at 396 mg/dl
    2 The patient has a 3-cm laceration of his left eye
    3 The patient is complaining of shortness of breath
    4 A distraught family member is crying in the hallway

119. The primary reason that adverse drug reactions occur frequently in elderly patients is because older adults have a:
    1 Higher percentage of body water
    2 Higher percentage of lean muscle
    3 Lower percentage of body fat
    4 Higher percentage of body fat

120. A nurse is evaluating the effectiveness of a patient's IV therapy. Which of the following symptoms would lead the nurse to suspect the patient may have circulatory overload?
    1 Bounding pulse, dyspnea, cough
    2 Pain, edema, erythema at the infusion site
    3 Pain, edema, a palpable venous cord at the infusion site
    4 Fever, chills, purulent discharge from the IV insertion site

121. When applying sterile gloves, the nurse is careful to:
    1 Handle only the outside of each glove
    2 Pick the first glove up by the inside of the cuff
    3 Keep the gloves on the sterile field throughout the procedure
    4 Insert fingers under the outside cuff to apply the first glove

122. While preparing to administer digitalis to a newly admitted patient, the nurse counted an apical pulse rate of 52 beats per minute. The nurse would be correct to:
    1 Give the drug as usual
    2 Omit the drug and report it to the physician
    3 Give the patient one half the dosage
    4 Give the drug but with twice as much water as usual

123. When contributing to the nursing care plan, the nurse knows that an example of a short-term goal is:
    1 Assist patient in ROM exercises
    2 Patient will transfer from bed to chair this week
    3 Patient will return to previous level of functioning
    4 Physical activity will improve muscle tone and function

124. An 11-year-old female patient has an order for prochlorperazine (Compazine) 4 mg IM. On hand is Compazine 10 mg/ml. The nurse gives this patient _____ ml.

125. Using Clark's rule, answer the following problem:
    Child's weight: 30 lb
    Average adult dose: 10 mg
    What is the child's dose?
    Clark's rule: Weight in pounds × adult dose/150

PART 1 ANSWERS AND RATIONALES

1. Comprehension, assessment, physiological integrity (b).

    4 An increase in potassium can result in cardiac irregularities.

    1 An increase in calcium has side effects, but they are not as serious as is an increase in potassium.

    2 An increase in chloride does not have significant side effects.

    3 An increase in sodium has side effects, but they are not as serious as is an increase in potassium.

2. Knowledge, assessment, physiological integrity (a).

    2 This is true. In dark-skinned persons, pressure areas appear darker. With blanching, these areas appear gray.

    1 This is descriptive in light-skinned persons.

    3 This is a sign of pressure, not blanching.

    4 This may be a sign of pressure.

3. Knowledge, assessment, physiological integrity (a).

    4 Celiac disease is a basic defect of metabolism, leading to impaired fat absorption.

    1 Celiac disease does not affect absorption of proteins.

    2 Celiac disease does not affect absorption of carbohydrates.

    3 Celiac disease does not affect absorption of vitamins.

4. Application, implementation, physiological integrity (b).

    4 Because of the neuropathy that can occur in patients with diabetes, they are more sensitive to the cold and can get frostbite more easily.

    1 This is an abrasion and, if cared for properly, should not become infected.

    2 Substantial data are not given to warrant the need for an x-ray examination at this time.

    3 Rebound swelling should not occur if the time of the cold application is no longer than 20 to 30 minutes.

5. Knowledge, implementation, safe, effective care environment (a).

    2 Two persons to assist will maintain safety and provide assistance should the patient become dizzy.

    1 One person cannot provide adequate assistance in the case of a fall.

    3 Giving a narcotic will relieve any pain but may contribute to potential falls.

    4 The patient should never dangle alone for the first time postoperatively; this is extremely unsafe.

6. Comprehension, assessment, physiological integrity (b).

    1 Severe tachypnea seen in bronchiolitis is a contraindication for oral feedings.

    2 Bronchiolitis normally causes tachycardia.

    3, 4 These are not contraindications for oral fluids.

7. Knowledge, planning, health promotion and maintenance (a).

    2 Nicotine is a potent vasoconstrictor, and the further narrowing of the arterial walls will worsen peripheral vascular disease.

    1 Smoke causes hypertension, not hypotension.

    3 Smoke does irritate the lungs, but this is not the mechanism by which it worsens peripheral vascular disease.

    4 Smoke does not decrease the RBC count.

8. Application, assessment, physiological integrity (a).

    2 These are signs of hyperkalemia.

    1 These are vague, generalized signs and symptoms.

    3 These are signs of fluid imbalance.

    4 These are signs of fluid deficit.

9. Comprehension, assessment, physiological integrity (b).

    1 Accidental removal of the parathyroid glands can lead to tetany because the glands secrete a hormone that regulates calcium balance.

    2 A seizure is possible in tetany but is not one of the initial symptoms.

    3 This is not associated with parathyroid removal.

    4 Although respiratory compromise is a potential problem with a thyroidectomy, loss of the gag reflex is not associated with parathyroid removal.

10. Comprehension, assessment, physiological integrity (a).

    1 These are the early symptoms of prostatitis.

    2 This is related and may indicate a urinary tract infection. General.

    3, 4 This is a routine part of any general health history.

11. Application, planning, physiological integrity (b).

    4 Persons with pulmonary disease are at risk for acidosis, secondary to CO_2 retention.

    1 This does not warrant checking within the next hour.

    2, 3 Data are insufficient to support this assumption.

12. Comprehension, knowledge, safe, effective care environment (a).

    2 The client will be able to get out of bed and pivot into a chair with no weight bearing on the affected leg.

    1 Bed rest is not needed and increases the risk of deep-vein thrombosis.

    3 Full weight bearing is not appropriate immediately postoperative.

    4 No skeletal traction is used for this type of procedure.

13. Comprehension, implementation, psychosocial integrity (b).

    3 The purpose of an arthroscopy is to improve joint function and limit the amount of pain.

    1 This does not alleviate the patient's anxiety, and although a surgeon may need to speak to the patient, the nurse should answer the patient's question to the best of his or her ability.

    2 Having an arthroscopy will most likely postpone the need for a knee replacement, but it may not eliminate the need for a knee replacement at a later time.

    4 This procedure will not cure degenerative joint disease, but it will alleviate some of the symptoms.

14. Comprehension, assessment, physiological integrity (b).

    2 Hypocalcemia can occur after a thyroidectomy resulting from inadvertent removal of parathyroid tissue. The signs and symptoms of this complication are numbness and tingling of fingertips, toes, and lips; carpopedal spasms; tachycardia; tachypnea; and hypertension.

    1 Hyperglycemia is not a usual consequence of thyroid surgery, and the signs and symptoms are polydipsia, polyuria, and polyphagia.

    3 Hyperkalemia is not a usual consequence of thyroid surgery, and the signs and symptoms would include cardiac rhythm disturbances.

    4 Thyroid storm can occur postsurgically, but it is characterized by severe tachycardia, severe hypertension, and hyperthermia.

15. Comprehension, implementation, health promotion and maintenance (c).

2 Obesity increases strain on weight-bearing joints; reduction of weight minimizes some of the presenting symptoms.

1 This does not reduce joint strain but does maintain existing ROM.

3 This will provide comfort but will not reduce strain.

4 This does not control strain but will aid in pain control.

16. Application, assessment, physiological integrity (a).

2 The standard assessment model for any emergency situation is always ABC—airway, breathing, and circulation. The patient must have an open airway to have effective breathing, and effective breathing must be present to have effective circulation.

1, 3, 4 These sequences are incorrect.

17. Application, implementation, physiological integrity (b).

4 This direction allows the fluid left in the space to consolidate and lessens the possibility of mediastinal shift.

1, 2, 3 These are inappropriate; they increase risk of mediastinal shift when placed on unaffected side.

18. Comprehension, assessment, physiological integrity (a)

2 Fluid balance and removal of excess fluids is one of the primary goals of dialysis. Comparing predialysis and postdialysis weights will measure the effectiveness of therapy.

1 Benadryl is not routinely given for dialysis.

3 Urinalysis is not necessary because blood tests are used to measure kidney function.

4 Patients do not need to be NPO.

19. Comprehension, assessment, physiological integrity (b).

4 Cerebral palsy is a disorder that affects the motor centers of the brain; it is usually caused by birth trauma or head trauma.

1 This is a chromosomal abnormality.

2 This is an S-shaped curvature of the spine.

3 This is an infection of the bone.

20. Comprehension, planning, physiological integrity (a).

4 Comatose patients can still hear what is being said and may react physiologically.

1, 3 No data are available to support these.

2 The family may be upset by bad news, but that is not the reason to avoid bedside conversation.

21. Knowledge, planning, psychosocial integrity (a).

3 It aids in family grieving and allows the family to feel useful.

1 No evidence exists to support the prolongation of the dying process.

2 Actually, it increases the workload because the nurse must assist the family and their psychosocial needs.

4 Family members often want to help and do not view it as work.

22. Application, assessment, physiological integrity (b).

2 Normal urine should be a clear, yellow liquid. Differences in color and clarity may signify body fluid imbalance.

1 Normally, urine is slightly aromatic.

3 The specific gravity of urine is normally low.

4 The presence of RBCs in a urine sample would signify kidney disease.

23. Knowledge, implementation, physiological integrity (a).

2 The inner cannula is removed and hydrogen peroxide used to break up the dried mucus.

1 Q-tips are never used because they can leave behind tiny cotton fibers, which can be inhaled.

3, 4 The outer cannula is never removed.

24. Comprehension, assessment, physiological integrity (c).

2 These are symptoms of rubeola.

1 Symptoms of chickenpox include a clear, vesicular rash, fever, irritability, and pruritus.

3 Symptoms of mumps include enlarged parotid glands and fever, with no rash.

4 Symptoms of rubella do not include a high fever or white spots at the back of the throat.

25. Comprehension, planning, physiological integrity (b).

3 This is an appropriate discharge instruction; Kegel exercises help strengthen the perineal floor muscles.

1 This is an unsafe instruction that may cause further bleeding.

2 This is an unsafe instruction; fluids should be encouraged to 10 to 12 glasses a day.

4 This is an unsafe instruction; any increased redness of the urine should be reported because it may indicate hemorrhage.

26. Comprehension, planning, physiological integrity (a).

3 It takes longer to inspire or expire air because of age-related physiological changes.

1 This is not a proven fact for older adults.

2 This is not a proven correlation.

4 Overall respiratory muscle structure and function decrease in older adults.

27. Knowledge, assessment, physiological integrity (b).

A Wilms' tumor is found only in the kidney and kidney area.

28. Comprehension, evaluation, physiological integrity (b).

3 The presence of meat in this patient's system will cause the Hemoccult test to be positive, whether or not blood is actually in his stool. The patient should be free of red meat for 2 to 3 days for the test to be considered accurate.

1 Ingestion of coffee should have no bearing on the test results.

2 The gelatin should not cause the developer slide to turn blue, which would indicate the presence of blood.

4 Lots of fiber should not have any bearing on the results of the test.

29. Application, implementation, physiological integrity (b).

3 A dietary record will assist the nurse in determining problem areas.

1 This intervention will promote salivation but does not affect food or caloric intake.

2 This intervention will promote elasticity of the skin but does not affect food or caloric intake.

4 This is an appropriate intervention for the diagnosis altered nutrition: more than body requirements.

30. Comprehension, assessment, physiological integrity (b).

2 These are classic symptoms of an infant with pyloric stenosis.

1 Symptoms of Hirschsprung's disease include constipation, abdominal distention, bile-stained mucous and emesis, and inadequate weight gain.

3 Symptoms of esophageal atresia include excessive salivation and drooling, coughing and choking during feedings, and regurgitation of all feedings.

4 Symptoms of intussusception appear suddenly and include pallor, vomiting, stools with blood and mucous, drawing up of the legs and crying out caused by sharp colicky pain, and signs of shock.

31. Comprehension, implementation, physiological integrity (b).
2 For the proper laboratory tests to be completed, all voided urine must be collected.
1 In a 24-hour urine specimen, all urine is collected that the patient voids in a 24-hour period.
3 No discernible reason exists to insert a retention catheter, unless the patient is incontinent.
4 All urine is sent to the laboratory in one large, dark container.

32. Comprehension, planning, physiological integrity (b).
2 The patient has difficulty swallowing and will need special feeding precautions taken.
1 Facial exercises will not assist in helping the patient swallow.
3 The patient may or may not have difficulty forming words; however, if dysphagia is present, then special feeding precautions must be instituted.
4 This may be necessary and needs to be determined, but the plan of care needs to address the swallowing difficulty.

33. Comprehension, implementation, physiological integrity (b).
3 Hemianopsia is blindness of one half of the visual field. For the patient to maximize eyesight, scanning the environment is necessary.
1 This will further blind the patient.
2 Both eyes have lost one half the vision.
4 The problem is not dry corneas.

34. Knowledge, assessment, physiological integrity (a).
1 In the assessment phase, the nurse observes the physiological, psychosocial, health, and safety needs of clients.
2 Teaching is part of nursing intervention.
3 Prioritizing problems is part of the planning phase.
4 Collaborating to determine a plan of care if part of the planning phase.

35. Comprehension, assessment, physiological integrity (b).
4 The patient may be unable to expel all urine fully from the bladder. Further assessment is indicated to assess the fullness of the urinary bladder, but this response is the best indicator that the patient may need the catheter.
1 Without further data, this would not indicate that the patient needs the catheter.
2 The urinary bladder should be palpated to assess fullness. Consuming large amounts of fluids is not an indication that the catheterization is necessary.
3 The patient's bladder is most likely empty if the incontinent episode occurred. Further assessment is necessary.

36. Knowledge, planning, physiological integrity (c).
4 Nitroprusside (Nipride) is preferred because of its quick vasoactivity and short half-life.
1 Propranolol hydrochloride (Inderal) is a maintenance drug for hypertension.
2 Enalapril maleate (Vasotec) is primarily used for maintenance therapy for hypertension.
3 Nifedipine (Procardia) is used as a maintenance drug for hypertension.

37. Application, assessment, psychosocial integrity (b).
2 Collecting data concerning normal home practices allows the nurse to plan care effectively for the patient and is a priority.
1 Whether this is necessary has not been ascertained.
3 This may not be possible, and the nurse must communicate effectively with the patient.
4 This is appropriate; however, the nurse must first establish communication with the patient.

38. Application, implementation, physiological integrity (c).
1 This response best describes the reason for the runny nose and watery eyes, which is the question posed by the patient.
2 This is not clearly established, and it does not answer the patient's question.
3 This may be a normal reflex; however, the patient is asking why it happens during hay fever season.
4 This is true, but it does not describe the reason for the watery eyes and runny nose.

39. Application, implementation, physiological integrity (b).
This is correct: 7.5 mg/x × 2 ml/10 mg = 1.5 ml.

40. Knowledge, planning, physiological integrity (b).
3 Dried fruits are excellent sources of iron.
1 Milk and dairy products contain very little iron.
2 Refined cereals have had much of the valuable nutrients removed.
4 These are good sources of vitamin A, not iron.

41. Comprehension, planning, physiological integrity (c).
4 Dobutrex increases cardiac contractility. Decreased contractility is the basic mechanism of heart failure.
1 Intropin at doses greater than 5 µg/kg/min cause vasoconstriction and increases arterial blood pressure. This would increase afterload, making the already weak heart work harder. Doses less than 5 µg/kg/min would increase renal artery perfusion. Neither dose would directly improve myocardial contractility.
2 Lasix would increase the urinary output and decrease preload, but it would not directly increase myocardial contractility.
3 Nipride causes vasodilation and is used to treat hypertensive crisis.

42. Application, implementation, physiological integrity (b).
3 Newer medications decrease gastric acid secretion. A well-balanced diet provides nutrients for healing.
1 Dairy products provide only temporary relief and have a high fat content.
2 No longer is indicated.
4 Eating three full meals is better. Any food intake produces acid.

43. Comprehension, implementation, physiological integrity (c).
1 Because the patient is having difficulty swallowing, this position will create a gravity force for downward motion of food.
2 This position would put him in danger of injury if he should fall.
3 This position would not help his dysphagia.
4 This position would not help.

44. Comprehension, evaluation, physiological integrity (b).
4 In general, ventricular arrhythmias are the most dangerous and potentially life threatening.
1 A sinus arrhythmia may cause difficulty, but it is generally not life threatening.

2 An atrial arrhythmia is not as dangerous compared with a ventricular arrhythmia.

3 An AV nodal arrhythmia can cause serious consequences but is not as dangerous compared with a ventricular arrhythmia.

45. Application, planning, safe, effective care environment (b).

2 E. coli–related illness is prevented by ensuring that red meats are thoroughly cooked.

1 Botulism is prevalent in improperly canned foods.

3 This may prevent infection; however, it is indicated in preventing salmonellosis.

4 Eggs contribute to infections caused by Salmonella.

46. Application, implementation, physiological integrity (a).

1 Positioning the patient on the side lessens the danger of aspiration of secretions.

2, 3, 4 These are not practical and might cause injury to the patient in a postictal state.

47. Comprehension, assessment, physiological integrity (a).

2 Meat and dairy products are the main source of protein in the diet.

1 Green, leafy vegetables and dried fruits can be good sources of iron.

3 Bread and cereals can provide many B-complex vitamins.

4 Many fruits and vegetables can be good sources of vitamins A, D, E, and K.

48. Analysis, evaluation, physiological integrity (b).

1 The muscle rigidity caused by the involuntary contraction of striated muscles may inhibit fluid voluntary movement. This results in the "cogwheel" jerking motor contractions that are a characteristic manifestation of this disease.

2 Movement may appear weak, especially when the patient is fatigued.

3 The tremors associated with Parkinson's disease usually lessen with voluntary movement.

4 The goal is to get and keep the patient as physically active as long as possible.

49. Application, implementation, physiological integrity (b).

4 Research studies have indicated that a link may exist between omega-3 fatty acids and a low incidence of heart disease.

1 This is not a true statement. Fatty acids are essential to the diet.

2 No evidence exists that this necessary. The patient merely requires information from the nurse.

3 No evidence exists to support this.

50. Knowledge, planning, physiological integrity (a).

4 Mineral oil is indigestible and will carry fat-soluble vitamins with it as it leaves the body.

1 Mineral oil is not irritating, but it is also not a good idea, as previously indicated.

2 This does not add calories, but it is indigestible, and its action on fat-soluble vitamins makes it a poor choice.

3 Mineral oil has no calories, because it is not digested by the body.

51. Analysis, evaluation, physiological integrity (b).

1 An unexpected change has occurred in the patient's condition, especially with the confusion; the physician must therefore be notified.

2 This would be negligent.

3 Reality orientation is in order but is not a priority.

4 Older adults do not absorb drugs the same as younger adults do. However, simply observing would be negligent given that the physician has to be kept current; the medication may not be causing the confusion.

52. Application, implementation, physiological integrity (a).

4 This equipment may be necessary if the enlarged epiglottis completely obstructs the airway.

1 Any examination of the throat may lead to laryngospasm.

2 The child with epiglottis has difficulty swallowing.

3 Warm steam is not a method of treatment in epiglottis.

53. Knowledge, implementation, physiological integrity (b).

3 Recommendations are that smokers increase their vitamin C by 100 mg/day.

1 Vitamin A is fat soluble and can be toxic in mega doses.

2 Vitamin K is synthesized by the body.

4 Vitamin B has not been shown to be deficient in smokers.

54. Comprehension, assessment, safe, effective care environment (b).

1 This is the first priority question.

2, 3, 4 These questions ask for information that is not important at this time.

55. Comprehension, assessment, physiological integrity (c).

2 The patient is experiencing an aura, which can appear as any sensory sensation. An aura is a precursor to a seizure. The nurse will have her immediately lie down to protect her from injury should she fall.

1 The nurse would note her comments later but needs to stay with her at this point; a psychiatrist need not be contacted.

3 IV Valium would probably be given but only with an order.

4 Her physician would be called to inform him or her of the seizure, but this would be done later.

56. Comprehension, evaluation, physiological integrity (b).

3 Approximately 60% of the total calories in the diet should come from carbohydrates. Of this amount, 40% should come from complex forms such as pastas and whole grains. They break down more slowly than do simple sugars, thus providing a steadier blood level.

1 Approximately 15% of carbohydrates come from simple sugars, such as those found in fruit or milk.

2 Artificial sweeteners should be used only in moderation.

4 Adolescents find support with peers, and they must spend time with them. Healthy choices can be made at most fast-food restaurants.

57. Knowledge, application, safe, effective care environment (b).

4 Popcorn is a choking hazard for young children.

1 Apples are appropriate for toddlers.

2 Toddlers should drink whole milk to help promote growth and energy metabolism.

3 Chocolate cake is not a hazard, although it is not very nutritious.

58. Analysis, evaluation, physiological integrity (c).

1 One of the purposes of the four-bottle technique is to observe the color changes in the urine to assess for blood over time. Normally, the urine lightens in color as bleeding decreases. Therefore the oldest specimen is discarded, which would be the one to the left.

2, 3, 4 These choices do not follow proper procedure for such a technique; refer to the rationale for #1.

59. Comprehension, implementation, psychosocial integrity (b).
   2 This is the most therapeutic.
   1 This will have a negative effect.
   3 Previous unacceptable behavior should be challenged and integrated into current behavioral activities.
   4 This is not therapeutic.

60. Comprehension, implementation, physiological integrity (b).
   1 Many antibiotics, including ampicillin, decrease the effects of Ortho-Novum 1/50 and other oral contraceptives.
   2 Blood sugar should be checked; ampicillin can cause a false-positive urine sugar result.
   3 The full course of antibiotics should be completed to decrease the chances of a superinfection.
   4 A rash is indicative of an allergic reaction and is to be observed for but is not an expected effect of treatment.

61. Application, evaluation, psychosocial integrity (b).
   4 Additional information is needed to provide the necessary care for this patient.
   1 This does not help the current situation.
   2 This is false reassurance.
   3 This does not help solve the situation.

62. Application, assessment, psychosocial integrity (b).
   2 Denial is common when diagnosed with a potentially fatal disease.
   1 Repression is a response to a painful experience.
   3 Fantasy is unacceptable behavior.
   4 Rationalization is using a "good" reason to explain behavior.

63. Application, implementation, physiological integrity (b).
   1 Cranial nerve I (olfactory) is assessed following the technique described. A normal finding occurs when the person correctly identifies odors presented.
   2 Cranial nerve II (optic) is the nerve that controls sight.
   3 Cranial nerve III (otic) is the oculomotor nerve.
   4 Cranial nerve VII (facial) is the facial nerve and provides symmetry of facial movement.

64. Comprehension, implementation, psychosocial integrity (b).
   2 The nurse must be able to deal with his or her own feelings first.
   1 Standard Precautions are all that is required.
   3 This is not a priority.
   4 This is not the first thing to do.

65. Analysis, implementation, physiological integrity (c).
   4 A change in neurological status may indicate increased intracranial pressure. A thorough neurological assessment is indicated. Placing the head of bed in a slightly elevated position will aid in decreasing the pressure rise. The physician should be notified immediately in case emergency interventions are required.
   1 This is an inappropriate and negligent action.
   2 In suspected increased intracranial pressure, the head of the bed is slightly elevated to decrease intracranial pressure.
   3 Preparing the patient for emergency surgery may be indicated, but the nurse must begin with assessment of the patient's status and subsequent notification of the physician.

66. Application, evaluation, physiological integrity (a).
   3 Patients usually show improvement in 2 to 4 weeks.
   1, 2 This is not long enough to see the desired effect.
   4 Seeing improvement should not take this long.

67. Comprehension, evaluation, physiological integrity (c).
   3 Prednisone is given to decrease inflammation.
   1, 2, 4 Prednisone is not used for these reasons in the treatment of rheumatic fever.

68. Knowledge, assessment, health promotion and maintenance (b).
   An infant normally triples his or her birth weight by 12 months of age.

69. Knowledge, assessment, physiological integrity (a).
   1 Assessment data relevant to seizure disorder includes obtaining a complete history, medication history, and allergy history. Data collection should be specific to the seizure disorder, such as onset, duration, behavior before and after, type of body movements, loss of consciousness, incontinence, and awareness of seizure afterward.
   2 Diet and exercise history is not specific to the seizure disorder.
   3 Social and educational levels are not relative to this disorder.
   4 Work history is not relative to this disorder.

70. Comprehension, implementation, physiological integrity (b).
   2 Patient teaching should include instructing the patient in the importance of wearing a Medic-Alert bracelet, tag, or other medical identification. The person is taught to avoid situations known to trigger seizures, such as flashing or blinking lights, stress, or lack of sleep.
   1 This response is an expected outcome of the nursing and medical treatment plan.
   3 Persons with a diagnosis of seizure disorders are frequently evaluated many times throughout the year and should be encouraged to keep follow-up medical appointments, as well as appointments to have blood drawn for laboratory work.
   4 This response supports social stigmas associated with epilepsy. Individuals in the community need education regarding seizure disorders. Individuals with a seizure disorder are encouraged to live normal lives.

71. Comprehension, implementation, psychosocial integrity (b).
   1 This helps identify the content of the delusion.
   2 Logic cannot be used to explain delusions.
   3 Do not leave the patient alone.
   4 Do not imply that the patient is wrong.

72. Application, implementation, physiological integrity (b).
   2 This is a toxic level. The dose should be held and the physician notified.
   1, 3 The level is already toxic.
   4 Xanax is an antianxiety medication and will not substitute for lithium.

73. Comprehension, implementation, physiological integrity (b).
   1 An appropriate nursing action in the administration of TPN is to weigh the patient daily, monitor blood glucose levels regularly to assess the patient's ability to metabolize concentrated glucose, and wean gradually to avoid a sudden drop in blood sugar.
   2 This response reflects a lack of knowledge relevant to the rationale for administering TPN. The patient may express hunger sensations but may be physiologically compromised, requiring TPN for nutritional support.

3 Monitoring liver, renal, and cardiovascular function is required of any patient receiving fluids but is not specific to the administration of TPN.

4 This response is incorrect; refer to #1.

74. Application, implementation, physiological integrity (b).

   1 This can cause hypertensive crisis.

   2 The medicine can be taken on an empty stomach.

   3 It is taken in the morning or may be multiple doses.

   4 This is not necessary.

75. Comprehension, implementation, psychosocial integrity (b).

   2 This is a realistic, feasible approach.

   1 Blanket approval is unrealistic.

   3 She should begin to learn to tolerate separation.

   4 This is unrealistic and leads to mistrust.

76. Comprehension, planning, psychosocial integrity (b).

   1 This is the best response; it helps develop trust.

   2 This is not a good reason to stay. In this response, the nurse, rather than the patient, is the focus. This does not foster trust.

   3 This is false reassurance.

   4 This puts the patient on the defensive.

77. Comprehension, planning, psychosocial integrity (b).

   1 The effect of conscious sedation requires careful monitoring of the airway; therefore the risk for ineffective breathing pattern is appropriate.

   2 This response is a goal statement.

   3 This response is a nursing intervention.

   4 This response is an evaluation statement.

78. Application, implementation, psychosocial integrity (c).

   2 Being dependable is necessary for the patient to trust and feel secure; contracted time with the patient is for that patient only; terminating a session early is a patient response that the nurse should understand and anticipate.

   1 This is inappropriate; the patient has to assume responsibility for his behavior.

   3 Contracted time with the patient is time for that patient only; the nurse should remain for the duration of the contracted time.

   4 This is inappropriate; the focus is always the patient, not the nurse.

79. Comprehension, evaluation, psychosocial integrity (b).

   2 Patients who are less depressed have more energy to commit suicide.

   1, 3 The opposite is true.

   4 Patients may not verbalize suicide plans.

80. Knowledge, assessment, physiological integrity (a).

   3 The posterior fontanel closes by this age.

   1 This develops at 6 to 7 months of age.

   2 This develops at 8 to 9 months of age.

   4 This occurs at 7 to 8 months of age.

81. Application, implementation, physiological integrity (a).

   3 This position promotes venous return.

   1, 2 These positions may increase intracranial pressure.

   4 This position causes flexion of the hips and perhaps the neck.

82. Application, assessment, physiological integrity (b).

   2 Bleeding is a serious side effect of anticoagulant therapy. Nursing measures focus on monitoring for signs of active bleeding.

   1 This is a common side effect of any medication. Hematemesis would be of serious concern.

3 This is not a common side effect of this class of medications and is not suggestive of bleeding.

4 This is a common side effect of many medications.

83. Application, implementation, physiological integrity (b).

   1 Weight should be measured at the same time each day, in the same clothing.

   2 Not enough information is given to assume this. The patient may be taking medication several times a day or at irregular intervals.

   3 Daily weights are a more accurate measurement of fluid retention.

   4 Daily weights will indicate early fluid retention, avoiding symptoms of advancing congestive heart failure.

84. Application, implementation, health promotion and maintenance (b).

   3 Increased fluid intake decreases the tenacity of respiratory secretions, making sputum removal easier.

   1 Low hydration makes respiratory secretions tenacious and difficult to expel.

   2 Tracheal suctioning is invasive and should be used only if the patient is unable to expel secretions independently.

   4 Postural drainage relies on gravity to assist with expulsion of secretions. Affected lung areas vary and must be vertical for this to occur.

85. Application, implementation, physiological integrity (a).

   1 Persons taking this anticonvulsant are especially prone to developing gingival hyperplasia.

   2 This is inappropriate and is not relative to the situation presented; see #4.

   3 This is inappropriate and is not a patient responsibility.

   4 Adequate rest and diet are important. Answer #1 is individualized to the situation and is the better choice.

86. Comprehension, evaluation, physiological integrity (b).

   3 Nitroglycerine has a vasodilating effect and is often the cause of headaches, at least in the initial period of therapy.

   1 Tylenol normally alleviates headache discomfort.

   2 Lanoxin is a cardiotonic and does not normally cause headache.

   4 Potassium chloride is used to counter the side effect of hypokalemia and does not cause headaches.

87. Comprehension, assessment, physiological integrity (b).

   1 Increased respiratory rate, chest tightness, and hypoxemia are signs of complications following a thoracentesis and should be reported to the physician immediately.

   2 Respiratory rate would be increased, as would the pulse; hypotension would be noted.

   3 Bradycardia is not an early sign of respiratory distress. Low blood pressure may occur secondary to removing a volume of fluid and should be monitored. A dry, hacking cough is usually not indicative of respiratory distress.

   4 A normal sinus rhythm indicates adequate cardiac function, normotension reflects blood pressure within normal limits, and ventilation is the act of moving air into and out of the lungs.

88. Comprehension, assessment, health promotion and maintenance (b).

   2 These are the classic signs of cardiogenic shock.

   1 Fever and bounding pulse are not normally seen in patients with cardiogenic shock.

3 High blood pressure is not a normal symptom in cardiogenic shock.

4 Hot, dry skin is not normally seen in patients with cardiogenic shock.

89. Knowledge, assessment, physiological integrity (a).

3 Assessment begins with first determining responsiveness.

1 Activation of the emergency medical system occurs after responsiveness is determined.

2, 4 These actions are initiated only after determining responsiveness.

90. Application, implementation, physiological integrity (b).

3 The Holter monitor will record a tracing of the heart during various activities and is compared with activities that the patient is documenting as well.

1 A glucometer evaluates capillary blood sugar levels.

2 Urines are used to evaluate various conditions but not heart activity during exertion.

4 This study evaluates blood flow through a carotid artery or extremity.

91. Comprehension, knowledge, physiological integrity (a).

2 Injuries at or above C5 result in quadriplegia.

1 Emotions remain intact; however, grief and mourning reactions and depression frequently occur.

3 Desire remains; however, it may be affected by emotional reactions to the trauma and its effects.

4 Speaking ability remains intact.

92. Application, implementation, physiological integrity (b).

1 This steroidal medication is usually used for this specific type of meningitis.

2, 3, 4 These drugs are not used for treating *H. influenzae* type B meningitis.

93. Comprehension, planning, health promotion and maintenance (b).

2 Injury can lead to infection. The tissues are already compromised of oxygen and nutrients; certain positions (legs crossed, knees flexed) hamper circulation.

1, 3, 4 These measures can lead to greater compromise in circulation and burns.

94. Comprehension, implementation, physiological integrity (b).

4 Bag-valve-mask ventilation or Ambu ventilation provides oxygen to correct the hypoxia.

1 Chest tubes only drain the pleural space.

2 Cricothyroid puncture would be indicated if injury to the upper airway has occurred.

3 Trendelenburg position may assist with fluid drainage but will not help correct hypoxia; it may also cause dyspnea.

95. Comprehension, assessment, physiological integrity (b).

4 These are early signs reflecting the heart's attempt to compensate through tachycardia. Yawning is the body's way to take deep breaths to increase oxygen to the brain.

1 These are signs of prolonged or severe oxygen deprivation.

2 Wheezing is not usually present. Bradycardia and confusion are later signs.

3 These are later signs of severe hypoxemia.

96. Application, implementation, safe, effective care environment (a).

2 This maintains an intact drainage system. The urine specimen will not likely become contaminated.

1 This disrupts the patency of the system and increases likelihood of contamination and a urinary tract infection.

3 Urine collecting in the drainage bag is likely to have organisms present, thereby giving inaccurate test results.

4 These are unnecessary actions and increase risk to the patient of acquiring trauma or infection, or both.

97. Application, planning, physiological integrity (a).

60 mg = 1 gr 60 × 5 = 300 mg/tablet: 2 tablets = 600 mg.

98. Comprehension, implementation, psychosocial integrity (a).

3 This is an emotional change that is common after a CVA. Emotional lability may or may not be appropriate to the situation.

1 This is common but normal.

2 This is inappropriate and encourages a negative behavior-modification technique. The patient has emotional lability.

4 This is inappropriate. The patient is not acting this way on purpose.

99. Comprehension, evaluation, physiological integrity (a).

4 This question seeks more data and demonstrates attentive listening. Beets, blackberries, rhubarb, and some medications may turn the urine red or orange.

1 Milk increase is unnecessary. Liquids should normally be approximately 2000 ml/day. This response gives a quick fix.

2 This response offers false reassurance and is belittling the patient's concern.

3 This response does show the nurse is listening. The nurse is seeking more data; however, #4 is individualized and therefore a better choice.

100. Comprehension, assessment, health promotion and maintenance (b).

4 As individuals age, the action of the sweat and oil glands become less active; daily bathing is therefore not required.

1 Body odor may not diminish, although perspiration does.

2 This may not be true of all older adults.

3 This is not a true statement.

101. Application, assessment, health promotion and maintenance (b).

2 These are the classic symptoms of hyperthyroidism.

1 These symptoms are typical of hypothyroidism.

3 These are not indicative of thyroid disease.

4 These symptoms are caused by a slowed metabolic rate and are seen in hypothyroidism.

102. Application, planning, safe, effective care environment (c).

1 This allows the nurse to perform skills completely yet decreases the amount of time that the nurse must spend in the radioactive environment.

2 Entering the patient's room frequently exposes the nurse to the radioactive environment: the implant should not be visible for the nurse to assess.

3 This increases the amount of time the nurse spends in the radioactive environment.

4 Although decreasing the loneliness of an isolated patient is important, this measure would increase the amount of time the nurse is in the radioactive environment.

103. Comprehension, planning, physiological integrity (a).
    2 This is the physiological action of the pharmacological therapy.
    1 This is true of any medication.
    3 This is true, but it is not the appropriate rationale.
    4 This may occur after multiple consecutive missed doses.

104. Knowledge, implementation, physiological integrity (a).
    1 Massaging the area and avoiding repeated pressure will enhance circulation.
    2, 3, 4 These are inappropriate nursing actions for pressure areas.

105. Comprehension, evaluation, safe, effective care environment (b).
    4 These foods will increase the amount of bulk and fiber in the diet.
    1 Although fruit juices do contain some fiber, the dairy products will constipate the individual.
    2 Meat, cheese, and poultry products will not increase fiber in the diet.
    3 Processed carbohydrates and milk products will not combat constipation.

106. Application, planning, safe, effective care environment (b).
    3 The Centers for Disease Control and Prevention recommends using Standard Precautions at all times.
    1 In emergency situations, patients are often not able to provide accurate information.
    2 This is highly impractical and inappropriate.
    4 Relying only on the obvious is inappropriate.

107. Knowledge, assessment, physiological integrity (b).
    4 Rheumatic fever is a chronic disease caused by a streptococcal infection.
    1 It is not caused by a fungus.
    2 It is not caused by Staphylococcus bacteria.
    3 It is not caused by a virus.

108. Comprehension, assessment, psychosocial integrity (a).
    3 Denial is indicated by the patient's inability to recognize the seriousness of his act and his belief that he can go home.
    1 Sublimation is the process by which negative impulses are channeled into more acceptable outlets.
    2 Projection is the placing of unacceptable impulses onto another person.
    4 Regression is the moving back to an earlier time or developmental level during periods of stress.

109. Comprehension, evaluation, safe, effective care environment (b).
    2 Hardwood floors may pose a risk for slippage, especially if scatter rugs are used.
    1 An electric stove is safer compared with a gas stove.
    3 Nonglare lighting assists older adults in reading.
    4 Elevated toilet seats may assist older adults in transferring to and from the toilet.

110. Knowledge, evaluation, health promotion and maintenance (b).
    3 Circulatory changes cause drug distribution in older adults to be altered, thereby increasing the chances for adverse drug reactions.
    1 Older adults do not excrete drugs more effectively.
    2 This statement is not true; some muscle wasting occurs.
    4 Absorption is altered, but it is the result of decreased gastric motility.

111. Knowledge, assessment, physiological integrity (a).
    4 This is a correct assessment.
    1 These are not likely to be delusions.
    2 This is unlikely.
    3 This is incorrect; symptoms may worsen.

112. Knowledge, implementation, physiological integrity (a).
    2 Vomiting from acute alcoholism can cause aspiration, and the depressed central nervous system can lead to respiratory arrest.
    1 Shock is associated with delirium tremens, not acute alcoholism.
    3 This is appropriate for mild alcohol withdrawal; acute alcoholism requires observation.
    4 Disulfiram (Antabuse) may be recommended as part of an aftercare program for the alcoholic who has already undergone withdrawal.

113. Application, implementation, physiological integrity (b).
    2 This allows the older adult, who may have dry mucous membranes, to swallow the medications more easily.
    1 The head of the bed should be at 60 to 90 degrees.
    3 Medications given in this manner may not be compatible and may be overwhelming.
    4 Medications should never be mixed with the patient's food.

114. Comprehension, planning, safe, effective care environment (b).
    3 Advance directives include living wills and health care proxies (durable power of attorney).
    1 Guardianship is established by the courts.
    2 Organ donation is not included under advance directives.
    4 Active euthanasia is currently illegal in the United States, and passive euthanasia includes "do not resuscitate" (DNR) orders.

115. Knowledge, implementation, physiological integrity (b).
    3 An arrest in an adult is usually caused by a cardiac arrhythmia such as ventricular fibrillation. Early defibrillation is necessary to revive the patient.
    1 Prolonged lack of oxygen in either the child or the adult will cause brain damage; this is not the correct explanation.
    2 Children need to be ventilated as quickly as possible because an arrest in a child usually results from choking or suffocation. The child may revive quickly after CPR is initiated.
    4 Adults can be resuscitated many times, especially if defibrillation is done early. The rescuer must always try, unless the patient has obviously been without oxygen for a long time.

116. Knowledge, implementation, physiological integrity (b).
    3 The vastus lateralis is the recommended muscle and site to be used for a patient this age.
    1 The deltoid muscle is not developed enough to safely give an IM injection in a patient this age.
    2 The gluteus maximus should not be used because it is not developed enough, and the sciatic nerve and artery are in this area.
    4 The patient should be over age 2 years to use the ventrogluteal area.

117. Knowledge, assessment, health promotion and maintenance (b).
    2 Cataracts, which are easily removed, cause more blindness than any other disorder.

1 Glaucoma can cause blindness if not treated.

3 Presbyopia is the result of the normal changes of aging.

4 Macular degeneration causes blindness; however, more individuals suffer from cataracts.

118. Comprehension, assessment, psychosocial integrity (b).

2 In early Alzheimer's disease, short-term memory, which spans a few minutes or hours, is impaired.

1 This is long-term memory, which is usually preserved in early Alzheimer's disease.

3 This is benign forgetfulness, which is usually limited to trivial matters, and tends to occur in all individuals at some time in their life.

4 This is an example of immediate memory, which is not impaired in early Alzheimer's disease.

119. Knowledge, assessment, physiological integrity (b).

1 Follow the rule of nines.

Left leg = 18%

Right leg = 18%

Right arm = 9%

Total = 45%

2, 3, 4 These do not follow the rule of nines.

120. Knowledge, assessment, health promotion and maintenance (b).

3 The changes in this portion of the brain diminish the ability of older adults to produce a fever in response to an inflammatory agent.

1 Aging changes normally increase the older adult's pain threshold.

2 Cardiovascular aging changes do not increase erythema.

4 Older adults generally have normal to subnormal temperature levels.

121. Comprehension, evaluation, physiological integrity (b).

1 Victim should be observed for laryngeal and tracheal edema because the degree of inhalation burns is unknown.

2, 3, 4 These are characteristic of third-degree burns; it was previously determined that the victim has second-degree burns.

122. Application, implementation, physiological integrity (c).

3 The area should be covered with a dressing to reduce the risk of infection until it can be evaluated.

1 A splint can put pressure on the fracture site, causing further injury.

2 Although this is not totally inappropriate, the victim might be allergic to the ointment; the best action is to apply a dressing.

4 Attempting to return the bone might cause further injury.

123. Comprehension, planning, psychosocial integrity (b).

4 Surrounding the patient with familiar objects will increase a feeling of recognition in the new facility.

1 Bringing along familiar objects will not increase the attention span of the individual.

2 Although the familiar objects will be calming, they will not decrease dementia behaviors.

3 The objects would most likely facilitate long-term memory, if they facilitate memory at all.

124. Comprehension, implementation, physiological integrity (a).

1 Stop the flow of the IV fluids to prevent further swelling and report to charge nurse.

2, 3, 4 These are inappropriate responses that will not correct the stated situation.

125. Application, assessment, physiological integrity (b).

1 Wheezing and respiratory distress are symptoms of an anaphylactic reaction to the bee sting.

2, 3, 4 Although wheezing and respiratory distress are common with these disorders, the precipitating event was the bee sting.

PART 2 ANSWERS AND RATIONALES

1. Application, implementation, physiological integrity (b).
   2 Keeping the head of the bed below 30 degrees will reduce shearing of the skin.
   1 A turning schedule that is adhered to will be most effective.
   3 Incorrect information is being given.
   4 This is inappropriately stated; additionally, nerve endings may be compromised, and pain may not be present.

2. Analysis, evaluation, physiological integrity (c).
   1 Health care professionals generally agree that elderly people with diabetes are best managed by maintaining a fasting blood glucose in the 100- to 140-mg/dl range and postprandial glucose in the 120- to 180-mg/dl range.
   2, 3, 4 This is incorrect information; therefore learning has not occurred.

3. Application, assessment, health promotion and maintenance (b).
   4 These are common manifestations of hypertension in patients.
   1 Nausea and vomiting are not common symptoms of hypertension.
   2 Increased urination is not a common finding in patients with hypertension.
   3 These are not common assessment findings for a patient with hypertension.

4. Application, planning, physiological integrity (b).
   3 If mucus is too thick for the patient to expectorate, aerosol treatments would help.
   1 This is appropriate, but may not be as effective or act as quickly as #3.
   2 These actions would relieve the throat irritation but would not assist in making his cough productive.
   4 This is inappropriate. The high humidity may make breathing more difficult.

5. Comprehension, planning, physiological integrity (c).
   4 Normal changes of aging include reduction in total body water and muscle mass, which results in a greater risk of adverse drug reactions. Digoxin is a water-soluble drug and is distributed in smaller compartments, placing the older adult at risk for drug toxicity.
   1 In the older adult, a water-soluble drug is distributed into smaller compartments, causing an increased risk of drug toxicity.
   2 In the older adult, digoxin is more likely to accumulate to toxic levels in association with physiological changes.
   3 Digoxin dosing in the older adult is usually smaller than the dose prescribed for the younger adult because of a decrease in total body water and muscle mass and an increase in total body fat.

6. Application, assessment, health promotion and maintenance (b).
   2 Both of these conditions create regurgitation of blood back through the mitral valve, causing murmurs.
   1 Angina is not a common assessment finding in valvular disease.
   3 Syncope is not normally a finding in these types of valvular disease.
   4 Hypertension may be an underlying condition, but it is not specifically associated with either of these diseases.

7. Application, implementation, physiological integrity (b).
   4 Coughing when supine may be associated with left-sided heart failure.
   1 Decreased appetite may be caused by a variety of factors.
   2 Respirations should be documented, although easy, regular respirations are normal.
   3 This may have a variety of causes.

8. Comprehension, implementation, physiological integrity (b).
   3 The funduscopic examination is useful in examining the retina of the eye for changes that are suggestive of those accompanying hypertension.
   1 A vision screen tests only visual acuity.
   2 A tonometer test evaluates pressure within the eye and is useful in monitoring glaucoma.
   4 A visual fields examination evaluates peripheral vision and is useful in monitoring glaucoma and in evaluating neurological problems.

9. Comprehension, planning, physiological integrity (b).
   2 A firm surface provides support so that the heart is adequately compressed between the sternum and spine.
   1 The speed of compressions is not affected by the surface composition.
   3 The risk of breaking the xyphoid process is dependent on the hand position on the chest wall.
   4 Palpation of landmarks is not affected by the surface composition.

10. Knowledge, implementation, physiological integrity (b).
    4 A healthy weight-loss diet should include a variety of foods, as well as exercise.
    1 This is true, but it does not completely answer the question.
    2 A variety of nutrients are needed for a healthy diet.
    3 This is true, but it does not completely answer the question.

11. Knowledge, assessment, health promotion and maintenance (b).
    2 Metabolism slows in the older person; therefore fewer calories are needed.
    1 Frequently, the tolerance to fat is less, and it is harder to digest.
    3 Fluid intake should be increased to help eliminate waste products.
    4 Vitamin and mineral intake should be maintained and perhaps increased to account for decreased absorption.

12. Comprehension, planning, physiological integrity (b).
    4 Quadriceps muscles must be strengthened to allow for ambulation.
    1 Extension and abduction should prevent possible dislocation of the prosthesis but does not strengthen muscles.
    2 Passive ROM to the ankle will prevent joint freezing but does not strengthen muscles.
    3 Active ROM to the ankle will prevent joint freezing but does not strengthen muscles.

13. Knowledge, planning, physiological integrity (b).
    3 Lactose intolerance refers to the inability to digest milk sugar (lactose) because of a deficiency of the enzyme lactase.
    1 This contains no lactose.

2 This does not contain lactose and thus does not need to be avoided.

4 These foods contain no lactose.

14. Comprehension, implementation, physiological integrity (b).

4 This prevents bacterial spread into the wound.

1 Pressure on a wound diminishes bleeding; it would interfere with wound cleansing.

2 Forceful wound irrigation disrupts healing tissue.

3 Scrubbing disrupts healing tissue.

15. Comprehension, assessment, physiological integrity (a).

4 In acute glomerulonephritis, an immune response occurs, which damages the kidney and reduces glomerular filtration. This results in fluid volume excess, which is characterized by periorbital edema, lung crackles, distension of neck veins, and weight gain.

1 Typically, fever is characteristic of inflammation, infection, or injury. A person with glomerulonephritis can exhibit a fever, but this is not the result of the decreased GFR.

2 Thirst is characteristic of fluid volume deficit, not excess.

3 Polyuria is urination of large volumes, which does not occur with decreased GFRs.

16. Application, implementation, physiological integrity (c).

3 These are symptoms of an allergic reaction; this action removes the allergen while preserving the IV line.

1 This causes the patient pain and undue risk if the IV must be restarted.

2 This causes the patient undue risk and pain; it will not correct the problem, and if the allergic reaction worsens, an IV line may be needed quickly.

4 This is not a normal reaction, and the nurse cannot apply medication without an order.

17. Application, assessment, physiological integrity (c).

3 The symptoms indicate air embolism. Placing the patient in this position prevents the embolism from moving from the right atrium.

1 Despite the respiratory symptoms, this is a circulatory emergency, and the patient needs to be positioned to prevent further injury.

2 TPN ports should be reconnected after the patient is positioned.

4 Placing the patient in high-Fowler's position allows embolism dispersal to vital organs and will not diminish the patient's distress.

18. Knowledge, implementation, physiological integrity (b).

4 Oxygen has a drying effect on mucous membranes.

1 Ventilating oxygen through water will not reduce its combustibility.

2 The patient's level of oxygen absorption is related to liter flow, not humidity.

3 Particle contamination is not a factor in oxygen therapy.

19. Comprehension, evaluation, physiological integrity (b).

3 The outcome of care related to less-than-normal nutrition would be stable body weight, indicating maintenance of nutritional status.

1 Moist mucous membranes would be an appropriate outcome of care for dehydration.

2 Absence of diarrhea would be an appropriate outcome of care for altered gastrointestinal status: diarrhea.

4 Normal body temperature would be an appropriate outcome of care for altered body temperature: higher than normal.

20. Knowledge, implementation, safe, effective care environment (a).

3 Formula hang time should not exceed 8 hours because bacteria will multiply in the feeding once it is opened and kept at room temperature.

1 One day's supply of formula may require 16 to 20 hours of infusion time, providing an environment for bacteria growth.

2 More than one can of formula can be hung for efficiency, as long as the solution is not open at room temperature for more than 8 hours.

4 A 2-hour time frame is inefficient and unnecessary.

21. Application, implementation, physiological integrity (b).

4 An accurate intake and output record is necessary for correct calculation of the patient's fluid replacement needs.

1 Mouth care is an important comfort measure for the patient undergoing gastrointestinal suction, but it is not as critical compared with intake and output amounts.

2 Thorough skin care of the nares is important for skin integrity, but fluid balance is more critical.

3 Turning and positioning the patient may promote better gastrointestinal drainage and will prevent decubitus formation, but fluid balance is more critical.

22. Comprehension, evaluation, physiological integrity (c).

3 Cardiac arrhythmias are a serious consequence of potassium deficiency. Diuretics can cause hypokalemia.

1 This can indicate a deficiency of vitamin C.

2 This can be caused by a deficiency of riboflavin.

4 This can indicate a deficiency of niacin or B-complex vitamins.

23. Application, implementation, physiological integrity (b).

2 This degree allows for the best circulation and drainage of central nervous system fluid.

1 This is not enough elevation.

3 This is too much elevation.

4 This would be uncomfortable and may promote flexion of the neck, which would increase pressure.

24. Knowledge, assessment, health promotion and maintenance (b).

1 These are symptoms of a deficiency of vitamins C and B$_{12}$. The aging process may increase the need for these nutrients because of impaired absorption and decreased intake.

2 Symptoms are not typical of these deficiencies.

3 These are fat-soluble vitamins and are stored in the liver.

4 The symptoms are not typical of these vitamin deficiencies.

25. Application, evaluation, physiological integrity (b).

4 Edema found above the catheter is indicative of infiltration.

1 Poor skin turgor is a symptom of dehydration.

2 Redness at the site is a symptom of infection or phlebitis.

3 Warmth at the insertion site is indicative of infection or phlebitis.

26. Knowledge, planning, health promotion and maintenance (a).

2 Absence of prenatal care precludes early detection so that the condition can be watched and controlled.

1 Hypertensive drugs were discovered and used for primary hypertension and were adopted for use by obstetricians; this is a poor answer.

3 This is controversial; recent studies reveal that it may have no effect.

4 PIH may occur at any age; the number of pregnancies is of more concern, that is, whether this is the first baby; although PIH is more likely in adolescents or older women, this is not the best possible answer.

27. Comprehension, evaluation, physiological integrity (b).
4 The high salt content in the lunchmeat and potato chips would contribute to edema formation.
1 Although eggs contain salt, this food choice would not be as likely to contribute to edema.
2 Tuna fish and cantaloupe are low-salt food choices that should not contribute to edema.
3 Although the French fries may be salted, this food choice is less likely to contribute to edema compared with the salami and potato chips.

28. Knowledge, assessment, health promotion and maintenance (b).
1 The primitive Moro reflex is still present at 3 weeks of age.
2, 4 Vocalizations and holding the head erect are behaviors that can be observed in the 2-month-old infant. This infant does not have the neuromuscular development to perform these behaviors.
3 Recognizing familiar faces occurs at approximately 3 months. Before this time, younger infants may start to recognize familiar voices.

29. Application, implementation, physiological integrity (a).
3 This helps prevent muscle cramping.
1 This promotes circulation and helps prevent thrombophlebitis.
2 This relieves urinary incontinence.
4 This prevents anemia.

30. Application, planning, physiological integrity (b).
3 Milkshakes or nutritional supplements can supply the patient with anorexia additional calories and nutrients without overwhelming the person.
1 This overwhelms the person, makes him or her feel too full, and is not encouraged for patients with anorexia.
2 Taking pain medication before meals will allow a pain-free dining experience that may encourage the patient to eat more.
4 Fruits and vegetables are nutritious but should not be eaten in exclusion of protein or other foods.

31. Application, implementation, physiological integrity (b).
3 This is the best answer.
1 These relieve perineal discomfort.
2 These provide temporary relief at best.
4 This is improper advice.

32. Application, implementation, safe, effective care environment (b).
2 *Streptococcus pneumoniae* is the most common cause of meningitis and a common cause of upper respiratory infections. It may result in meningitis caused by extension of the infection into the central nervous system. Only good hand washing is needed.
1 Strict isolation is not required for the streptococcal organism but is for meningococcal meningitis to prevent transmission of the organism.
3 Meningitis transmission usually does not occur through wounds.
4 Respiratory precautions are necessary only as a part of strict isolation for meningococcal meningitis.

33. Comprehension, assessment, health promotion and maintenance (b).
3 This should resolve in 5 days.
1 This plantar reflex is normal for a year.
2 This should disappear in 3 to 4 weeks.
4 This is normal; sleep patterns vary widely.

34. Comprehension, planning, health promotion and maintenance (c).
1 This provides reassurance and explanation.
2 Levels of perception of pain differ; therefore they do not promise that "no pain" will occur.
3 This test takes from 20 minutes to over an hour.
4 This is untrue; most women will never need this test.

35. Comprehension, planning, health promotion and maintenance (b).
1 A balance of all nutrients provides a favorable environment for the developing fetus.
2 An adequate amount of calories is needed for protein utilization and fat metabolism.
3 Fluid intake facilitates the clearance of creatinine, urea, and other waste products of fetal and maternal metabolism.
4 A well-balanced diet is recommended for adequate metabolism.

36. Comprehension, planning, physiological integrity (b).
4 Evaluating each pregnancy individually will be necessary.
1 This would be possible but not guaranteed.
2 Pregnancy lasts only approximately 40 weeks.
3 A high-risk pregnancy would generally require starting weekly visits sooner.

37. Knowledge, planning, safe, effective care environment (c).
1 A disulfiram (Antabuse)-type reaction can occur, causing severe nausea and vomiting.
2, 4 No significant literature reports this occurring.
3 Because the two substances should not be taken together, this answer is not correct.

38. Comprehension, assessment, health promotion and maintenance (b).
1 This is appropriate for an infant at 24 weeks.
2 This is appropriate for a full-term infant.
3 This is appropriate at 16 weeks.
4 This is appropriate at 20 weeks

39. Comprehension, planning, physiological integrity (a).
1 As a result of the decreased glandular function of the skin in older adults, they have dryer, thinner, and extremely fragile skin. Older adults also tolerate extreme heat and extreme cold poorly.
2 Hot water can damage the skin, causing scalds.
3 This is not frequent enough.
4 Cold water would cause chilling and discomfort.

40. Application, planning, safe, effective care environment (b).
3 Monitoring vital signs is within the nursing assistant's scope of practice.
1 Documentation should be done by the individual who cared for the residents, presumably the nurse.
2 Administering medications is not within the scope of the nursing assistant.
4 The nurse should provide the input concerning the resident's care.

41. Comprehension, implementation, physiological integrity (c).
3 Fluid intake of at least 2400 ml should be encouraged to prevent crystalluria; the nurse should use terms the

patient will understand (3 quarts rather than 3 liters or 3000 ml).

1 Acyclovir (Zovirax) helps reduce the duration of the lesions but does not eradicate the virus.

2 The patient should be encouraged to complete the full prescribed course of the medication.

4 The medication will not protect a sexual partner from contracting the virus. The patient should be instructed to use condoms for or abstain from sexual intercourse.

42. Application, implementation, safe, effective care environment (b).

4 This is priority emergency care; the patient must have an intact airway before any other assessment can begin.

1 This may cause injury before the assessment.

2, 3 This is done after the patient's airway is secured.

43. Comprehension, planning, physiological integrity (b).

4 Nonselective beta-adrenergic blocking agents may affect the beta$_1$ receptors, leading to bronchoconstriction or bronchospasm, producing dyspnea.

1 Stimulation, rather than blocking, of the adrenergic receptors causes nervousness.

2 Photophobia is a result of pupil dilation as occurs with adrenergic stimulation, not blocking.

3 An increase in heart rate is caused by the simulation, rather than the blocking, of adrenergic receptors.

44. Application, assessment, physiological integrity (b).

2 The best way to assess for this patient problem is to actually watch the patient perform the activity.

1 Although helpful, this will not provide as much information as would watching the patient perform the activity.

3 This is an assessment that the nurse is capable of making.

4 This is descriptive, but it still does not provide as much information as would watching him perform the task.

45. Application, implementation, physiological integrity (c).

3 With an unconscious victim, the priority is the airway. To open the airway, the victim first has to be properly positioned.

1, 2, 4 These actions, though appropriate, are not done first, as indicated in the rationale for #3.

46. Application, planning, safe, effective care environment (b).

4 This is a true statement.

1 Medicare covers only some of the expenses, such as those that would necessitate highly skilled care.

2 Medicare generally covers skilled nursing services, some of which do not last 1 or 2 years.

3 Social Security payments will assist in paying for long-term care, but Medicaid pays for most of the care.

47. Comprehension, planning, physiological integrity (b).

2 Quadriceps-setting exercises improve the strength of muscles needed for walking.

1, 3, 4 These actions will not strengthen muscles, as indicated in #2.

48. Comprehension, implementation, physiological integrity (b).

1 Regular insulin is administered either intravenously or subcutaneously to treat the elevated blood glucose.

2 This is the recommended treatment for hypoglycemia.

3 An IV infusion should be initiated with a normal saline solution, not a dextrose solution.

4 Blood potassium levels should be monitored, but this is not a treatment.

49. Application, evaluation, physiological integrity (c).

3 Potassium is needed to allow the body to use insulin to metabolize glucose.

1, 2, 4 These electrolytes do not work with metabolism of glucose and insulin.

50. Application, implementation, physiological integrity (a).

3 The hemodynamic instability following burn injury must be stopped to proceed with airway, breathing, and circulation and to prevent further trauma to the victim.

1 The situation does not indicate that CPR is necessary.

2, 4 These are appropriate but not priorities.

51. Comprehension, planning, physiological integrity (a).

2 Thromboembolic problems are a postoperative complication of hip surgery. Low-dose aspirin reduces the risks of this complication.

1 This dose is too low for an antiinflammatory effect.

3, 4 These are not the primary purpose behind such an order.

52. Comprehension, assessment, psychosocial integrity (b).

2 The acute stage, disorganization, immediately follows sexual assault and is either verbally expressed or hidden. Regardless of the manner of expression, the survivor experiences feelings of shock, restlessness, anger, guilt, confusion, and fear.

1, 3 These usually follow acute disorganization and precede reorganization.

4 Reorganization indicates that the survivor has put the event in perspective and moves toward some degree of recovery.

53. Comprehension, planning, physiological integrity (a).

3 The patient's nonverbal responses may indicate pain or discomfort associated with the exercise.

1 The joint should not be exercised past the point of pain or stiffness to prevent joint injury.

2 Each exercise should be repeated at least two to five times; the number of repetitions varies among patients.

4 The exercises should be performed in a consistent order to prevent overlooking a joint.

54. Application, implementation, psychosocial integrity (b).

2 This behavior can be caused by anxiety over the unknown biopsy results.

1 This would be insulting to the patient.

3 The nurse needs to acknowledge the behavior.

4 The nurse needs to address the behavior.

55. Comprehension, assessment, physiological integrity (b).

2 This is a frequent symptom with prostate enlargement.

1 This is more common with bladder carcinoma or upper urinary tract infection.

3 This is more common with a urinary tract infection.

4 This symptom is vague; nausea may occur with various disease states.

56. Comprehension, planning, psychosocial integrity (b).

4 Exercise will help the patient burn calories and use energy.

1, 2 These require the patient to be still and concentrate.

3 This is not as good a choice and may be too focused.

57. Application, implementation, safe, effective care environment (a).

4 Nurses always write the orders as the physician gives orders and then repeat the orders for verification.

1 Orders are written as given then repeated for verification.

2 Telephone orders are signed by the nurse receiving the order with the physician counter-signing the order within a specified time period.

3 The steps are to write the orders as the physician is giving the order, verify the orders, then make sure the patient's name appears on the order sheet. The next of kin is not information found on the order sheet.

58. Comprehension, assessment, psychosocial integrity (b).

1 Compulsive behavior helps the patient cope with the anxiety.

2 This is normal, not an obsession.

3, 4 These do not address specific activities.

59. Application, evaluation, physiological integrity (b).

2 Postural drainage helps drain sections of the lung, aids in coughing and removing secretions, and improves breathing.

1 High-Fowler's position (45- to 90-degree elevation) is most effective in relieving dyspnea.

3 Fluids should be forced to liquefy secretions.

4 Patient should have rest and conserve energy.

60. Knowledge, evaluation, physiological integrity (a).

1 Sedation is a common side effect of Haldol.

2 Weight gain is more common.

3 Dry mouth is not a common side effect.

4 Agitation is seen with an overdose.

61. Comprehension, assessment, physiological integrity (a).

1 Circulation and sensation are periodically assessed to determine the presence of pressure areas that may obstruct circulation and nerve pathways.

2, 3, 4 These are inappropriate actions.

62. Application, planning, physiological integrity (b).

4 Diminished caliber or force (or both) of urinary stream and a feeling of incomplete bladder emptying are common complaints.

1, 2 These are more common with urinary tract infections.

3 This is unrelated to the situation.

63. Knowledge, planning, safe, effective care environment (a).

1 The gold standard for administering medications is the five rights: the right drug, dose, patient, route, and time.

2 Five rights are presented in this response, although many consider the documentation as the sixth right.

3 Hospital policy should be followed but is not considered one of the components in the standard.

4 This is an inaccurate response.

64. Comprehension, assessment, psychosocial integrity (b).

1 Safety is always a number one priority.

2 Ability to perform self-care is unknown.

3 This is a problem but not as much a priority compared with safety.

4 He is hearing voices, but safety is more important.

65. Application, assessment, physiological integrity (b).

4 This is correct. The creatinine clearance increases as renal function diminishes.

1, 2, 3 These may be indications of renal function, anemia, or infection, but not GFR.

66. Application, implementation, safe, effective care environment (b).

1 This victim requires immediate medical care.

2 This is appropriate but not the first priority.

3 This is inappropriate; the victim needs immediate medical care.

4 Referring a victim to a physician does not put the nurse at legal risk; *not* referring a victim to a physician can result in legal action being initiated against the nurse.

67. Comprehension, assessment, physiological integrity (b).

2 Although any stimulation can cause this phenomenon to occur, the most common are a full bladder, full bowel, and wrinkled sheets.

1, 3, 4 Skin stimulation may be a stimulus and needs to be done gently, as when taking vital signs. Visitors may unknowingly cause a draft, which may stimulate this reaction.

68. Comprehension, assessment, physiological integrity (b).

1 Hypoventilation reduces O_2 to the alveoli and reduces CO_2 elimination. The retained CO_2 then combines with water to form an excess of carbonic acid (H_2CO_3), decreasing the blood pH. As a result, concentration of hydrogen ions in body fluids, which directly reflects acidity, increases.

2 The lungs excrete CO_2 and water. The rate of excretion of CO_2 is controlled by the respiratory center in the medulla of the brain. If increased amounts of CO_2 or hydrogens are present, the respiratory center stimulates an increased rate and depth of breathing.

3, 4 The lungs excrete CO_2 and water, which are byproducts of cellular metabolism.

69. Comprehension, planning, physiological integrity (c).

1 This is an outcome-criteria statement.

2 This is a nursing intervention.

3 This is an appropriate nursing diagnosis.

4 This is an appropriate evaluation statement.

70. Knowledge, planning, physiological integrity (a).

1 15:2 is correct for two-rescuer CPR.

2 This would be too few compressions for two-rescuer CPR.

3 This would be too few ventilations for two-rescuer CPR.

4 This would be too few ventilations and too few compressions for two-rescuer CPR.

71. Application, planning, physiological integrity (c).

3 Assessment of motor function includes muscle movement, size, tone, strength, and coordination of muscle groups.

1 Cranial nerve VIII is responsible for hearing; cranial nerves IX and X are responsible for the gag reflex and ability to speak. Cranial nerve XI allows the person to raise the shoulders, and cranial nerve XII allows movement of the tongue.

2 Body positioning is evaluated during the inspection portion of the assessment; mental status and level of consciousness are assessed throughout the examination and are not specific to motor function.

4 Intellectual functions and speech patterns are components of a neurological examination but are not included in the motor function assessment.

72. Comprehension, planning, physiological integrity (b).

4 Cheese and crackers provide enough complex carbohydrates to sustain the person through the activity.

1 This provides a rapid form of glucose that would not sustain the person.

2 This rapidly acting form of glucose is best taken during a hypoglycemic episode.

3 A can of soda, sweetened, would not sustain the person through the activity.
73. Comprehension, implementation, physiological integrity (b).
   2 Rest and avoidance of heaving lifting or strenuous activity promote healing and decrease intraabdominal pressures to the puncture site. Heavy lifting or strenuous exercise may precipitate a bleeding episode. Large volumes of blood can be lost should bleeding occur; therefore prompt medical attention is required.
   1 The bandage can be changed in 24 hours; the puncture is expected to be sore for several days, however progressive.
   3 Tub baths are contraindicated until the puncture site is healed because of placing undue stress at the puncture site.
   4 Driving and climbing stairs are contraindicated for 24 hours following catheterization because of an increased risk of bleeding.
74. Application, planning, safe effective and safe, effective care environment (b).
   3 Chicken salad is a protein food and would be restricted in someone with elevated ammonia levels.
   1 Pretzels would not be restricted for a person with this diagnosis.
   2 Although cheese does contain some protein, chicken salad would more likely be restricted.
   4 A bowl of ice cream is mostly fat and carbohydrates and would not be restricted.
75. Knowledge, assessment, physiological integrity (b).
   2 CK-MB is found mainly in cardiac muscle and rises 4 to 12 hours after infarction, peaks in 24 hours, and returns to normal in 3 to 4 days.
   1 The white blood cell count may be elevated by the third day because of the inflammatory response. This test is not specific, however, to myocardial infarction.
   3 This is a test used primarily to screen for disseminated intravascular coagulation (DIC).
   4 This is a test useful in the diagnosis of several disorders: anemia, cardiomyopathy, congestive heart failure, delirium tremens, hypothyroidism, inflammation, leukemia, muscle injury, myxedema, pulmonary infarction, and renal infarction. LDH will be elevated 24 to 48 hours after infarction, peaks in 3 to 6 days, and returns to normal in 7 to 14 days.
76. Comprehension, implementation, physiological integrity (b).
   4 The patient should be placed in low- or semi-Fowler's position to decrease strain on the sutures.
   1 The supine position would lead to increased edema of the neck, which would compromise the patient's airway.
   2 Placing the patient in left lateral Sims' position has no benefit.
   3 Trendelenberg's position would compromise the airway and place undue strain on the suture line.
77. Comprehension, assessment, physiological integrity (c).
   3 With left-sided heart failure, blood becomes backed up in the lungs causing crackles or fluid in the lungs.
   1 Nausea is not normally associated with heart failure.
   2 An extra heart sound (S3) may be heard, but it is not the sound of a murmur.
   4 Right ventricular heart failure would result in peripheral edema.

78. Comprehension, planning, physiological integrity (b).
   4 Oral agents are useful in treating diabetes when some beta-cell function still exists.
   1 Obesity is not a measurement for beta-cell function.
   2 The liver clears most agents, but this fact is unrelated to the need for functioning beta cells.
   3 Type 1 diabetes usually is associated with no beta-cell function.
79. Knowledge, implementation, health promotion and maintenance (a).
   4 At this age, the baby should be able to follow bright lights and moving objects.
   1 Vision is 20/100 at 1 year of age. Because vision is not yet normal, this is the age at which babies keep bumping into things.
   2 Visual acuity is approximately 20/300, and babies can see only at a very close range.
   3 By 9 to 10 months of age, depth perception is developing.
80. Application, planning, physiological integrity (a).
   1 The patient is at high risk for a decubitus ulcer. Sensory loss prevents perception of pain and pressure, the warning signs of tissue injury. If the patient is able, encourage patient involvement.
   2 This is inappropriate; adequate calcium intake is essential for all individuals.
   3 This is inappropriate and is not relative to the situation.
   4 This is not individualized to persons with sensory or motor loss.
81. Application, implementation, physiological integrity (b).
   3 The clot may dislodge itself; bright-red or darker color may indicate hemorrhage.
   1 This would cause painful bladder spasms.
   2 This may increase the patient's anxiety. The coughing may also increase the patient's discomfort.
   4 This may increase the patient's discomfort. He is already at risk for fluid and electrolyte imbalance because of absorption of the irrigation fluid.
82. Knowledge, implementation, safe, effective care environment (a).
   2 Chlorpromazine makes skin sensitive to sunlight.
   1 This is related to MAOIs.
   3, 4 These are not related.
83. Knowledge, assessment, physiological integrity (a).
   1 This answer is accurate. Other behaviors include sleepiness, very short attention span, and the person is able to respond verbally. Patient fends off painful stimuli with purposeful movement.
   2 This is descriptive of deep coma state.
   3, 4 These answers are descriptive of stuporous state.
84. Comprehension, planning, physiological integrity (a).
   1 Pattern is essential with retraining.
   2 The patient need not understand the program for the program to be successful.
   3 Laxatives are never used with bowel retraining.
   4 Regular days and times must be strictly followed to establish a pattern.
85. Comprehension, implementation, physiological integrity (a).
   3 These are known as hyperosmolar drugs. Mannitol (Osmitrol) is an example. These agents draw water from the edematous brain.
   1 These should be used carefully; they may mask level of consciousness or cause respiratory distress.

2 These may be ordered if nausea is present.

4 These may be ordered if open wound is caused by trauma.

86. Application, implementation, physiological integrity (a).

   3 These will not increase systemic blood pressure because they are not resistive.

   1, 2 These are unsafe; they cause sudden increase in blood pressure and intracranial pressure.

   4 This is unsafe and may cause flexion of hips or neck, or both. Both of these positions may cause sudden increase in intracranial pressure.

87. Knowledge, implementation, physiological integrity (b).

   1 The first step in treating hemorrhage is to apply pressure for at least 6 minutes.

   2 Application of ice is not an emergency measure.

   3 Elevating the affected part aids in controlling the bleeding but would not stop the bleeding.

   4 This action would have no effect on occipital bleeding.

88. Application, implementation, safe, effective care environment (b).

   3 This is correct according to the 1993 changes instituted by the American Heart Association.

   1 This is incorrect; eight back blows and eight chest thrusts were never a recommended sequence for obstructed airway in an infant.

   2 This is incorrect; six back blows and six chest thrusts were never a recommended sequence for obstructed airway in an infant.

   4 This is incorrect; four back blows and four chest thrusts were the recommended sequence for obstructed airway in an infant *before the changes instituted early in 1993.*

89. Comprehension, implementation, physiological integrity (a).

   3 Hydration and lying flat for 4 to 6 hours help individuals who may develop a spinal headache. This response addresses her concerns and gives a plan of action.

   1 This is not a proven fact. Some individuals will develop a headache.

   2 Staying prone versus supine does not give any additional benefit. It may increase patient's apprehension because she may be fearful of moving. This is not a comfortable position to maintain.

   4 While advances have occurred in medicine this response does not allay the individual's apprehension about getting a headache following the procedure.

90. Application, planning, physiological integrity (b).

   1 Delayed wound healing is common in older adults because of nutritional problems.

   2, 3, 4 These intervention are appropriate, regardless of the patient's age.

91. Comprehension, assessment, physiological integrity (a).

   4 An immediate physical observation of a person burned in the area of the face is assessment of respiration (difficulty, rate, sound).

   1, 2, 3 These are not immediate physical observations during an emergency.

92. Comprehension, evaluation, physiological integrity (a).

   3 Being able to perform activities of daily living indicates that activity tolerance is increasing.

   1 Anxiety is most likely related to being unable to breathe.

2 This is related to a knowledge deficit diagnosis.

4 This is related to an ineffective airway clearance problem.

93. Comprehension, implementation, physiological integrity (c).

   4 This action will prevent further injury to the fingers.

   1, 2 These actions are contraindicated.

   3 The frostbitten parts should not be used.

94. Comprehension, implementation, physiological integrity (a).

   3 The splint should be applied above and below the fracture.

   1, 2 Although this is important, no indications of these problems exist.

   4 Although the fracture should be elevated, lying flat is unnecessary.

95. Application, implementation, physiological integrity (c).

   1 The priority is always airway, breathing, and circulation.

   2 Although important, this is not the priority.

   3 This is necessary and important but not the priority.

   4 A person cannot breathe unless the airway is patent.

96. Comprehension, implementation, physiological integrity (b).

   3 As long as 12 weeks may be required for antidepressants to achieve their full therapeutic effect.

   1 Fluids need not be limited while taking antidepressants.

   2 Dry mouth and orthostatic hypotension are common, bothersome side effects of antidepressants.

   4 If the first antidepressant fails to control depression, other effective medications are available.

97. Knowledge, planning, physiological integrity (b).

   1 Chewing and daily ear hygiene aid in the removal of cerumen.

   2 This may be necessary; however, it subjects the patient to a procedure that can be prevented through health-promoting habits.

   3 This allows for hydration, but it is not directly related to cerumen buildup.

   4 This may damage the hearing aid.

98. Knowledge, planning, safe, effective care environment (c).

   2 Alternatives to restraints should be tried before resorting to restraints.

   1 Restraints are to be used only for a specific period.

   3 Restraints should be removed at least every 2 hours to allow for activities of daily living.

   4 Restraints should be tied with knots that can be quickly released and secured to parts of the bed that move with the patient.

99. Comprehension, planning, physiological integrity (b).

   2 Ambulation stimulates circulation and prevents the formation of thrombi, besides aiding in breaking up clots.

   1 This is to relieve pain, promote healing, and prevent infection.

   3 Splinting helps diminish pain and discomfort.

   4 Keeping urinary functions at a maximum aids in promoting involution, and offering stool softeners relieves initial pain and discomfort during the postpartum period.

100. Application, planning, physiological integrity (c).

   1 Focusing specifically on rehabilitation and the elements involved and rationale should expedite recovery by gaining the patient's cooperation.

   2 This is common in normal preoperative teaching.

3 This information would be given to any individual before surgery.

4 This is common information for any individual before surgery.

101. Knowledge, implementation, physiological integrity (a).

2 This is the first priority.

1 This is not first priority.

3 The physician knows; it is not necessary to do test unless the nurse is asked to do so.

4 Pads are not used during labor and delivery.

102. Application, assessment, physiological integrity (b).

3 Diaphoresis is one of the first symptoms of hypoglycemia. Hypoglycemia would result when taking insulin without eating or from a sudden increase in activity or body demands, such as during illness, surgery, or stress.

1 Polydipsia is a symptom of hyperglycemia.

2 This is a late sign of both hyperglycemia and hypoglycemia. The nurse needs to assess for early signs to intervene before this occurs.

4 This is a symptom of hyperglycemia.

103. Application, assessment, physiological integrity (b).

3 As the heart fails, circulating blood backs up into the pulmonary tree; a sign of congestion is crackles in the lung bases.

1 Although fluid does build up in pneumonia, given the patient's history, the crackles most likely signify the beginning of heart failure.

2 Dysrhythmias are not assessed by listening to lung sounds. A heart monitor, change in vital signs, or patient symptoms will alert the nurse to this complication.

4 This does not normally manifest itself as crackles in the lungs. Increased complaints of chest pain or changes in vital signs would alert the nurse to an extension of the myocardial infarction.

104. Comprehension, assessment, physiological integrity (a).

3 These signs are normal for a 2-day-old newborn.

1 This is a full-term infant thus she cannot be premature.

2 No indication in the situation exists that the infant is premature.

4 Nothing abnormal is reported in the situation.

105. Comprehension, planning, physiological integrity (b).

1 Safety should come first. In this patient's case, use of Maslow's hierarchy of needs is appropriate.

2 Safety should be the first priority.

3 Answer #1 is the better choice. The situation did not indicate that pain was present. Assessment of respiratory function would be more appropriate and more individualized.

4 Safety should be the first priority.

106. Knowledge, assessment, physiological integrity (b).

4 The hemoglobin is decreased, not increased, in sickle cell crisis.

1, 2, 3 These are common symptoms of sickle cell crisis.

107. Knowledge, assessment, physiological integrity (a).

3 Toxic levels (laboratory value of theophylline 20 μ/ml) are accompanied by these signs. The patient may also have palpitations or develop seizures.

1, 2, 4 These are not typical side effects of theophylline and bronchodilators.

108. Application, assessment, physiological integrity (b).

4 Excessive urination is one of the classic signs and symptoms that blood sugar levels may be abnormal.

1 Refusing to bathe is no indication that diabetes is out of control.

2 A cough does not indicate that diabetes needs to be checked.

3 One diarrhea stool last week does not need further assessment.

109. Comprehension, assessment, health promotion and maintenance (b).

1 Neck pain, decreased neck mobility caused by pain, and upper extremity motor or sensory changes are common symptoms.

2 This may be a symptom of lumbar involvement.

3 This may also be a symptom of lumbar involvement.

4 Muscle atrophy of this group is not a finding when the cervical region is involved.

110. Application, implementation, physiological integrity (b).

4 Some diuretics, such as Lasix, are ototoxic and can cause tinnitus and dizziness.

1 This is most unlikely; the tinnitus should not affect her ability to drive.

2 This would not alleviate the patient's concern and is an untrue statement.

3 The tinnitus is caused by the ototoxicity of the diuretic.

111. Knowledge, evaluation, physiological integrity (b).

1 Ditropan acts by exerting a direct antispasmodic effect on smooth-muscle tissue, such as that found in the bladder.

2 Cholinergic drugs are helpful with an atonic bladder.

3 Propantheline bromide is used for complaints of urinary frequency and urgency.

4 Trimethoprim sulfamethoxazole is an antiinfective.

112. Comprehension, assessment, physiological integrity (b).

4 Anticoagulants can cause blood to be present in urine.

1 Diuretics alter the urine quantity output.

2 Pyridium will alter the urine color to a red or orange color but will not test positive for blood.

3 Macrodantin alters the color of urine to a harmless brown.

113. Knowledge, implementation, physiological integrity (a).

3 Sternal compression is performed approximately the width of one finger below the nipple level.

1, 2 These positions are too high.

4 This is the position for children and adults.

114. Application, assessment, health promotion and maintenance (b).

4 These are common assessment findings in peritonitis.

1 This symptom is common in several conditions but not in peritonitis.

2 Reduced urine output may occur as a late symptom if the infection is not controlled.

3 Frequent stool or diarrhea is not a common assessment finding.

115. Knowledge, assessment, physiological integrity (a).

2 Cholesterol is found in blood and body cells, especially brain and nerve tissue.

1 It should not nor can it be eliminated totally from the diet.

3 It is necessary for normal body functioning.

4 It is mainly through animal sources—meat, eggs, saturated fats.

116. Application, implementation, physiological integrity (a).

3 The patient is displaying signs of hypovolemia. Initial measures would be those for treating shock. Turning the patient on the side helps prevent aspiration.

1 Monitoring vital signs is important; application of a cool cloth is a later measure.

2 Sips of water are inappropriate if patient is going into shock.

4 Decreasing the room temperature is not relative to the situation; turning the patient on the side helps prevent aspiration.

117. Comprehension, planning, psychosocial integrity (c).

1 Modesty and sensitivity are of prime importance to this age group.

2, 4 This is part of the normal admission procedure for any age group.

3 This is not the case for this age group.

118. Application, planning, physiological integrity (b).

3 This complaint can be life threatening and is a priority.

1 This blood glucose level does need to be corrected; however, respiratory status takes priority.

2 This small laceration will need to be attended to at some time; however, the shortness of breath is of primary importance.

4 While it is important to keep the family calm and informed, the patient's complaints of "shortness of breath" is priority.

119. Comprehension, assessment, physiological integrity (c).

4 Older adults have a higher percentage of body fat, which affects the metabolism and storage of medications.

1 Older adults have a lower percentage of body water.

2 Older adults have a decrease in lean muscle mass.

3 Older adults have a higher percentage of body fat.

120. Comprehension, evaluation, physiological integrity (c).

1 Bounding pulse, dyspnea, and cough are symptoms of heart failure caused by the inability of the heart to pump excessive IV fluid volume.

2 These are symptoms of IV infiltration.

3 These are symptoms of phlebitis.

4 These are symptoms of a systemic infection.

121. Comprehension, implementation, safe, effective care environment (b).

2 Handling the glove on the inside guarantees that the nurse's bare, nonsterile hand will not contaminate the sterile exterior of the glove.

1 Contamination occurs if the nurse's nonsterile hand touches the sterile exterior of the glove.

3 Keeping the gloves on the sterile field throughout the gloving procedure risks contamination of the field.

4 Contamination occurs if the nonsterile hand touches the outside of the glove.

122. Application, assessment, safe, effective care environment (a).

2 Pulse rate is below 60 beats/minute.

1, 3, 4 These can lead to adverse reactions.

123. Application, planning, safe, effective care environment (b).

2 This is an expected outcome of the nursing action that should occur within a short period.

1 This is a nursing intervention; it outlines the actual nursing activity.

3 This is a long-term goal, outlining the overall purpose of the nursing action.

4 This is a rationale because it explains why the action is being implemented.

124. Application, implementation, physiological integrity (a).

DD = 4 mg DH = 10 mg V = 1 ml DD/DH = 4 mg/10 mg × 1 ml = 0.4 ml.

125. Application, implementation, safe, effective care environment (a).

Weight in pounds (30) × adult dose (10 mg)/150 = 300/150 = 2 mg.

Part 1

This examination contains individual questions, the majority of which relate to clinical situations. Read all questions carefully. Each question has only *one best answer*.

Test time allotment (Part 1): approximately 2 hours

Answers and rationales begin on p. 651.

1. The preoperative injection order reads, "Meperidine (Demerol) 35 mg and Atropine 0.1 mg IM." The meperidine is supplied at 50 mg/ml, and the atropine at 0.2 mg/ml. What volume of meperidine and atropine should the nurse administer?
   1 Meperidine 0.35 ml, atropine 0.5 ml
   2 Meperidine 0.6 ml, atropine 0.4 ml
   3 Meperidine 0.7 ml, atropine 0.5 ml
   4 Meperidine 0.85 ml, atropine 0.1 ml

2. Nursing intervention for the child in sickle cell crisis is directed primarily toward:
   1 Maintaining active range of motion
   2 Oxygen therapy
   3 Administering blood
   4 Maintaining adequate hydration

3. A nurse is assessing a patient's intravenous (IV) site and administration set. Which of the following requires corrective action by the nurse?
   1 The IV site is clean and dry
   2 Fluid is in the IV container
   3 The tubing was changed 5 days ago
   4 No swelling or redness is present at the site

4. Which bandage turn should the nurse use when wrapping a joint, such as the elbow?
   1 Figure-of-eight
   2 Recurrent
   3 Spiral
   4 Circular

5. A patient is in respiratory alkalosis. Which of the following would assist this patient to increase his arterial carbon dioxide partial pressure ($PaCO_2$)?
   1 Suctioning
   2 Postural drainage with cupping and clapping
   3 Administering oxygen via nasal cannula
   4 Using a rebreathing mask

6. A patient who performs home glucose testing tells the nurse that she can never seem to get enough blood from her finger to do the test. Which of the following methods should the nurse recommend that the patient try so as to increase blood flow to the fingertips?
   1 "Milk the finger down toward the fingertips."
   2 "Hold your fingers in the air for a few minutes before the test."
   3 "Apply a warm, moist compress over the fingers a few minutes before the test."
   4 "Collect blood from more than one finger to get enough blood for the test."

7. A patient who is recovering from a respiratory condition is confined to bed rest. In which of the following positions should the nurse place the patient to facilitate the best respiratory effort?
   1 Sims'
   2 Supine
   3 Low-Fowler's
   4 High-Fowler's

8. A patient was recently admitted to the hospital for treatment of congestive heart failure. Her admitting blood pressure was 188/96 mm Hg. She has been taking Monopril 30 mg every day for 3 days. Now, she must take her dose of Monopril. The nurse finds her diaphoretic, pale, and weak. Her pulse is 96 beats per minute (bpm) and her blood pressure is 96/56 mm Hg. She is alert and talking. The nurse should first:
   1 Position her in a supine position with her legs elevated
   2 Call the physician
   3 Administer the Monopril
   4 Place her in a high-Fowler's position

9. A patient has been diagnosed with Guillian-Barre syndrome. He is unable to turn his head, and his shoulders are drooping. The nurse informs the physician that she suspects involvement of which of the following cranial nerves?
   1 VII
   2 V
   3 XI
   4 IX

10. Blood urea nitrogen (BUN) and creatinine levels are useful in determining if damage has occurred in the:
    1 Liver
    2 Kidneys
    3 Muscles
    4 Intestines

11. A patient has end-stage cancer secondary to cancer of the colon. He is having difficulty with pain control. The nurse should:
    1 Administer narcotics indiscriminately
    2 Assess the effect of each pain intervention with a 1-to-10 scale
    3 Instruct him on the use of guided imagery
    4 Increase his fluid allowance

12. Which of the following methods would be the best way for the nurse to determine the effectiveness of preoperative teaching?
    1 Have the patient verbalize what has been taught
    2 Have the patient take a written, comprehensive quiz
    3 Ask the patient to teach another patient how to do the skill
    4 Ask the patient to perform the skill for you, describing each step

13. A patient has a history of tonic-clonic seizures. Which of the following would best describe an aura that she may experience immediately before a seizure?
    1 Extreme anxiety
    2 Brief loss of consciousness
    3 Automatic repetitive movements
    4 Sensation of weakness or numbness

14. Which of the following immediate postoperative orders would a nurse question for a patient who has received spinal anesthesia?
    1 Encourage fluids
    2 Bathroom privileges in the mornings
    3 Clear fluids, advance diet as tolerated
    4 Keep head of bed elevated at 45 degrees

15. Which of the following facts reported by a patient with Parkinson's disease would indicate to the nurse that the patient has a basic understanding of his disease process?
    1 Autosomal dominant genetic disorder
    2 Progressive, fatal disease caused by a virus
    3 Chronic progressive hereditary disease of the nervous system
    4 Progressive damage to neurons that regulate and control movement

16. When a patient is stressed and the sympathetic nervous system is activated, the heart responds by:
    1 Slowing the conduction cycle
    2 Decreasing cardiac output
    3 Increasing cardiac output
    4 Stopping the beats

17. A nurse responds to a resident's call bell and finds the patient standing at the bedside in a puddle of urine, with his pajamas soaked. Which of the following is the most appropriate response by the nurse?
    1 "Not again. You may need to wear Attends from now on."
    2 "Now look what you've done. Let's go to the bathroom again."
    3 "Next time, wait for help before getting out of bed. That's why I'm here."
    4 "Let's go to the bathroom where you can wash up and put on clean pajamas."

18. When contributing to the nursing care plan, the nurse knows that an example of a short-term goal is:
    1 Assisting the patient in range-of-motion exercises
    2 The patient will transfer from bed to chair this week
    3 The patient will return to the previous level of functioning
    4 Physical activity will improve muscle tone and function

19. Which of the following activities is *most* appropriate for a patient with Alzheimer's disease who is demonstrating increasing difficulty with planning and decision making?
    1 Sorting the laundry
    2 Hoeing the garden
    3 Planning the dinner menu
    4 Writing out the grocery list

20. A pregnant patient delivers quickly and without complications. The patient's husband arrives and is taken to the recovery room to see his wife. After visiting with her for a while, he asks to see the baby. It would be *best* for the nurse to suggest that:
    1 He go to the nursery to see the baby and let his wife sleep
    2 He visit with his wife for a while, then go home and see both his wife and the baby the next morning
    3 The baby can be brought to the parents so they can begin the attachment process
    4 Both parents go to the nursery to see the baby

21. An 89-year-old patient is alert and active. During her annual physical examination, she complains of hemorrhoids and annoying constipation. Her physician instructs her to increase her fluid and dietary fiber intake. Which of the following snacks, if selected by the patient, would indicate that she can identify food sources that are high in fiber?
    1 Cucumbers
    2 Apple juice
    3 Bran cereal
    4 Small banana

22. A young female patient comes to the clinic stating that she has missed a menstrual period. During her visit, she tells the nurse that her last menstrual cycle was normal with a moderate amount of flow; it began on February 5 and ended February 11. Using Nagele's rule, the nurse is able to calculate that her estimated date of confinement (EDC) would be:
    1 November 18
    2 November 12
    3 November 4
    4 October 29

23. Which of the following measures should be reinforced in the discharge teaching plan for an older adult recovering from a total knee replacement?
    1 Full weight bearing on the affected leg
    2 Non–weight bearing on the affected leg
    3 Weight bearing only as tolerated by the patient
    4 Weight bearing only as prescribed by the physician

24. A 6-week-old infant is admitted for surgical repair of a cleft lip. Vital signs are temperature, 100.8°F (38.2°C); pulse rate, 90 bpm; respirations, 36/min; blood pressure, 70/35 mm Hg. Which vital sign is abnormal, and what should the nurse do about it?
    1 Respirations: call the anesthesiologist
    2 Pulse rate: notify the anesthesiologist
    3 Temperature: notify the admitting physician
    4 Blood pressure: notify the admitting physician

25. A 79-year-old nursing home resident is confused. Which of the following nursing measures would best reduce his confusion?
    1 Placing a weekly activity calendar in his room
    2 Speaking clearly, calmly, and in short sentences
    3 Leaving him alone and letting him do what he wants
    4 Explaining the planned daily activities to him each morning

26. An 86-year-old resident in a nursing home has rheumatoid arthritis, resulting in severe deformities of both hands. Her medications are prednisone (Prednisone) 5 mg oral (PO) daily and auranofin (Ridaura) 2 mg PO twice daily. The resident refuses her daily dose of prednisone. Which of the following actions should the nurse take?
    1 Chart the refusal in the nurses' notes and inform the head nurse
    2 Chart "*refused*" on the medication sheet and report it to the physician
    3 Return to the patient in 30 minutes and offer her the medication again
    4 Call the physician and get an order for an injectable adrenocorticosteroid

27. A female patient with Alzheimer's disease, who has been looking through the window at the garden outside, suddenly becomes agitated when another patient approaches. Which of the following actions is most beneficial?
    1 Offering a high-protein drink
    2 Sending the patient to her room
    3 Turning the day room television on
    4 Taking the patient for a walk outside

28. Identical twins and fraternal twins were delivered. Which of the following explanations distinguishes the type of twins delivered if one was a boy and the other a girl?
    1 Monozygotic or single ovum twins: union of one sperm and one ovum

2 Dizygotic or double ovum twins: union of two sperm and two ovum

3 Type of twins, either identical or fraternal, can be determined only by blood tests

4 Type of twins, either identical or fraternal, can be determined only by deoxyribonucleic acid (DNA) tests

29. Along with close monitoring, which nursing action is most essential to a patient scheduled for induction of labor?
1 Hydrating with oral fluids
2 Providing emotional support
3 Placing a "NO VISITORS" sign on the door
4 Keeping the room temperature at a low setting

30. The diagnosis of Hirschsprung's disease is usually confirmed by a:
1 Rectal biopsy
2 Upper gastrointestinal series
3 Esophagoscopy
4 Gastroscopy

31. To promote a safe environment for a patient who is blind, which of the following nursing measures is most appropriate?
1 Leaving the door ajar
2 Providing privacy at mealtime
3 Explaining the location of the call light
4 Rearranging the furnishings in the room

32. A 37-year-old male patient has been diagnosed with multiple sclerosis. To relieve fear and anxiety, which nursing action should be implemented *first?*
1 Establishing a routine schedule
2 Explaining the disease in detail
3 Initiating measures to prevent falls
4 Involving the family in the care plan

33. A 2-month-old newborn presents at the pediatrician's office with a 2-week history of paroxysmal abdominal cramping. Her mother states that her child has been fussy and cries as if she were in pain but has been tolerating normal amounts of formula. The infant has gained weight since her last visit. These signs and symptoms indicate:
1 Intussusception
2 Colic
3 Pyloric stenosis
4 Hirschsprung's disease

34. When using a heat lamp, the nurse should:
1 Keep the skin damp during treatment
2 Cover the lamp with a pillowcase after positioning it
3 Position the lamp 18 to 24 inches from the area being treated
4 Assess the patient every 30 minutes

35. An 18-month-old toddler has been diagnosed with developmental dysplasia of the right hip and will be hospitalized for surgery and application of a hip spica cast. Which of the following measures will be essential when caring for this child?
1 Avoiding administering pain medication as much as possible to prevent constipation
2 Limiting fluids so she will be less likely to get the cast wet when she voids
3 Informing the parents to prop her on pillows, with her legs down, when taking her home in the car
4 Assessing sensation, circulation, and motion of her feet and toes

36. Following a physician's order, which one of the medications listed would a nurse most likely administer to terminate status epilepticus in a patient?
1 Diazepam (Valium)
2 Doxazosin (Cardura)
3 Phenytoin (Dilantin)
4 Buprenorphine (Buprenex)

37. The most notable symptoms that a nurse would observe in a 13-month-old toddler with meningitis would be:
1 Weak or absent cry, coma
2 Bulging fontanel, irritability
3 Absent reflexes, rigid joints
4 Dilated and fixed pupils

38. A patient with a new colostomy should be instructed on methods to prevent skin breakdown, including which of the following?
1 Shaving the area clean with a regular razor before applying the pouch
2 Using tincture of benzoin as a skin barrier
3 Performing a patch test for allergies to new skin products
4 Washing the stoma area several times a day with soap and water

39. An 18-month-old toddler is admitted to the hospital for a bilateral myringotomy resulting from frequent occurrences of otitis media. This condition occurs more frequently in younger children than it does in older children because of the different position and shape of the child's:
1 Esophagus
2 Eustachian tubes
3 External ear canals
4 Tympanic membranes

40. A patient is admitted for a colon resection. During the admitting assessment, the patient explains that she has a history of malignant hyperthermia. The nurse would:
1 Administer dantrolene (Dantrium) before the surgery
2 Notify the anesthesiologist
3 Serve only cold foods and water preoperatively
4 Take her temperature and record

41. A nurse is caring for a child who weighs 25 lb. The usual dose for ampicillin for children is 100 mg/kg/day. Which of the following would be an appropriate order for this child?
1 Ampicillin 25 mg every 4 hours
2 Ampicillin 250 mg four times daily
3 Ampicillin 100mg every 6 hours
4 Ampicillin 100 mg four times daily

42. When applying antiembolism stockings, the nurse would apply the stockings:
1 Before the patient arises
2 2 hours after the patient arises
3 Following the patient's bath
4 While the patient is sitting in a chair

43. A patient has chronic renal failure. Which of the following laboratory results would the nurse anticipate being below normal?
1 Calcium levels
2 White blood cell count
3 Creatinine
4 BUN

44. A patient has undergone a cardiac catheterization this morning. Which of the following nursing interventions is most important during the first 4 to 6 hours after the procedure?
    1 Immobilizing the involved leg
    2 Maintaining the extremity used for the procedure in a flexed position
    3 Keeping the extremity elevated on at least two pillows
    4 Limiting the intake of fluids

45. A patient is admitted following a stroke, with damage to the right side of the brain and middle cerebral artery involvement. Which of the following behaviors are typical of this type of stroke?
    1 Aphasia
    2 Dysphasia
    3 Right-sided paralysis
    4 Inability to remember words

46. A nurse was exposed to active tuberculosis last week. She had a purified protein derivative (PPD) test done immediately after discovery of exposure, but she knows she will need to be retested to see if she is positive for the infection. The second PPD test should be done:
    1 1 week later
    2 1 month later
    3 3 months later
    4 12 months later

47. A 19-year-old student has had a nephrectomy. The physician recommends that he withdraw from being an active member of the college football team. The reason for this recommendation is that:
    1 At least a year is required to recover from surgery
    2 Major back, abdominal, and flank muscles have been compromised
    3 He might injure the remaining kidney during play
    4 The remaining kidney will not be able to meet the demands of his body

48. The three primary factors that influence the management of diabetes are:
    1 Diet, medication, rest
    2 Diet, rest, exercise
    3 Diet, medication, exercise
    4 Rest, exercise, medication

49. A patient is admitted for possible obstructive urinary retention caused by an enlarged prostate gland. The nurse is preparing him for a cystourethroscopy with balloon dilation. When preparing him for the procedure and in planning his care, the nurse should inform him to expect:
    1 Impotence
    2 Significant pain
    3 General anesthesia
    4 A Foley catheter

50. A patient is admitted to the emergency room with diabetic ketoacidosis (DKA), the most common cause of which is:
    1 Stress
    2 Infection
    3 Not enough food
    4 Too much insulin

51. A patient who had a mastectomy for breast cancer is receiving prednisone as part of her therapy. The nurse will instruct her to observe for which of the following side effects?
    1 Hypotension
    2 Weight gain
    3 Dehydration
    4 Increase in muscle mass

52. The nurse is assigned to ambulate a patient who is non–weight bearing on the right. Physical therapy taught her how to use a three-point crutch gait. Which of the following indicates that the patient is performing the gait correctly?
    1 The patient advances the crutches then advances both legs
    2 The patient advances the crutches and the right leg then advances the left leg
    3 The patient advances the right crutch with the left foot then advances the left crutch with the right foot
    4 The patient advances the left crutch followed by the right foot then the right crutch followed by the left foot

53. A 48-year-old patient has chronic obstructive pulmonary disease (COPD) and is overweight. She has a chronic cough, brings up copious amounts of mucopurulent sputum, and at times, experiences bronchospasm. These are assessment findings of:
    1 Asthma
    2 Lung cancer
    3 Emphysema
    4 Chronic bronchitis

54. While the nurse is preparing to apply antiembolism stockings, the patient states, "Boy, the back of my calf really hurts." What should the nurse do?
    1 Assess the patient for Homans' sign
    2 Apply the stocking as assigned
    3 Tell the patient that the stockings will help the pain
    4 Check the patient's Babinski reflex

55. In a patient suspected of having benign prostatic hypertrophy, the common, most frequent and disturbing signs to assess for are:
    1 Dysuria, nocturia
    2 Flank pain, chills
    3 Bladder stones, malaise
    4 Hematuria, groin discomfort

56. The nurse is teaching an individual with asthma the proper use of his Azmacort inhaler. He is ordered to take two puffs twice a day and remember to:
    1 Rinse the mouthpiece at least twice a week
    2 Exhale quickly before inhaling the medication
    3 Avoid shaking the container before inhalation
    4 Wait 30 seconds to 2 minutes between puffs

57. The patient with an arteriovenous fistula and graft in the left forearm receives hemodialysis three times a week. The nurse should plan to:
    1 Monitor intake and output hourly
    2 Keep the patient on bed rest
    3 Irrigate the fistula every 4 hours
    4 Take blood pressure on right arm

58. During a nutrition-related seminar, individuals on a sodium-restricted diet are cautioned to read labels to determine the content of added:
    1 Monosaccharides
    2 Sodium and iron
    3 Sodium and monosodium glutamate
    4 High-density lipoproteins

59. A patient has a wound infection. The physician prescribes ampicillin (Aminopenicillin) 250 mg PO twice a day and

probenecid (Benemid) 250 mg PO twice a day. The purpose of the probenecid is to:
1 Reduce the risk of an anaphylactic reaction
2 Promote metabolism of the ampicillin
3 Prevent an increase in the uric acid level
4 Increase the effect of the ampicillin

60. Which of the following meals should the nurse recognize as appropriate for a patient on a moderate sodium-restricted diet?
1 Macaroni and cheese, cookies
2 Corned beef, cabbage, bread, fresh fruit
3 Barbecued chicken, fresh corn, fresh fruit
4 Lobster, baked potato, canned peaches

61. The physician orders spironolactone (Aldactone) 50 mg every morning to treat a patient with congestive heart failure. What patient teaching should be provided?
1 Use a salt substitute to decrease sodium intake
2 Increase foods such as bananas and oranges in her diet
3 Change positions slowly when moving from lying to standing
4 Maintain a record of monthly weights

62. The childhood disease that exhibits symptoms of lethargy, muscle pain, polyarthritis, and chorea, and is diagnosed by using the Jones criteria is:
1 Cystic fibrosis
2 Rheumatic fever
3 Muscular dystrophy
4 Infectious mononucleosis

63. The physician orders tetracycline (Sumycin) 500 mg daily to treat a patient's acne. Patient teaching for this individual should include instructions to:
1 Take the medication with yogurt to prevent diarrhea
2 Wear sunscreen to prevent a photosensitivity reaction
3 Take the medication in the morning with her vitamin and mineral supplement
4 Continue taking the medication for 2 days after the acne lesions subside

64. Characteristics of an infant diagnosed as failure to thrive (FTT) include:
1 No interest in toys
2 Distrust of human contact
3 Sociable smile at 2 months
4 Weight below the twenty-fifth percentile

65. The nurse is providing discharge teaching for a patient following hospitalization for a myocardial infarction. One of his discharge prescriptions reads, "Nitrostat (nitroglycerine) 0.4 mg SL up to 3 doses every 5 min prn for angina." How should the nurse explain this prescription to the patient?
1 "You should place one, two, or three of these tablets under your tongue when you have chest pain. How many you use depends on the severity of the pain."
2 "When you have chest pain, you can place one tablet under your tongue every 5 minutes until the pain is relieved, up to a maximum of three tablets."
3 "You should take one of these tablets every 5 minutes when you have chest pain and before activities that precipitate chest pain but no more than three tablets."
4 "You can take up to three of these tablets with a full glass of water when you have chest pain."

66. A patient presents to the emergency room with pain from acute diverticulitis. Which of the following foods from the patient's 24-hour food history would have aggravated the ulcer?
1 Broiled fish, rice
2 Steak, French fries
3 Green salad with raw vegetables
4 Baked potato, steamed vegetables

67. A nurse is planning a diet for a patient who was newly diagnosed with diabetes mellitus. The patient is of the Hindu faith. Which of the following factors is most important to consider when planning this patient's diet?
1 Protein needs may be difficult to meet
2 The patient will not eat any fruits or vegetables
3 The patient will not likely enjoy any of the foods on the plan
4 The exchange lists for the American Dietary Association diet will need to be modified

68. A 44-year-old patient with advanced multiple sclerosis is weak and dysphagic. To prevent respiratory complications, the nurse should:
1 Administer supplemental oxygen when the patient attempts to cough and clear her lungs
2 Provide the patient with an opportunity to talk about her anxiety to ease breathing
3 Inform the patient of the benefits of vitamin therapy to improve respiratory function
4 Sit the patient upright with head flexed forward toward the sternum while eating

69. A nurse is doing a patient education program for individuals who are at high risk for developing diabetes mellitus. Which of the following cardinal symptoms of the condition will the nurse include in her program?
1 Polyuria, polydipsia, polyphagia
2 Clammy skin, tremors, confusion
3 Headache, high blood pressure, nosebleeds
4 Lethargy, slowed mental processes, hypotension

70. A mother of a 2-week-old newborn is nervous about his feedings. The nurse's advice to her should include which of the following?
1 "Begin infant cereal at 1 month of age."
2 "Do not give honey to the baby until he is at least 1 year old."
3 "Add sugar or salt to foods if he finds something unpalatable."
4 "Delay giving egg yolk to the baby until he is a year old because of a possible allergic reaction."

71. A nurse is providing care to a patient with a tracheostomy. Which of the following actions poses the most risk to the patient?
1 Suctioning
2 Cleansing the stoma
3 Cleansing the tracheotomy ties
4 Cleansing the inner cannula

72. A patient is admitted with a left fractured tibia and fibula. The nurse assesses capillary filling to the left toes to determine adequate:
1 Arterial peripheral circulation
2 Venous peripheral circulation
3 Neurological functioning
4 Cardiac output

73. Preoperatively, which diet would be given to a patient who is scheduled for a cholecystectomy to prevent further recurrence of abdominal discomfort?
    1 Hamburger, French fries, milkshake
    2 Avocado salad, cookies, chocolate milk
    3 Lamb, mashed potatoes, ice cream, coffee
    4 Broiled chicken, boiled potatoes, canned peaches, skim milk

74. Individuals with glaucoma or benign prostatic hyperplasia (BPH) should be cautioned relative to taking which of the following medications?
    1 Atropine sulfate
    2 Etodolac (Lodine)
    3 Furosemide (Lasix)
    4 Dopamine hydrochloride (Intropin)

75. Of the following medications, which one reverses the effects of morphine sulfate?
    1 Hydromorphone hydrochloride (Dilaudid)
    2 Acetylcysteine sodium (Mucomyst)
    3 Naloxone hydrochloride (Narcan)
    4 Epinephrine hydrochloride

76. Which of the following menus best meets a postoperative patient's needs for a vitamin specific to tissue healing?
    1 Liver, mashed potatoes, carrots
    2 Roast pork, egg noodles, baked squash
    3 Baked chicken, white rice, sliced peaches
    4 Swiss steak in tomato sauce, mashed potatoes, strawberries

77. Which of the following should the nurse encourage a patient with diabetes to carry on his or her person at all times?
    1 Gum
    2 Candy
    3 Water
    4 Crackers

78. A concern of the nurse who is caring for a patient who tested positive for human immunodeficiency virus (HIV) is to provide adequate education. The nurse should explain how the patient can prevent:
    1 Acquired immunodeficiency syndrome (AIDS)
    2 Pneumonia
    3 Hypotension
    4 Opportunistic infections

79. The nurse knows that which of the following reverses the effect of heparin-sodium therapy?
    1 Warfarin sodium (Coumadin)
    2 Naloxone hydrochloride (Narcan)
    3 AquaMEPHYTON (vitamin K)
    4 Protamine sulfate

80. A patient with Meniere's disease is experiencing severe vertigo. Which of the following instructions can the nurse give to help the patient manage the vertigo?
    1 Wear dark glasses
    2 Listen to soft music
    3 Avoid sudden movements
    4 Rest on the involved side

81. A patient with rheumatoid arthritis complains to the nurse that she is in a great deal of pain, and all the physician did was "give me some aspirin." Which of the following responses would best increase the knowledge base of the patient?
    1 "The physician wants to start you on a low-dose pain reliever."

2 "I am sure that the doctor put you on salicylates because of their ability to relax skeletal muscles."
    3 "The aspirin interrupts the nerve transmission of pain and will reduce your discomfort."
    4 "The antiinflammatory properties of the aspirin will reduce the inflammation in your joints."

82. A pregnant patient has been experiencing morning sickness and is concerned that she will be unable to meet the increased caloric needs of pregnancy. Which of the following food groups should the nurse advise the patient to increase by one serving to meet the caloric demands of the pregnancy?
    1 Meats
    2 Starches
    3 Milk and dairy
    4 Fruits and vegetables

83. A patient has an IV infusing at a rate of 1000 ml every 8 hours. How many ml will have infused in 7.5 hours?
    _____ ml

84. A patient has a medical diagnosis of respiratory acidosis. The nursing diagnosis is activity intolerance. Which of the following activities is most directly aimed at his nursing diagnosis?
    1 Suctioning him every 2 hours and as needed (PRN)
    2 Planning activities to provide rest periods in between
    3 Encouraging fluid intake by offering fluids every 2 hours
    4 Doing postural drainage with cupping every 2 to 4 hours

85. A nursing assistant is assessing an unconscious patient with acute lymphoblastic leukemia. Which of the following modes of temperature assessment should the nurse instruct the nursing assistant to use?
    1 Oral
    2 Rectal
    3 Tympanic
    4 Axillary

86. A patient has a cast on his left leg. The nurse will assess him for neurovascular compromise. When monitoring an individual for neurovascular integrity, capillary refill should be less than:
    1 1 second
    2 2 seconds
    3 3 seconds
    4 4 seconds

87. In a patient with a nursing diagnosis of knowledge deficit related to transurethral resection of the prostate (TURP), the expected outcome is that the patient will describe activity restrictions. Which of the following teaching points is most appropriate?
    1 Avoid straining while trying to pass hard stool for 4 to 6 weeks by using stool softeners as necessary.
    2 Do Kegel perineal exercises every 4 to 6 hours for the next 2 weeks.
    3 Report any dribbling that occurs in the next 2 weeks.
    4 Monitor appearance of urine and report if urine is persistently bright red.

88. Signs of compromised neurovascular integrity include which of the following?
    1 Increase in red blood cells
    2 Warmness of the involved extremity
    3 Tingling and numbness in the involved extremity
    4 Confusion

89. Adolescence begins when:
    1 The growth rate increases rapidly
    2 Secondary sex characteristics appear
    3 The child develops a positive self-image
    4 The child starts to be attracted to the opposite sex
90. The patient has been maintaining an acid ash diet and has been instructed to avoid certain medications and foods. Which of the following can the patient consume?
    1 Salt substitutes
    2 Antacids
    3 Sulfa drugs
    4 NutraSweet
91. The nurse is concerned that a patient who had an appendectomy 3 days ago is developing a paralytic ileus. The nurse should observe for:
    1 Increased bowel sounds
    2 Sudden relief of pain
    3 Abdominal distention
    4 Severe headache
92. According to Erikson's theory of psychosocial development, preschool children are in the stage of:
    1 Trust vs. mistrust
    2 Industry vs. inferiority
    3 Autonomy vs. shame and doubt
    4 Initiative vs. guilt
93. A patient has asthma and has been using an inhaler. He takes beta-adrenergic agonists metaproterenol (Alupent) or albuterol (Proventil) but complains that he does not like the side effects these inhaled medications cause. To which of the following common side effects is the patient referring?
    1 Itching, peripheral edema
    2 Nervousness, dizziness
    3 Nausea, vomiting
    4 Bruising, increased appetite
94. A patient has gastroesophageal reflux disorder (GERD) and emphysema. She has a nursing diagnosis of ineffective airway clearance related to expiratory airflow obstruction. Based on this nursing diagnosis, the nurse should plan to observe the patient for:
    1 Retained secretions
    2 Pitting edema of the lower extremities
    3 Chronic fatigue
    4 Dyspnea on exertion
95. A patient with COPD and pneumonia is unable to walk 20 feet without becoming dyspneic. His pulse oximeter reading drops to 79% with activity. His nursing diagnosis is activity intolerance related to insufficient oxygen to meet body requirements. Which of the following goals would be a appropriate for activity intolerance?
    1 Lips are cyanotic after ambulation
    2 Pulse returns to baseline within 30 minutes after walking
    3 Oxygen saturation remains greater than 90% after walking
    4 Respiratory rate returns to baseline within 30 minutes of ambulation
96. The patient sustained a gashing head wound when hit by a car. The wound required cleansing and 24 sutures. The nurse is assessing wound status. Three key factors that affect would healing are:
    1 Condition of the patient, type of wound, degree of contamination

2 Age of the patient, type of wound, skill of closure
    3 General nutritional status, age of wound, degree of contamination
    4 Location of the wound, degree of cleansing, type of suture used for closure
97. A patient is experiencing problems related to dysphagia. A teaching session is scheduled to discuss ways to promote adequate swallowing without choking. The best technique to use is to instruct the patient to:
    1 Tuck his chin and swallow
    2 Lie down immediately after eating
    3 Drink plenty of water with his meals
    4 Hyperextend his head and swallow
98. A patient has a history of urinary tract infection (UTI). The nurse is doing patient education and should stress the need to:
    1 Take tub baths daily
    2 Avoid sexual intercourse
    3 Avoid perfumed feminine hygiene products
    4 Increase her daily orange juice to eight 8-oz glasses
99. The important thing a nurse can do in the prevention and treatment of cerebrovascular accident (CVA) is to:
    1 Make the public aware of the signs and symptoms and what to do when they occur
    2 Make health care providers more aware of the need to treat within the first 60 minutes
    3 Encourage patients to contact their physician as soon as they suspect that they are having a stroke
    4 Refer the patient immediately to a neurosurgeon
100. A patient is admitted for obstructive urinary retention. When planning care for this patient, the nurse would expect him to have which of the following complaints?
    1 Dysuria
    2 Nocturia
    3 Increased thirst
    4 Diminished force of urinary stream
101. The patient, age 3, has an order for sulfisoxazole (Gantrisin) 750 mg PO every morning. On hand, the nurse has sulfisoxazole 0.5 g/5ml. The nurse should administer _____ to the patient.
102. The nurse is caring for a patient who was burned 72 hours ago. He has partial-thickness burns to 24% of his body surface and begins to excrete large amounts of urine. The nurse should monitor for signs and symptoms of:
    1 Infection
    2 Electrolyte disturbances
    3 Respiratory obstruction
    4 Shock
103. A patient had a CVA 2 days ago, received nutrients via IV infusion, and has progressed to diet as tolerated. The nurse assesses that he has an intact gag reflex, although he does cough when given water to drink. The best approach for the nurse to take to assist this patient to swallow is to:
    1 Make sure suction equipment is available during feedings
    2 Ensure that the patient is in a semi-Fowler's position with his head hyperextended during meals
    3 Place the patient in a semi-Fowler's position, with head flexed slightly forward, and provide soft food
    4 Insist that his food be pureed, liquefied, and bland

104. When assessing a patient at the onset of severe anaphylaxis, the breath sounds that indicate occlusion of the upper airways are:
    1 Wheezes
    2 Crackles
    3 Rhonchi
    4 Friction rubs

105. The nurse in an assisted living facility has been assisting a resident who has a lower motor neuron disorder similar to multiple sclerosis. The nurse is aware that in giving care, she must remember that dysfunction in the lower motor neuron pathways result in:
    1 Spasticity
    2 Hypertonia
    3 Hypertrophy
    4 Flaccidity

106. Which of the following nursing actions will minimize venous stasis?
    1 Ambulation
    2 Leg massage
    3 Sitting with knees crossed
    4 Placing pillows under the knee in a position of comfort

107. Symptoms of celiac disease include which of the following?
    1 Constipation, anorexia, malnutrition
    2 Malnutrition, distended abdomen, craving for sweets
    3 Distended abdomen, constipation, anorexia
    4 Bulky greasy stools, distended abdomen, malnutrition

108. A patient has a history of renal calculi and is admitted to the hospital with gross hematuria and severe colicky left flank pain. In planning care for this patient, the nurse gives the highest priority to which of the following nursing diagnoses?
    1 Pain related to inflammation and urinary blockage
    2 Altered skin integrity related to immobility
    3 Hypertension related to fluid overload
    4 Altered health maintenance related to lack of information about kidney stones

109. A 23-year-old patient has been diagnosed with prostatitis and is started on antibiotics. Which of the following should the nurse include in the teaching plan?
    1 He should take the antibiotics until he feels better
    2 Because this cannot be spread to his sexual partner, a condom need not be used
    3 He should avoid having bowel movements for at least 3 days
    4 He should avoid sexual arousal during the period of acute inflammation

110. The patient has come into the clinic with complaints of repeated episodes of Meniere's disease. The chief symptom this patient experiences during an acute episode is:
    1 Vertigo
    2 Ear pain
    3 Headache
    4 Sudden hearing loss

111. If the tuberculosis (TB) bacteria are walled off by capsules within the lung, the patient should still understand that it is possible to:
    1 React negatively to the TB skin test
    2 Be highly contagious
    3 Continue to have active symptoms of TB
    4 Have the bacteria break out and return to an active infection state

112. A patient has just returned from the operating room after having nasal surgery. Although the patient has nasal packing in place, the nurse must observe for signs of bleeding. Which of the following actions by the nurse would be the most appropriate to detect signs of possible bleeding?
    1 Observing for frequent swallowing
    2 Checking stools for occult blood
    3 Observing for discoloration around the eyes
    4 Checking capillary refill

113. The nurse would suspect circulatory overload in a patient receiving IV therapy if which of the following were observed?
    1 Fever, chills
    2 Confusion, headache
    3 Bounding pulse, dyspnea, cough
    4 Pain, edema, erythema at the infusion site

114. The nurse is watching a patient who has no history of epilepsy for the possibility of seizures. Besides head trauma, which of the following can be considered a secondary cause of seizures?
    1 History of cigarette smoking
    2 Obesity with a sedentary lifestyle
    3 Weight loss of 5% in the last month
    4 Chemical changes from medications

115. During the assessment phase of the nursing process, the nurse should be alert for cardinal signs and symptoms of respiratory dysfunction, including:
    1 Dyspnea
    2 Skin turgor
    3 Red, burning eyes
    4 Complaints of headache

116. A patient comes in to the clinic concerned about his infected foot. He has had emphysema for the last 5 years. The physician believes that this patient is in acidosis and orders arterial blood gas assessments. A patient with this history can develop acidosis resulting from:
    1 Carbon dioxide retention
    2 Hyperventilation
    3 Malnourishment
    4 Decreased activity

117. A patient is admitted with diabetes mellitus. While performing routine checks at midnight, the nurse finds her lethargic, trembling, perspiring, and complaining of a headache. The nurse notifies the charge nurse and performs which of the following actions?
    1 Perform an electrocardiogram
    2 Administer 5 units of regular insulin IV
    3 Give orange juice
    4 Perform a blood glucose monitoring test

118. When planning care for a patient with an infection, the nurse must remember that fever and profuse perspiration:
    1 Increase the body's need for fluids
    2 Increase urinary output
    3 Result in a rise in serum electrolytes
    4 Decrease the respiratory rate

119. Which of the following acid-base disturbances would be the most characteristic of a patient with acute asthma?
    1 Respiratory acidosis
    2 Metabolic acidosis

3 Respiratory alkalosis

4 Metabolic alkalosis

120. Which of the following actions by the nurse best helps to decrease the possibility of the intracranial pressure from increasing in a patient recovering from cranial surgery?

1 Encouraging the patient to perform deep-breathing and coughing exercises

2 Performing endotracheal suctioning every 4 hours prn

3 Maintaining bed in a high-Fowler's (90-degree) position

4 Spreading interventions evenly throughout the day

121. Which of the following is an appropriate short-term goal for the nursing diagnosis of pain?

1 To be pain free by discharge

2 To be free of constipation by discharge

3 To have a pain rating scale of less than 3 after analgesics are administered

4 To have a pain rating scale of greater than 5 after analgesics are administered

122. Drugs affect the urinary tract in several ways. During patient assessment, the nurse would expect a change in the normal characteristics and quantity of urine if the patient stated that he was taking:

1 Calcium channel blockers

2 Anticoagulants

3 Diuretics

4 Antihistamines

123. After surgery to remove a brain tumor, a patient is conscious but lethargic. The nurse asks the patient to move her extremities to check for paralysis, as well as to check for the patient's:

1 Ability to hear

2 Desire to do well

3 Willingness to cooperate

4 Ability to respond to and follow commands

124. A 2-year-old patient is diagnosed with leukemia. The most common signs and symptoms of leukemia related to bone marrow involvement are:

1 Anemia, infection, bleeding

2 Headache, papilledema, irritability

3 Muscle wasting, weight loss, fatigue

4 Decreased intracranial pressure, psychosis, confusion

125. Measures that are used to help prevent hepatic coma (hepatic encephalopathy) are:

1 Giving soapsuds enemas

2 Reducing protein in the diet

3 Performing iced saline lavages

4 Reducing carbohydrates in the diet

Part 2

This examination contains individual questions, the majority of which relate to clinical situations. Read all questions carefully. Each question has only *one best answer*.

Test time allotment (Part 2): approximately 2 hours

Answers and rationales begin on p. 660.

1. During the last decade, health care trends have caused nursing care to be:
   1 Greatly diminished in scope
   2 More focused on treatment of illness
   3 Less concentrated in the acute-care setting
   4 Based on technology rather than on treatment

2. A patient is scheduled to begin a 24-hour urine collection for creatinine clearance at 8:00 AM. The nurse asks the patient to void at 8:00 AM. What should the nurse do with this urine?
   1 Send it to the laboratory for a urinalysis
   2 Pour it into the 24-hour collection container
   3 Discard it
   4 Test it for glucose and ketones

3. In a managed-care environment, the nurse has an ethical responsibility to the patient to:
   1 Provide only allowable services
   2 Assume the role of patient advocate
   3 Interpret insurance coverage for the patient
   4 Determine the level of care based on insurance benefits

4. When feeding a patient with dysphagia, the nurse knows that it is best to:
   1 Provide the patient with thin liquids
   2 Combine different food textures in one bite
   3 Instruct the patient to swallow twice with each bite of food
   4 Offer foods that the patient can pick up easily

5. A patient who has just undergone cataract repair to the left eye is recovering in the same-day surgery unit and is being served lunch. How can the nurse best assist this patient?
   1 Offer to feed the patient
   2 Remove all hot foods from the tray
   3 Describe the tray in clock fashion to the patient
   4 Place the tray so that the patient does not have to strain to reach it

6. Oxygen therapy for the newborn must be administered with caution to prevent:
   1 Ophthalmia neonatorum
   2 ABO incompatibility
   3 Respiratory distress syndrome
   4 Retrolental fibroplasia

7. A patient with insulin controlled diabetes mellitus, residing in a long-term care facility, tells the nurse that she has been vomiting during the night and is now feeling weak and lightheaded. Which of the following nursing interventions would take priority?
   1 Taking her blood pressure
   2 Performing a glucometer test
   3 Instructing her to remain in bed today
   4 Having her maintain a clear fluid diet for the day

8. A new patient needs instructions about the proper administration of Synthroid. Patient teaching should include which one of the following?
   1 Withholding medication and calling the physician if pulse rate is below 60 bpm
   2 Taking the medication at bedtime
   3 Discontinuing drug therapy when all symptoms have subsided
   4 Withholding medication and calling the physician if the pulse rate is over 100 bpm

9. When working in a long-term care facility, which one of the following actions would be considered unethical?
   1 Reporting UAPs for sneaking food out of the kitchen on a break
   2 Going to the dementia unit and looking at a resident's (your neighbor's) chart
   3 Calling a resident's husband to come sit with her because she asked you to
   4 Asking the business office to lock up $400 that you found under a resident's pillow

10. A patient is admitted for surgery, and the physician orders insertion of an indwelling Foley catheter. The nurse needs to take which of the following precautions while performing this procedure?
    1 Reverse isolation
    2 Medical asepsis
    3 Surgical asepsis
    4 Proper hand washing

11. While assisting an elderly nursing home resident with a bath, the nurse observes that his skin is dry and he has been scratching his skin. A priority in planning care for this resident is to:
    1 Avoid bathing the resident
    2 Call the physician
    3 Avoid the use of soap
    4 Apply a medicated lotion

12. A patient who has been having irregular heart rhythms has orders written for the nurses to take apical-radial pulses. Which of the following statements best describes this procedure?
    1 The nurse counts the apical pulse for 1 minute, then counts the radial pulse for 1 minute
    2 One nurse counts the apical pulse for 1 minute while a second nurse counts the radial pulse for 1 minute, both using the same watch
    3 One nurse counts the apical pulse for 1 minute while another nurse counts the radial pulse for 1 minute, each using his or her own watch
    4 A nurse counts the apical and radial pulses simultaneously for 1 minute

13. During a sterile dressing change, the nurse should dispose of the soiled dressings:
    1 In the dirty utility room
    2 In the patient's bedside trashcan
    3 On the sterile waterproof barrier
    4 In a waterproof container away from the sterile field

14. A patient is receiving oxygen therapy at 8 liters per minute continuously via a simple facemask. Which of the following symptoms would alert the nurse as being an early sign of oxygen toxicity?
    1 Fever
    2 Excessive mucus production
    3 Dry cough
    4 Moist breath sounds

15. A 32-year-old woman has been admitted for induction of labor. During the early stages of labor, the patient complains of feeling faint, particularly in the supine position.

The nurse would:

1 Take the patient's blood pressure
2 Place the patient in Trendelenburg's position
3 Turn the patient on her left side
4 Begin preparation for an operative delivery

16. When caring for an patient with AIDS who is on zidovudine (AZT), the nurse needs to monitor the patient for toxic effects of the medication. These toxic effects would include:

1 Stomatitis, fever
2 Painful peripheral nerves
3 Headache, fatigue
4 Painful peripheral nerves, anemia

17. A patient has just undergone a lumbar puncture and questions why he must remain flat in bed for several hours. The nurse's best response is:

1 "You are less likely to fall if you remain quiet today."
2 "It is easier for the nurses to check for any complications this way."
3 "This position prevents any increased blood loss from the spinal area."
4 "This position allows your body to readjust pressure around your brain."

18. A nurse is assisting a physician perform a physical examination in the clinic. Which of the following signs should the nurse recognize as a potential clinical sign of poor nutrition?

1 Feeling of fatigue after exercise
2 Sleeping 8 to 10 hours every night
3 Complaints of chronic constipation
4 Smooth reddish-pink mucous membranes

19. When caring for an individual with AIDS, the nurse must follow Standard Precautions, which include:

1 Sterile gloves and gown
2 Gloves when in contact with blood or any body fluids
3 Mask and gloves at all times when caring for any HIV-positive client
4 Gloves at all times when in contact with any patient in the hospital

20. An elderly patient has had a urinary catheter in place for 1 month. During a routine urinalysis, results indicated that the patient has an infection caused by *Escherichia coli.* Given the patient's history, the nurse suspects that the infection is a(an):

1 Secondary infection
2 Nosocomial infection
3 Autoimmune reaction
4 Antibiotic resistant strain

21. When evaluating a patient for possible pulse deficit, the nurse will need:

1 The assistance of a second nurse
2 An understanding of systolic murmur
3 The cooperative assistance of the patient
4 The availability of an electrocardiograph machine

22. A nurse is using wet-moist saline dressings to débride a patient's stage III decubitus ulcer. The patient asks the purpose of using this type of dressing. Which of the following is the nurse's best response?

1 "The wet dressing soothes the damaged tissue."
2 "The wet dressing keeps the wound from getting infected."

3 "The saline is eventually absorbed into the body, promoting healing."
4 "The drying of the dressing helps remove any drainage or dead skin."

23. When teaching a patient the procedure for collecting stools for occult blood, the nurse should include which of the following?

1 Diarrhea stools are unacceptable sources for this examination
2 The specimen should be kept warm until delivery to the laboratory
3 Small samples should be taken from two separate areas of the stool
4 The specimen should only be obtained from stool areas containing blood

24. Which of the following postprocedure orders should the nurse expect after a patient receives a barium enema?

1 NPO for 3 days
2 Straight cath, PRN
3 Remain flat in bed until the next morning
4 Cleansing enemas until clear

25. A 97-year-old patient is hospitalized for treatment of a fractured hip. On admission, she is noted to have poor skin turgor, and her son states that she has not been drinking much before her fall. Of the following nursing diagnoses, which should receive the highest priority by the nurse who is providing care to the patient?

1 Altered family processes related to stress of hospitalization evidenced by ineffective communication between family members
2 Risk for impaired gas exchange caused by recent surgery and limited mobility
3 Risk for skin breakdown related to limited mobility
4 Fluid volume deficit related to limited oral intake evidenced by poor skin turgor and concentrated urine

26. A patient is being admitted to a long-term care facility inquires why he must undergo a routine TB test. The nurse should respond by advising the patient that:

1 It is a rule that all patients admitted have to have one
2 He will need to take the issue up with his primary physician
3 He needs to take the screening examination whether he likes it or not
4 This is a routine screening examination that is used to safeguard the resident's health

27. The physician orders meperidine (Demerol) 20 mg with atropine 0.08 mg intramuscularly (IM) as a preoperative medication. The meperidine is supplied at 50 mg/ml, the atropine at 0.2 mg/ml. The nurse should draw up a total volume of:

1 0.4 ml
2 0.8 ml
3 1.0 ml
4 1.2 ml

28. Which of the following diet modifications would the nurse recommend for a woman who is experiencing nausea and vomiting during early pregnancy?

1 Increase fat content
2 Increase protein foods
3 Frequent small meals and snacks
4 Increase beverages with meals

29. Heparin sodium is ordered for a patient because of the potential for developing a blood clot caused by immobility. To correctly administer heparin, the nurse would:
   1 Administer the heparin deep IM
   2 Aspirate before administering the heparin to ensure the injection is not in a blood vessel
   3 Administer the heparin in the same site each time
   4 Refrain from massaging the area after the injection

30. A patient has been receiving theophylline (Aminophylline) 80 mg IV every hour for exacerbation of acute asthma. He states he is feeling "jittery." His pulse is 120 bpm, respirations are 22 breaths per minute, and his lungs are clear to auscultation. The physician has ordered a theophylline level to be drawn. Which of the following titers are within therapeutic range?
   1 4 mg/dl
   2 14 mg/dl
   3 26 mg/dl
   4 34 mg/dl

31. A patient is concerned with the amount of cholesterol in his bloodstream because he eats a lot of high-fat food. The nurse knows that cholesterol:
   1 Is a derivative of amino acids
   2 Can contribute to atherosclerosis
   3 Supplements should be taken every day
   4 Is necessary for the body to metabolize vitamin C

32. The order is to give heparin sodium 25,000 units in 1000 ml of IV fluid at a rate of 40 ml/hr. How many units of heparin sodium per hour will the patient be receiving?
   _____ units per hour

33. A patient is placed on a low-fat diet because of hyperlipidemia. Which of the following food listings would be acceptable for this patient?
   1 Whole milk, steak, rice, cake
   2 Liver, fried potatoes, avocado salad
   3 Skim milk, fish, tapioca pudding with fruit
   4 Pork chops, mashed potatoes with gravy, a roll

34. Warfarin sodium (Coumadin) therapy is regulated by which of the following laboratory tests?
   1 Partial fibrinogen time (PFT)
   2 Prothrombin time (PT)
   3 Partial thromboplastin time (PTT)
   4 Bleeding time

35. Which of the following factors may be the most important for the nurse to consider when planning an adequate diet for healthy persons?
   1 Geographic locale
   2 Culture and religion
   3 Family health history
   4 Dietary guidelines and recommendations

36. Which of the following drugs should not be administered through a nasogastric tube?
   1 Digoxin (Lanoxin) tablets
   2 Potassium chloride (Klor) elixir
   3 Acetaminophen (Tylenol) tablets
   4 Theophylline anhydrase (Theo-Dur) tablets

37. Nursing interventions related to postoperative care of the patient who has just had a thyroidectomy performed include:
   1 Immediately reporting a moderate drop in body temperature to less than 98.6° F, heart rate less than 80 bpm, lethargy
   2 Placing the patient in the Fowler's position, supporting head with sand bags, obtaining vital signs every 2 to 4 hours
   3 Reporting any signs of redness or discomfort to the physician
   4 Assessing for hypercalcemia, return of voice, restlessness

38. Which of the following is the major function of the lymphatic system?
   1 Destroys enzymes
   2 Manufactures erythrocytes
   3 Filters and aids in blood clotting
   4 Localizes infections and filters foreign cells

39. A newly admitted patient has a history of convulsions. The nurse is in the patient's room when suddenly he states, "I smell roses." The nurse understands that the patient may be experiencing a(n):
   1 Aura
   2 Olfactory hallucination
   3 Petit mal seizure
   4 Pleasant aroma from his flowers

40. A patient is admitted with obstruction of the bile duct. The nurse alerts the patient that his stools may appear:
   1 Tarry
   2 Very watery
   3 Clay colored
   4 Full of mucus

41. The nursing diagnosis for a 65-year-old patient who is 3 days postoperative hip replacement is potential for infection related to surgical incision. Identify the data that best reflects an evaluation statement.
   1 Temperature 100.9° F; white blood cell count 12,000/mm³; incision with small amount of redness, moderate swelling
   2 Temperature 99.0° F; white blood cell count 13,000/mm³; incision red with small amount of drainage
   3 Temperature 99.0° F; white blood cell count 9800/mm³; incision with redness and swelling with small amount of serosanguineous drainage
   4 Temperature 98.6° F; white blood cell count 10,000/mm³; incision red; large amount of swelling with purulent drainage

42. Immunity occurring in the early months of an infant's life results from the functioning of which gland?
   1 Pineal
   2 Thymus
   3 Thyroid
   4 Pituitary

43. A nurse is caring for a patient in skin traction. Which of the following nursing interventions would be most important?
   1 Assessing neurovascular status
   2 Encouraging liberal fluid intake
   3 Encouraging a diet high in carbohydrates and vitamins
   4 Limiting the patient's activities to maintain effectiveness of the traction

44. The nurse is planning to teach a patient how to administer his insulin injections. Which goal would indicate that the nurse expects the patient to exhibit learning in the psychomotor domain?
   1 The patient will correctly explain how to administer his insulin injection by next Tuesday

2 The patient will correctly state the importance of taking his insulin at the same time every day by next Tuesday

3 The patient will correctly demonstrate administration of his insulin by next Tuesday

4 The patient will correctly identify the sites for insulin administration by next Tuesday

45. Which of the following statements about central hyperalimentation (total parenteral nutrition) administration is most appropriate?
1 Can be given via the antecubital vein
2 Should be given very slowly
3 Can cause rebound hypoglycemia
4 Can be given via a central venous access catheter

46. A patient is recovering from a comminuted fracture of the patella. On the second postoperative day, the surgeon is concerned that the patient may have developed osteomyelitis. Which of the following assessment data may indicate this condition?
1 Chest pain, dyspnea
2 Edema, pain, drainage
3 Numbness, delayed capillary refill
4 Paresthesia, bluish skin around the knee

47. One complication that is more common in cesarean section deliveries is ileus with abdominal distention. To reduce the likelihood of this complication, the nursing care plan for a patient who has had a cesarean section should include:
1 A well-balanced diet with adequate bulk
2 Splinting of the abdomen when deep breathing and coughing
3 Early ambulation
4 Kegel exercises

48. A nurse is caring for a patient who has had chemotherapy. The patient's white blood cell count is 0.2 mm/cm^3. The primary concern of the nurse would be to:
1 Protect the patient from infection
2 Instruct the patient to wear a facemask
3 Implement contact isolation precautions
4 Encourage participation in group activities to build the immune system

49. Aerosol treatment, chest physiotherapy, and postural drainage are ordered for children with cystic fibrosis to:
1 Decrease respiratory effort and mucus production
2 Dilate the bronchioles and clear secretions
3 Increase efficiency of the diaphragm and gas exchange
4 Stimulate coughing and arterial oxygen consumption

50. An active patient who has been complaining of difficulty dressing, weight loss, fatigue, and progressive muscle weakness is diagnosed amyotrophic lateral sclerosis (ALS). When planning care for a patient with ALS, a priority nursing intervention would include:
1 Increased periods of exercise
2 Alternative means of communication
3 Clear airway maintenance
4 Facilitating adjustment (coping) to the diagnosis

51. A patient is admitted to the hospital with the diagnosis of cirrhosis of the liver related to alcohol abuse and malnutrition. He is jaundiced, has ascites, and has recently experienced dyspnea. A nursing assistant asks the nurses what causes the ascites. Which of the following is the most correct statement by the nurse?
1 The fluid is caused by cardiovascular hypertension

2 Low levels of albumin cause fluid to collect in the abdomen

3 The fluid is accumulating because of a large obstruction of the patient's common bile duct

4 The patient is producing a large amount of ammonia, which causes the fluid collection

52. A patient is scheduled for surgery. What is the responsibility of the nurse with regard to the surgical consent form?
1 The nurse should obtain the patient's signature on the form
2 The nurse should witness the patient's signature on the form
3 The nurse should check that the signed consent form is on the patient's chart before surgery
4 The nurse should be sure that the patient understands what he is signing

53. A 60-year-old woman with a history of osteoarthritis presents to a clinic for a short-stay cataract removal. An important piece of information for the nurse to obtain in planning his care is the patient's:
1 Hobbies and interests
2 Food likes and dislikes
3 Use of alcohol and tobacco
4 Use of a cane or walker

54. A hospitalized patient was recently diagnosed with lung cancer. While the nurse is providing care, the patient states, "If someone had only warned me that I would get lung cancer, I would have stopped smoking years ago." The nurse recognizes that this statement reflects which coping mechanism?
1 Compensation
2 Rationalization
3 Sublimation
4 Repression

55. A patient who is now clinically stable following a myocardial infarction is admitted on Monday to an extended-care facility. The registered nurse identifies the following nursing diagnosis: activity intolerance related to low oxygen saturation evidenced by dyspnea after ambulating 10 feet. What is an acceptable goal for this nursing diagnosis?
1 The patient will exhibit an oxygen saturation level of 95% by Saturday
2 The patient will use oxygen by nasal cannula before and after ambulating
3 The patient will ambulate 12 feet without dyspnea by Saturday
4 The patient will exhibit pink skin and mucous membranes by Wednesday

56. A patient has been diagnosed with acromegaly. The nurse is aware that this condition is caused by an overproduction of:
1 Prolactin
2 Cortisol
3 Growth hormone
4 Thyroid hormone

57. The nurse is preparing to administer a dose from the following order: meperidine (Demerol) 75 mg IM every 4 hours PRN. What is it most important for the nurse to check before preparing the dose?
1 The date and time that the order was written
2 The time when the last dose of the medication was given
3 The amount of the medication that is left on hand
4 The effect of the last dose of the medication

58. A patient is taking ipratropium (Atrovent), an anticholinergic agent, for a respiratory condition. The nurse might expect the patient to exhibit which of the following adverse effects?
    1 Bradycardia
    2 Diarrhea
    3 Dry mouth
    4 Pupil constriction

59. When instructing a female patient about antibiotic therapy, the nurse should alert the patient concerning the possibility of getting candidiasis as a secondary infection. For which of the following symptoms should the nurse tell the patient to be alert?
    1 High fever, swollen lymph glands
    2 Itching, cream cheese–like white discharge
    3 Chancres that develop outside the vagina
    4 Excessive bleeding occurring in the absence of a period

60. The patient with a hiatal hernia and reflux syndrome is having discomfort lying in a supine position and complains of having trouble sleeping. An appropriate suggestion by the nurse would be to:
    1 Remove high-acid food from the diet
    2 Suggest a hot cup of cocoa before retiring for the night
    3 Suggest that the head of the bed be raised up on blocks
    4 Recommend a glass of milk and a sandwich just before going to bed

61. The nurse is assessing for signs of active TB in a patient who is in respiratory isolation. Which of the following best describes signs and symptoms of active TB?
    1 Night sweats, dyspnea, weakness
    2 Wheezing, insomnia, productive cough
    3 Dyspepsia, being cold, fatigue
    4 Loss of appetite, bloody stools

62. In planning the nursing care of a patient with Addison's disease, a priority of the nursing care is to:
    1 Provide diversional activities
    2 Protect the patient from stress and exertion
    3 Plan a well-balanced diet with nourishing snacks
    4 Permit all activity as desired by the patient

63. A patient with second- and third-degree burns over 40% of his body is being treated by the open method. Which of the following interventions is most appropriate in his care?
    1 Wearing sterile gloves to apply the topical antimicrobial agents
    2 Keeping the room temperature between 65° and 70° F for patient comfort
    3 Providing a high-protein, high-fat diet to meet increased nutritional demands
    4 Elevating his arms on two pillows to prevent contractures

64. The nurse just received laboratory results on her patient who is in acute renal failure. Which of the following statements accurately describes the laboratory findings common to patients in acute renal failure?
    1 Increased BUN and decreased creatinine levels
    2 Increased BUN and creatinine levels
    3 Increased calcium levels and decreased BUN
    4 Decreased BUN and potassium levels

65. A patient with cholelithiasis is experiencing right upper quadrant pain after eating a meal that was high in fat and asks the nurse for an explanation of how his diet can precipitate pain. The most appropriate response by the nurse would be:
    1 "Foods high in fat are harder to digest."
    2 "The ducts from the liver and pancreas become obstructed."
    3 "Obstructed bile flow limits the amount of bile available to emulsify fat."
    4 "There is an inadequate absorption of both fat and soluble vitamins."

66. Drugs can affect the urinary tract in several ways, even to the point of being nephrotoxic. Assessment of a patient's current and past use of medications, including over-the-counter drugs and herbs, is important. During a patient assessment, the nurse would expect possible kidney problems if the patient gave a history of taking:
    1 Imipramine (Tofranil)
    2 Nitrofurantoin (Macrodantin)
    3 Nifedipine (Adalat)
    4 Ibuprofen (Advil, Motrin)

67. An indication that cord prolapse has occurred following rupture of an expectant mother's membranes would be related to which observation?
    1 Decreased fetal heart rate
    2 Increased fetal heart rate
    3 Continuous leakage of fluid
    4 Protrusion of the cord by 10 inches

68. A patient who recently returned to the unit after a bronchoscopy starts to wheeze and appears frightened. The nurse's most appropriate response to the patient's obvious concern is:
    1 "Wheezing frequently occurs after this type of test."
    2 "This is a sign that the local anesthetic is wearing off."
    3 "This means that your gag reflex is returning."
    4 "I will notify your physician that this is occurring."

69. The nurse is caring for a patient in diabetic ketoacidosis (DKA). Which of the following insulins should the nurse expect to administer in the acute phase of this condition?
    1 Lente
    2 NPH
    3 Regular
    4 Glucotrol

70. A patient was admitted 2 days ago with acute renal failure secondary to a severe infection. The infection has improved but the patient continues to have an output below 30 ml/hr. The nurse should instruct him that his diet will be:
    1 High carbohydrate, low protein, low potassium
    2 High carbohydrate, high protein, supplementary potassium
    3 Low carbohydrate, low protein, high potassium
    4 Low carbohydrate, high protein, low potassium

71. A patient experienced a pulmonary embolus and was immediately started on IV heparin. The goal is to maintain the PTT at:
    1 One half to one times normal
    2 One and one half to two times normal
    3 Two to three times normal
    4 Three to four times normal

72. A patient who had a cerebrovascular accident (CVA) has paresis of her left side and weighs 90 kg, is incontinent of urine, and perspires heavily. The nurse instructs the nursing assistant to:
    1 Pull the patient up in bed at least once a shift

2 Keep the patient off the affected side when positioning her

3 Get help to move and reposition the patient

4 Lower the temperature in the room

73. A patient who had a right below-the-knee amputation is 3 days postoperative. She has no signs of infection and is doing well; however, she states that the pain she felt preoperatively continues to be present. She also states that, at times, it feels as though her right lower leg is floating in mid air. The nurse should obtain an order for:

1 A narcotic analgesic for pain prn

2 Massage therapy to the residual limb

3 The application of cold to the residual limb

4 A transcutaneous electrical nerve stimulation unit

74. A known alcohol and substance user comes to the emergency room with a hand laceration. He has not consumed any alcohol or taken any drugs for the last 3 days. He starts having hallucinations. This is most likely caused by withdrawal from:

1 Alcohol

2 Hallucinogens

3 Narcotics

4 Stimulants

75. A 75-year-old woman with hypertension has a history of passing out on arising in the morning. The nurse should:

1 Have her sit on the side of the bed for a few minutes before standing

2 Advise her to take a multivitamin daily

3 Call the physician

4 Increase her fluid intake

76. Which individual is at greatest risk to suffer from heat stroke?

1 9-month-old girl

2 23-year-old man

3 37-year-old woman

4 51-year-old man

77. A patient is 2 days postoperative from extensive abdominal surgery and is using the incentive spirometer as directed. The nurse notices crackles in the posterior right lower lobe. The nurse has him cough and deep breathe and should:

1 Assess his lung sounds before and after deep-breathing and coughing exercises

2 Notify respiratory therapy to check his SAT level

3 Measure his vital signs before the deep-breathing and coughing exercises

4 Position him in a semi-Fowler's position for the exercises

78. The nurse is driving in a rural area on an isolated country road and sees a child, approximately 12 to 15 years of age, lying in the middle of the road, with an overturned bicycle not far away. Which of the following nursing actions should she take immediately?

1 Keep driving to the nearest gas station and telephone for an ambulance

2 Turn around and go back to the nearest main highway and hail a police car

3 Proceed with a rapid clinical assessment, with emphasis on airway, breathing, and circulation

4 Check with local authorities for specifics on the state's Good Samaritan law

79. A 40-year-old woman is admitted to the emergency department bleeding profusely from an injury on the lower portion of her right arm. Emergency management of hemorrhage requires the nurse to implement which of the following actions first?

1 Apply pressure to the bleeding area

2 Apply a pressure dressing to the bleeding area

3 Elevate the injured area

4 Immobilize the injured area

80. A patient with COPD is admitted to the hospital for an acute episode of respiratory distress. Which type of oxygen mask is the most appropriate for the nurse to administer oxygen to this patient?

1 Venturi mask

2 Non-rebreather mask

3 Partial-rebreather mask

4 Simple mask

81. A woman who is postmenopausal and not taking estrogen should have a calcium intake of:

1 1200 mg/day

2 1000 mg/day

3 1500 mg/day

4 2000 mg/day

82. According to the Patient Self-Determination Act, information about advance directives is given to patients when they are:

1 Admitted to the hospital

2 Involved in a life-threatening crisis

3 Discharged into a home health agency

4 Willing to discuss the issue with the physician

83. According to Erikson's theory of life stages, older adults spend a great deal of the latter part of their life managing the task of:

1 Intimacy vs. isolation

2 Ego integrity vs. despair

3 Generativity vs. stagnation

4 Identity vs. role confusion

84. The proper way to interpret a Mantoux skin test is to measure the amount of:

1 Erythema in mm

2 Induration and erythema in mm

3 Induration in mm

4 Lipohypertrophy in mm

85. A patient presents to the emergency department with acute myocardial infarction. A family member states that the patient has been depressed since his retirement 3 months ago. Which of the following factors may be contributing to the patient's current health status?

1 An inability to "let go" of work problems

2 Excitement caused by the prospect of retirement

3 Excess stimulation from new friends and activities

4 Stress over loss of income and change in daily routine

86. Many researchers believe that sudden infant death syndrome (SIDS) may be related to a brain stem abnormality in the regulation of cardiorespiratory control. Other recent studies have demonstrated that an increased risk of SIDS is present in infants who:

1 Breast-feed rather than bottle-feed

2 Sleep in the prone position

3 Are older than 10 months of age

4 Use a pacifier while they sleep

87. The nurse is planning care for a patient who has been admitted for observation with a possible skull fracture. The nurse must observe for the possibility of changing levels of consciousness caused by a venous bleed. Which type of hematoma is being described?
    1 Intracerebral
    2 Epidural
    3 Subarachnoid
    4 Subdural

88. A patient has an order for an IV of 1000 ml D5.45 normal saline to be infused over 8 hours. If the IV infusion set delivers 10 gtt/ml, at what rate should the nurse infuse the IV fluid?
    1 8 gtt/min
    2 13 gtt/min
    3 16 gtt/min
    4 21 gtt/min

89. The physician prescribes phenelzine (Nardil), a monoamine oxidase inhibitor (MAOI), for a patient with a diagnosis of depression. What should the nurse teach the patient about this medication?
    1 Limit foods that are high in potassium
    2 Avoid foods that are high in tyramine
    3 Avoid exposure to direct sunlight
    4 Expect to notice a therapeutic response within 3 days

90. The nurse administers meperidine hydrochloride (Demerol) 100 mg IM for pain. The nurse should plan to monitor the patient for which condition?
    1 Diarrhea
    2 Hypertension
    3 Respiratory depression
    4 Hypoglycemia

91. A 76-year-old patient is being discharged 2 days after a cholecystectomy. A family member inquires why he is being discharged so soon after surgery. Which of the following responses by the nurse accurately defines the trend in today's managed health care system?
    1 "Why don't you ask the physician to keep him longer?"
    2 "Because of insurance requirements, we can't keep patients too long after simple surgery."
    3 "Home health agencies need older adults to return home so they can be taken care of at home."
    4 "Patients are given a certain length of time to recuperate in the hospital, but most recovery is done at home."

92. An employee who works in a laboratory splashed a chemical into her eyes. Her co-workers irrigated her eyes with plain water and then brought her to the emergency clinic. The patient is complaining of "burning" in the eyes. Both eyes and the surrounding tissue are reddened. The physician orders that each eye be irrigated with 1000 ml of normal saline. The patient is placed in a reclining position in preparation for the irrigation. The nurse should direct the flow of fluid:
    1 From the outer canthus to the inner canthus
    2 From the inner canthus to the outer canthus
    3 Directly on the center of the eyeball
    4 Indirectly and slowly from the lower lid

93. A 95-year-old man is returning home with his daughter, who is concerned that her home is not safe for her father. List four safety hazards that could pose a possible problem for this man.
    1 _____.
    2 _____.
    3 _____.
    4 _____.

94. When preparing to give an injection of NPH and regular insulin, the nurse knows to mix the two insulins in the same syringe to:
    1 Potentiate the action of the NPH insulin
    2 Potentiate the action of the regular insulin
    3 Avoid two injections
    4 Prolong the effects of both insulins

95. A patient receiving hemodialysis has been connected for 20 minutes and complains to the nurse that he is having some chest pain. The nurse observes that the patient is anxious, has a cough, and has respirations of 28 breaths per minute. The nurse should:
    1 Check the needle insertion site and continue the procedure
    2 Clamp the venous line and stop the pump
    3 Position the patient on his right side for 10 minutes
    4 Have the patient stand up and take his blood pressure

96. An agitated, delusional resident is receiving haloperidol (Haldol) because of extreme acting out behavior. The nurse is concerned because of this drug's side effects. The nurse asks the nursing assistants to alert her if the patient exhibits:
    1 Increased urine output
    2 Jaundice and lethargy
    3 Confusion and dizziness
    4 Headache and swollen glands

97. Diagnosis of nephrotic syndrome in a child is based on:
    1 Symptoms of edema, hyperalbuminemia, tea-colored urine
    2 Results of renal ultrasound, proteinuria, increased levels of protein in the blood
    3 Increased proteinuria, edema, decreased serum protein, renal biopsy
    4 Edema of face and abdomen, positive renal MRI, increased serum protein

98. A patient has a serum potassium level of 7.2 mEq/L. Which of the following substances will most likely be ordered?
    1 Potassium chloride (Kay Ciel)
    2 Sodium polystyrene sulfonate (Kayexalate)
    3 Bananas
    4 Strawberries

99. An adolescent who exhibits changes in behavior patterns, an increase in school absences, a decrease in academic performance, and starts to spend time with people other than his regular friends may be showing signs of:
    1 Manic depression
    2 Bulimia
    3 Drug abuse
    4 Schizophrenia

100. A patient with a history of an extremely stressful lifestyle underwent coronary bypass surgery a week ago. The multidisciplinary team decided that he needs to learn stress-management strategies. The principle behind this recommendation is that:
    1 A reduction in stress will decrease cardiac workload
    2 Stress-reduction exercises are good for persons who have had major surgery
    3 Relaxation enhances the flow of blood to the periphery
    4 Exercise increases the blood flow to the heart

101. Projectile vomiting in an infant is a classic sign of:
    1 Intussusception
    2 Celiac disease
    3 Tracheoesophageal fistula
    4 Pyloric stenosis

102. When assessing a patient who is dying from cancer for pain relief, the nurse should first focus his or her assessment on:
    1 Medication for the pain
    2 Quality of the pain
    3 Source of the pain
    4 Duration of the pain

103. Retinoic acid is used in the treatment of:
    1 Acne vulgaris
    2 Tinea corporis
    3 Pediculosis
    4 Ringworm

104. The physician orders ampicillin 300 mg intravenous piggyback (IVPB). Ampicillin is supplied as 500 mg/2 ml. What volume of ampicillin would the nurse draw up from the vial? _____ ml

105. The patient reports to the nurse that the medication she is taking for her UTI has stopped the frequency and urgency she had been experiencing. Which of the following medications works in this manner?
    1 Trimethoprim/sulfamethoxazole (TMP/SMZ) (Bactrim)
    2 Hyoscyamine (Anaspaz)
    3 Ciprofloxacin (Cipro)
    4 Amoxicillin (Amoxil)

106. A patient is admitted with hyperemesis gravidarum. Initially, her diet should consist of:
    1 Dry toast, tea
    2 Low-fat foods three times a day
    3 High protein foods six times a day
    4 IV fluids of glucose, electrolytes, vitamins

107. A hereditary musculoskeletal disorder that exhibits symptoms of gradual muscle weakness, a "waddle" gait, and difficulty standing and sitting is known as:
    1 Multiple sclerosis
    2 Cerebral palsy
    3 Developmental hip dysplasia
    4 Muscular dystrophy

108. A patient, age 17 months, is admitted to the hospital with a diagnosis of meningitis. Which of the following findings would be noted relative to the patient's cerebrospinal fluid (CSF)?
    1 Reduced protein level
    2 Elevated glucose level
    3 Reduced pressure
    4 Cloudy

109. An infant weighing 11 lb has been ordered to receive morphine sulfate 0.5 mg subcutaneously (SQ) for postoperative pain. The normal dose of morphine is 0.1 mg/kg. The ordered dose of morphine is:
    1 Too low, based on the weight of the infant
    2 Too high, based on the weight of the infant
    3 Inappropriate; morphine should not be given SQ
    4 Correct, based on the weight of the infant

110. The physician has ordered an IV of D5.2 normal saline to be infused at 100 ml/hr. If the IV tubing delivers 10 gtt/ml, at what rate would the nurse infuse the IV fluid?
    1 10 gtt/min
    2 12 gtt/min
    3 16 gtt/min
    4 18 gtt/min

111. An X-linked recessive disorder of metabolism that results in a delayed coagulation of blood is known as:
    1 Sickle cell anemia
    2 Thalassemia major
    3 Hemophilia
    4 Leukemia

112. A patient has diabetes insipidus, and his physician has ordered vasopressin. The nurse should expect to see:
    1 A decrease in blood pressure
    2 An increase in abdominal distention
    3 A decrease in urinary output
    4 An elevation in temperature

113. During the initial assessment of an 8-year-old boy who has nephrotic syndrome, the nurse should expect to see:
    1 Absence of tears
    2 Increased urine output
    3 Flushed skin
    4 Scrotal edema

114. A patient who has angina complained of chest pain to his wife, who then called 9-1-1. The patient has sublingual nitroglycerine ordered PRN. The emergency medical technician, a nurse, has administered 3 tablets at 5-minute intervals over a 15-minute period. The most appropriate action by the nurse will be to:
    1 Monitor the patient's blood pressure
    2 Hold the nitroglycerine until she hears from the physician
    3 Increase the dose to two tablets every 5 minutes while waiting for the physician
    4 Wait 5 minutes and administer the fourth tablet while waiting for the physician

115. A patient is receiving oral anticoagulants. The nurse should instruct him to:
    1 Limit the amount of turnip greens, broccoli, and kale in his diet
    2 Use a disposable razor when shaving to avoid the chance of infection
    3 Take an extra aspirin daily to potentiate the effects of the anticoagulant
    4 Use a hard-bristled toothbrush to massage and toughen the gums

116. When using an inhaler that contains albuterol (Proventil), the patient should be instructed to:
    1 Open his mouth and hold the inhaler 1 to 2 inches away
    2 Use the inhaler when he is extremely short of breath
    3 Wash the inhaler after every use in warm, soapy water
    4 Use mouthwash after each use

117. Daily head circumference measurements are important nursing interventions postoperatively for the child with a:
    1 Wilms' tumor
    2 Seizure disorder
    3 Ventriculoperitoneal shunt
    4 Spinal cord injury

118. Primitive newborn reflexes disappear to:
    1 2 weeks of age
    2 6 to 8 weeks of age
    3 3 months of age
    4 5 months of age

119. An 18-year-old woman is seen in the clinic and is diagnosed with anorexia nervosa. Her symptoms would most likely include:
    1 Dysmenorrhea
    2 Periods of hyperactivity
    3 Tachycardia
    4 Diarrhea

120. The most serious complication of rheumatic fever is:
    1 Endocarditis
    2 Pneumonia
    3 Arthritis
    4 Meningitis

121. The morning after a vaginal birth, the patient's hemoglobin is 10.9 g/dl. The nurse expects the mother to experience:
    1 Dizzy spells
    2 Unstable vital signs
    3 Difficulty performing small tasks
    4 Managing basic care of herself and her infant

122. The nurse is admitting a child with a diagnosis of trisomy 21. Another term for this genetic condition is:
    1 Hurler's syndrome
    2 Cri du chat syndrome
    3 Turner's syndrome
    4 Down syndrome

123. A 2-week-old newborn has been admitted to the hospital with a diagnosis of possible hydrocephalus. Which assessment would be most important for the nurse to make?
    1 Daily weight
    2 Frequent neurovascular checks
    3 Specific gravity on all urine output
    4 Daily head circumference measurement

124. During a myasthenia crisis a patient may experience several problems. Which is likely to necessitate an immediate response?
    1 Respiratory distress
    2 Slower speech rate
    3 Difficulty chewing food
    4 Weakness of arms and legs

125. The nurse has an order to administer ampicillin 425 mg IVPB. Ampicillin is supplied as 1 g/4 ml. How much should the nurse withdraw from the vial?
    _____ ml

PART 1 ANSWERS AND RATIONALES

1. Application, implementation, physiological integrity (c).

   3 Meperidine: DD = 35 mg

   D = 50 mg

   V= 1 ml

   $$\frac{DD}{DH} = \frac{35\ mg}{50\ mg} \times 1\ ml = 0.7\ ml$$

   Atropine: DD = 0.1 mg

   DH = 0.2 mg

   V = 1 ml

   $$\frac{DD}{DH} = \frac{0.1\ mg}{0.2\ mg} \times 1\ ml = 0.5\ ml$$

   1, 2, 4 These are not the correct doses.

2. Comprehension, implementation, physiological integrity (b).

   2 Oxygen therapy to prevent tissue deoxygenation is of primary importance in sickle cell crisis.

   1 This is part of the treatment for children with chronic sickle cell disease.

   3 This may be part of the treatment in chronic sickle cell disease.

   4 Hydration is important in treating sickle cell crisis; however, oxygen therapy ranks first in order of importance.

3. Application, assessment, physiological integrity (b).

   3 This is too long for IV tubing to hang without being changed; IV tubing is normally changed every 2 to 3 days. The nurse needs to hang a new IV bag and tubing to decrease the incidence of infection.

   1 The IV site is not infected; no action is required.

   2 Fluid in the IV container signifies that enough is being infused into the patient, depending on the flow rate. If the tubing does not need changing, the bag would not need to be changed.

   4 This is a normal IV site; no action is needed.

4. Knowledge, implementation, physiological integrity (a).

   1 The figure-of-eight turn allows the bandage to lay smoothly and provides support for the joint.

   2 The recurrent turn is used to cover distal areas, such as the head, a digit, or a stump.

   3 The spiral turn is used on cylindrical parts, such as the forearm.

   4 The circular turn is used to anchor the beginning and end of the bandage.

5. Comprehension, implementation, physiological integrity (c).

   4 This is the purpose of a rebreathing mask.

   1, 2, 3 These are appropriate interventions for a patient in respiratory acidosis.

6. Application, implementation, physiological integrity (c).

   3 Application of heat should dilate the blood vessels of the fingers and increase blood flow to the area.

   1 Milking the finger may cause an inaccurate reading on the machine.

   2 This will prevent blood from reaching the fingertips; fingers can be held downward to facilitate filling.

   4 This practice is not only painful, but it may also affect the accuracy of the reading.

7. Application, planning, physiological integrity (b).

   4 The patient in the high-Fowler's position is sitting virtually upright, which facilitates the greatest chest expansion.

   1 This side-lying position will not allow the patient to achieve full chest expansion.

2 This flat position will not maximize the patient's chest expansion.

   3 The low-Fowler's position is not high enough to maximize chest expansion.

8. Comprehension, assessment, physiological integrity, (c).

   1 The patient is exhibiting excessive hypotension and going into shock. An important measure is to get the blood to her head to maintain consciousness. Her blood pressure has undergone a marked change since admission. A patient who is receiving antihypertensives should have blood pressure monitored regularly and compared with the admitting baseline.

   2, 3 The nurse will call the physician after the patient is immediately attended to. She will hold the Monopril because this is the source of the problem. The dosage may need adjustment.

   4 This position would take blood away from the brain and place the patient at risk for loss of consciousness.

9. Knowledge, assessment, physiological integrity (c).

   3 The accessory nerve (spinal accessory) has two branches and is a motor nerve. One branch controls the trapezius and the sternocleidomastoid. The trapezius functions to raise and pull back the shoulder and extend the head. The sternocleidomastoid flexes the neck and rotates the head.

   1 Involvement of the facial nerve will decrease the ability of the patient to wrinkle the forehead or close the eyes.

   2 Involvement of the trigeminal nerve will cause the patient to have loss of facial sensation, forehead, and temples; he will also have problems chewing.

   4 The glossopharyngeal nerve (cranial nerve IX) controls taste, secretions of the parotid gland, and swallowing.

10. Knowledge, implementation, physiological integrity (b).

    2 Elevated BUN and creatinine levels indicate damage to the kidneys.

    1 These levels are not indicators of liver function.

    3 Damaged muscles do not result in elevated BUN and creatinine levels.

    4 These levels cannot determine damage to the intestines.

11. Comprehension, evaluation, physiological integrity (c).

    2 Assessing the effects of each intervention will serve as a guideline for subsequent interventions to everyone involved in his care.

    1 Medications, including narcotics, are never used indiscriminately.

    3 Guided imagery can be useful for mild pain but not for moderate or severe pain.

    4 Increasing his fluid intake would have no effect on pain control.

12. Comprehension, evaluation, safe, effective care environment (c).

    4 A return demonstration of the skill coupled with verbalizations of the steps is considered the best way of evaluating the knowledge base of the individual.

    1 The patient may be able to tell you what he or she has learned but be unable to perform the task or skill.

    2 Taking a quiz is anxiety producing for patients and will evaluate only the knowledge base of the individual, not the skill base.

    3 Although this would be an excellent way to determine the effectiveness of the teaching, asking a patient to teach another patient is generally anxiety producing and inappropriate.

13. Knowledge, assessment, safe, effective care environment (a).
    4 This is a typical example of an aura.
    1 This may likely be seen in the preictal phase, before the aura.
    2 This occurs after the aura and during the seizure.
    3 These may be seen with partial seizures and are termed *automatisms.*

14. Comprehension, evaluation, physiological integrity (b).
    4 Normally, individuals who have had spinal anesthesia are to remain flat for a specified length of time after surgery (4 to 6 hours) to prevent spinal headache.
    1 This is an appropriate order.
    2 Generally, surgical patients can get out of bed after 4 to 6 hours of lying flat.
    3 This order allows patients to advance their diet as they tolerate fluids.

15. Comprehension, evaluation, psychosocial integrity (b).
    4 This is the only remark that describes Parkinson's disease.
    1 This describes Huntington's disease.
    2 This describes Creutzfeldt-Jakob disease.
    3 This describes Huntington's disease.

16. Knowledge, assessment, physiological integrity, (b).
    3 The sympathetic nervous system increases heart rate, thereby increasing cardiac output (heart rate times stroke volume).
    1 The sympathetic nervous system speeds up heart rate rather than slowing it down.
    2 The sympathetic nervous system increases heart rate and cardiac output.
    4 The sympathetic nervous system does not cause cardiac arrest.

17. Application, implementation, psychosocial integrity (b).
    4 This is the only response that conveys dignity and respect for the resident.
    1 This response is humiliating and degrading.
    2 This response demeans the resident.
    3 Chastising the resident demeans the resident's dignity.

18. Application, planning, safe, effective care environment (b).
    2 This is an expected outcome of the nursing action that should occur within a short period.
    1 This is a nursing intervention; it outlines the actual nursing activity.
    3 This is a long-term goal, outlining the overall purpose of the nursing actions.
    4 This is the rationale for reaching the goal; it explains why the action is being implemented.

19. Application, planning, psychosocial integrity (b).
    2 Hoeing is a repetitive action that does not require decision making or planning.
    1 Sorting laundry has some measure of decision making.
    3 Too much planning is involved in this activity.
    4 The patient will become frustrated because of the inability to plan the grocery list.

20. Comprehension, implementation, psychosocial integrity (b).
    3 Promoting attachment of the family to the infant is important and is best done by providing an environment in which the family is able to touch the infant and to interact as a unit.
    1, 2, 4 These do not promote family interaction and sharing.

21. Comprehension, evaluation, health promotion and maintenance (b).
    3 Bran cereal has a higher fiber content compared with any of the other sources.
    1 Cucumbers have a low fiber content.
    2 Apple juice contains low fiber content.
    4 Bananas contain some fiber but not as much compared with the bran cereal.

22. Application, assessment, health promotion and maintenance (b).
    2 Using Nagele's rule, add 7 days to the first day of the last menstrual period, then subtract 3 months.
    1 This calculation incorrectly started using the last day of the menstrual cycle.
    3 This calculation incorrectly subtracted 7 days instead of adding 7 days.
    4 This date has no relation to the application of Nagele's rule.

23. Comprehension, planning, physiological integrity (b).
    4 Weight-bearing limits are always determined by the physician and depend on the surgical technique used, the patient's postoperative condition, and type of prosthesis.
    1 Full weight bearing is not normally ordered; this is determined by the physician.
    2 Physicians do not normally order this, but once again, it must be ordered by the physician.
    3 Patient tolerance is important, but progress must be made in physical therapy, which the physician will order.

24. Comprehension, implementation, safe, effective care environment (c).
    3 If a patient scheduled for the operating room has an elevated temperature, the admitting physician should be notified.
    1 Respirations are within normal limits; the physician should be notified of abnormal vital signs, not the anesthesiologist.
    2 Pulse is within normal limits; the physician should be notified of abnormal vital signs, not the anesthesiologist.
    4 Blood pressure is within normal limits.

25. Application, planning, psychosocial integrity (b).
    2 By using short sentences and speaking clearly, short-term memory is maximized.
    1 This is too much information for the resident to remember.
    3 This does not support the resident's cognitive function.
    4 This is too much information given to him at one time.

26. Application, implementation, physiological integrity (b).
    3 The individual need not take the daily medication at exactly 9:00 AM. She may have mood swings and may take the medication at a later time.
    1 This may eventually be the correct course of action, but the patient should be offered the medication first.
    2 Doing this eventually is important but not until the resident has been offered the medication.
    4 This would be the last course of action and would be done only after repeatedly trying to get the resident to take the oral form of the medication.

27. Comprehension, implementation, psychosocial integrity (b).
    4 A form of distraction may provide relief from the current situation.
    1 This is not a remedy for this situation.

2 The patient may get lost on the way to her room and does not need to be isolated.

3 Excess stimulation may add to her agitation.

28. Knowledge, assessment, health promotion and maintenance (b).

2 Because the patient delivered a boy and a girl, they must be fraternal or unidentical; if they had been the same sex, the placenta and sacs would have to be identified.

1 Monozygotic twins are always the same sex.

3 Blood tests are not the *best* answer; a nurse should know the status by identifying the placenta and the sacs.

4 DNA tests are not the *best* answer; a nurse should know the status by identifying the placenta and the sacs.

29. Application, implementation, psychosocial integrity (a).

2 Maintaining a caring attitude is important.

1 It would depend on how well she is progressing and if orders were received.

3 This is not routinely done unless requested.

4 The temperature should be kept at a level that is comfortable for the patient; it is not the top priority.

30. Comprehension, implementation, health promotion and maintenance (b).

1 This test, along with a barium enema, is used to confirm Hirschsprung's disease.

2, 3, 4 These tests are not used to confirm the diagnosis of Hirschsprung's disease.

31. Knowledge, planning, safe, effective care environment (a).

3 The patient will be able to call the nurse when the need arises; it will help relieve anxiety and may prevent an accident.

1 Leaving the door ajar is dangerous; it should be left all the way open or be closed.

2 Eating alone is not essential for the patient, unless this is a personal request.

4 Accidents may be avoided if the patient is informed of any rearrangement of furnishings.

32. Application, implementation, psychosocial integrity (b).

4 Talking with the family first is important so they can be involved first-hand with care issues.

1 Although this is important, it is not the first thing that should be done.

2 This may be done later based on the needs of the patient and family.

3 After the care plan has been developed, this may be a priority.

33. Comprehension, assessment, physiological integrity (b).

2 The infant with colic demonstrates these signs and symptoms.

1 Signs and symptoms of intussusception begin suddenly and include vomiting and bloody stools.

3 Signs and symptoms of pyloric stenosis include projectile vomiting and weight loss.

4 Signs and symptoms of Hirschsprung's disease include abdominal distention, vomiting, and inadequate weight gain.

34. Knowledge, implementation, safe, effective care environment (a).

3 This delivers adequate heat and will not damage skin from this distance.

1 Skin should be kept dry during treatment.

2 The lamp should be uncovered.

4 The patient is assessed every 10 minutes while the heat lamp is in use.

35. Application, planning, physiological integrity (b).

4 Assessing sensation, circulation, and motion in affected extremities is necessary for all children in a cast.

1 Children having pain should be medicated for pain as needed.

2 Fluids should be encouraged; the cast can be kept dry by careful diapering and padding of the cast.

3 The child will need an adapted car seat to take her home safely.

36. Application, implementation, physiological integrity (b).

1 This is the medication used to terminate status epilepticus.

2 This is used to treat hypertension.

3 This medication is used for control and maintenance of seizures but is not the drug of choice for status epilepticus.

4 This is an opioid analgesic for management of moderate-to-severe pain.

37. Comprehension, assessment, physiological integrity (b).

2 These signs are the most notable because they are caused by increased intracranial pressure, a serious complication of meningitis.

1 The child's cry would be shrill and high-pitched.

3, 4 These are not signs of meningitis.

38. Application, implementation, physiological integrity (b).

3 The patient with a colostomy is at increased risk for peristomal skin breakdown. All skin-care products should be evaluated for allergic reaction. A patch test should be performed on an area of the abdomen away from the stoma.

1 If shaving is necessary, an electric razor should be used. A blade increases the risk of irritation or cuts.

2 Tincture of benzoin is drying to the skin and is not an effective barrier.

4 Soaps should be avoided, except when showering.

39. Comprehension, assessment, health promotion and maintenance (b).

2 The eustachian tubes are shorter and wider in the young child than they are in the older child, which allows for easier introduction of bacteria.

1, 4 The shape and position of these do not affect otitis media.

3 The external ear canals are basically the same shape and in the same position in young and older children.

40. Comprehension, implementation, physiological integrity (c).

2 Malignant hyperthermia is caused by an idiosyntric reaction to drugs and anesthetics administered during surgery.

1 Dantrium is given after malignant hyperthermia occurs.

3 This would have no effect on the occurrence.

4 Routine admitting vital signs are taken, not just the temperature. This action would have no effect on the potential problem.

41. Application, implementation, physiological integrity (b).

2 25 lb = 11.3 kg

100 mg × 11.3 kg/day = 1130 mg/day

$$\frac{1130 \text{ mg}}{4 \text{ doses}} = 282 \text{ mg}$$

Appropriate order = 250 mg four times daily

1, 3, 4 These are not appropriate orders for this child.

42. Application, implementation, physiological integrity (a).
   1 They are applied before feet and legs have a chance to swell.
   2 The patient's legs will be collecting fluid through gravity and a decrease in venous return after they arise.
   3 The stockings may be removed for the bath and reapplied immediately after.
   4 The legs would be in a dependent position, and venous return would be decreased; lying down is better.

43. Comprehension, assessment, physiological integrity (b).
   1 Because vitamin D cannot be converted to its biologically active form, which is needed for calcium reabsorption, hypocalcemia may develop.
   2 White blood cell count is usually decreased.
   3, 4 Both creatinine and BUN levels increase because of excessive amounts of nitrogenous wastes accumulating in the blood.

44. Application, implementation, physiological integrity (c).
   1 Immobilization promotes clot formation around the catheter insertion site.
   2, 3 The extremity is maintained in an extended position to promote circulation to the area and to enhance clot formation at the insertion site.
   4 Clients may have fluids after the procedure.

45. Comprehension, assessment, physiological integrity (b).
   4 This the deficit that frequently occurs in right-sided damage and is distressful for the patient.
   1, 2, 3 These are deficits with left-sided brain damage.

46. Application, assessment, physiological integrity (c).
   3 2 to 3 months are required after exposure to *Mycobacterium tuberculosis* for an infected person to develop skin sensitivity to PPD.
   1, 2 These would be too soon.
   4 Waiting this long is not recommended and would cause needless anxiety.

47. Comprehension, planning, physiological integrity (b).
   3 Trauma to the remaining kidney would place the patient's renal function at risk. He should not be allowed to play contact sports ever again.
   1, 2 Approximately 1 year is required for the major back, abdominal, and flank muscles to heal, but this is not the reason for withdrawal from the football team. However, heavy lifting should be avoided for that year.
   4 Only one kidney is needed to meet the body's demand for kidney function.

48. Knowledge, planning, physiological integrity (b).
   3 A balance of these three factors is necessary for the control of diabetes. The blood glucose level in diabetes mellitus is naturally elevated. Eating a diet low in simple carbohydrates is important. Because the body does not make enough insulin, a supplement has to be given; or in the case of type 2 diabetes, a stimulant is given in the form of a medication to enhance the production of more insulin to meet the body's needs. If a patient exercises excessively or becomes inactive without adjustments being made in the other two factors (diet and medication), then the body will be either hyperglycemic or hypoglycemic. Exercise uses glucose. Diet adds glucose to the system; insulin uses glucose. The three factors have to be in balance.
   1, 2, 4 Rest is important to everyone. However, an individual with diabetes must maintain proper balance of

the three factors indicated in #3 to maintain control of this condition. Refer to the rationale for #3.

49. Application, planning, physiological integrity (b).
   4 An indwelling catheter may be in place for up to 24 hours related to possible edema of the urethra and to decrease the possibility of infection and discomfort. A three-way Foley may be used if bladder irrigation is desired.
   1, 2 These statements increase anxiety for the patient and are not usually true in these procedures.
   3 These procedures are usually done under local anesthesia.

50. Application, assessment, health promotion and maintenance (b).
   2 Infection increases metabolism and increases the demand for insulin.
   1 This may affect glucose levels, but it is not a primary cause.
   3, 4 These would cause hypoglycemia.

51. Comprehension, evaluation, physiological integrity (b).
   2 Weight gain frequently occurs because of the increase in appetite and fluid retention.
   1 Hypertension is more apt to occur related to fluid retention.
   3 Fluid retention is more apt to occur, not dehydration.
   4 Muscle mass will atrophy with extended use of cortisones, and the patient's strength will weaken.

52. Knowledge, evaluation, physiological integrity (a).
   2 This describes the three-point crutch gait.
   1 This technique is the swing-through crutch gait.
   3 This statement describes the two-point crutch gait.
   4 This technique describes the four-point crutch gait.

53. Application, assessment, physiological integrity (b).
   4 These symptoms are consistent with those of chronic bronchitis.
   1, 3 Although these are forms of COPD, these symptoms may not be present.
   2 These symptoms may be present in this disease process, but it is not a form of COPD.

54. Application, assessment, physiological integrity (b).
   1 The patient's pain may be related to a blood clot (deep-vein thrombosis); a positive Homans' sign is indicative of a blood clot.
   2 The nurse should ensure that the possibility of a blood clot has been ruled out. The action of the stockings may dislodge the clot into general circulation.
   3 If the pain is related to a blood clot, the stockings will not help the pain and may contribute to a pulmonary embolism.
   4 Babinski's reflex is part of the neurological assessment and has nothing to do with calf pain.

55. Knowledge, assessment, physiological integrity (a).
   1 Awakening at night to void is most common. Pain on urination is a sign of cystitis that most men find disturbing.
   2 These may result if a UTI develops because of stasis of urine.
   3 These may develop; however, they are not common signs.
   4 Hematuria may result from blood vessels that have been overstretched. Groin pain is not present in most men.

56. Application, planning, physiological integrity (b).
   4 Waiting 30 seconds to 2 minutes between puffs gives the medication time to disperse.

1 Rinsing the mouthpiece daily minimizes the presence of bacteria.

2 The patient should exhale slowly so that the airway is completely empty when the medication enters.

3 The container should be shaken for 3 to 5 seconds to allow thorough mixing of the medication.

57. Application, implementation, physiological integrity (a).

   4 Taking the blood pressure in the left arm may cause compression or occlude the fistula, or both. Any compression, tight clothing, or carrying objects with arm bent should be avoided.

   1 Fluids may be restricted. Some patients may have urine output. Hourly monitoring is usually not appropriate.

   2 To do this is unnecessary; patients are discharged with this in place.

   3 This is inappropriate and is not according to procedure.

58. Comprehension, planning, health promotion and maintenance (b).

   3 Individuals should look for both sodium and monosodium glutamate when reading labels.

   1 Individuals on a sodium-restricted diet may consume monosaccharides.

   2 Iron is not restricted on a sodium-restricted diet.

   4 High-density lipoproteins, a type of fat in the bloodstream, are not listed on nutrition labels.

59. Comprehension, planning, physiological integrity (b).

   4 Probenecid, an antigout agent, decreases the excretion of penicillin antibiotics, thereby prolonging the action and increasing the effect of the ampicillin.

   1 Probenecid will not reduce the risk of anaphylaxis.

   2 Probenecid reduces the excretion of penicillin antibiotics and does not affect the metabolism.

   3 This is the action of probenecid when it is used to treat gout; however, in this case, it is used to prolong the action of the ampicillin.

60. Comprehension, assessment, physiological integrity (b).

   3 These foods are low in sodium.

   1 Macaroni and cheese are high in sodium.

   2 Corned beef is high in sodium.

   4 Lobster and canned peaches are high in sodium.

61. Application, implementation, physiological integrity (b).

   3 Postural hypotension is a common side effect of diuretics that causes a transient but symptomatic drop in blood pressure.

   1 Most salt substitutes contain potassium chloride and should be avoided when a client is taking a potassium-sparing diuretic, such as spironolactone.

   2 These foods are high in potassium, which can lead to hyperkalemia.

   4 The patient should be taught to maintain a record of daily rather than monthly weights. Daily fluctuations provide a reflection of fluid status.

62. Comprehension, assessment, physiological integrity (a).

   2 The Jones criteria are used only to diagnose rheumatic fever.

   1, 3 These are hereditary diseases.

   4 This is a viral disease diagnosed by the symptoms and the Monospot test.

63. Knowledge, planning, physiological integrity (b).

   2 Photosensitivity (increased sensitivity to ultraviolet radiation), a frequent adverse reaction to tetracycline, causes the patient to develop sunburn more readily than is usual.

In addition to sunscreen, the nurse might teach the patient to wear protective clothing and to avoid tanning beds.

   1 Yogurt helps replace some of the normal flora that are often destroyed by antibiotic therapy; however, the calcium in yogurt binds with the tetracycline, forming an insoluble complex that will not be absorbed into circulation.

   3 The iron and other minerals in the supplement bind with the tetracycline, forming an insoluble complex that will not be absorbed into circulation.

   4 The patient should continue to take the medication until ordered to do so by the physician.

64. Knowledge, assessment, physiological integrity (b).

   2 The infant with FTT is distrustful of people.

   1 The infant with FTT prefers inanimate objects, such as toys.

   3 This is a characteristic of a healthy infant.

   4 This can be caused by other medical conditions or prematurity.

65. Application, implementation, physiological integrity (b).

   2 This explanation clearly describes when and how the client is to take the medication.

   1 This explanation does not clearly describe how the client is to take the medication.

   3 This explanation describes how to carry out the prescription but does not inform the client to stop taking the tablets if the pain subsides. In addition, Nitrostat is indicated for treatment of acute angina, not prophylaxis of anginal attacks.

   4 Aside from being an incomplete explanation of the order, this explanation describes taking the medication by the wrong route.

66. Application, evaluation, physiological integrity (b).

   3 Raw foods such as vegetables and salad would contribute to the pain the patient is experiencing.

   1 These foods are generally bland; when cooked, they would not aggravate diverticulitis.

   2 These foods would not stimulate pain.

   4 This may contribute to pain but not to the degree that raw, high-fiber foods would.

67. Application, planning, physiological integrity (b).

   1 Members of the Hindu faith are vegetarians; meeting protein needs of the patient may be difficult.

   2 Fruits and vegetables are not restricted in the Hindu diet.

   3 If cultural considerations are given, the patient should enjoy his meal plan choices.

   4 The exchange lists will not need to be modified, although creative approaches to planning for protein intake will be necessary.

68. Comprehension, implementation, physiological integrity (c).

   4 An upright position with head flexed toward sternum improves swallowing, thereby reducing the risk of aspiration—the key respiratory complication in patients with dysphagia.

   1 Supplemental oxygen may improve blood oxygen level but does not prevent the respiratory complication of aspiration.

   2 No indication in this question of an abnormal breathing pattern exists.

   3 Vitamin therapy may help with healing and tissue function but will not prevent aspiration.

69. Application, planning, health promotion and maintenance (b).
    1 Increased urination, increased thirst, and increased hunger are the cardinal symptoms of diabetes mellitus.
    2 These are the symptoms of hypoglycemia.
    3 These are not the cardinal signs of diabetes mellitus but are indicative of hypertension.
    4 These symptoms are not indicative of diabetes mellitus but can be indicative of anemia.

70. Application, planning, health promotion and maintenance (b).
    2 Honey contains botulism spores, which can be a problem for very young children.
    1 Current thinking holds that rice cereal should be started at 4 to 6 months of age.
    3 The baby should not become accustomed to the taste of additives that have little nutritional value.
    4 Most allergies to eggs are caused by the white, not the yolk.

71. Comprehension, implementation, physiological integrity (b).
    3 Changing the trach ties poses the most risk because the patient might cough out the trach, thereby losing the patency of the airway.
    1 Suctioning should pose limited risk if performed in a safe manner.
    2 Limited risk, cleansing the stoma does not directly effect the airway.
    4 As long as the trach ties are in place, cleansing the inner cannula should not pose a risk.

72. Comprehension, assessment, physiological integrity (a).
    1 A check of capillary filling, also known as the blanching test, is done to determine adequate arterial blood flow. Slow or no capillary filling would be indicative of compartment syndrome.
    2 An obstruction of venous peripheral circulation would be exhibited by edema.
    3 Impaired neurological function, such as in compartment syndrome, would be exhibited by paralysis and sensory loss.
    4 Although capillary filling is affected by cardiac output, that is not what the nurse is assessing in this case. The nurse is looking for signs and symptoms of compartment syndrome.

73. Knowledge, planning, physiological integrity (b).
    4 A low-fat diet is recommended to avoid aggravating gallbladder disease. These items are acceptable on a low-fat diet.
    1 These are high-fat foods.
    2 The avocado salad and chocolate milk are especially high in fat.
    3 Ice cream is high in fat.

74. Comprehension, planning, physiological integrity (b).
    1 Atropine sulfate can increase intraocular pressure and precipitate urinary retention.
    2 Etodolac (Lodine) is a nonsteroidal antiinflammatory drug (NSAID) and not usually contraindicated for persons with these disorders.
    3 Furosemide (Lasix) is a diuretic and not usually contraindicated for persons with these disorders.
    4 Dopamine hydrochloride (Intropin) is an alpha- and beta-adrenergic and not usually contraindicated for persons with these disorders.

75. Knowledge, planning, physiological integrity (a).
    3 Naloxone hydrochloride (Narcan) is the narcotic antagonist used to reverse the effects of morphine sulfate.
    1 Hydromorphone hydrochloride (Dilaudid) is an opioid analgesic.
    2 Acetylcysteine sodium (Mucomyst) is a mucolytic that is used as an acetaminophen antidote.
    4 Epinephrine hydrochloride is a sympathomimetic drug.

76. Comprehension, planning, physiological integrity (c).
    4 The tomato sauce, mashed potatoes, and strawberries are all good sources of vitamin C, which is the vitamin especially needed for tissue healing.
    1 Mashed potatoes are the only source of vitamin C in this food group.
    2 None of these foods provide a source of vitamin C.
    3 None of these foods provide a good source of vitamin C.

77. Application, planning, physiological integrity (b).
    2 The patient with diabetes should carry a fast source of glucose with them at all times. Candy has the most simple sugar content and is easy to carry and use.
    1 Gum does not have as much sugar as does candy and would not work as quickly.
    3 Water is important for patients with diabetes to consume but will not correct insulin shock, which is the life-threatening emergency that candy corrects.
    4 Crackers are complex carbohydrates and are not a rapid enough source of sugar.

78. Application, implementation, physiological integrity (b).
    4 The patient may have a weakened immune system and should avoid the risk of infection.
    1 HIV-positive patients can develop AIDS, and no fail-safe way is available to prevent it.
    2 Although a specific pneumonia is commonly seen in AIDS, prevention goes beyond this one problem.
    3 Preventing infection is of primary concern over preventing hypotension.

79. Knowledge, planning, physiological integrity (b).
    4 Protamine sulfate reverses the effect of heparin sodium.
    1 Warfarin sodium (Coumadin) is an anticoagulant.
    2 Naloxone hydrochloride (Narcan) is a narcotic antagonist.
    3 AquaMEPHYTON (vitamin K) reverses the effects of warfarin sodium (Coumadin).

80. Comprehension, implementation, physiological integrity (b).
    3 Lying immobile and keeping the head in one position will minimize the vertigo.
    1 Dark glasses may prevent migraines or light halos but not vertigo.
    2 Soft music is soothing but will not diminish vertigo.
    4 Resting will help vertigo, but the side on which the patient rests does not matter.

81. Application, implementation, physiological integrity (b).
    4 The antiinflammatory properties of aspirin decrease joint inflammation and pain.
    1 The primary purpose of aspirin therapy is to decrease joint inflammation. The nurse does not know the dose of the aspirin or the agenda of the physician.
    2 Aspirin does not relax skeletal muscles.
    3 Aspirin is given to reduce inflammation in joints.

82. Comprehension, planning, health promotion and maintenance (b).

2 Frequent small, low-fat meals and snacks consisting of easily digested energy-yielding foods such as carbohydrates (starches) are more easily tolerated by patients experiencing morning sickness.

1, 3, 4 Adding extra servings of these foods would increase foods that are more difficult to digest and are therefore not easily tolerated by patients experiencing morning sickness.

83. Application, evaluation, physiological integrity (b).

1000 ml/8 hours = 125 ml/hour; 125 ml/hour × 7.5 hours = 937.5 ml or 938 ml.

84. Comprehension, implementation, physiological integrity (b).

2 This allows for time to recover and rest.

1, 3, 4 These are more appropriate if the nursing diagnosis indicated a respiratory problem.

85. Application, planning, safe, effective care environment (c).

3 The tympanic mode would pose the least chance for injury and bleeding for the patient.

1 Oral temperatures should not be taken on an unconscious patient because of the chance for injury to the mucous membranes.

2 A rectal temperature may damage the rectal mucosa and cause bleeding.

4 Although this method is safe, axillary temperatures are less accurate compared with tympanic temperature.

86. Knowledge, assessment, physiological integrity (b).

3 Prolonged capillary refill time indicates diminished capillary perfusion; thus it should not take longer than 3 seconds.

1, 2 Capillary refill in 1 or 2 seconds is acceptable; it should not take longer than 3 seconds.

4 Refer to rationale for the correct response (#3).

87. Application, planning, physiological integrity (b).

1 Straining may initiate bleeding.

2, 3, 4 These are inappropriate for the expected outcome.

88. Knowledge, assessment, physiological integrity (b).

3 The decrease in circulation to the involved extremity causes tingling and numbness.

1, 4 These are not factors in compromised neurovascular integrity.

2 The extremity would feel cool.

89. Comprehension, assessment, health promotion and maintenance (b).

2 This is when adolescence is considered to begin in each child's life.

1 This occurs more than once in childhood.

3 Developing a self-image is part of adolescence, but it may be positive or negative during the teenage years.

4 Adolescent boys are often attracted to adolescent girls at an earlier age than the girls are attracted to the boys.

90. Application, planning, physiological integrity (c).

4 NutraSweet has no known effect on urine acidity.

1, 2 Antacids and salt substitutes cause the urine to become alkaline.

3 Sulfa drugs require an alkaline urine for maximal drug absorption.

91. Comprehension, assessment, physiological integrity (b).

3 Because of manipulation of the intestines, the patient may experience a reflex paralysis of the ileus. When peristalsis is stopped, the intestines continues to produce gas. The gut also are not moving the contents along its pathway, which results in abdominal distention. Paralytic ileus typically occurs 3 to 5 days postoperatively.

1 The patient with a paralytic ileus will have decreased or absent bowel sounds.

2 The pain may be localized, sharp, or intermittent.

4 Headache is not a result of paralytic ileus.

92. Knowledge, assessment, health promotion and maintenance (a).

4 Preschooler children are at the stage when they are learning how to interact with other people, as well as learning proper behavior; this helps them develop a sense of initiative and accomplishment.

1 This is the stage of infants.

2 This is the stage of school-age children.

3 This is the stage of toddlers.

93. Application, assessment, physiological integrity (b).

2 These are common side effects of this classification; they are also common side effects of the methylxanthine derivatives. Other side effects include palpitations, changes in blood pressure, tachycardia, headache, and muscle tremors.

1 These are not identified as common side effects for any of the classifications of medications used to threat asthma.

3 These may be associated with large doses of chlorambucil, a drug used in treating neoplastic diseases.

4 These are associated with antiinflammatory agents that may be given for asthma.

94. Application, planning, physiological integrity (b).

1 Retained secretions would indicate her difficulty in removing them caused by an ineffective cough. Adventitious breath sounds may also be present.

2 This is a symptom of altered tissue perfusion.

3, 4 These complaints by the patient reflect an activity intolerance.

95. Application, planning, physiological integrity (b).

3 Pulse oximetry monitors the actual oxygen content in the blood. A reading of 90% or greater from 79% would indicate that the patient's body is tolerating the activity and is better able to meet the body's oxygen requirements.

1 Cyanosis indicates poor oxygenation to the tissues.

2, 4 These are later signs indicating activity tolerance. A better indication would be the return of these rates to baseline within 1 to 5 minutes.

96. Comprehension, assessment, health promotion and maintenance (b).

1 These are the key factors. General nutritional state, age, and any chronic disease state co-existing can influence the rate of wound healing.

2, 3, 4 Skill of closure, mental awareness, and type of suture are not key factors.

97. Application, implementation, physiological integrity (b).

1 This technique allows for smoother passage of food into the stomach because the trachea is partially closed; therefore food is less likely to be aspirated into the lungs.

2 This is inappropriate and may cause aspiration of food into the lungs.

3 Liquids should be thickened to assist with swallowing difficulties.

4 Hyperextension of the neck is uncomfortable and may increase the possibility of aspiration.

98. Knowledge, implementation, physiological integrity (a).
    3 These patients should avoid douching, using feminine sprays, and using perfumed feminine hygiene products because these products would increase incidence of UTI in the patient.
    2 Voiding is recommended after sexual intercourse.
    1 Showers are recommended instead of tub baths.
    4 8-ounce glasses of water and caffeine-free, noncarbonated beverages are recommended. A diet that acidifies the urine is recommended, including cranberry juice. A consistent fluid intake of 2 liters a day is also recommended.

99. Application, planning, health promotion and maintenance (c).
    1 Increased public awareness regarding signs and symptoms and what to do in the event of a CVA will relay the importance of seeking prompt medical attention; "time is brain"
    2 Health care providers understand the need to treat promptly so as to facilitate recovery. To best decrease delays in seeking treatment, the general public needs to be more knowledgeable because ignorance prevents patients from seeking treatment.
    3, 4 When a stroke is suspected, the first course of action is to call 9-1-1.

100. Application, planning, physiological integrity (b).
    4 Diminished caliber or force (or both) of urinary stream and a feeling of incomplete bladder emptying are common complaints.
    1, 2 These are more common with UTI.
    3 This is unrelated to the situation.

101. Application, implementation, physiological integrity (b).
    DD = 750 mg
    DH = 0.5 g (500 mg)
    V = 5 ml
    $$\frac{DD}{DH} = \frac{750 \text{ mg}}{500 \text{ mg}} \times 5 \text{ ml} = 7.5 \text{ ml} = 1 \tfrac{1}{2} \text{ tsp}$$

102. Comprehension, assessment, physiological integrity (c).
    2 Polyuria that occurs 72 hours after a burn indicates the diuretic phase of burn recovery. The nurse should monitor for electrolyte disturbances (sodium and potassium), which often accompany massive diuresis.
    1 Signs and symptoms of skin infection are fever, redness, and swelling.
    3 Signs and symptoms of respiratory obstruction are shortness of breath, dyspnea, and wheezing.
    4 Signs and symptoms of shock are hypotension, tachycardia, and oliguria.

103. Application, implementation, physiological integrity (b).
    3 This position and the soft-textured foods decrease the risk of aspiration.
    1 Suction equipment should be available; however, positioning and the type of foods provided will help the patient more with the actual swallowing.
    2 Hyperextension of the neck serves to increase the possibility of aspiration.
    4 Pureeing, liquefying, or providing a diet of bland foods is unnecessary. The goal is to offer the patient as normal a diet as possible.

104. Knowledge, assessment, physiological integrity (a).
    1 Wheezes are produced by airflow through narrow airways as in bronchospasm of anaphylaxis.
    2 Crackles are produced by fluid in the bronchioles and alveoli, are usually caused by pulmonary edema.
    3 Rhonchi are produced when fluid or mucus blocks the larger airways, such as with infection.
    4 Friction rubs are caused by pleural inflammation.

105. Application, implementation, physiological integrity (b).
    4 With lower motor neuron pathways, disruption in the myoneural junction and muscles occur, resulting in flaccidity; muscle weakness may also be noted.
    1, 2 Upper motor neuron lesions lead to spasticity and hypertonia.
    3 Hypertrophy, the enlargement of muscle mass, usually occurs from overuse.

106. Knowledge, planning, physiological integrity (a).
    1 Ambulation is the most effective way of keeping blood circulating and preventing pooling of blood in the extremities.
    2 Leg massage is contraindicated because it may loosen a clot that is already formed and create an embolus.
    3 Sitting with knees crossed cuts off venous return and contributes to venous stasis.
    4 Pillows under the knees cut off venous return and contribute to venous stasis.

107. Knowledge, assessment, physiological integrity (b).
    4 These are all common symptoms of celiac disease.
    1, 3 Constipation is not a symptom of celiac disease.
    2 An appetite for sweets is not a sign of celiac disease.

108. Comprehension, planning, physiological integrity (b).
    1 The top priority in this client's care is pain management.
    2 Altered skin integrity may not occur because no indication exists that the client is immobile.
    3 No indication exists in this scenario that hypertension is occurring.
    4 The priority problem during the acute phase is pain relief. Discharge teaching, if necessary, will be a priority at the end of the acute episode.

109. Application, implementation, physiological integrity (b).
    4 Sexual arousal causes vasodilation and increases patient discomfort.
    1 Antibiotics should be taken for the full prescribed time.
    2 Of the four most common forms of prostatitis, nonbacterial prostatitis may occur after a viral illness, or it may be associated with other sexually transmitted diseases, particularly in the young adult. This patient is started on antibiotics, which implies that this is an acute or chronic bacterial prostatitis. A condom will protect the partner from infection.
    3 Constipation and bearing down to pass a hard stool increase patient discomfort. Stool softeners are often prescribed to provide relief from painful symptoms.

110. Application, assessment, physiological integrity (b).
    1 Characteristically, vertigo or the sensation of spinning is a chief complaint with Meniere's disease.
    2, 3 Ear pain is usually not described; however, a feeling of fullness or headache may be an accompanying complaint.
    4 Hearing loss would be gradual.

111. Comprehension, planning, safe, effective care environment (b).
    4 A compromised immune system or other stress can cause the capsule to open and release active TB bacteria.
    1 The TB skin test would be positive because antibodies have been formed against the TB bacteria.

2 To be contagious, the disease must be active.

3 Walling off the TB bacteria eliminates the active symptoms.

112. Application, implementation, physiological integrity (b).

1 Drainage trickling down the posterior pharynx may be exhibited by frequent swallowing, belching, and hematemesis. The nurse should use a flashlight when assessing the back of the throat.

2, 4 These are very late signs for bleeding from this type of surgery.

3 This would be expected from this type of surgery.

113. Comprehension, assessment, physiological integrity (b).

3 An increase in blood volume can result in hypertension, bounding pulses, and pulmonary edema (dyspnea, cough).

1 This indicates possible systemic infection.

2 These indicate central nervous system involvement or hypoxia.

4 This indicates local infection.

114. Comprehension, assessment, physiological integrity (b).

4 Some drugs are known to lower the seizure threshold. Other secondary causes of seizures are cerebral ischemia, such as in a CVA, or fever.

1, 2, 3 These states have not been identified as potential risk factors for seizures.

115. Application, assessment, physiological integrity (b).

1 Labored breathing is considered a cardinal symptom.

2 Skin turgor does not relate to a respiratory dysfunction.

3, 4 These may also be accompanying complaints but are not considered to be cardinal symptoms.

116. Comprehension, assessment, physiological integrity (c).

1 Carbon dioxide is trapped in the alveoli, which is the basic problem in emphysema. Respiratory acidosis occurs when the lungs cannot exhale carbon dioxide adequately. As a result, the PaCO2 and carbonic acid increase and pH decreases.

2 Hyperventilation causes the rapid blowing off of carbon dioxide.

3, 4 These are potential effects of emphysema not the basic cause of acidosis.

117. Comprehension, implementation, physiological integrity (b).

4 These signs and symptoms, in addition to the admitting diagnosis, are the most characteristic of hypoglycemia. To confirm this assessment, the nurse would perform a blood glucose monitoring test.

1 The first suspicion should be hypoglycemia, not a heart problem.

2 Giving insulin can worsen the hypoglycemia.

3 Giving orange juice is the second priority after the glucose test to confirm the problem.

118. Comprehension, planning, physiological integrity (b).

1 Fever increases the body's energy expenditures, and profuse perspiration causes fluid loss, resulting in the body's increased need for fluids. If fluids are not replaced, dehydration will occur.

2, 3, 4 The opposite of these occur because of fluid loss. Respirations increase with fever.

119. Comprehension, assessment, physiological integrity (c).

1 The narrowing of the airways traps carbon dioxide. This buildup of carbon dioxide produces carbonic acid, and the net result is respiratory acidosis.

2 The metabolic system is not involved in this acute respiratory problem.

3 High carbon dioxide levels result in acidosis, not alkalosis.

4 The metabolic system is not involved in this acute respiratory problem.

120. Application, implementation, physiological integrity (b).

4 Intracranial pressure (ICP) is the pressure produced by the brain tissue, cerebral spinal fluid (CSF), and blood volume within the skull. When the nurse allows the patient to rest between nursing activities, it helps keep the ICP within 5 to 15 mm Hg. Too much activity may increase metabolic demands that would alter the balance of the three components, which determine ICP and the brain's inherent compensatory capability.

1, 2 Coughing, suctioning, laying flat, bearing down, or the Valsalva maneuver may cause ICP to rise.

3 Avoiding neck and hip flexion is necessary. Maintaining the patient's neck, hips, and knees in alignment helps promote venous flow. The high-Fowler's position causes flexion. A semi-Fowler's position improves cerebral perfusion and allows for gravity to drain fluid from the brain.

121. Comprehension, planning, physiological integrity (b).

3 This goal is measurable and attainable over a short period.

1 This goal is unrealistic and long term.

2 This goal has nothing to do with the diagnosis.

4 A pain rating scale of greater than 5 is not an acceptable goal.

122. Application, assessment, physiological integrity (b).

3 Diuretics increase the quantity and alter the characteristics of the urine.

1, 4 These may affect the ability of the bladder or sphincter to contract or relax normally.

2 Anticoagulants may cause hematuria.

123. Comprehension, assessment, physiological integrity (a).

4 The ability to respond and follow commands assesses the return of normal cerebral cortex function after brain surgery.

1 Hearing is an assessment of the eighth cranial nerve and not overall brain function.

2, 3 These relate to the patient's attitude, not physiological function.

124. Comprehension, assessment, physiological integrity (b).

1 These symptoms of leukemia result directly from changes in the bone marrow.

2 These symptoms are caused by leukemic effects on the nervous system that lead to increased ICP.

3 These symptoms result from the body's increasing need to meet the metabolic needs of the leukemic cells.

4 These are not symptoms of leukemia.

125. Comprehension, planning, health promotion and maintenance (c).

2 Hepatic coma is caused by an inability to metabolize ammonia and other substances. Proteins are avoided because one of their breakdown products is ammonia.

1 Soaps-suds enemas will not help prevent hepatic coma.

3 Iced saline lavages are used for gastrointestinal hemorrhaging, not hepatic coma.

4 Carbohydrates are necessary in the diet to provide energy for healing.

PART 2 ANSWERS AND RATIONALES

1. Comprehension, evaluation, safe, effective care environment (a).

    3 The movement toward cost reduction has shifted health care delivery out of hospitals and into long-term care, home care, and skilled nursing facilities.

    1 The scope of nursing practice has increased with technological advances in health care.

    2 The focus of all health care delivery has moved to wellness promotion rather than illness treatment.

    4 Nursing remains patient centered. Treatment is more technology based but still involves direct contact with the patient by the nurse.

2. Knowledge, implementation, physiological integrity (a).

    3 The specimen is discarded to ensure that all of the urine in the container was collected during a 24-hour period. The voiding at 8:00 AM contained urine that was collected since the last voiding and would make the collection period longer than 24 hours.

    1 The nurse would not send the specimen for urinalysis unless a physician's order to do so is given.

    2 Adding the urine to the collection container would include urine outside of the 24-hour collection period.

    4 Although creatinine clearance reflects kidney function and the fact that renal impairment is a complication of diabetes mellitus, the information given does not indicate that the patient has diabetes. Additionally, no mention is made of an order to test the urine for glucose and ketones.

3. Application, implementation, safe, effective care environment (b).

    2 The nurse protects the patient's best interests in all care situations.

    1 Allowable services may not always meet the patient's needs.

    3 The nurse is not the representative of the insuring agency.

    4 Level of care is based on patient needs, not allowable benefits.

4. Application, implementation, physiological integrity (a).

    3 Instructing the patient to swallow twice for each bite of food helps ensure that food is swallowed and reduces the risk of choking.

    1 Thickened liquids are generally tolerated better compared with thin liquids by individuals with dysphagia.

    2 Combining more than one texture in a bite predisposes the patient to choking.

    4 Offering finger foods does not address swallowing problems associated with dysphagia; this type of food is more likely to cause choking than would softer foods fed from the tip of a spoon.

5. Application, implementation, physiological integrity (b).

    3 This allows the patient to be independent and feed herself.

    1 This denies the patient's independence.

    2 This denies the patient full nourishment and is unnecessary if precautions are taken.

    4 This does not address the patient's impaired vision.

6. Knowledge, planning, health promotion and maintenance (b).

    4 Oxygen therapy for the newborn must be administered with great caution to prevent retrolental fibroplasia.

    This condition is caused by high levels of oxygen concentration and may result in blindness.

    1 Ophthalmia neonatorum is a purulent conjunctivitis and keratitis of the newborn resulting from exposure of the eyes to chemical, chlamydial, bacterial, or viral agents.

    2 ABO incompatibility is a hereditary condition that causes blood destruction in the fetus or the newborn; it is classified as a hemolytic disease of the newborn.

    3 Respiratory distress syndrome is an acute lung disease of the newborn caused by a deficiency of pulmonary surfactant.

7. Application, implementation, physiological integrity (c).

    2 Blood glucose levels are a significant assessment for individuals with diabetes, especially during illness.

    1 Although helpful, this is not a priority for this patient at this time.

    3 This may not be indicated for this particular patient, and the glucometer takes precedence.

    4 This may not be indicated; further assessment data is needed.

8. Comprehension, implementation, safe, effective care environment (b).

    4 A high pulse rate such as this may indicate that too much thyroid hormone

    1 This is not a standard aspect of teaching for thyroid medication.

    2, 3 These are not part of the teaching protocol for this type of medication.

9. Comprehension, evaluation, safe, effective care environment (b).

    2 The resident's chart is private and the nurse should not view the chart unless involved in direct patient care.

    1 This is inappropriate behavior and must be reported.

    3 This is an inappropriate intervention based on the patient's wishes.

    4 This is a most appropriate action; the incident requires further investigation.

10. Knowledge, implementation, safe, effective care environment (a).

    3 In a hospital setting, insertion of a Foley catheter must always be done using sterile technique.

    1 Reverse isolation is not appropriate in this case.

    2 Medical aseptic technique can be used by patients in their home setting.

    4 Good hand washing is always a priority, but insertion of a Foley catheter must be done with sterile technique.

11. Application, planning, health promotion and maintenance (b).

    3 Soap has a drying effect on the skin of older adults.

    1 The resident must be clean.

    2 No indication exists that this is a medical issue.

    4 This requires a physician's order; nursing interventions should be tried first.

12. Comprehension, assessment, health promotion and maintenance (a).

    2 Two nurses count simultaneously to compare the number of beats produced by the heart with the number of beats that are perfused to peripheral circulation; using the same watch ensures accuracy.

    1 By not counting the beats simultaneously, the nurse is unable to compare the number of beats produced with the number of beats perfused.

3 Two nurses count simultaneously to compare the number of beats produced with the number of beats perfused; using different watches may affect accuracy.

4 One nurse cannot accurately count the apical and radial beats simultaneously if a pulse deficit is present.

13 Application, implementation, safe, effective care environment (a).

4 This prevents contamination of the environment with wound drainage.

1 The nurse cannot leave the patient's bedside during a sterile procedure.

2 Leaving soiled dressing materials in the bedside trash creates odor problems and the potential for spread of pathogens.

3 This contaminates the sterile field.

14. Knowledge, evaluation, health promotion and maintenance (a).

3 Dry cough is an early sign of oxygen toxicity.

1 Although fever might indicate the presence of infection associated with the effects of oxygen toxicity on the mucosal lining, it is not an early sign of the condition.

2 Excessive mucus production may result from the ongoing effects of oxygen toxicity, but it is a later sign of the condition.

4 Moist breath sounds may result from the ongoing effects of oxygen toxicity, but this too is a later sign of the condition.

15. Application, implementation, physiological integrity (b).

3 Failure of venous return of blood from the legs and pelvis may be caused by compression of the inferior vena cava by the uterus while the patient is in a supine position during labor. Turning the patient on her left side relieves the pressure on the inferior vena cava and is the best and simplest nursing measure for comfort and relief.

1, 2, 4 These are inappropriate nursing actions that are unnecessary and would not correct the situation.

16. Knowledge, evaluation, physiological integrity (c).

3 These symptoms, along with malaise and fever, are those of toxicity that a patient on zidovudine (AZT) may experience.

1 These are toxic effects of dideoxycytidine (ddC).

2 Painful peripheral nerves are caused by the drug dideoxyinosine (ddI).

4 These symptoms are caused by dideoxythymidine (d4T).

17 Comprehension, implementation, physiological integrity (b).

4 Approximately 4 to 6 hours are required for spinal fluid pressure to stabilize following lumbar puncture; fewer neurological side effects occur if bed rest is maintained during this period.

1 Falling may occur because of vertigo, but this explanation is not as inclusive compared with answer #4.

2 The nursing staff's convenience is not a reason for remaining flat.

3 Although the position may limit spinal fluid leakage, little or no blood loss should occur from the procedure.

18. Knowledge, assessment, physiological integrity (b).

3 Recurrent constipation can indicate a problem with nutrition.

1 Feeling fatigue is normal after exercise.

2 This is a normal pattern.

4 This is normal for healthy mucous membranes.

19. Application, implementation, safe, effective care environment (a).

2 Standard Precautions advise that gloves are to be worn whenever the nurse comes into contact with blood or any body fluid.

1 Wearing sterile gloves is unnecessary; they cannot be kept sterile anyway. A gown is not necessary unless the patient is also in wound or drainage isolation.

3 A mask is not necessary unless the patient with AIDS has active TB or an methicillin-resistant *Staphylococcus aureus* infection.

4 Gloves are not necessary unless the nurse will come into actual contact with any body secretion.

20. Comprehension, evaluation, safe, effective care environment (b).

2 The catheter most likely was the reservoir for the infection.

1 No indication exists that a primary infection is present.

3 UTI is not normally caused by an autoimmune response.

4 No evidence exists that the patient received antibiotics.

21. Comprehension, planning, safe, effective care environment (b).

1 The pulse deficit examination requires one nurse to take the radial pulse while the second nurse takes the apical pulse.

2 Pulse deficit does not determine systolic murmur.

3 The assistance of a second nurse is more useful than patient cooperation.

4 The electrocardiograph is a diagnostic tool that measures electrical currents in the heart; it is not needed to measure pulse deficit.

22. Application, implementation, physiological integrity (b).

4 The term *débride* means to cleanse a wound, which is the purpose of this type of dressing.

1 The dressing may soothe the tissue, but this is not the purpose of the dressing.

2 Unless impregnated with an antibiotic solution, the dressing has no antiinfective qualities.

3 The saline evaporates from the dressing, and as it dries, the gauze adheres to the tissue that needs to be removed.

23. Knowledge, implementation, safe, effective care environment (a).

3 This procedure increases the likelihood of detecting occult blood in the stool.

1 Diarrhea stools are acceptable sources provided they are not contaminated with urine.

2 Stools for ova and parasites must be kept warm and delivered to the laboratory immediately.

4 Occult blood is hidden or unseen blood.

24. Comprehension, planning, physiological integrity (b).

4 Because of the barium in the bowel, cleansing enemas will be ordered to decrease the chance of fecal impaction from the barium.

1 Unless further procedures are ordered, the patient should not have to be NPO for any excessive length of time.

2 This is not an order that is normally associated with a barium enema.

3 A patient who has had a routine barium enema need not remain flat in bed.

25. Application, planning, safe, effective care environment (b).

4 The need for nutrition and hydration falls under physiological needs, which are the most basic of needs and therefore receive the highest priority when planning care.

1   Altered family processes falls under love and belonging needs, which are two levels up from the basic needs, according to Maslow's hierarchy of needs.

2   Although the need for oxygenation is also a basic physiological need, an actual problem is given a higher priority compared with a potential problem.

3   Skin integrity is part of the safety and protection needs, which is one level above the basic physiological needs. In addition, an actual problem is given a higher priority compared with a potential problem.

26.   Comprehension, implementation, health promotion and maintenance (b).

   4   Most long-term care facilities routinely test for TB on admission; this is a routine screening done to protect other residents in the facility.

   1   This does not validate the patient's concern nor explain the rationale for the test.

   2   This response appears to be antagonistic and does not help the patient.

   3   Once again, this response will only antagonize the patient and does not explain the reason for the test.

27.   Application, implementation, safe, effective care environment (b).

   2   Meperidine: DD = 20 mg DH = 50 mg V = 1 ml DD/DH = 20 mg/50 mg × 1 ml = 0.4 ml

   Atropine: DD = 0.08 mg DH = 0.2 mg V = 1 ml DD/DH = 0.08 mg/0.2 mg × 1 ml = 0.4 m /0.4 ml 0.4 ml = 0.8 ml

   1, 3, 4   These are not the correct amounts.

28.   Comprehension, implementation, health promotion and maintenance (b).

   3   Frequent small meals and snacks will not overfill the stomach, causing distension, discomfort, and nausea.

   1   The feeling of fullness from eating fats may increase nausea and vomiting.

   2   Increased protein foods will not alleviate the nausea and vomiting associated with pregnancy.

   4   Drinking beverages with meals will cause excessive gastric filling, contributing to nausea and vomiting.

29.   Application, implementation, safe, effective care environment (b).

   4   Massaging after administering the heparin can cause bleeding in the tissue.

   1   Heparin is usually given subcutaneously.

   2   Aspirating can cause bleeding in the tissue.

   3   All injection sites should be rotated.

30.   Knowledge, assessment, physiological integrity (c).

   2   The therapeutic range for theophylline is 10 to 20 mg/dl.

   1   This is subtherapeutic.

   3   This level is above the therapeutic range.

   4   This level is toxic.

31.   Knowledge, assessment, physiological integrity (a).

   2   Excessive cholesterol can contribute to the development of fatty plaques in the arteries (atherosclerosis).

   1   Cholesterol is a complex, fat-related substance.

   3   Supplements need not be taken because the body can synthesize cholesterol.

   4   Cholesterol is a major factor in the manufacture of vitamin D in the body.

32.   Application, implementation, physiological integrity (b).

   1000 units per hour is correct. 25,000 units ÷ 1000 ml = 25 units per ml; 25 units per ml × 40 ml per hour = 1000 units per hour.

33.   Comprehension, evaluation, physiological integrity (b).

   3   This meal has the lowest fat content.

   1   Whole milk and cake have a high fat content, and if the steak is not lean, it will also have excess fat.

   2   These foods are high in fat.

   4   These foods are higher in fat compared with fish, skim milk, and pudding with fruit.

34.   Knowledge, planning, physiological integrity (a).

   2   This test measures the extrinsic pathway of the clotting process and is used to regulate warfarin sodium (Coumadin) therapy.

   1   No such test exists.

   3   This test helps regulate heparin sodium therapy.

   4   This test is used for assisting in the diagnosis of bleeding disorders, not in regulating therapy of anticoagulants.

35.   Application, assessment, physiological integrity (c).

   2   Culture and religion shape the food likes and dislikes of the individual, and any plan that does not incorporate foods from the culture or religion might not be followed.

   1   Geographical region is important; however, culture and religion may be the most important.

   3   Family health history may cause the nurse to be concerned in planning a diet to prevent certain disorders, such as heart disease and cancer; however, these diets may not be followed if attention is not given to culture and religion.

   4   Although important to consider, the individual will more likely comply with the diet plan if personal choices are given consideration.

36.   Comprehension, planning, physiological integrity (b).

   4   Theophylline anhydrase (Theo-Dur) should not be given via a nasogastric tube because it is an extended-release medication.

   1   Other than checking the apical heart rate before administering, this route is acceptable.

   2   Other than giving with 3 to 4 ounces of juice, this route is acceptable.

   3   Although Tylenol elixir would be easier to take compared with tablets, this route is acceptable.

37.   Application, implementation, safe, effective care environment (c).

   2   The Fowler's position facilitates breathing and decreases swelling of the operative site; sandbags relieve tension on suture lines; frequent monitoring of vital signs allows for early intervention should complications arise.

   1   A complication of a thyroidectomy is a thyroid crisis, which causes a sudden increase in thyroxine. Signs of thyroid crisis are body temperatures as high as 106° F or higher, an increased heart rate of 200 bpm or greater, increased respiratory rate, apprehension, and restlessness. If the crisis is not arrested, death may occur.

   3   Redness, some swelling, and discomfort at the operative site are expected.

   4   Tetany secondary to hypocalcemia is a possible complication of the surgery secondary to accidental removal of the parathyroid glands.

38.   Knowledge, planning, physiological integrity (a).

   4   The lymphatic system drains excess fluids through a series of filters, lymph nodes, where bacteria and foreign bodies are trapped and destroyed.

1   The lymphatic system destroys bacteria.
2   Erythrocytes are manufactured in the red bone marrow of the long bones.
3   Clotting of blood is aided by platelets.

39. Comprehension, assessment, safe, effective care environment (a).

   1   Many patients experience an aura or unusual sensory perception before having a seizure.
   2   Hallucinations may be auditory or visual and are mental stimuli not based in reality.
   3   Petit mal seizures are usually confined to children without an associated aura. Petit mal is classified as a brief loss of consciousness.
   4   This in unrelated to seizure activity.

40. Comprehension, implementation, physiological integrity (b).

   3   With blockage of the bile duct, little bile enters the small intestine, causing the stool to appear clay colored as bile gives stool its characteristic color.
   1   Tarry stools are a sign of gastrointestinal bleeding.
   2   This is common in individuals having food poisoning or influenza.
   4   This is not a common finding in gallbladder disease.

41. Knowledge, evaluation, physiological integrity (b).

   3   The data support absence of infection, with normal physiological responses expected after surgery.
   1   The data suggest that the patient has developed an infection.
   2   The data suggest that the patient has developed an infection, especially with a white blood cell count of 13,000/mm^3
   4   A reddened incision site with purulent drainage indicates the presence of an infection.

42. Knowledge, planning, physiological integrity (a).

   2   The thymus gland produces T cells, which protect the infant during the first few months of life.
   1   The pineal gland secretes melatonin, which may regulate sexual dysfunction.
   3   The thyroid gland influences body metabolism.
   4   The pituitary gland secretes many substances that affect health promotion and maintenance, protect the body in stressful situations, and promote reabsorption of water.

43. Application, planning, physiological integrity (b).

   1   This action takes priority. If the patient's neurovascular status is compromised, the patient may lose a limb.
   2   Although important, this is not the most important nursing intervention.
   3   Maintenance of diet is important, but it is not the most important factor in this list.
   4   Activity that is within the limits of the patient's traction should be encouraged.

44. Application, planning, safe, effective care environment (b).

   3   The psychomotor domain of learning involves physically performing a task or skill.
   1   Stating or explaining information that has been provided indicates learning in the cognitive domain.
   2   Stating the importance of doing something is cognitive learning. Applying the knowledge in life situations indicates learning in the affective domain.
   4   Identification indicates learning at the cognitive domain.

45. Comprehension, planning, physiological integrity (c).

   4   Because the glucose concentration of central hyperalimentation is greater than 10%, it should be administered

via a central venous access catheter to prevent vein irritation and possible extravasation into the surrounding tissue.
   1   Because the glucose concentration of central hyperalimentation is greater than 10%, it should be administered via a central venous access catheter, not via the antecubital vein. See rationale for correct response (#4).
   2   These solutions can infuse at rates of 75 to 100 ml/hr.
   3   These solutions can cause hyperglycemia initially. Rebound hypoglycemia can occur if the infusion is discontinued abruptly.

46. Application, assessment, physiological integrity (b).

   2   These are classic symptoms of osteomyelitis.
   1   These symptoms may signal a pulmonary emboli.
   3   These symptoms may indicate neurovascular impairment.
   4   These are symptoms of neurological impairment.

47. Comprehension, planning, physiological integrity (b).

   3   Early ambulation helps promote the return of intestinal peristalsis, thereby decreasing the likelihood of ileus.
   1   Until bowel sounds are present, the patient should not receive solid food.
   2   Splinting of the abdomen will do nothing to promote normal bowel function.
   4   Kegel exercises promote urinary control and do not affect the intestines.

48. Application, planning, safe, effective care environment (b).

   1   A white blood cell count of 0.2 is indicative of immunosuppression. The immunocompromised patient is unable to resist foreign agents and is susceptible to overwhelming infection.
   2   The nursing staff wears facemasks to prevent the spread of microorganisms to the patient.
   3   Protective isolation precautions are indicated.
   4   Patients with immunosuppression are encouraged to avoid groups of people because this increases their risk of infection.

49. Knowledge, assessment, physiological integrity (a).

   2   The main function of aerosolized bronchodilators and chest physiotherapy is to dilate the bronchioles and loosen and move secretions out of the lungs.
   1   Nothing has been shown to be effective in decreasing mucus production.
   3   Efficiency of the diaphragm is not a problem in cystic fibrosis.
   4   Although chest physiotherapy may stimulate coughing to some degree, it is not done to increase oxygen consumption.

50. Application, planning, psychosocial integrity (b).

   4   A patient who is newly diagnosed with ALS needs support from family and health care professionals. Of the responses listed, this is a priority at this time.
   1   Periods of exercise are necessary, but they would not be increased. Adequate periods of rest are a necessity for this patient.
   2, 3   These are unrelated to the situation at this time; they are a priority during later stages of the disease.

51. Comprehension, implementation, safe, effective care environment (c).

   2   Decreased albumin levels alter the hydrostatic pressure in the liver's portal circulation, forcing fluid into the abdominal cavity.

1 Hypertension may contribute to portal hypertension but does not cause ascites.

3 This may cause jaundice but should not cause ascites.

4 Ammonia levels may be elevated, but this does not cause ascites.

52. Knowledge, assessment, safe, effective care environment (a).

3 The nurse, as part of the preoperative routine, ascertains that the signed consent form is on the chart.

1 The physician and anesthesiologist should obtain the patient's signature after explaining the procedure to the client.

2 The nurse sometimes witnesses the consent form, but it is not a responsibility of the nurse.

4 The surgeon and anesthesiologist are responsible for ascertaining that the patient understands what he is signing.

53. Application, assessment, physiological integrity (c).

4 Given that the patient will be staying a short time, this information appears to be the most pertinent because the nurse will need to ascertain how the patient will ambulate before and after surgery.

1 This data would not be particularly relevant at this time.

2 Although this is important to note, the nurse will need to assess how the patient will ambulate given that the priority for the short stay will be on rapid recovery.

3 Although this information is very important, it is not the most pertinent at this time.

54. Knowledge, assessment, psychosocial integrity (b).

2 The patient is relieving himself of his responsibility to quit smoking by placing the blame on people who should have warned him about the consequences.

1 Compensation is striving for excellence in one area to make up for a weakness in another area.

3 Sublimation involves replacing an unacceptable or unrealistic action with an acceptable alternative.

4 Repression means that the person forgets about the situation that is causing stress.

55. Application, planning, physiological integrity (b).

3 This goal is realistic, contains an observable behavior, includes a target date, and addresses the manifestation of the nursing diagnosis.

1 This goal addresses the cause rather than the manifestation of the nursing diagnosis.

2 This statement is a dependent nursing intervention rather than a goal statement.

4 Although this statement describes a desired outcome for a patient with dyspnea, it does not address the manifestation of the nursing diagnosis.

56. Comprehension, assessment, physiological integrity (a).

3 An increase in growth hormone after the epiphyseal plates close leads to acromegaly.

1 Prolactin is not associated with acromegaly.

2 Cortisol is made by the adrenal cortex and will produce Cushing's syndrome if it is overproduced.

4 An overproduction of thyroid hormone is referred to as hyperthyroidism.

57. Application, assessment, physiological integrity (a).

2 The nurse should check to be sure that the medication has not been given in the last 4 hours.

1 Narcotic orders may, by institutional policy, have automatic stop dates; the discontinuation date should be determined and noted when the order is transcribed.

3 Because schedule II drugs must, by law, be accounted for, the amount left on hand should be checked. This is done with change-of-shift narcotic counts and when the medication is signed out after preparing and administering the dose.

4 The effect of the last dose should be checked when the dose peaks rather than immediately before the next dose.

58. Comprehension, evaluation, physiological integrity (b).

3 Anticholinergic agents reduce secretions, resulting in dry mouth.

1 Anticholinergic agents tend to increase heart rate.

2 Anticholinergic agents reduce gastrointestinal motility, resulting in constipation.

4 Anticholinergic agents cause pupil dilation.

59. Application, implementation, health promotion and maintenance (b).

2 These are the common symptoms of candidiasis.

1 This is not common in candidiasis, but it is common of some systemic infections.

3 This is common in genital warts.

4 Although a cause for concern, these are not symptoms associated with candidiasis.

60. Application, implementation, health promotion and maintenance (b).

3 Elevating the head of the bed will reduce pressure on the cardiac sphincter, reducing the chance of esophageal reflux.

1 This suggestion will not reduce bedtime discomfort.

2 This will worsen the symptoms; eating or drinking within 3 hours of going to bed is not recommended.

4 This will cause worsening of the symptoms; see rationale for #2.

61. Comprehension, assessment, physiological integrity (b).

1 Symptoms of active TB include a cough lasting longer than 2 weeks, fever, night sweats, malaise, irritability, weakness, fatigue, and dyspnea.

2 These symptoms may be present in asthma or chronic bronchitis.

3 Feeling cold, tired, and having stomach upset may reflect a gastrointestinal problem, anemia, or anxiety.

4 Bloody stools may reflect a gastrointestinal problem.

62. Application, planning, physiological integrity (c).

2 Stress and exertion can overwhelm the patient and increase the risk of an addisonian crisis.

1 Although important, planning diversional activities does not take precedence in this case.

3 Providing a well-balanced diet is always important for the nurse, but reducing stress is the priority in this plan of care.

4 Activity must be planned and moderated for this patient.

63. Application, implementation, physiological integrity (b).

1 Sterile technique is necessary because of the loss of the body's first line of defense—intact skin.

2 The room temperature should be closer to 80° to 85° F.

3 A diet high in protein and carbohydrates is appropriate for any burned patient.

4 When positioning extremities, the nurse must consider the possibility of flexion contracture.

64. Comprehension, assessment, physiological integrity (b).

2 In acute renal failure, potassium, BUN, and creatinine increase because of the kidneys' inability to filtrate,

resulting in an accumulation of nitrogenous wastes in the blood.

1, 3, 4 See rationale for #2. The BUN increases, the creatinine increases, potassium is increased, and calcium is decreased.

65. Comprehension, implementation, physiological integrity (c).

3 **Bile is needed to emulsify fat. When fat requires bile for emulsification, the gallbladder contracts in an effort to release the bile to be used in this process. A diseased gallbladder that must contract causes a sensation of pain.**

1 Foods high in fat require bile released by the gallbladder to aid in the emulsification process.

2 The duct leading from the liver to the gallbladder may become blocked, but it is less likely to involve the pancreas in most acute presentations.

4 Although a portion of this statement is true, this does not explain the mechanism by which pain is produced.

66. Application, assessment, physiological integrity (b).

4 **These are NSAIDs, which may be nephrotoxic.**

1 This is an tricyclic antidepressant that may be prescribed for urinary incontinence.

2 This drug is a urinary antiseptic that may change the urine's color.

3 Calcium channel blockers may affect the ability of the bladder or sphincter to contract or relax normally.

67. Comprehension, assessment, physiological integrity (b).

1 **Fetal distress is present and is a sign of cord prolapse following rupture of the membranes.**

2 The opposite is true because the fetal heart rate decreases.

3 Amniotic fluid may continue to leak and is not an indication of cord prolapse.

4 No specific length of cord protrusion makes this answer correct; the cord may be hidden inside, with the presenting part against it.

68. Application, implementation, psychosocial integrity (b).

4 **This may indicate bronchospasm and laryngospasm.**

1 Wheezing is not usual; it may indicate complications.

2 Wheezing is abnormal; it is not a usual indication that the anesthesia is wearing off.

3 Return of the gag reflex does not include wheezing.

69. Application, planning, physiological integrity (b).

3 **Regular insulin is fast acting and is used in the acute phase.**

1 Lente is an intermediate-acting insulin that is not used in the acute phase of DKA.

2 NPH is an intermediate-acting insulin and may be used after the acute phase is passed.

4 This is an oral agent and is not used in the acute phase of DKA.

70. Comprehension, planning, physiological integrity (c).

1 **The diet is high in carbohydrates, usually 2500 to 3000 calories per day, to prevent the breakdown of fats that would produce ketosis; it is low in protein to reduce the BUN. Potassium is restricted because patients in renal failure retain potassium and are at risk for hyperkalemia.**

2, 3, 4 These diets are inappropriate for this patient and would further compromise the patient's condition. See rationale for #1.

71. Knowledge, planning, physiological integrity (c).

2 **One and one half to two times the amount of the control is considered thin enough to prevent further clot formation with minimal risk for undue bleeding.**

1 This would present a risk for clot formation.

3, 4 These would present a high risk of hemorrhage.

72. Application, planning, physiological integrity (a).

3 **The incontinence, perspiration, and weight put her at risk for a pressure ulcer.**

1 This is not appropriate and would also require assistance; shearing forces can cause breakdown.

2 She can be positioned on her left side with appropriate support.

4 This is inappropriate and may predispose her to complications.

73. Application, implementation, physiological integrity (c).

4 **Stimulation of a different site may override the phantom sensation.**

1 Narcotics are not effective for phantom limb pain.

2 Massage therapy might be ordered after 2 weeks.

3 Cold would increase phantom limb pain.

74. Application, implementation, physiological integrity (c).

1 **Hallucinations are a symptom of alcohol withdrawal.**

2, 3, 4 Hallucinations are not symptoms of withdrawal from these drugs.

75. Application, implementation, physiological integrity (a).

1 **The patient is experiencing orthostatic hypotension, which results in her blood pressure dropping on standing. Having her sit up before standing will allow her circulation to stabilize to her brain.**

2 This will have no effect on her orthostatic hypotension.

3 This is not necessary at this point. Her blood pressure needs to be evaluated lying, sitting, and standing before calling. She may need a lower dose.

4 This would not help her orthostatic hypertension but may increase her hypertension, which can be harmful.

76. Knowledge, evaluation, health promotion and maintenance (a).

1 **Heat stroke is more likely in the very young and older adults.**

2, 3, 4 These age groups are not as likely to develop heat stroke.

77. Application, evaluation, physiological integrity (b).

1 **This helps the nurse evaluate the effectiveness of the deep-breathing and coughing exercises.**

2 Nurses usually have a pulse oximeter on the unit for spot checks of a client's blood oxygen levels.

3 This is not necessary.

4 He should be positioned in the highest position possible so as to not interfere with gas exchange.

78. Comprehension, assessment, physiological integrity (b).

3 **Emergency nursing calls for a rapid clinical assessment, with emphasis on airway, breathing, circulation, establishing priorities, and then beginning lifesaving measures.**

1 Although calling for help is important, it is not the priority.

2 This is not a priority action.

4 The Good Samaritan law provisions should be known before traveling out of the home state.

79. Comprehension, implementation, physiological integrity (a).

1 **These are correct interventions for hemorrhage, but the priority is to stop or control the bleeding.**

2 This is an appropriate intervention after bleeding is under control.

3 After applying the pressure dressing, the health care professional should elevate the affected part to further aid in controlling hemorrhage.

4 Movement stimulates circulation; immobilization will also aid in controlling hemorrhage.

80. Application, planning, safe, effective care environment (b).

1 The Venturi mask is correct; it can provide precise concentrations of oxygen through a noninvasive route and avoids risk of suppressing the patient's hypoxic drive to breathe.

2, 3, 4 These masks do not provide precise oxygen concentrations, which can suppress the patient's hypoxic drive to breathe.

81. Knowledge, planning, physiological integrity (b).

3 Older women need an increased intake to compensate for decreased absorption, thereby decreasing the symptoms of osteoporosis.

1 Individuals up to the age of 24 should receive 1200 mg per day because bone mass is forming.

2 Adults should receive 1000 mg per day to maintain bone mass and to prepare for postmenopausal losses.

4 This level is not recommended for any age group by the National Osteoporosis Association.

82. Comprehension, assessment, safe, effective care environment (b).

1 The Patient Self-Determination Act stipulates that information concerning advance directives be given to patients on their admission to the hospital.

2 Giving patients information during this time would be too late.

3 The information should be given when the patient is admitted into an acute-care facility.

4 This is not always a comfortable issue, and patients may postpone the decision

83. Knowledge, assessment, health promotion and maintenance (b).

2 Older adults spend the latter part of their life dealing with the issues of ego integrity and despair. If the elderly patient reflects on his life and is pleased with the events, then the ego remains intact. If the patient is not happy with his life, then he will despair because it cannot be changed.

1 This is the task stage for early adulthood.

3 Adults (middle age) manage the tasks of generativity and stagnation.

4 Adolescents deal with the tasks of identity and role confusion.

84. Analysis, evaluation, physiological integrity (b).

3 The amount of induration (hardness and or elevation) in mm at the greatest diameter is the proper method; 0 to 4 mm is insignificant; 5 to 10 mm may be significant; greater than 10 mm is considered significant.

1 The amount of erythema (redness) is not helpful in interpretation.

2 Only the amount of induration is used for interpretation.

4 The Mantoux test is intradermal. Lipohypertrophy occurs in the subcutaneous layer of the skin and is usually related to multiple subcutaneous injections.

85. Comprehension, assessment, health promotion and maintenance (b).

4 Stress over the loss of a work-related role may have contributed to the patient's current health problem.

1 No indication from the family or patient exists that this is the problem because the patient is retired.

2 The patient may be excited to retire; however, the family member states that the patient has been depressed.

3 It is unlikely that the patient has met new friends or has been involved in activities since he has been depressed.

86. Knowledge, evaluation, physiological integrity (b).

2 Several studies have demonstrated that infants sleeping prone are at a greater risk for SIDS.

1, 4 These are not applicable to SIDS.

3 The peak age for SIDS is 2 to 4 months.

87. Comprehension, planning, physiological integrity (b).

4 Subdural hematomas are usually caused by venous bleeding; 50% are associated with skull fractures.

1 With intracerebral hematomas, bleeding occurs in the parenchymal tissue; it may be caused by head trauma or secondary to hypertensive bleeding.

2 Epidural hematomas generally result from arterial bleeding.

3 Subarachnoid hematomas usually result secondary to rupture of intracranial aneurysms, atrioventricular malformation, or hypertensive bleed.

88. Knowledge, implementation, physiological integrity (b).

4 This is the correct rate of infusion.

$$\frac{1000\ ml}{8\ hr} = 125\ ml/hr$$

$$\frac{125\ ml/hr}{60\ min/hr} = 2.1\ ml/min$$

2.1 ml/min × 10 gtts/ml = 21 gtts/min

1, 2, 3 These rates are too slow.

89. Comprehension, planning, physiological integrity (b).

2 Tyramine stimulates the production of norepinephrine (a monamine), which elevates blood pressure. Because this drug inhibits the action of monamine oxidase and therefore blocks the destruction of norepinephrine, the patient's blood pressure may rise to critical levels.

1 Potassium levels do not affect the action or effects of MAOIs.

3 MAOIs do not increase the patient's risk of sunburn.

4 At least 1 to 4 weeks are required for the therapeutic effects of an MAOI to be evident.

90. Comprehension, planning, physiological integrity (a).

3 Meperidine hydrochloride and other narcotic analgesics tend to depress the respiratory center located in the medulla oblongata.

1 Narcotic analgesics commonly lead to slowing of peristalsis, predisposing the client to constipation rather than diarrhea.

2 Narcotic analgesics usually lower blood pressure.

4 Narcotic analgesics have no effect on blood sugar.

91. Application, implementation, safe, effective care environment (b).

4 This response correctly summarizes the trend of managed care within the health care system.

1 This does not answer the family member's question.

2 A cholecystectomy may not be simple for an older adult, and this statement does not correctly define diagnostic-related groups.

3 Although home health care providers visit individuals after discharge (if needed), this is not the major reason for short hospital stays.

92. Application, implementation, safe, effective care environment (b).

2 Eyes are irrigated from the inner to the outer canthus because the inner canthus may absorb the chemical into the patient's system. Catching the overflow from the outer canthus rather than from the side of the face is also easier. The chemical may also be breathed into the nose if it is draining toward the inner canthus.

1 This is an inappropriate direction of irrigating fluid; see rationale for #2.

3 Irrigating directly onto the eyeball would be painful, and the fluid would drain into the inner canthus.

4 Although the fluid should be directed along the lower conjunctiva, it is more important that it be directed from the inner to the outer canthus.

93. Comprehension, evaluation, safe, effective care environment (b).

Poor lighting in and around stairs

Hardwood floors

Scatter rugs

Gas stove

94. Application, implementation, physiological integrity (a).

3 Giving two injections increases the risk for lipodystrophy (hypertrophy of subcutaneous tissue) or lipoatrophy (atrophy of subcutaneous tissue).

1, 2, 4 NPH and regular insulin mix well; mixing will have no effect on their respective actions.

95. Comprehension, assessment, physiological integrity (c).

2 The patient is exhibiting signs and symptoms of air embolism. As little as 10 ml of air can be significant. Clamping the line and stopping the pump can stop the infusion of air.

1 Monitoring the insertion site is necessary throughout the dialysis procedure but is not a priority in this case.

3 When air embolism is suspected, the patient is positioned on the left side, with the feet elevated for 30 minutes, which prevents air from going to the head. Rather, the air is trapped in the right atrium and the right ventricle where it is kept away from the pulmonary circulation.

4 This is an inappropriate action; see the rationale for #3.

96. Application, planning, physiological integrity (b).

2 Because the liver metabolizes Haldol, jaundice may develop. The antipsychotic nature may cause excessive lethargy.

1 Haldol normally causes urinary retention as a side effect.

3 These are not normally considered as side effects.

4 These are not significant side effects of Haldol.

97. Knowledge, assessment, physiological integrity (c).

3 These are signs and symptoms of nephrotic syndrome.

1 Nephrotic syndrome includes hypoalbuminemia.

2, 4 Nephrotic syndrome is diagnosed via renal biopsy; levels of protein in the blood are decreased.

98. Comprehension, planning, physiological integrity (b).

2 Sodium polystyrene sulfonate (Kayexalate) will most likely be ordered to decrease the serum potassium level. The normal serum potassium level range is 3.8 to 5.5 mEq/L.

1 This is a potassium supplement and would increase the serum potassium [+]level.

3 Bananas are a source of potassium and should not be encouraged at this time.

4 Strawberries are a source of potassium and should not be encouraged at this time.

99. Comprehension, assessment, health promotion and maintenance (b).

3 These are the typical signs of an adolescent who is abusing drugs or alcohol.

1, 2, 4 These are not all typical signs of this disease.

100. Comprehension, planning, physiological integrity (c).

1 Stress causes the release of epinephrine, which, in turn, increases the heart rate while constricting blood vessels and raising blood pressure. This increases the demands on the heart and can lead to failure.

2 Stress-reduction exercises are good for anyone, not only for those who have had surgery. This answer is too general.

3 Relaxation will direct the flow of blood away from the periphery.

4 Exercise would be a part of the treatment for managing stress but is not the principle behind the recommendation.

101. Knowledge, assessment, physiological integrity (b).

4 The symptom of projectile vomiting is a classic sign of pyloric stenosis.

1 Symptoms appear suddenly and include pallor, sharp colicky pain, vomiting, stools with blood and mucus, and signs of shock.

2 Symptoms appear between the ages of 1 and 5 and include chronic diarrhea with bulky, greasy, foul smelling stools, anaruia, distended abdomen, and muscle wasting.

3 Symptoms include excessive salivation and drooling, coughing and choking during feeding, and regurgitation of all feedings.

102. Application, implementation, physiological integrity, (b).

3 Pain is not always the result of tissue destruction. Pain from different sources requires different interventions.

1 This might be a consideration but not the first consideration.

2, 4 These are considerations but not the first focus of the initial assessment.

103. Application, implementation, physiological integrity (b).

1 Retinoic acid is commonly used in combination with benzoyl peroxide in the treatment of acne vulgaris.

2, 4 Tinea corporis and all forms of ringworm are treated with antifungal creams or ointments.

3 Pediculosis is treated with a pediculicide shampoo.

104. Application, implementation, safe, effective care environment (b).

DD = 300 mg

DH = 500 mg

V = 2 ml

DD/DH = 300 mg/500 mg × 2 ml = 1.2 ml

105. Analysis, evaluation, physiological integrity (c).

2 This is an example of an antispasmodic that may be given for UTI to decrease frequency and urgency.

1, 3, 4 These are antimicrobials that may be used to treat UTI; they may have this effect indirectly.

106. Comprehension, planning, physiological integrity (a).

4 This form of intake would be the choice until oral food and fluids are tolerated.

1 This diet is not recommended until nausea and vomiting subside.

2 The patient is not able to tolerate this diet on admission.

3 Frequent feedings are not advised because of the patient's intolerance of food.

107. Knowledge, assessment, physiological integrity (b).

4 These are all characteristic signs of muscular dystrophy.

1 Onset occurs in young adults. Symptoms include ataxia paresthesia, numbness, tingling, weakness, and loss of muscle tone, and fatigue.

2 Symptoms include abnormal muscle tone and coordination, delays in development, hearing and vision impairment, seizures, and mental retardation in some cases.

3 Symptoms include limited hip abduction, apparent shortening of the femur, asymmetry of gluteal and thigh folds.

108. Knowledge, assessment, physiological integrity (b).

4 The CSF of a child with meningitis is cloudy because of the increased white blood cell count.

1 Meningitis causes an increased protein level.

2 Meningitis causes a decreased glucose level.

3 The CSF pressure increases in meningitis.

109. Application, intervention, physiological integrity (c).

4 This is the correct dose.

2.2 lb = 1 kg; 11 pounds × 2.2 pounds = 5 kg

DD = 0.1 mg/kg

0.1 mg × 5 kg = 0.5 mg

1, 2 These responses are incorrect; the dose is neither too high nor too low.

3 Morphine can be given via SQ, IM, IV, and via epidural routes.

110. Knowledge, implementation, safe, effective care environment (b).

3 This is the correct rate of infusion.

1, 2 This rate is too slow.

4 This rate is too fast.

111. Knowledge, assessment, physiological integrity (b).

3 This clotting disorder is known as hemophilia.

1 Autosomal disease which causes breakdown of red blood cells carrying an abnormal hemoglobin.

2 A genetic disorder resulting in abnormal hemoglobin synthesis.

4 A term given to a group of malignant diseases of the bone marrow and lymphatic system.

112. Comprehension, assessment, physiological integrity (b).

3 Diabetes insipidus is caused by a deficiency of antidiuretic hormone (ADH). Vasopressin acts as replacement therapy for ADH, which acts in the renal tubules to increase the reabsorption of water back into the blood. Therefore the amount of urine formed is decreased.

1 This would be a side effect and not an expected outcome.

2 Abdominal distention would decrease.

4 This should not effect temperature.

113. Comprehension, assessment, physiological integrity (b).

4 Scrotal edema, along with edema to the face, extremities, and abdomen, are common signs of nephrotic syndrome.

1 This is a sign of severe dehydration.

2 A child with nephrotic syndrome exhibits decreased urinary output.

3 The skin is very pale in a child with nephrotic syndrome.

114. Application, implementation, physiological integrity (b).

1 Nitroglycerine increases blood pressure; therefore blood pressure should be monitored while administering nitroglycerine.

2, 3, 4 Recommendations suggest transporting the person to the nearest emergency room after three tablets.

115. Application, implementation, physiological integrity (b).

1 These foods have high amounts of vitamin K, which will decrease the effect of the anticoagulant. These foods should be eaten in small amounts.

2 An electric razor should be used to avoid nicking the skin and bleeding.

3 Aspirin will increase the effects of the anticoagulant and should not be taken without a physician's order.

4 A soft-bristled toothbrush should be used to avoid damage and subsequent bleeding of the gums.

116. Knowledge, implementation, physiological integrity (b).

1 This is the proper method for using an inhaler.

2 The inhaler should be used as ordered and before the individual becomes this short of breath.

3 This is unnecessary with inhalers; if a spacer is used, then cleaning is recommended.

4 Some individuals may find this comforting, but it is not required for the therapeutic effect.

117. Application, implementation, physiological integrity (b).

3 Nursing care of the child after a ventriculoperitoneal shunt should include head circumference measurements to help determine if the shunt is draining CSF properly.

1, 2, 4 These are not necessary postoperative nursing interventions for this disorder.

118. Knowledge, assessment, health promotion and maintenance (b).

4 Primitive reflexes (grasp, tonic neck, and so forth) disappear between 4 and 5 months of age.

1, 2 Primitive reflexes remain strong at these ages.

3 Primitive reflexes are still present but fading.

119. Comprehension, assessment, physiological integrity (b).

2 This is a symptom of the condition.

1 Amenorrhea, not dysmenorrhea, is commonly seen in these patients.

3 Bradycardia and hypotension are common, probably because of the state of starvation.

4 Constipation, not diarrhea, is a symptom of anorexia nervosa.

120. Comprehension, assessment, safe, effective care environment (c).

1 This is the most common, serious complication of rheumatic fever. The endocardium and valves become inflamed and are often permanently damaged.

2 This is not a common complication of rheumatic fever.

3 Arthritis is a symptom of rheumatic fever but not the most serious complication.

4 This is not a complication of rheumatic fever.

121. Comprehension, evaluation, physiological integrity (b).

4 A slight drop in hemoglobin is normal, and the mother is able to care for herself and her infant.

1 This is not usually associated with a slight drop in hemoglobin.

2 Unless other problems are identified, vital signs are generally normal.

3 Performing basic tasks is usually within her realm and not a problem.

122. Knowledge, assessment, physiological integrity (a).

4 This is another name for trisomy 21.

1 Hurler's syndrome is a genetic condition transmitted as an autosomal-recessive trait that produces severe mental retardation.

2 Cri-du-chat syndrome (cat-cry syndrome) is a rare congenital disorder recognized at birth by a kitten like cry caused by a laryngeal anomaly.

3 Turner's syndrome is a chromosomal anomaly seen in about 1 in 3000 live female births, characterized by the absence of one X chromosome.

123. Application, assessment, physiological integrity (b).

4 This is the most important assessment to make on a child with hydrocephalus.

1, 3 These are not important assessments to make on this child.

2 Frequent neurological checks may be necessary, not neurovascular checks.

124. Comprehension, assessment, physiological integrity (b).

1 Respiratory distress would need immediate attention.

2 This is associated with the disease but is not a priority need.

3 This problem needs to be met but does not take precedence.

4 The needs resulting from this problem can be met later.

125. Application, implementation, physiological integrity (b).

DD = 425 mg

DH = 1 g (1000 mg)

C = 4 ml

$$\frac{DD}{DH} = \frac{425 \text{ mg}}{1000 \text{ mg}} \times 4 \text{ ml} = 1.7 \text{ ml}$$

APPENDICES

Activity Intolerance: Insufficient physiological or psychological energy to endure or complete required or desired daily activities

Risk for Activity Intolerance: The state in which an individual is at risk of experiencing insufficient physiological or psychological energy to endure or complete required or desired daily activities

Impaired Adjustment: Inability to modify lifestyle/behavior in a manner consistent with a change in health status

Ineffective Airway Clearance: Inability to clear secretions or obstructions from the respiratory tract to maintain a clear airway

Latex Allergy Response: An allergic response to natural latex rubber products

Risk for Latex Allergy Response: At risk for allergic response to natural latex rubber products

Anxiety: A vague uneasy feeling of discomfort or dread accompanied by an autonomic response (the source often nonspecific or unknown to the individual); a feeling of apprehension caused by anticipation of danger; an alerting signal that warns of impending danger and enables the individual to take measures to deal with threat

Death Anxiety: Apprehension, worry, or fear related to death or dying

Risk for Aspiration: At risk for entry of gastrointestinal secretions, oropharyngeal secretions, solids, or fluids into tracheobronchial passages

Risk for Impaired Parent/Infant/Child Attachment: Disruption of the interactive process among parent/significant other, child, and infant that fosters the development of a protective and nurturing reciprocal relationship

Autonomic Dysreflexia: Life-threatening, uninhibited sympathetic response of the nervous system to a noxious stimulus after a spinal cord injury at T7 or above

Risk for Autonomic Dysreflexia: At risk for life-threatening, uninhibited sympathetic response of the nervous system, post spinal shock, in an individual with spinal cord injury or lesion at T6 or above (has been demonstrated in patients with injuries at T7 or T8)

Disturbed Body Image: Confusion in mental picture of one's physical self

Risk for Imbalanced Body Temperature: At risk for failure to maintain body temperature within normal range

Bowel Incontinence: Change in normal bowel habits characterized by involuntary passage of stool

Effective Breast-Feeding: Mother-infant dyad/family exhibits adequate proficiency and satisfaction with the breast-feeding process

Ineffective Breast-Feeding: Dissatisfaction or difficulty a mother, infant, or child experiences with the breast-feeding process

Interrupted Breast-Feeding: Break in the continuity of the breast-feeding process as a result of inability or inadvisability to put baby to breast for feeding

Ineffective Breathing Pattern: Inspiration and/or expiration that does not provide adequate ventilation

Decreased Cardiac Output: Inadequate blood pumped by the heart to meet metabolic demands of the body

Caregiver Role Strain: Difficulty in performing family caregiver role

Risk for Caregiver Role Strain: Caregiver is vulnerable for perceived difficulty in performing the family caregiver role

Impaired Verbal Communication: Decreased, delayed, or absent ability to receive, process, transmit, and use a system of symbols

*Readiness for Enhanced Communication: A pattern of exchanging information and ideas with others that is sufficient for meeting one's needs and life's goals and can be strengthened

Decisional Conflict (specify): Uncertainty about course of action to be taken when choice among competing actions involves risk, loss, or challenge to personal life values

Parental Role Conflict: Parent experience of role confusion and conflict in response to crisis

Acute Confusion: Abrupt onset of a cluster of global, transient changes and disturbances in attention, cognition, psychomotor activity, level of consciousness, and/or sleep and wake cycle

Chronic Confusion: Irreversible, long-standing, and/or progressive deterioration of intellect and personality characterized by decreased ability to interpret environmental stimuli, decreased capacity for intellectual thought processes; manifested by disturbances of memory, orientation, and behavior

Constipation: Decrease in normal frequency of defecation accompanied by difficult or incomplete passage of stool and/or passage of excessively hard, dry stool

Perceived Constipation: Self-diagnosis of constipation and abuse of laxatives, enemas, and suppositories to ensure a daily bowel movement

Risk for Constipation: At risk for a decrease in normal frequency of defecation accompanied by difficult or incomplete passage of stool and/or passage of excessively hard, dry stool

Ineffective Coping: Inability to form a valid appraisal of the stressors, inadequate choices of practiced responses, and/or inability to use available resources

*New nursing diagnoses, 2003.

From North American Nursing Diagnosis Association International: *Nursing diagnoses: definitions and classification 2003-2004,* Philadelphia, 2003, NANDA International.

Defensive Coping: Repeated projection of falsely positive self-evaluation based on a self-protective pattern that defends against underlying perceived threats to positive self-regard

*****Readiness for Enhanced Coping:** A pattern of cognitive and behavioral efforts to manage demands that is sufficient for well being and can be strengthened

Ineffective Community Coping: Pattern of community activities (for adaptation and problem solving) that is unsatisfactory for meeting the demands or needs of the community

Readiness for Enhanced Community Coping: Pattern of community activities for adaptation and problem solving that is satisfactory for meeting the demands or needs of the community but can be improved for management of current and future problems/stressors

Compromised Family Coping: Usually supportive primary person (family member or close friend) provides insufficient, ineffective, or compromised support, comfort, assistance, or encouragement that may be needed by the patient to manage or master adaptive tasks related to his/her health challenge

Disabled Family Coping: Behavior of significant person (family member or other primary person) that disables his/her capacities and the patient's capacities to effectively address tasks essential to either person's adaptation to the health challenge

Readiness for Enhanced Family Coping: Effective management of adaptive tasks by family member involved with the patient's health challenge, who now exhibits desire and readiness for enhanced health and growth in regard to self and in relation to the patient

*****Risk for Sudden Infant Death Syndrome:** Presence of risk factors for sudden death of an infant under 1 year of age

Ineffective Denial: Conscious or unconscious attempt to disavow the knowledge or meaning of an event to reduce anxiety/fear, but leading to the detriment of health

Impaired Dentition: Disruption in tooth development/eruption patterns or structural integrity of individual teeth

Risk for Delayed Development: At risk for delay of 25% or more in one or more of the areas of social or self-regulatory behavior, or in cognitive, language, gross or fine motor skills

Diarrhea: Passage of loose, unformed stools

Risk for Disuse Syndrome: At risk for deterioration of body systems as the result of prescribed or unavoidable musculoskeletal inactivity

Deficient Diversional Activity: Decreased stimulation from (or interest or engagement in) recreational or leisure activities

Disturbed Energy Field: Disruption of the flow of energy surrounding a person's being that results in a disharmony of the body, mind, and/or spirit

Impaired Environmental Interpretation Syndrome: Consistent lack of orientation to person, place, time, or circumstances over more than 3 to 6 months, necessitating a protective environment

Adult Failure to Thrive: Progressive functional deterioration of a physical and cognitive nature; the individual's ability to live with multisystem diseases, cope with ensuing problems, and manage his/her care are remarkably diminished

Risk for Falls: Increased susceptibility to falling that may cause physical harm

Dysfunctional Family Processes—Alcoholism: Psychosocial, spiritual, and physiological functions of the family unit are chronically disorganized, which leads to conflict, denial of problems, resistance to change, ineffective problem solving, and a series of self-perpetuating crises

Interrupted Family Processes: Change in family relationships and/or functioning

*****Readiness for Enhanced Family Processes:** A pattern of family functioning that is sufficient to support the well being of family members and can be strengthened

Fatigue: An overwhelming sustained sense of exhaustion and decreased capacity for physical and mental work at usual level

Fear: Response to perceived threat that is consciously recognized as a danger

*****Readiness for Enhanced Fluid Balance:** A pattern of equilibrium between fluid volume and chemical composition of body fluids that is sufficient for meeting physical needs and can be strengthened

Deficient Fluid Volume: Decreased intravascular, interstitial, and/or intracellular fluid; refers to dehydration, water loss alone without change in sodium

Excess Fluid Volume: Increased isotonic fluid retention

Risk for Deficient Fluid Volume: At risk for experiencing vascular, cellular, or intracellular dehydration

Risk for Imbalanced Fluid Volume: At risk for a decrease, increase, or rapid shift from one to the other of intravascular, interstitial, and/or intracellular fluid; refers to body fluid loss or gain, or both

Impaired Gas Exchange: Excess or deficit in oxygenation and/or carbon dioxide elimination at the alveolar-capillary membrane

Anticipatory Grieving: Intellectual and emotional responses and behaviors by which individuals, families, communities work through the process of modifying self-concept based on the perception of potential loss

Dysfunctional Grieving: Extended, unsuccessful use of intellectual and emotional responses by which individuals, families, communities attempt to work through the process of modifying self-concept based on the perception of loss

Delayed Growth and Development: Deviations from age-group norms

Risk for Disproportionate Growth: At risk for growth above the ninety-seventh percentile or below the third percentile for age, crossing two percentile channels; disproportionate growth

Ineffective Health Maintenance: Inability to identify, manage, and/or seek out help to maintain health

Health-Seeking Behaviors (specify): Active seeking (by a person in stable health) of ways to alter personal health habits and/or the environment to move toward a higher level of health

Impaired Home Maintenance: Inability to independently maintain a safe growth-promoting immediate environment

Hopelessness: Subjective state in which an individual sees limited or no alternatives or personal choices available and is unable to mobilize energy on own behalf

Hyperthermia: Body temperature elevated above normal range

Hypothermia: Body temperature below normal range

*New nursing diagnoses, 2003.
From North American Nursing Diagnosis Association International: *Nursing diagnoses: definitions and classification 2003-2004,* Philadelphia, 2003, NANDA International.

Disturbed Personal Identity: Inability to distinguish between self and nonself

Reflex Urinary Incontinence: Involuntary loss of urine at somewhat predictable intervals when a specific bladder volume is reached

Stress Urinary Incontinence: Loss of less than 50 ml of urine occurring with increased abdominal pressure

Total Urinary Incontinence: Continuous and unpredictable loss of urine

Urge Urinary Incontinence: Involuntary passage of urine occurring soon after a strong sense of urgency to void

Risk for Urge Urinary Incontinence: At risk for involuntary loss of urine associated with a sudden, strong sensation or urinary urgency

Disorganized Infant Behavior: Disintegrated physiological and neurobehavioral responses to the environment

Risk for Disorganized Infant Behavior: Risk for alteration in integrating and modulation of the physiological and behavioral systems of functioning (i.e., autonomic, motor, state, organizational, self-regulatory, attentional-interactional systems)

Readiness for Enhanced Organized Infant Behavior: A pattern of modulation of the physiologic and behavioral systems of functioning (i.e., autonomic, motor, state, organizational, self-regulatory, attentional-interactional systems) in an infant that is satisfactory but that can be improved resulting in higher levels of integration in response to environmental stimuli

Ineffective Infant Feeding Pattern: Impaired ability to suck or coordinate the suck-swallow response

Risk for Infection: At increased risk for being invaded by pathogenic organisms

Risk for Injury: The state in which an individual is at risk of injury as a result of environmental conditions interacting with the individual's adaptive and defensive resources

Risk for Perioperative-Positioning Injury: At risk for injury as a result of the environmental conditions found in the perioperative setting

Decreased Intracranial Adaptive Capacity: Intracranial fluid dynamic mechanisms that normally compensate for increases in intracranial volumes are compromised, resulting in repeated disproportionate increases in intracranial pressure in response to a variety of noxious and nonnoxious stimuli

Deficient Knowledge (specify): Absence or deficiency of cognitive information related to specific topic

*Readiness for Enhanced Knowledge (specify): The presence or acquisition of cognitive information related to a specific topic that is sufficient for meeting health-related goals and can be strengthened

Risk for Loneliness: At risk for experiencing vague dysphoria

Impaired Memory: Inability to remember or recall bits of information or behavioral skills; may be attributed to pathophysiological or situational causes that are either temporary or permanent

Impaired Bed Mobility: Limitation of independent movement from one bed position to another

Impaired Physical Mobility: Limitation in independent, purposeful physical movement of the body or of one or more extremities

Impaired Wheelchair Mobility: Limitation of independent operation of wheelchair within environment

Nausea: A subjective unpleasant, wavelike sensation in the back of the throat, epigastrium, or abdomen that may lead to the urge or need to vomit

Unilateral Neglect: Lack of awareness and attention to one side of the body

Noncompliance: Behavior of person and/or caregiver that fails to coincide with a health-promoting or therapeutic plan agreed on by the person (and/or family and/or community) and health care professional; in the presence of an agreed-on, health-promoting or therapeutic plan, person or caregiver's behavior is fully or partially nonadherent and may lead to clinically ineffective or partially ineffective outcomes

Imbalanced Nutrition, Less than Body Requirements: Intake of nutrients insufficient to meet metabolic needs

Imbalanced Nutrition, More than Body Requirements: Intake of nutrients that exceeds metabolic needs

*Readiness for Enhanced Nutrition: A pattern of nutrient intake that is sufficient for meeting metabolic needs and can be strengthened

Risk for Imbalanced Nutrition, More than Body Requirements: At risk for an intake of nutrients that exceeds metabolic needs

Impaired Oral Mucous Membrane: Disruption of the lips and soft tissue of the oral cavity

Acute Pain: Unpleasant sensory and emotional experience arising from actual or potential tissue damage or described in terms of such damage (International Association for the Study of Pain); sudden or slow onset of any intensity from mild to severe with an anticipated or predictable end and a duration of less than 6 months

Chronic Pain: Unpleasant sensory and emotional experience arising from actual or potential tissue damage or described in terms of such damage (International Association for the Study of Pain); sudden or slow onset of any intensity from mild to severe, constant or recurring without an anticipated or predictable end and a duration of greater than 6 months

*Readiness for Enhanced Parenting: A pattern of providing an environment for children or other dependent person(s) that is sufficient to nurture growth and development and can be strengthened

Impaired Parenting: Inability of the primary caretaker to create, maintain, or regain an environment that promotes the optimum growth and development of the child

Risk for Impaired Parenting: Risk for inability of the primary caretaker to create, maintain, or regain an environment that promotes the optimum growth and development of the child

Risk for Peripheral Neurovascular Dysfunction: At risk for disruption in circulation, sensation, or motion of an extremity

Risk for Poisoning: Accentuated risk of accidental exposure to or ingestion of drugs or dangerous products in doses sufficient to cause poisoning

Post-Trauma Syndrome: Sustained maladaptive response to a traumatic, overwhelming event

Risk for Post-Trauma Syndrome: At risk for sustained maladaptive response to a traumatic, overwhelming event

---

*New nursing diagnoses, 2003.

From North American Nursing Diagnosis Association International: *Nursing diagnoses: definitions and classification 2003-2004*, Philadelphia, 2003, NANDA International.

Powerlessness: Perception that one's own action will not significantly affect an outcome; a perceived lack of control over a current situation or immediate happening

Risk for Powerlessness: At risk for perceived lack of control over a situation and/or one's ability to significantly affect an outcome

Ineffective Protection: Decrease in the ability to guard self from internal or external threats such as illness or injury

Rape-Trauma Syndrome: Sustained maladaptive response to a forced, violent sexual penetration against the victim's will and consent

Rape-Trauma Syndrome, Compound Reaction: Forced violent sexual penetration against the victim's will and consent; includes an acute phase of disorganization of the victim's lifestyle and a long-term process of reorganization of lifestyle that develop as a result of the attack or attempted attack

Rape-Trauma Syndrome, Silent Reaction: Forced violent sexual penetration against the victim's will and consent; includes an acute phase of disorganization of the victim's lifestyle and a long-term process of reorganization of lifestyle that develop as a result of the attack or attempted attack

Relocation Stress Syndrome: Physiological and/or psychosocial disturbance following transfer from one environment to another

Risk for Relocation Stress Syndrome: At risk for physiological and/or psychosocial disturbance following transfer from one environment to another

Ineffective Role Performance: Patterns of behavior and self-expression that do not match the environmental context, norms, and expectations

Bathing/Hygiene Self-Care Deficit: Impaired ability to perform or complete bathing/hygiene activities for self

Dressing/Grooming Self-Care Deficit: Impaired ability to perform or complete dressing and grooming activities for self

Feeding Self-Care Deficit: Impaired ability to perform or complete feeding activities

Toileting Self-Care Deficit: Impaired ability to perform or complete own toileting activities

*Readiness for Enhanced Self-Concept: A pattern of perceptions or ideas about the self that is sufficient for well being and can be strengthened

Chronic Low Self-Esteem: Long-standing negative self-evaluation/feelings about self or self-capabilities

Situational Low Self-Esteem: Development of a negative perception of self-worth in response to a current situation (specify)

Risk for Situational Low Self-Esteem: At risk for developing negative perception of self-worth in response to a current situation (specify)

Self-Mutilation: Deliberate self-injurious behavior causing tissue damage with the intent of causing nonfatal injury to attain relief of tension

Risk for Self-Mutilation: At risk for deliberate self-injurious behavior causing tissue damage with the intent of causing nonfatal injury to attain relief of tension

Disturbed Sensory Perception (specify visual, auditory, kinesthetic, gustatory, tactile, olfactory): Change in the amount or patterning of incoming stimuli accompanied by a diminished, exaggerated, distorted, or impaired response to such stimuli

Sexual Dysfunction: Change in sexual function that is viewed as unsatisfying, unrewarding, or inadequate

Ineffective Sexuality Pattern: Expressions of concern regarding own sexuality

Impaired Skin Integrity: Altered epidermis and/or dermis

Risk for Impaired Skin Integrity: At risk for skin being adversely altered

Sleep Deprivation: Prolonged periods of time without sleep (sustained natural, periodic suspension of relative consciousness)

Disturbed Sleep Pattern: Time-limited disruption of sleep (natural, periodic suspension of consciousness) amount and quality

Readiness for Enhanced Sleep: A pattern of natural, periodic suspension of consciousness that provides adequate rest, sustains a desired lifestyle, and can be strengthened

Impaired Social Interaction: Insufficient or excessive quantity or ineffective quality of social exchange

Social Isolation: Aloneness experienced by the individual and perceived as imposed by others and as a negative or threatening state

Chronic Sorrow: Cyclical, recurring, and potentially progressive pattern of pervasive sadness experienced (by a patient, caregiver, individual with chronic illness or disability) in response to continual loss, throughout the trajectory of an illness or disability

Spiritual Distress: Impaired ability to experience and integrate meaning and purpose in life through a person's connectedness with self, others, art, music, literature, nature, or a power great than oneself

Risk for Spiritual Distress: At risk for an altered sense of harmonious connectedness with all of life and the universe in which dimensions that transcend and empower the self may be disrupted

Readiness for Enhanced Spiritual Well Being: Ability to experience and integrate meaning and purpose in life through connectedness with self, others, art, music, literature, nature, or a power great than oneself

Risk for Suffocation: Accentuated risk of accidental suffocation (inadequate air available for inhalation)

Risk for Suicide: At risk for self-inflicted, life-threatening injury

Delayed Surgical Recovery: Extension of the number of postoperative days required to initiate and perform activities that maintain life, health, and well being

Impaired Swallowing: Abnormal functioning of the swallowing mechanism associated with deficits in oral, pharyngeal, or esophageal structure or function

Effective Therapeutic Regimen Management: Pattern of regulating and integrating into daily living a program for treatment of illness and its sequelae that is satisfactory for meeting specific health goals

Ineffective Therapeutic Regimen Management: Pattern of regulating and integrating into daily living a program for treatment of illness and the sequelae of illness that is unsatisfactory for meeting specific health goals

---

*New nursing diagnoses, 2003.

From North American Nursing Diagnosis Association International: *Nursing diagnoses: definitions and classification 2003-2004,* Philadelphia, 2003, NANDA International.

*Readiness for Enhanced Therapeutic Regimen Management: A pattern of regulating and integrating into daily living program or programs for treatment of illness and its sequelae that is sufficient for meeting health-related goals and can be strengthened

Ineffective Community Therapeutic Regimen Management: Pattern of regulating and integrating into community processes programs for treatment of illness and the sequelae of illness that are unsatisfactory for meeting health-related goals

Ineffective Family Therapeutic Regimen Management: Pattern of regulating and integrating into family processes a program for treatment of illness and the sequelae of illness that is unsatisfactory for meeting specific health goals

Ineffective Thermoregulation: Temperature fluctuation between hypothermia and hyperthermia

Disturbed Thought Processes: Disruption in cognitive operations and activities

Impaired Tissue Integrity: Damage to mucus membrane, or corneal, integumentary, or subcutaneous tissues

Ineffective Tissue Perfusion (specify type: renal, cerebral, cardiopulmonary, gastrointestinal, peripheral): Decrease in oxygen resulting in the failure to nourish the tissues at the capillary level

Impaired Transfer Ability: Limitation of independent movement between two nearby surfaces

Risk for Trauma: Accentuated risk of accidental tissue injury (e.g., wound, burn, fracture)

Impaired Urinary Elimination: Disturbance in urine elimination

*Readiness for Enhanced Urinary Elimination: A pattern of urinary functions that is sufficient for meeting eliminatory needs and can be strengthened

Urinary Retention: Incomplete emptying of the bladder

Impaired Spontaneous Ventilation: Decreased energy reserves result in an individual's inability to maintain breathing adequate to support life

Dysfunctional Ventilatory Weaning Response: Inability to adjust to lowered levels of mechanical ventilator support that interrupts and prolongs the weaning process

Risk for Other-Directed Violence: At risk for behaviors in which an individual demonstrates that he/she can be physically, emotionally, and/or sexually harmful to others

Risk for Self-Directed Violence: At risk for behaviors in which an individual demonstrates that he/she can be physically, emotionally, and/or sexually harmful to self

Impaired Walking: Limitation of independent movement within the environment on foot

Wandering: Meandering, aimless or repetitive locomotion that exposes the individual to harm; frequently incongruent with boundaries, limits, or obstacles

*New nursing diagnoses, 2003.
From North American Nursing Diagnosis Association International: *Nursing diagnoses: definitions and classification 2003-2004,* Philadelphia, 2003, NANDA International.

APPENDIX B

NANDA International Taxonomy I and Taxonomy II Nomenclature Conversion Classified by Human Response Pattern

Taxonomy I Nursing Diagnoses	Taxonomy II Nursing Diagnoses
Exchanging	
Altered nutrition: more than body requirements	Imbalanced nutrition: more than body requirements
Altered nutrition: less than body requirements	Imbalanced nutrition: less than body requirements
Altered nutrition: risk for more than body requirements	Risk for imbalanced nutrition: more than body requirements
Risk for infection	Risk for infection
Risk for altered body temperature	Risk for imbalanced body temperature
Hypothermia	Hypothermia
Hyperthermia	Hyperthermia
Ineffective thermoregulation	Ineffective thermoregulation
Dysreflexia	Autonomic dysreflexia
Risk for autonomic dysreflexia	Risk for autonomic dysreflexia
Constipation	Constipation
Perceived constipation	Perceived constipation
Diarrhea	Diarrhea
Bowel incontinence	Bowel incontinence
Risk for constipation	Risk for constipation
Altered urinary elimination	Impaired urinary elimination
Stress incontinence	Stress urinary incontinence
Reflex urinary incontinence	Reflex urinary incontinence
Urge incontinence	Urge urinary incontinence
Functional urinary incontinence	Functional urinary incontinence
Total incontinence	Total urinary incontinence
Risk for urinary urge incontinence	Risk for urge urinary incontinence
Urinary retention	Urinary retention
Altered tissue perfusion (specify type)	Ineffective tissue perfusion (specify type)
Risk for fluid volume imbalance	Risk for imbalanced fluid volume
Fluid volume excess	Excess fluid volume
Fluid volume deficit	Deficient fluid volume
Risk for fluid volume deficit	Risk for deficient fluid volume
Decreased cardiac output	Decreased cardiac output
Impaired gas exchange	Impaired gas exchange
Ineffective airway clearance	Ineffective airway clearance
Ineffective breathing pattern	Ineffective breathing pattern
Inability to sustain spontaneous ventilation	Impaired spontaneous ventilation
Dysfunctional ventilatory weaning response	Dysfunctional ventilatory weaning response
Risk for injury	Risk for injury
Risk for suffocation	Risk for suffocation
Risk for poisoning	Risk for poisoning
Risk for trauma	Risk for trauma
Risk for aspiration	Risk for aspiration
Risk for disuse syndrome	Risk for disuse syndrome
Latex allergy response	Latex allergy response
Risk for latex allergy response	Risk for latex allergy response
Altered protection	Ineffective protection
Impaired tissue integrity	Impaired tissue integrity
Altered oral mucous membrane	Impaired oral mucous membrane
Impaired skin integrity	Impaired skin integrity
Risk for impaired skin integrity	Risk for impaired skin integrity

Taxonomy I Nursing Diagnoses	Taxonomy II Nursing Diagnoses
Exchanging—cont'd	
Altered dentition	Impaired dentition
Decreased adaptive capacity: intracranial	Decreased intracranial adaptive capacity
Energy field disturbance	Disturbed energy field
Communicating	
Impaired verbal communication	Impaired verbal communication
Relating	
Impaired social interaction	Impaired social interaction
Social isolation	Social isolation
Risk for loneliness	Risk for loneliness
Altered role performance	Ineffective role performance
Altered parenting	Impaired parenting
Risk for altered parenting	Risk for impaired parenting
Risk for altered parent/infant/child attachment	Risk for impaired parent/infant/child attachment
Sexual dysfunction	Sexual dysfunction
Altered family processes	Interrupted family processes
Caregiver role strain	Caregiver role strain
Risk for caregiver role strain	Risk for caregiver role strain
Altered family processes: alcoholism	Dysfunctional family processes: alcoholism
Parental role conflict	Parental role conflict
Altered sexuality patterns	Ineffective sexuality patterns
Valuing	
Spiritual distress (distress of the human spirit)	Spiritual distress
Risk for spiritual distress	Risk for spiritual distress
Potential for enhanced spiritual well-being	Readiness for enhanced spiritual well being
Choosing	
Ineffective individual coping	Ineffective coping
Impaired adjustment	Impaired adjustment
Defensive coping	Defensive coping
Ineffective denial	Ineffective denial
Ineffective family coping: disabling	Disabled family coping
Ineffective family coping: compromised	Compromised family coping
Family coping: potential for growth	Readiness for enhanced family coping
Potential for enhanced community coping	Readiness for enhanced community coping
Ineffective community coping	Ineffective community coping
Ineffective management of therapeutic regimen: individuals	Ineffective therapeutic regimen management
Noncompliance (specify)	Noncompliance (specify)
Ineffective management of therapeutic regimen: families	Ineffective family therapeutic regimen management
Ineffective management of therapeutic regimen: community	Ineffective community therapeutic regimen management
Effective management of therapeutic regimen: individual	Effective therapeutic regimen management
Decisional conflict (specify)	Decisional conflict (specify)
Health-seeking behaviors (specify)	Health-seeking behaviors (specify)
Moving	
Impaired physical mobility	Impaired physical mobility
Risk for peripheral neurovascular dysfunction	Risk for peripheral neurovascular dysfunction
Risk for perioperative positioning injury	Risk for perioperative positioning injury
Impaired walking	Impaired walking
Impaired wheelchair mobility	Impaired wheelchair mobility
Impaired transfer ability	Impaired transfer ability
Impaired bed mobility	Impaired bed mobility
Activity intolerance	Activity intolerance
Fatigue	Fatigue
Risk for activity intolerance	Risk for activity intolerance
Sleep pattern disturbance	Disturbed sleep pattern
Sleep deprivation	Sleep deprivation

Taxonomy I Nursing Diagnoses	Taxonomy II Nursing Diagnoses
Moving—cont'd	
Diversional activity deficit	Deficient diversional activity
Impaired home maintenance management	Impaired home maintenance
Altered health maintenance	Ineffective health maintenance
Delayed surgical recovery	Delayed surgical recovery
Adult failure to thrive	Adult failure to thrive
Feeding self-care deficit	Feeding self-care deficit
Impaired swallowing	Impaired swallowing
Ineffective breast-feeding	Ineffective breast-feeding
Interrupted breast-feeding	Interrupted breast-feeding
Effective breast-feeding	Effective breast-feeding
Ineffective infant feeding pattern	Ineffective infant feeding pattern
Bathing/hygiene self-care deficit	Bathing/hygiene self-care deficit
Dressing/grooming self-care deficit	Dressing/grooming self-care deficit
Toileting self-care deficit	Toileting self-care deficit
Altered growth and development	Delayed growth and development
Risk for altered development	Risk for delayed development
Risk for altered growth	Risk for disproportionate growth
Relocation stress syndrome	Relocation stress syndrome
Risk for disorganized infant behavior	Risk for disorganized infant behavior
Disorganized infant behavior	Disorganized infant behavior
Potential for enhanced organized infant behavior	Readiness for enhanced organized infant behavior
Perceiving	
Body image disturbance	Disturbed body image
Chronic low self-esteem	Chronic low self-esteem
Situational low self-esteem	Situational low self-esteem
Personal identity disturbance	Disturbed personal identity
Sensory/perceptual alterations (specify)	Disturbed sensory perception (specify)
Unilateral neglect	Unilateral neglect
Hopelessness	Hopelessness
Powerlessness	Powerlessness
Knowing	
Knowledge deficit (specify)	Deficient knowledge (specify)
Impaired environmental interpretation syndrome	Impaired interpretation syndrome
Acute confusion	Acute confusion
Chronic confusion	Chronic confusion
Altered thought processes	Disturbed thought processes
Impaired memory	Impaired memory
Feeling	
Pain	Acute pain
Chronic pain	Chronic pain
Nausea	Nausea
Dysfunctional grieving	Dysfunctional grieving
Anticipatory grieving	Anticipatory grieving
Chronic sorrow	Chronic sorrow
Risk for violence: directed at others	Risk for other-directed violence
Risk for self-mutilation	Risk for self-mutilation
Risk for violence: self-directed	Risk for self-directed violence
Post-trauma syndrome	Post-trauma syndrome
Rape-trauma syndrome	Rape-trauma syndrome
Rape-trauma syndrome: compound reaction	Rape-trauma syndrome: compound reaction
Rape-trauma syndrome: silent reaction	Rape-trauma syndrome: silent reaction
Risk for post-trauma syndrome	Risk for post-trauma syndrome
Anxiety	Anxiety
Death anxiety	Death anxiety
Fear	Fear

Taxonomy I Nursing Diagnoses	Taxonomy II Nursing Diagnoses
	New to Taxonomy II
	Readiness for enhanced communication
	Readiness for enhanced coping
	Readiness for enhanced family processes
	Readiness for enhanced fluid balance
	Readiness for enhanced knowledge (specify)
	Readiness for enhanced nutrition
	Readiness for enhanced parenting
	Readiness for enhanced self-concept
	Readiness for enhanced sleep
	Readiness for enhanced therapeutic regimen management
	Readiness for enhanced urinary elimination
	Risk for falls
	Risk for powerlessness
	Risk for relocation stress syndrome
	Risk for situational low self-esteem
	Risk for sudden infant death syndrome
	Risk for suicide
	Self-mutilation
	Wandering

From North American Nursing Diagnosis Association International: *Nursing diagnoses: definitions and classification 2003-2004*, Philadelphia, 2003, NANDA International.

HEALTH PERCEPTION–HEALTH MANAGEMENT PATTERN

Health-seeking behaviors (specify)
Ineffective health maintenance (specify)
Ineffective therapeutic regimen management (specify area)
Risk for ineffective therapeutic regimen management (specify area)
Effective therapeutic regimen management
Ineffective family therapeutic regimen management
Ineffective community therapeutic regimen management
Health-management deficit (specify area)
Risk for health-management deficit (specify area)
Noncompliance (specify)
Risk for noncompliance (specify area)
Risk for infection (specify type/area)
Risk for injury (trauma)
Risk for falls
Risk for perioperative positioning injury
Risk for poisoning
Risk for suffocation
Ineffective protection (specify)
Disturbed energy field

NUTRITIONAL-METABOLIC PATTERN

Imbalanced nutrition: more than body requirements **or Exogenous obesity**
Imbalanced nutrition: risk for more than body requirements **or Risk for obesity**
Imbalanced nutrition: less than body requirements **or Nutritional deficit** (specify type)
Adult failure to thrive
Ineffective breast-feeding
Interrupted breast-feeding
Effective breast-feeding
Ineffective infant feeding pattern
Impaired swallowing (uncompensated)
Nausea
Risk for aspiration
Impaired oral mucous membrane (specify)
Impaired dentition
Deficient fluid volume
Risk for deficient fluid volume
Excess fluid volume
Risk for imbalanced fluid volume
Impaired skin integrity
Risk for impaired skin integrity **or Risk for skin breakdown**

Pressure ulcer (specify stage)
Impaired tissue integrity (specify type)
Latex allergy response
Risk for latex allergy response
Ineffective thermoregulation
Hyperthermia
Hypothermia
Risk for imbalanced body temperature

ELIMINATION PATTERN

Constipation
Perceived constipation
Intermittent constipation pattern
Risk for constipation
Diarrhea
Bowel incontinence
Impaired urinary elimination
Functional urinary incontinence
Reflex urinary incontinence
Stress incontinence
Urge incontinence
Risk for urinary urge incontinence
Total incontinence
Urinary retention

ACTIVITY-EXERCISE PATTERN

Activity intolerance (specify level)
Risk for activity intolerance
Fatigue
Deficient diversional activity
Impaired physical mobility (specify level)
Impaired bed mobility (specify level)
Impaired transfer ability (specify level)
Impaired wheelchair mobility
Impaired walking (specify level)
Wandering
Risk for disuse syndrome
Risk for joint contractures
Total self-care deficit (specify level)
Bathing/hygiene self-care deficit (specify level)
Dressing/grooming self-care deficit (specify level)
Feeding self-care deficit (specify level)
Toileting self-care deficit (specify level)
Developmental delay: self-care skills (specify level)
Delayed surgical recovery
Delayed growth and development

From Gordon M: *Manual of nursing diagnosis,* ed 10, St. Louis, 2002, Mosby.
Boldface type indicates diagnoses developed by the author and found to be useful in clinical practice but are not reviewed by NANDA International.

Risk for delayed development
Risk for disproportionate growth
Impaired home maintenance (mild, moderate, severe, potential, chronic)
Dysfunctional ventilatory weaning response
Impaired spontaneous ventilation
Ineffective airway clearance
Ineffective breathing pattern
Impaired gas exchange
Decreased cardiac output
Altered tissue perfusion (specify type)
Autonomic dysreflexia
Risk for autonomic dysreflexia
Disorganized infant behavior
Risk for disorganized infant behavior
Potential for enhanced organized infant behavior
Risk for peripheral neurovascular dysfunction
Decreased intracranial adaptive capacity

SLEEP-REST PATTERN

Disturbed sleep pattern (specify type)
Sleep deprivation
Delayed sleep onset
Sleep-pattern reversal

COGNITIVE-PERCEPTUAL PATTERN

Pain (specify location)
Chronic pain (specify location)
Pain self-management deficit (acute, chronic)
Uncompensated sensory loss (specify type and degree)
Sensory overload
Sensory deprivation
Sensory/perceptual alterations (specify)
Unilateral neglect
Knowledge deficit (specify)
Disturbed thought processes
Attention-concentration deficit
Acute confusion
Chronic confusion
Impaired environmental interpretation syndrome
Uncompensated memory loss
Impaired memory
Risk for cognitive impairment
Decisional conflict (specify)

SELF-PERCEPTION–SELF-CONCEPT PATTERN

Fear (specify focus)
Anxiety
Mild anxiety
Moderate anxiety
Severe anxiety (panic)
Anticipatory anxiety (mild, moderate, severe)
Death anxiety
Reactive depression (specify situation)
Risk for loneliness
Hopelessness
Powerlessness (severe, moderate, low)
Risk for powerlessness
Situational low self-esteem
Risk for situational low self-esteem

Chronic low self-esteem
Disturbed body image
Disturbed personal identity
Risk for self-directed violence

ROLE-RELATIONSHIP PATTERN

Anticipatory grieving
Dysfunctional grieving
Chronic sorrow
Ineffective role performance (specify)
Unresolved independence-dependence conflict
Social isolation or Social rejection
Impaired social interaction
Developmental delay: social skills (specify)
Relocation stress syndrome
Risk for relocation stress syndrome
Interrupted family processes (specify process)
Dysfunctional family process: alcoholism
Impaired parenting (specify)
Risk for impaired parenting (specify)
Parental role conflict
Weak parent-infant attachment
Risk for impaired parent/infant/child attachment
Parent-infant separation
Caregiver role strain
Risk for caregiver role strain
Impaired verbal communication
Developmental delay: communication skills (specify)
Risk for other-directed violence

SEXUALITY-REPRODUCTIVE PATTERN

Ineffective sexuality patterns
Sexual dysfunction
Rape-trauma syndrome
Rape-trauma syndrome: compound reaction
Rape-trauma syndrome: silent reaction

COPING–STRESS-TOLERANCE PATTERN

Ineffective coping
Avoidance coping
Defensive coping
Compromised family coping
Disabled family coping
Readiness for enhanced family coping
Ineffective community coping
Readiness for enhanced community coping
Ineffective denial
Impaired adjustment
Post-trauma syndrome
Risk for post-trauma syndrome
Support system deficit
Risk for suicide
Self-mutilation
Risk for self-mutilation

VALUE-BELIEF PATTERN

Spiritual distress (distress of the human spirit)
Readiness for enhanced spiritual well being
Risk for spiritual distress

APPENDIX D Common Drug Interactions

Drug Category/ Representative Drugs	Interacting Drug or Substance	Effect
Antibiotics		
Macrolides (azithromycin, clarithromycin, dirithromycin, erythromycin)	Blood thinners (warfarin)	May enhance blood thinning effects
	Ergot alkaloids (ergotamine, methysergide)	Increased risk of toxicity
	HMG-CoA reductase inhibitors (lovastatin, pravastatin, simvastatin)	Toxic effects on muscle and severe muscle damage may occur
Penicillins (ampicillin, amoxicillin)	Antiseizure drugs (carbamazepine)	May increase toxicity of carbamazepine
	Birth control pills (norethindrone with ethinyl estradiol)	May interfere with birth control pills and result in unplanned pregnancy or menstrual problems
	Tetracyclines (doxycycline, tetracycline)	May interfere with effects of penicillins
Sulfonamides (trimethoprim/ sulfamethoxazole, sulfamethizole)	Blood thinners (warfarin)	May enhance blood-thinning effects
	Blood thinners (warfarin)	May increase blood-thinning effects
Tetracyclines (doxycycline, tetracycline)	Antacids (aluminum or magnesium containing)	Effects of tetracyclines may be reduced; separate by 3-4 hrs
	Penicillins (ampicillin, amoxicillin)	May interfere with effects of penicillins
	Barbiturates (pentobarbital, phenobarbital, secobarbital)	May decrease effects of doxycycline; consider alternative tetracycline
Antidepressants		
Lithium	Sodium chloride (salt)	Low-salt diet or sudden changes in diet may cause lithium to build up
	Thiazide diuretics (hydrochlorothiazide)	May cause lithium toxicity
	Weight-loss agents (sibutramine)	May cause serious nervous system reactions
	Loop diuretics (furosemide)	May cause lithium toxicity
	ACE inhibitors (captopril, enalapril)	May cause lithium toxicity
MAOIs (isocarboxazid, phenelzine, tranylcypromine)	TCAs (amitriptyline, desipramine, doxepin, imipramine, nortriptyline)	Severe seizures and death may result; separate by at least 14 days
	SSRIs (citalopram, fluoxetine, fluvoxamine, paroxetine, sertraline)	Serious effects on nervous system; possibly life threatening
	Sulfonylureas (glipizide, glyburide, tolbutamide)	May cause extremely low blood sugar
	Insulin	May cause extremely low blood sugar
	Dextromethorphan	May affect nervous system
	Tyramine-containing foods (avocados, bananas, beer, wine, caffeine, chocolate, cheese, liver, fava beans, fermented meats, canned figs, pickled herring, pineapple, raisins, sauerkraut, soy sauce, yeast extract, yogurt)	May cause severe and possibly fatal high blood pressure; warning signs are headache, vomiting, fever, and increased blood pressure
	Selective 5-HT1 receptor agonists (naratriptan, rizatriptan, sumatriptan, zolmitriptan)	Increased risk of serious heart problems
	Painkillers: narcotic analgesics (codeine, meperidine)	May cause severe and possibly life-threatening reaction

Drug Category/ Representative Drugs	Interacting Drug or Substance	Effect
Antidepressants—cont'd		
	Weight-loss agents (sibutramine)	May cause serious nervous system reactions
SSRIs (citalopram, fluoxetine, fluvoxamine, paroxetine, sertraline)	TCAs (amitriptyline, desipramine, doxepin, imipramine, nortriptyline)	Toxic effects may occur
	MAOIs (isocarboxazid, phenelzine, tranylcypromine)	May cause serious effects on nervous system, possibly life threatening
	Selective 5-HT1 receptor agonists (naratriptan, rizatriptan, sumatriptan, zolmitriptan)	May cause serious nervous system reactions
	Weight-loss agents (sibutramine)	May cause serious nervous system reactions
TCAs (amitriptyline, desipramine, doxepin, imipramine, nortriptyline)	Alcohol	May cause extreme drowsiness
	Antiseizure agents (carbamazepine)	Effects of antiseizure drug may be increased
	MAOIs (isocarboxazid, phenelzine, tranylcypromine)	Severe seizures and death may result; separate by at least 14 days
	Narcotic analgesics (codeine, meperidine, oxycodone, propoxyphene)	May depress nervous system, slow breathing, and lower blood pressure
	SSRIs (citalopram, fluoxetine, fluvoxamine, paroxetine, sertraline)	Toxic effects may occur
Antidiabetic Agents		
Insulin	Beta-adrenergic blockers (pindolol, propranolol)	May mask symptoms of low blood sugar, especially with nonselective beta blockers
	Birth control pills (norethindrone with ethinyl estradiol)	May increase risk of high blood sugar
	MAOIs (isocarboxazid, phenelzine, tranylcypromine)	May cause extremely low blood sugar
	Alcohol	May cause low blood sugar
Sulfonylureas (glipizide, glyburide, tolbutamide)	Histamine H2-antagonists (cimetidine, famotidine, nizatidine, ranitidine)	May cause low blood sugar
	Alcohol	May cause stomach upset, headaches, low blood sugar
	Beta-adrenergic blockers (metoprolol, propranolol)	May mask symptoms of low blood sugar; may increase or decrease blood sugar
	MAOIs (isocarboxazid, phenelzine, tranylcypromine)	May cause extremely low blood sugar
	Salicylates (aspirin, aspirin-containing compounds)	May cause low blood sugar
Antihyperlipidemic Agents		
Fibric acids (clofibrate, gemfibrozil)	HMG-CoA reductase inhibitors (lovastatin, pravastatin, simvastatin)	May have toxic effects on muscle and cause severe muscle damage
	Blood thinners (warfarin)	May increase blood-thinning effects and cause serious bleeding
HMG-CoA reductase inhibitors (lovastatin, pravastatin, simvastatin)	Macrolides (azithromycin, clarithromycin, dirithromycin, erythromycin)	May have toxic effects on muscle and cause severe muscle damage
	Fibric acids (clofibrate, gemfibrozil)	May have toxic effects on muscle and severe muscle damage
Antiseizure agents (carbamazepine, phenytoin)	Alcohol	May cause drowsiness
	Birth control pills (norethindrone with ethinyl estradiol)	May interfere with birth control pills and result in unplanned pregnancy
	TCAs (amitriptyline, desipramine, doxepin, imipramine, nortriptyline)	May increase or decrease effects of antiseizure drug; may increase CNS effects; dosage may need adjusting

Drug Category/ Representative Drugs	Interacting Drug or Substance	Effect
Barbiturates (pentobarbital, phenobarbital, secobarbital)	Macrolides (azithromycin, clarithromycin, dirithromycin, erythromycin)	May increase toxicity of carbamazepine
	Alcohol	May increase effects of drug, cause drowsiness, stop breathing, or cause blood pressure to drop too low
	Birth control pills (norethindrone with ethinyl estradiol)	May interfere with birth control pills and result in unplanned pregnancy
	Blood-thinners (warfarin)	May decrease blood-thinning effects
	Tetracyclines (doxycycline)	May decrease effects of doxycycline; consider alternative tetracycline
	Beta-adrenergic blockers (metoprolol, propranolol)	May decrease effects of beta-blockers
Benzodiazepines (alprazolam, chlordiazepoxide, clonazepam, diazepam)	Alcohol	Increased effects on CNS: drowsiness, confusion
	Narcotic analgesics (codeine, meperidine, oxycodone, propoxyphene)	May cause drowsiness and confusion
Birth control pills (norethindrone with ethinyl estradiol)	Antiseizure agents (carbamazepine, phenytoin)	May interfere with birth control pills and result in unplanned pregnancy; may decrease effects of antiseizure drugs
	Barbiturates (pentobarbital, phenobarbital, secobarbital)	May interfere with birth control pills and result in unplanned pregnancy
	Insulin	May increase risk of high blood sugar
	Penicillins (ampicillin, amoxicillin)	May interfere with birth control pills and result in unplanned pregnancy or menstrual problems
	Tobacco (smoking)	Increases chance of blood clots, stroke, and heart attack
Blood Pressure Drugs		
ACE inhibitors (captopril, enalapril)	Potassium preparations	Increases potassium levels
	Digitalis glycosides (digoxin)	May increase digoxin levels
	Lithium	May cause lithium toxicity
Beta-adrenergic blockers (propranolol, metoprolol)	Sulfonylureas (glipizide, glyburide, tolbutamide)	May mask symptoms of low blood sugar; may increase or decrease blood sugar
	Insulin	May mask symptoms of low blood sugar, especially with nonselective beta blockers
	Barbiturates (pentobarbital, phenobarbital, secobarbital)	May decrease effects of beta-blockers
	Digitalis glycosides (digoxin)	May cause extremely slow heartbeat, possibly heart block
	Calcium channel blockers (diltiazem, verapamil)	May increase effects on heart contractility
	Thiazide diuretics (hydrochlorothiazide)	May cause extremely low blood pressure
	Loop diuretics (furosemide)	May cause extremely low blood pressure
Calcium channel blockers (diltiazem, verapamil)	Beta-adrenergic blockers (metoprolol, propranolol)	May increase effects on heart contractility
	Thiazide diuretics (hydrochlorothiazide)	May cause low blood pressure
	Loop diuretics (furosemide)	May cause low blood pressure
Loop diuretics (furosemide)	Beta-adrenergic blockers (metoprolol, propranolol)	May cause extremely low blood pressure
	Digitalis glycosides (digoxin)	Can cause irregular heartbeat and extremely low blood pressure
	Lithium	May cause lithium toxicity
	Thiazide diuretics (hydrochlorothiazide)	May cause low blood pressure

Drug Category/ Representative Drugs	Interacting Drug or Substance	Effect
Blood Pressure Drugs—cont'd		
Thiazide diuretics (hydrochlorothiazide)	Digitalis glycosides (digoxin)	Can cause irregular heartbeat and extremely low blood pressure
	Lithium	May cause lithium toxicity
	Loop diuretics (furosemide)	May cause low blood pressure
Blood thinners (heparin)	Blood thinners (warfarin)	May increase risk of bleeding
	Salicylates (aspirin, aspirin-containing compounds)	Increases risk of internal bleeding
	NSAIDs (etodolac, ibuprofen, naproxen, oxaprozin)	May cause internal bleeding or ulcers
Blood thinners (warfarin)	Acetaminophen, acetaminophen-containing combinations	High doses of acetaminophen may increase blood-thinning effects
	Barbiturates (pentobarbital, phenobarbital, secobarbital)	May decrease blood-thinning effects
	Blood thinners (heparin)	May increase risk of bleeding
	Penicillins (ampicillin, amoxicillin)	May enhance blood-thinning effects
	Salicylates (aspirin, aspirin-containing compounds)	Increases risk of internal bleeding
	NSAIDs (etodolac, ibuprofen, naproxen, oxaprozin)	May cause internal bleeding or ulcers
	Sulfonamides (trimethoprim/ sulfamethoxazole, sulfamethizole)	May increase blood-thinning effects
	Thyroid hormones (thyroid, levothyroxine)	May increase blood-thinning effects
	Vitamin K– containing foods and products	May decrease blood-thinning effects
	Macrolides (azithromycin, clarithromycin, dirithromycin, erythromycin)	May enhance blood thinning effects
	Fibric acids (clofibrate, gemfibrozil)	May increase blood-thinning effects and cause serious bleeding
Erectile dysfunction agents (sildenafil)	Nitrates (amyl nitrate, isosorbide dinitrate, isosorbide mononitrate, nitroglycerin)	Severe, possibly life-threatening drop in blood pressure
Heart Drugs		
Digitalis glycosides (digoxin)	Beta-adrenergic blockers (metoprolol, propranolol)	May cause extremely slow heartbeat, possibly heart attack
	Calcium channel blockers (diltiazem, verapamil)	May increase digoxin levels, increasing risk of toxicity
	Thiazide diuretics (hydrochlorothiazide)	Can cause irregular heartbeat and extremely low blood pressure
	Loop diuretics (furosemide)	Can cause irregular heartbeat and extremely low blood pressure
	ACE inhibitors (captopril, enalapril)	May increase digoxin levels
Nitrates (amyl nitrate, isosorbide dinitrate, isosorbide mononitrate, nitroglycerin)	Erectile dysfunction agents (sildenafil)	Severe, possibly life-threatening drop in blood pressure
Histamine H2-antagonists (cimetidine, famotidine, nizatidine, ranitidine)	Sulfonylureas (glipizide, glyburide, tolbutamide)	Risk of low blood sugar
	Blood thinners (warfarin)	May increase effect of warfarin; possible bleeding risk, particularly with cimetidine
Migraine Drugs		
Ergot alkaloids (ergotamine, methysergide)	Macrolides (azithromycin, clarithromycin, dirithromycin, erythromycin)	Increases risk of toxicity
	Selective 5-HT1 receptor agonists (naratriptan, rizatriptan, sumatriptan, zolmitriptan)	Increases risk of serious heart problem

Drug Category/Representative Drugs	Interacting Drug or Substance	Effect
Migraine Drugs—cont'd		
	Weight-loss agents (sibutramine)	May cause serious nervous system reactions
Selective 5-HT1 receptor agonists (naratriptan, rizatriptan, sumatriptan, zolmitriptan)	SSRIs (citalopram, fluoxetine, fluvoxamine, paroxetine, sertraline)	May cause serious nervous system reactions
	MAOIs (isocarboxazid, phenelzine, tranylcypromine)	Increases risk of serious heart problems
	Ergot alkaloids (ergotamine, methysergide)	Increases risk of serious heart problems
	Weight-loss agents (sibutramine)	May cause serious nervous system reactions
Painkillers		
Acetaminophen, acetaminophen-containing combinations	Alcohol	May cause liver damage
	Blood thinners (warfarin, heparin)	High doses of acetaminophen may increase blood-thinning effects
Narcotic analgesics (codeine, meperidine, oxycodone, propoxyphene)	Alcohol	May depress nervous system, slow breathing, and lower blood pressure
	MAOIs (isocarboxazid, phenelzine, tranylcypromine)	May cause severe and possibly fatal reaction
	TCAs (amitriptyline, desipramine, doxepin, imipramine, nortriptyline)	May depress nervous system, slow breathing, and lower blood pressure
	Benzodiazepines (alprazolam, diazepam, chlordiazepoxide, clonazepam)	May cause drowsiness and confusion
	Weight-loss agents (sibutramine)	May cause serious nervous system reactions
NSAIDs (etodolac, ibuprofen, naproxen, oxaprozin)	Alcohol	May cause internal bleeding or ulcers
	Blood thinners (warfarin, heparin)	May cause internal bleeding or ulcers
	Salicylates (aspirin, aspirin-containing compounds)	May cause stomach upset without relieving pain; may cause internal bleeding or ulcers
Salicylates (aspirin, aspirin-containing compounds)	Alcohol	May cause internal bleeding or ulcers
	Sulfonylureas (glipizide, glyburide, tolbutamide)	May cause low blood sugar
	Blood thinners (warfarin, heparin)	Increases risk of internal bleeding
	NSAIDs (etodolac, ibuprofen, naproxen, oxaprozin)	May cause stomach upset without relieving pain; may cause internal bleeding or ulcers
Thyroid hormones **Weight-loss agents (sibutramine)**	Blood thinners (warfarin)	May increase blood-thinning effects
	Lithium	May cause serious nervous system reactions
	Ergot alkaloids (ergotamine, methysergide)	May cause serious nervous system reactions
	Selective 5-HT1 receptor agonists (naratriptan, rizatriptan, sumatriptan, zolmitriptan)	May cause serious nervous system reactions
	Dextromethorphan	May cause serious nervous system reactions
	MAOIs (isocarboxazid, phenelzine, tranylcypromine)	May cause serious nervous system reactions
	SSRIs (citalopram, fluoxetine, fluvoxamine, paroxetine, sertraline)	May cause serious nervous system reactions

Drug Category/ Representative Drugs	Interacting Drug or Substance	Effect
Weight-loss agents (sibutramine)—cont'd		
	Narcotic analgesics (codeine, meperidine, oxycodone, propoxyphene)	May cause serious nervous system reactions

HMG-CoA, Beta-hydroxy-beta-methylglutaryl-CoA; *ACE,* angiotensin-converting enzyme; *MAOI,* monoamine oxidase inhibitor; *TCA,* tricyclic antidepressant; *SSRI,* serotonin-specific reuptake inhibitor; *CNS,* central nervous system; *NSAID,* nonsteroidal antiinflammatory drug.
From *Mosby's medical, nursing, and allied health dictionary,* ed 6, St. Louis, 2002, Mosby. Updated by Jennifer L. McQuade, Pharm.D.

APPENDIX E
Tables of Weights, Measures, Pharmacology and Clinical Calculations

Metric System

Length	Weight	Volume
meter (m) basic unit	gram (g or gm) basic unit	liter (L) basic unit
1 micrometer (μm) = 0.000001 meter	1 microgram (mcg or μg) = 0.000001 gram	1 milliliter (ml)* = 0.001 liter
1 millimeter (mm) = 0.001 meter	1 milligram (mg) = 0.001 gram	1 centiliter (cl) = 0.01 liter
1 centimeter (cm) = 0.01 meter	1 centigram (cg) = 0.01 gram	1 deciliter (dL) = 0.1 liter
1 decimeter (dm) = 0.1 meter	1 decigram (dg) = 0.1 gram	1 dekaliter (Dl) = 10 liters
1 dekameter (Dm) = 10 meters	1 dekagram (Dg) = 10 grams	1 hectoliter (Hl) = 100 liters
1 hectometer (Hm) = 100 meters	1 hectogram (Hg) = 100 grams	1 kiloliter (kl) = 1000 liters
1 kilometer (km) = 1000 meters	1 kilogram (kg) = 1000 grams	

Apothecary System

Weight	Volume
20 grains (gr) = 1 scruple	60 minims = 1 fluidram
3 scruples = 1 dram	8 fluidrams = 1 fluidounce
8 drams = 1 ounce	16 fluidounces = 1 pint (pt)
12 ounces = 1 pound (lb)	2 pints = 1 quart (qt)
	4 quarts (qt) = 1 gallon (C, Cong, or gal)

Household Equivalents and Other Commonly Used Equivalents (Approximate)

Volume	Weight	Volume
1 teaspoonful (tsp) = 5 milliliters (ml)	1 grain (gr) = 60 to 65 milligrams (mg)	1 minim = 0.06 milliliter (ml)
1 dessertspoonful = 10 milliliters (ml)	15 grains (gr) = 1 gram (g)	16 minims = 1 milliliter (ml)
1 tablespoonful (tbsp) = 15 milliliters (ml) or ½ ounce (oz)	1 kilogram (kg) = 2.2 pounds (lb)	1 fluidram = 1 teaspoonful (tsp)
1 teacupful = 120 milliliters (ml) or 4 ounces		1 fluidounce (f[dram]) = 30 milliliters (ml)
1 cupful = 240 milliliters (ml) or 8 ounces		1 pint (pt) = 500 milliliters

*1 ml is considered equivalent to 1 cubic centimeter (cc).

FORMULAS FOR DRUG CALCULATIONS

Surface area rule:

$$\text{Child dose} = \frac{\text{Surface area } (m^2)}{1.73 m^2} \times \text{Adult dose}$$

Calculating strength of a solution:

Solution strength:

$$\frac{X}{100} =$$

Desired solution:

$$\frac{\text{Amount of drug desired}}{\text{Amount of finished solution}}$$

Calculation of medication dosages

Formula method:

$$\frac{\text{Amount ordered}}{\text{Amount on hand}} \times \text{Vehicle*} = \text{Number of tablets, capsules, or amount of liquid}$$

*Vehicle is the drug form or amount of liquid containing the dosage. Amounts used in calculation by formula must be in same system.

Ratio—proportion method:

1 tablet : tablet in mg on hand :: x tablet order in mg
Know or have :: Want to know or order
Multiply means and extremes, divide both sides by known amount to get X. Amounts used in equation must be in same system.

Dimensional analysis method:

$$\text{Order in mg} \times \frac{1 \text{ tablet or capsule}}{\text{What 1 tablet or capsule is in mg}} = \text{Tablets or capsules to be given}$$

If amounts are in different systems:

$$\text{Order in mg} \times \frac{1 \text{ tablet or capsule}}{\text{What 1 tablet or capsule is in g}} \times \frac{1}{1000 \text{ mg}} = \text{Tablets or capsules to be given}$$

(From Skidmore-Roth: *Mosby's 1997 nursing drug reference,* St. Louis, 1997, Mosby.)

IV FLOW RATE FORMULAS

Use the following formulas to calculate IV flow rates

$$\text{Flow rate (ml/hr)} = \frac{\text{Desired dose (mg/min)} \times 60 \text{ (min/hr)}}{\text{Drug concentration (mg/ml)}}$$

$$\text{Or} = \frac{\text{Desired dose (}\mu\text{g/kg/min)} \times 60 \text{ (min/hr)} \times \text{wt (kg)}}{\text{Drug concentration (}\mu\text{g/ml)}}$$

$$\text{Or} = \frac{\text{Drip rate (drops/min)} \times 60 \text{ (min/hr)}}{60 \text{ (drops/ml)}}$$

$$\text{Drip rate (drops/min)} = \frac{\text{Total volume to be infused (ml)} \times \text{drop factor (drops/ml)}}{\text{Total time for the infusion (min)}}$$

$$\text{Or} = \frac{\text{Drops/ml}}{60 \text{ (min/hr)}} \times \frac{\text{Volume to be infused (ml/hr)}}{1}$$

(From Thompson JM: *Quick reference for clinical nursing,* ed 2, St. Louis, 1997, Mosby.)

APPENDIX F   Common Communicable Diseases

To prevent the spread of infection, any person with symptoms suggestive of a communicable disease should be kept away from others. Measures for control of communicable diseases are established either by law or by regulation in various states and communities. Because these may vary, practical nurses should keep in touch with local health authorities and cooperate with them in preventing the spread of disease.

Disease and Synopsis of Symptoms	Incubation Period	Mode of Transmission	Period of Communicability
Actinomycosis Chronic disease most frequently localized in jaw, thorax, or abdomen; septicemic spread with generalized disease may occur. Lesions are firmly indurated areas of purulence and fibrosis.	Irregular; probably years after colonization in oral tissues, plus days or months after precipitating trauma and actual penetration of tissues.	Contact from person to person as part of normal oral flora.	Time and manner in which *Actinomyces israelii* becomes part of normal flora is unknown.
Amebiasis Infection with a protozoan parasite that exists in two forms: the hardy, infective cyst and the more fragile, potentially invasive trophozoite. Parasite may act as a commensal or invade tissues, giving rise to intestinal or extraintestinal disease.	Variation: from a few days to several months or years. Commonly 2 to 4 weeks.	Contaminated water or food containing cysts from feces of infected persons, often as complication of another infection such as shigellosis.	During period of cyst passing, which may continue for years.
Ascariasis (Roundworm Infection) Helminthic infection of small intestine. Symptoms are variable, often vague or absent, or ordinarily mild; live worms, passed in stools or regurgitated, are frequently first recognized sign of infection.	Worms reach maturity approximately 2 months after ingestion of embryonated eggs.	By ingestion of infective eggs from soil contaminated with human feces containing eggs, but not directly from person to person.	As long as mature female worms live in intestine. Maximum life span of adult worms is under 18 months; however, female produces up to 200,000 eggs a day that can remain viable in soil for months or years.
Balantidiasis Disease of colon characteristically producing diarrhea or dysentery accompanied by abdominal colic, tenesmus, nausea, and vomiting.	Unknown; may be only a few days.	By ingestion of cysts from feces of infected hosts; in epidemics, mainly by fecally contaminated water.	As long as infection persists.
Candidiasis (Moniliasis, Thrush, Candidosis) Mycosis usually confined to superficial layers of skin or mucous membranes	Variable; 2 to 5 days in thrush of infants.	Through contact with excretions of mouth, skin, vagina, and especially feces from patients or carriers;	Presumably for duration of lesions.

Disease and Synopsis of Symptoms	Incubation Period	Mode of Transmission	Period of Communicability
Candidiasis (*Moniliasis, Thrush, Candidosis*)—cont'd			
with patients who have oral thrush, intertrigo, vulvovaginitis, paronychia, or onychomycosis.		from mother to infant during childbirth; and by endogenous spread.	
Carditis, Coxsackie (*Viral Carditis, Enteroviral Carditis*) Acute or subacute myocarditis or pericarditis, which occurs as the only manifestation, or may occasionally be associated with other manifestations.	Usually 3 to 5 days.	Fecal-oral or respiratory droplet contact with infected person.	Apparently during acute stage of disease.
Chickenpox, Herpes Zoster (*Varicella Shingles*) Acute generalized viral disease with sudden onset of slight fever, mild constitutional symptoms, and a skin eruption that is maculopapular for a few hours, vesicular for 3 to 4 days, and leaves a granular scab.	From 2 to 3 weeks; commonly 13 to 17 days.	From person to person by direct contact, droplet, or airborne spread of secretion of respiratory tract of chickenpox cases or of vesicle fluid of patients with herpes zoster.	As long as 5 days but usually 1 to 2 days before onset of rash and not more than 6 days after appearance of first crop of vesicles.
Cholera Acute intestinal disease with sudden onset, profuse watery stools, occasional vomiting, rapid dehydration, acidosis, and circulatory collapse. Death may occur within a few hours.	From a few hours to 5 days, usually 2 to 3 days.	Through ingestion of food or water contaminated with feces or vomitus of infected persons or with feces of carriers.	Thought to be for duration of stool-positive stage, usually only a few days after recovery. Carrier stage may last for several months.
Conjunctivitis, Acute Bacterial Clinical syndrome beginning with lacrimation, irritation, and hyperemia of the palpebral and bulbar conjunctivae of one or both eyes, followed by edema of lids, photophobia, and mucopurulent discharge.	Usually 24 to 72 hours.	Contact with discharges from conjunctivae or upper respiratory tract of infected persons through contaminated fingers, clothing, or other articles.	During course of active infection.
Conjunctivitis, Epidemic Hemorrhagic (*Apollo 11 Disease*) Virus infection with sudden onset of pain or sensation of a foreign body in eye. Disease rapidly progresses (1 to 2 days) to full case of swollen eyelids, hyperemia of the conjunctivae, often with a circumcorneal distribution, seromucous disease, and frequent subconjunctival hemorrhages.	1 to 2 days, or even shorter.	Through direct or indirect contact with discharge from infected eyes and possibly by droplet infection from persons with virus in throat.	Unknown, but assumed to be for period of active disease, usually 1 to 2 weeks.
Dermatophytosis A. Ringworm of scalp and beard (tinea capitis, tinea kerion, favus). Begins as	10 to 14 days.	Direct or indirect contact with articles infected with hair from	As long as lesions are present and viable fungus persists on contaminated materials.

Disease and Synopsis of Symptoms	Incubation Period	Mode of Transmission	Period of Communicability
Dermatophytosis—cont'd			
small papule and spreads peripherally, leaving scaly patches of temporary baldness. Infected hairs become brittle and break off easily. Kerions sometimes develop.		humans or infected animals.	
B. Ringworm of nails (tinea unguium, onychomycosis). Chronic infectious disease involving one or more nails of hands or feet. Nail thickens, becoming discolored and brittle with an accumulation of caseous-appearing material beneath nail.	Unknown.	Presumably by direct extension from skin or nail lesions of infected persons. Low rate of transmission.	Possibly as long as infected lesion is present.
C. Ringworm of groin and perianal region (dhobie itch, tinea cruris).	4 to 10 days.	Direct or indirect contact with skin and scalp lesions of infected persons or animals.	As long as lesions are present and viable fungus persists on contaminated materials.
D. Ringworm of the body (tinea corporis). Characteristically appears as flat, spreading, ring-shaped lesions. Periphery is usually reddish, vesicular, or pustular and may be dry and scaly or moist and crusted.	Unknown.	Fungus transmitted through direct contact; person to person or from animal to person.	As long as lesions are present and fungus is viable.
E. Ringworm of the foot (tinea pedis, athlete's foot). Scaling or cracking of skin, especially between toes, or blisters containing watery fluid are characteristic. In severe cases, vesicular lesions appear on various parts of body.	Unknown.	Direct or indirect contact with skin lesions of infected persons or contaminated floors or shower stalls.	As long as lesions are present and viable spores persist on contaminated materials.
Diphtheria Characteristic lesion marked by patch or patches of grayish membrane with surrounding dull red inflammatory zone. Throat is moderately sore in faucial diphtheria, with cervical lymph nodes enlarged and tender; occasionally swelling and edema of neck.	2 to 5 days, sometimes longer.	Contact with patient or carrier; more rarely with articles soiled with discharges from lesions of infected persons. Raw milk has been a vehicle.	Variable, until virulent bacilli have disappeared from discharge and lesions. Usual period is 2 to 4 weeks, but chronic carriers may shed organisms for 6 months or more.
Gastroenteritis, Viral A. Epidemic viral gastroenteritis.	24 to 48 hours; in volunteer studies with	Unknown; probably by fecal-oral route.	During acute stage of disease and shortly thereafter.

Disease and Synopsis of Symptoms	Incubation Period	Mode of Transmission	Period of Communicability
Gastroenteritis, Viral—cont'd			
Usually self-limited mild disease that often occurs in outbreaks with clinical symptoms of nausea, vomiting, diarrhea, abdominal pain, myalgia, headache, malaise, low-grade fever, or a combination thereof.	Norwalk agent, range was 10 to 51 hours.	Several recent outbreaks strongly suggest food-borne and water-borne transmission.	
B. Rotavirus gastroenteritis (sporadic viral gastroenteritis of infants and children). Sporadic severe gastroenteritis of infants and young children characterized by diarrhea and vomiting, often with severe dehydration and occasional deaths.	Approximately 48 hours.	Probably fecal-oral and possibly respiratory routes.	During acute stage of disease and later while virus shedding continues. Virus is not usually detectable after eighth day of illness.
Giardiasis (Giardia Enteritis, Lambliasis) Protozoan infection principally of upper small bowel; often asymptomatic, it may also be associated with a variety of intestinal symptoms such as chronic diarrhea; steatorrhea; abdominal cramps; bloating; frequent loose, pale, greasy, malodorous stools; fatigue; and weight loss.	In a water-borne epidemic in United States, clinical illnesses occurred 1 to 4 weeks after exposure; average 2 weeks.	Localized outbreaks occur from contaminated water supplies. By ingestion of cysts in fecally contaminated water and occasionally by fecally contaminated food.	Entire period of infection.
Hepatitis, Viral A. Viral hepatitis A (infectious hepatitis, epidemic hepatitis, epidemic jaundice, catarrhal jaundice, type A hepatitis). Onset is usually abrupt, with fever, malaise, anorexia, nausea, and abdominal discomfort, followed within a few days by jaundice.	From 15 to 50 days, depending on dose; average 28 to 30 days.	Person to person by fecal-oral route. Common-vehicle outbreaks have been related to contaminated water and food.	Studies indicate maximum infectivity during latter half of incubation period, continuing for a few days, after onset of jaundice.
B. Viral hepatitis B (type B hepatitis, serum hepatitis). Onset is usually insidious, with anorexia, vague abdominal discomfort, and nausea and vomiting, sometimes arthralgias and rash, often progressing to jaundice. Fever may be absent or mild.	Usually 45 to 160 days, average 60 to 90 days. Variation is related in part to amount of virus in inoculum, mode of transmission, and host factors.	HB_sAg, the infectious agent, has been found in virtually all body secretions, but only blood, saliva, and semen have been shown to be infectious. Transmission usually by percutaneous inoculation of infected blood and blood	From several weeks before onset of symptoms through clinical course of disease; carrier stage can last for years.

Disease and Synopsis of Symptoms	Incubation Period	Mode of Transmission	Period of Communicability
Hepatitis, Viral—cont'd			
		products; contaminated needles, syringes, and IV equipment.	
C. Hepatitis, non-A, non-B (non-B transfusion-associated hepatitis, hepatitis C). Chronic infection may be symptomatic or asymptomatic. Differential diagnosis depends on exclusion of hepatitis types A and B.	2 weeks to 6 months, model 6 to 8 weeks.	Most common posttransfusion hepatitis in United States and is more common when paid donors are used. Percutaneous transmission documented and other modes similar to those of hepatitis B virus are suspected.	Degree of immunity following infection is not known.
Herpangina, Hand-Foot-and-Mouth Disease, Acute Lymphonodular Pharyngitis *Herpangina*—grayish papulovesicular pharyngeal lesions on an erythematous base. *Hand-foot-and mouth disease*—more diffuse oral lesions on buccal surfaces of cheeks, gums, and tongue. *Acute lymphonodular pharyngitis*—lesions are firm, raised, discrete, whitish to yellowish nodules.	3 to 5 days for herpangina and hand-foot-and-mouth disease; 5 days for acute lymphonodular pharyngitis.	Direct contact with nose and throat discharges and feces of infected (possibly asymptomatic) persons and by droplet spread.	During acute stage of illness and longer because virus persists in stools for as long as several weeks.
Herpes Simplex Viral infection characterized by localized primary lesion, latency, and a tendency to localized recurrence. In perhaps 10% of primary infections, overt disease may appear as illness of varying severity marked by fever and malaise lasting 1 week or more.	2 to 12 days.	HSV type 1: direct contact with virus in saliva of carriers. HSV type 2: sexual contact.	Secretion of virus in saliva has been reported for as long as 7 weeks after recovery from stomatitis. Patients with primary lesions are infective for approximately 7 to 12 days, with recurrent disease for 4 days to 1 week.
Influenza Acute viral disease of respiratory tract characterized by fever, chilliness, headache, myalgia, prostration, coryza, and mild sore throat. Cough is often severe and protracted.	Usually 24 to 72 hours.	By direct contact through droplet infection; probably airborne among crowded populations in enclosed spaces.	Probably limited to 3 days from clinical onset.
Measles (Rubeola, Hard Measles, Red Measles, Morbilli) Acute, highly communicable viral disease with prodromal fever, conjunctivitis, coryza, bronchitis, and Koplik's spots on the buccal mucosa. A characteristic red blotchy rash appears on third to seventh day, beginning on face, becoming generalized,	Approximately 10 days varying from 8 to 13 days from exposure to onset of fever; approximately 14 days until rash appears; uncommonly longer or shorter human normal immune globulin (IG), given later than third day of incubation	By droplet spread or direct contact with nasal or throat secretions of infected persons. Measles is one of most readily transmitted communicable diseases.	From slightly before beginning of prodromal period to 4 days after appearance of rash; communicability is minimal after second day of rash.

Disease and Synopsis of Symptoms	Incubation Period	Mode of Transmission	Period of Communicability
Measles—cont'd			
lasting 4 to 7 days and sometimes ending in branny desquamation. Leukopenia is common.	period for passive protection, may extend the incubation period to 21 days instead of preventing disease.		
Meningitis, Meningococcal (Cerebrospinal Fever, Meningococcemia) Characterized by sudden onset of fever, intense headache, nausea and often vomiting, stiff neck, and frequently a petechial rash with pink macules or, very rarely, vesicles. Delirium and coma often appear; occasional fulminating cases exhibit sudden prostration.	Varies from 2 to 10 days, commonly 3 to 4 days.	By direct contact, including droplets and discharges from nose and throat of infected persons, more often carriers than cases.	Until meningococci are no longer present in discharges from nose and throat. If organisms are sensitive to sulfonamides, meningococci usually disappear from nasopharynx within 24 hours after institution of treatment. Not fully eradicated from oronasopharynx by penicillin.
Meningitis, Haemophilus (Meningitis caused by Haemophilus influenzae) Most common bacterial meningitis in children ages 2 months to 3 years in the United States. Otitis media or sinusitis may be precursor. Almost always associated with bacteremia. Onset is sudden with symptoms of fever, vomiting, lethargy, and meningeal irritation.	Probably short— within 2 to 4 days.	By droplet infection and discharges from nose and throat during infectious period. May be purulent rhinitis. Portal of entry is most commonly nasopharyngeal.	As long as organisms are present, which may be for prolonged period even without nasal discharge.
Mononucleosis, Infectious (Glandular Fever, EBV Mononucleosis) Characterized by fever, sore throat (often with exudative pharyngotonsillitis), and lymphadenopathy (especially posterior cervical). Jaundice occurs in approximately 4% of infected young adults and splenomegaly in 50%. Duration is from 1 to several weeks.	From 4 to 6 weeks.	Person-to-person spread by oropharyngeal route via saliva. Spread may also occur via blood transfusion to susceptible recipients.	Prolonged; pharyngeal excretion may persist for 1 year after infection; 15% to 20% of healthy adults are oropharyngeal carriers.
Mumps (Infectious Parotitis) Acute viral disease characterized by fever, swelling, and tenderness of one or more salivary glands, usually parotid and sometimes sublingual or submaxillary glands.	Approximately 2 to 3 weeks, commonly 18 days.	By droplet spread and by direct contact with saliva of an infected person.	Virus has been isolated from saliva from 6 days before salivary gland involvement to as long as 9 days thereafter; but height of infectiousness occurs approximately 48 hours before swelling begins. Urine may be positive for as long as 14 days after onset of illness.
Paratyphoid Fever Frequently generalized bacterial enteric	1 to 3 weeks for enteric fever; 1 to 10 days	Direct or indirect contact with feces or	As long as infectious agent persists in excreta, which is from

Disease and Synopsis of Symptoms	Incubation Period	Mode of Transmission	Period of Communicability
Paratyphoid Fever—cont'd			
infection, often with abrupt onset, continued fever, enlargement of spleen, sometimes rose spots on trunk, usually diarrhea, and involvement of lymphoid tissues of mesentery and intestines.	for gastroenteritis.	urine of patient or carrier. Spread by food, especially milk, milk products, and shellfish. Flies may be vectors.	appearance of prodromal symptoms, throughout illness, and for periods up to several weeks or months. Commonly 1 to 2 weeks after recovery.
Pediculosis (Louse Infestation) Infestation of head, hairy parts of body, or clothing with adult lice, larvae, or nits (eggs), which results in severe itching and excoriation of scalp or scratch marks on body.	Under optimal conditions, eggs of lice hatch in 1 week and reach sexual maturity in approximately 2 weeks.	Direct contact with infected person and indirectly by contact with personal belongings, especially clothing and headgear. Crab lice are usually transmitted through sexual contact.	Communicable as long as lice remain alive on infested person or in clothing, and until eggs in hair and clothing have been destroyed.
The Pneumonias			
A. Pneumococcal pneumonia. Acute bacterial infection characterized by sudden onset with single shaking chill, fever, pleural pain, dyspnea, cough productive of "rusty" sputum and leukocytosis.	Not well determined; believed to be 1 to 3 days.	By droplet spread; by direct oral contact or indirectly, commonly through articles freshly soiled with respiratory organisms.	Presumably until discharges of mouth and nose no longer contain virulent pneumococci in significant numbers. Penicillin will render patient noninfectious within 24 to 48 hours.
B. Mycoplasmal pneumonia (primary atypical pneumonia). Predominantly afebrile lower respiratory infection. Onset is gradual with headache, malaise, cough often paroxysmal, and usually substernal pain (not pleuritic). Sputum, scant at first, may increase later.	14 to 21 days.	Probably by droplet inhalation, direct contact with infected person or with articles freshly soiled with discharges of nose and throat from acutely ill and coughing patient.	Probably less than 10 days; occasionally longer with persisting febrile illness or persistence of the organisms in convalescence (as long as 13 weeks is known).
C. Pneumocystis pneumonia (interstitial plasma cell pneumonia). Acute pulmonary disease occurring early in life, especially in malnourished, chronically ill, or premature infants. Characterized by progressive dyspnea, tachypnea, and cyanosis; fever may not be present.	Analysis of data from institutional outbreaks among infants indicates 1 to 2 months.	Unknown.	Unknown.
D. Chlamydial pneumonia (pertussoid eosinophilic pneumonia). Subacute pulmonary disease occurring in early infancy, primarily in	Not known, but pneumonia may occur in infants from 1 to 18 weeks of age (more commonly between 4 and 12 weeks).	Presumed to be vertically transmitted from infected cervix to infant during birth, with resultant	Unknown, but length of nasopharyngeal excretion can be at least 2 months.

Disease and Synopsis of Symptoms	Incubation Period	Mode of Transmission	Period of Communicability
The Pneumonias—cont'd			
infants of mothers with infection of uterine cervix with causative organism.		nasopharyngeal infection.	
Poliomyelitis (infantile paralysis) Acute viral infection whose symptoms include fever, malaise, headache, nausea, vomiting, and stiffness of neck and back with or without paralysis.	Commonly 7 to 14 days for paralytic cases, with a range from 3 to possibly 35 days.	Direct contact through close association. In rare instances milk, foodstuffs, and other fecally contaminated materials have been incriminated as vehicles. Fecal-oral is major route when sanitation is poor, but during epidemics and when sanitation is good, pharyngeal spread becomes relatively more important.	Not accurately known. Cases are probably most infectious during first few days after onset of symptoms.
Respiratory Disease (Excluding Influenza)			
A. Acute febrile respiratory disease. Viral diseases of respiratory tract characterized by fever and one or more constitutional reactions such as chills or chilliness, headache, general aching, malaise, and anorexia; in infants by occasional gastrointestinal disturbances.	From a few days to 1 week or more.	Directly by oral contact or by droplet spread, indirectly by hands or other materials soiled by respiratory discharges of infected person.	For duration of active disease; little is known about subclinical or latent infections.
B. Common cold (acute coryza). Acute catarrhal infections of upper respiratory tract characterized by coryza, sneezing, lacrimation, irritated nasopharynx, chilliness, and malaise lasting 2 to 7 days. Fever is uncommon in children and rare in adults.		Presumably by direct oral contact or by droplet spread; indirectly by hands and articles freshly soiled by discharges of nose and throat of infected person.	
Rubella (German Measles) A. Congenital rubella. Mild febrile infectious disease with diffuse punctate and macular rash. Sometimes resembling that of measles, scarlet fever, or both. May be few or no constitutional symptoms in children but adults may experience 1- to 5-day prodrome characterized by low-grade fever, headache, malaise, mild coryza, and conjunctivitis. As many as	From 16 to 18 days, with a range of 14 to 21 days.	Contact with nasopharyngeal secretions of infected person. Infection is by droplet spread or direct contact with patients and indirect contact.	For approximately 1 week before and at least 4 days after onset of rash. Highly communicable. Infants with congenital rubella syndrome may shed virus for months after birth.

Disease and Synopsis of Symptoms	Incubation Period	Mode of Transmission	Period of Communicability
Rubella—cont'd			
20% to 50% of infections may occur without evidence rash; overall 50% are not recognized. B. Erythema infectiosum (fifth disease). Mild nonfebrile erythematous eruption occurring as epidemics among children. Characterized by striking erythema of cheeks, reddening of skin, and lacelike serpiginous rash of body. C. Exanthema subitum (roseola infantum). Acute illness of probable viral cause characterized by high fever that suddenly appears and lasts 3 to 5 days. A maculopapular rash on trunk and later on rest of body ordinarily follows lysis of fever.			
Shigellosis (Bacillary Dysentery) Acute bacterial disease primarily involving large intestine characterized by diarrhea accompanied by fever, nausea, sometimes vomiting, cramps, and tenesmus. In severe cases, stools contain blood, mucus, and pus.	1 to 7 days, usually 1 to 3 days.	By direct or indirect fecal-oral transmission from patient or carrier. Infection may occur after ingestion of very few organisms.	During acute infection and until infectious agent is no longer present in feces, usually within 4 weeks of illness.
Staphylococcal Disease A. Staphylococcal disease in community, boils, carbuncles, furuncles, impetigo, cellulitis, abscesses, staphylococcal septicemia, staphylococcal pneumonia, osteomyelitis, endocarditis. Staphylococci produce variety of syndromes with clinical manifestations that range from single pustule to impetigo to septicemia to death. Lesion or lesions containing pus are primary clinical finding, abscess formation is typical.	Variable and indefinite; commonly 4 to 10 days.	Major site of colonization is anterior nares. Autoinfection is responsible for at least one third of infections. Person with draining lesion or any purulent lesion or who is asymptomatic (usually nasal) carrier of pathogenic strain. Airborne spread is rare.	As long as purulent lesions continue to drain or carrier state persists.
B. Staphylococcal disease in hospital nurseries, impetigo, abscess of breast.	Commonly 4 to 10 days but may occur several months after colonization.	Spread by hands of hospital personnel is primary mode of transmission within	Same.

Disease and Synopsis of Symptoms	Incubation Period	Mode of Transmission	Period of Communicability
Staphylococcal Disease—cont'd			
Characteristic lesions develop secondary to colonization of nose or umbilicus, conjunction, circumcision site, or rectum of infants with pathogenic strain.		hospitals; to a lesser extent, airborne.	
C. Staphylococcal disease in medical and surgical wards of hospitals. Lesions may from simple furuncles or stitch abscesses to extensively infected bedsores or surgical wounds, septic phlebitis, chronic osteomyelitis, fulminating pneumonia, endocarditis, or septicemia.	Variable and indefinite. Commonly 4 to 10 days.	Major site of colonization is anterior nares. Autoinfection is responsible for at least one third of infections. Person with a draining lesion or any purulent lesion or who is an asymptomatic (usually nasal) carrier of a pathogenic strain. Airborne spread is rare.	As long as purulent lesions continue to drain or carrier state persists.
Streptococcal Sore Throat Fever, sore throat, exudative tonsillitis or pharyngitis, and tender anterior cervical lymph nodes.	Short, usually 1 to 3 days, rarely longer.	Transmission results from direct or intimate contact with patient or carrier, rarely by indirect contact through objects or hands. Nasal carriers are particularly likely to transmit diseases.	In untreated uncomplicated cases 10 to 21 days; in untreated conditions with purulent discharges, weeks or months.
Syphilis, Nonvenereal Endemic Acute disease of limited geographical distribution characterized clinically by eruption of skin and mucous membranes, usually without evident primary sore.	2 weeks to 3 months	Direct or indirect contact with infectious early lesions of skin and mucous membranes. Congenital transmission does not occur.	Until moist eruptions of skin and mucous patches disappear—sometimes several weeks or months.
Trachoma Communicable keratoconjunctivitis characterized by conjunctival inflammation with papillary hyperplasia, associated with vascular invasion of cornea, and in later stages by conjunctival scarring that may eventually lead to blindness.	5 to 12 days (based on volunteer studies).	By direct contact with ocular discharges and possibly mucoid or purulent discharges of nasal mucous membranes of infected persons or materials. Flies *(Musca sorbens)* may contribute to spread of disease.	As long as active lesions are present in the conjunctivae and adnexal mucous membranes.
Tuberculosis Mycobacterial disease. Initial infection usually goes unnoticed; tuberculin sensitivity appears within a few weeks; lesions commonly heal, leaving no residual changes except pulmonary or tracheobronchial lymph node calcification. May progress to pulmonary tuberculosis or, by lymphohematogenous dissemination of bacilli, to	From infection to demonstrable primary lesion, approximately 4 to 12 weeks. Whereas subsequent risk of progressive pulmonary or extrapulmonary tuberculosis is greatest within 1 or 2 years after infection, it may persist for a lifetime as latent infection.	Exposure to bacilli in airborne droplet nuclei from sputum of persons with infectious tuberculosis. Bovine tuberculosis results from exposure to tubercular cattle and ingestion of unpasteurized dairy products.	As long as infectious tubercle bacilli are being discharged.

Disease and Synopsis of Symptoms	Incubation Period	Mode of Transmission	Period of Communicability
Tuberculosis—cont'd			
produce miliary, meningeal, or other extrapulmonary involvement.			
Typhoid Fever (Enteric Fever, Typhus Abdominalis) Systemic infectious disease characterized by sustained fever, headache, malaise, anorexia, relative bradycardia, enlargement of spleen, rose spots on trunk, nonproductive cough, constipation more common than diarrhea, and involvement of lymphoid tissues.	Depends on size of infecting dose; usual range 1 to 3 weeks.	By food or water contaminated by feces or urine of patient or carrier.	As long as typhoid bacilli appear in excreta; usually first week throughout convalescence; variable thereafter. Approximately 10% of untreated patients will discharge bacilli for 3 months after onset of symptoms; 2% to 5% become permanent carriers.
Whooping Cough (Pertussis) Acute bacterial disease involving tracheobronchial tree. Initial catarrhal stage has insidious onset with irritating cough that gradually becomes paroxysmal, usually within 1 to 2 weeks, and lasts for 1 to 2 months.	Commonly 7 days; almost uniformly within 10 days and not exceeding 21 days.	Primarily by direct contact with discharges from respiratory mucous membranes of infected persons by airborne route, probably by droplets. Frequently brought into home by older sibling.	Highly communicable in early catarrhal stage before paroxysmal cough stage. For control purposes, communicable stage extends from 7 days after exposure to 3 weeks after onset of typical paroxysms in patients not treated with antibiotics; in patients treated with erythromycin, period of infectiousness extends only 5 to 7 days after onset of therapy.
Sexually Transmitted Diseases			
Acquired Immunodeficiency Syndrome (AIDS) Acute viral infection characterized by breakdown and failure of immune system, opening body to often lethal infections and disorders such as Kaposi's sarcoma, pneumonia, and meningitis. Symptoms begins with fever, weight loss, fatigue, shortness of breath, diarrhea, and neurological disorders.	Variable.	By direct sexual contact and transmission of semen, saliva, blood, or other body fluids; also by blood transfusion or contaminated syringes.	For duration of infection.
Chancroid (Ulcus Molle, Soft Chancre) Acute, localized, genital infection characterized by single or multiple painful necrotizing ulcers at site of inoculation, frequently accompanied by painful inflammatory swelling and suppuration of regional lymph nodes. Extragenital lesions have been reported.	From 3 to 5 days, up to 14 days.	By direct contact with discharges from open lesions and pus from buboes; suggestive evidence of asymptomatic infections in women. Multiple sexual partners and uncleanliness favor transmission.	As long as infectious agent persists in original lesion or discharging regional lymph nodes; usually until healed— a matter of weeks.

Disease and Synopsis of Symptoms	Incubation Period	Mode of Transmission	Period of Communicability
Conjunctivitis, Inclusion (*Swimming Pool Conjunctivitis, Paratrachoma*) In the newborn, acute papillary conjunctivitis with abundant mucopurulent discharge. In children and adults, acute follicular conjunctivitis with preauricular lymphadenopathy, often with superficial corneal involvement.	5 to 12 days.	During sexual intercourse; genital discharges of infected persons are infectious.	While genital infection persists; can be longer than 1 year in women.
Cytomegalovirus Infections, Congenital Cytomegalovirus Infection, Cytomegalic Inclusion Disease Most severe form of disease occurs in perinatal period, following congenital infection, with signs and symptoms of severe generalized infection especially involving central nervous system and liver.	Information inexact; 3 to 8 weeks following transfusion with infected blood; 3 to 12 weeks after birth.	Intimate exposure to infectious secretions or excretions. Virus is excreted in urine, saliva, cervical secretions, breast milk, and semen.	Virus is excreted in urine or saliva for months and may persist for several years following primary infection.
Gonococcal Infections A. Gonococcal infection of genitourinary tract (gonorrhea, gonococcal urethritis). *Men*—purulent discharge from anterior urethra with dysuria appears 2 to 7 days after infecting exposure. *Women*—few days after exposure initial urethritis or cervicitis occurs, frequently so mild as to pass unnoticed. approximately 20% of patients have uterine invasion at the first, second, or later menstrual period with symptoms of endometritis, salpingitis, or pelvic peritonitis.	Usually 2 to 7 days, sometimes longer.	By contact with exudates from mucous membranes of infected persons, almost always result of sexual activity.	May extend for months if untreated, especially in women who are frequently asymptomatic. Specific therapy usually ends communicability within hours except with penicillin-resistant strains.
B. Gonococcal conjunctivitis neonatorum (gonorrheal ophthalmia neonatorum). Acute redness and swelling of conjunctiva of one or both eyes, with mucopurulent or purulent discharge in which gonococci are identifiable by microscopic and cultural methods.	Usually 1 to 5 days.	Contact with infected birth canal during childbirth.	While discharge persists if untreated; for 24 hours following initiation of specific treatment.

Disease and Synopsis of Symptoms	Incubation Period	Mode of Transmission	Period of Communicability
Granuloma Inguinale (*Donovanosis*) Mildly communicable, nonfatal, chronic and progressive, autoinoculable bacterial disease of skin and mucous membranes of external genitalia, inguinal, and anal region. Small nodule, vesicle, or papule is present.	Unknown.	Presumably by direct contact with lesions during sexual activity.	Unknown and probably for duration of open lesions on skin or mucous membranes.
Herpes Simplex Viral infection characterized by localized primary lesion, latency, and a tendency to localized recurrence. In perhaps 10% of primary infections overt disease may appear as illness of varying severity marked by fever and malaise lasting 1 week or more.	2 to 12 days.	HSV type 1: direct contact with virus in saliva of carriers. HSV type 2: sexual contact.	Secretion of virus in saliva has been reported for as long as 7 weeks after recovery from stomatititis. Patients with primary lesions are infective for approximately 7 to 12 days, with recurrent disease for 4 days to 1 week.
Lymphogranuloma Venereum (*Lymphogranuloma Inguinale, Esthiomene, Climatic Bubo, Tropical Bubo*) Venereally acquired infection, beginning with painless evanescent erosion, papule, nodule, or herpetiform lesion on penis or vulva, frequently unnoticed. Regional lymph nodes undergo suppuration followed by extension of inflammatory process to adjacent tissues.	Usually 7 to 12 days, with a range of 4 to 21 days to primary lesion. If bubo is first manifestation, 10 to 30 days, sometimes several months.	Direct contact with open lesions of infected persons usually during sexual intercourse.	Variable, from weeks to years, during presence of active lesions.
Syphilis, Venereal (*Lues*) Acute and chronic treponematosis characterized clinically by primary lesion, secondary eruption involving skin and mucous membranes, long periods of latency, and late lesions of skin, bone, viscera, and central nervous and cardiovascular systems. Papule appears 3 weeks after exposure at site of initial invasion; after erosion, most common form is indurated chancre.	10 days to 10 weeks, usually 3 weeks.	By direct contact with infectious exudates from obvious or concealed moist early lesions of skin and mucous membrane, body fluids, and secretions of infected persons during sexual contact.	Variable and indefinite during primary and secondary stages and also in mucocutaneous recurrences; some cases may be intermittently communicable for 2 to 4 years.
Trichomoniasis Common disease of genitourinary tract, characterized in women by vaginitis, with small	4 to 20 days, average 7 days.	By contact with vaginal and urethral discharges of infected persons during sexual intercourse and	For duration of infection.

Disease and Synopsis of Symptoms	Incubation Period	Mode of Transmission	Period of Communicability
Trichomoniasis—cont'd			
petechial or sometimes punctate hemorrhagic lesions and profuse, thin, foamy, yellowish discharge with foul odor; frequently asymptomatic. In men, infectious agent invades and persists in prostate, urethra, or seminal vesicles, but rarely produces symptoms or demonstrable lesions.		possibly by contact with contaminated articles.	
Urethritis, Chlamydial Urethritis, Nongonorrheal and Nonspecific Sexually transmitted urethritis of men caused by chlamydial agent. Clinical manifestations are usually indistinguishable from gonorrhea but are often milder and include opaque discharge of moderate or scanty quantity, urethral itching, and burning on urination. Infection of women results in cervicitis and salpingitis.	5 to 7 days or longer.	Sexual contact.	Unknown.

HB,Ag, Hepatitis B surface antigen; *IV,* intravenous; *HSV,* herpes simplex virus; *EBV,* Epstein-Barr virus.
Modified from *Mosby's medical nursing and allied health dictionary,* ed 5, St Louis, 1998, Mosby.

Index

Note: Page numbers followed by a lowercase t indicate tables, lowercase b indicates boxes, and f indicate figures.